# Neale's Disorders OF THE FOOT

## EIGHTH EDITION

**Edited by**

**Paul Frowen** MPhil, FCHS, FCPodMed, DPodM
Head of Wales Centre for Podiatric Studies, Principal Lecturer, Podiatry, University of Wales Institute, Cardiff, UK

**Maureen O'Donnell** BSc(Hons), FChS, FPodMed, DPod M, Dip Ed
Podiatrist; Formerly Programme Leader, Senior Lecturer, Division of Podiatric Medicine and Surgery, Glasgow Caledonian University, Glasgow, UK

**Donald L Lorimer** B Ed (Hons), MChS, FCPodMed, DPod M
Podiatrist, Former Head of School, Durham School of Podiatric Medicine; Past Chairman of Council The Society of Chiropodists and Podiatrists; Former Co-ordinator Joint Quality Assurance Committee of the Society of Chiropodists and Podiatrists/Health Professions Council; Health Professions Council Partner, UK

**Gordon Burrow** DPodM, BA, AdvDipEd, FChS, MPhil, FCPodMed, MSc, CMIOSH, FHEA
Podiatrist, Senior Lecturer, Department of Diagnostic Imaging, Operating Department Practice, Podiatry and Radiotherapy, School of Health, Glasgow Caledonian University, Glasgow, UK

**Foreword by**

**Val Brewster**

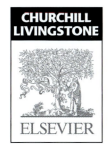

Edinburgh London New York Oxford Philadelphia St Louis Sydney Toronto 2010

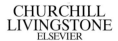

© 2002, Elsevier Limited. All rights reserved.
© 2006, Elsevier Limited. All rights reserved.
© 2011, Elsevier Limited. All rights reserved.

ISBN 978-0-7020-4470-0
Formerly 978-0-7020-3029-1

**British Library Cataloguing in Publication Data**
A catalogue record for this book is available from the British Library

**Library of Congress Cataloging in Publication Data**
A catalog record for this book is available from the Library of Congress

**Notices**
Knowledge and best practice in this field are constantly changing. As new research and experience broaden our understanding, changes in research methods, professional practices, or medical treatment may become necessary.

Practitioners and researchers must always rely on their own experience and knowledge in evaluating and using any information, methods, compounds, or experiments described herein. In using such information or methods they should be mindful of their own safety and the safety of others, including parties for whom they have a professional responsibility.

With respect to any drug or pharmaceutical products identified, readers are advised to check the most current information provided (i) on procedures featured or (ii) by the manufacturer of each product to be administered, to verify the recommended dose or formula, the method and duration of administration, and contraindications. It is the responsibility of practitioners, relying on their own experience and knowledge of their patients, to make diagnoses, to determine dosages and the best treatment for each individual patient, and to take all appropriate safety precautions.

To the fullest extent of the law, neither the Publisher nor the authors, contributors, or editors, assume any liability for any injury and/or damage to persons or property as a matter of products liability, negligence or otherwise, or from any use or operation of any methods, products, instructions, or ideas contained in the material herein.

*The Publisher*

Printed in China

# Contents

# Web Contents
## and Evolve information

## Videos

### Assessing foot function

Assessing foot function 1
   Frontal Plane Calcaneal Position
Assessing foot function 2
   Malleolar Position
Assessing foot function 3
   'Too many toes'
   Medial Longitudinal Arch Profile
Assessing foot function 4
   Lateral Malleolar Curvature
   Hallux Dorsiflexion Test
Assessing foot function 5
   Tip-Toe Test

### Regional examination techniques

Limb length discrepancy 1
Limb length discrepancy 2
Palpation of the knee
Patellar apprehension test
Cruciate ligament test
Valgus stress test
The Knee: Muscle power
Rectus femoris contracture test
90-90 Test
Examination of the Foot and ankle
   The Foot and Ankle: Muscle Power
   Forefoot Compression Test
   Directed functional tasks

### Observational gait analysis

Anterior and Posterior Views
Lateral and Medial Views

### Summary

## Powerpoint Slides

Chilling and Chilblains
Exostosis at the base of the first metatarsal
Padding and Strapping
Mechanical Therapy used in Podiatry
Subungual Haematoma
Contact Dermatitis
Corn and Callus over the head of the first
   metatarsophanageal joint
Cutaneous Horn
Gouty tophi
Granuloma
Haglund's deformity
Onychogryphosis
Onychomycosis
Padding and Strapping
Periungual haematoma
Pustules
Talipes Equino Varus
Raynaud's Phenomenon
Systemic Lupus Erythematosis (SLE)

## Image Bank

### Questions

# Foreword

In 1981 when my grandfather, Donald Neale, completed the 1st edition of his book 'Common Foot Disorders' he would never have imagined that the book would become the academic heavyweight that the 8th edition is today. His work always played a part in my life, from my visits to him at the Edinburgh Foot Clinic (usually for treatment of my verrucae) to my fascination with the gruesome photographs that were always on his desk. My grandfather was so proud of me when I started nursing but I wish he had known that I was to have a career change and follow in his footsteps shortly after his death in 1997. His dedication to his family and the profession was absolute and his hard work was a major contributor to the progression of the profession.

The original title of 'Common Foot Disorders' is no longer suitable for this book which has developed to meet the increased scope of practice of the podiatrist, the ever evolving curriculum for students and the CPD requirements for practitioners. A vast range of foot disorders and systemic related pathologies including, rheumatology, vascular disorders, dermatology and diabetes are covered in detail. Whilst the text is thorough it is enhanced by explicit diagrams, tables and photographs. Some of the foot conditions and related disorders are not necessarily seen in everyday clinical practice but recognition, diagnosis, referral and management is a requirement for today's clinicians and this book meets these needs. A Clinical Companion and an interactive Web Base is now available with the 8th edition.

The 8th edition is an invaluable source of references and updated material for practitioners and other health care professionals. It continues to focus on, and deliver, updated learning material for students and comprehensively covers topics required for their clinical experience, examinations and assessments. The web pages include video clips and self assessment multiple-choice questions all of which are clinically relevant to students and practitioners. Several chapters have been altered, amalgamated or streamlined to reflect current practice. Leprosy and Tropical Diseases have been combined, Musculoskeletal Disorders updated and there is a new slant on the chapter dealing with the podiatric problems of the elderly patient. Therapeutic footwear is now an addition within the footwear chapter and the medical emergencies chapter is very appropriate to current podiatric practice.

The addition of the clinical companion and web based interactive material is a huge step forward. The clinical companion is based on the main book and is an excellent resource for a quick reference clinical tool or revision, with concise information which is easy to access and is very relevant to the clinical situation. To have such a variety of learning tools is excellent; it helps to consolidate information in a memorable and interesting way.

The 8th edition continues to extend the work started by my grandfather 30 years ago. It clearly reflects the great strides which have been made in the profession since the first edition.

I am certain that all podiatry practitioners will find this an invaluable and informative book.

Valerie Brewster
Private Practitioner
Bearsden Foot Clinic

# Preface
## to Eighth Edition

The first edition of this text was produced by Donald Neale in 1981, with a view to develop a book which incorporated the many diverse bodies of medical and biological knowledge that are essential components of the profession of podiatry. Prior to this most of the literature that had been specifically developed for the profession had been written in the years preceding World War 2 and whilst revised to reflect changes in practice were very much embedded in the fourth decade of the twentieth century.

Neale's Disorders of the foot, has incrementally evolved since the first edition which represented UK podiatric practice in the late 1970s. Notably in the first edition, local anaesthesia, nail surgery and surgical procedures (other than those carried out by orthopaedic surgeons) were not included. These omissions were rectified within the second and third editions of the book.

Podiatric practice and education has developed significantly within the past 30 years both in respect of scope of practice and educational changes that were required to support practice. All approved programmes of Podiatry in the UK are now normally at honours degree level or above. Increasing numbers of podiatrists now have higher degrees and this has contributed to the breadth of the evidence base upon which best practice is founded. The text has similarly developed edition by edition in an effort to reflect the changes and in this the eighth edition in addition to the re-writing and revisions of chapters the opportunity to utilise web based media has also been taken.

The seven previous editions of the text have endeavoured to be a focus for the knowledge base of the profession whilst giving emphasis to the place it holds within the wider field of patient care. Similarly the eighth edition strives to continue this role and many chapters have been revised or rewritten and a number of new contributors have provided a fresh approach to some of the content.

The layout and content of chapters has caused much thought and there have been a number of changes which place some elements in more logically clinically related locations and where possible duplication of information has been minimised. The need for the text to provide for the needs of both the student podiatrist and the practitioner has been at the forefront of our deliberations and it is hoped that the eighth edition continues to provide a ready reference from assessment to diagnosis and management.

The common cutaneous conditions such as corn and callous have been displaced from the chapter which deals with dermatological conditions and the chapter on nail disorders has been expanded to include cutaneous disorders. The chapter on podiatric management of the elderly has been rewritten and focuses on the elderly patient's journey in relation to a host of conditions which may affect the foot and the specific issues that relate to caring for the older patient. Much of the chapter on orthoses has been modified and now is more reflective of current therapies and paradigms whilst continuing to reflect traditional techniques which remain part of contemporary practice.

The podiatrists increasing role in the prescription and supply of therapeutic footwear is addressed by an additional section within the chapter that relates to footwear and will add additional relevance. Furthermore, the podiatrist's role in health promotion has also been recognised and the chapter on patient education has been substantially revised to reflect this.

The material that is based on the web has allowed enhancement of information by making material available with video and a greater number of images and presentations. Patient examination techniques and gait analysis are available as videos and a range of self assessment questions are also available. It is hoped that when necessary updates may be possible using this medium. In a new departure, a companion to this text has also been created which is intended to provide for quick and easy reference within the clinical environment.

Paul Frowen
2010

# Preface
## to First Edition

Most books about the feet have naturally enough been written by medical authors for medical readers and they have dealt mainly with the major deformities and acute traumatic injuries and with their surgical management. Most everyday foot troubles, however, develop from biomechanical anomalies which only gradually become symptomatic, though they may ultimately be quite disabling in their cumulative effects. They only seldom reach the physician or surgeon and are generally treated by chiropodists, for whom there has recently been a relative dearth of literature. This book has been compiled to help to fill that need and it has been written with a clinical orientation.

There is abundant evidence that the common foot disorders cause a great deal of pain and disability. Numerous surveys have shown how prevalent they are among all groups of the population from school children to the elderly. They require specialized knowledge and skills for their effective management. The evolution and development of a chiropodial profession specializing in this field is sufficient testimony to the need.

In the UK, the training of a state registered chiropodist is broadly based on the medical sciences. It equips him/her to provide a comprehensive service of diagnosis and treatment virtually from the cradle to the grave and to identify those cases which require medical or surgical investigation and treatment. The scope of practice of the chiropodist has steadily enlarged within recent years and his/her therapeutic methods have become more efficient and durable. Developments in the field of mechanical therapy and the capacity to undertake minor surgical procedures under local anaesthesia have particularly increased his/her range and effectiveness.

It is in the public interest that this expansion should continue since it is a wasteful use of other costly skills and facilities if physicians and surgeons are unnecessarily burdened with cases within the competence of chiropodists. Heavy demands on hospital beds and operating theatres place a premium on effective methods of foot care which obviate or postpone the need for admission to hospital or which enhance post-operating care.

The diagnosis and management of the common foot disorders require the application of a variety of manual skills which cannot be taught or learnt solely from books. Such practical techniques as clinical examination, operating, and applying dressings can be mastered only through repeated practice under the guidance of clinical teachers. While they are all necessarily based on scientific principles, their application to individual cases is more art than science. There is no way of acquiring such skills other than by instruction from expert clinicians and practice in the techniques involved. It is impracticable to attempt to include much detailed instruction of that kind in a general text and it is properly left to the clinical teacher who has the dominant role in establishing the required levels of practical expertise. This book attempts no more than to encapsulate current concepts on the origins, diagnosis and conservative management of the common foot disorders, while relating this particular field to the general medical and surgical conditions which bear directly upon it. The willing cooperation of so many different disciplines in its preparation is indicative of such collaboration in the clinical field.

D. N.
Edinburgh, UK, 1981

# Acknowledgements

The editors are indebted and grateful to the authors who have contributed to this revised edition and are most pleased that Mrs Valerie Brewster (Donald Neale's Granddaughter) was able to provide the foreword. Her personal references provided a touching insight into the man originally responsible for this text. We would also like to offer our thanks to Ian Mathieson and Sarah Curran for their commitment in providing the videos for the website. We are also most appreciative of the help and assistance provided by Ms Nicola Lally, Mr Robert Edwards, Ms Nayagi Athmanathan and Sarena Wolfaard in the development and production of this edition.

# Contributors

**Asra Ahmad,** BSc (Hons), MChS
Podiatrist, Southwark Foot Health Services,
London, UK

**James A Black,** MChS, DPodM
Podiatrist, Private Practitioner Glasgow,
Clinical Associate at the Orthopaedic Foot Clinic,
Western Infirmary,
Glasgow, UK

**Jacqueline Saxe Buchman,** D.P.M.
Podiatrist, Diplomat, American Board of Podiatric Surgery,
Diplomat, American Board of Podiatric Orthopedics and Primary
Podiatric Medicine,
Associate Professor of Podiatric Medicine,
Barry University School of Graduate Medical Sciences, Florida,
United States of America,
Assistant Director of Residency Training,
Mercy Hospital,
Miami, Florida USA

**Gordon Burrow,** MPhil, MSc, BA, FChS, DPodM, MIOSH, MILT
Podiatrist, Senior Lecturer, Department of Diagnostic Imaging,
Operating Department Practice, Podiatry and Radiotherapy,
School of Health,
Glasgow Caledonian University,
Glasgow, UK

**Robert Campbell,** MSc, MChS, DPodM
Podiatrist, Formerly Senior Lecturer, Post-Registration Masters
Framework Co-ordinator,
Division of Podiatric Medicine and Surgery,
Glasgow Caledonian University,
Glasgow, UK

**Bev Durrant,** MSc BSc PgCert LTHE
Senior Lecturer,
Division of Podiatry,
University of Brighton,
Eastbourne, East Sussex, UK

**Michael E Edmonds,** MB, FRCP
Consultant Physician,
Diabetic Department,
Kings College Hospital,
London, UK

**Brian M Ellis,** PhD, MSc, BA, FChS
Podiatrist, Director,
Dr William M. Scholl Podiatric Research and Development Fund;
Head of Department,
Department of Diagnostic Imaging, Operating Department Practice,
Podiatry and Radiotherapy,
School of Health,
Glasgow Caledonian University, Glasgow, UK;
Former Head of Department of Podiatry,
Queen Margaret University College,
Edinburgh, UK

**Jeffrey Evans,** MSc BA FCPodS MChS DPodM
Senior Lecturer in Podiatry & Fellow in Podiatric Surgery,
Wales Centre for Podiatric Studies,
Cardiff School of Health Sciences,
University of Wales Institute,
Cardiff, UK

**J Douglas Forrest,** BSc (Hons), MChS, D Pod M
Podiatrist, Senior Teacher, Department of Podiatry,
Southern General Hospital,
Glasgow, UK

**Dr Krishna Goel,** MD, DCH, FRCP(Lond, Edin and Glasg), Hon
FRCPCH
Formerly Honorary Senior Lecturer,
Department of Child Health,
University of Glasgow,
Scotland, UK
Consultant Paediatrician,
Royal Hospital for Sick Children,
Glasgow, Scotland, UK

**Robert James Hardie,** DPodM, MChS, FCPodS, LRPS, LBPPA
Consultant Podiatric Surgeon – Castle Point & Rochford Primary
Care Trust,
UK

**Farina Hashmi,** PhD, FCPodMed, BSc(hons) Podiatry, BSc(Hons)
Biochemistry
Senior Lecturer/ Research Coordinator,
Division of Podiatry,
University of Brighton School of Health Professions,
Eastbourne, UK

**Phillip Helliwell,** PhD, FRCP
Consultant Rheumatologist and Senior Lecturer,
Academic Unit of Musculoskeletal Disease,
School of Medicine,
University of Leeds, UK

**Margaret Johnson,** PhD, MChS, DPodM
Podiatrist, Assistant Director of Curriculum,
New College,
Durham, UK

**Donald L Lorimer,** B Ed (Hons), FCPodMed, MChS, DPod M
Podiatrist, Former Head of School,
Durham School of Podiatric Medicine;
Past Chairman of Council The Society of Chiropodists and
Podiatrists;
Former Co-ordinator Joint Quality Assurance Committee of the
Society of Chiropodists and Podiatrists/Health Professions Council;
Health Professions Council Partner,
UK

**Tom Lucke,** MA, MBBS, FRRCP
Consultant Dermatologist,
Royal Cornwall Hospital,
Truro, England, UK

**Peter Madigan,** BEd, FCPod(S)
Podiatric Surgeon,
Department of Diagnostic Imaging, Operating Department Practice,
Podiatry and Radiotherapy,
School of Health,
Glasgow Caledonian University, Glasgow, UK

**Ian Mathieson,** PhD, FCPodMed
Senior Lecturer,
Wales Centre for University of Wales, Institute,
Cardiff School of Health Sciences,
University of Wales Institute Cardiff, UK

**Jonathan McGhie,** MBChB, FRCA, FFPMANZCA, FFPMRCA
Consultant in Anaesthesia & Pain Medicine,
Gartnavel General Hospital,
Glasgow, Scotland

**Alistair McInnes,** BSc(Hons), FCPodMed, D. Pod. M. PG Cert LTHE
Senior Lecturer,
School Of Health Professions,
University of Brighton, UK

**Janet McInnes,** MChS, BSc(Hons) Podiatry, D.PodM, PGCE
Deputy Head of School and Head of Division of Podiatry,
School Of Health Professions,
University of Brighton, UK

**Jean Mooney,** PhD, MA, BSc (Hons), FChS, FCPodS
Podiatrist, Private Practitioner,
Formerly Senior Teacher,
London Foot Hospital, and Senior Lecturer,
University of East,
London, UK

**Colin Munro,** MD FRCP (Glasgow)
Consultant Dermatologist,
Southern General Hospital,
South Glasgow University Hospitals NHS Trust,
Glasgow, UK

**Maureen O'Donnell,** BSc(Hons), FChS, FPodMed, DPod M, Dip Ed
Podiatrist, Formerly Programme Leader, Senior Lecturer,
Division of Podiatric Medicine and Surgery,
Glasgow Caledonian University,
Glasgow, UK

**Anthony Redmond,** PhD, MSc, MChS
Podiatrist, Arthritis Research Campaign Lecturer,
Academic Unit of Musculoskeletal Disease,
School of Medicine,
University of Leeds, UK

**David T Roberts**
Consultant Dermatologist formerly Southern General Hospital,
South Glasgow University Hospitals NHS Trust,
Glasgow, UK

**Pamela M Sabine,** MA, FChS, FCPodS, FCPodMed
Consultant Podiatric Surgeon, Director of Specialist Services and
Head of Podiatric Surgery,
Allied Health Professions Representative,
South East Essex PCT;
Past Chairman of Council of the Society of Chiropodists and
Podiatrists;
Former Registrant Member of the Health Professions Council;
Former CHAI Reviewer,
Essex
UK

**Michael Graham Serpell,** MB ChB, ECFMG, FRCA, FCPodS,
FFPMRCA
Senior Lecturer,
University Department of Anaesthesia,
University of Glasgow,
Glasgow, Scotland
Consultant,
Anaesthesia,
Intensive Care & Pain Management,
Gartnavel General Hospital,
Glasgow, Scotland

**Anne Shirley,** MSc, DPodM, MChS, PGCE
Lecturer,
Wales Centre for Podiatric Studies,
Cardiff School of Health Sciences,
University of Wales Institute Cardiff, UK

**Christine M Skinner,** BSc (Hons) D Pod M, MChS
Senior Lecturer, Programme Organiser, Podiatry,
Department of Diagnostic Imaging, Operating Department Practice,
Podiatry and Radiotherapy,
School of Health,
Glasgow Caledonian University,
Glasgow, UK

**Kate Springett,** PhD, FChS, DPodM
Podiatrist, Head of Department of Allied Health Professions,
Canterbury Christ Church University,
UK

**Jane Thomas,** MSc, RGN, RM, RHV, RNT
Dip N Wales,
Deputy Head of School,
Superintendent of Assessment,
Swansea University,
Swansea, UK

**John Thomson,** MD FRCP (Glasgow & Edinburgh) D.Obst.RCOG
Honorary FChS
Consultant Dermatologist,
Formerly Glasgow Royal Infirmary, Glasgow;
Locum Consultant Dermatologist,
Argyle and Clyde and Lanarkshire Health Authority,
Scotland, UK

**Wendy Tyrrell,** MEd, FHEA, DPodM, MChS, FCPod Med
Until September 2008 Director of Research & Enterprise and Principal
Lecturer,
Cardiff School of Health Sciences,
University of Wales Institute Cardiff,
Cardiff, UK

**James Watkins,** BEd, MA, PhD
Professor of Biomechanics,
School of Engineering,
Swansea University,
Singleton Park,
Swansea, Wales, UK

**Gordon F Watt,** DPodM. MChS Podiatrist
Lecturer,
Department of Diagnostic Imaging, Operating Department Practice,
Podiatry and Radiotherapy,
School of Health,
Glasgow Caledonian University, Glasgow, UK

**Anne Whinfield,** BSc(Hons) MChs DPodM
Former Honorary Research Fellow,
Department of Primary Care,
Kings College School of Medicine,
London, UK
Former  Lead in Advanced Therapies, Research and Development,
Foot Health Services,
Lambeth PCT,
London, UK

# Chapter 1

# Examination and diagnosis in clinical management

*Gordon Burrow*

*'Use the past as a mirror when studying the present; there can be no present without the past.'*

*'Watching others do something is easy; learning to do it yourself is hard.'*

*'To experience is better than to be told; seeing for oneself is better than hearing from others.'*

Chinese proverbs (Wanheng & Xiaoxiang 1996)

## INTRODUCTION

Communications are the most useful/vital component part of clinicians' skills, allowing them to manage patients effectively and efficiently. It is apparent that, in a litigious society, failure to communicate to, with and about our patients is a primary cause of many cases against practitioners. It is failure to communicate with the patient from the start, in our history taking, that may lead to misdiagnoses, poor management strategy or poor compliance by the patient. Failure to communicate properly what occurred during the consultation phase, and to document the management strategy and agreement by the patient in the case record leads to many cases of complaint, disciplinary procedures or litigation by patients against podiatrists.

The process by which clinicians gain, analyse or interpret the information that the patient imparts to them is, by and large, an invisible process, but it gives visible and resultant shape to the data compiled throughout the consultation and clinical interactions. 'Clinical thinking' is a name given to that invisible process (Bates 1995). It is a process demonstrated and observed during training but developed and honed by experience and continuous professional development of clinical and academic skills. It is a skill that is acquired rather than taught, as it is very much based on clinical experience and judgement.

## GATHERING DATA

From the initial referral letter, or initial contact with the patient in the surgery, the practitioner continually observes, asks open-ended questions and uses additional methods to encourage the patient to divulge his or her story.

This process of taking a podiatric history comprises many constituent parts and in American terms is the 'clerking process'. To many students it is a daunting experience, requiring the collection of information, which often needs restructuring to make sense of the vast amount of data obtained from both the history and the examination. The student/practitioner requires an open, enquiring approach to this process, within a systematic framework, to ensure that the all-important information is gleaned in an efficient and effective manner.

During the process the student/practitioner needs to encourage the patient to divulge information. This encouragement may take numerous forms (Bates 1995):

- Facilitation – actions, postures or words communicating the practitioner's interest in the patient: may take the form of leaning forward, ensuring eye contact, a gentle touch to a particular spot.
- Reflection – a word or phrase the patient has used is repeated back to them.
- Clarification – requesting the patient to give more meaning to what he or she has said, to ensure that the practitioner's interpretation matches that of the patient.
- Empathy – recognition of the patient's feelings through the practitioner's words or actions.
- Ask about feelings – ask what the patient felt about the pain, discomfort, event or symptom.
- Interpretation – put into words what the practitioner has deduced/inferred/interpreted about what the patient has said to them, to ensure there is no misunderstanding.
- Confrontation – state something about the patient's responses (feelings, behaviour) which is inconsistent with other symptoms or signs.

The interview/consultation is potentially the most powerful, sensitive instrument at the command of the podiatrist, and yet it is probably the most misused or misunderstood aspect of our practice.

The patient has become the focus of NHS attention, and as patient-based clinical methods are paramount, the interview/consultation has taken on even greater importance. Most clinicians still rely on the gathering of information from the patient as the prime means of making a diagnosis and deciding on a management strategy for treating the condition or complaint. Technology and instrumentation or tests *assist* in the process but communication is still the primary basis of the process. The physical examination is based on the information gleaned, and helps to confirm an initial working hypothesis or diagnosis and to enable the clinician to make the best use of resources such as tests, diagnostic equipment, time and expertise. It also demonstrates a professional approach to the patient, and is both an efficient and an effective use of scarce resources.

It is routine practice that a patient's history is obtained before undertaking a physical examination. Remember, however, that informed consent is required for a practitioner to obtain information and prior to performing a physical examination. It is prudent to ask the patient whether he or she is willing to divulge information to you by explaining *why and how* the consultation will be conducted.

After the physical examination it may be necessary to conduct a further specific examination or to undertake more robust tests, or to refer elsewhere for further opinion. Although these are explained as separate areas, they should be viewed as dynamic intertwined processes. Taking the history is usually the first, and perhaps most important, aspect of the assessment of and interaction with a patient. It is a gathering of data that is not just about the specific complaint that brought the patient to the surgery and upon which the podiatrist will make the diagnosis. It is a learning experience for the practitioner about the patient, about how the patient experiences and views his or her symptoms, and perhaps about the patient's expectations of treatment. It also allows the patient to have a learning experience about the practitioner. Thus it is the building block or foundation of future trust and a professional patient–practitioner relationship.

## TAKING A COMPREHENSIVE PODIATRIC HISTORY

The purpose of a consultation is twofold.

First, it allows the patient to present the problem to the podiatrist, which is a therapeutic process in itself.

Secondly, it enables the podiatrist to sort out the nature of the problem (diagnosis) and decide on any further course of action that might be needed.

There are four key skills to history taking:

- active listening
- soliciting attribution
- providing support
- establishing agreement.

The manner in which a podiatrist talks with, rather than to, a patient while taking the history, establishes the foundation for good care. Listen carefully; respond skilfully and empathetically (Bates 1995) – the active listening stage. The podiatrist needs to learn what exactly is bothering the patient, what symptoms he or she has experienced, and what the patient thinks the trouble may be, how or why it happened and what the hoped-for outcome is. As the information is given, the podiatrist formulates hypotheses or a range of potential diagnoses. Do not attempt to plump for a diagnosis straight off, as this may close the mind to other signs and symptoms that do not fit with that hypothesis. The hypothesis/examination, or history taking, starts immediately the patient is introduced in the waiting room and the practitioner greets the patient. Too often practitioners miss the opportunity to observe patients unobtrusively while they are relaxed and apparently unobserved – from the time they are called to the time when the patient feels the consultation starts (i.e. when they are sitting on the patient's chair). Significant opportunities for gait analysis are missed. The standard approach is to elicit the history before any physical examination (Marsh 1999) but this misses opportunities to observe patients in the waiting area without them knowing they are being observed.

The atmosphere and setting of the assessment is as important as the examination itself. The patient should be assured of absolute confidentiality, and the assessment should not be rushed. Each patient expects, and deserves, full attention to and sympathy for their problems. The patient should feel confident in the podiatrist's diagnostic abilities, but also in their empathy, understanding and motivation. 'The history is the most important part of the patient's assessment as it provides 80% of the information required to make a diagnosis' (Marsh 1999).

Assessment forms the basis for any planned intervention (Baker 1991), providing the baseline upon which subsequent intervention is measured and outcomes compared. Systematic, ongoing assessment is vital, to monitor and evaluate the success of care and detect new or different problems from those presented initially. This forms the basis of evidence-based practice and care. However, prior to any form of assessment, the patient's consent to treatment and giving of personal information should be sought.

There are two types of consent: tacit and informed consent. Consent is defined as 'to give assent or permission; accede; agree. It is voluntary acceptance of what is planned or done by another, agreement as to opinion or course of action' (Readers Digest 1987). *Tacit consent* is the act of non-verbal or written agreement to treatment, while *informed consent* is the act of making a rational consent to treatment based on all the facts provided (Ricketts 1999). If a patient agrees to come to the podiatrist's surgery, removes their socks and shoes, and sits in the chair expecting treatment, they are tacitly agreeing to the podiatrist undertaking some form of examination. However, when a specific form of treatment/examination is proposed, informed consent is required from the patient to ensure their compliance with and agreement to that form of treatment/examination taking place. Again, this comes down to communication. Patients should be aware of why a podiatrist requires certain information, such as current medication, previous illness, previous drug therapy, surgery etc., otherwise the patient may not see the relevance and not divulge the information – potentially leading to misdiagnoses as a consequence of the incomplete information upon which the diagnosis is based. The podiatrist cannot do every possible test on every patient, and therefore intelligent use of the history may shorten the examination and yet make it more informative (DeMeyer 1998).

## ELEMENTS OF THE HISTORY

The examination will consist of:

- introductory information
- chief complaints
- past history
- current health status
- family/social history
- psychosocial history
- review of systems.

### Introductory information

Introductory information includes the date of the history taking, identifying data or demographics (age, sex, ethnicity, place of birth, marital status, occupation, religion), source of referral (if any), source and reliability of the history. The history taking then proceeds to a discussion of the patient's chief complaints. It is necessary to discuss with the patient why these particular pieces of information are required, especially as nowadays people are more attuned to discrimination for various reasons. Careful thought should be given as to why these pieces of information are really needed. Age can lead to vital clues as to which condition it is most likely to be, given that some foot pathologies are more likely to occur in early childhood, but the effects may produce other pathologies in later life. Furthermore, women are more at risk of some disorders than others; for example, rheumatoid disease is three times more likely in women than in men at a given age. The patient's place of birth may lead to a diagnosis of a rarer form of systemic disease than would otherwise be suggested by the current place of residence; for example, someone now resident in the UK, but who was born and spent most of their early childhood in the Indian subcontinent, may have developed Hansen's disease – a condition not normally associated with the UK. Marital status may provide assurance that the correct phrases and forms of address are used, and that no *faux pas* are made by the podiatrist leading to a breakdown in communications, for example, where children are concerned. Occupation is possibly the most easily explained question, as it may give vital clues to the amount of load or trauma the foot is undergoing, or specific conditions to which the foot is exposed. Religion, perhaps, will help to guide practitioners through some areas leading to non-compliance with management plans, or the inability of the person to communicate certain vital clues to diagnoses. Communication skills are required throughout, ensuring tact, diplomacy and empathy.

## Chief complaints – soliciting contribution

This is the main focus of the history and the prime reason why the patient has presented to the practitioner. A detailed and thorough investigation of the current concern is vital, and comprises two essential but combined parts: the patient's account of the symptoms (ensure that it is the patient's view and not that of another, such as a carer or parent), that is the subjective symptoms; and the objective signs – those detected by the skill of the practitioner. The main aim is to obtain a comprehensive, succinct account of the patient's perspective of the presenting symptom(s). There is a need to allow patients sufficient opportunity to describe their symptoms for themselves. The practitioner needs to practise patience and take care not to interrupt inappropriately. If the patient starts to drift, that is the time to interrupt and take control of the situation. Ask specific questions to obtain detail – the interrogative stage of the history taking. If the history is complicated, reflect on the information and recount it back to the patient, to ensure that he or she agrees with your interpretation. Attempt to be systematic and objective. Look for other supporting evidence to the interpretation, ensuring that questions are posed in a simple, unambiguous manner, without technical or medical jargon.

## Past medical history

This includes information about the patient's general state of health, childhood illnesses (remember the age of the patient and his or her country of birth), adult illnesses, psychiatric illness, accidents and injuries, and operations and hospitalisations. This information will help you gauge the patient overall, and how he or she views health and disease. It is also important to gain outline information of what investigations have been made during previous hospital admissions or at clinics, so reducing duplication of effort. Procedures or operations should be listed chronologically to help with future additions – they should be collected and reported with dates where possible. There is the need to pursue problems that are related to the underlying present condition or complaint.

## Drug/medication history

It is advisable to request this information before the first appointment by advising the patient to present with a list of current medication (prescribed and over-the-counter medicine) and dosage. The drug history may give an indication of current illness. It is important to include home remedies, vitamin/mineral supplements, borrowed medicines, as well as prescription-only medicines (POMs) and over-the-counter (OTC) drugs. The drugs may be the cause of the symptoms (some cases of peripheral neuropathy may be induced by drug therapy), or the withdrawal of a drug therapy may be the reason why symptoms are now apparent (e.g. if the patient has suddenly stopped taking diuretics and suffers from swollen and painful ankles). Details should be obtained about possible drug allergies, to inform any decision about the continuation of a drug therapy. Also ask about other allergies such as hay fever, eczema, asthma, or to latex.

## Social history

It is important to establish how the disease or complaint and patient interact at a functional level. Try to establish what the patient's normal daily activities are and how his or her complaint has affected them. Smoking and alcohol consumption are the factors most frequently asked about in this regard, but it is essential that judgements are not implied by the manner in which the questions are asked. It is more difficult but equally important that the use of other related substances is also investigated.

## Family history

Information about the health and age of other family members can be useful, particularly where there may be a genetic link to disorders. It may be appropriate to identify age or cause of death of family members such as parents or grandparents.

## Review of systems

- *General* – identify factors such as height, weight, recent weight changes, fatigue or fever.
- *Skin* – look for rashes, lumps, sores, itching, dryness, colour changes, or changes in hair or nails. These may indicate systemic conditions such as diabetes or rheumatoid disease.
- *Respiratory* – signs of asthma, bronchitis, emphysema or past history of tuberculosis.
- *Cardiac* – heart trouble, high blood pressure, rheumatic fever, heart murmurs, chest pain, palpitations and results of any heart tests.
- *Urinary* – frequency of urination, polyuria, nocturia, burning pain on urination.
- *Endocrine* – thyroid trouble, heat or cold intolerance, excessive sweating, excessive hunger or thirst.
- *Haematological* – anaemia, easy bruising or bleeding, past transfusions and possible reactions.
- *Neurological* – fainting, blackouts, seizures, weakness, paralysis, numbness, tingling, tremor, involuntary movements.
- *Peripheral vascular* – intermittent claudication, leg cramps, varicose veins.
- *Musculoskeletal* – muscle or joint pains, stiffness, arthritis, gout, backache.

## ATTRIBUTES OF SYMPTOMS

Patients may complain of symptoms that are local (e.g. to the foot or toe) or general (e.g. abnormal gait or more widespread aches and pains). Specific detailed questions by the practitioner can elicit the signs of the complaint. This should be a clear, chronological narrative which includes the onset of the problem, the setting in which it manifests, the means by which it presents, and any treatment that has been tried. The principal symptoms should be described using seven basic attributes (Bates 1995):

- location
- quality
- quantity or severity
- timing (onset, duration, frequency)
- setting
- factors which aggravate or relieve
- associated manifestations.

The amount of time spent on each component depends on a number of factors: the communication skills of the patient, underlying problem(s) and the listening skills of the practitioner. It is difficult to know when to interrupt and when to allow the patient to continue before stepping in and asking probing closed questions. It is essential, however, that the full circumstances of the presenting complaint are obtained.

Once the various symptoms have been described, it is good practice to undertake a brief review of the symptoms (Marsh 1999) using a systems enquiry method. This may help to arrange the thoughts of the practitioner, highlight missing information, or give guidance as to how to perform the physical examination in a logical sequence of actions. It is basically a screening method for establishing the areas that require detailed physical examination. When the presenting complaint appears to involve only one system, that system is promoted in importance in the examination and a detailed history of the presenting complaint and a more detailed physical examination of that system are made.

## PERFORMING THE PHYSICAL EXAMINATION

How complete should a physical examination of a patient be? This is a common question raised by students as well as experienced practitioners. There is growing concern over how much should be assessed and, therefore, how much should be recorded. There is a growing number of pieces of equipment that many podiatrists are starting to use for routine measurements within their practice. However, concern must be raised about the apparent overreliance on sophisticated equipment, which may have a place in some specialist settings but which, on the whole, is too expensive to become necessary in all clinics. Clinicians should rely first on the physical signs and symptoms to indicate whether a more detailed or rigorous assessment is required, and thereafter refer the patient for the specialist tests, or carry these out themselves at another time. In the majority of cases the simple routine consultation, which consists of physical examination together with the ability to use the assessment tools that we all have (i.e. use of the eyes, ears, hands, nose and common sense), should be sufficient. If more sophisticated equipment is to be used, then practitioners require adequate training not only in the use of the equipment but also in the interpretation of the findings. Doppler ultrasound, which enables the sounds of the foot pulses to be identified and recorded, is becoming a routine practice. However, in untrained hands, this equipment can be used incorrectly and diagnoses may be either wrongly interpreted or missed altogether. The equipment may make podiatrists look more professional and more sophisticated. However, the ability to use the equipment correctly, interpret the results accurately and record clearly is something that should be taken seriously.

Therefore, the answer to the question as to how complete an examination should be depends on the signs and symptoms at presentation. The examination and assessment should be related exclusively to the complaint the patient presents with, unless it is thought that a complete and full examination is required to exclude or include other signs and symptoms noticed during the question phase of the assessment process. For patients who have symptoms related to a specific body part (or foot region), a more limited examination may be more appropriate (Bates 1995).

It is the duty of the practitioner to select the relevant methods to assess the problems as precisely and efficiently as possible. The symptoms, along with the demographic data (age, sex, occupation and previous history) collected, influence that selection and determine what examination is required. Knowledge of disease patterns, and the

practitioner's previous knowledge and experience of other conditions also influence the decision. These are all component parts of the clinical thinking, or reasoning, process. When undertaking the physical examination, a sequence that maximises the practitioner's efficiency while minimising the patient's efforts, yet allows thoroughness by the practitioner, is the best. Two important details need to be considered: the positioning and the exposure of the patient.

*'Ideally, the whole limb being examined ought to be exposed, but in practice it is usually sufficient only to expose the leg from above the knee distally.' (Anderson & Black 1997)*

This level of exposure should give the practitioner sufficient sight of the main areas of complaint, without requiring exposure that the patient might feel is not justified for a podiatric examination. It is important to be able to palpate and see the knee during the examination, whether the patient is seated or standing (weight bearing). Thus, where possible, trousers should be rolled up to expose the full knee and patella. It is also important that both legs and knees are visible, even when the patient is complaining of problems in only one foot. Comparison, one with the other, is a vital source of data gathering. In most cases patients are examined in a semi-supine position and are positioned at a higher level than the practitioner. However, where a more accurate biomechanical examination is required, the prone or supine position may be adopted. Whatever the position, it should not be uncomfortable for the patient for the duration of that examination. The patient must be able to be relaxed in the position chosen or false data may be gathered. According to Anderson and Black (1997) it is good practice, and ensures that nothing is missed, to adopt a systematic set pattern for the examination, proceeding from the superficial (skin and soft tissues) to the deep structure (bone and joints) and from the local to the general.

The sequence of a comprehensive examination should be: a general survey, mental status, skin, musculoskeletal system, cardiovascular and neurological systems, followed by specific peripheral neurological and vascular systems and the important aspect of footwear (see Ch. 18).

The purpose of this chapter is not to give detailed information about the physical examination, but rather to provide an overview of those aspects likely to be performed in routine clinical practice. More detailed books are available (Merriman & Turner 2002) and there are various journal articles on each aspect of the process.

The general survey should give an overall impression of the patient's general attributes, but these may vary according to socioeconomic status, nutrition, genetic makeup, early illness, gender, and the country and era of birth. The overview should encompass areas such as:

- apparent state of health – robust, acutely or chronically ill, frail
- signs of distress – laboured breathing, wincing, limping, sweatiness, trembling
- skin colour – pallor, cyanosis, jaundice, rashes, and bruises
- height and build – tall, short, muscular, disproportionate, symmetrical (e.g. Turner's syndrome, child may be of short stature)
- weight by appearance or measurement – emaciated, slender, plump, fat, obese, (although what is the appropriate weight is controversial)
- posture, motor ability and gait – posture, which aids breathing, or pain, ataxia, limp, and paralysis – does the patient walk easily, confidently, balanced?
- dress, grooming, and personal hygiene – excessive amount of clothing may mean hypothyroidism, long sleeves may be to cover rashes or needle marks. Is the patient wearing unusual

jewellery, such as copper bands which might indicate arthritis? Is personal hygiene reflective of the patient's mood, personality, lifestyle, occupation and socio-economic grouping?

- facial expressions – observe these throughout the encounter, during the physical examination (immobile face of Parkinsonism; grimacing when certain areas are touched)
- odour of body or breath – breath odour of alcohol, acetone (diabetes).

## Mental status

The patient's mental status should be observed throughout the consultation, and the appropriateness of behaviour and the ability of the patient to comply with any management plan suggested should be noted. Level of consciousness can be evaluated by observing the patient's responses to verbal and tactile stimuli and their alertness during the interview or clerking process. For example, this may indicate lethargy or stupor. During the short walk to the surgery from the waiting area, and while seated during the interview, the practitioner should observe the patient's posture and motor behaviour and look for restlessness, agitation, bizarre postures, immobility or involuntary movements, along with pace, range, character and appropriateness of movements. The patient's dress, grooming and personal hygiene can be evaluated in terms of neglect or fastidiousness. The facial expressions during rest and interactions should be observed for anxiety, depression, elation, anger or withdrawal. The mood of the patient should also be assessed to gauge the level of happiness, elation, indifference or anxiety. All may give clues as to how the patient views the current problem, how it is affecting his or her daily activities and how the patient may respond to suggestions about altering behaviour patterns adversely affecting their feet (e.g. inappropriate footwear).

## Skin (see also Chs 2 and 3)

Look and observe, touch and palpate skin over the foot and lower limb and observe the following:

- texture: coarse, fine, dull or shiny, smooth or rough
- colour: cyanosis, jaundice, changes in melanin, pallor, erythema, pigmentation, gangrene
- temperature: cool, warm, distinctly hot, normal temperature gradient
- humidity: moist, dry, oily, areas of maceration, dryness associated with hypothyroidism, oiliness in acne
- elasticity: mobility, ease with which a fold of skin can be moved, decreased oedema
- hyperkeratosis: corns and callus formation, sites, texture, quality
- hair: presence, absence, quantity, thickness, distribution, texture
- integrity: fissures (especially heel or interdigital clefts), ulcers, abrasions
- dermatoses (eczema, psoriasis)
- surgical interventions: scars, infections.

It is important to note any lesions, their anatomical location, whether they are generalised or localised, their arrangement (linear, clustered, dermatomal), the type (macule, papule, bulla, tumour, etc.) along with colour (red, brown, white, mauve) and whether raised or indurated.

## Nails (see also Ch. 3)

Inspect and palpate these, identifying:

- structure – ridged, cracked, thickened
- extent – overgrown, onychogryphotic, stunted, ingrowing, chewed, picked

- colour – cyanosis, pallor
- shape – club, excessive curvature
- subungual abnormality – swelling, pigmentation
- lesions – paronychia, onycholysis.

## Swellings

Palpate and inspect any swellings, and note:

- tenderness – local or radiating
- consistency – hard, firm, soft, fluctuant
- adherence to underlying structures – to skin, underlying soft tissues, bone
- transillumination – does swelling transilluminate to light?
- temperature.

## Musculoskeletal system (see also Ch. 8)

The musculoskeletal system should be assessed using a screening method to ensure that lower limb manifestations of systemic disorders are encompassed within the assessment process. This assessment will include an inspection of the joints and the surrounding tissues, and observation of the following:

- Ease and range of motion – assess for limitation in movement, but also any unusual increase in mobility of the joint, which might lead to instability. Range of motion varies between individuals and decreases with age (Fig. 1.1).
- Signs of inflammation and swelling in or around the joint. The swelling may involve the synovium, which feels soft and boggy, or doughy to the touch, or it may produce excessive synovial tissue fluid within the joint space. Palpable bogginess suggests synovitis; palpable joint fluid indicates effusion in the joint. Synovitis and joint fluid may well coexist. Swelling may originate outside the joint itself and may come from the bone, tendons, tendon sheaths, bursae or fat. Trauma to any of these structures produces swelling. Tenderness in or around the joint should be investigated and assessed. An attempt should be

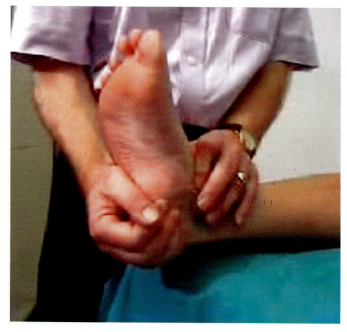

**Figure 1.1** Testing the range of motion – in this case the ankle joint.

made to define the specific anatomical structure that is tender, as trauma may also cause tenderness. Arthritis, tendinitis, bursitis and osteomyelitis all produce symptoms of tenderness. Increased heat can be assessed using the back of the hand or fingers to compare the joint with the corresponding one of the opposite foot or, if both joints are involved, with similar joints or tissues near them. This gives a better indication of whether the increased heat is localised or generalised. It may also lead to better diagnosis of the problem. For example, rheumatoid disease may manifest as generalised increased heat in the more proximal joints and soft tissues surrounding the joints, compared to osteoarthritis. Redness of the overlying skin over a tender joint suggests gout or septic arthritis, but is possibly the least common sign of inflammation of the joint (Bates 1995).

- Condition of the surrounding tissues – look for signs such as muscle atrophy, subcutaneous nodules and skin changes.
- Crepitus or crepitation, a palpable, sometimes audible, crunching or grating produced on movement of a joint or tendon. A fine, soft crepitus might be experienced over inflamed joints, whereas a coarser crepitus suggests roughened articular cartilage, as found in osteoarthritis.
- Any musculoskeletal deformities, including abnormal curvature of the spine. Deformities such as those due to malalignment of bones (genu varum, valgum) or those produced by restricted range of motion (e.g. Dupytren's contracture) may lead to lower limb and foot biomechanical abnormalities, or interfere with the way in which the patient manages his or her foot problems.

When examining a patient with a suspected musculoskeletal problem and presenting with painful joints it is important that the practitioner is gentle and moves the joint slowly. It is a difficult balance to achieve between being gentle and not being afraid to cause some discomfort in order to ensure proper examination to uncover the true cause of the complaint.

Each joint complex within the foot should be assessed individually, comparing one side with the other. Thus the ankle, subtalar and midtarsal joint complexes should all be assessed and compared with the corresponding joint complex on the other limb, and an assessment should be made of the range of motion normally expected for that complex, giving due regard to the age and sex of the patient. The first and fifth ray (Fig. 1.2) should be included in this assessment, and the foot should also be viewed holistically (i.e. both weight bearing and non-weight bearing). Where rheumatoid disease is suspected, it

may be necessary to make an individual assessment of the metatarsal joints by gripping the forefoot across the metatarsal heads and squeezing gently transversely.

## Footwear (see also Ch. 18)

Footwear gives a variety of clues as to diagnosis, and therefore it should also be examined during the patient's first visit. Footwear should initially be checked for size, shape, style, suitability for the patient's foot and occupation and indications of (abnormal) wear marks. Abnormal wear on the soles and heels of the footwear will give some indication as to the gait and weight-bearing patterns of the gait cycle. Inspection of the outer sole and insole can also provide valuable clues about the relative pressures occurring during the foot-flat and take-off phases that occur during mid- and forefoot postures. The shape or distortion of the upper also gives important data as to abnormal frontal plane motion. Abnormal wear of the sole, such as a circular pattern across the forefoot, suggests a rotational element or circumduction of the forefoot on the rearfoot typical of a rearfoot varus. Some wear patterns might suggest particular gait patterns (Anderson & Black 1997):

- Heel wear:
  - excessive wear at rear edge along entire edge – calcaneal gait, as in calcaneal gait of spina bifida
  - excessive wear at anterior edge – *excessively* pronated foot or broken shank
  - excessive wear at lateral edge – supinated foot occurring in pes cavus, painful first ray (postoperatively)
  - excessive wear at medial edge – *excessively* pronated foot.
- Heel and sole wear:
  - excessive wear on lateral side – supinated foot from pes cavus, weakness of evertor muscles such as peroneal, as in peroneal muscular atrophy
  - excessive wear on medial side – *excessively* pronated foot
  - lateral heel to medial sole –if excessive may be the result of externally rotated leg or forefoot abduction
  - lateral heel to lateral sole – leg might be internally rotated or there may be forefoot abduction
  - medial heel to medial sole – *excessively* pronated foot.
- Sole wear:
  - excessive across whole of tread – pes cavus
  - excessive at tip – drop foot, spastic flat foot, result of neurological disease affecting dorsiflexors
  - excessive under hallux – hallux rigidus or limitus
  - excessive under lateral side – metatarsus adductus.

Deformity at heel counters, which may suggest excessive pronation or supination, should also be noted.

## Vascular assessment (see also Ch. 12)

As podiatry moves to evidence-based systems of healthcare, podiatrists need to produce evidence that vascular assessment of presenting patients is beneficial. This does not mean the use of more sophisticated equipment, but the clinical ability to diagnose accurately possible risk factors from signs and symptoms and simple evaluative tests. Those patients potentially at risk of lower limb amputation and receiving podiatric care are nearly four times less likely to undergo such amputation than those not receiving podiatric care (Sowell et al 1999). However, it is essential podiatrists do not depend solely on equipment to make their diagnoses, but instead rely mainly on their clinical and physical examination skills. Equipment is expensive, the results obtained are liable to misinterpretation, and there are problems of validity and reliability.

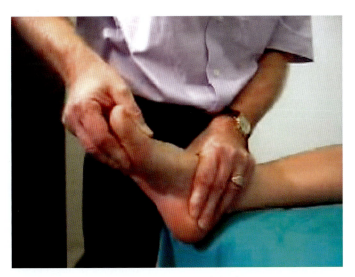

**Figure 1.2** Examination of the movement of the first ray.

The vascular section of the patient history and the physical examination is vitally important, and a misdiagnosis of vascular disease may result in significant morbidity (Nelson 1992). Podiatrists must be acutely aware of the potential limb loss, gangrene, ulceration and infection attributed to underlying arterial disease, and therefore the need for a peripheral vascular evaluation. Infection management, wound management and preoperative assessment, all require appropriate evaluation of the vascular status of podiatric patients. Hoffman (1992) suggests that 'with non-invasive arterial evaluation, the clinician must have a diagnosis in mind before initiating the testing, know exactly what data need to be documented, and be able to question the validity of what is being recorded'. Podiatrists understand the need for a sufficient vascular supply and thus must have the ability to evaluate that supply, ensuring that there is sufficient flow entering the leg or foot to sustain normal nutrition, to heal an existing ulcer or to sustain nutrition following surgery, depending on other factors, such as age.

Pain is a common symptom of vascular disease. The three components of the vascular 'tree' – arterial, venous and lymphatic – all have differing manifestations and pain severity. It is imperative that practitioners differentiate between the different types of pain, and differentiate between 'rest pain' and the night cramps of a venous disorder. The patient with rest pain complains of intense burning in the toes, the severity increasing with coldness or when the foot or leg is elevated; they may state that they obtain relief by putting the foot into the dependent position by hanging the limb out of the bed. This severe, persistent pain is associated with ulceration or gangrene, and is indicative of a more severe arterial disease. A sudden or abrupt onset of severe pain may suggest an acute arterial or venous obstruction. In the acute arterial occlusion the pain is immediate and persistent. It may be accompanied by a sensation of coldness, tingling and numbness distally to the occlusion site. On the other hand, the pain associated with venous occlusion is similar to that of phlebitis, which is characterised by a severe ache over the involved vein. There may also be an accompanying burning or swelling of the ankle and foot.

The 'classic' pain normally found with chronic arterial insufficiency is termed 'intermittent claudication'. This symptom is transient, is usually induced by exercise and is characteristically described as cramp, ache, tiredness or tightness of the associated muscles (usually the calf, but it can be the buttocks or the small intrinsic muscles of the foot). The main diagnostic criterion is that rest relieves the pain. The clinician must differentiate between orthopaedic and neurological conditions producing pain and the pain of intermittent claudication. Claudication distance can be evaluated using external factors, such as the distance the patient can walk by counting the number of lamp posts, or between two known landmarks, or clinically by the use of a treadmill. The latter allows variations of speed and of slope, and this helps in determining which factors make the situation worse. This allows the clinician to guide the patient as to what pace to take and what characteristics of the landscape to avoid (e.g. advising the patient to find routes that avoid hills). The ischaemia from acute or chronic arterial occlusion will ultimately lead to ischaemic neuropathy. The pain associated with this is sharp and shooting but poorly localised in nature.

The ability to heal is of paramount importance, especially where elective surgery is considered. Thus the clinician must be able to hypothesise and predict healing ability. Normally, adequate blood flow equates with healing ability. However, certain conditions – such as anaemia, alcoholism, uncontrolled diabetes, some connective tissue diseases and poor nutrition – refute this general assumption. Poor nutrition may be found in the elderly or alcoholics, and may result from inadequate oxygenation. Simple questions such as 'How quickly does your skin normally heal after it has been damaged?' should be used alongside a visual inspection of skin. It is important to realise that the physical examination should correlate with the signs and symptoms described by the patient. Where there is a lack of correlation, a double check or further more detailed investigations may be warranted. For example, pedal pulses may be absent, but on its own this sign may be insignificant; similarly, the presence of pedal pulses does not necessarily indicate adequate pedal perfusion.

The most significant findings aiding clinicians to diagnose the presence of peripheral arterial disease are abnormal pedal pulses, a unilaterally cool extremity, prolonged venous filling time and a femoral bruit. Other physical signs help determine the extent and distribution of the disease, but findings such as abnormal capillary refill time, foot discoloration, atrophic skin and hairless extremities are unhelpful to diagnosis. Within the pedal pulses the absence or diminution of the posterior tibial pulses is a more accurate indicator than is an absent dorsalis pedis pulse (Criqui et al 1985).

Palpation of pedal pulses is crucial (Nelson 1992) but clinical experience indicates that there is lack of precision associated with these pulses (Kazmers et al 1996). Each clinician has a different ability to palpate these pulses. In the foot the pedal pulses to be palpated are the posterior and anterior tibial and the dorsalis pedis. The dorsalis pedis pulse is palpated lateral to the extensor hallucis tendon at the base of the first metatarsal; the anterior tibial pulse is found at the front of the ankle; while the posterior tibial pulse is located below and behind the medial malleolus, with the foot slightly inverted. Unfortunately there is no standardisation of gradation of pulses or how they are recorded. Thus confusion exists as to how they should be recorded, with adjectives and verbs being used to describe the quality, rhythm and rate of the pulses as well as the amplitude. The most frequently used scale is (Kidawa 1993, Nelson 1992):

0/4 – absence of pulses
1/4 – weak (may suggest impairment)
2/4 – normal
3/4 – full
4/4 – bounding (may suggest aneurysm).

Baker (1991), suggests that pulses should be recorded as normal, decreased or absent. He does, however, anticipate a fourth category, where pulses are greater than expected. As the assessment is subjective, it is probable that these descriptions are all that is required.

Clinicians demonstrate fair to almost perfect agreement when stating a pulse was present or absent, but disagreement occurs when attempting to distinguish between normal and reduced pulses. Where both pedal pulses are absent there is more likelihood of vascular disease than when only one is absent (Reich 1934, cited in McGee & Boyko 1998). This is because where the dorsalis pedis pulse is absent, the posterior tibial pulse will act as a collateral supply, and vice versa. The reproducibility and accuracy of pulse palpation can be increased by undertaking the assessment under unhurried, good, quiet conditions.

The foot and lower extremities should also be inspected, taking account of colour, texture of skin, trophic changes, hair growth, oedema and ulceration. For further information on vascular disease, see Chapter 5.

Oedema of the lower leg or foot can be the result of a variety of diseases. An assessment of whether the oedema is unilateral or bilateral may suggest if it is local or regional in the former or systemic if the latter. It must also be differentiated by palpation. Is it pitting (i.e. soft in nature, leaving a depression after 15–30 s) or indurated (non-pitting)? Oedema associated with systemic disease is generally pitting, occurring bilaterally and involving the whole leg or foot to the level of the toes. Swelling of venous origin may also be pitting, but it is usually unilateral, and the oedema of varicosity or venous stasis is

**Table 1.1** Signs and symptoms of peripheral vascular disease

| Arterial insufficiency | Venous insufficiency |
|---|---|
| **Acute** | |
| Pain – severe, steady | Steady, moderate to severe |
| Cold pallid limb | Skin warm, may be mottled, cyanotic |
| Diminution/loss of sensory and motor function | No significant neurological deficit |
| Absent pulsation beyond embolus | Pulses present or diminished |
| Veins collapsed | Veins filled (legs dependent) |
| No swelling (unless ischaemia advanced) | Usually moderate to severe swelling, with tenderness over veins and muscles |
| **Chronic** | |
| Intermittent claudication progressing to rest pain with severe ischaemia | Aching, heavy-legs sensation, muscle cramps |
| Extremity cool, distal pulses diminished | Prominent, superficial veins, warm feet |
| Delayed healing of minor traumatic lesions | Pigmentation, oedema of lower leg |
| Atrophy of skin, loss of hair on toes | Haemosiderosis, soft pitting oedema disappears overnight, unless of longstanding, when it becomes fibrosed, harder and firmer |
| Pallor when elevated, rubor when dependent | Scaling, thickening and scarring of skin |
| Ulceration, superficial gangrene | Ulceration around ankle, medial malleolus |

**Table 1.2** The ankle–brachial index (ABI)

| Pressure/ABI | Indicator |
|---|---|
| 0.9–1.00 | Normal |
| 0.5–0.9 | Claudicators |
| < 0.5 | Ischaemia |
| 0.1–0.2 | Impending gangrene |

obvious due to bulging varicosities of the perforating veins just above the medial malleolus during weight bearing. There may also be haemosiderosis or brownish pigmentation around the site.

Ulceration may be one of the first external signs and symptoms of arterial disease. Ischaemic or arterial ulcers are usually painful and are found on the anterior or lateral lower leg above the ankle, whereas venous ulcers are usually painless and found on the medial lower leg just above the medial malleolus. Table 1.1 highlights the differential diagnosis between arterial and venous insufficiency.

Where pedal pulses are not palpable Doppler studies may help. The Doppler scanner is one of a number of non-invasive evaluation techniques available to some podiatrists. The Doppler can be used to extend clinical examination by detecting pulses over a very wide range. Therefore it is primarily useful for measuring distal blood pressures. The use of the Doppler scan has become more widespread in podiatric practice, but the successful use of this device depends on a number of factors. The tip of the Doppler probe must be coupled to the skin using an ultrasound-coupling medium, and the angle of the probe to the artery is important. The correct range of this angle has been reported to be from 45° to 60°, but there is debate about whether this angle is to the skin or to the artery (Baker 1991, Hoffman 1992). Whatever the angle, the probe should be placed in the direction of the heart. Light application of the probe to the skin surface is sufficient to ensure good detection in most cases. If excessive pressure is applied, occlusion of the artery is possible. Arteries and veins generate characteristic signals, which must be differentiated. The normal distal artery has a biphasic or triphasic sound, with a brisk systolic upstroke followed by a less prominent early and mid-diastolic component (Baker 1991). In occlusive arterial disease the systolic component may be less prominent, with few or no diastolic parts. In severe disease there may be only one continuous sound. Large and medium veins produce a low-frequency sound, which has often been likened to that of wind blowing through trees (Baker 1991). The slower the blood flow, the lower the audible pitch.

The most common use of Doppler is to measure the ankle–brachial index (ABI) or ankle–arm index (AAI). Ankle blood pressure should be approximately 90% of the brachial artery systolic pressure (Nelson 1992). The ABI is usually classified as shown in Table 1.2.

To measure the pressure at the ankle, the cuff is placed around the ankle of a supine patient with the foot at the same level as the heart. The sounds through a pedal vessel are located and the cuff is slowly inflated until no sounds are detected. The cuff is then slowly deflated until a sound is heard, and the pressure of the ankle cuff is noted. The arm, or brachial, pressure is also noted. The ankle measurement is divided by the brachial reading and the resultant figure (the ABI) is recorded. However, care needs to be used when interpreting the results of the ABI. If the ABI is 1 there is good flow velocity, this indicates only the adequacy of blood flow at the ankle level. It does not indicate adequacy of any flow below this level. In diabetes, in particular, there may be distal occlusions in the foot, and thus ankle blood flow cannot be used to estimate blood flow in the foot (Hoffman 1992). The ABI can be falsely elevated in the presence of calcifications of arteries. Thus both the sounds noted with the Doppler and the ABI should be considered prior to assuming that a correct ABI has been noted. Where, for example, the ABI is 1.2 but there is a low-pitched, long, swishing sound on the Doppler, an assumption that there is some calcification is more likely to be correct.

Other sophisticated techniques, such as photoplethysmography, Perthe's test, the Brodie/Trendelenberg test, percussion and thermography, may be used to measure various components of the vascular system, but this is usually the realm of either researchers or more specialist clinical areas.

## Neurological assessment (see also Ch. 6)

Ziegler (1985) stated that there is 'in all clinical medicine a subtle competition between the value of information given us by increasingly sophisticated instruments and that by our own eyes, ears and hands'. This is true of neurology and the neurological examination: 'It still requires the skills of the clinician to be attuned to signs and symptoms within the history which suggests that further neurological tests might be advised to identify the problem or cause of these symptoms.' As DeMeyer (1998) states: 'Since the examiner cannot do every possible test on every patient, intelligent utilisation of the history may shorten the examination yet make it more informative.'

The way in which a neurological examination is conducted will depend on the age of the patient and the presenting complaint. Green (1974) suggests that there is a trinity required in examination of the elderly:

- patience
- a capacity to repeat parts of the examination gently
- a sense of humour.

In a child the neurological examination may be handicapped by lack of cooperation, and thus observation may provide the most information (Bernstein 1987, Singh 1978). Singh (1978) suggests it is not generally feasible to have a scheme of examination for infants. Height, weight, ambulatory status and general activity level may be required information in children (Bernstein 1987), but it is good practice to record these data for all patients.

The history and the physical examination are vitally important components of the evaluation, often determining the diagnosis and the need to plan further diagnostic tests (Magee 1977). Although gait is discussed later, the patient should be observed as he or she walks into the clinic and as the history is taken. Thus, again, observation is highlighted as a key component, with the diagnostic tools of our ears and eyes being the mainstay of the examination. The most vital, and often forgotten, part of any neurological examination is communication. Inform the patient about what each test is, what is required of them, and why it is being carried out.

## Motor system

The main aims of examining the motor system are to:

- identify any lesions
- ascertain whether the lesion is an *upper motor neuron* (UMN) or a *lower motor neuron* (LMN) lesion
- locate the anatomical site
- consider the differential diagnosis of lesions at that site.

The examination should follow a routine:

- inspection
- palpation
- assessment of motor tone
- assessment of power
- assessment of reflexes
- assessment of coordination
- assessment of gait

not necessarily in this order.

### Inspection

Inspection of the patient begins as soon as he or she is called in the waiting area. The clinician should observe as he or she is walking towards them, looking for abnormalities of posture, gait or coordination or involuntary movements. Inspect for wasting, and note symmetry, looking specifically for distribution. Note any fasciculations (a spontaneous contraction of muscles, usually of small muscle fibres) that imply an LMN lesion (e.g. motor neuron disease or a 'slipped disc' (prolapsed disc)). Look also for tremors, and note whether these are fine or coarse, and whether they occur at rest or during movement (intention tremor).

### Palpation and assessment of tone

Palpate the muscles and muscle groups, looking at the muscle bulk and for tenderness (suggesting a myositis); also at this point note the tone. This evaluation is subjective and will require experience. Attempt to identify hypertonia (high resistance then sudden release – usually UMN) or hypotonia (LMN and cerebellar lesions).

### Assessment of power

Assess the muscles individually or as a group. Muscle power should be classified using the Medical Research Council (MRC) grade (Table 1.3). When a weakness is found or suspected, attempt to classify the origin as UMN or LMN.

**Table 1.3** Medical Research Council (MRC) classification of muscle power (adapted from Marsh 1999)

| Grade | MRC grade of muscle strength |
|---|---|
| 0 | No movement |
| 1 | Flicker of movement visible |
| 2 | Movement possible – gravity eliminated |
| 3 | Movement possible against gravity, but no resistance |
| 4 | Movement against resistance possible, but it is weak (can be divided into 4+ or 4−) |
| 5 | Normal |

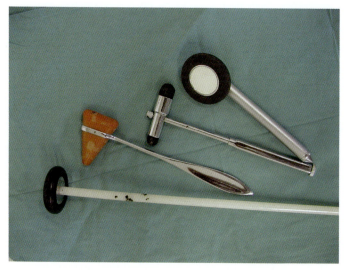

**Figure 1.3** A variety of hammers available for testing reflexes.

### Assessment of reflexes

Podiatrists should test the knee and ankle reflexes. According to DeMeyer (1998) neurologists persistently misname the muscle stretch reflexes (MSRs) 'deep tendon reflexes'. The MSR response should be elicited using a tendon hammer (Fig. 1.3). The MSRs tested by podiatrists are the quadriceps reflex, which assesses the fourth lumbar nerve (L4), and the Achilles reflex. Comparison of the reflex should be made with the corresponding one on the opposite limb and with 'normal'. The response should be recorded as normal, brisk, reduced or absent. If the reflex is absent, attempt to produce it by reinforcement methods – ask the patient to interlock fingers and pull them apart while attempting to elicit a response in the knee (Jendrassik's manoeuvre) (Merck Manual 1997).

The Babinski reflex is tested using moderate pressure, not light stroking, as this may produce only a tickle response rather than a reflex. If this test is inadequate then the Chaddock reflex test can be performed (DeMeyer 1998, Magee 1977). This involves stroking the side of the foot with a blunt instrument and looking for the same extensor response of the hallux as occurs in the Babinski response. The result should be recorded as either a normal plantar response (hallux and toes curl and claw plantarly), reduced or absent, or a Babinski response (hallux extends dorsally, the toes may or may not also fan out). However, it should be noted that a Babinski response is a normal finding in infants up to 18 months of age (Bernstein 1987).

## Assessment of coordination

The lower limbs are assessed using the heel–shin test. Ask the patient to place his or her right heel on the left shin and slide it up and down the shin, and then to repeat the test on the other side using the alternate limb.

## Motor and sensory system functions

It is only necessary to perform muscle testing for strength, size and symmetry. In the foot this will normally involve testing of the dorsiflexors, plantarflexors and invertors and evertors.

Observation during the examination will demonstrate evidence of atrophy, fasciculations and involuntary movements, along with the symmetry of one leg/foot/side to the other. Passive movements of the various muscle groups can determine fluidity of movement and will elicit lead-pipe rigidity (basal ganglia disorder) or clasp-knife should movements (pyramidal tract disorders).

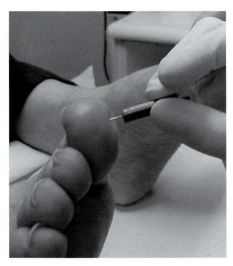

**Figure 1.4** Demonstrating the use of the Neurotip: testing sensation for sharp and blunt.

## Sensory investigations

Patients are normally aware of some change in sensation and may describe numbness, paraesthesia or altered sensation, which will indicate a sensory pathology or dysfunction. Examination of the sensory system is part of the routine examination. An attempt should be made to identify the modality of loss and also its distribution (i.e. correlate it with a dermatome or a sensory peripheral nerve).

### Light touch

Dab a cotton wool ball onto the skin lightly. If an area of sensory diminution is suggested, attempt to map this out. Start from the area of decreased sensation and progress to an area of normal sensation.

### Pin prick

As pain and temperature run in the same tract (spinothalamic), it is necessary to perform only one of the tests rather than both, unless some concern or questions remain having performed one test. Magee (1977) suggested using the pain test and leaving temperature, as does Marsh (1999). However, DeMeyer (1998) suggests that in the screening neurological examination the clinician test first for temperature and reserve the pin prick test for cases where there is a neurological problem or sensory findings (Fig. 1.4).

### Vibration

The posterior column is the location of sensing position and vibration. These are evaluated at the ankle and distal aspects of the hallux. Vibration can be grossly evaluated using a 128 Hz tuning fork at the malleolus or the medial border of the hallux (Fig. 1.5). Patients should be aware of a buzzing sensation (Marsh 1999). The patient should close his or her eyes and indicate when they can no longer feel the sensation. More precise and recordable measurements are obtained by using a Rydel–Seiffer tuning fork with a graduated scale (Fig. 1.6)

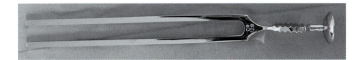

**Figure 1.5** Normal 128 Hz or middle C tuning fork. It measures gross vibration sense but gives no scalar quantifiable data.

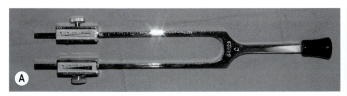

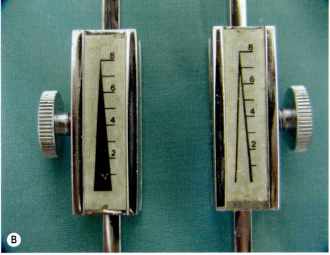

**Figure 1.6** Rydel–Seiffer (RS) tuning fork with a graduated scale (A). Scalar measurement and quantifiable data from the RS tuning fork (B).

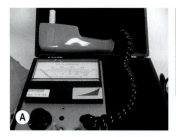
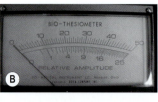

**Figure 1.7** A biothesiometer (A) and the scalar reading area (B).

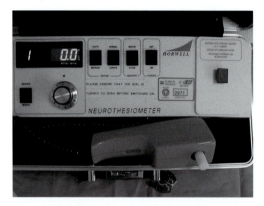

**Figure 1.8** A neurothesiometer. It uses a battery pack but has a vibration head similar to that of a biothesiometer.

**Table 1.4** Upper and lower motor neuron disease: differential diagnosis

| Differentiating factor | Upper motor neuron | Lower motor neuron |
| --- | --- | --- |
| Location of weakness | Lesion in brain; pyramidal distribution (distal, weak extensors in arms, weak flexors in legs) Lesion in cord: variable, depending on location | Depends on lower motor neurons involved (which segment, root or nerves) |
| Muscle tone | Spasticity increased in flexors in arms and extensors in legs | Flaccidity |
| Muscle bulk | Atrophy of disuse | Atrophy which is marked |
| Reflexes | Increased, Babinski reflex present | Decreased, absent |
| Fasciculations | Absent | Present |
| Clonus (rhythmic, rapid, alternating muscle contraction and relaxation brought on by sudden, passive tendon stretching) | Frequently present | Absent |

or, better, the biothesiometer (Fig. 1.7) or neurothesiometer (Fig. 1.8). However, the latter two are fairly expensive pieces of equipment and should be reserved for those either undertaking research or conducting examinations in those with a degradable sensory dysfunction such as diabetes.

In elderly patients, reduced perception of vibration, pain and touch at the ankle and a diminished ankle reflex are not necessarily clinically significant. Testing of more sophisticated sensory functions, such as stereognosis and two-point discrimination, is unnecessary for a routine clinical neurological survey.

In evaluating the motor and sensory systems the aim is to determine the anatomical site or pathway affected, localising the lesions or disorder to the peripheral nerves, nerve roots, spinal cord, brainstem, basal ganglia or cerebral hemispheres. It may also be possible to differentiate between single or multiple lesion disorders. Table 1.4 outlines the main characteristics of differential diagnosis between upper motor neuron lesions (central nervous system) and lower motor neuron lesions (peripheral nervous system).

Similarly, the motor examination and gait analyses localise lesions to the neuromuscular junctions or to a particular muscle.

One further test, which has become more frequently used by podiatrists, is the monofilament test (Semmes–Weinstein monofilament). This test is used to predict foot ulceration, especially in diabetes (Armstrong et al 1998, Bell-Krotoski et al 1995, Bell-Krotoski & Tomancik 1987, Kumar et al 1991, Olmos et al 1995, van Vliet et al 1993, Weinstein 1993). Semmes–Weinstein monofilaments can be purchased as a set of 20 pressure-sensitive nylon filaments attached to a lucite rod, or as single unit (Neuropen, Owen Mumford,

Woodstock, Oxford, UK) or in a pack of three (Bailey Instruments, UK). The Neuropen has a 10 g or 15 g retractable, interchangeable monofilament as well as a calibrated neurotip. The set of three monofilaments is in a boxed set of 1 g, 10 g and 75 g monofilaments, each on a lucite rod. These monofilaments have a standardised length and thickness enabling them to buckle at reproducible forces ranging from 0.0045 g to 447 g (Olmos et al 1995). This allows the amount of pressure being applied to cause buckling to be a constant force for that particular rod. The monofilament is applied perpendicular to the skin surface, and pressure is applied slowly until the monofilament bends. At that point the practitioner should request the patient to state whether they are able to determine any sensation of pressure. The 5.067 log monofilament (10 g) has been proven to be the level of pressure providing protective sensation against foot ulceration (Birke & Sims (1986) and Halar et al (1987) as cited in Olmos et al (1995)). As with any device, there are some known idiosyncrasies that a practitioner should take into account when using monofilaments and when interpreting the data obtained. Van Vliet et al (1993) found that pressure thresholds vary significantly with the duration of contact of the monofilament, thus requiring practitioners to maintain a consistent protocol when using these devices. These filaments are used to test the pressure at various places on the foot (Fig. 1.9).

The sites tested may vary (Armstrong et al 1998, Bell-Krotoski et al 1995) but the area of dermatomes of the foot should be covered. Another problem noted when using monofilaments is slippage when

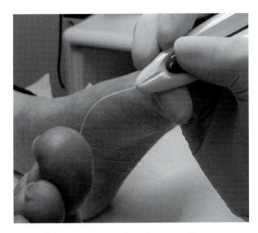

**Figure 1.9** Use of the Semmes–Weinstein mono-filament to test for pressure – a 10 g filament.

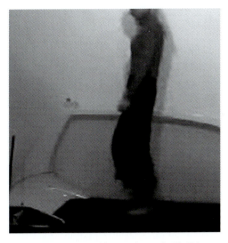

**Figure 1.10** Gait analysis using video and treadmill. Using patients fully clad can lead to problems of identification.

the filament is applied to the skin, which causes some disruption to the testing. However, this has been corrected for by the modification incorporated in the newer Weinstein Enhanced Sensory Test (WEST) (Weinstein 1993). These filaments are used daily in diabetes clinics, and together with other diagnostic or predictor factors help podiatrists to reduce possible ulceration and pressure lesions in diabetics. They are useful screening tools.

When a podiatrist detects an abnormality but is unsure of its origin they should refer the patient to a neurophysiologist for further studies and advanced testing of the nervous system. The ability of the podiatrist to determine when a patient needs to be referred is crucial to good patient management.

## Gait

Analysis of gait is rudimentary and should be carried out routinely when first seeing the patient. It is best to observe the gait when the patient is unaware of being observed. The analysis can be either by simple observation or by means of various measuring devices and mechanical methods. However, most practitioners will need to rely on observation as the primary method of analysis. Observation gives data about the full gait cycle, while mechanical methods usually determine the forces and pressures through the plantar of the foot. The use of a treadmill allows the cadence to be controlled, and the patient and practitioner are in a static position while undertaking a dynamic sequence of events. Video recording enables more subtle changes or patterns to be viewed and repeated, but this is not always available. Gait analysis using video and a treadmill is shown in Figure 1.10. A long, well-lit corridor is usually sufficient for gait analysis, but experience is needed to view minor changes and compensations from more than one angle. Gait analysis requires a holistic approach to the patient, and practitioners should look at each body segment in turn, and preferably from the front, back and one side. With informed consent, and a chaperone, it is best to view a patient in a semi-undressed state (Fig. 1.11). Most of the mechanical methods are confined to use by researchers or by specialist clinicians, due to cost, experience and time factors. Although the following gives a brief outline of some of the methods available, it is by no means an exhaustive list and detailed reviews by independent researchers should be viewed prior to purchasing any equipment. The methods are subdivided into static and dynamic methods. The information obtained from using these methods is in addition to the basic knowledge obtained in the general observation and examination, and in general

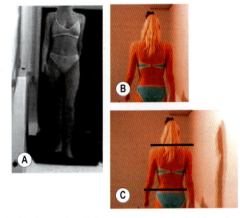

**Figure 1.11** Having gained informed consent, and with a chaperone, it is best to view a patient in a semi-undressed state (A). Rear view (B), and detailed segmental view (C), of the subject.

does not in itself lead to a diagnosis, but rather aids in making the diagnosis or is used to confirm it.

### Static evaluation

The *plantarscope* shows how the plantar surface of tissues blanches on loading. It consists of a safety-glass platform over an angled mirror, allowing the clinician to view the plantar surface of the foot. The *podometer* is more elaborate, and combines measurements of foot size and calcaneal deviation with the reflected image. The *pedobaroscope* is an internally lit sheet of glass with a plastic or card interface (Anderson & Black 1997). The patient stands on the interface and reflected light produces a grey-scale image, which is stored digitally or a hard copy produced for analysis.

### Dynamic evaluation

Possibly the simplest device is a sheet of black paper. The feet are dusted with chalk and the patient walks the length of the sheet or roll of paper. The resultant footprints give an indication of pressure areas, an outline of the footprint and weight-bearing surface, the angle and base of gait, as well as stride length.

The *Harris and Beath mat* is a rubber mat with ridges forming squares crossed by smaller squares which, when inked and overlaid with paper, allow the footprint to be left on the paper. The highest pressures are recorded.

The *dynamic pedobarograph* is a variant of the pedobaroscope and is used as a research tool. The resolution of this device is excellent but careful analysis of the results is required, and this takes experience and time. There are numerous commercially available devices of this type. One of these is the Musgrave foot pressure gait analysis system, which gives relatively good resolution of the pressure distribution of the plantar of the foot in real-time mode as well as static impressions. The pictorial results can be used for a variety of different analyses, and the device has become quite sophisticated. However, the system needs to be housed in a walkway. It has the advantage of giving highly visible pictures which enable discussion and visualisation of the problems with patients (Figs 1.12 and 1.13).

The *Kistler force plate* provides information about the forces acting through various joints and through the foot in all three axes. The interpretation of the resulting 'stick' figures is complex, requiring expertise and experience, and therefore this is definitely a tool for the researcher.

This is very much the case for these and other in-shoe pressure devices, which are too numerous to detail. In most cases the devices are upgraded or new versions and new devices are coming onto the market, all claiming to be repeatable, reliable and giving valid measurements, as well as ease of use.

For most clinicians, observation of gait and a Harris and Beath mat or other pressure-sensitive paper device will be sufficient.

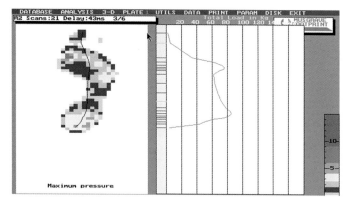

**Figure 1.12** Musgrave visual representation of centre of load of a typical rheumatoid disease patient.

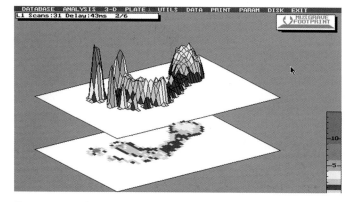

**Figure 1.13** A three-dimensional visual representation showing maximum pressures in a rheumatoid patient.

## Other soft tissues

Some clinical signs should be given greater importance than others. The most important of all clinical signs is that of the inflammatory process, classically described as rubor, calor, dolor and tumor – redness, warmth, pain and swelling. Loss of function is another classic sign of the inflammatory process. Again, accurate recording of the features will enhance clinical practice. The record card should indicate:

- if acute, chronic, or subacute
- if infected, whether localised, and if suppurating or resolving
- if infected and spreading, the other tissues involved (cellulitis, lymphadenitis, lymphangitis)
- if pus is produced, the colour, texture and fluidity– this will enable comparison between streptococcal and staphylococcal infections.

The treatment of an acute or subacute inflammatory lesion takes priority over a deformity, while a spreading infection requires immediate referral for further investigation and management (Anderson & Black 1997).

## Biomechanical examination

Assessment of the joint complexes of the foot and ankle and their relationships to the lower extremity and spinal column are vital to any diagnosis of foot problems of a structural or functional nature. Motion of any joints within their normal range should be pain-free and unrestricted. Pain, crepitus, restricted movement or excessive motion may suggest a joint pathology. Deformity affecting either of the osseous components of the joint, or tenderness affecting the surrounding structures on palpation may also indicate pathology. The various complexes of the foot and ankle should be assessed and examined individually.

## Further investigations

Some simple further tests may be initiated by podiatrists to enable a more reliable diagnosis and a suitable management plan to be conducted. These tests require taking samples of various constituent parts of the body, and it is necessary to communicate to the patient why these samples are needed and what information is expected to be obtained from them.

### Discharge

Bacteriological examination of pus and other wound discharge may help diagnose the particular infective agent present, enabling the practitioner to establish the most appropriate management plan. It is of paramount importance to establish the nature of the organisms present in wounds when the level of risk to the patient is high. Thus, high-risk diabetics with vascularly compromised or insensitive feet should clearly have the identity of any infective agent established as a matter of urgency. Where streptococcal or anaerobic organisms are suspected and the wound is not healing, it is vital to identify the organisms to ensure an appropriate management plan.

### Skin and nail

Research has demonstrated (McLarnon et al 1999, Millar et al 1996) that nails with suspected fungal infection must be mycologically examined prior to reduction by nail drill, as this process carries risks in terms of respiratory and ocular effects for the podiatrist. Scrapings can be examined for fungal infection, and should be collected when there is any suspicion of contamination by fungi. Scrapings are collected by scraping the edge of the skin lesion with a scalpel. The scrapings are placed in some form of container for transport to an approved laboratory. Scrapings are also taken from the affected nail at the advancing edge or the distal aspect of the nail and these too are placed in a transport container. It is important that, when mycotic nail infections are to be treated, (a) the fungus is identified prior to drilling or reduction, and (b) appropriate personal protective equipment is utilised during the reduction process.

## APPLYING CRITICAL THINKING TO THE INFORMATION GATHERED

Data gathered through the above processes may be either partial or complete, but all data require analysis. This is achieved using the following steps:

- Identify the abnormal findings, including the symptoms, physical signs and any laboratory test findings.
- Cluster or organise these findings into a logical group or groups.
- Localise the findings anatomically – the clinician may have to settle for a body region (e.g. the foot) or a system (e.g. musculoskeletal), or may be able to define the exact nature and location (spring ligament).
- Interpret the findings in terms of the probable process:
  - *pathological* – abnormality in body structure (processes such as inflammatory, traumatic, toxic, vascular)
  - *pathophysiological* – abnormality in function
  - *psychopathological* – disorder of mood or thinking.
- Attempt to interpret the findings and cluster them to form a hypothesis or probable diagnosis. Select the most specific data that fit a hypothesis and make inferences about structures and processes against the conditions that are likely to produce them. A patient may have described tenderness and a general ache of the feet, that they are tired, or have to rest, or that the pain is worst first thing in the morning but gradually diminishes as the day progresses. Signs may show an enlargement of the metatarsal area, with swelling of a boggy nature. On attempting a transverse metatarsal test the patient may have complained of extreme pain. The letter of referral suggested a raised erythrocyte sedimentation rate (ESR) but not much else. Using selection of the data and inferences about the pathological process a hypothesis of rheumatoid disease may be reached. This will require a sound knowledge and experience, and continuous professional development is essential to further learning about abnormalities and diseases.
- Eliminate any hypothesis that fails to explain the findings. The patient has some enlargement in the distal joints of the fingers but it is not symmetrical, although they have some swelling symmetrically of the more proximal joints. Although osteoarthritis may be a cause of the distal enlargement, it does not account for the more proximal swelling and the symmetry of the problem in the patient's feet.
- Weigh the probability of a different hypothesis or diagnosis according to:
  - the match with the findings
  - the statistical probability of a given disease in a patient of this age, sex, race, habits, lifestyle, locality and other variables
  - the timing of the patient's illness.
- Test the diagnosis. This may require further history, additional physical examination or laboratory tests. The clinician may require consultation with, or referral to, other specialists.
- Establish a working definition of the problem.

## DEVELOPMENT OF THE DIAGNOSIS

Establish a problem list and name each problem for the patient's record. This may be that the patient has:

- rheumatoid disease
- forefoot pain and discomfort (metatarsalgia)
- a biomechanical anomaly such as ligamentous laxity of the subtalar joint complex ligaments.

From this list, organise a plan to manage the problems both individually and holistically. For each active problem requiring attention, develop a plan, which may have three component parts: diagnostic, therapeutic and educational. It is best practice to include the patient in making the plans, as failure to do so may lead the patient to be non-compliant. The goals, attitudes, economic means, as well as competing responsibilities affect the practicality, acceptability and wisdom of the plan, and involving the patient from the very beginning improves the chances of success.

## CREATING THE RECORD

The patient's record is not just a record of what was done to the patient by the practitioner – it is a legal documentation of the consultation process (see also Ch. 16). There are certain legal, ethical and professional requirements for podiatric records. (In the UK these are laid down by the Health Professions Council (HPC), Society of Chiropodists and Podiatrists (SCP) and Department of Health (DoH); there are corresponding appropriate bodies in other countries.) The record documents the findings, the assessment of the nature and causes of the problem, the diagnostic conclusions as well as the plan for the management of the patient and their condition(s). The record should be accurate, clear, well organised, up to date and legible. It should emphasise important features and omit the irrelevant. Data not recorded are lost, but data buried in trivia can be overlooked. Record all positive data that contributed to the assessment, and describe the negative data, such as the absence of a sign or symptom, if this has affected or enabled a diagnosis. Remember that a patient is entitled to ask to see their health record; therefore, stick to factual information and avoid litigious phrases about the patient.

A good record leads to good communication between the practitioner and the patient and between other professionals who may participate in the patient's care. It is also helps in medicolegal cases.

Abbreviations and symbols used should be those commonly used and understood (SCP 1999), and measurements should be in centimetres and not obtuse inaccurate schemes of measurement such as 'pea-sized'. Where appropriate, diagrams add greatly to the clarity of records (Bates 1995).

The SOAPE system is a well-established recording method, and ensures accuracy and completeness of data for each consultation. The method consists of writing the letters perpendicularly down the record card, and adding information in the following scheme:

S = symptoms described by the patient
O = objective signs observed by the practitioner
A = action taken that day
P = plan of management for patient as agreed between the two parties
E = evaluation of previous treatment given, and thus a synopsis of how the management plan is progressing.

## CASE STUDY 1.1 RHEUMATOLOGY REFERRAL

A young female patient aged 31 years, with an office occupation, presents to a podiatrist with a letter from her GP. The letter invites the podiatrist to see and advise about a metatarsalgia the patient has been experiencing for a few weeks.

On the day of the consultation the patient explains that she has experienced pain in the forefoot across the 'ball' of her foot. She has noticed it in both feet, recently, with sometimes what she thinks is swelling of both feet. The pain is worse in the morning and takes about an hour or so to lessen. Recently, she has had difficulty walking up stairs and has taken to using the lift in her office building rather than taking the one flight of stairs. She has noticed that her hands have become sore and tender, especially over her small finger joints, and using the keyboard has become more difficult. She says she has no other complaints.

On examination you notice that her feet are swollen and feel hot to the touch over the metatarsal areas. Palpation of the areas suggests some swelling, and they are tender to the touch. Her hands also display some swelling across the metacarpophalangeal joints and the proximal interphalangeal joints. Both hands and feet appear to be bilaterally involved, with symmetry across the joints affected. When you lightly grasp the metatarsal heads just proximal to them and squeeze the foot she gasps in pain and is obviously distressed by the technique.

She is referred to the rheumatologist with a possible diagnosis of rheumatoid disease, which is confirmed a few weeks later with a positive rheumatoid factor in her blood serum.

## CASE STUDY 1.2 DIABETES MELLITUS

A male patient, 46 years of age, presents with problems with cutting nails, a history according to the GP's letter of ingrown toenails and infections not responding well to antibiotics.

The patient is 1.67 m tall and says that he weighs about 95 kg. He states that his problems have persisted over the last 6 months or so, during which time he has had difficulty cutting his nails – after cutting them they seem to become infected on a regular basis. He has had numerous courses of antibiotics but they do not seem to clear the infection. On examination it is noticed that the great toe is swollen and inflamed, with pus exuding but no sign of a spur.

Further questioning suggests a history on his mother's side of the family of diabetes and his father was also a diabetic. This suggests that the patient should be questioned about his diet, his weight gain, his social drinking and work.

Recently, the patient has noticed that he cannot concentrate for as long as usual, and that he is drinking 'quite a lot of water' more often at his place of work, but has put this down to the office being too hot. His weight has been steadily increasing in the past year but he has put this down to 'middle-age spread' and lack of exercise.

The symptoms suggest type 2 diabetes and the patient is referred back to his GP who conducts the necessary tests with a positive result.

## REFERENCES

Anderson EG, Black JA 1997 Examination and assessment. In: Lorimer D et al (eds) Neale's common foot disorders: diagnosis and management. Churchill Livingstone, Edinburgh.

Armstrong DG, Lavery LA, Vela SA et al 1998 Choosing a practical screening instrument to identify patients at risk for diabetic foot ulceration. Archives of Internal Medicine 158:289–292.

Baker JD 1991 Assessment of peripheral arterial occlusive disease. Critical Care Nursing Clinics of North America 3(3):493–498.

Bates B 1995 A guide to physical examination and history taking, 6th edn. Lippincott, Philadelphia.

Bell-Krotoski J, Tomancik E 1987 The repeatability of testing with Semmes–Weinstein monofilaments. Journal of Hand Surgery [Am] 12(1):155–161.

Bell-Krotoski JA, Fess EE, Figarola JH, Hiltz D 1995 Threshold detection and Semmes–Weinstein monofilaments. Journal of Hand Therapy 8(2):155–162.

Bernstein AL 1987 Neurologic examination in children. Clinics in Podiatric Medicine and Surgery 4(1):11–20.

Criqui MH, Fronek A, Klauber MR et al 1985 The sensitivity, specificity, and predictive value of traditional clinical evaluation of

peripheral arterial disease: results from non-invasive testing in a defined population. Circulation 71(3):516–522.

DeMeyer W 1998 Pointers and pitfalls in the neurologic examination. Seminars in Neurology 18(2):161–168.

Green D 1974 Neurologic examination of the elderly. New York State Journal of Medicine 74(6):969–972.

Hoffman AF 1992 Evaluation of arterial blood flow in the lower extremity. Clinics in Podiatric Medicine and Surgery 9(1):19–56.

Kazmers A, Koski MF, Groehn H et al 1996 Assessment of non-invasive lower extremity arterial testing versus pulse exam. American Surgeon 62(4):315–319.

Kidawa AS 1993 Vascular evaluation. Clinical Podiatric Medicine and Surgery 10(2):187–203.

Kumar S, Fernando DJS, Veves A et al 1991 Semmes–Weinstein monofilaments: a simple, effective and inexpensive screening device for identifying diabetic patients at risk of foot ulceration. Diabetes Research and Clinical Practice 13(1–2):63–67.

McGee SR, Boyko EJ 1998 Physical examination and chronic lower-extremity ischemia: a critical review. Archives of Internal Medicine 158(12):1357–1364.

McLarnon NA, Burrow JG, Aidoo KE 1999 Ocular risk to podiatrists from human toe nails. Unpublished work, PhD thesis, Glasgow Caledonian University.

Magee KR 1977 The neurologic workup by the primary care physician. Postgraduate Medicine 61(3):77–80, 83–86.

Marsh J 1999 History and examination, Mosby's crash course. Mosby, London.

Merck Manual Medical Library, Online medical Library 1997 found at www.merck.com/MMPE/index.html.

Merriman LM, Turner W 2002 Assessment of the lower limb, 2nd edn. Churchill Livingstone, Edinburgh (ISBN 0-443-071128).

Millar NA, Burrow JG, Hay J, Stevenson R 1996 Putative risks of ocular infection for chiropodists and podiatrists. Journal of British Podiatric Medicine 51(11):158–160.

Nelson JP 1992 The vascular history and physical examination. Clinics in Podiatric Medicine and Surgery 9(1):1–17.

Olmos PR, Cataland S, O'Dorisio TM et al 1995 The Semmes–Weinstein monofilaments as a potential predictor of foot ulceration in patients with non-insulin dependent diabetes. American Journal of the Medical Sciences 309(2):76–82.

Ricketts P 1999 Did you consent to treatment? http://www.pfiworld1.cwc.net/GPQ/patient1.htm.

Singh M 1978 Neurologic examination of an infant. Indian Journal of Paediatrics 45(371):3086–3089.

The Society of Chiropodists and Podiatrists Guidelines on Minimum Standards of Clinical Practice 1999 SCP, London.

The Readers Digest Universal Dictionary 1987. Readers Digest Association Limited, London.

van Vliet D, Novak CB, Mackinnon SE 1993 Duration of contact time alters cutaneous pressure threshold measurements. Annals of Practical Surgery 31(4):335–339.

Wanheng C, Xiaoxiang L 1996 Wisdom in Chinese Proverbs, Asiapac Books, Singapore (ISBN 981-3068-27-2).

Weinstein S 1993 Fifty years of somatosensory research: from the Semmes–Weinstein monofilaments to the Weinstein Enhanced Sensory Test. Journal of Hand Therapy 6(1):11–22.

Ziegler DK 1985 Is the neurologic examination becoming obsolete? Neurology 35(4):559.

# Chapter | 2 |

# The skin and nails in podiatry

*Kate Springett and Margaret Johnson*

## KEYWORDS

Chilblains
Chronic wounds (ulcers)
Corns and callus
Differential diagnosis of foot infection
Disorders of sweating
Fissures
Juvenile plantar dermatosis
Human foot
Infections
Inflammation
Management of chronic wounds
Structure and function of the skin
Systemic treatment of foot and nail infections
Treatment of fungal foot and nail infections
Viral infections
Vitiligo
Eponychium
Granulation tissue
Growth and development
Hippocratic
Hyponychium
Involution
Lovibond's angle
Matrix
Onychauxis
Onychocryptosis
Onychocytes
Onychodermal band

Clinical observation of the skin and nails is an important aspect of the process of assessment and diagnosis of the patient, and the many indicators provided by these easily observed structures can very quickly point the way to an accurate diagnosis.

## AFFECTATIONS OF THE SKIN

The skin provides an insight into the well-being of the individual as a whole as well as the peripheral tissue status. It can provide diagnostic indicators of various systemic disorders, such as pruritus (itchiness) with chronic liver disease or bullae (blisters) with an adverse drug reaction. It provides an indication of the quality of the peripheral tissues, both superficial and deep. The skin will show physical changes, for example in the microcirculation in diabetes, that are also likely to be occurring in the deeper tissues not visible to the clinician. If the skin shows poor tissue viability then it is likely that deeper tissues are in a similar state.

Changes with age are normal, for example fine to coarse wrinkling, mottled hyperpigmentation and yellowing (Gnaidecka & Jemec 1998). Xerosis (fine, dry scales) with actinosis (skin plaques) and elastosis (altered elasticity) are associated with photo damage (Diridollou et al 2001). Skin cancers are covered later in this chapter.

Often, the medical, social and family history in addition to the history of the skin complaint provides a clear indication of the nature of the problem. Observation and clinical tests provide further information. A clear diagnosis is not always possible, as the presentation may not be classic. However, the lack a of definitive diagnosis cannot be used as an excuse for not managing the condition, as symptomatic management should be undertaken until further tests facilitate a differential diagnosis of the condition.

All the following sections assume that the history has been taken, including the drug history. It is good practice to work towards evidence-based care for patients, and it is appropriate to review the results of monitoring and evaluation and modify practices as necessary (Feder et al 1999, Hurwitz 1999), and according to the contemporary literature. However, lack of evidence in the literature of the effectiveness of a particular treatment should not be taken to mean that it is ineffective and thus not to be used (Ryan 1998).

## STRUCTURE AND FUNCTION OF THE SKIN

The skin is the largest of the body's organs and has a number of roles, which include protection, interaction with the environment and homeostasis (Freinkel & Woodley 2001). Three main components of the skin, the epidermis, the dermoepidermal junction (DEJ, basement membrane) and the dermis, are further divided into layers. The epidermis is a stratified squamous keratinising epithelium (MacKie 2003), the outermost layer of which (the stratum corneum) forms the primary barrier for the body. This layer is not an inert structure but is capable of releasing growth factors when traumatised (McKay & Leigh 1991), a point which should be emphasised to discourage patients from rubbing overvigorously when self-treating callus.

The epidermis is avascular, though enervated, and is separated from the dermis by the undulating DEJ. The dermis provides the secondary barrier to the body through its vascular supply, tissue structure and immunological role. The base of the dermis also undulates, and is bounded by adipose tissue and fascia, then muscle.

## ACUTE INFLAMMATION

Human tissues respond to trauma by a complex series of events that have yet to be fully understood. This trauma may be mechanical, thermal, photo or chemical, or brought about through allergic or autoimmune events. If blood vessels have been injured, damaged platelets will activate the clotting cascade. Damaged tissues will release chemical messengers (Table 2.1), which start the inflammatory process. In health, sequential phases of proliferation, maturation and repair of the damaged tissue follow inflammation.

Blood cells and platelets, the immune system and nerves (Tortora et al 2005), chemical transmitters, and tissue cells such as macrophages are among the tissues and systems involved in inflammation. The molecular and cellular events during inflammation flow into and overlap with one with the other (Dealey 2005). Initially, neutrophils arrive, followed by macrophages, lymphocytes and then fibroblasts, which lay down collagen. Epithelial cells migrate on from wound edges over the newly laid down dermis and healing is complete. Healing by first intention will close over 2–5 days; a wound healing by second intention will take longer, the time taken depending on the tissue area that needs to be filled in and covered. The predominance and sequence of mediator release will allow different types of inflammatory response to occur.

The classic and clinical features of inflammation are redness (rubor), heat (calor), swelling (tumour) and pain (dolor); loss of function is sometimes included in this list. These features are brought about through chemical/inflammatory mediators released from damaged tissues (Table 2.1). The main effects of these mediators are on the blood supply, causing vasodilation (redness and heat) and increased blood-vessel permeability that allow plasma proteins and immunoglobulins to pass easily into the tissues (increased fluid interstitially causes swelling). Pressure on nerve endings from the interstitial fluid and the effect of some inflammatory mediators such as substance P and prostaglandins (e.g. PGE1) cause pain.

The mainstay of management for acute inflammation and pain management in healthy individuals is rest, ice, compression and elevation (RICE) (Brown 1992, Humphreys 1999). This should be adapted for different patients and different situations (see also Chs 4, 13 and 16). It is essential to identify the cause of the acute inflammation and, if possible, remove it and inform the patient of the cause so that they can avoid the situation in the future. The therapeutic aim in acute inflammation is to allow it to occur but to control its excesses and keep the phases as short as possible. Therapeutic ultrasound (Hart 1998) and low-level laser therapy (Halery et al 1997) have a part to play in management, along with the application of soothing and cooling substances such as witch hazel and lavender and camomile oils (Hitchen 1987). Controversy exists over the use of orthodox anti-inflammatory drugs (e.g. ibuprofen) in acute inflammation but analgesics (e.g. paracetamol) may help in controlling pain.

## CHRONIC WOUNDS (ULCERS)

Ulcers (Fig. 2.1) occur where a predisposing condition impairs the ability of the tissue to maintain its integrity or heal from damage. They may be superficial or deep, extending to bone, and may track under the tissues such that there is an extensive area of damage not visible on the skin's surface. Generally, chronic wounds take weeks to months to heal, and some may take years. All require careful and informed assessment (Wall 1997) and management, which will change as the wound changes. As with any break in the skin barrier, chronic wounds can become infected (Dealey 2005).

### Assessment of chronic wounds

It is essential to take a holistic approach to assessing and managing chronic wounds. Risk assessment scores may be calculated (e.g. Waterlow score) to identify those particularly at risk of developing chronic wounds (Dealey 2005). After assessing and obtaining the history of general health and peripheral status (e.g. blood supply (Baker & Rayman 1999), neurological status), specific enquiry about the wound can start.

The features of the skin generally, and that surrounding the wound, the nature of the wound margins and base, and the type of exudate (Jones 2005, Phillips et al 1998) in the wound and on the dressing must be assessed and recorded for monitoring and evaluation purposes. Swabs for culture and sensitivity may be taken if infection is present, but are likely to contain skin contaminants and therefore to be of limited use. Information obtained about the patient and wound will lead to diagnosis of the type of chronic wound (Table 2.2). The wound may be measured across the diameter, or margin traced on a sterile film; photographs can be stored in the patient's notes, and non-invasive methods such as ultrasound imaging (Rippon et al 1998) used to measure and record wound progress.

Assessment tools for chronic wounds should be used only for what they are designed to do; the Wagner classification is for diabetic ulcer-

---

**Table 2.1** Some chemical/inflammatory mediators that cause the features of inflammation

| | |
|---|---|
| Histamine<br>Kinins<br>Prostaglandins<br>Leucotrienes | From a variety of sources, including mast cells, macrophages, platelets |
| Complement component<br>Plasma<br>Cytokines | Have differing functions according to predominance and sequence of release, so different types of inflammatory response occur |

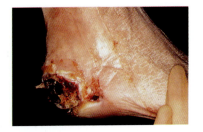

**Figure 2.1** A pressure sore on a heel is a chronic wound where tissue damage may be far more extensive than is apparent on the surface. Tissue at all levels down to bone may be involved.

**Table 2.2** Possible causes and types of ulcer

| Cause | Type of ulcer |
|-------|---------------|
| Impaired venous drainage | Venous (varicose) ulcer<br>Ischaemic ulcer |
| Metabolic/endocrine disorder with complications of neuropathy | Neuropathic ulcer |
| Combinations of all three of the above | Mixed aetiology ulcer |
| Persistent mechanical stress | Pressure sore (decubitus ulcer) |
| Malignancy | Rodent ulcer, fungating wound |
| Genetic disorder, e.g. sickle-cell anaemia | Ulcer |

---

Box 2.1  **A suggested protocol for the treatment of bacterial infections of the skin**

- Any open lesions should be cleaned with warm hypertonic saline solution or irrigated with sterile normal saline (Lawrence 1997), all at body temperature (Cameron & Leaper 1987, Springett 1989) and using an aseptic/non-touch technique.

- If the wound is chronic, slough may be present and it will be necessary to physically debride this to allow healing (Jones 1998) to occur – autolysis (e.g. by using a hydrogel or hydrocolloid dressing). Other methods, such as biotherapy (application of maggots), have been reported as having some success (Bale 1998).

- A swab for culture and sensitivity can be taken from deep in the wound if necessary, and appropriate antibiotics prescribed.

- Low-adherence dressings with hypoallergenic (acrylic adhesive) strapping can be used, or dressings designed for specific applications such as hydrogels, providing no anaerobes are present.

- A protective (and insulatory) pad may be adhered to the skin over the sterile dressing so movement of the pad is minimal and cannot impinge on the damaged area. Any removable pad should have toe-loops and metatarsal straps firm enough to keep the pad in position, but not so tight as to slow blood flow, as this also increases blood viscosity, further impeding flow (Ryan 1991), and oedema will make loops tighter still. Any apertures or 'U's in a replaceable pad should be large enough to allow movement tolerance, otherwise it will disrupt tissues further. Accurately and appropriately prescribed and manufactured orthoses can be of long-term help.

- The patient should be given verbal and written information relating to re-dressings, information about what adverse changes to look for in the infected area and what to do if infection occurs (e.g. remove dressing, warm hypertonic saline footbath, re-dress and contact for an urgent appointment or contact their GP). Some indication of prognosis and detailed discussion with the patient is essential.

- Footwear needs to be large enough to accommodate all dressings and orthoses.

- It may be appropriate to consider referral to other healthcare professions and agencies if, during the assessment, other problems come to light, especially if these affect resolution of the infection, for example for dietary help (Lewes 1998), for surgical debridement, GP or hospital doctor, district or practice nurse, tissue viability nurse specialist, or if bed rest is required.

- Once the skin has returned to 'normal for that patient' and symptoms have cleared the condition may be considered resolved, although in an 'at-risk' patient further monitoring is required as the probability of recurrence is high.

---

ation and has shortcomings (Armstrong & Peters 2001). Staging systems for pressure ulceration include risk assessment (Royal College of Nursing 2001). Diagnosing the cause of ulceration (e.g. ischaemia, malignancy) is essential to direct management of the patient, the peripheral tissues, the wound margins and the base of the wound (Romanelli and Flanagan 2005).

## Pathogenesis of chronic wounds

This is a developing and exceedingly complex area, involving many body systems and tissues that are also affected by the underlying medical disorder (Hoffman 1997, Renwick et al 1998). These include the immune system, the nerve system, the vascular system (Wall 1997), and the nutritional status (Lewes 1998), physical mobility and mental agility of the patient.

However, in general terms, the tightly controlled sequential process of normal inflammation is disrupted and out of sequence in chronic wound healing. Furthermore, the various phases of wound healing can occur at the same time in the wound. Chronic wounds are frequently colonised by bacteria, and healing can be delayed through infection when the bacteria present begin to have a pathological effect on tissue.

## Management of chronic wounds

The primary aim of management is to prevent the development of chronic wounds, as these are painful and distressing for the patient and are costly to manage (Bale et al 1998). Early identification of skin change is therefore essential, requiring the patient and clinician to be aware of the skin, and the patient to be armed with knowledge of what to do. This will include avoiding extremes of temperature or wearing ill-fitting footwear, avoiding going barefoot, wearing protective clothing around the feet and legs when gardening or shopping, as well as 'first aid' knowledge of how to clean and dress wounds (Box 2.1).

It is essential to recall that the patient's general health and drug therapy may inhibit an inflammatory response to infection, so the practitioner must be alert for other evidence of infection such as increase in exudate, smell of exudate or increase in pain. If infection does occur, systemic antibiotics may be used (Sheppard 2005), with particular care being paid to tissues of bacterial resistance, biofilm information (Hardy 2002) and the presence of methicillin-resistant *Staphylococcus aureus* (MRSA). There is controversy about antiseptic use (Drosou et al 2003); antiseptics can have a cytotoxic effect on tissues (Enoch & Harding 2003) and affect microcirculation (Langer et al 2004), although there is increasing use of povidone iodine and silver sulphadiazine.

Management of chronic wounds is primarily according to the aetiology and site. Sites of increased mechanical stress must be protected and offloaded with padding, orthoses, footwear adaptations or scotch cast boots and, if necessary, bed rest. Compression is a key issue in managing venous ulcers (Royal College of Nursing 1998). Wound and protective dressings take up space in footwear and this must be accommodated for to avoid further and different problems. Generally, the patient should be encouraged to rest with the limb raised as often as possible, avoiding overloading at risk sites, and if necessary hospital admission arranged. This advice needs to be adapted for each patient;

elevating an ischaemic limb may not be tolerable, or indeed appropriate, in every case.

If a wound does develop, then the information outlined in the section under bacterial infection should be employed (Box 2.1). Additionally, slough (soft, yellowish, stringy, sometimes shiny, dead tissue) or necrotic tissue (hard, black dead tissue) should be debrided to allow healing to occur (Bale 1998). The podiatrist may achieve this through careful use of a scalpel and non-touch technique and/or with dressings designed for this purpose (e.g. hydrogels, dextranomer beads or larval therapy (Bale 1998). Occasionally, bony sequestrae (loose fragments of bone) may be present and require removal, possibly surgically. Callus and corn tissue should be removed (Jones 1998) and possibly mobilisation of joints undertaken to adjust tissue loading (Springett & Greaves 1995).

Chronic wounds change with time, and management should change accordingly. For example, if copious exudate is present a highly absorptive dressing (e.g. hydrocolloid wafer) would be used, but when the wound changes to produce little exudate a low-absorption dressing (e.g. alginate) would be selected. Controlling maceration is important to prevent tissue excoriation and further complications, including infection (White & Cutting 2004). The range of wound dressings is vast (Thomas 1997), some being available on the drug tariff while others may be purchased through the pharmacist. Each dressing has specific information about use, removal and re-dressing. Other treatments include grafting and cultured dermal grafting (Falanga 2005), use of growth factors (Graham 1998), long-term use of antibiotics, possibly antiseptics (Drossu et al 2003), therapeutic ultrasound (Hart 1998) and low-level laser therapy (Halery et al 1997).

Patients may need to be seen daily or at intervals appropriate to the management needs, according to the nature of the wound, dressing used or whether they are re-dressing the lesions themselves. It may be necessary to involve the help of the district or practice nurse, or refer for specialist advice from professional colleagues, including podiatrists, physiotherapists, nutritionists, a tissue viability nurse specialist or a doctor.

## SCARRING

During the post-injury healing process (Dealey 2005) collagen is laid down by fibroblasts, creating a relatively avascular seal. Wounds healing by first intention will usually leave minimal scars, while those healing by second intention will develop noticeable scars. In chronic wounds, the prolonged, abnormal activity of fibroblasts (Phillips et al 1998) and abnormal sequencing of growth factors usually lead to marked scarring, such as the atrophie blanche seen in healed venous ulceration.

Scarring on the dorsum of the foot causes little problem unless it adheres to underlying tissue. Plantar scarring can produce discomfort, as scar tissue does not have the biomechanical characteristics of normal skin.

Very gentle, superficial massage (Field et al 1998) with essential oils (Baker 1998) can provide some relief and reduction in tissue adhesion. Use of ultrasound (Hart 1998) and low-level laser therapy (Halery et al 1997) can help with collagen realignment during wound healing and even in an established scar.

Keloid is a much raised prominent scar which involves adjacent tissues and is seen in black skin ten times more frequently than in white skin.

Hypertrophic scarring is broader than normal scars and elevated above the surrounding skin; it is red, sometimes painful and sometimes with contracture. Keloid or hypertrophic scarring may

be excised, but often recurs following surgery. Sub-scar injection of a corticosteroid can reduce pain; electrostimulation and compression with a silicone sheet or polymer gel can help with pain and minimise scarring. Skin grafts may be undertaken (Fowler 1998).

## BURNS

The skin can be damaged through thermal, photo and chemical burns. Thermal injury can be minor to severe according to the depth of tissue damage and the percentage of surface area injured. Superficial burns involve only the epidermis, while partial thickness burns extend into the dermis. In full-thickness burns, the epidermis and dermis are destroyed, and muscle and bone may be involved.

Boiling water scalds and accidents with hot water bottles are frequent causes of burn injury to the foot, particularly when heat injury is not perceived because of neuropathy or if sleeping tablets are taken. The skin may blister, and this will take differing times to heal according to the depth of injury and the patient's general health. Sunburn can cause severe immediate effects of pain and blistering, as well as long-term skin malignancy (Gnaidecka & Jemec 1998).

First aid for burns is to apply cold to the area, and to keep it cool and covered to minimise risk of bacterial infection. There are various proprietary products available for relief of symptoms. Severe burns will require hospital treatment. Wound contracture after burns is a serious complication, and massage (Field et al 1998) with use of snug-fitting compression with polymer gels can help. Low-level laser therapy and therapeutic ultrasound may also be beneficial.

Chemical burns usually arise through spillage and inadvertent contact with the substance. This requires immediate irrigation of the site with water, hypertonic saline solution, buffer solution or neutraliser (if the burn chemical is acidic use an alkali such as sodium bicarbonate; if alkali, use a weak acid such as vinegar; if phenol, use glycerine). If burning is severe, hospital treatment will be required.

## ATROPHY

Atrophic skin lacks nutrition owing to a poor blood supply due to a systemic or peripheral disorder, or to a lack of nutrient intake because of poor diet or malabsorption syndromes. Atrophic skin is thin, mechanically weak and has poor viability (i.e. if it is damaged it will heal slowly, if at all). Nails usually show changes due to atrophy.

Management includes identifying and managing the primary cause, perhaps with referral. Otherwise, prevention of skin injury is paramount, with health education for the patient about management of injuries, for example cleaning the wound, dressing with a clean or sterile low-adherent gauze and, if severe, seeking help from a suitably qualified healthcare professional (Box 2.1).

## CHILBLAINS AND CHILLING

This is a seasonal, vasospastic condition affecting the young and old; generally the mid-age group is less affected (Cribier et al 2001) (Case study 2.1). This cold injury, when resolving, may be mistaken for unusual callus or old blisters. There may be an underlying medical condition complicating the problem, such as systemic sclerosis.

## CASE STUDY 2.1 **HOW CHILLING CAN LEAD TO TISSUE ATROPHY AND SCARRING**

A female patient in her late sixties had been prone to chilblains all her life. Each winter brings a return of painful chilled feet. On most toes there are scars and there are tailor's bunions from prior episodes of long-term chilling and chronic inflammation. Her general health is good and she does not have predisposing factors such as systemic sclerosis. At the time of her visit to the podiatrist the weather was warm and her feet had patches of hard, scaly skin with slight cyanosis, and there were brown speckles on the skin at the old chilblain sites.

In chilling, the blood vascular system is abnormal, with prolonged vasospasm after exposure to cold and change in blood rheology – flow characteristics (Ryan 1991) – thus tissue perfusion with oxygen and nutrients, and metabolite removal is poor. Chronic inflammation occurs instead of the tightly controlled sequential process of inflammation, so repair and resolution is disrupted. 'Out-of-sequence' events occur and for an abnormal duration; for example, fibroblast activity (Phillips et al 1998) will be prolonged with a consequent increase in collagen deposition, giving the clinical appearance of scarring.

Scar tissue is relatively avascular and does not have the mechanical (viscoelastic) behaviour of normal skin, and is thus less able to withstand further mechanical stress and becomes injured more readily. The patient is always concerned that each podiatrist she consults recognises these skin changes, that they are not mistaken for callus, and attempts made to remove it result in bleeding, sometimes with slow healing and occasional infection. There is little in the literature to provide evidence of good practice to help manage the condition. Development of clinical guidelines such as these are resource-intensive (Feder et al 1999). However, lack of evidence should not stop the use of empirical methods, the use of which over time has been demonstrated to have some success (Ryan 1998).

The most important treatment for the patient was the prevention of chilling, which was achieved by avoiding extremes of temperature, using thermal/insulating insoles, offloading mechanical stress at vulnerable points, and wearing footwear large enough for thicker socks in winter.

When chilblains did develop, it was important to encourage the inflammatory process to maintain its normal sequence and to have each phase as short as possible. Various treatment modalities were considered and a proprietary anti-chilblain preparation was selected so that it could be purchased easily by the patient.

Chilblains occur most commonly in the winter, and are about 2 cm in diameter, are usually discoloured and may itch or be painful. The discoloration changes according to the stage of the chilblain. Initially the area of cold damage is white due to vasoconstriction (Ryan 1991). Later, following delayed vasodilation and consequent tissue damage, the site shows a bright red (erythematous) inflammatory reaction. A few hours later the site becomes swollen and bluish (cyanotic) with prolonged vasodilation. As the lesions resolve over days to weeks, the skin may wrinkle, look shiny and scale. If the chilblain site is traumatised the lesion may become broken and take some weeks to heal.

Chilling or tissue damage from cold may result in extensive areas of the foot being affected, with similar changes occurring as in chilblains that are localised.

Management requires minimising exposure to extremes of temperature and rapid temperature change, minimising mechanical stress and arranging for an optimal healing rate to be achieved. Insulating footwear may need to be a size bigger than normal; adding insulating materials to footwear also requires sufficient space, otherwise the tissues will be constricted, depriving them of local blood flow, which will make the situation worse. Topical preparations can be applied according to the 'stage' of the chilblain; a cooling, soothing preparation (e.g. witch hazel) can be used to control the inflammatory response in the erythematous stage. In the cyanotic phase, a rubefacient (e.g. weak iodine solution, but check for allergy, or tincture of benzoin) may help to stimulate superficial blood flow. Homeopathic and herbal preparations (Kerschott 1997) such as calendula and peppermint oil can help at any stage, along with very gentle superficial soft-tissue massage (Baker 1998) (except in the case of broken chilblains). There are various proprietary chilblain creams, containing active ingredients such as methyl salicylate or capsaicin, aimed at dealing with the chilblain in all its phases. When the chilblain is broken it is essential to keep it free from infection and to protect tissues from mechanical stress by using padding and suitable dressings. In the past, ichthammol was used to optimise healing, but is rarely used today. It is not clear whether therapies such as ultrasound and low-level laser therapy have a helpful role in managing chilling or at which stage they may be most useful.

## INFECTIONS AND THE SKIN

In health, the skin has very effective mechanisms for keeping infection (bacterial, viral, fungal) (Freinkel & Woodley 2001) out of the body, both through the primary skin barrier at the base of the stratum corneum and through the immune system. Bacterial and viral infections of the skin can develop if there is a break in the skin (wound) or if the pathogen is able to penetrate the skin barrier. Wounds are frequently colonised by bacteria, and are said to be infected when these microorganisms exert a pathological effect (Hardy 2002). Ulcers are chronic wounds that fail to heal in the expected time (Phillips et al 1998), and bacterial infection is one of the common causes of delayed healing. The very elderly and malnourished, those with a systemic disorder such as rheumatoid arthritis or diabetes mellitus, or those whose drug therapies affect their immune system are particularly at risk of infection.

Fungal infections (e.g. tinea pedis) may have a secondary overlay of bacterial infection, and vice versa. Parasites (Swinscoe 1998), such as fleas and ticks in temperate climates, and jigger worm and tumbu bug in tropical areas, cause itching, and the bites and burrows can become secondarily infected (see Ch. 7). Bacterial and viral infections are discussed below, followed by a section on parasites. Mycotic infections are covered elsewhere in this chapter.

### Bacterial infections

#### Systemic bacterial infections

Systemic bacterial infection (septicaemia) can cause marked generalised erythema (redness), pruritus (itching) and scaling (scalded skin syndrome) (Fig. 2.2) in the skin. Deep, localised and spreading infection (cellulitis) will show similar skin changes and pain (Humphreys 1999), perhaps also with lymphangitis (red lines of inflamed lymphatics) and lymphadenitis (lymph nodes inflamed).

#### Common skin bacteria and resultant conditions

The most important skin pathogens are *Staphylococcus aureus* and beta-haemolytic streptococci (Hardy 2002). *Staphylococcus aureus* generally forms demarcated yellowish pustules due to the formation of a fibrin wall in the periphery of the involved area containing the pus (Veien

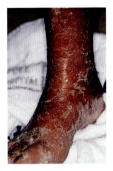

Figure 2.2 Scalded skin syndrome seen in septicaemia, a large area of infected tissue, or in some adverse drug reactions.

1998). Beta-haemolytic streptococci cause erysipelas and spread rapidly; infected wounds show an eroded margin and liquid, transparent, straw- to yellow-coloured exudate due to bacterial production of enzymes such as hyaluronidase (Veien 1998).

Bacterial exotoxins can cause skin diseases (e.g. impetigo, erysipelas) (MacKie 2003). Bacterial superantigens and proteolytic toxins can sustain cutaneous inflammation through attenuation of T-cell responses (Leung 1998), and are important in skin diseases such as eczema and atopic dermatitis. *Corynebacterium minutissimum*, which causes erythrasma (moist interdigital fissuring), is particularly associated with sweating and is therefore treated primarily by controlling sweat. *Pseudomonas aeruginosa*, which produces a greenish pigment that discolours the skin and dressings (Veien 1998), and *Proteus* species are the chief Gram-negative bacilli in feet. These latter pathogens are especially prevalent with occlusion, and cause skin damage by releasing powerful proteolytic enzymes. All these pathogens may be present in chronic wounds.

## Features of cutaneous infections

Cutaneous bacterial infections (Hardy 2002) have different features according to the infecting pathogen and the health of the host. People who are immunocompromised, immunosuppressed or who have poor peripheral vascular supply and/or microcirculation will have a subdued response to infection and will show lessened or few signs of inflammation. People with disorders such as diabetes mellitus are particularly susceptible to infection (Jude & Boulton 1998) owing to the multisystem effects of these conditions. It is important to assess the patient, obtain the history and carry out relevant tests to help with diagnosis and prognosis (Wall 1997).

The degree of inflammatory response (redness, heat, pain, swelling), features of the lesion, and the nature of any exudate provide clinical diagnostic indicators of the pathogen. It is worth looking at and noting the smell, the nature and the volume of exudate of the wound bed as well as that of the exudate on the dressing (Lawrence 1997).

It is essential to be aware that infection may be present when clinical features are inhibited through disease processes or effects of therapeutic drugs such as steroids and that infection will delay healing.

## Management of bacterial infection in the skin

The algorithm shown in Figure 2.3 helps with decision-making in the management process. The patient should contribute to the development of a management plan, which is specific to each individual (Hayry 1998).

Optimal management of bacterial infections requires a cost-effective approach coupled with prompt management to give speedy

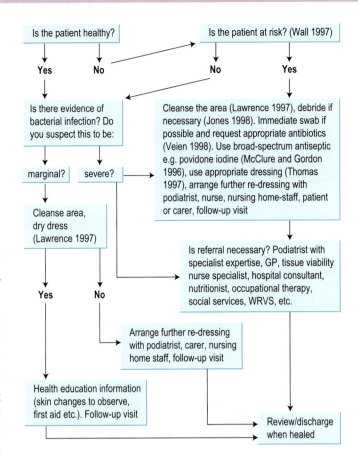

Figure 2.3 Outline algorithm for managing skin infection.

resolution of the problem in order that the patient's distress is minimal. Waiting for microbiological swab results (for culture and sensitivity) may not allow this ideal to be met. Prescription and use of a broad-spectrum antibiotic (Table 2.3), and perhaps a topical antiseptic, while awaiting the laboratory report (culture and sensitivity) and selection of a specific antibiotic is necessary. Bacterial resistance (e.g. to MRSA) is a major problem today (Dealey 2005, Sheppard 2005). Bacterial resistance to antiseptics has also been reported (Irizarry 1996, Leelaporn et al 1994, Littlejohn 1992), and if using an antiseptic it is necessary to ensure that a sufficient volume of antiseptic is applied and that re-dressing is frequent enough to maintain a bactericidal environment in any wound. Antiseptics can delay healing (Cameron & Leaper 1987) and are probably applied most appropriately only when infection is present (Springett 1989).

## Viral infections

Systemic viral infections can cause skin changes, such as HIV and Kaposi's sarcoma, and Coxsackie virus (chickenpox) and papular, urticarial (itchy) rash. The skin can also be infected by viral organisms such as molluscum contagiosum, which is usually seen in children, herpes simplex (cold sores) and the human papilloma virus (HPV), which causes warts. Generally, viral skin infections are difficult to treat and a number of different strategies may be employed, including medicinal plant extracts (Abad et al 1997). Molluscum contagiosum is treated by topical application of iodine/povidone iodine and keeping the child separated from others to minimise the potential for spread. Herpes simplex outbreak is treatable with aciclovir, a topical anti-inflammatory and low-level laser therapy. Information relating to warts is given below.

**Table 2.3** Antimicrobials currently in use for bacterial infections of the skin (Lawrence & Bennett 1992, Veien 1998, BNF)

| Infection | Treatment |
|---|---|
| *Staphylococcus* species e.g. impetigo, cellulitis | Systemic antibiotics: flucloxacillin, fuscidic acid, dicloxacillin, azithromycin, erythromycin, co-amoxiclav<br>Topical antibiotics: mupirocin, fuscidic acid<br>Antiseptics: chlorhexidine, povidone iodine<br>Topical: silver sulphadiazine |
| *Streptococcus* species, e.g. infected ulcer | Systemic antibiotics: penicillin, erythromycin, clindamycin, phenyloxymethylpenicillin |
| Beta-haemolytic *Streptococcus*, e.g. infected burns | Systemic antibiotics: phenyloxymethylpenicillin |
| *Pseudomonas aeruginosa* | Systemic antibiotics: ciprofloxacin, ticarcillin + clavulanic acid, azlocillin, piperacillin |

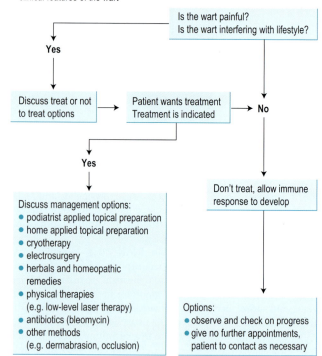

**Figure 2.4** Algorithm for management of warts on the foot.

## Verrucae/warts

There are a number of human papilloma viruses (HPVs), which cause different clinical features and infect different body sites (Bunney et al 1992). The virus causes hyperplasia of the stratum spinosum and thus a localised increased bulk of tissue within the skin. Generally, warts affect children of school age, which may be related to frequency of exposure to this ubiquitous virus. Exposure to the virus may be in the communal, barefoot environment of school changing rooms, as well as being the first time that the body has encountered the pathogen. An older person who has recently taken up a sport and uses communal changing rooms may also develop verrucae. The spread of the lesion is impossible to predict as it depends, among other factors, upon the individual's susceptibility to the virus (Pray 2005).

HPVs causing warts in the foot include:

- HPV1 – single, deep plantar warts
- HPV2 – mosaic warts
- HPV2, 4, 60 – raised warts.

Clinically there is no need to type the virion, except to note that the management of these lesions is according to the health of the owner, clinical features and any special requirements.

## Clinical features of verrucae (warts)

### Single plantar wart (verruca)

The patient's age, lesion site and history will give clues to the viral aetiology. Very new single plantar warts may be mistaken for seed corns or a foreign body in the skin. Established verrucae have a rough, cauliflower-like surface, sometimes with black dots of thrombosed capillaries. Verrucae appear encapsulated in the skin, can appear to push the skin striae to one side and, when pinched, cause a sharp pain (as can a neurovascular corn or a foreign body such as a splinter). Pain can occur with plantar warts, and is usually described as being a throbbing pain when first standing on the foot, or off-loading. The bulk of the wart is palpable and this may give an indication of lesion depth. Regressing warts may show the black dots changing into radiat-

ing lines, the area may be more painful and the skin of the wart may change to a slight yellow-orange colour. Restoration of the skin to normal is considered to be an indication of wart resolution.

### Mosaic warts

Mosaic warts look as though single, more shallow plantar warts have coalesced to form a mass of warty tissue. The site can vary – plantar, interdigital, peri- and subungual. They can be painful and their cosmetic appearance may cause distress.

## Management

Pain and cosmetic appearance may cause treatment to be considered (Fig. 2.4). Health professionals have an obligation to explain management options to patients and ultimately leave the choice to the patient (Hayry 1998). However, the currently generally held recommendation is to allow the body's immune system time to recognise the virus and it will resolve spontaneously (Powell 1998), although the timescale may be long. A recent Cochrane Review (Gibbs et al 2003) found from the few clinical studies that could be included that salicylic acid was effective, more so than cryotherapy. The evidence base is still poor and practitioners rely on their experience in the absence of advice. However, certain topical preparations should be avoided (see below).

Almost all wart treatments rely on destruction of the wart tissue with an increased opportunity for the HPV antigen to be presented to the immune system (Powell 1998), and possibly release of nitric oxide analogues/precursors to have an antitumour effect. Sublesion injection of bleomycin is an expensive treatment option (Schuwen & Meigun 1996). After any wart treatment patients must be given advice to remove the dressing if necessary (e.g. pain, suspected infection), have a warm, hypertonic saline footbath for about five minutes, re-dress with a dry dressing, and contact their GP for an urgent appointment (see Ch. 27).

It is medicolegally and ethically essential to ensure that the patient is fully aware of this advice.

### Topical preparations for wart treatment

Topical preparations for wart treatment (Table 2.4) include monochloroacetic acid and trichloroacetic acid, which, for therapeutic classification purposes, are termed 'caustics'. Salicylic acid in strengths from 40% to 75% ointment in white soft paraffin (keratolytic) may be used alone or with monochloroacetic acid in saturated solution. In this case the wart tissue becomes macerated (white, soggy) and hopefully cleaves away from normal skin after one or two treatments. Pyrogallic acid paste is currently less commonly used for treating warts, and has the potential for causing an allergic response and stains the skin brown. Generally all these treatments need to be repeated one to two times a week, and the patient has to keep the dressing on and dry for the duration. Trichloracetic acid may be used alone or usually with silver nitrate (75% or 95%), another caustic which forms a grey/brown/black eschar (scab-like cover). This combination usually requires repeating every two weeks or so, for six or more visits, to be effective. Overenthusiastic application of any of the strong caustics can cause ulceration (see Ch. 16).

For home use, there is a wide range of topical proprietary preparations, which should be used as per the instructions supplied with the product. Homeopathic methods include Thuja paint (Chatterjee & Jana 1993) (Thuja tablets are also available, but are outside the scope of podiatry practice to recommend) and herbals such as Kalanchoe

leaves and Tea tree oil (Hitchen 1987). Dermabrasion (Chapman & Visaya 1998) may also be used (see Ch. 16).

### Electrosurgery

Often this method of treating warts is considered when all else fails, as it entails giving a local anaesthetic, perhaps as an ankle block to avoid plantar infiltration, followed by tissue excision and/or electro-desiccation (Brown 1992) and wound healing. However, it is worth considering early on in the decision algorithm, as it is quick, does not require frequent return visits and postoperative discomfort is usually minimal. Complications include postoperative infection and scarring. This method is probably contraindicated in those whose race characteristics predispose them to marked scarring (see Ch. 16).

---

**CASE STUDY 2.2 VERRUCAE: TO TREAT OR NOT TO TREAT?**

A 15-year-old girl had an asymptomatic but large plantar wart (verruca) on the plantar aspect of the third metatarsal joint. The patient had not had warts previously. The medical history and assessment of physical state revealed nothing abnormal, but the patient was due to take a series of examinations over the next few weeks. In addition to these factors, an assessment of the patient's psychosocial aspects was made, together with recreational commitments and the patient's reaction to pain. The wart site, size and pain perceived were recorded in the patient's case notes for monitoring and evaluation purposes.

The option of not treating the verruca was discussed with the patient and her parent, together with an outline of treatment options. These included topical application of caustics of varying strengths (see Table 2.4), dermabrasion (Chapman & Visaya 1998), cryotherapy, electrosurgery (Brown 1992) and complementary therapies such as kalanchoe leaves and Thuja paint.

In view of the impending examinations the patient and her parent elected to have no treatment and to arrange a further appointment if they wished after 3 months (Bunney et al 1992).

---

## Parasitic infestations

As people travel more widely and insects travel with imported goods, so the range of parasites seen has altered. Lice (Pediculosis) can infest different body sites and cause itching where they feed, as can scabies (*Sarcoptes scabei*) where they burrow in the skin (Smith 1999). Both organisms are visible with a good hand lens and are transferred by close contact with an affected person. The practice nurse, school medical service or local pharmacist will know the current recommended insecticide and have leaflets offering information on prevention of infestation. Skin hypersensitivity may develop through the antiparasitic effect of forms of nitric oxide released by the skin in response to parasitic invasion. Secondary bacterial infection may occur following scratching.

Lumps and bumps and scratches in the skin that have no obvious explanation need to be looked at carefully along with a full history to help diagnosis of parasites caught in tropical climates (e.g. tumbu bug and hookworm) (Swinscoe 1998). Specific treatments are required for each parasite, and it is necessary to investigate these with the help of the GP, pharmacist and literature. Scratching and poor treatment can result in bacterial infection. The best method of management is to prevent infection by ensuring that all washed clothing is thoroughly ironed to heat-destroy larvae, avoiding going barefoot across open ground, etc.

| Table 2.4 Topical agents for the treatment of plantar warts | |
|---|---|
| **Caustics and keratolytics** | **Properties/mode of use** |
| Monochloroacetic acid | Saturated solution painted on (see Ch. 16) |
| Trichloroacetic acid | Saturated solution as above, but more commonly used as 10% solution (see Ch.16) |
| Salicylic acid | Keratolytic 40%; 60% paste with mask around verruca (see Ch. 16); lesser and varying percentages in proprietary wart treatment products |
| Silver nitrate | 75% and 95%, if moistened too much prior to use will be diluted and have reduced action; paint on perhaps with etching of wart surface with a scalpel or a file first |
| Proprietary products | Contain caustics/keratolytics in various formulations, often with collodion to provide a flexible seal covering the lesion |
| **Herbal and homeopathic remedies** | |
| *Thuja* | Tincture is painted on once or twice a day |
| Kalanchoe leaves | Leaves are slit longitudinally with juicy area placed on the verruca. |
| Tea tree oil | Paint on daily and cover |

## VITILIGO

The abnormal pigmentation in this condition is particularly obvious in dark-skinned people, and as a differential diagnosis is leprosy there may be some concern over the condition. Other differential diagnoses include pityriasis versicolor and postinflammatory hypopigmentation. There is a familial association in this autoimmune disorder. Currently, treatment is reassurance and use of cosmetic camouflage; PUVA may be used.

## DISORDERS OF SWEATING

Too much sweat (hyperhidrosis) or too little sweat (anhidrosis) secreted by the eccrine glands in the skin will cause changes in the skin's mechanical strength. This will give rise, respectively, to moist fissures, usually interdigitally, and dry fissures around the heel. Both forms of fissure may develop complications of superimposed fungal or bacterial infection, especially if the dermis is exposed. With hyperhidrosis there is an increased potential for bacterial infection causing characteristic malodorous feet (bromidrosis). Sweat rash can develop, consisting of tiny vesicles secondary to duct blockage, causing tension and damage in the tissues with a resultant inflammatory response.

Excess sweating may indicate a medical disorder (e.g. hyperthyroidism), while anhidrosis may suggest poor tissue nutrition, perhaps due to poor diet, malabsorption syndromes or peripheral vascular disease (Table 2.5). A previously undiagnosed but suspected underlying medical disorder should be referred for further investigation.

Symptomatic management of hyperhidrosis includes use of sweat-absorbing insoles, changing and airing footwear frequently, application of astringents (e.g. surgical spirit, potassium permanganate footbaths), antiperspirants (e.g. aluminium chloride) and deodorants. In severe cases, a surgical or chemical sympathectomy may be contemplated, or in severe sweating injections of botulinum toxin (Krogstad et al 2005) can be undertaken.

Symptomatic management of anhidrosis involves restoring normal stratum corneum water content (Potts 1986) by use of emollients and barrier creams, and the application of hydrocolloid wafers (Springett et al 1997) or films. Dry skin and associated itch or stinging may be helped by topical combination formulations containing moisturisers and antipruritics (Yosipovitch 2004) as found in a number of cosmetic bases. Avoiding sling-backed shoes and wearing correctly fitting footwear will reduce tension on skin and hence fissuring. Heel cups of a polymer gel or silicone will maintain heel tissue contours, thus minimising tension stress around the heel margins. Also, transepidermal water loss (TEWL) will be reduced, thus maintaining skin hydration.

## FISSURES

Fissures can be moist or dry cracks in the epidermis at sites where the skin is under tension, and may extend to and involve the dermis, with the potential for infection. The fissure usually develops at 90° to the direction of the tension stress (Vincent 1983). The common site for moist fissures is interdigitally and for dry fissures around the heel margins. Systemic and peripheral states that affect skin quality (e.g. peripheral vascular disease, rheumatoid arthritis, systemic sclerosis, dermatitis, ichthyosis, psoriasis, tinea pedis) can make fissures worse.

Management requires removal of the cause if possible (e.g. removal of the allergen, treating tinea pedis with an antifungal (Ch. 16)). Optimising epidermal strength is beneficial by controlling the stratum corneum water content. This is achieved by hydrating anhidrotic (dry) skin with emollients or hydrocolloid dressings (Springett et al 1997), or dehydrating hyperhidrotic (sweaty) skin with an astringent (e.g. IMS or an antiperspirant such as aluminium chloride). If necessary, the fissure can be closed with medical-grade acrylic glue, adhesive skin closure, hydrocolloid wafer or strapping. Bacterial infection may complicate this condition and require additional treatment.

## CORNS AND CALLUS

Callus (callosity, mechanically induced hyperkeratosis) is a yellowish plaque of hard skin, and a corn is an inverted cone of similarly hard skin (Table 2.6) that is pushed into the skin. Both conditions are

**Table 2.6** The different forms of corn and some differential diagnoses

| Type | Site | Appearance |
|---|---|---|
| Hard corns (heloma durum) | Over bony prominences and plantar metatarsal heads (Merriman et al 1986) | Darkish yellow, hard core pushing into the skin sometimes covered with callus, may be mistaken for new warts or foreign body |
| Soft corns (heloma molle) | Interdigital | White soggy mass with indented centre, may be mistaken for tinea pedis |
| Seed corns (heloma miliare) | On areas of weight bearing | Single or clusters of small corns |
| Fibrous corns | Areas taking high load | Long-standing corns tied down to underlying structures, may be mistaken for scars |
| Vascular and neurovascular corns | Areas taking high load, particularly torsion | As for fibrous corns, with vascular elements visibly intertwined in epidermal tissue; painful on direct pressure; may be mistaken for scar or verruca |

**Table 2.5** Causes of anhidrosis and hyperhidrosis

| Some causes of anhidrosis | Some causes of hyperhidrosis |
|---|---|
| Hypothyroidism | Hyperthyroidism |
| Autonomic neuropathy | Anxiety |
| Increasing age (Gnaidecka & Jemec 1998) | Heat |
| Peripheral vascular disease | Eating hot and spicy foods |
| Systemic sclerosis | Pain |
| Deficiency states | |

associated with excess intermittent mechanical stress (shear, friction, pressure, torsion and tension), which results in abnormal keratinisation (Springett 1993, Thomas et al 1985). These conditions may be painful, and the subsequent antalgic gait can overstress other body structures giving rise to more proximal conditions and effects on lifestyle. Often cosmesis provokes requests for treatment. In those at risk, the presence of corns and callus can predispose to ulceration (Jones 1998). Corns and callus may be present for a number of years, with the mode age of onset being in the sixth decade and slightly earlier for women than men. Corns and callus are rarely seen in those less than 16 years old. Those developing corns and callus when less than 30 years old, as a guide, require foot function to be assessed and managed carefully.

## Pathogenesis of corns and callus

Excess mechanical stress and duration of loading of tissue during gait at foot–ground, foot–shoe or toe–toe interfaces damages the skin. This may be due to abnormal foot function, such as excess pronation causing overloading of second and third metatarsal heads (Potter 2000). The increased load and duration of loading of the tissues in this area, with the frequently observed abductory twist at toe-off, overstresses the skin (Springett 1993) and this trauma stimulates a local release of growth factors (McKay & Leigh 1991). The stratum corneum is not inert and is capable of releasing growth factors, as do the viable epidermis and dermis, one of the resultant effects being a rapid epidermal transit rate and insufficient time for keratinocytes to mature normally (Thomas et al 1985). The physical and biochemical changes in skin result in callus and corn formation, and slight fibrosis in the dermis with changes in the subjacent microvasculature (Springett 1993). Histologically, callus appears to be in the continuum of forming corns (Springett 1993). Biochemically, the fatty acid content of callus (McCourt 1998) and seed corns (O'Halloran 1990) appears to be similar to that in normal skin. As calloused skin has an altered structure, it is less efficient at withstanding mechanical stress, subjacent tissues can be damaged more easily and so the problem of callus formation perpetuates (Springett & Merriman 1995).

## Management of corns and callus

Successful management requires removal of the cause followed by treatment aimed at reducing pain and restoring normal skin function. If there is a biomechanical aetiology, this needs assessing and managing with orthoses and exercises, or surgery. If poor-fitting shoes are the cause, then suitable footwear advice must be given, along with goal-setting and agreement with the patient. For adults, it is important that the inside of the shoe is about 1 cm longer than the foot and there is some space available in width and depth across the ball of the foot and toes. A smooth inside to footwear avoids causing problems such as blisters in the short term and corns and callus in the long term. Heel height may be varied to achieve different foot function to avoid overloading one particular site. A method of attaching the shoe to the foot is best in order to minimise friction and shear stress, but this is not always achievable.

Poor-quality skin may be associated with a medical disorder or poor nutrient intake; if the latter, then referral for dietary advice may be relevant.

Podiatric symptomatic management involves callus reduction and corn enucleation with a scalpel to reduce pain. This dermatological condition is particularly important when the epidermis is glycated (Hashmi 2000), for example in diabetes. Pads, either adhesive or replaceable, can be used to reduce the duration of tissue loading and redistribute mechanical stress, and manage pain (e.g. a holed or U-shaped pad of semi-compressed felt; or a cushion such as a plantar cover of open-cell foam). To absorb shear, orthoses and other devices (e.g. a toe pad of a polymer gel, silicones, tubifoam) may be used. Pads may also be used to change foot function temporarily, to observe the effects before translating to an orthotic device (e.g. a shaft pad for the fourth metatarsal head can be used to change the alignment of this structure against the fifth toe, to treat an interdigital corn between the fourth and fifth toes – see Ch. 16).

Topical preparations (Table 2.7) may be used to reduce callus and corn hardness or bulk, providing there are no contraindications such as poor peripheral tissue status or a medical disorder such as diabetes or rheumatoid arthritis. Some preparations are available as over-the-

**Table 2.7** Topical products* and instrumentation for podiatric use in treating corns and callus

| Topical therapeutic product classification | Example |
|---|---|
| **Callus** | |
| *Keratolytic callus* | Salicylic acid (12.5%) in collodion BP |
| ***Keratoplastic callus*** | |
| Emollient | Urea cream (10%)<br>Aqueous cream, E 45 cream |
| Dressing | Hydrocolloid wafer to hydrate skin optimally (Springett et al 1997), polymer gel pad, strapping or fleecy web |
| **Corns** | |
| *Keratolytic corns* | |
| Caustic | Salicylic acid (12.5%) in collodion BP<br>Salicylic acid (20% or 40%) paste or plaster (contained in many proprietary 'medicated' corn products) |
| Dressing | Silver nitrate (75% or 95%)<br>Viscogel (acrylic gel)<br>Polymer gel pad |
| Physical therapy | Low-level laser therapy, therapeutic ultrasound |
| Caustic | As above |
| *Fibrous corns* | |
| Dressing | As above |
| Caustic | Saturated phenol solution as preoperative analgesic (apply for 5 min, irrigate profusely with alcohol to dilute, then operate) |
| *Neurovascular corns* | |
| Analgesic | Ametop, EMLA creams under occlusion preoperatively |
| Keratolytic | As above |
| Physical therapy | As above |
| Dressing | As above |

*Caustics and keratolytics are contraindicated in those at risk. Some products may contain allergens such as lanolin.

counter products, as are various callus-debriding devices. Minor surgery (electrodesiccation) can be undertaken to treat corns (Whinfield & Forster 1997). The cavities of well-enucleated corns may be filled with a polymer gel, silicone or acrylic gel (e.g. Viscogel) to discourage further corn formation.

Lesion progress can be measured or traced around, dated and recorded in the patient's notes. Pain analogue scales are useful. Non-invasive measurement of lesion depth and tissue changes may be achieved using ultrasound imaging (Rippon et al 1998). Data so gathered can be evaluated to provide evidence of the success (or otherwise) of treatments tried for patients generally, thus contributing to the knowledge base of the profession and evidence of best practice.

## BURSITIS

Inflammation of a congenital or adventitious (acquired) bursa is termed bursitis (Klenerman 1991). This may be aseptic and acute, infected and acute, or chronic bursitis. The clinical features (signs and symptoms) of inflammation of differing degrees of severity and history (including that of recent changes in footwear) should lead to the diagnosis. Any site that has been exposed to intermittent mechanical stress, particularly shear and friction, is likely to become inflamed, and thus common sites for bursitis include the medial aspect of the first metatarsal head and lateral side of the fifth metatarsal, the dorsal interphalangeal joints and the retrocalcaneal area. Differential diagnosis includes gout, insect bites, rheumatoid nodules, cysts, injury and infection.

There is little in the literature to support the approach to managing bursitis, but this lack of reporting should not be misunderstood to mean lack of evidence for empirical treatments being of benefit to patients (Ryan 1998). Management requires removal of the cause of the problem, so if footwear is the cause then this must be changed to a type that fits the foot and does not rub. Foot function should be assessed for biomechanical abnormality, followed by management (including orthoses and mobilisation (Menz 1998)) to minimise shear and friction at this site, but without overloading adjacent tissues or body segments.

'First aid' short-term treatment includes managing pain (Izzo et al 1996) while also recalling the patient's general health and peripheral status. Anti-inflammatory preparations (orthodox treatments such as topical ibuprofen or complementary therapies such as arnica and calendula) and physical therapies including low-level laser therapy, therapeutic ultrasound or footbaths (see Ch. 16) can help in acute bursitis. Chronic bursitis may benefit from a 're-sequencing' of the inflammatory process by use of topical rubefacients (e.g. weak iodine solution), therapeutic ultrasound (but note the proximity of the target tissue to bone) or contrast footbaths (see Ch. 16). Pain and discomfort may be improved with topical agents such as capsaicin (Nurmikko & Nash 1998), witch hazel or aluminium acetate solution BP. Infected bursitis will almost definitely require systemic antibiotics. Occasionally, a sinus may develop and in this case an aseptic technique is essential when debriding overlying epidermal tissue; management is then directed towards creating the optimum environment for healing.

In all forms of bursitis, protection from mechanical stress is essential and may be achieved by changing or adapting footwear, providing replaceable or adhesive protective pads or covering with a polymer gel material that will absorb shear instead of the tissues. In chronic bursitis, 'tying' down the tissues firmly with fleecy web or polymer film enlarges the area over which shear, torsion and friction may be dissipated, thus reducing mechanical stress in the problem area. Prognosis is good if diagnosis and management is correct. An aseptic condition will subside promptly, requiring perhaps two or three follow-up visits a few weeks apart, but will recur if the primary cause is not removed.

## THE SKIN AS AN INDICATOR OF PSYCHOLOGICAL DISTURBANCE

Some people bite their nails habitually, but picking them to destruction (onychotillomania) may be considered problematic. Cigarette burns on reachable areas of skin should also be observed carefully. Munchausen's syndrome (repeated fabrication of illness) can take many different forms; a key indicator is either inconsistent symptoms from visit to visit, or symptoms that are inconsistent with the disorder the patient feels themselves to have.

Skin disorders may cause psychological problems, sometimes severe (Cotteril & Cunliffe 1997), as the failure of skin in cosmesis and function becomes intimately related to a sense of failure as a human.

## THE NAIL IN HEALTH AND DISEASE

The human nail is a hard plate of densely packed keratinised cells which protects the dorsal aspect of the digits and greatly enhances fine digital movements of the hands. Nails are descendants of claws used for digging and fighting, but now only serve as a protection for the digit and to assist in basic behaviour such as scratching and picking up small objects.

The nail is a flat, horny structure, roughly rectangular and transparent. It is the end product of the epithelial component of the nail unit, the matrix. The nail plate moves with the nail-bed tissues to extend unattached as a free edge, growing past the distal tip of the finger or toe. The nail bed is normally seen through the plate as a pink area due to a rich vascular network. A paler, crescent-shaped lunula is seen extending from the proximal nail fold of the hallux, thumb and some of the larger nails. At the lunula, the nail is thin and the epidermis is thicker, so that the underlying capillaries cannot be seen. It is less firmly attached to the bed at this point and light is reflected from the interface between the nail and the bed, making the lunula appear white.

In profile, the nail plate emerges from the proximal nail fold at an angle to the surface of the dorsal digital skin. This angle is commonly called Lovibond's angle (Fig. 2.5A) and should be less than 180°. Only in abnormal circumstances, for example clubbing, is this angle greater (Fig. 2.5B).

The nail grooves mark the limit of the nail, are separated into proximal, distal and lateral grooves (sulci), and are best seen when the nail is avulsed. The nail plate covers the distal groove situated at the hyponychium, and lying immediately proximal is a thin pale translucent line known as Terry's onychodermal band (Fig. 2.6).

The proximal nail fold (PNF) is an extension of the skin of the surface of the digit and lies superficial to the matrix, which is deeper in the tissues. It has a superficial and deep epithelial border, the latter not being visible from the exterior. The PNF extends its stratum corneum onto the nail plate as a cuticle, which remains adhered for a short distance before being shed. The function of the cuticle is unclear – it may prevent bacterial access to the thinner and more delicate tissues of the ventral PNF epidermis or it may help in forming a smooth nail surface.

The superficial skin of the PNF, extending from the distal interphalangeal joint to the nail plate, is devoid of hair follicles and is thinner than the dorsal skin of the digit. At the tip of the PNF, adjacent

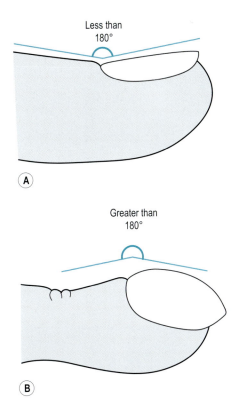

**Figure 2.5** (A) Lovibond's angle. (B) Clubbing.

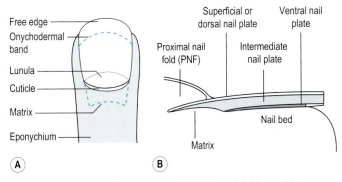

**Figure 2.6** Structure of the human nail. (A) Superficial layer. (B) Deep layer.

to the cuticle, capillary loops can be seen and, if proliferative, can be associated with certain disease states (e.g. lupus erythematosus, dermatomyositis, phototoxic conditions).

The ventral PNF is thinner than the superficial PNF; it does not have epidermal ridges and may be the portal of entry for bacteria and/or irritating chemicals, which produce chronic paronychia. It is continuous with the matrix epithelium but has a stratum granulosum that may be differentiated on staining.

## Embryonic development and nail growth

The earliest anatomical sign of nail development occurs on the surface of the digit of the embryo at week 9, appearing as a flattened rectangular area. The primary nail field is outlined by grooves, which are the forerunners of the proximal and distal grooves and lateral sulci (Zaias & Alvarez 1968). The nail field mesenchyme differentiates into the

nail unit structures, and the fully keratinised nail is complete in week 20 of gestation. Toenail formation usually occurs 4 weeks later than that of the corresponding fingernail.

The theories proposed to explain the formation and growth of the human nail have polarised between a single source of matrix production from the lunula (Achten 1982, Norton 1971, Zaias & Alvarez 1968) and a trilamellar structure where, in addition to the lunula, the nail bed and proximal nail fold contribute as the nail plate grows out (Hashimito et al 1966, Jarrett & Spearman 1966, Johnson et al 1991, Lewin 1965, Lewis 1954, Samman & Fenton 1995).

Zaias (1990) stated that the nail plate is a uniform structure produced solely by the matrix, with onychocytes genetically directed diagonally and distally, and not shaped or redirected by the PNF. The proximal portions of the matrix form the superficial nail plate, and the distal matrix forms the deepest portion of the plate. As the nail produced from the lunula is in advance of that from the proximal matrix, this supports the theory that nail plate shape is related to lunula shape. Zaias (1990) also demonstrated a direct relationship between nail plate thickness and the length of the matrix.

However, the exact structure of the nail plate is still disputed, as Achten (1982) claimed that nail embedded in paraffin and stained using the periodic acid–Schiff method (PAS), toluidine blue and the sulfydryl groups reveals three layers with differential staining. The most proximal cells of the matrix form the superficial layer of the nail, while the distal cells form the deeper nail layer, which is thicker (Fig. 2.6). As the nail grows distally and comes to rest on the nail bed distal to the lunula, a thin layer of keratin from the bed attaches to the undersurface of the nail. Achten argued that this keratin does not form an integral part of the nail, but migrates with it, and remains firmly attached to it even when the nail is surgically avulsed. Measurements of progressive thickness of the nail from the proximal lunula to the point of detachment at the onychodermal band have shown that about 19% of nail mass is formed by the nail bed as the nail grows out along it (Johnson et al 1991).

The nail bed has a surface with numerous parallel longitudinal ridges that fit closely into a similar pattern on the underside of the nail plate, thus ensuring a very strong cohesion between the two surfaces.

The three nail layers are often described as the dorsal, intermediate and ventral nail plates, and each is physiochemically different. Seen in transverse and longitudinal sections, the cells of the nail plate are arranged regularly and interlock like roof tiles, with the main axis horizontal. In the superficial layer, cells are flatter and closer together, and in the nail bed they are more polyhedral and less regularly arranged.

It is thought that the layers stain differently due to variations in the composition of the main polypeptide chains and the number of lateral bonds in the keratin molecule (Achten 1982). The more numerous the lateral bonds, the fewer free radicals are available to combine with different stains. In softer keratin there is less bonding, and therefore more staining (Fig. 2.7). Studies on the chemical composition of nails show moderately high concentrations of sulphur, selenium, calcium and potassium.

## Blood supply and innervation

In the foot, the nail is supplied by two branches of the dorsal metatarsal artery and two branches of the plantar metatarsal artery, lying at the laterodorsal and lateroplantar areas of each toe. They form an anastomosis at the terminal phalanx, the plantar arteries supplying the pad of the toe and the nail bed.

Innervation of the proximodorsal area of the nail and bed is provided by two small branches from the dorsal nerves (superficial pero-

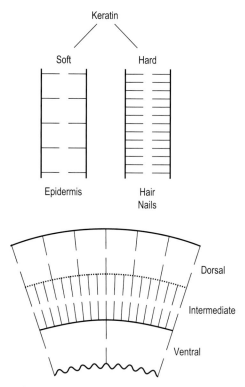

Figure 2.7 Polypeptide chain composition in the human nail.

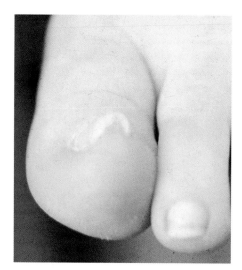

Figure 2.8 Involution.

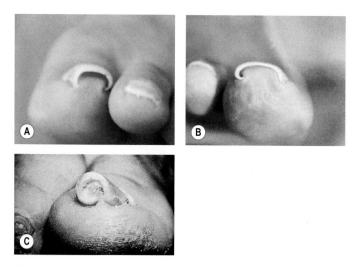

Figure 2.9 Types of involution. (A) Tile-shaped. (B) Plicatured. (C) Pincer.

neal (fibular), deep peroneal (fibular) and sural), while the medial and lateral plantar nerves provide a medial and lateral branch to each toe to supply the plantar skin, and extend to supply the anterodistal area of the nail bed and superficial skin.

Growth of the nail is continuous throughout life, the rate being greatest in the first two decades when the nail plate is thin (Hamilton et al 1955). The rate of growth decreases with age, and ultimately in the elderly the nail plate loses colour and may thicken and develop longitudinal ridges. The normal development of the nail depends on the matrix and nail bed having an adequate nerve and blood supply, and interference with either will affect growth. Some systemic disorders may cause a reduction or an increase in the growth rate. Other factors that, either directly or indirectly, have a detrimental effect on the development and growth of the nail are trauma, infection, nutritional deficiencies and some skin diseases. Congenital and inherited factors are not common.

Nail growth is continuous throughout life, with peak rates of elongation in the age range 10–14 years and a steady decline in growth rate after the second decade (Hamilton et al 1955); therefore, periodic cutting is necessary, and incorrect performance of this task leads to onychocryptosis (ingrowing toe nail), one of the most painful conditions affecting nails. The free edge of a nail should never be cut so short as to expose the nail bed, but should be cut straight across or slightly convex with all rough and sharp edges smoothed. The overall aim should be to ensure that the nail complies with the shape of the toe.

## INVOLUTION (PINCER, OMEGA NAIL)

This term describes a nail that increases in transverse curvature along the longitudinal axis of the nail, reaching its maximum at the distal part (Fig. 2.8). Three types of this condition exist (Fig. 2.9), and they produce a variety of symptoms.

Tile-shaped nails often occur in association with yellow nail syndrome, affecting both fingers and toenails. The nail increases in transverse curvature, while the lateral edges of the nail remain parallel (Baran et al 1991). The condition rarely produces symptoms.

Plicatured nails occur where the surface of the plate remains flat while one or both edges of the nail form vertical parallel sides hidden by the sulcus tissue. Toenails and fingernails are affected and the condition causes considerable pain in the foot if the nail is thickened and subjected to shoe pressure, with the development of onychophosis.

Pincer (omega, trumpet) nail dystrophy shows transverse curvature, which ranges from a minimal asymptomatic in-curving to involution so marked that the lateral edges of the nail practically meet, forming a cylinder or roll; hence the names for this deformity. Lateral compression of the nail may result in strangulation of the soft nail bed tissues and the formation of subungual ulceration as the circulation to the nail bed and matrix is reduced. In all stages of the condition, the sulcus may become inflamed and may ulcerate, causing considerable pain.

## Aetiology

Although the precise cause of involution is unknown, in toenails it is often associated with constriction from tight footwear or hosiery. In fingernails, an association with osteoarthritic changes in the distal interphalangeal joint has been shown (Zaias 1990), and heredity may play a part, particularly where all nails are affected (hidrotic ectodermal dysplasia, yellow nail syndrome). Some severe cases of involution have an underlying exostosis of the terminal phalanx, which must be excised.

## Treatment

In minor degrees, involution produces little or no discomfort and the main consideration is to ensure that the nail is cut so that it conforms to the length and shape of the toe. The in-curved edges, if thickened, should be reduced and advice given about correctly fitting footwear and hosiery.

More severe cases may be treated conservatively with careful clearing of the sulcus and the fitting of a nail brace. This is made from a short piece of 0.5-mm gauge, stainless steel wire which applies a slight upward and outward tension to the nail edges to correct them gradually. The nail must be of adequate length to allow correct fitting of the side arms of the brace, and good contact of the nail plate with the nail bed is essential to allow effective tension for correction.

The brace is formed using a piece of wire approximately 1.5 cm longer than the width of the nail. At the middle of the length of the wire, a U-shaped loop is formed in the horizontal plane so that the open end of the loop faces towards the free edge of the nail. With round-nosed pliers, a small hook is made at each end of the wire, lying in the frontal plane and being large enough to accept the thickness of the nail edges. The ends of the wire must be rounded and filed smooth before finally fitting. Each arm of the brace from the hook to the central loop is shaped to conform to the curvature of the nail (Fig. 2.10).

The brace is applied by engaging each hook over the appropriate edge of the nail, and tension is achieved by closing the long side of the loop as far as possible, without applying so much tension that the nail splits. A light packing of cotton wool and suitable antiseptic (e.g. Betadine solution) may be inserted into each sulcus if necessary. The brace should be kept in position for at least one month and then reassessed for the correction achieved, which is assessed by calliper measurements; tension can be adjusted throughout the period of the treatment.

Other derivatives of the nail brace are now available in plastic and are adhered to the nail directly, exerting tension upwards and outwards because of their preformed shape, or via rubber bands fitted to small plastic hooks. These are reported to be very successful where good adherence is achieved.

Severe and painful involution is likely to require a unilateral or bilateral partial nail avulsion with destruction of the matrix. Where lateral compression causes painful nail bed constriction and ulceration, a total nail avulsion with matrix destruction is the only means of providing relief.

If an underlying subungual exostosis is detected, this needs to be surgically excised (see Ch. 21).

## ONYCHOCRYPTOSIS (INGROWING TOENAIL)

Onychocryptosis is a condition in which a spike, shoulder or serrated edge of the nail has pierced the epidermis of the sulcus and penetrated the dermal tissues. It occurs most frequently in the hallux of male adolescents and may be unilateral or bilateral. Initially, it causes little inconvenience, but as the nail grows out along the sulcus the offending portion penetrates further into the tissues and promotes an acute inflammation in the surrounding soft tissues, which often become infected (paronychia).

The skin becomes red, shiny and tense and the toe appears swollen. There is throbbing pain, acute tenderness to the slightest pressure and a degree of localised hyperhidrosis. The continued penetration of the nail spike prevents normal healing by granulation of the wound in the sulcus, and a prolific increase of granulation tissue is common (hypergranulation). This excess tissue, together with the swollen nail folds, overlaps the nail plate, sometimes to a considerable extent, partially obscuring it (Fig. 2.11). Because infection is almost always present, pus may exude from the point of penetration in the sulcus and may be seen as a pocket lying beneath the sulcus epidermis or beneath the nail plate.

Zaias (1990) describes three stages of the condition, with individual treatment regimens for each stage:

- *Stage I* is the first sign of ingrowing, with minimal injury to the sulcus tissue but with symptoms of pain, slight swelling,

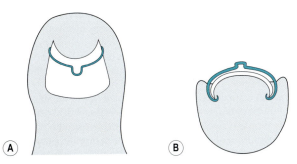

**Figure 2.10** Involution. (A) Nail brace in position, dorsal view. (B) Nail brace in position, transverse view.

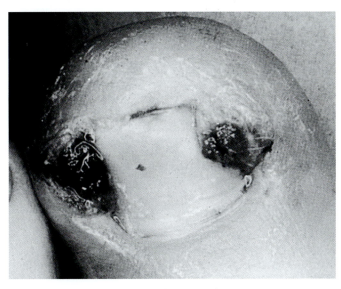

**Figure 2.11** Onychocryptosis with hypergranulation.

33

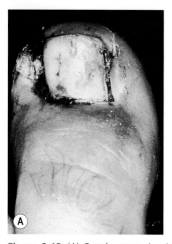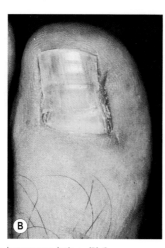

**Figure 2.12** (A) Onychocryptosis with hypergranulation. (B) Same case as in (A), 8 weeks after partial nail avulsion. The nail plate is permanently flattened and narrowed after excision of the involuted nail edges.

oedema, varying degrees of redness and hyperhidrosis. Elevation of the nail with non-absorbent cotton wool corrects the condition in 7–14 days.

- *Stage II* demonstrates acute pain, erythema, hyperhidrosis, and granulation tissue from the ulcerated sulcus tissue, a seropurulent exudate and a fetid odour. The latter may be the result of Gram-positive or colonic bacterial growth on the surface of the granulation tissue. Topical high-potency steroids or intralesional corticosteroid injection of 2 mg/ml triamcinolone acetonide are reported to clear the granulating tissue, and the condition clears with further cotton wool packing as in stage I.
- *Stage III*. The symptoms present in stage III are those described for stage II, with the addition of an epidermal overgrowth of the granulation tissue, thus making elevation of the nail out of the sulcus impossible. Surgical intervention with excision or cauterisation of the granulation is recommended (Fig. 2.12).

## Aetiology

The most common predisposing factors are faulty nail cutting, hyperhidrosis and pressure from ill-fitting footwear, although any disease state that causes an abnormal nail plate (e.g. onychomycosis, onychorrhexis) may promote piercing of the sulcus tissue by the nail.

If a nail is cut too short, the corners cut obliquely, or if it is subjected to tearing, normal pressure on the underlying tissue is removed, and without that resistance the tissue begins to protrude. As the nail grows forward, it becomes embedded in the protruding tissue. Tearing of the nails has a similar effect to cutting obliquely across the corners of the nail plate. Both are likely to result in a spike of nail left deep in the sulcus, especially if the nail is involuted. Any spike left at the edge of the nail increases the risk of sulcus penetration as the nail grows forward. Maceration of the sulcus tissue is commonly due to hyperhidrosis in adolescent males but may also arise from the overuse of hot footbaths in the young or elderly. Moist tissue is less resistant to pressure from the nail such as that caused by lateral pressure from narrow footwear or abnormal weight-bearing forces (e.g. pronation, hallux limitus) and as compression forces the lateral nail fold to roll over the edge of the nail plate, the sulcus deepens and the nail may penetrate the softened tissues.

Hamilton et al (1955) showed that the nails of adolescent males increased in lateral width disproportionately to the increase in length of the nail plate. This, together with hyperhydrated tissues, abnormal foot function and/or pressure from footwear may lead to onychocryptosis. However, the relationship between toenail length and width in adolescents has not been investigated further.

## Treatment

If the onychocryptosis is uncomplicated by infection, the penetrating splinter may be located by careful probing and then removed with a small scalpel or fine nippers. Extreme care must be taken to avoid further injury to the sulcus and to ensure that a spike of nail is not left deep in the sulcus. The edge of the nail can be smoothed with a Black's file, although this should be avoided if the nail plate is extremely thin or shows signs of onychorrhexis. The area is then irrigated with sterile solution and dried thoroughly. It should then be packed firmly with sterile cotton wool or gauze, making sure that it is inserted a little way under the nail plate to maintain its elevation. An antiseptic astringent preparation, such as Betadine, is applied to the packing and the toe is covered with a non-adherent sterile dressing and tubular gauze.

It is sometimes necessary to make use of an interdigital wedge to relieve pressure on the distal phalanx from the adjacent toe. In approximately 3–5 days the nail should again be inspected and re-packed, and then again at appropriate intervals until the nail has regained its normal length and shape. If there is associated hyperhidrosis, this requires an appropriate treatment regimen while the onychocryptosis is being treated.

When onychocryptosis is complicated by infection and suppuration is present, it is important to remove the splinter of nail, facilitating drainage and allowing healing to take place. Hot footbaths of magnesium sulphate solution or hypertonic saline solution may be used to reduce the inflammation and localise the sepsis before removal of the splinter is attempted.

Location and removal of the penetrating nail may cause considerable pain and, if there are no contraindications, a local anaesthetic should be given. The injection should be made at the base of the toe, well away from the infected area. After the splinter has been removed, the edge of the nail should be left smooth, and the area irrigated thoroughly with a sterile solution and dried carefully. A light packing of sterile gauze or cotton wool with a suitable broad-spectrum antiseptic agent can be applied and the toe covered with a sterile non-adherent dressing and tubular gauze.

The patient should be advised to rest the foot and, if necessary, to cut away the upper of the slipper or shoe to remove all pressure from the toe. The patient should return the following day for renewal of the dressings, and this must be continued until the sepsis is cleared.

If hypergranulation tissue is present, it may be excised when the splinter of nail is removed, taking care to control the profuse bleeding that often results following excision. Small amounts of granulation tissue may be reduced by repeated applications of silver nitrate, taking care to avoid its introduction into the sulcus.

Following this treatment the prognosis is good, but the patient must be given clear guidance on the predisposing factors so that they can avoid recurrence. If the condition does not respond, it is likely that there is still a small nail splinter embedded in the sulcus, and further careful investigation must be undertaken to locate the remaining piece of nail. Where it is obvious that the onychocryptosis results from a minor involution of the nail, the application of a nail brace will flatten out the nail plate and reduce the involution. If conservative treatment of severe involution does not provide long-term relief, nail surgery will invariably be necessary. This involves partial or complete avulsion of the nail and the destruction of part or the whole of the nail matrix (see Ch. 23).

## SUBUNGUAL EXOSTOSIS

Subungual exostosis (Fig. 2.13) is a small outgrowth of bone under the nail plate near its free edge or immediately distal to it. Most frequently, it occurs on the hallux in young people, is slow growing and is a source of considerable pain in the later stages. Trauma is a major causative factor (Baran et al 1991), although this is disputed by some authors (Cohen et al 1973). Repeated trauma, although slight, from shoes which are too short, too shallow or excessively high-heeled, is a common finding in podiatric practice.

As the outgrowth increases, the nail becomes elevated and displaced from the nail bed and the tumour may emerge from the free edge or destroy the nail plate. If the nail is eroded, the nail bed tissue ulcerates and may become infected. The protuberance offers a hard resistance to pressure and there is usually a clear line of demarcation around the area. As the exostosis increases, a fissure may develop at the edge of this line of demarcation, with a serous or purulent exudate.

The epidermis covering the tumour becomes stretched and thinned and takes on a bright red colour that blanches on pressure. When the exostosis protrudes distal to the free edge, the bright red gives way to a more yellow coloration, which must be differentiated from subungual heloma and psoriasis. Accurate diagnosis of this condition requires x-ray examination, which shows trabeculated osseous growth, expansion of the distal portion and a radiolucent fibrocartilage cover.

### Pathology

Following an injury to the periosteum of the distal phalanx, a periostitis occurs. Initially, there is an outgrowth of cartilage, which later ossifies.

### Treatment

Temporary relief may be given by means of protective padding and advice on footwear, but surgical excision is always the most satisfactory treatment (see Ch. 21).

## SUBUNGUAL HELOMA (CORN)

As the term implies, a subungual heloma is the development of a nucleated keratinised lesion under the nail plate. It may occur on any part of the nail bed. As the lesion increases in size, it detaches the nail from the nail bed and is seen clinically as a small area of onycholysis, although it assumes a yellowish grey colour. The colour does not change under pressure, and this distinguishes a subungual heloma from a subungual exostosis. A further aid to diagnosis is that a subungual heloma will yield slightly to pressure, while the subungual exostosis presents hard resistance. Once the condition is fully established, pain in the area is acute, and may prevent wearing of shoes with an enclosed toe box. Even slight pressure from bedclothes will elicit extreme, sharp pain.

### Aetiology

- Trauma, which may be slight but prolonged, from shoes which are too short or too shallow, or sometimes from high-heeled shoes which produce abnormal pressure on the nail plate.
- Forefoot deformity, such as hallux limitus/rigidus with hyperextension of the hallux, or overlying toes in association with hallux abductovalgus; each incurs increased pressure from the shoe onto the nail plate, resulting in keratinisation of that particular part of the nail bed.

### Treatment

If the heloma is near the free edge, an area of the nail plate can be removed to enable it to be enucleated. A suitable antiseptic emollient can then be applied together with protective padding, if necessary, and the dressing held in place with tubular gauze.

Where the heloma is located towards the proximal half of the nail, it is necessary to carefully reduce the nail thickness overlying the lesion with a nail drill. Care must be taken not to drill into nail bed tissue. The remaining thin shell of nail can then be removed with a scalpel and the area enucleated and dressed as before.

It may be necessary to repeat treatment, especially if the heloma forms proximally, and it is essential to eliminate the cause or provide permanent protection to prevent recurrence, pain and the possible formation of an aseptic necrosis. Modification of footwear may accommodate the deformity, but there are cases where nail surgery is indicated.

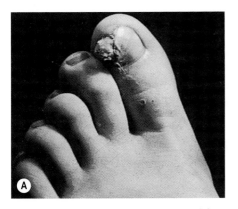
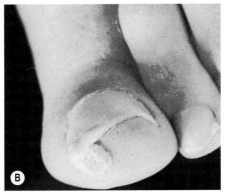
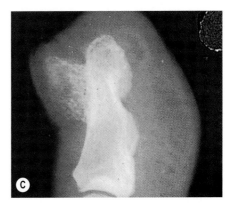

**Figure 2.13** (A, B) Subungual exostoses. (C) X-ray shows elevation of nail plate by exostosis.

## SUBUNGUAL MELANOMA

A variant of acral melanoma, this condition can be confused with subungual haematoma, but careful examination of the physical signs and a detailed history will reduce the likelihood of misdiagnosis.

### Aetiology

The term 'longitudinal melanonychia' is used to describe single or multiple longitudinal pigmented bands within the nail plate. The aetiology of these bands is varied and includes:

- racial variation – 77% of African-Americans over 20 years of age, and approximately 15% of Japanese individuals, present with this melanocyte activity
- repeated trauma to the matrix from picking or chewing
- post-inflammatory melanonychia (e.g. lichen planus, chronic radiodermatitis)
- endocrine disease (e.g. Addison's, pregnancy, HIV infection)
- naevus
- melanoma of the nail matrix.

Most patients with melanoma have a fair complexion, with light hair and blue or hazel coloured eyes. No sex predominance has been identified, and the mean age of onset is 55–60 years. The hallux (and the thumb) are the most likely sites to develop tumours.

Subungual melanoma manifests as an insidious pigmented spot in the matrix, nail bed or plate, or a longitudinal band of variable width in the nail plate. The latter often has a straight edge, which is clearly seen along the plate. Either pigmented area may show one or more of several characteristics:

- Variation in colour of the pigmented spot or band from brown to black; colour may be homogenous or irregular. Seldom painful.
- Pigment may spread to surrounding periungual tissues (Hutchinson's sign) and, although an important indicator of subungual melanoma, it is not a totally accurate predictor of melanoma.
- Eventual dystrophy and destruction of the nail plate.

Diagnosis has until recently been made almost exclusively following biopsy of the matrix and/or nail bed tissues, and this is often painful and disfiguring. The possibility of tumour or melanoma still provokes fear in most patients, and the need for early diagnosis and treatment is important. Dermoscopy, or epiluminescence microscopy, of nail pigmentation is a relatively new modality and it is proving useful in discriminating between suspect lesions that should undergo nail apparatus biopsy and less suspect ones that can be left to follow-up (Baran et al 2003). Less complex and less expensive than ultrasonography and magnetic resonance imaging (MRI), dermoscopy is particularly useful for pigmented nail lesions and vascular abnormalities seen in scleroderma and systemic lupus erythematosus. Semiological patterns allow differentiation between haematoma, racial discoloration, drug-induced pigmentation and nail tissue naevus.

### Treatment

Subungual melanoma has a poor prognosis, with up to 50% of patients dying within 5 years of the diagnosis. Delay in diagnosis contributes significantly to poor prognosis, as does the stage of the disease. Level I and II melanomas can be adequately treated by wide local excision with repair of the resultant defect by skin grafts. If the melanoma is more advanced then amputation is advised, but there is lack of agreement on the need for elective lymph node dissection.

## ONYCHAUXIS (HYPERTROPHIED NAIL)

This is an abnormal, but uniform, thickening of the nail, increasing from the nail base to the free edge, which is commonly seen in podiatric practice. It may be accompanied by slight brown colour changes in the nail plate and enlargement of the sulci due to the thickened lateral edges of the nail. Often, only the nail of the hallux is affected but the disorder may appear in other nails. The excessive growth makes nail cutting difficult and this is often neglected, with the result that subsequent shoe pressure may cause pain and discomfort. Unremitting pressure from footwear may lead to the development of subungual aseptic necrosis, especially in the elderly. A differential diagnosis must be made from pachyonychia congenita, in which all the nails are affected and nail bed hypertrophy is a major feature.

### Aetiology

Onychauxis occurs following damage to the nail matrix, for which there may have been one or more of several causes:

- single major trauma from a heavy blow or severe stubbing, or repeated minor trauma from shallow shoes or pressure from footwear on long and neglected nails
- fungal infection of the nails and chronic skin diseases such as eczema, psoriasis and pityriasis rubra pilaris
- poor peripheral circulation, especially in the elderly
- some systemic disturbance (e.g. Darier's disease); this may be suspected when several or all of the nails are affected.

### Pathology

Trauma to the nail matrix results in the excess production of onychocytes, and the nail becomes progressively thicker as it grows along the nail bed. Why this increased production is permanent is as yet unresolved, as very little research into the condition has been undertaken. Rayner (1973) reported that the proximal nail fold was shortened and everted and therefore unable to exert pressure on newly formed cells, but also that there was a greater vascularity of the nail fold and nail matrix areas, together with an enlarged artery a short distance proximal to the angle of the nail matrix. Furthermore, it was shown that the nail matrix produced an epidermal-type keratin, which increased the thickness of the nail plate and resulted in a thicker but softer intermediate nail layer.

Baran et al (1991) described hyperplasia of subungual tissues, seen in histological sections, as homogeneous oval-shaped amorphous masses surrounded by normal squamous cells and separated from each other by empty spaces (positive PAS stain).

### Treatment

Irrespective of the cause, the nail should be reduced in size to as near normal as possible at each visit, in order to relieve pain caused by pressure on the nail bed tissues. Footwear should be examined for correct fitting but, as the damage to the matrix is irreversible, regular treatment is necessary. In some cases where the cause is linked to a skin disease such as eczema, stabilisation of the skin condition results in a remarkable improvement in the nails of both the hands and the feet (Fig. 2.14a and b).

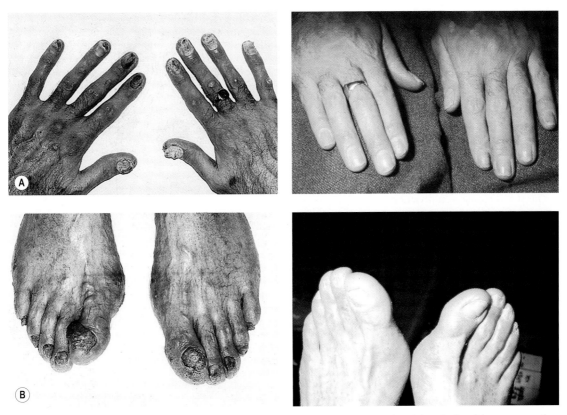

**Figure 2.14** Onychauxis with eczema. Hands before (A) and after (B) treatment of eczema. Feet before (C) and after (D) treatment of eczema.

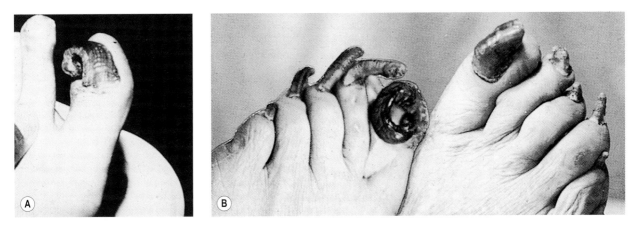

**Figure 2.15** Onychogryphosis.

If the patient is young and the condition is confined to one toenail only, and if there is no contraindication, avulsion of the nail and destruction of the matrix provide the most satisfactory treatment.

## ONYCHOGRYPHOSIS (RAM'S HORN, OSTLER'S TOE)

Onychogryphosis is readily distinguishable from onychauxis because, as well as hypertrophy, there is gross deformity of the nail, which develops into a curved or ram's horn shape (Fig. 2.15a). The nail is usually a dark brown or yellowish colour, with both longitudinal and transverse ridges on its surface. Commonly, only the great toe is affected because, from its size and prominence, it is the one most prone to injury – but the condition may also arise in other toes.

### Aetiology

Any one of the aetiological factors involved in the development of onychauxis may be the cause, but by far the commonest cause is a single major trauma arising from a heavy blow or a severe stubbing of the toe. It is sometimes the result of neglect and the consequent increasing impaction from footwear against the lengthening nail. This may cause the nail's free edge to penetrate the soft tissues of the affected toe and perhaps also of the adjacent toe, resulting in an area of ulceration.

## Pathology

It is believed that the spiral-like appearance of onychogryphosis is due to an uneven production of cells from the nail matrix, the damaged side of the matrix producing cells at a slower rate (Zaias 1990). However, if the faster-growing side determines the direction of the deformity, it would be unlikely that the same side would be damaged in each nail. The most commonly seen deviation in onychogryphosis is towards the median of each foot (Fig. 2.15b) and the most probable explanation for this is shoe pressure.

## Treatment

Palliative treatment consists of reduction of the hypertrophy, taking care to prevent haemorrhage from any nail bed tissue that has been caught up in the malformed nail. Throughout this treatment, it is important to hold the toe firmly to avoid excessive pull on the underlying soft tissue. Footwear should be examined to ensure adequate fitting. This treatment, if repeated at regular intervals, is usually sufficient to give the patient freedom from discomfort. In a young person, especially when only one toe is affected and when palliative measures have been tried, avulsion with matrix destruction is the most satisfactory method of providing long-term relief.

## ONYCHOPHOSIS

Onychophosis is a condition in which callus and/or the formation of an heloma occurs in the nail sulcus, which may result in the sulci becoming swollen and inflamed. In a mild case the effect is little more than irritating, but it can develop to a degree where even slight pressure to the nail plate or the sulcus wall gives rise to acute, sharp pain. There may be associated hypertrophy of the shoulders of the nail plate.

## Aetiology

- Lateral pressure from constricting footwear or from an adjacent toe which has some structural abnormality (e.g. hallux abductovalgus).
- Unskilled nail cutting, particularly if the lateral edges of the nail have been left rough or jagged, which may irritate the epithelium of the sulcus and give rise to callus or heloma formation.
- Unnecessarily harsh probing of the sulcus may lead to excessive thickening of the stratum corneum.

## Treatment

It is sometimes necessary to soften onychophosis to facilitate its removal. This may be achieved by the application of a soak of hydrogen peroxide (10 vol.) left in situ for several minutes; the callus can then be carefully cleared with a small scalpel and checked for the presence of corns, which must be enucleated.

If removal is not possible after such a soak, it may be necessary to pack the sulcus with a keratolytic, such as 10–15% salicylic acid in collodium, and left in situ for no more than 7 days. Reduction of the callus and full enucleation can then be carried out, leaving a smooth edge to the nail plate. If the lateral edge of the nail is thickened, this should be reduced with a Black's file or a pencil burr. Depending on the skin texture, an antiseptic astringent or an emollient should then be applied and cotton wool packing inserted between the nail edge and the sulcus.

If it is necessary to reduce pressure from an adjacent toe, an interdigital wedge, made from semicompressed felt or a long-lasting silicone material, may be inserted. Footwear should always be examined to ensure adequate fitting, and advice on the care of the nails should be given.

## PARONYCHIA

Paronychia and onychia frequently occur together. The former is characterised by inflammation of the tissues surrounding the nail plate, and the latter by inflammation of the matrix and the nail bed. Both may be acute or chronic conditions and are always potentially serious as they arise most commonly from either a bacterial infection or a systemic disease. Acute paronychia begins with local redness, swelling and throbbing pain at the side of the nail; gentle lateral compression of the digit produces a droplet of pus at the lateral or posterior fold. Chronic paronychia develops insidiously and may not be noticed by the patient. Redness and mild swelling of the proximal nail fold are the earliest signs, which progress slowly to resemble a semicircular cushion around the base of the nail (Fig. 2.16). The cuticle is detached and eventually the nail shows transverse ridging and becomes friable, which may cause shedding of the entire nail plate, beginning at the proximal margin.

## Aetiology

Any traumatic incident to the toe that might facilitate the entry of bacteria or a foreign body into the tissues can predispose to paronychia. There are many causes, which include severe stubbing of the toe, slight injury to the periungual tissue, unskilled treatment with a scalpel and untreated ingrowing toenail. The condition may be a manifestation of some systemic disease, such as diabetes mellitus, collagen vascular disease, sarcoidosis or vasculitis.

There is always the possibility that the infection will become widespread, and therefore it is advisable to suggest that the patient consult a physician. Spreading infection is particularly likely when more than one nail is affected. Chronic paronychia most often occurs in the fingernail, particularly among persons whose occupation entails regular immersion of their hands (e.g. bar staff, fishmongers, confectioners), thus rendering them more likely to infection, even after slight trauma. Young women are more susceptible to the condition.

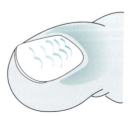

**Figure 2.16** Paronychia with swelling of the proximal nail fold (PNF) and transverse ridging of the nail plate.

## Pathology

Once bacteria or some other foreign body have gained access into the tissues, the natural defensive reaction of the body induces a local inflammatory response in the area, which becomes red, swollen and extremely painful. The oedema separates the nail fold from the proximal nail plate, allowing further ready access to bacteria, which are commonly of the staphylococcal or streptococcal type. Infection leads to the formation of pus, which may be expressed from the nail fold. The yeast *Candida albicans* can also infect the tissue (See Ch. 3).

## Treatment

Paronychia should always be regarded as potentially serious and it must be ascertained whether the condition is acute or chronic.

Acute paronychia is mainly the result of local trauma, and treatment is directed primarily towards the prevention of infection, if this is not already present, and towards the reduction of inflammation and congestion. Cold compresses of Burow's solution every 4 hours for 24 hours should be applied to relieve congestion. This is followed by an application of an antiseptic agent and a suitable protective dressing. The treatment should be repeated at frequent intervals until the symptoms subside. It is important that the patient be advised to rest the foot as much as possible and avoid the causative action, if it is practicable to do so. Usually, if infection is not present, the condition will resolve satisfactorily.

If infection is present, the first principle is to promote drainage of any pus by means of a hot antiseptic footbath, repeated at home at 4-hourly intervals, or by surgically removing the nail plate. Arrangements should be made for the patient to obtain appropriate systemic antibiotic therapy from the doctor, while podiatric dressings continue at frequent intervals. Drainage, once established, must be maintained until all pus has been cleared. The insertion of a piece of sterile ribbon gauze, to prevent premature closure of the wound, will assist this process. Once complete drainage has been achieved the lesion can be thoroughly cleaned with a sterile saline solution and dried. To promote healing, an antiseptic of wide antibacterial spectrum should be applied and covered by a sterile dressing. Such treatment is usually adequate, but the condition may progress to become chronic, when further medical advice should be sought.

## ONYCHIA

Onychia is an inflammation of the matrix and nail bed and frequently originates from paronychia. The clinical features of both conditions are similar, and they should always be regarded as serious. Local infection will cause suppuration, which produces a discoloration of the overlying nail plate (yellow, brown, black or green, depending on the infecting organism). A throbbing pain, which increases in severity, is the common symptom, relief being obtained only by drainage of the pus.

## Aetiology

- Any traumatic incident that introduces bacteria or a foreign body into the tissues; the condition will probably be confined to one toe.
- Any one of a number of systemic diseases; it is likely that several of the toes will be affected.

## Pathology

Onychia can, and often does, result from paronychia (see above) and the pathology is similar. Bacterial invasion results in a purulent infection, which collects beneath the nail plate, causing pressure and onycholysis (seen as separation of the nail from the nail bed).

## Treatment

Immediate relief of acute pain will be obtained by removal of as much as necessary, or even all, of the nail plate to provide drainage of the underlying pus. Once this has been achieved, the further treatment is the same as for paronychia.

## ONYCHOLYSIS

Onycholysis is defined as separation of the nail from its bed at its distal end and/or its lateral margins (Baran et al 2003). It may be idiopathic or secondary to systemic and cutaneous diseases, or it may be the result of local causes. Air entering from the distal free edge gives a greyish-white appearance to the nail plate and forms variably shaped areas of detachment. If a sharp sculptured edge is present, it is likely to be self-induced by harsh manicuring. Onycholysis is more common in fingernails than toenails, and affects women more frequently than men.

## Aetiology

- Idiopathic – Baran et al (1991) suggested that idiopathic onycholysis in women and sculptured onycholysis are probably the same condition.
- Systemic disease, such as poor peripheral circulation, thyrotoxicosis and iron-deficiency anaemia.
- Cutaneous diseases, which include psoriasis, eczema and hyperhidrosis.
- Drug-induced, due to the administration of bleomycin, retinoids, chlorpromazine, tetracyclines or thiazides.
- Local causes, such as trauma, where only one nail will be affected, or local infections (e.g. fungal, bacterial, viral). External irritants also result in onycholysis, the most common being prolonged immersion in hot water with added detergents, solvents such as petrol and cosmetic nail polishes.

## Pathology

Separation of the nail is usually symptomless, but as the condition progresses the space becomes filled with hard keratinous material from the exposed nail bed. The increased subungual pressure caused by this excess tissue may give rise to inflammation and very rarely becomes liable to infection.

## Treatment

If a systemic cause is suspected, the patient should be advised to consult a physician. The single most important step in the treatment of onycholysis is to remove all of the detached nail at each visit. This prevents trauma from hosiery and bedclothes, allows possible mycotic material to be taken from the most proximal lytic area for culture, allows the nail bed to dry out where *Candida albicans* is the infecting organism, and permits application of a suitable antifungal preparation at the active edge of the disease (see Ch. 3). Within 3–4 months the nail should resume a normal, fully attached appearance (Zaias 1990).

## ONYCHOMADESIS (ONYCHOPTOSIS, APLASTIC ANONYCHIA)

This condition involves spontaneous separation of the nail, beginning at the matrix area and quickly reaching the free edge. The separation is often accompanied by some transient arrest of nail growth, characterised by a Beau's line.

### Aetiology

- Trauma, resulting in a subungual haematoma, or from repeated minor trauma (e.g. sportsman's toe).
- Serious generalised diseases (e.g. bullous dermatoses, lichen planus or drug reactions).
- Local inflammation (e.g. paronychia or irradiation).
- Defective peripheral circulation or prolonged exposure to cold.
- It may be an inherited disorder (dominant), and shedding will occur periodically.

### Treatment

If a newly formed subungual haematoma is present, treatment should be aimed at relieving pressure, which may necessitate puncturing the nail.

For those cases where trauma can be excluded, the podiatrist can merely protect the nail with simple tubular gauze dressings or an acrylic resin plate, which prevents snagging on bedclothes and hosiery until the nail regrows fully.

## ONYCHATROPHIA (ANONYCHIA)

The term 'onychatrophia' is used to describe a nail that has reached mature size and then undergoes partial or total regression. The term 'anonychia' is reserved to describe a nail that has failed to develop. However, the two conditions are difficult to differentiate.

Damage to the nail matrix resulting in onychatrophia is caused by lichen planus, cicatricial pemphigoid, severe paronychia, epidermolysis bullosa dystrophica or severe psoriasis. Anonychia occurs with rare congenital disorders, for example nail–patella syndrome.

## ONYCHORRHEXIS (REED NAIL)

This condition presents as a series of narrow, longitudinal, parallel superficial ridges. The nail is very brittle, and splitting at the free edge is common. Ridging naturally becomes more prominent with age, but can be initiated by lichen planus, rheumatoid arthritis and peripheral circulatory disorders.

## BEAU'S LINES

First described by Beau in 1846, these transverse ridges or grooves reflect a temporary retardation of the normal growth of the nail. They first appear towards the proximal nail fold (PNF) and move towards the free edge as the nail grows. The distance of the groove from the PNF indicates quite accurately the length of time since the illness or trauma (nail growth being about 1 mm/week).

### Aetiology

Any condition or disease that may temporarily affect nail production from the matrix can be responsible. A single groove is usually the result of a severe febrile illness, although single grooves have also been noted postnatally and in many other non-specific events. When the transverse ridges are due to paronychia or repeated minor trauma, they often have a rhythmic, rippling appearance.

### Treatment

No specific treatment, other than reassurance, is necessary, as the nail condition will resolve once the aetiological factor has been removed.

## HIPPOCRATIC NAILS (CLUBBING)

'Hippocratic nail' is the term used to describe an exaggerated longitudinal curvature of the nail, sometimes extending over the apex of the toe, which gives the digit a 'clubbed' appearance. The disorder is usually associated with some long-standing pulmonary or cardiac disorder, and has been linked with thyroid disease, cirrhosis and ulcerative colitis (Fig. 2.17).

## KOILONYCHIA (SPOON-SHAPED NAIL)

This condition is seen more frequently in fingernails than toenails. The normal convex curvature is lost and, instead, it becomes slightly concave or spoon-shaped. In infancy, koilonychia is a temporary physiological condition, but there is a proven correlation between koilonychia and iron-deficiency anaemia. Thin nails of any origin, occupational softening and congenital forms are all aetiological factors (Fig. 2.18).

## ONYCHOMYCOSIS (TINEA UNGUIUM)

Onychomycosis is a fungal infection of the nail bed and nail plate. Fungi are microscopic vegetable organisms possessing no chlorophyll, which can exist only by utilising other organic matter for food. Certain groups of fungi, which are generally classified as dermatophytes, possess the ability to metabolise keratin and thereby grow and prolif-

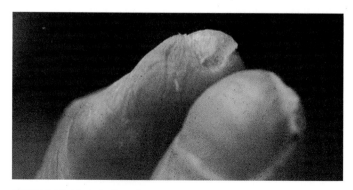

**Figure 2.17** Hippocratic nail.

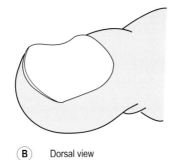

**Figure 2.18** Koilonychia (spoon-shaped nail). (A) Apical view. (B) Dorsal view.

erate in the presence of protein. The human nail and its nail bed provide an exceedingly suitable environment in which the dermatophytes can flourish, and once these fungi have established themselves in that situation, the condition is known as 'onychomycosis'. Because dermatophytes can utilise keratin as a source of food, it follows that any one or all of the nails will be liable to attack.

Zaias (1990) first described three distinct types of fungal invasion, and this has recently been expanded to four (Baran et al 2003):

- Distal lateral subungual onychomycosis (DLCO) is the most common and often affects the skin of the palms and soles as well as the nails. Toenails are more frequently affected than finger nails, and show distal subungual hyperkeratosis, onycholysis which appears yellow-white, and longitudinal streaks when the disease is spreading.
- Proximal subungual onychomycosis (PSO) is caused by moulds (e.g. *Scopulariopsis brevicaulis*), and presents as an area of leuchonychia in the proximal portion of the nail with a normal surface to the nail plate as the fungal elements are located in the ventral portion of the proximal plate. Periungual tissues are often inflamed and a differential diagnosis must be made to rule out bacterial infection. In advanced cases a purulent discharge may be present.
- Superficial onychomycosis is most commonly due to *Trichophyton mentagrophytes* var. *interdigitale* and affects only toenails. The nail plate shows small, white, friable opaque patches that can be easily scraped away, hence the name 'white superficial onychomycosis'.
- Endonix onychomycosis is rare and is due to *Trichophyton soudanese* and *T. violaceum*. The nail plate is diffusely opaque and white, and it is common for plantar tissues to be involved. There is no onycholysis or subungual hyperkeratosis.

Fungally infected toenails often become thickened and quite brittle, and in some cases take on a yellowish brown colour. Left untreated, the nail becomes more friable and develops a 'worm-eaten' or porous appearance.

## Aetiology

It is not always possible to pinpoint the actual source of the infection, but one of the predisposing factors is failure to maintain a good standard of foot hygiene. Hyperhidrosis, communal showers, failure to dry the feet thoroughly following sporting activities, and spread of an existing skin infection are all factors to be considered.

## Pathology

Of the dermatophytes associated with onychomycosis, the most frequently identified in practice are *Trichophyton rubrum* and *T. interdig-*

*itale*. Infection usually commences at the distal edge of the nail and gradually spreads over the entire nail plate and nail bed. Eventually, the nail plate becomes onycholytic as subungual debris increases. White marks, indicating fissuring, may appear on the nail plate.

## Treatment

Advice must also emphasise the possible spread of the infection via towels, hosiery and shoes, together with vigilant attention to drying and general personal hygiene. Superficial onychomycosis can be treated with any topical antifungal agent; this is particularly useful when systemic treatment is contraindicated. The areas of affected nail should be thinned as far as is practicable prior to the application of the topical preparation in order to facilitate its full potential. Amorolfine nail lacquer (5%) has proved successful if treatment is continuous for more than 6 months. It is therefore very important that a full explanation of the treatment regimen is given to the patient, as success will depend largely on patient compliance. Topical therapies need to be continued for many months until clearance is achieved.

Dermatophyte onychomycosis requires systemic antifungal therapy. Griseofulvin has been disappointing – with side-effects that cause the patient to discontinue treatment after a short time – and ketaconazole is now rarely used because of its hepatotoxicity. The new systemic antimycotic therapies such as fluconazole, itraconazole and terbinafine have been shown to reach the affected nail in a short time after the start of treatment and then to stay in the nail for periods of 2–6 months after the completion of the drug. This reservoir effect allows the drug to take effect in a shorter period and to prevent relapse. Patients should, however, be advised to continue a regimen of topical application of antifungals to previously affected areas after cure with systemic therapy to reduce the chance of relapse.

Advice must also emphasise the possible spread of the infection via towels, hosiery and shoes, together with vigilant attention to drying and general personal hygiene.

## LEUCONYCHIA

This is characterised by white markings on the nail in lines (striata), dots (punctata) or extending over the entire nail plate (totalis). They usually indicate minor trauma, for example as a result of short shoes or sporting activities, but rarely result from an illness.

## YELLOW NAIL SYNDROME

In this disorder the rate of nail growth reduces greatly and sometimes almost ceases. All the nails become a yellowish green colour; they also thicken and display an increased longitudinal curvature, with some evidence of onycholysis. The condition is almost always associated with some underlying respiratory or lymphoedema abnormality. Spontaneous recovery occurs in 30% of cases, and the use of intravenous vitamin E is said to give beneficial results (Zaias 1990).

## PTERYGIUM

Pterygium is adhesion of the eponychium to the nail bed following destruction of the matrix due to diminished circulation or some systemic disease. The entire nail plate is eventually shed.

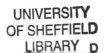

# REFERENCES

Abad M, Bermejo P, Villar A et al 1997 Antiviral activity of medicinal plant extracts. Phytotherapy Research 11(3):198–202.

Achten G 1982 Histopathology of the nail. In: Pierre M (ed.) The nail. G.E.M. Monograph 5. Churchill Livingstone, Edinburgh.

Armstrong D, Peters E 2001 Classification of wounds of the diabetic foot, Current Diabetes Reports 1:233–238.

Baker J 1998 Essential oils: a complementary therapy in wound management. Journal of Wound Care 7(7):355–357.

Baker N, Rayman G 1999 Clinical evaluation of Doppler signals. Practical Diabetes 2(1):22–23.

Bale S, Hagelstein S, Banks V, Harding K 1998 Costs of dressings in the community. Journal of Wound Care 7(7):327–330.

Baran R, Barth JH, Dawber RPR 1991 Nail disorders. Common presenting signs, differential diagnosis and treatment. Martin Dunitz, London.

Baran R, Dawber RPR, Hanecke E et al 2003 A text atlas of nail disorders. Techniques in investigation and diagnosis, 3rd edn. Martin Dunitz, London.

Brown JS 1992 Minor surgery. Chapman & Hall, London.

Bunney M, Benton C, Cubie H 1992 Viral warts – biology and treatment. Oxford Medical Publications, Oxford.

Cameron S, Leaper D 1987 Antiseptic toxicity of open wounds. Care Science and Practice 5(2):19–20.

Chapman C, Visaya G 1998 Treatment of multiple verrucae by triggering cell-mediated immunity – a clinical trial. British Journal of Podiatry 1(3):89–90.

Chatterjee A, Jana B 1993 Cytological effect of Thuja occidentalis in homeopathic preparations. Homeopathy International 7(1):14.

Cohen HJ, Franck SB, Minkin W, Gibbs RC 1973 Subungual exostosis. Archives of Dermatology 107:431–432.

Cotteril J, Cunliffe W 1997 Suicide in dermatology patients. British Journal of Dermatology 137(2):246–250.

Cribier B, Djeridi N, Peitre B 2001 A histologic and immunohistochemical study of chilblains. Journal of the American Academy of Dermatology 45(6):924–929.

Dealey C 2005 The care of wounds, 3rd edn. Blackwell Scientific, Oxford.

Diridollou S, Vabre V, Berson M, et al 2001 Skin ageing: changes of physical properties of human skin in vivo. International Journal of Cosmetic Science 23(6):353.

Drosou A, Fallabella A, Kirsnet R 2003 Antiseptics on wounds: an area of controversy. Wounds 15(5):149–166

Drossu A, Fallabella A, Kirsnet R 2003 Antiseptics on wounds: an area of controversy. Wounds 15(5):149–166.

Enoch S, Harding K 2003 Wound bed preparation: the science behind the removal of barriers to healing. Wounds 15(7):213–229.

Falanga V 2005 Advanced treatments for non-healing chronic wounds. http://www.worldwidewounds.com/2005/april/Falanga/Advanced-Treatments-Chronic-Wounds.html.

Feder G, Eccles M, Grol R et al 1999 Using clinical guidelines. British Medical Journal 318(7185):728–730.

Field T, Peck M, Krugman S et al 1998 Burn injuries benefit from massage therapy. Journal of Burn Care and Rehabilitation 19(3):241–244.

Fowler A, 1998 Split thickness skin graft donor sites. Journal of Wound Care 7(8):399–402.

Freinkel R, Woodley D (eds) 2001 The biology of skin. Parthenon, London.

Gibbs S, Harvey I, Sterling JC 2003 Local treatments for cutaneous warts. Cochrane Database Systematic Review 2003;3.

Gnaidecka M, Jemec G 1998 Chronological and photo ageing due to accumulative effects of UVR. British Journal of Dermatology 139(5):815–821.

Graham A 1998 The use of growth factors in clinical practice. Journal of Wound Care 7(9):464–466.

Halery S, Lubart S Reuveni H, Grossman N 1997 Infra-red (780 nm) low level laser therapy for wound healing, in vivo and in vitro studies. Laser Therapy 9(4):159–164.

Hamilton JB, Terada H, Meistler GE 1955 Studies of growth throughout the life span in Japanese: growth and size of nails and relationships to age, sex, heredity and other factors. Journal of Gerontology 10:401–415.

Hardy S 2002 Human microbiology. Lifeline Series. Taylor & Francis, London.

Hart J 1998 The use of ultrasound in wound healing. Journal of Wound Care 7(1):25–28.

Hashimito K, Gross BG, Nelson R, Lever WF 1966 The ultrastructure of the skin of human embryos. III. The formation of the nail in 16–18 week-old embryos. Journal of Investigative Dermatology 40:143–145.

Hashmi F 2000 Non-enzymatic glycation and the development of plantar callus. British Journal of Podiatry 3(4):91–94.

Hayry M 1998 Ethics Committees, principles and consequences. Journal of Medical Ethics 24:81–85.

Hitchen D 1987 Wound care and the aromatherapist. Journal of Tissue Viability 3(2):56–57.

Hoffman D 1997 Leg ulceration with mixed arterial and venous disease. Journal of Wound Care 6(2):53–55.

Humphreys W 1999 The red painful foot – inflammation or ischaemia. British Medical Journal 318(7188):53–55.

Hurwitz B 1999 Legal and political considerations of clinical practice guidelines. British Medical Journal 318(7184):661–664.

Irizarry L 1996 Reduced sensitivity of Staphylococcus aureus to cetylpyridium chloride and chlorhexidine. Chemotherapy 42:248–252.

Izzo K, Aravabhumi S, Nieres R 1996 An algorithmic approach to diagnosis and treatment of chronic benign lower extremity pain. Lower Extremity 3(3):155–176.

Jarrett A, Spearman RIC 1966 The histochemistry of the human nail. Archives of Dermatology 94:652–657.

Johnson M, Comaish JS, Shuster S 1991 Nail is produced by the nail bed: a controversy resolved. British Journal of Dermatology 125:27–29.

Jones J 2005 Winter's concept of moist wound healing: a review of the evidence and impact on clinical practice. Journal of Wound Care 14(6):273.

Jones V 1998 Debridement of diabetic foot lesions. Diabetic Foot 1(3):88–94.

Jude E, Boulton A 1998 Foot problems in diabetes mellitus. British Journal of Podiatry 1(4):117–120.

Kerschott J 1997 The complementary use of homeopathic preparations in primary care practice. Biomedical Therapy 15(2):47–52.

Klenerman L 1991 The foot and its disorders. Blackwell Scientific, Oxford.

Krogstad AL, Skymme A, Pegenius G et al 2005 No compensatory sweating after botulinum toxin treatment of palmar hyperhidrosis. British Journal of Dermatology 152(2):329–333.

Langer S, Sedigh Salakdeh M, Goertz O et al 2004 The impact of topical antiseptics on skin microcirculation. European Journal of Medical Research 9(9):449–454.

Lawrence D, Bennett P 1992 Clinical Pharmacology, 7th ed. Churchill Livingstone, Edinburgh.

Lawrence J 1997 Wound irrigation. Journal of Wound Care 6(1):23–26.

Leelaporn A, Pualsen I, Tennent J et al 1994 Multidrug resistance to antiseptics and disinfection in coagulase-negative staphylococci. Journal of Medicine and Biology 40:214–230.

Leung AKC 1998 Pruritis in children. Journal of the Society for Promotion of Health 118(5):280–286.

Lewes B 1998 Nutrient intake and risk of pressure sore development in older patients. Journal of Wound Care 7(1):31–33.

Lewin K 1965 The normal finger nail. British Journal of Dermatology 77:421–430.

Lewis BL 1954 Microscopic studies of fetal and mature nail and surrounding soft tissue. Archives of Dermatology 70:732–747.

Littlejohn T 1992 Substrate energetics of antiseptics and disinfectant resistance in Staphylococcus aureus. FEMS Microbiology Letters 95:259–266.

McCourt F 1998 Normal plantar stratum corneum and callus. An analysis of fatty acids. British Journal of Podiatry 1(3):98–101.

McKay IA, Leigh IM 1991 Epidermal cytokines and their roles in cutaneous wound healing. British Journal of Dermatology 124:513–518.

MacKie R 2003 Clinical dermatology – an Oxford core text, 5th edn. Oxford University Press, Oxford.

Menz H 1998 Manipulative therapy of the foot and ankle: science or mesmerism? The Foot 8:68–74.

Merriman L, Griffiths C, Tollafield D 1986 Plantar Lesion Patterns. Chiropodist 42:145–148.

Nurmikko T, Nash T 1998 Control of chronic pain. British Medical Journal 317(7170):1438–1441.

Norton LA 1971 Incorporation of thymidine-methyl-H³ and glycine-2-H³ in the nail matrix and bed of humans. Journal of Investigative Dermatology 56:61–68.

O'Halloran N 1990 A biomechanical investigation into the cholesterol content of seed corns. BSc dissertation, University of Brighton.

Phillips T, Al-Amoudi H, Leverkus M, Park H-Y 1998 Effect of chronic wound fluid on fibroblasts. Journal of Wound Care 7(10):527–532.

Potter J 2000 Regrowth patterns of plantar callus. The Foot 10(3):144–148.

Potts RO 1986 Stratum corneum hydration: experimental techniques and interpretation of results. Journal of Society of Cosmetic Chemists 37:9–33.

Powell J 1998 Papillomavirus research and plantar warts. The Foot 8(1):26–32.

Pray WS 2005 Treatment of warts. US Pharmacist. http://www.medscape.com/viewarticle/505452.

Rayner VR 1973 An investigation into nail hypertrophy. Chiropodist September:288–302.

Royal College of Nursing 1998 The management of patients with chronic venous leg ulcer. Recommendations for assessment, compression therapy, cleansing, debridement, dressing, contact sensitivity, training, education and quality assurance. http://www.nelh.nhs.uk/guidelinesdb/html/LegUlcer-front.htm.

Royal College of Nursing 2001 Pressure ulcer risk assessment and prevention. http://www.nhs.uk/guidelinesdb/html/PrUlcer-recs.htm.

Renwick P, Vowden K, Willkinson D, Vowden P 1998 The pathophysiology and treatment of diabetic foot lesions. Journal of Wound Care 7(2):107–110.

Rippon M, Springett K, Walmsley R et al 1998 Ultrasound assessment of skin and wound tissue: comparison with histology. Skin Research and Technology 4:147–154.

Romanelli M, Flanagan M 2005 Wound bed preparation for pressure ulcers http://www.worldwidewounds.com/2005/july/Romanelli/Wound-Bed-Preparation-Pressure-Ulcer.html.

Ryan T 1991 Cutaneous circulation. In: Goldsmith L (ed.) Physiology, biochemistry and molecular biology of the skin. Oxford University Press, New York.

Ryan T 1998 Evidence based medicine: a critique. Journal of Tissue Viability 8(2):7–8.

Samman PD, Fenton DA 1995 The nails in disease, 5th edn. William Heinemann, London.

Schuwen Z, Meigun Z 1996 Bleomycin sulfate in the treatment of mosaic plantar verrucae: a follow up study. Journal of Foot and Ankle 35(2):169–172.

Sheppard SJ 2005 Antibiotic treatment of diabetic foot ulcers. Journal of Wound Care 14(6):260–263.

Smith AG 1999 Skin infections of the foot. The Foot 9(2):56–59.

Springett K 1989 Prophylactic use of antiseptics. The Chiropodist 4:118–120.

Springett K 1993 The influences of forces generated during gait on the clinical appearance and physical properties of skin callus. Doctoral thesis, University of Brighton.

Springett K, Greaves S 1995 Case study: a multidisciplinary approach to prevent foot ulceration. Journal of Tissue Viability 5(1):32–33.

Springett K, Merriman L 1995 Assessment of the skin and its appendages. In: Merriman L, Tollafield D (eds) Assessment of the lower limb. Churchill Livingstone, Edinburgh.

Springett K, Deane M, Dancaster P 1997 Treatment of corns, calluses and heel fissures with a hydrocolloid dressing. Journal of British Podiatric Medicine 52(7):102–104.

Swinscoe M 1998 Skin infections of the foot. The Foot 9(2):56–59.

Thomas S, Dykes P, Marks R 1985 Plantar hyperkeratosis: a study of callosities and normal plantar skin. Journal of Investigative Dermatology 85:394–397.

Thomas S, Dykes P, Marks R 1997 Plantar hyperkeratosis: a study of callosities and normal plantar skin. Journal of Investigative Dermatology 85:394–397.

Tortora G, Kemnitz C, Jenkins G 2005 Anatomy and physiology: from science to life, 1st edn, John Wiley, Chichester.

Veien N 1998 The clinician's choice of antibiotics in the treatment of bacterial skin infection. British Journal of Dermatology 139(Suppl 52):3–36.

Vincent J 1983 Structural biomaterials. Macmillan, London.

Wall B 1997 Assessment of the ischaemic foot in diabetes. Journal of Wound Care 6(1):32–38.

Whinfield A, Forster M 1997 Effect of electrodessication on pain intensity associated with chronic heloma durum. The Foot 7:224–228.

White RJ, Cutting KF 2004. Maceration of the skin and wound bed by indication. In: White RJ (ed.) Trends in wound care. Quay Books, London.

Yosipovitch G 2004 Dry skin and impairment of barrier function associated with itch – new insights. International Journal of Cosmetic Science 26(1):1–7.

Zaias N (ed.) 1990 In: The nail in health and disease, 2nd edn. Appleton and Lange, Norwalk, CT.

Zaias N, Alvarez J 1968 The formation of the primate nail. An autoradiographic study in the squirrel monkey. Journal of Investigative Dermatology 51(2):120–136.

## FURTHER READING

Baden HP 1987 Diseases of the hair and nails. Year Book Medical Publishers, Chicago, IL.

Baran R, Dawber RPR 1984 Diseases of the nails and their management. Blackwell, Oxford.

Baran R, Dawber RPR, Levene GM 1991 A colour atlas of the hair, scalp and nails. Wolfe, London.

Burton JL 1991 Textbook of dermatology, 5th edn. Blackwell, London.

# Chapter | 3 |

# Dermatological conditions of the foot and leg

*Tom Lucke, Colin Munro, David T Roberts, John Thomson and Maureen O'Donnell*

## KEYWORDS

Acquired keratoderma

Adnexal tumours

Blistering disorders

Causes of tumours

Classification of tumours

Contact dermatitis

Cutaneous metastatic tumours

Dermatophyte infection

Eczema (dermatitis)

Epidermal and dermal naevi

Epidermal tumours

Fibrous tumours

Juvenile plantar dermatosis

Inflammation

Laboratory diagnosis of dermatophyte infection

Pigmented skin lesions

Pompholyx

Psoriasis

Reiter's disease

Swellings

Systemic treatment of foot and nail infections

Tinea incognito

Treatment of fungal foot and nail infections

Tumours

Vascular tumours

## Inflammatory skin diseases

Several chronic inflammatory skin diseases commonly involve the feet. A podiatrist should be able to recognise the clinical features of the most common skin diseases and be aware of appropriate management and referral criteria.

## PSORIASIS AND RELATED DISORDERS

Psoriasis is a chronic inflammatory skin condition with a prevalence of about 2% of the UK population (Griffiths & Barker 2007). It can affect any age group, including children, but onset is commonest in early adulthood and late middle age. The disease is characterised by increased turnover of the epidermis, but the pathogenesis involves abnormalities in T-lymphocyte function and increased vascularity, as well as proliferation and altered differentiation of keratinocytes. There

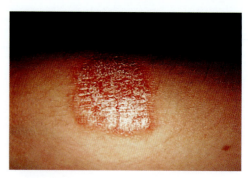

**Figure 3.1** A typical plaque of chronic plaque psoriasis. These plaques are normally found on the limbs.

is clear evidence to suggest that susceptibility to psoriasis is inherited; a number of genetic loci have been implicated but the precise genetic basis of the disease is not yet known (Ortonne 1999).

Chronic plaque psoriasis is the most characteristic form. Patients present with circumscribed itchy patches of thick, scaly, red skin often prominent on the elbows, knees and scalp, although any body site can be affected (Fig. 3.1). Other variants include:

- *guttate* psoriasis, in which multiple small patches of psoriasis erupt acutely after a streptococcal throat infection
- *erythrodermic* psoriasis, a rare medical emergency in which more than 80% of the skin becomes red and inflamed
- *pustular* psoriasis, in which numerous sterile pustules stud the surface of affected skin and patients may become systemically unwell.

Psoriasis can be triggered or exacerbated by a number of factors, which include: trauma (psoriasis appearing at sites of injury such as operative scars is called the Köbner phenomenon); drugs, such as lithium or hydroxychloroquine; infection, particularly the streptococcal pharyngitis, which triggers guttate psoriasis (see above); and stress, which does appear to be important in disease exacerbations in some patients. As with many chronic diseases, patients with severe psoriasis have increased cardiovascular morbidity, and are more prone to psychological problems, including alcoholism. About 40% of women with psoriasis improve during pregnancy while 15% deteriorate.

The severity of psoriasis can be assessed by the PASI (psoriasis area and severity index) score. This is useful in measuring objective response in clinical trials, in which 75% improvement (PASI 75) is a commonly used an endpoint. However, the PASI is mainly a measure of extent and fails to take account of many other factors; it is often supplemented by the Dermatology Life Quality Index (DLQI).

The feet are commonly involved in psoriasis. Typical pink or red plaques with a superficial layer of fine silvery white scale may be seen on the dorsum of the foot, while more hyperkeratotic, fissured skin is seen on the plantar surface, particularly at sites of pressure. Psoriasis commonly also causes nail dystrophy, including separation of the nail plate from the nail bed (onycholysis) or subungual hyperkeratosis. Fine indentations or pitting of the nail plate may also be seen; this is more prominent on fingernails. Psoriatic arthritis may be an additional problem, and can present with pain and decreased mobility in the axial skeleton and the small joints of the hands and feet. A rare mutilating form of arthritis can result in significant resorption of bone in the digits.

Differentiating plantar psoriasis from other causes of acquired plantar keratoderma (thickening of the plantar skin), such as eczema, lichen planus and fungal infection, is often difficult. It is therefore important to look for typical signs of psoriasis at other sites and to enquire about a positive family history of the disease.

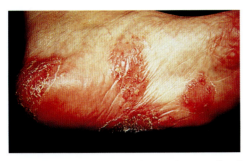

**Figure 3.2** Palmoplantar pustulosis. Fresh pustules are yellow but they become green and then brown with age.

## Treatment

Regular emollients reduce scaling and fissuring, and keratolytics such as 5% salicylic acid in Vaseline or 50% propylene glycol in water treat hyperkeratosis. The numerous active topical treatments available include vitamin D analogues such as calcipotriol, topical steroids, coal-tar-based preparations, dithranol (anthralin), an anthraquinone compound, and vitamin A derived drugs (retinoids).

Patients may benefit from treatment with ultraviolet B (UVB) phototherapy, or photochemotherapy using an oral or topical photoactive drug (a psoralen) in combination with ultraviolet A (PUVA). This treatment can be localised by using hand and foot irradiation units. More severe cases may require treatment with drugs such as the oral retinoid acitretin, or immunosuppressive agents such as methotrexate or ciclosporin (Warren & Griffiths 2008). The latter two agents in particular carry significant toxicity risks for bone marrow, liver or kidney, and all long-term systemic agents for psoriasis necessitate monitoring. Patients with severe psoriasis not suitable for these drugs or who respond poorly may be treated with biological agents (Smith et al 2005). These include the TNF-alpha antagonists etantercept, infliximab, and adalimumab. These agents carry the risks of immunosuppression, and are currently very expensive. Biological agents with other targets are licensed or under development for psoriasis and psoriatic arthropathy.

## Palmoplantar pustular psoriasis (PPP)

Many patients with this chronic inflammatory disorder of the palms and soles have no other features of psoriasis and hence there is some debate as to whether it is a true subtype of the disorder. It typically presents with red scaly hyperkeratotic palmar and plantar skin studded with sterile pustules (Fig. 3.2). Fresh pustules initially appear yellow and subsequently dry to leave brown discoloration. Extensive plantar disease can result in pain on weight-bearing. PPP is more common in middle-aged women and is strongly associated with cigarette smoking. The differential diagnosis includes acute infected eczema, dermatophyte fungal infection and Reiter's disease (see below). Treatment of PPP is similar to that of psoriasis but the disease is often resistant to many of the available therapeutic options (Eriksson et al 1998).

## REITER'S DISEASE

This is a reactive disorder in which arthritis, urethritis, conjunctivitis and inflammatory mucocutaneous disease are triggered by urogenital or gut infections. It is most commonly seen in young men in whom it often follows *Chlamydia trachomatis* urethritis.

The classic cutaneous finding is keratoderma blenorrhagicum, a psoriasis-like eruption that usually affects the soles of the feet and may not appear for several months after the onset of arthritis and conjunctivitis. Affected patients have thick, 'limpet-like' hyperkeratoses with a dull yellow discoloration or a more acute pustular rash.

Patients with active systemic disease may require treatment with immunosuppressive drugs such as methotrexate or azathioprine, which may also improve the cutaneous features of the disease. Application of emollients and keratolytics may reduce the plantar keratoderma.

## PITYRIASIS RUBRA PILARIS (PRP)

This is a rare group of disorders characterised by hyperkeratosis of hair follicles, widespread erythema and palmoplantar keratoderma. The cause of PRP is unknown.

In the classic form, erythema surrounding individual hair follicles spreads out to become confluent, although there are typically islands of spared normal-appearing skin. The erythema has a distinctive orange-yellow hue, which is particularly prominent in the hyperkeratotic skin of the palms and soles. The disorder is often difficult to differentiate from psoriasis. Patients are generally treated with bland emollients, although many subsequently require the addition of systemic agents such as acitretin or methotrexate. Response to treatment is often poor but the disease generally resolves spontaneously (Griffiths 1980).

## ECZEMA (DERMATITIS) AND RELATED DISORDERS

Dermatitis is an inflammatory skin disease that may be caused by a number of factors. For most purposes the terms 'eczema' and 'dermatitis' are synonymous. Acute dermatitis is characterised by redness, scaling and weeping, often with vesiculation (tiny fluid-filled blisters). In contrast, chronic dermatitis is characterised by excoriation (scratch marks) and thickening of the skin known as 'lichenification'. Common categories of eczema include those described below.

> ## CASE STUDY 3.1 ECZEMA/DERMATITIS – OUTLINE OF DIFFERENTIAL DIAGNOSIS AND MANAGEMENT
>
> A boy aged 8 years and a keen swimmer had to stop this activity as he developed thin plantar skin on both feet which fissured easily, becoming painful and prone to infection. There was no family history of similar problems, but his mother recalled that he developed a red itchy rash (urticaria) the previous summer. He had treated it with a number of topical preparations without success. Previously the skin problem had occurred around the toes but now the site and skin changes followed the shoe/skin contact line, which suggested an allergy to the dye and/or adhesive in the footwear. Differential diagnosis included tinea pedis, hyperhidrotic skin (sweaty skin that dries quickly on exposure, becoming dry and scaly – xerosis), juvenile plantar dermatosis and atopic dermatitis (Leung 1998). Laboratory microscopy and culture of scrapings showed no evidence of fungal infection.
>
> The treatment was symptomatic, as no clear diagnosis was evident. Fissures were closed with adhesive skin closures or medical-grade acrylic glue (with prior patch testing, although this cannot be relied

upon). While waiting for the laboratory report, the patient's mother spent some time isolating the suspected allergen. The patient's socks were washed in water only, all topical applications were stopped and the shoes suspected of being implicated were not worn for 5 weeks to allow the apparent hypersensitivity to subside. There was a marked improvement after 2 weeks and a gradual introduction of the suspected allergens identified a particular pair of shoes, which were discarded. The patient could have been referred to the allergy clinic for tests, but this simple method of identifying a potential allergen was an attractive option given the time delay in referral.

Further aspects of management to prevent recurrence included distancing the patient's skin from potential allergens, and the control of any hyperhidrosis. Water enhances percutaneous absorption of many topical substances, and a sweaty environment provides an opportunity for enhanced bacterial colonisation of the skin and increased potential for bacterial superantigen associated with atopy (Leung 1998). The boy's mother contacted the shoe manufacturers to enquire about products used in manufacture; a barrier cream was applied to the patient's feet (e.g. silicone). Sweat-absorbing socks and charcoal-impregnated insoles were also used by the patient.

It is difficult to say whether one or all of these management methods were responsible for the success in the relief of the patient's symptoms. In this particular case it was neither good clinical practice nor ethical to withhold treatment to determine which was the most successful.

## Atopic eczema

This is a common, chronically relapsing skin disease with a genetic predisposition and a rising prevalence in the population. It is often associated with the other atopic diseases, asthma and hay fever. Onset is usually in infancy, and about 60% of children are clear of dermatitis by the age of 10 years. In a minority, eczema persists into adult life, and others may present for the first time later in life. The cause is complex and multifactorial, but a major underlying factor is a defective skin barrier. Many patients with atopic eczema carry null mutations in the epidermal barrier protein filaggrin (Sandilands et al 2007). Defects in the skin barrier may be responsible for the altered immune reactivity to common environmental allergens such as the house dust mite. Atopic eczema can affect any body site but is particularly common on the flexural surfaces of limbs and on the face. Involvement of the feet is less common, although the ankles are often affected (Fig. 3.3). Patients with defects in filaggrin are more likely to show hyperlinearity and hyperkeratosis of the palms and soles.

### Treatment

The mainstay of treatment is a combination of regular emollients (moisturisers) and topical corticosteroid ointments or creams. These vary in potency from the mild hydrocortisone, to the more potent synthetic fluorinated corticosteroids, which in prolonged use cause skin atrophy. Topical immunosuppressive agents (tacrolimus, pimecrolimus) are a more recent alternative to topical corticosteroids. Anti-inflammatory pastes containing tars such as ichthammol, or zinc, are particularly effective in settling eczema of the feet and ankles. Affected skin is often infected by *Staphylococcus aureus*, and antiseptic or topical or oral antibiotic may be needed. Patients with severe chronic eczema may require treatment with immunosuppressive drugs such as azathioprine or ciclosporin; phototherapy is also used (Brehler et al 1997).

## Contact dermatitis

Contact dermatitis can be subdivided into patients who have a hypersensitivity reaction to specific allergens (*allergic contact dermatitis*) and those who have a non-specific reaction to irritants (*irritant contact dermatitis*), but the two often coexist.

Irritant contact dermatitis is usually the result of non-allergic, chemical damage to the skin. This may occur acutely, for instance after exposure to acids or alkalis, but is more commonly the result of cumulative exposure to a variety of irritants such as soaps, detergents and even water. Workers in jobs where wet work is common are particularly prone to irritant contact dermatitis. Some workers are far more prone to the effects of irritants than others, although the reason for this is not clear. The hands are the most common site of irritant contact dermatitis.

Allergic contact dermatitis is an important cause of dermatitis of the feet. Patients may become sensitised (allergic) to a wide variety of allergens present in footwear, hosiery and even topical medicaments (Fig. 3.4). In footwear dermatitis, the commonest sources of allergens are chrome (used in leather tanning), rubber vulcanising agents, adhesives (e.g. colophony) and textile dyes. On repeated exposure to such allergens, a contact dermatitis develops. Sometimes a distinctive pattern of dermatitis, with a sharp demarcation between normal and affected skin, will point to allergic contact hypersensitivity as a possible cause.

Patch testing with standardised concentrations of allergens may identify the source of allergic contact dermatitis. This procedure involves application of a series of allergens to the back under adhesive tape. Patches are removed after 48 hours and reactions read at 48 and 96 hours; positive tests are identified as individual red papular or vesicular reactions. In assessing footwear dermatitis, patch tests with samples from different parts of a patient's shoe may be useful (Cockayne et al 1998).

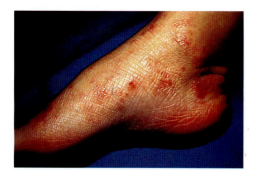

**Figure 3.3** A 3-year-old child of with severe atopic eczema showing erythema and coarse skin markings (lichenification) of the feet.

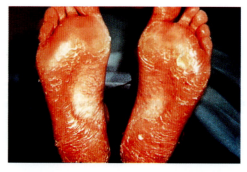

**Figure 3.4** Allergic contact dermatitis of the soles of the feet due to sensitivity to mercaptobenzothiazole, a rubber additive.

## Stasis and varicose eczema

Chronic venous or lymphatic insufficiency may cause dermatitis. The classic distribution of venous or varicose eczema is on the gaiter area of the leg (lower shin and calf), although it can also extend onto the foot. There is often a history of varicose veins or of deep vein thrombosis. Oedema, increased pigmentation (haemosiderin deposition), purpura and ulceration are often present with the dermatitis. Chronic venous hypertension causes distended veins to develop a fibrin cuff, which inhibits movement of fluid, nutrients and metabolites (Hoffman 1997), resulting in poor tissue viability and mechanical weakness (Dealey 2005). Atrophie blanche (white, scarred skin) may be present, and such skin is especially vulnerable to ulceration.

Dermatitis may also complicate chronic oedema due to cardiac or renal insufficiency, obesity, immobility or lymphatic disease. Often these are present in combination. In lymphoedema a firm non-pitting oedema is present, and dilated lymph vessels may give a cobbled appearance to the skin; there may also be a wary hyperkeratosis of the feet. Lymphoedematous legs are vulnerable to recurrent cellulitis, which in turn causes further lymphatic damage.

Allergic contact dermatitis may complicate up to 50% of cases of stasis dermatitis, with hypersensitivity to preservatives and other ingredients in topical medicaments and rubber in bandages being common. The treatment of choice is graduated elastic compression in the form of bandaging or stockings.

## Pompholyx

This is a striking acute vesicular type of dermatitis that affects the palms (cheiropompholyx) and the soles of the feet (podopompholyx). The aetiology of pompholyx is unclear, although some studies have suggested a prevalence of atopy in up to 50% of sufferers. Patients complain of intense itching and discomfort and examination reveals multiple tiny vesicles that look like sago grains (Fig. 3.5). The role of contact allergy in pompholyx is debated, although some investigators believe that ingested nickel may be a factor in nickel-sensitive patients. Treatment is aimed at drying the acute, weeping vesicles with potassium permanganate soaks and reducing the inflammatory component with potent topical steroid creams (Burton & Holden 1998).

### Juvenile plantar dermatosis

This is probably a type of irritant plantar dermatitis that occurs almost exclusively in children aged between 3 and 14 years and is more common in atopics. It presents with fissured, dry dermatitis on the forefoot and heel, with a typical glazed red appearance (Fig. 3.6). Again, the cause is not clear although there have been suggestions that excess humidity in shoes made from modern non-porous materials, such as trainers, might be responsible. The differential diagnosis includes allergic contact dermatitis and fungal infection. Most cases clear spontaneously but some patients benefit from regular emollients and avoidance of synthetic footwear. Cork insoles are anecdotally of value (Lemont & Pearl 1992).

## LICHEN PLANUS

Lichen planus (LP) is an intensely itchy inflammatory skin condition which appears to be immunologically mediated, although the exact cause is not clear. Some cases are associated with adverse reactions to drugs such as gold, while other cases have been reported in patients infected with hepatitis B and C viruses.

Patients classically present with itchy, polygonal, violaceous, flat-topped papules covered with superficial white lines known as Wickham's striae. Papules may coalesce into plaques, and lesions can appear in lines of trauma (another example of the Koebner phenomenon). The rash can affect any body site, although lesions on the wrists and ankles are particularly common. In addition, LP can cause nail dystrophy, scarring alopecia and can affect oral and genital mucosa.

LP can affect plantar skin and the lesions are often not characteristic of LP lesions at other sites. A spectrum of disease may be seen ranging from a few discrete papules at the margin of the foot to widespread hyperkeratosis with fissuring and ulceration (Fig. 3.7).

LP is usually a self-limiting disease, although it may occasionally persist for years. The treatment of choice for widespread, severe disease is systemic steroids, although more limited disease may respond well to potent topical steroids. Hyperkeratotic plantar involvement should be treated with combinations of keratolytics, such as salicylic acid, and potent topical steroids. Oral steroids or ciclosporin can be added in difficult cases (Boyd & Neldner 1991).

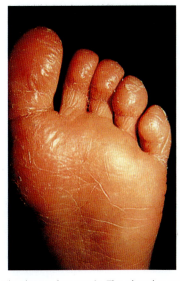

**Figure 3.6** Juvenile plantar dermatosis. The glazed appearance of the plantar forefoot is typical but is often more erythematous and may extend to the dorsa of the toes.

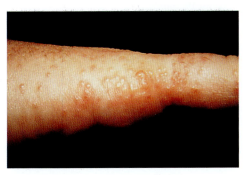

**Figure 3.5** Acute vesicular dermatitis (pompholyx).

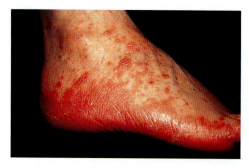

**Figure 3.7** Papules and confluent lesions of lichen planus showing the typical violaceous colour.

## ICHTHYOSIS

'Dry skin', or ichthyosis, of varying degrees is common in the population. Skin becomes more rough and scaly with age due to a reduction in lipid synthesis, and this may be exacerbated by medications or disease. Genetically determined types of ichthyosis also occur, of which the commonest is ichthyosis vulgaris, due to homozygosity for null mutations in the stratum corneum keratin filament aggregating protein filaggrin (Sandilands et al 2007). Other genetic causes include a lack of cholesterol processing due to steroid sulfatase deficiency in X-linked ichthyosis. Ichthyosis affecting the feet may be manifest by both hyperkeratosis and hyperlinearity.

## KERATODERMAS

Plantar skin is characterised by a markedly thickened outer horny layer, or stratum corneum, that provides a functional advantage in protecting the foot against the effects of chronic trauma. This becomes particularly apparent when comparing the feet of people who walk barefoot with those who do not. In addition to this physiological spectrum in the thickness of plantar skin, there are a number of pathological disorders that result in plantar hyperkeratosis or *keratoderma*. It is not uncommon for podiatrists to see patients presenting with plantar keratoderma, and this section will attempt to classify this heterogeneous group of disorders and define their clinical features and the options available for treatment.

Broadly speaking, the palmoplantar keratodermas (PPKs) can be divided into inherited or acquired varieties, the latter being associated with inflammatory skin diseases such as eczema or psoriasis (see above), or a variety of other or uncertain aetiologies.

### Inherited palmoplantar keratodermas

This is a group of rare genetic skin diseases that are characterised by variable degrees of palmar and plantar hyperkeratosis, often in association with other clinical features that make up a syndrome. There have been a number of attempts to classify these diseases based on the pattern of hyperkeratosis (diffuse, focal or punctate), histological features, mode of inheritance and, more recently, by identifying the underlying gene mutation. The latter technique may provide evidence for the molecular basis of these diseases and may have practical implications for both future prenatal diagnosis and gene-targeted therapy.

A detailed review of all the inherited PPKs is beyond the scope of this text, and interested readers are directed to reviews such as that by Kimyai-Asadi et al (2002).

For practical, clinical purposes it is helpful to classify inherited PPKs according to the pattern of hyperkeratosis and the presence or absence of other associated diseases (Table 3.1).

### Aetiology

Recent research has identified mutations in a variety of mainly structural genes of the epidermis that have been found in different patterns of keratoderma. These include keratins, a group of structural proteins with a range of properties that are expressed in specific patterns in different areas of the skin. Other keratodermas are due to mutations in proteins involved in cell adhesion, and in forming the cornified envelope, the waterproof outer layer of the epidermis.

### Clinical features

The features of some inherited PPKs are outlined in Table 3.1, and some examples are shown in Figure 3.8. The severity of these diseases varies both within and between affected families. Keratoderma tends to be more prominent in the weight-bearing areas of plantar skin and can result in discomfort on walking and abnormalities of gait. In addition, patients may complain of malodour as a result of bacterial degradation of the thick keratin layers. Keratoderma which extends to the dorsa of the digits may result in constricting bands and even autoamputation of digits (Fig. 3.9).

Although thickening of plantar skin is common, features that suggest a keratoderma of genetic origin include: early onset or a positive family history of keratoderma; an extensive or unusual pattern; thickening of the skin of other areas such as the elbows, knees and wrists; and other clinical features such as abnormalities of the hair, nails and teeth or a history of deafness. If an inherited PPK is likely then referral to a dermatologist may be appropriate.

In a few families with an inherited PPK there is an associated increased risk of developing some internal malignancies. In a few families, focal keratoderma is associated with a high risk of oesophageal cancer (the Howel–Evans syndrome).

### Treatment

Patients should be advised on the regular use of topical keratolytics such as salicylic acid 5–10% in white soft paraffin or 35–70% propylene glycol. Occlusion with polythene increases the efficacy of keratolytics and can be used in combination with manual paring or abrasion with a pumice stone. Oral vitamin A derived drugs (retinoids) are particularly helpful for some patients but may result in increased pain in affected skin. Surgery has an occasional role for patients with focal keratoderma. Keratoderma may be complicated by dermatophyte fungal infections, and skin scrapings should be sent for mycological culture if this is suspected.

### CASE STUDY 3.3 **KERATIN MUTATION**

A 6-month-old child developed blistering and hyperkeratosis of the feet as she began to weight bear. Her mother was affected by life-long hard skin of the hands and feet. Genetic investigation showed them to have a mutation in keratin 9. This intermediate filament protein is specifically expressed in palmoplantar epidermis, and the mutation causes structural weakness and a hyperkeratotic response.

**Table 3.1** Examples of inherited palmoplantar keratoderma and their causes (Judge et al 2004)

| Pattern of keratoderma | Disease | Inheritance | Other features | Genetic basis |
|---|---|---|---|---|
| Diffuse | | | | |
| | Epidemolytic PPK (Vörner) | Autosomal dominant, well demarcated symmetrical involvement of palms and soles; marked redness at edge of keratoderma; epidermolysis present on histology | No | Mutation in keratin 9 gene |
| | Mutilating keratoderma with ichthyosis | Autosomal dominant: onset in infancy; honeycomb-like keratoderma; constrictions may form on digits | Ichthyosis | Mutation in loricrin gene |
| | Mutilating keratoderma with deafness (Vohwinkel) | Autosomal dominant: onset in infancy; honeycomb-like keratoderma; constrictions may form on digits | Hearing loss | Specific mutation in gap Junction B 2 (connexin 26) gene |
| Focal and striate | | | | |
| | Focal non-epidermolytic palmoplantar keratoderma | Autosomal dominant: onset in infancy | Oral leucokeratoses | Keratin 16 |
| | Pachyonychia congenita Type I (Jadassohn–Lewandowsky) | Autosomal dominant. Hyperkeratosis over pressure points, palms and soles | Type I; orogenital, laryngeal and follicular hyperkeratosis, nail and hair abnormalities | Type I; keratin 6 or 16 gene mutation |
| | Type II (Jackson–Lawler) | No associated malignancy | Type II; nail and teeth abnormalities; cysts, bushy eyebrows | Type II; keratin 6b or 17 gene mutation |
| | Howell–Evans Syndrome (tylosis) | Focal PPK; perifollicular papules | Oral hyperkeratosis; oral and oesophageal carcinoma | Linked to 17q24 |
| | Striate keratoderma (Siemens) | Autosomal dominant: onset in infancy, extension onto elbows and knees | No | Mutation in desmoglein 1 or desmoplakin |
| Punctate | | | | |
| | Punctate PPK, (Buschke–Fischer–Brauer) | Autosomal dominant; develops at ages 12–30 years; multiple tiny punctate keratoses on palms and soles coalescing to diffuse keratoderma over pressure points | Variable nail abnormalities | Unknown |

## Acquired keratoderma

### Keratoderma climactericum

This disorder occurs predominantly in obese postmenopausal women. It presents with erythema and hyperkeratosis over the weight-bearing areas of the heel and forefoot. Patients are often asymptomatic, although pain on walking can be a problem if there is extensive involvement. The disorder has been described in younger women following oophorectomy, suggesting that reduction in endogenous oestrogens may be important in the aetiology. Treatment with emol-lients and keratolytics may be of some benefit (Deschamps et al 1986).

### Acrokeratosis paraneoplastica (Bazex's syndrome)

This is a rare cause of acquired keratoderma that is associated with some internal malignancies. It is more common in men and typically presents with erythema and scaling on the extremities (ears, nose, hands and feet). With time the eruption becomes more generalised

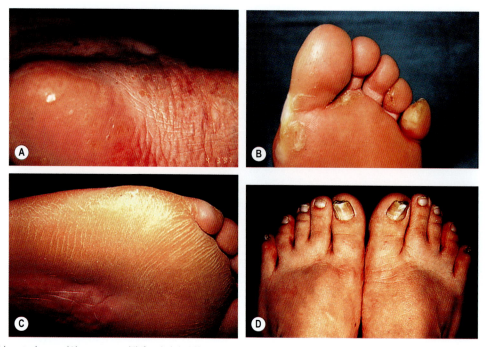

**Figure 3.8** Patterns of keratoderma: (A) punctate; (B) focal; (C) diffuse. (D) Focal keratoderma is seen with a hypertrophic nail dystrophy in pachyonychia congenita.

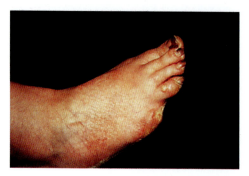

**Figure 3.9** Vohwinkel's keratoderma (mutilating keratoderma with deafness). A toe has been lost due to the formation of a constricting band ('pseudo-ainhum').

and more hyperkeratotic, with keratoderma on the hands and feet. Successful treatment of the underlying malignancy often leads to resolution of the disorder (Bolognia 1995).

### Keratoderma and hypothyroidism

Palmar and plantar hyperkeratosis have been reported in association with hypothyroidism. Treatment with thyroxine replacement may result in clinical improvement (Hodak et al 1986).

## Blistering disorders

Blistering has many causes, including bacterial or viral infections, insect bites and inflammatory skin disorders. Traumatic blistering of the feet is common and is particularly prevalent in recreational sports, such as hill walking and jogging, which impart recurrent shearing mechanical forces to the plantar skin. Poorly fitting or inappropriate footwear may exacerbate the problem. In addition, there is a group of rare skin disorders that are characterised by blistering as a result of inherited abnormalities in a variety of key structural skin proteins.

## EPIDERMOLYSIS BULLOSA: THE INHERITED MECHANOBULLOUS DISORDERS

Epidermolysis bullosa (EB) encompasses a spectrum of disorders characterised by skin fragility and blistering following mild mechanical trauma. Recent research into EB has identified the molecular basis for a number of the diseases, opening up the possibility for prenatal diagnosis and gene-targeted therapy in the future.

EB can be broadly divided into three groups of diseases on the basis of the ultrastructural level of the blister formation.

- In *EB simplex* the plane of cleavage is through the basal keratinocyte layer of the epidermis. It is usually due to defects in the keratin intermediate filaments of this cell layer. Several variants include the *Weber–Cockayne* variety, in which non-scarring blisters predominantly affect palmar and plantar skin (Fig. 3.10). The condition typically worsens in warm weather, particularly in childhood.

- In *junctional EB* separation is at the upper level of the dermoepidermal junction in the lamina lucida. Both skin and oral mucosa may be affected by blisters and erosions that heal with scars. In the *Herlitz* variant (lethal junctional EB), many affected children die in infancy with overwhelming infection.

- In *dystrophic EB* separation is below the lower level of the dermoepidermal junction, the lamina densa, due to defects in the collagenous fibrils which anchor the epidermis to the dermis. Blistering generally starts in infancy and affected patients have a relentlessly progressive course with scarring following minimal trauma and eventual fusion and resorption of the fingers and toes. Growth retardation and anaemia may result from blistering and strictures in the oesophagus (Fine et al 1991, Mellerio 1999).

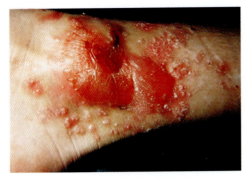

**Figure 3.10** Dystrophic epidermolysis bullosa. In this mild case of dystrophic epidermolysis bullosa there is a defect in the collagens underlying the skin leading to easy blistering.

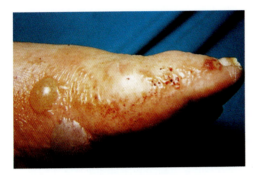

**Figure 3.11** Bullous pemphigoid. On palmoplantar skin this can produce multilocular vesicles resembling pompholyx as well as larger tense blisters.

## AUTOIMMUNE BLISTERING DISORDERS

Disease mediated by autoantibodies against target antigens in the epidermis or its basement layer results in increased skin fragility or blistering. The commonest autoimmune blistering disorder is bullous pemphigoid, in which proteins of the basement membranes are attacked. This causes the whole epidermis to lift off, producing an intact firm blister. On the feet, the blisters may be more vesicular, resembling those of pompholyx (Fig. 3.11). In the various forms of pemphigus, antibodies are directed against adhesion molecules within the epidermis, and the result is friable blisters or erosions. Both of these conditions are commonest in the elderly, and require aggressive treatment with high doses of oral corticosteroids or other immunosuppressive agents.

## Tumours

'Tumor' in Latin simply means a swelling. This, on the foot, could include some corns, verruca plantaris, boils, etc. By usage and wont, the anglified version 'tumour' (American 'tumor') is applied to new growths or neoplasms (Table 3.2). Customarily, these are divided into benign or malignant, which is obviously a vitally important distinction. In the skin, perhaps more so than other systems, these margins can be indistinct. Some tumours are initially premalignant but inexorably transform if neglected. Some normally benign lesions may become malignant. Some apparently aggressive malignancies may

**Table 3.2** Classification of skin tumours

| Tumour type | Degree of malignancy | Examples |
|---|---|---|
| Epidermal tumours | Benign | Seborrhoeic keratoses |
| | Premalignant | Bowen's disease |
| | Malignant | Basal cell carcinoma |
| | | Squamous cell carcinoma |
| | | Cutaneous metastatic tumours |
| Pigmented skin tumours | Benign | Freckle |
| | | Lentigo |
| | | Congenital naevus |
| | | Benign acquired naevus |
| | | Speckled and lentiginous naevus |
| | | Becker's naevus |
| | | Epidermal and dermal naevi |
| | Premalignant | Spitz naevus |
| | | Dysplastic naevus |
| | Malignant | Malignant melanoma |
| Vascular tumours | Benign | Pyogenic granuloma |
| | | Glomus tumour |
| | Malignant | Kaposi's sarcoma |
| Fibrous tumours | Benign | Acquired fibrokeratoma |
| | | Dermatofibroma |
| | Malignant | Dermatofibrosarcoma protuberans |
| Adnexal tumours | Benign | Eccrine poroma |
| Other structures | Benign | Leiomyoma (smooth muscle) |
| | | Subungual exostosis (bone) |
| | | Myxoid cyst (joint) |
| | | Ganglion (joint) |
| | | Bursitis (joint) |
| | | Piezogenic pedal papules (fat) |
| | | Neurofibromatosis (nerve) |

spontaneously involute. Malignancy usually implies the ability to spread, or metastasise, to distant sites by blood or lymphatic vessels. However, lesions such as basal cell carcinoma in the skin may be locally malignant and destructive, but virtually never metastasise.

Nevertheless, the concept of benign or malignant is a useful working one, provided that the limitations are appreciated and the compartments are not considered too watertight.

Tumours of cells in the epidermis, dermis, appendages, etc. are numerous. Some are very rare. Some virtually never affect the feet. Thus the ones discussed in this section are not exhaustive and selection has been made. Some 'tumours', that is swellings, have been included because they might be mistaken for true neoplasms. Some tumours of deeper structures are described, as they may present as a foot swelling.

Any podiatric procedure should include visual and clinical examination of the foot skin and subcutaneous structures (see Ch. 1). The podiatrist is often the person most likely to diagnose foot tumours.

For the patient, ageing, if it brings eyesight problems, obesity and/or arthritis, can make their feet a 'lost world'. Doctors can be curiously reluctant to examine the feet. Most medical examination couches and their lighting are better geared to visualisation of the upper half of the patient. The daunting prospect of the time involved in the removal of the patient's tights, multi-laced boots, etc. in a busy surgery can be a deterrent.

## CAUSES OF SKIN TUMOURS

The cause of many skin tumours is unknown. Understandably, research has mainly concentrated on malignant tumours. A number of factors have been identified as being important. These include external agents and the host's genetic makeup.

In 1775, Sir Percival Pott noted an increase in scrotal cancers in chimney sweeps. This was the first realisation of the skin carcinogenicity of soot, pitches and tars. This finding has been confirmed in animal experimentation and in other occupations over the centuries. Other substances, including arsenic, nitrogen mustard and psoralens, have been added. It has been discovered that the agent may have the same property even if taken systemically. This is especially so with arsenic, immunosuppressants, etc.

Areas of long-continued skin damage, such as leg ulcers, burns and tuberculosis infections, may undergo malignant transformation. More recently, the damage due to radiation has been appreciated. Many of the early medical pioneers of x-radiation developed skin tumours, usually on the hands, because they were unaware of the need for protection. A number of skin tumours are linked to excess exposure to ultraviolet (UV) radiation, mainly in the 280–320 nm wavelength range.

Much more recently, the importance of some infecting viruses has been appreciated. A number can produce tumours in animals, either in the natural situation or experimentally. In the human, the papilloma virus (especially types 16/18) promotes malignancy in the female genitalia and cervix. A herpes virus is established in some cases of Kaposi's sarcoma and a retrovirus in some T-cell lymphomas. This is a developing field and other associations may soon be found.

The host's resistance depends on genetic individuality, modified by lifestyle, occupation, etc. The Celtic races have skin that tends to burn rather than tan, rendering them more vulnerable to UV-radiation-induced tumours. UV radiation, inter alia, can damage the cellular DNA. Normally, there is a repair system that mops up this damaged DNA. When this is defective, cancer can develop. This happens predominantly in the disease xeroderma pigmentosum, which is rare in the UK but more common in Asia.

Cell growth is a very complicated procedure. Normally genes accelerate it forward at an appropriate speed. If these are altered, they can change to transforming genes or oncogenes (i.e. cancer-producing genes). If viruses are involved they may hijack the normal genes. The oncogenes, formed for whatever reason, may thus inappropriately speed the cells along, proliferating in abnormal forms. The brakes applied in the normal system are via the suppressor genes. Of the tumour suppressor genes involved in human skin cancer, p53 tumour suppressor gene is possibly the most important. When this is inactivated by limitation or inhibition, the brakes fail and the lesion progresses abnormally quickly.

Because of their easy accessibility, skin tumours are easier to investigate than systemic ones. There are bound to be many discoveries in the future.

## EPIDERMAL TUMOURS

### Seborrhoeic keratosis

Seborrhoeic keratosis (synonyms: senile or seborrhoeic wart, basal cell papilloma) is one of the commonest tumours found. They are benign but can mimic malignant tumours Their incidence increases with advancing age. They tend to cluster on the trunk, but any body surface, including the feet, can be involved. There are several varieties. One type, stucco keratoses, generally affects the legs and ankles.

#### Aetiology

This is unknown.

#### Clinical features

The commonest type of seborrhoeic keratosis is found on the trunk. There are usually a number of lesions at various stages of development. Initially, they are small papular lesions with a slight increase in pigmentation. They become larger, usually up to about 1 cm in diameter, tending to darken, sometimes until they are almost black. Some can become very large, up to 10 cm or more. The edge is distinct and may slightly overhang the surrounding normal skin. The degree of pigmentation is variable but is usually homogeneous throughout any individual lesion. The surface is rough and wart-like, and at times can become extremely heaped up and thickened. Small circumscribed round areas on the surface are characteristic and known as horn cysts. The surface colour is matt and lacklustre (Fig. 3.12).

On palpation they can feel rather greasy – hence the 'seborrhoeic' in the name. Horn cysts give them a simultaneous warty feel. On the extremities they tend to be flatter. Some can be irritated by clothing, etc., and secondary infection can supervene.

Some may spontaneously involute, but the natural history is for slow development to a certain size. Normally at least several other lesions can be found. At times, massive numbers can erupt rapidly. This is called the sign of Leser–Trélat. It has been much disputed as to whether this is a sign of underlying malignancy (Lindelöf et al 1992).

Stucco keratosis is the name given to a type usually seen on the legs and ankles. They are usually white or grey and smaller. They rarely exceed 3–4 mm. The crusting is easily detachable.

Seborrhoeic keratoses can usually be easily diagnosed by careful examination, but may be confused with viral warts and other hyperkeratotic lesions. The various pigmented lesions may at times need to be excluded.

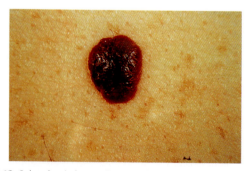

**Figure 3.12** Seborrhoeic keratosis. Note distinct margin, homogeneous colour and scattered horn cysts.

## Histology

Keratinocytes resembling basal cells gather in the epidermis. Increased numbers of melanocytes may contribute to the darkening colour. Concentric whorls of keratin form the keratin cysts.

## Treatment

This is usually indicated for cosmetic reasons or because the lesion is catching and becoming irritated.

Seborrhoeic keratoses are superficial and usually entirely epidermal. They are ideally suited for treatment with liquid nitrogen and usually require only a short application of this. They will curette off easily, and this has the merit of being able to obtain histology, which is always needed if there is diagnostic doubt. The reddish area left will slowly return to normal.

## Bowen's disease

Bowen's disease (Kossard & Rosen 1992) is an intradermal carcinoma in situ which can slowly progress towards a squamous cell carcinoma. Sun damage, arsenic exposure and papilloma virus have all been suggested as causes.

## Clinical features

Bowen's disease as described in the foreign literature has a predilection for the head and neck but the general view in the UK is of a preponderance to affect the lower leg. The usual picture is of a slowly enlarging reddish, scaly patch with definite margins (Fig. 3.13). This can be mistaken for psoriasis, but a careful history and examination should differentiate. Some of the patches may be more crusted or raised (Fig. 3.14).

The differential diagnosis includes basal cell carcinoma, squamous cell carcinoma, malignant melanoma or eczema. If there is doubt, histological examination is essential. Rarely, a nail bed or periungual variant has been described (Sau et al 1994). If neglected, there is a slow progression to squamous cell carcinoma, which is reckoned to occur in approximately 5%.

## Histology

The entire epidermis is replaced by very abnormal looking keratocytic cells. These exhibit nuclear atypia with numerous abnormal mitoses. There is premature keratinisation, which leads to intraepidermal pink horn cysts. The basement membrane remains intact until malignancy supervenes.

## Treatment

In the early stages it can respond to the topical application of 5-fluorouracil (Efudix) which selectively destroys the abnormal cells. A shallow ulcerated area is left, which thereafter heals. Cryotherapy, photodynamic therapy, topical imiquimod or excision are all options.

## Basal cell carcinoma

Basal cell carcinoma (synonyms: rodent ulcer, basal cell epithelioma) (Leffell & Fitzgerald 1999) is the commonest skin tumour, certainly of the white races. Close on one million occur annually in the USA. They are, however, extremely rare on the foot, and especially the plantar surface, where only about 22 have been described (Roth et al 1995). Even fewer peri- or subungual ones have been noted. A certain number occur on the leg.

## Clinical features

The incidence of basal cell carcinoma increases with age. The commonest site is on the face, which may suggest a solar aetiology. However, many occur in areas where there is little or no UV exposure.

The typical history is of a small lesion developing and extending very slowly over months or years. From time to time it crusts and the patient thinks it is healing. The crust comes off with a little bleeding and this cycle often repeats itself, with slow peripheral growth. The outline is round or oval, with a raised or rolled border. This is often pinkish and slightly nodular and is likened to a string of pearls. Over this edge are usually seen dilated telangiectatic vessels (Fig. 3.15). The centre may ulcerate or be more raised and dome-shaped. Locally, they may be very large and destructive, eroding down to the deep structures – hence 'rodent' ulcer.

Those on the lower leg can be less characteristic (Fig. 3.16), and the differential diagnosis between them and Bowen's disease, squamous cell carcinoma, malignant melanoma or vascular lesions may be difficult. They virtually never metastasise.

Some patients have multiple lesions and some of those suffer from the naevoid basal cell carcinoma syndrome (Gorlin's syndrome). There are several features of this, but with reference to the feet and

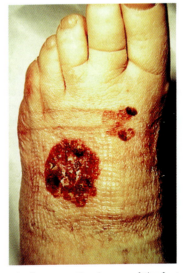

Figure 3.14 Bowen's disease on the dorsum of the foot. Well-demarcated area. Somewhat unusually superadded infection has caused increased crusting.

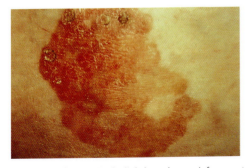

Figure 3.13 Bowen's disease. Red, slightly scaly, psoriaform patch.

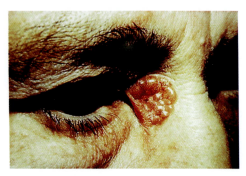

**Figure 3.15** Basal cell carcinoma (rodent ulcer). Typical site showing the raised border, like a string of pearls, with telangiectasic vessels crossing it.

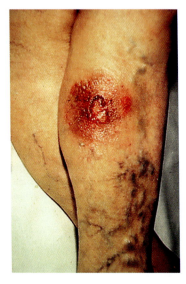

**Figure 3.16** Basal cell carcinoma (rodent ulcer) on the leg. Surrounding redness is atypical and due to a contact dermatitis.

hands, small pits or depressions may be seen on the plantar and palmar surfaces.

## Histology

Cells resembling those of the basal cell layer or appendages appear to 'bud' down from that layer. They form spherical masses of very uniform cells in the dermis. Characteristically the cells at the periphery of these spheres line up in a regular arrangement known as pallisading. The masses are surrounded by a fibrous stroma.

## Treatment

Most are best surgically excised. Curettage, cryotherapy, photodynamic therapy or radiation can be employed. Topical imiquimod can be effective, especially in the superficial ones.

## Squamous cell carcinoma

Cutaneous squamous cell carcinoma (Kwa et al 1992, Salasche et al 1993) arises from the skin keratinocytes. It is the second commonest skin tumour after basal cell carcinoma. It may affect any area of the skin. It is relatively rare on the foot, although an orthopaedic study

suggested that, of the soft-tissue tumours encountered, it was the commonest (Ozedmir et al 1997). A rare variant, verrucose carcinoma, largely targets the foot.

### Aetiology

Numerous factors leading to squamous cell carcinoma have been described (Kwa et al 1992). The host's age, natural skin colour, and immune and genetic status are all important. Thus there is an increased incidence of squamous cell carcinoma in those immunosuppressed by drugs or human immunodeficiency virus (HIV)/acquired immune deficiency syndrome (AIDS). Similarly, those unable to naturally protect their skin, such as albinos with no pigment or those whose DNA repair mechanisms are impaired, as in xeroderma pigmentosum, are at risk. External agents are also important. Scrotal carcinoma was described in 1775 in chimney sweeps from ingrained soot and tar. Over the ensuing centuries, many other outside factors that may contribute to squamous cell carcinoma have been described. Some skin lesions are known to be premalignant, for example Bowen's disease (carcinoma in situ) or actinic keratoses. An area of chronic irritation, including leg ulcers, may progress to squamous cell carcinoma (Hill et al 1996).

Human papilloma virus is a powerful carcinogen in genital carcinoma, but its role in the skin is more uncertain (Sasaoka et al 1996). Contamination with tars, heavy mineral oils, hydrocarbons, etc. continues to be a problem in some industries.

Exposure to UV radiation is a definite factor, as witnessed by the problems encountered by fair-skinned immigrants to very sunny climates, as found in Australia, etc. The feet are usually relatively protected, but one variant of squamous cell carcinoma was described in elderly Japanese on the dorsa of unprotected feet (Toyama et al 1995).

X-radiation is also carcinogenic. Repeated damage from radiant heat may provoke erythema ab igne, and rarely may progress to squamous cell carcinoma. Arsenic exposure has been incriminated.

### Clinical features

Squamous cell carcinoma may present in very many different ways. Thus, in any unusual or non-responsive skin condition the possibility of it should be borne in mind, otherwise it may be missed.

- There may be pre-existing host or intrinsic factors that would render the patient more liable to develop it.
- A chronic skin disease such as actinic keratosis, Bowen's disease, leg ulcers, burns, etc. always has the potential to transform to malignancy, and this should be borne in mind.
- The lesion of squamous cell carcinoma is more likely to present in a sun-exposed area, but no site is immune.
- It may take various forms. It can start as a reddish plaque, mimicking eczema or dermatitis. The edges would tend to be more irregular and the lesion more indurated. Some commence or progress to a nodule of variable size, the surface of which is usually raw and does not epithelialise. It may have a tendency to ooze serosanguinous fluid.
- Some squamous cell carcinomas ulcerate. The ulcer is usually irregular in shape, with undermined ragged edges. The base is covered with a dirty yellowish green slough (Figs 3.17, 3.18).
- Squamous cell cancers of the nail are often misdiagnosed. The feet are less commonly affected than the hand, and when so it is usually the hallux (Dalle et al, 2007).

The vast majority of squamous cell carcinomas are only locally aggressive, but if neglected, they can spread to the draining lymph nodes

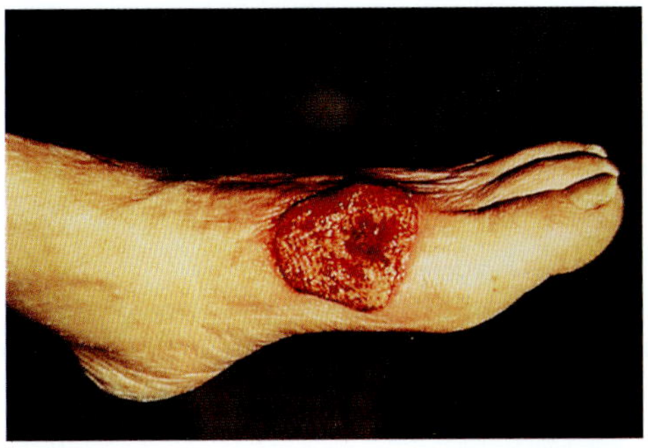

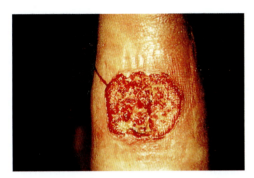

Figure 3.17 Ulcerated squamous cell carcinoma of the foot. Irregular undermined edge.

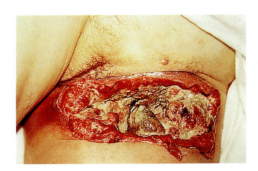

Figure 3.19 Metastasis of squamous cell carcinoma to the groin lymph nodes with subsequent breakdown.

Figure 3.18 Squamous cell carcinoma on the shin. There is an irregular outline with an undermined edge and a dirty, sloughy base.

and thence to other areas (Lund & Greensboro 1965) (Fig. 3.19). This takes a variable time. Head and neck, genital and large tumours all spread more quickly.

### CASE STUDY 3.4 **DIAGNOSIS OF ULCERATED AREA**

A 70-year-old man presented with a symptomless, irregular, ulcerated area on the dorsum of his left foot. He was of Celtic extraction, but had spent most of his working life as a lifeguard on an Australian beach. What is the likeliest diagnosis and appropriate treatment?

The answer is squamous-cell carcinoma. The Celtic races are more likely to suffer sun damage. The dorsum of the foot is a relatively unusual area, but in his work he is likely to have been more exposed to the sun. It would be essential that a biopsy and surgical excision be undertaken as soon as reasonably possible.

## Squamous cell carcinoma variant: verrucose carcinoma of the foot

Verrucose carcinoma (synonyms: epithelioma or carcinoma cuniculatum) (Seehafer et al 1979) may appear at any site but it has a special predilection for the plantar aspect of the foot. Initially it may resemble a simple verruca plantaris. It progresses relatively slowly and may become nodular. At this stage the differential diagnosis would include many nodular foot lesions. With time, the tumour bulk increases and becomes soggy and foul smelling, having been likened to an over-ripe orange. It has a marked tendency to burrow under the skin surface, the sinuses appearing at a slightly distant site from the main lesion

– hence the 'cuniculatum' denoting a resemblance to rabbit burrows. These rarely metastasise.

### Histology

In squamous cell carcinoma the epidermal cells are malignant and manifest in a variety of ways, from large, well-differentiated cells with some individual cell keratinisation, to bizarre, abnormal cells with little or no resemblance to epidermal cells. While in situ, they are contained by the basement membrane to within the epidermis. Sooner or later they 'break through' into the dermis, initially often in fine filaments, but later in broad masses.

Verrucose carcinoma is a well-differentiated tumour, but it may have minimal changes suggesting malignancy at the start.

With all suspected squamous cell carcinomas, clinical suspicion should override an apparently normal biopsy. The cancer may not have manifested itself histologically or the sample may have missed the diagnostic part. Therefore, always keep an open mind and be prepared to re-biopsy on several occasions if clinical doubt persists.

### Treatment

Prevention should be practised. Measures would include control of UV exposure, radiation, etc. If possible, potentially premalignant lesions should be treated. Particular care in monitoring those at risk for genetic reasons is desirable. This is especially expedient in the immunosuppressed and transplanted patient. Immunisation programmes for young girls in Scotland have commenced. Hopefully, this will reduce the future incidence of genital skin and cervical cancers. The programme may be extended to boys and others later.

In the patient with established squamous cell carcinoma, surgical excision of the region with histological confirmation is therefore the best option. If there is suspicion of lymph node involvement, a suitable dissection should also be undertaken.

In the few patients where surgery is not an option, cryotherapy, laser, photodynamic therapy or intralesional injections have all been suggested. If the patient continues to be at risk, long-term follow-up is necessary.

### CASE STUDY 3.5 **SEQUELAE OF LONG-TERM VARICOSE ULCERATION**

A 58-year-old man asks you about a vascular lesion on his ankle during a podiatry session. He has gross varicose veins with pigmentation around the ankle. He has had a small varicose ulcer near the area for years. He works as a forester. What might be developing?

There are a number of possibilities. Trauma from his work might lead to a pyogenic granuloma. The long-standing ulcer may undergo malignant transformation to a squamous-cell carcinoma. Malignant melanoma on the lower leg may be hypomelanotic or amelanotic. Ideally, histology examination should be undertaken in the near future.

# CUTANEOUS METASTATIC DISEASE

Neoplasms beginning in another tissue may spread to the skin by direct extension or as local or distant metastases (Lookingbill et al 1990, Schwartz 1995). These lesions may occur in a patient with known malignant disease or be the first manifestation of the underlying tumour. Skin malignancies themselves, notably melanoma, may also metastasise to other areas of the skin.

## Clinical features

There have been several very large surveys of many thousands of patients. Skin involvement as the first sign of cancer is rare (0.8%), and this was equally divided between direct extension, local and remote metastases.

In patients presenting with a tumour elsewhere, skin involvement at that time was found in 1.3%. In all patients with cancers, the skin involvement seems to be of the order of 5%. The skin involvement may come from many initial sites and, in a significant number, no primary site can be identified.

The non-skin tumours that most commonly spread to the skin are breast, colon and rectum, ovary and prostate. There is a wide range of skin lesions. With direct spread from, for example, breast, there may be an apparent nipple or areolar eczema in Paget's disease, which arises from an intraduct carcinoma (Fig. 3.20). Other breast tumours may spread and grow into the skin, hardening it to resemble a metal breastplate (carcinoma en cuirasse). This may occur in tumours from other sources. Many other types of lesion occur. Small nodules are perhaps the commonest. They often appear to be under the skin, pushing up from below and splaying out the normal cutaneous markings (Fig. 3.21). Indurated erythema, telangiectic plaques or non-healing ulcers are among descriptions of other presentations.

When the skin metastasis comes from another skin tumour, malignant melanoma is the commonest cause. The metastases will often mimic the original tumour.

Any suspicious lesion should be biopsied.

## Histology

This is usually identical to that of the original tumour. However, at times it can be unclassifiable. This is particularly so in highly aggressive anaplastic lesions.

## Treatment

The treatment is essentially that of the primary lesion. In a few instances treatment of the skin lesion by surgery, radiation or chemotherapy may be considered.

# PIGMENTED SKIN LESIONS

Skin colour is largely, although not entirely, due to melanin pigment produced by melanocytes (Bleehen 1998, MacKie 1998, Rhodes 1999). These cells originate from the neural crest and are found in the skin from the eighth fetal week onwards. The melanocytes are the basic factory unit. The rate of production of pigment is influenced by many factors. Ethnic background and sun exposure are two obvious influences.

The melanocyte produces a pigment-containing package – the melanosome – which is transferred to the keratinocyte. The melanocyte is a dendritic cell, which can interdigitate with and 'service' about three dozen keratinocytes. This entire complex is called the melanin unit.

The melanocytes are normally situated in the basal epidermal layer and comprise approximately 6% of these cells in covered sites. This rises to 15% in sun-exposed areas.

## Naevus

A naevus is the term used to designate a non-malignant growth. Its use is mainly, although not exclusively, confined to skin lesions. They can be classified under headings such as epidermal, dermal, subcutaneous, vascular, etc. Pigmented naevi (in lay terminology, moles) form a large group.

## Classification of pigmented lesions

- Freckles
- Lentigo
- Congenital naevus
- Benign acquired naevus
- Becker's naevus
- Spitz naevus
- Malignant melanoma.

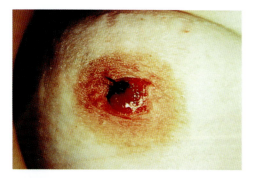

**Figure 3.20** Paget's disease of the nipple representing surface spread of an intraduct carcinoma.

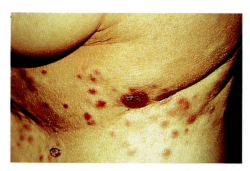

**Figure 3.21** Cutaneous nodules pushing up from below. These are secondaries from a primary breast cancer.

## Freckles

Freckles (synonyms: ephelis, ephelide) are common, especially in red-haired persons of Celtic extraction. In size, they are up to 2–3 mm. They tend to be familial. Freckles require UV radiation to develop and usually appear in sun-exposed areas at the age of 3–5 years. Thereafter, they fluctuate in colour intensity in response to sunlight. There is no increase in melanocyte numbers, but these produce more and slightly unusual melanosomes.

Treatment is unnecessary, although these populations are statistically more liable to malignant melanomas. This may be due to them having a similar phenotype and pigmentation profile to adults at risk (McLean & Gallagher 1995).

## Lentigo

Lentigos are flat, brownish/black lesions, of which the common 'age' or 'liver' spots on the dorsa of the hands are examples. They may be induced by sun (solar or actinic changes) but, unlike freckles, tend to fade with UV protection. The lesions can get quite large, up to 25 mm or more and, although the margins can be somewhat ragged, the overall pigmentation is homogeneous with no clumping. They may respond to cryotherapy.

Variants occur in relation to other UV stimuli. Photochemotherapy plus PUVA leads to PUVA lentigos, and sun-bed usage to very large, dark, freckle-like lesions with a slightly irregular edge.

Lentigos show an increase in normal melanocytes, which are arranged along the basal layer.

The sun-bed and PUVA lentigos indicate skin damage and such patients may be at later risk of developing malignant melanoma.

## Congenital melanocytic naevus

Congenital melanocytic naevus (synonym: congenital naevomelanocytic naevus) should, by definition, be present at birth, and about 1% of neonates have these. However, rather similar lesions can develop up to a few years postpartum and may be included under this title. It may be that some of these contain the naevus cells, but for whatever reason they delay in producing the pigment. The lesion probably forms between the second and sixth uterine months.

It is traditional to classify these naevi according to size: under 1.5 cm is small, 1.5 cm to 20 cm is medium, and over 20 cm is large.

### Clinical features

Congenital melanocytic naevi are usually brown to black in colour. The skin markings can be seen traversing the lesion and may be more pronounced than normal. In many cases, hair of an inappropriate terminal type will develop with time. The surface of the lesion may be smooth, ranging to warty or lobular. An irregular edge may cause concern, but the pigmentation in this area, and throughout the main lesion, is relatively homogeneous. They grow disproportionately slowly with age, compared with the increase in body size (Fig. 3.22).

### Histology

Melanocytes are increased in the basal cell area. There is often a gap with a relatively normal area and clumps of naevoid melanocytes in the lower dermis. These seem to have a predilection for skin appendages.

### Treatment

The true incidence of congenital melanocytic naevi developing malignancy is disputed, but it is generally agreed that the larger they are the

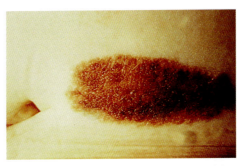

**Figure 3.22** Congenital melanocytic naevus lateral to umbilicus. Despite irregularities of the edge and colour skin markings are intact and there is hair growth within the lesion.

more likely is this complication. However, the large congenital melanocytic naevi affecting the extremities seem to be immune from this (DeDavid et al 1997). Nonetheless, monitoring of all these lesions is advised. Serial photography is advocated.

Small lesions may be excised for cosmetic reasons. The larger the lesion, the more disfiguring it is, but perversely, the more difficult it is to remove. Regular monitoring and attempts at cosmetic camouflage are perhaps the best options.

## Acquired melanocytic naevus

An acquired melanocytic naevus (synonym: acquired naevocytic naevus) is an abnormality, but it is an abnormal person who never has any of these. They affect both sexes and appear at intervals throughout life, from shortly after birth. Small numbers present, peaking in incidence around the teens, then falling off in old age.

The melanocytic naevus cells have been the subject of long debate as to their origin. They may be entirely located at the dermoepidermal junction forming junctional naevi. Junctional naevi may represent a stage in the development of compound naevi. This progression is often arrested in areas such as the palms, soles and genitalia, where they can remain for a long time. If junctional changes persist and dermal ones develop, the lesions are called 'compound naevi', of which there are various histological variants. There may be closely packed melanocytic naevus cells in the dermis, mainly in the upper papillary layers, in contradistinction to the appearance in congenital naevi.

If the junctional changes are absent, the lesion is termed an 'intradermal naevus'.

### Clinical features

Acquired melanocytic naevi occur in both sexes, with an increased prevalence in black skin (Fig. 3.23). Junctional naevi are the commonest on palms, soles and genitalia. They are usually flat and only a few millimetres in diameter, being round or oval. The colour varies from brown to dark black. Occasionally, stippling can be seen, often with the aid of magnification. The individual, darker areas have a smooth outline. The skin markings are not disturbed. With time, in areas other than the palms and soles, etc., they usually progress toward compound naevi.

Compound naevi are usually dome-shaped papules with a light to dark colour, which is usually homogeneous. Coarse hair may grow through the lesion. Occasionally, there can be a circle of increased pigmentation around the periphery, which may be postinflammatory hyperpigmentation from trauma. The nail matrix may be affected by

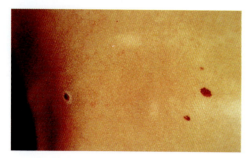

**Figure 3.23** Typical benign acquired naevi. They are multiple with a clearly demarcated edge and the colour is homogeneous.

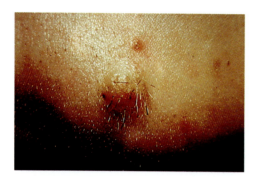

**Figure 3.24** Intradermal naevus. Note the relative lack of pigmentation and the growth of hair.

junctional or compound naevi, with a marked preponderance of the former. Longitudinal melanonychia may occur (Tosti et al 1996).

---

### CASE STUDY 3.6 **POSSIBLE MELANOCYTIC NAEVUS**

A 20-year-old woman noted a brown spot on her right sole. It measured about 2 mm in diameter. She was reasonably sure that it had not been there 4 months ago. She was on the oral contraceptive. On examination, the pigmentation was homogeneous, the margin was distinct, the lesion round and the skin markings uninterrupted. What should you do?

The answer is to reassure her. The history and examination suggest a benign acquired melanocytic naevus. In view of the apparently fairly rapid history, she should be reviewed in a few months to see if any change has occurred. The oral contraceptive pill is not relevant.

---

## Intradermal naevi

With the disappearance of the junctional component, pigmentation tends to fade. In intradermal naevi, the lesion is often a flesh-coloured papule. Hair may grow through it (Fig. 3.24).

## Histology

In the junctional naevus, small collections of melanocytes or 'packets' seem almost to be inserted between the epidermis and dermis. Thereafter, some appear to travel into the upper dermis, either as packets or columns. This forms the compound naevus. When the junctional activity fades, the lesion becomes an intradermal naevus. There is often a zone of normal dermis between the lesion and the epidermis.

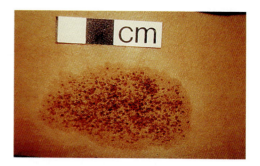

**Figure 3.25** Speckled and lentiginous naevus (naevus spilus).

The melanocytic naevus cells have nuclei of similar size to normal melanocytes. They have abundant, slightly eosinophilic cytoplasm. There are many histological variants.

## Treatment

It is manifestly impossible to remove all naevi and, indeed, this would be undesirable. Surgical removal can be carried out for cosmetic reasons or if the physical location is such that constant irritation occurs. The patient must be aware that formal surgical excision will inevitably result in a scar. This scar may be more noticeable and disfiguring than the original lesion. This is particularly so in the young teenager or adult, with firm elastic skin. It is especially relevant to lesions on the trunk, and in particular on the back.

Some of the protuberant lesions may be improved by a shave biopsy. This will not remove any hair growth and, if there is deeper pigmentation, it may recur and darken. That the lesion will not regrow cannot be guaranteed.

Acceptance of the lesion as a 'beauty spot' or cosmetic camouflage techniques are other options.

If there is any doubt whatsoever that the lesion may be a malignant melanoma, excision, or at least a diagnostic biopsy, should be carried out. If there is less doubt and these procedures are deemed to be liable to be mutilating, then assiduous monitoring is essential.

## Speckled and lentiginous naevus

Speckled and lentiginous naevus (synonym: naevus spilus) (Rhodes 1999, Stewart et al 1978) is considered relatively rare, although an Australian survey found a prevalence of 2% (Rivers et al 1995). Originally called naevus spilus (from *spilus* = dot), this name has become confused in the literature, especially when tardus (i.e. late developing) is added as naevus spilus tardus. Some reckon this to be equal to Becker's naevus.

## Clinical features

The lesion usually develops in childhood on the extremities, but other areas can be affected. It is a light brown macular area that may measure up to 10 cm in diameter. Spots, which may be very dark, develop within this (Fig. 3.25).

## Histology

The macular area has increased melanocytes, like a lentigo, and the dark areas show melanocytic naevoid cells in the epidermis and dermis.

## Treatment

The natural history is unclear, but there are sporadic reports of malignant melanoma developing. If surgically reasonable, excision may be the best option.

Otherwise, close monitoring with photographic records should be undertaken. Laser treatment has been suggested.

## Becker's naevus

Becker's naevus (Monckton et al 1965, Vincent 1999) is a fairly common lesion, occurring in about 1 in 2000 young men and a fifth of that in females. It is pigmented, but there are few or no changes in the melanocytes.

### Clinical features

It usually appears in the late teens or early adult life, gradually becoming more obvious. The usual site to be involved is the shoulder, but other areas, including the leg, have been described.

It is often large in area (over 20 cm diameter) with a markedly indented geographic outline. Within it, there can be white island areas about the size of a fingertip. Normally, coarse, darkish hairs develop within the patch. They remain for life.

### Histology

There is little or no increase in melanocytes. There may be melanosomal abnormalities.

### Treatment

Becker's naevus is usually too large for surgical removal. Future laser developments may prove useful but, at present, cosmetic camouflage appears to be the solution.

## Spitz naevus

Spitz naevus (Casso et al 1992) is a benign melanocytic lesion, akin to a compound naevus. However, the histology can be very similar to that of malignant melanoma, and pathologists asked to look at it without an adequate history can be forgiven for diagnosing the latter. In the past, benign juvenile melanoma was used to describe these naevi, but it is a term best not used, to avoid confusion.

### Clinical features

Spitz naevi usually occur in young people up to the age of 20 years. The head, neck and leg are common locations, although anywhere may be affected. They are usually asymptomatic, dome-shaped, firm nodules, which are pink, red or tan in colour (Fig. 3.26). The natural history is unclear.

### Histology

The lesions contain a mixture of spindle and epithelioid cells. They are usually compound naevi, and highly atypical looking melanocytes are found in the epidermis and the dermis. Differentiation from malignant melanoma can be a real challenge, even for an experienced histopathologist.

### Treatment

There are some variations in opinion, but most believe that complete excision is best.

## Dysplastic naevi

Synonym: clinically atypical naevus. Some patients have naevi, often multiple, which exhibit clinical and/or histological features

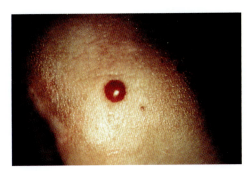

**Figure 3.26** Spitz naevus. Firm reddish papule.

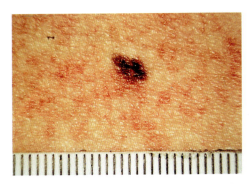

**Figure 3.27** Dysplastic naevus. This shows the difficulty in distinguishing this lesion from a malignant melanoma. The borders and colour heterogeneity are not so marked as in malignant melanoma. If in any doubt, further investigation or excision is necessary.

that are unusual and worrying (Sagebiel 1989, Slade et al 1995). These can occur in some families or in isolation. Many different names have been applied to these. They prove a difficult management problem.

### Clinical features

By definition, these are clinically atypical lesions and thus the great concern is to try to differentiate them from malignant melanoma. It is difficult to convey a word picture. They may occur in any sites, either singly or sometimes in vast numbers. They tend to be larger than benign naevi, often more than 5 mm in diameter. They are roughly round or oval, with some asymmetry. The border is irregular, but often fuzzy, rather than sharper, larger projections of the malignant melanoma. There may be a collarette of increased pigmentation. Colour variegation within the lesion is common, but more 'twin tone' in contradistinction to the multiple variations seen in malignant melanoma (Fig. 3.27).

The actual areas of pigmentation have more regular edges. Skin markings are usually uninterrupted.

The natural history is difficult to assess. Some may disappear, but all in all there is an increased chance of melanoma developing, which may be up to 70 times (Halpern et al 1993). This is most marked in those with multiple lesions and a family history of malignant melanoma.

### Histology

The microscopic changes may be found with or without clinical atypia and may be reported by the pathologist as dysplastic. As with the clinical situation, there is a kaleidoscope of variation within the histology. The cardinal changes are an irregular proliferation of melanocytes, singly or in packets along the basal cell layer. There is elongation of the rete ridges. The melanocytes themselves show variable atypia.

## Treatment

Any dysplastic naevi that cause clinical concern should be excised, along the same lines as for malignant melanoma. If there is less concern, then they may be left. If they are multiple and there is a family history of malignant melanoma, regular careful supervision is required. General photographic views plus individual close-ups are invaluable.

## Malignant melanoma of the skin

A cutaneous malignant melanoma (Grin-Jorgensen et al 1991, Langley et al 1999, MacKie 1998) arises from melanocytes in the epidermis. Similar tumours may occur in other tissues (e.g. the eye). It is vitally important for the patient and/or practitioner to diagnose the melanoma early, when a cure can easily be effected. Missing it until it is in later stages will greatly increase the chances that it will lead to the patient's death. There has been a tremendous increase in the incidence of the tumour in the last 50–60 years. It has been reckoned that in the USA the individual risk of an invasive melanoma increased from 1 in 1500 in 1935 to 1 in 75 in 2000.

## Aetiology

The main causative factor for malignant melanoma seems to be sun exposure, although some still seem less convinced. A single or a few burning episodes in the child or the young adult seems to be more provocative than longer term outdoor unprotected activity. Thus the culture in the western world of sun tanning by natural or artificial means, more holidays in the sun and scantier clothing may all play a part.

Some people are more at risk than others. The red-headed, freckled, Celtic races are a particular example. They tend to burn in the sun easily and their voluntary or enforced migration to sunnier climates has been responsible for an 'epidemic' of malignant melanoma in, for example, Australia.

There are differences in incidence in different occupations and socio-economic groups. Some of these may be dependent upon affordability of holidays, outdoor exposed working, etc.

In a few cases there is an apparent hereditary tendency to develop malignant melanoma. Skin type, lifestyle, geographical domicile, etc. all influence this.

There was an initial marked increase in malignant melanoma in females compared with males, although the incidence is now rising disproportionately in the latter. Differences in dress patterns may have been important.

Patients with some pre-existing pigmented lesions are at more risk of malignant melanoma. These include some dysplastic naevi and acral pigmented lesions. A personal history of a previous malignant melanoma renders the patient more at risk of developing a second primary lesion.

## Clinical features

Some malignant melanomas produce little or no pigment and are termed hypomelanotic or amelanotic melanomas. They pose particular difficulties in diagnosis. Most, however, retain the facility of pigment production. A careful history and meticulous examination in good light are essential. A changing lesion should be paid particular attention. There are many devices marketed to help visualisation, some of which are very expensive. Much can be achieved with a spot-light and some magnification, even using a hand lens. In most medical locations an auroscope is available and, used without the ear piece, this gives light and some magnification. Sometimes the application to the surface of the lesion of a little mineral oil will alter the refraction and allow the clinician to see a little deeper into the epidermis. Appearances on plantar surfaces may be misleading (Akasu & Sugiyama 1996).

Features that would cause concern in the pigmented cutaneous malignant melanoma are mainly related to irregularity. This irregularity of the outline, the border and its pigmentation, colour of the lesion and the skin marking are all ominous features. Increasing size to more than a pencil thickness (i.e. about 7 mm), bleeding, discharging and itching, can all be added.

An ABCD checklist has been suggested:

A = asymmetry of the outline
B = border irregularity
C = colour variegation
D = diameter enlargement.

It must be stressed that no system will be foolproof in the diagnosis of malignant melanoma. Very early lesions will not have developed the above features. A practitioner must realise that an evolving lesion may not be diagnosable at that moment in time, and the patient should not be deterred from seeking further advice if the lesion appears to change.

The prognosis depends vitally on the thickness of the melanoma. Those with a horizontal growth pattern are termed 'superficial spreading melanomas' and have a reasonably good outlook in general. On the other hand, those that grow vertically spread more rapidly into the lymphatics and blood vessels, metastasising earlier, with a consequently poorer prognosis. These are termed 'nodular melanomas'.

These and some other clinical types of malignant melanoma are recognised.

- *Lentigo malignant melanoma.* These are slow-growing lesions, usually on the face, commonly in the elderly. As the name suggests, it is a flat lentiginous lesion. It has an irregular border, colour variation and slowly extends. Ultimately, a central nodule may develop and it will become aggressive and spread (Fig. 3.28).
- *Superficial spreading melanoma.* This is the most commonly encountered type in the Caucasian. It can occur at any site, although statistically it is more likely on the male back or the

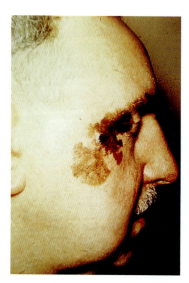

**Figure 3.28** Lentigo malignant melanoma.

female leg. It exhibits the irregular features detailed above. With time it may become raised, with palpable areas, and this will indicate transformation to a thicker, nodular type with a worse prognosis. Change in the colour, often in the centre, to a bluish colour, and even central clearing, should not be mistaken for a good sign. It usually means that the tumour is growing deeper and the change in colour is due to a physical light-scattering effect (Figs 3.29–3.31).

- *Nodular melanoma.* Malignant melanoma may commence ab initio as a nodular lesion with vertical growth. In other cases, it progresses from another type. The de novo type can appear anywhere, but the trunk and lower limb are commoner sites. Growth can be rapid and, more than any other form of malignant melanoma, this one is likely to be hypomelanotic or amelanotic. Thus the diagnosis may well be missed. A common misdiagnosis is a vascular lesion, due to the common raised, friable, oozing nature of these. There may be a ring of pigmentation on careful examination (Fig. 3.32).

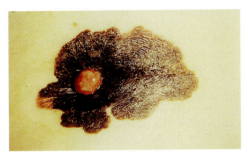

**Figure 3.29** Malignant melanoma. This exhibits asymmetry, an irregular border and colour variation. The main lesion is in a superficial spreading phase but the nodule represents vertical growth.

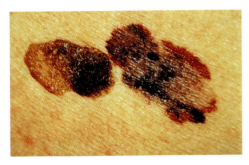

**Figure 3.30** Malignant melanoma on the left with irregularities of border and pigmentation. The serendipitous juxtaposition of a seborrhoeic keratosis on the right allows a comparison of features.

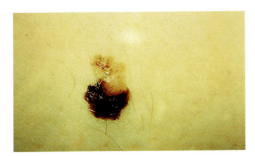

**Figure 3.31** Malignant melanoma on the ankle of a 21-year-old female. Jagged irregular border. over half of the lesion is almost amelanotic.

- *Acral lentiginous melanoma.* This variety is relatively uncommon in white skin, but more common in black and oriental skin (Kukita & Ishihara 1989). They start as a flat lentiginous area on the palms or soles or around nails, progressing in size more rapidly than other malignant melanomas and ultimately developing nodules. Thus they tend to have a poorer prognosis than that of other melanomas. Alternatively, the poorer prognosis may be due to a longer delay in diagnosis on a relatively non-visualised foot in the average patient.
- *Subungual melanoma.* These are a particularly difficult type to differentiate from benign melanonychia, subungual haematomas etc. The melanoma is usually proximal, and if the pigmentation involves the posterior nail fold (Hutchinson's sign) this is more ominous (Figs 3.33, 3.34).

Malignant melanoma can be an enigmatic and unpredictable disease. Very early lesions may spread. Nonetheless, there is usually a close correlation to the thickness of the tumour. The deeper the lesion penetrates the more liable it is to spread.

Metastases may take the form of nearby local nodules or spread to the local lymph nodes. Distant areas of skin, subcutaneous tissue and nodes may be affected. The visceral metastases affect, in descending frequency, the lungs, liver, brain, bone and intestines. All of these may occur many years after apparent cure.

Malignant melanoma may present as a distant metastasis. Sometimes the initial primary cannot be found. This may be due to the fact that, rarely, primary melanoma can spontaneously heal.

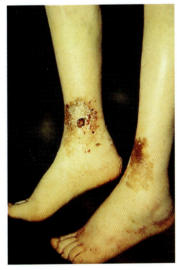

**Figure 3.32** Nodular malignant melanoma with local nodular metastases.

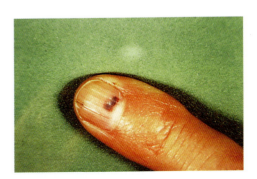

**Figure 3.33** Early subungual malignant melanoma.

**63**

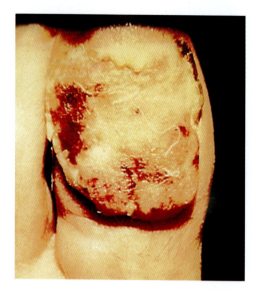

**Figure 3.34** Neglected subungual malignant melanoma. Hypomelanotic. Only a small rim of pigmentation can be seen.

In the examination of patients with pigmented lesions in general and malignant melanoma in particular, the keeping of meticulous records is mandatory. The history of the patient's observations and symptoms, a family history and a lifestyle for risk factors should be taken. On examination, measurements of the horizontal and vertical sizes, comments about the border, irregularity and colour variegation should be noted. If possible, the regional lymph nodes should be palpated.

Histology should be obtained if there is the slightest doubt about a lesion. There has been much controversy as to whether an incisional biopsy is likely to provoke spread and, to a certain extent, this still continues. Many authorities feel that there is no evidence for this. If possible, an excisional biopsy should be done, but there may be occasions when it is more expedient to send a part for diagnosis. Some feel that in thicker melanomas a biopsy of the main draining (sentinel) lymph node should be done. This can be identified by dye or radiation methods. This approach still remains controversial (Garcia & Poletti 2007).

---

**CASE STUDY 3.7 AREAS OF PIGMENTATION**

A 40-year-old labourer notices a brown subungual area on his right, second toe. He cannot remember any specific injury. On examination, a band of pigmentation is seen, extending throughout the length of the nail and onto the posterior nail cuticle. What action would you take?

The history and examination are highly suggestive of a subungual melanoma, and immediate fast-track referral for surgery is imperative.

---

## Histology

Malignant melanocytic cells invade the dermis. The cells vary in the degree of atypia, with cellular and nuclear enlargement and variation. There is often upward spread into other areas.

Stress has been placed on the importance of the thickness of the malignant melanoma, and the pathologist has a vital role to play

in the measurable assessment of this. Originally, this was done by measuring the invasion of the tumour in relation to other anatomical structures of the dermis. These were known as Clark's levels I–V:

I   only in the epidermis (i.e. in situ)
II  just into upper dermis
III significantly into upper dermis
IV  in deeper reticular dermis
V   into deep fat.

However, this can be difficult on certain sites, such as acral ones, and a micrometer measurement known as the Breslow thickness is now more often used. Using this, melanomas under 0.75 mm are considered to have a good prognosis. Over that, the outlook steadily declines with increasing thickness.

### Treatment

Prevention by removing all removable known causes is desirable. There have been many campaigns to warn of the dangers of sun exposure and to promote methods of sun protection. These need to continue.

Persons at risk from genetic problems, past history or due to at-risk pigmented lesions require careful monitoring.

In the suspected malignant melanoma, fast-track referring is essential.

In the event of malignant melanoma being diagnosed clinically or histologically, rapid and adequate excision at the primary site is of paramount importance. The exact surgical clearance margins are disputed but, in general, the thicker the lesion, the wider should be the margins.

If the regional lymph nodes are involved they should be excised.

Once the tumour has spread further, the prognosis is dire. Much work continues on the best chemotherapeutic regimen.

## Epidermal naevi

These are a collection of hamartomas or benign abnormalities. They are present from birth, but may not be clinically recognisable until later. Various classifications are suggested. Many lesions do not conform to these headings. Many are warty.

### Clinical features

Appearing at or after birth, the lesions develop slowly. Many are linear, probably along the path of embryonic development lines (Blaschko's lines).

Usually the surface becomes warty and pigmented, especially so on the limbs and palms and soles (Fig. 3.35).

Some become inflamed and intensely itchy. These may be designated inflammatory linear verrucose epidermal naevi (ILVEN).

### Histology

Many show hyperkeratosis with rising columns likened to church spires. Usually there is epidermal thickening. There is considerable variation.

### Treatment

They may be left. Surgical excision may occasionally be possible. If not, keratolytic softening agents and podiatry for foot lesions are options.

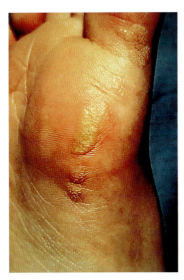

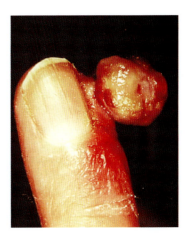

**Figure 3.36** Pyogenic granuloma. Note the constricted pedicle with a friable main lesion.

**Figure 3.35** Linear epidermal naevus (ILVEN) simulating a verruca plantaris.

## Dermal and subcutaneous naevi

Hamartomas may affect any of the dermal or subcutaneous structures. They may be isolated lesions or part of a syndrome (e.g. the tuberose sclerosis complex). Classification of dermal and subcutaneous naevi can be difficult, and infinite variations occur.

Usually they present clinically as a swelling. Often the diagnosis is obtained from the histology.

Treatment is dependent on the circumstances.

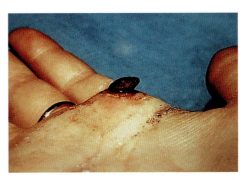

**Figure 3.37** Pyogenic granuloma following minor injury. Mushroom-like lesion.

## VASCULAR TUMOURS

### Pyogenic granuloma

Pyogenic granuloma (synonyms: granuloma pyogenicum, lobular capillary haemangioma) is a common lesion that usually follows an injury, which may or may not be remembered by the patient. In a paediatric survey, most gave no history of trauma (Patrice et al 1991). The injury may rarely be iatrogenic (e.g. after cryotherapy) (Kolbusz & O'Donoghue 1991).

### Clinical features

A friable vascular lesion develops rapidly at the site of a previous injury, or apparently spontaneously. There are, rarely, generalised forms of the disease that cannot be due to trauma and occasionally may have an underlying malignancy (Strohal et al 1991). Multiple ones may be triggered in severe acne on the site of active lesions where treatment is inaugurated with retinoids (Exner et al 1983). Paronychia has been described as a cause (Bouscarat et al 1998).

However, the commonest form is a single one. A usual history is of a thorn or pinprick injury followed by the development of a mushroom-type lesion, which bleeds on the slightest touch. Because of this, it is common to see evidence that the patient has covered the lesion with a protective dressing (Figs 3.36, 3.37).

Lesions occurring in restricted anatomical sites are constrained and may lose their mushroom-like appearance. An example of this would be in a nail fold (Fig. 3.38).

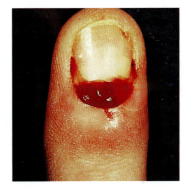

**Figure 3.38** Pyogenic granuloma in nail fold. The constrictive site alters typical features.

The lesion reaches a variable size, usually up to 1 cm, and then ceases growing. In long-established pyogenic granulomas there may be an attempt at epithelialisation, which may lessen the tendency to bleed. Some spontaneously involute. Some develop surrounding or satellite lesions of more pyogenic granulomas locally.

Pyogenic granuloma is usually an easy diagnosis to make and usually responds to treatment. However, it is vital not to miss a more sinister diagnosis, which some tumours may mimic. The greatest pitfall is the malignant melanoma, especially amelanotic or hypomelanotic ones (Elmets and Ceilley 1980).

Other tumours, such as Bowen's disease or squamous cell carcinoma (Mikhail 1985), verrucose carcinoma (Brownstein & Shapiro 1976), eccrine poroma (Pernia et al 1993) and metastatic lesions may confuse (Giardina et al 1996). Never remove tissue without first obtaining histological confirmation.

## Histology

The lesion is circumscribed and contains multiple capillaries, some very dilated (Lever & Schaumberg-Leuer 1990). There is considerable proliferation of endothelial cells. At the base, the epidermis tends to grow, leading to a collarette constricting the lesion and contributing to the 'mushroom stalk'.

## Treatment

The pyogenic granuloma is usually easy to curette. The tissue obtained should always be sent for histological examination. Curettage may need to be repeated on one or two occasions. Formal excision can be carried out.

---

### CASE STUDY 3.8 **FRIABLE NODULES**

A 15-year-old girl presents with a bleeding friable nodule at the side of her right hallux. She is keen on a martial art form, which necessitates her working out barefoot on a wooden floor. She says that she has noted some small glands on both groins and she has a family history of malignant melanoma. What is the likeliest diagnosis?

The answer is pyogenic granuloma from a minor injury to her foot. Malignant melanoma is rare at this age, but it would be important to consider this. Pyogenic granuloma should have a small stalk, like a mushroom, and it should be possible to curette this off. It would be imperative to send the tissue for histological examination. The finding of glands in the groins of young active persons is not uncommon, and the fact that she stated that these occurred in both groins is less worrying than if the glands had been on one side only.

---

## Glomus tumour

Glomus tumour (synonym: glomangioma) (Requena & Sangueza 1997) is rare and originates from the cells of smooth muscle, the normal function of which is to regulate temperature by acting as valves on arteriovenous anastomotic shunts. These are most profuse on the digits. Glomus tumours are commonest on the digits, although a multiple variety occurs.

## Clinical features

Preceding trauma has been implicated, but evidence is vague. There may be an increased incidence in musicians (Harvell & Maibach 1992).

A solitary glomus tumour is usually located in the periungual area, especially of the hands. It may occur at any age, although mostly in early adult life, and affects either sex. A small purplish nodule develops. It is usually only 5 mm in diameter and, if under the nail, can give it a purplish colour. The usual cardinal symptom is pain, which may be agonising and paroxysmal, sometimes triggered by minor pressure or temperature reduction.

The clinical history should suggest the diagnosis, but it can be confirmed in early stages by the use of magnetic resonance imaging (Drapé et al 1996), which may also be able to differentiate other tumours (Goettman et al 1994). Solitary lesions have been reported in other areas, such as the volar aspects of the hands and feet and also on the head and neck.

Multiple lesions are usually called 'glomangiomas' and occur as scattered blue dermal nodules. They are more common in childhood, although overall are very rare. Pain is not a feature of these.

## Histology

The single glomus tumour is composed of a nodule encapsulated in fibrous tissue. The glomus cells are filled with a large nucleus and a little cytoplasm surrounding vascular channels.

Multiple glomangiomas are not encapsulated and are more vascular.

## Treatment

Removal of a single lesion by surgery is the best option. Multiple lesions may be considered for laser treatment (Goldman 1978).

## Kaposi's sarcoma

Kaposi's sarcoma was originally described in 1872. This remained a rare tumour until almost a century later. It is now much more common and various types are recognised. These include a sporadic (or classic) type, African endemic, immunosuppressive-drug-induced and HIV-related. Whatever the type, it results in a tumour arising from mesenchymal cells of vascular or lymphocytic endothelium (Tappero et al 1993).

## Aetiology

Classic Kaposi's sarcoma was initially considered idiopathic. With the description of the African endemic disease, it was wondered if there was an infecting agent akin to that in Burkitt's lymphoma. The relative avalanche of cases in association with immunosuppression due to drugs or HIV infection led to further study, and human herpes virus number 8 has been found in all forms of the disease. It is not unique to this condition and it is likely that other cofactors are needed to enhance its propensity to lead to the disease (Dictor et al 1996, Kemény et al 1997).

## Clinical features

The classic or sporadic form mainly affects males over 60 years old, often of Jewish or Mediterranean extraction. The commonest affected site is the leg or foot, although lymph node and internal organs can be affected (Tappero et al 1993). It remains rare, one study finding only 163 cases in 20 years (Lospalluti et al 1995). In this series, the survival was 6–13 years. The disease often causes few clinical problems.

The African type has various forms, ranging from one similar to the classic type, through to a florid rapidly disseminating systemic variety. It can affect all ages.

Kaposi's sarcoma associated with immunosuppression was recognised in 1964 (Klein et al 1974), and there have been many reports since that time (La Parola et al 1997).

Kaposi's sarcoma associated with AIDS/HIV tends to be a very aggressive disease, with a survival time of up to 36 months (Lemlich et al 1987). Three-quarters had systemic involvement, especially affecting lymph nodes, the gastrointestinal tract and, to a lesser extent, the lungs.

The original skin changes of multiple bluish tumours looked rather like a bunch of grapes, located mainly on the extremities. As the new variants have been described, the spectrum of described skin lesions has extended considerably. Macular, papular, nodular and plaque forms have all been noted. Most of the forms have a purplish colour.

The differential diagnoses include malignant melanoma, glomus tumour, pyogenic granuloma, especially with satellites, sarcoid, etc. (Schwartz 1996).

## Histology

In early lesions, the changes may be subtle and difficult to discern. When fully developed, there are proliferations of small vessels, bundles of spindle cells and slit-like spaces, into which red blood cells haemorrhage (Lemlich et al 1987).

## Treatment

In the classic form in the elderly, if slow-growing, it may be expedient to do little or nothing. Local treatment for single or few lesions may include surgical removal, cryotherapy, laser, radiation or intralesional cytotoxic therapy (Tappero et al 1993). More aggressive systemic therapies with single or multi-drug therapy may be necessary.

Kaposi's sarcoma due to immunosuppression or drugs may resolve if these can be withdrawn (La Parola et al 1997). If the Kaposi's sarcoma is associated with AIDS/HIV, control of superinfection is well worthwhile, as is treatment of the HIV.

---

### CASE STUDY 3.9 **NODULES OF THE INSTEP**

A 30-year-old homosexual male comes in for treatment by a podiatrist on account of a plantar wart. Nearby you notice a group of purplish nodules, near his instep. What is the likely diagnosis?

The answer is Kaposi's sarcoma, related to HIV infection. Care should be taken for the operative's personal protection if there is any chance of contact with blood.

---

## FIBROUS TUMOURS

## Acquired fibrokeratoma

There is a group of fibrous lesions occurring on the distal extremities that have been reclassified and renamed over the years, resulting in a number of different names. An early description of the lesions, called 'acquired digital fibrokeratoses', was challenged in the ensuing discussion on account of their occurrence elsewhere and 'acral fibromatosis' suggested as a preferable name, but this does not seem to have caught on (Bart et al 1968). Other authors make the same point (Hare & Smith 1969, Kint et al 1985, Verallo 1968).

Some are designated 'periungual fibromatas' if around the nail (Baran et al 1996) where, if multiple, they can be called 'garlic clove tumours' (Steel 1965). The best term at present would appear to be 'acquired fibrokeratoma'.

Perhaps a separate heading should be kept for those periungual lesions in association with tuberose sclerosis (Koenen's tumours), although individually they are clinically and histologically similar to others (Kint & Baran 1988).

## Aetiology

On rather tenuous grounds, trauma is suggested as a cause (Bart et al 1968, Herman & Datnow 1974, Verallo 1968). However, in most recorded cases, no such history is obtainable.

## Clinical features

The lesions have a predilection for the digits, often near the joint, with the periungual area being very common (Verallo 1968). The rate of growth is usually slow, but they can appear in a few months (Kint et al 1985). The lesions are usually flesh-coloured or slightly translucent. They are usually projections slightly narrower at the base, widening out and then coming to a rather pointed end, which often has a hyperkeratotic tip with a reddish base. (Figs 3.39, 3.40) A hyperkeratotic collarette may be seen. Some are more plateau-like (Verallo 1968). Those around the nails commonly cause a groove or sulcus on the nail plate (Kint & Baran 1988) (Fig. 3.41). The differential diagnosis includes a supernumerary digit, dermatofibroma, osteoma or a pyogenic granuloma.

## Histology

There are variations, but often there are collagen bundles in the long axis of the lesion, interspersed with numerous capillaries (Kint et al 1985). There may be a mucopolysaccharide deposit between the

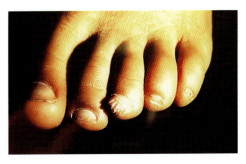

**Figure 3.39** 'Garlic clove' digital fibroma.

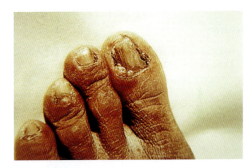

**Figure 3.40** Multiple digital fibromas in a patient with tuberose sclerosis complex.

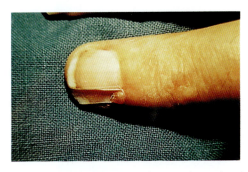

**Figure 3.41** Periungual fibroma producing a deep sulcus in the nail plate.

collagen bundles. This may account for the clinical translucent appearance.

## Treatment

Surgical excision is usually successful. Spontaneous clearing in an infantile variant has been described (Duran-McKinster et al 1993).

## Koenen's tumours

These are periungual fibromas that form one part of the condition now known as the 'tuberous sclerosis complex' (synonyms: epiloia, Bourneville disease). There are many features of the complex, which can be grouped into cutaneous, mental retardation and epilepsy. Skin problems include facial angiofibromas (adenoma sebaceum), pigmented leathery lesions (shagreen patches), hypopigmented areas (ash-leaf white macules) and Koenen's tumours. Infinite degrees of severity of the condition occur, and the Koenen's tumours may be the only manifestation at times. They appear more likely to recur after removal (Verallo 1968).

## Dermatofibroma

A dermatofibroma (synonyms: histiocytoma cutis, fibrous histiocytoma, sclerosing haemangioma) is a very common benign fibrous tumour, usually occurring on the extremities.

## Aetiology

These tumours have usually been attributed to minor trauma. A long-held belief that dermatofibromas were due to insect bites and a foreign-body reaction to the residual parts has not been confirmed (Evans et al 1989). They seem to be negative for p53 expression and CD34 (HPCA-1), which may help to distinguish them from malignant lesions (Diaz-Cascajo et al 1995, Kutzner 1993).

## Clinical features

Dermatofibromas can occur anywhere on the skin, but the limbs are the usual site. They may be flat, but more often are slightly protuberant (Fig. 3.42). Usually slow-growing and less than 1 cm in diameter, they can, on occasion, be giant and over 3 cm (Requena et al 1994).

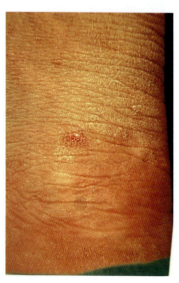

**Figure 3.42** Dermatofibroma on the heel.

They are usually flesh-coloured, but can have a yellowish tinge, mimicking xanthomata. This may be accentuated by cholesterol deposits (Hunt et al 1990). At times they are slightly pigmented. They may have a ring of enhanced pigmentation, probably in the nature of postinflammatory hyperpigmentation. On palpation, they are firm to hard, with the hardness extending beyond the visual lesion. In other words, the part seen is rather like the tip of an iceberg.

Normally they remain static for years, but some can become atrophic. Multiple lesions on the palms and soles have been described (Bedi et al 1976). Overlying basal cell carcinomas have been noted (Fujisawa et al 1991).

## Histology

There is a vascular network initially, with many histiocytes that are gradually superseded by fibroblasts and collagen. Haemosiderin may be present.

## Treatment

By and large, treatment is not required. If there is diagnostic doubt they should be biopsied or removed. Removal for this, cosmetic or pressure-effect reasons must be complete or regrowth occurs.

## Dermatofibrosarcoma protuberans

This is a rare tumour (Gloster 1996) that can be very aggressive locally.

## Clinical features

The dermatofibrosarcoma protuberans (DFSP) usually occurs in the trunk and only rarely on the hands and feet.

It commences as an indurated purplish-reddish or flesh-coloured plaque. Over time, which varies from several months to years, nodules develop. Locally malignant, it rarely metastasises.

## Histology

There is a dense, mat-like arrangement of cells with spindle-shaped nuclei. The overall pattern of the tumour cells is like a cartwheel.

## Treatment

Adequate wide excision is required, preferably with frozen-section assessment of clearance of operation (Moh's surgery).

## ADNEXAL TUMOURS

## Eccrine poroma

This was described as a benign tumour of the epidermal portion of the eccrine sweat gland in 1956 (Pinkus et al 1956). The same group described a malignant variant in 1963 (Pinkus & Mehregan 1963).

## Aetiology

An immunohistochemical study of cytokeratins helped to find associations between certain normal adnexal structures and the tumour cells. However, it could not determine whether the tumour cells were derived from the adnexal structures or undifferentiated pluripotent cells (Demirkesen et al 1995). The malignant tumours tended to be high expressors of the p53 protein (Tateyama et al 1995).

## Clinical features

The eccrine poroma is a relatively common tumour. It can occur at any age, although usually over 40 years, and affects both sexes (McKee 1994). More than a half are found in the sole or plantar surface of the toes. It usually appears as a solitary, non-tender, slightly red nodule. It may protrude or be pedunculated. The surface may be warty or ulcerated and bleeding (Moeller et al 1987). Rare variants, such as multiple lesions (eccrine poromatosis) (Goldner 1970) or linear lesions (Ogino 1976), have been described. Malignant forms are also rare. Only 27 cases were found in 31 years in a retrospective study in a large reference centre (Shaw et al 1982).

The common benign form should be easy to diagnose but may be confused with verrucae plantaris, fibromas, amelanotic melanoma, basal cell carcinoma or squamous cell carcinoma (Moeller et al 1987). It may become as large as 3 cm in diameter (McKee 1994). They may persist and remain benign for a very long time (Morris et al 1968).

## Histology

The tumour cells come from the outer layer of the upper dermal eccrine duct. They grow down as uniform cells with central nucleoli and prominent intercellular connections. There is a sharp boundary between the tumour cells and the epidermal cells(McKee 1994). The rare malignant forms range from showing Bowenoid change to frank malignancy with perineural and lymphatic infiltration (Shaw et al 1982).

## Treatment

In the benign form, surgical excision with an adequate margin is the preferred option (Goldner 1970). If the lesion is symptomless, the patient frail or the site surgically difficult, treatment need not be insisted upon if the tumour is benign. Any clinical or histological suspicion of malignancy necessitates a wide excision.

## OTHER STRUCTURES

## Leiomyoma

Leiomyomas (Fisher & Helwig 1963) are benign tumours that arise from smooth muscle cells. As such, they may occur in association with the muscle cells around hairs (piloleiomyoma), genitalia or veins (angioleiomyoma). They may be simple or multiple.

## Clinical features

Leiomyomas are uncommon. Only about 100 were reported in a review of the literature over a century and a quarter. However, they are often missed by the clinician and diagnosed by the pathologist. There appears to be a familial incidence (Verma et al 1973). Multiple lesions are more common than single ones. Leiomyomas are commonest on the extremities, especially the legs. A subungual leiomyoma has been described (Requena & Baran 1993) but is rare. Pain and tenderness are reported as the characteristics of the condition, but may be absent in some. Also, other conditions may be painful. The pain in leiomyomas may be spontaneous with a stabbing or burning sensation, or provoked by pressure. The severity is variable, but may be agonisingly severe. On examination, firm smooth, subcutaneous nodules are found, usually several millimetres in diameter, but rarely over a centimetre. They are pink to red in colour, fixed to the skin, but moveable over deeper structures.

## Histology

The tumour consists of muscle cells, which may be apparently normal in appearance (Mann 1970). There is evidence of nerve damage and distortion.

## Treatment

Solitary lesions may be able to be excised. Phenoxybenzamine (Venencie et al 1982), an alpha-adrenergic blocking agent, or nifedipine (Pulimood & Jacob 1997), a calcium-channel blocker, have been advocated to alleviate pain.

## Subungual exostosis

This lesion (Zimmerman 1997) is not a skin tumour but it is included here as it is commonly referred to as such. It is a benign, bony outgrowth from a terminal phalanx.

## Aetiology

A history of trauma may or may not be obtained.

## Clinical features

Females are affected twice as often as males. The hallux is the usual digit, but others can be affected. The lesion usually arises from the dorsal aspect of the terminal phalanx and appears under the distal edge of the nail plate, which it elevates but does not distort. There may be pain from pressure. On palpation, it is very hard. X-ray of the affected digit should be diagnostic, but should include an anteroposterior and a lateral view. In its early stages it may be cartilaginous, non-ossified and thus radiotranslucent.

## Histology

This shows trabecular bone with a cartilaginous cap.

## Treatment

Surgical removal is usually permanently curative. Outpatient procedures have been described (De Berker et al 1994).

## Myxoid cyst

Myxoid cyst (synonyms: mucoid cyst, pseudocyst) is a lesion that usually occurs around the distal aspect of a digit. They are very much more common on the fingers than on the toes.

## Aetiology

Myxoid cysts tend to be associated with degenerative joint disease. Thus, Heberden's nodes are commonly seen in association. A tiny thread-like channel connects the cyst to the joint space.

## Clinical features

The lesions appear usually on the skin covering the terminal phalanx. Toes can be affected, although much less commonly than the fingers.

While the commonest site is near the proximal nail folds, they can occur elsewhere round the nail, or at other sites. A small, translucent nodule appears (Fig. 3.43). If near the nail, it can cause pressure distortion with a sulcus developing. At times, some discharge, either spontaneously or after trauma, producing a rather sticky fluid.

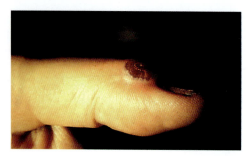

**Figure 3.43** Myxoid cyst.

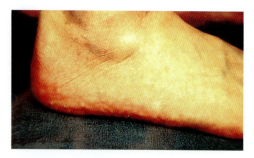

**Figure 3.44** Piezogenic pedal papules on the lateral border.

The symptoms are those related to the pressure effects. The distorted nail may catch or the lesion may cause pain on touch.

At times, depending on the site, they may transilluminate. Ultrasound or magnetic resonance imaging may help to resolve any diagnostic doubt.

## Histology

This shows a pseudocyst with a vague capsule. Within this, there are myxomatous changes.

## Treatment

Radical excision necessitates the identification of the connection to the joint, otherwise recurrence will occur. Local destructive means, such as cryotherapy (Dawber et al 1983), infrared coagulation (Kemmett & Colver 1994) or multiple needling, have been tried.

## Ganglia

A ganglion is a cystic swelling commonly formed near the wrist. They also occur on the feet. There is dispute as to whether they are a degenerative process or a benign tumour of the tendon sheath or joint capsule.

## Clinical features

On the foot, these are usually on the dorsum. In general, ganglia appear in early adult life. They may be symptomless or cause problems due to pressure. If a nerve is compressed, neurological symptoms may ensue.

## Histology

Ganglia are usually unilocular cysts with a thin wall of synovium and filled with synovial fluid.

## Treatment

They are benign and, if symptomless, may be left. They may disappear spontaneously or after a blow that ruptures them. If nerve damage or pressure effects are problems, excision may be needed. Surgery can be difficult and recurrences occur.

## Bursae

These are closed sacs, lined with synovial membrane, which are present in many parts of the body. Their aim is to prevent friction, usually between a tendon and a bony prominence. They may be present naturally or develop in response to a new challenge of this type. If such a sac becomes inflamed or infected it is termed 'bursitis'.

## Clinical features

A number of bursae are present normally around the foot, and others may develop. A common problem area is at the first metatarsophalangeal joint in the patient with hallux valgus. This can become inflamed and infected, causing considerable pain. Similar problems can occur in bursae situated in other areas. Another common site is near the Achilles tendon. Bursitis may complicate some autoimmune disorders.

## Treatment

This consists of treatment of any infection present and removal of friction by rest, appliances etc. In some cases, surgery may be required.

## Piezogenic pedal papules

Piezogenic pedal papules (synonym: painful piezogenic pedal papules) (Cohen et al 1970) are small papular lesions on the heel, provoked by pressure of standing (piezogenic = pressure generated). They can be painful.

## Clinical features

The flesh-coloured nodules typically appear on the heels when the patient stands and disappear when the pressure is removed. Usually they occur on the medial aspect of the heel, although they can affect the lateral aspect (Fig. 3.44).

## Treatment

Usually none is very feasible. Supportive heel pads may alleviate pain.

## Neurofibromatosis

Neurofibromatosis (synonym: von Recklinghausen's neurofibromatosis) (Zvulunov & Esterly 1995) is one of a mixed group of conditions affecting the skin and nerves – the neurocutaneous disorders. Since von Recklinghausen's original description, the condition has been split, mainly into neurofibromatosis 1 and neurofibromatosis 2, although other numbers are being added. The main skin involvement is in neurofibromatosis 1.

## Clinical features

Neurofibromatosis 1 is an autosomal-dominant, familial condition. It occurs in about 1 in 4000 persons. In neurofibromatosis 1 many

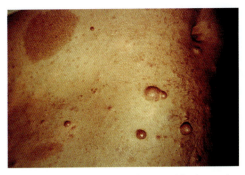

**Figure 3.45** Neurofibromatosis. Type 1 (von Recklinghausen) nodules, shagreen and café au lait patches are seen.

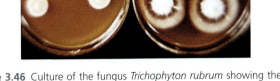

**Figure 3.46** Culture of the fungus *Trichophyton rubrum* showing the typical cotton-wool-like appearance.

systems can be affected. The skin changes can be divided into pigmentary and tumour ones.

The pigmentary changes start in childhood as smooth patches like milky coffee (café au lait), measuring over 15 mm in adults and numbering six or more. These changes can affect any area. Smaller, similar lesions resembling freckles aggregate in the axillae or groin. Axillary freckling is considered pathognomic of the condition. The tumorous lesions can be small and button-like. On palpation, they feel as though they can be pushed through the deep fascia. Larger subcutaneous lesions occur, which may be painful. (Fig. 3.45) Also, much larger nodular or diffuse plexiform neurofibromas can be present. These can all affect any area, including the foot.

The eye, skeletal structures and many other areas may be affected. The lesions can cause problems, either due to pressure effects or due to malignant transformation. The severity and extent of neurofibromatosis 1 can vary from minor to major involvement, even within one family.

Neurofibromatosis 2 is the other main variant, but is much rarer, affecting only 1 in 40 000. Skin lesions are rarer, but do include café au lait spots and tumours (Mautner et al 1997). The main problem is neurofibromas of the acoustic nerves.

## Histology

The café au lait spots are densely pigmented melanocytes. The neurofibromas are composed of loosely arranged spindle cells with pale cytoplasms. The cells are elongated and wavy.

## Treatment

Monitoring and genetic counselling form much of the management (Eichenfield et al 1997, Wolkenstein et al 1996).

Small numbers of neurofibromas may be amenable to surgical removal procedures for cosmetic reasons. Some cutaneous or visceral ones may need surgery due to pressure effects or suspicion of malignant transformation.

## Fungal infections of the feet and nails

Fungal infections constitute the most common dermatoses of the feet. About 20% of the population are likely to be affected at some time or other during their lives. Fungi are ubiquitous organisms, and well over 100 000 species have been described and are widely distributed in nature. They are very successful microorganisms and form a diverse group known as eukaryotes, which have definite cell walls but, unlike plants, contain no chlorophyll and are therefore incapable of produc-

ing their own nutrients. They thus exist as either parasites or saprophytes, which respectively depend upon living or dead organic material for nutrition. The majority of fungi are moulds, which are composed of a network of branching filaments and look rather like cotton wool in culture (Fig. 3.46). Yeasts, on the other hand, exist as single cells and their colonies are smooth-surfaced on culture.

Fungi are classified on the basis of their method of sexual reproduction and are divided into five groups or phyla, namely: chytridiomycetes, zygomycetes, ascomycetes, basidiomycetes and a group known as fungi imperfecti. Many human pathogens belong to this last group.

Fewer than 200 of the many thousands of species of fungi are recognised as human pathogens and many of these are pathogenic only in the face of a diminished host response. Therefore, many new fungal pathogens have been identified in recent times because of the advent of new diseases such as AIDS. In immunocompetent individuals only dermatophytes and *Candida* yeasts usually cause infection. A number of other saprophytic moulds and some yeasts may invade nail, but their role as primary pathogens is controversial and they may only affect previously damaged nail. However, this will be considered later in this chapter.

## DERMATOPHYTE INFECTION

Dermatophyte species are often classified according to their primary host. Hence, dermatophytes, which have man as a primary host, are called anthropophilic species; those which have an animal as a primary host are zoophilic; and those which primarily affect the soil but may infect either humans or animals are known as geophilic species. Fungal infections of the feet are almost always caused by anthropophilic species in developed societies. However, geophilic infection may occur in countries where the population regularly goes barefoot, but even then such infections are uncommon because geophilic dermatophytes are not so well adapted to survival on keratin as are their anthropophilic relatives. Zoophilic infections, which usually have a single animal species as a host, are relatively common in humans but usually affect the scalp, trunk or limbs but very rarely the feet. Indeed, if a zoophilic species is reported from a specimen taken from the foot or nail it is more likely to be due to laboratory error than a true infection.

Three varieties of dermatophyte, *Trichophyton rubrum*, *Trichophyton mentagrophytes* var. *interdigitalae* and *Epidermophyton floccosum*, are common pathogens of feet. *E. floccosum* generally accounts for less than 2% of all cases of foot infection and even a smaller number of nail infections. Many acute infections are caused by *T. mentagrophytes* var. *interdigitalae* but this variety often produces a brisk inflammatory response and may therefore be self-resolving. *T. rubrum* is by far the commonest pathogen seen in chronic infection because it is particularly well adapted to life on the human host and produces very little in the way of inflammatory response, and is therefore not likely to resolve spontaneously. Well over 80% of all nail infections are caused by *T. rubrum*.

## Epidemiology

Dermatophytes cause athlete's foot, or tinea pedis, which affects about 15% of the population. The prevalence rises to 25% or more in sportsmen who regularly use communal bathing facilities.

Although dermatophytes are not commensal organisms as such, they may produce very little in the way of clinical signs and can therefore be carried for long periods of time without the patient's knowledge. They are deposited on the floors of communal bathing places protected by small pieces of keratin and the average contamination rate in public swimming baths has been identified as being >100 fungal fragments/m² of floor space. In some areas, particularly steps, this has risen to figures as high as 700 fungal fragments/m² of floor. It is therefore easy to understand why fungal foot infection is so common, as each one of these fragments is capable of causing human infection. Although not highly pathogenic, dermatophytes are especially well adapted to life in the human host, and are therefore naturally difficult to eradicate. Disinfection of communal bathing places would seem an obvious method of disease control, but fungal elements are protected in small pieces of keratin and, therefore, a disinfectant that would penetrate keratin would be also likely to cause an acute dermatitis of the feet in users of such places and is thus not a feasible option. Swimming baths and other facilities that encourage users to walk through a trough of disinfectant are unlikely to contribute to solving the problems in that such a disinfectant is never going to be strong enough to do the job because of the damage it would cause to the feet. Regular hosing down of changing rooms and the surrounds of swimming pools etc. will reduce the carriage rate, but all floors can only be 'as clean as the users' feet' so this will not eradicate infection either.

Dermatophyte infection nearly always becomes established first in the toe clefts, although punctate infection of the sole can occur. The fourth toe cleft is nearly always infected first, and individuals with closed toe clefts are much more prone to infection than those with open clefts and this anatomical variation is well recognised. From the fourth toe cleft the disease can spread to all other toe clefts onto the soles and sides of the feet and sometimes onto the dorsum of the foot. From there, infection – of usually one hand – is often seen, although hand infection is much less usual than foot infection.

## Clinical types

### Toe cleft infection

The most common variety of fungal foot infection is tinea pedis or athlete's foot, which affects only the toe clefts. It is often confined to the fourth toe clefts and consists of maceration of the skin, often with the development of a single central fissure. Sometimes it is asymptomatic, but equally may produce itching and burning in the toe cleft. It may remain confined to the fourth toe cleft almost indefinitely or can spread to other clefts. There is little evidence as to why this is or is not so, and it is not easy to predict which individuals will develop spread out of the fourth cleft, but host defence mechanisms or frequency of use of communal bathing facilities probably have some part to play.

Secondary infections with yeasts or bacteria are common, although these will generally disappear with eradication of the dermatophyte

alone and are therefore secondary pathogens. Occasionally a Gram-negative bacterial infection may become established and often can persist alone.

## Moccasin tinea pedis

Spread from outwith the toe clefts onto the sole and sides of the foot may occur and this is known as moccasin tinea pedis because it is often confined to the sole and the sides of the foot in the distribution of a moccasin or loafer-type shoe (Fig. 3.47). This usually takes the form of a dry-type dermatitis reaction where scaling is often more pronounced than inflammation. In its early stages the disease is seen only in the region of the toe clefts as spread is relatively slow. Occasionally, a vesicopustular reaction can take place on the soles. Although moccasin tinea pedis is often bilateral, a unilateral picture raises greater suspicion of a fungal infection than, say, a dermatitis reaction secondary to contact. In advanced cases the dorsum of the foot can also become involved and even the lower part of the leg. In such cases classic anular lesions with raised scaly edges and healing centres are seen, hence the name ringworm.

Allergic reactions, often known as dermatophyte or id reactions, are well recognised. The commonest is a simple desquamation of the skin of the palms, which is usually asymptomatic, and non-inflamed. If a patient presents with sudden spontaneous peeling of the skin of the hands, the feet should always be examined. Treatment of the foot infection usually clears the hands as well. A blistering reaction on the soles, hands, or both is known as a podopompholyx, a cheiropompholyx (Fig. 3.48) or a cheiropodopompholyx, respectively. Again, fungi are rarely isolated from these blisters and this is an allergic response. The condition is sometimes so severe as to require a short

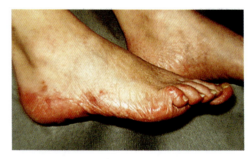

**Figure 3.47** Moccasin tinea pedis.

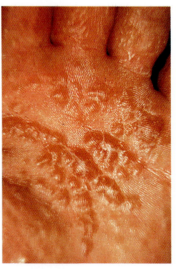

**Figure 3.48** Allergic cheiropompholyx secondary to tinea pedis.

course of systemic steroids but will usually settle down with treatment of the primary fungal infection.

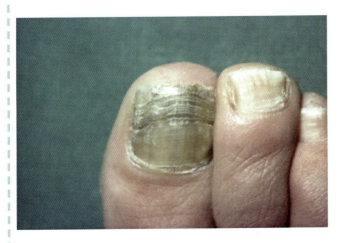
## DIFFERENTIAL DIAGNOSIS OF FOOT INFECTION

As mentioned previously, bacterial infection alone is an unusual reaction in the toe clefts but may occur with some Gram-negative species, and a specific infection called erythrasma caused by a corynebacterium can also occur. This has the unique quality of coral pink fluorescence under a Wood's light, and particularly inflamed toe clefts should always be examined in this fashion to exclude this infection, which responds to systemic antibiotics rather than antifungals. Psoriasis, pustular psoriasis, various types of dermatitis, plantar keratodermas and pitted keratolysis may all be confused with fungal infections of the soles, although, in truth, the clinical appearances are not especially similar and confusion is usually only to the uneducated eye.

Because the fourth toe cleft is nearly always initially affected, it can be said with some confidence that a normal fourth cleft precludes a fungal foot infection whatever else is wrong with the feet. This rule of thumb probably holds good in more than 99% of cases.

## NAIL INFECTION

Fungal nail infection may be caused by dermatophyte yeasts or non-dermatophyte moulds. It is accepted that dermatophytes are by far the predominant pathogens and probably account for more than 85% of all cases of fungal nail infection. This percentage is even higher in the toenails, where yeast infections are rarely seen. Yeasts, however, do much more often affect fingernails. The place of non-dermatophyte moulds in the pathogenesis of fungal nail infection is unclear. *Scytilidium dimidiatum*, previously known as *Hendersonula toruloidea*, is the only certain primary pathogen of nails in that it can also cause tinea pedis. This is a non-dermatophyte geophilic mould which is a tropical plant pathogen. It is generally seen in immigrants or visitors to the tropics and produces a typical black discoloration of the nails (Fig. 3.49). Other non-dermatophyte moulds that may occasionally be reported from mycology laboratories are probably secondary pathogens to previously damaged nail. It must be remembered that such previous damage is most likely to be due to a dermatophyte infection but other causes, notably onychogryphosis in the elderly, must be considered.

Fungal nail infection is a disease of insidious onset but thereafter there is relentless progression and it does not resolve spontaneously. Various surveys have found a prevalence of between 3% and 10% in western countries, and it is therefore likely to occur in 5–10% of the population. This makes it an especially common disease, and treatment is an important pharmaco-economic issue because of its high prevalence.

## Clinical types

There are various published clinical classifications of onychomycosis but the following is probably the most widely accepted:

- distal and lateral subungual onychomycosis (DLSO)
- superficial white onychomycosis (SWO)
- proximal subungual onychomycosis (PSO)
- total dystrophic onychomycosis (TDO)
- candidal onychomycosis (CO).

Some authorities add a further type, namely endonyx onychomycosis (EO). This variety is caused exclusively by *Trichophyton soudanense* and is exceedingly rare in the UK.

### Distal and lateral subungual onychomycosis (DLSO)

This is the commonest variety of onychomycosis and is almost exclusively caused by dermatophytes. Infection is initially a disease of the hyponichium, resulting in hyperkeratosis of the distal nail bed. It generally begins at the lateral edge of the nail, rather than the central portion, and spreads progressively proximally down the nail bed producing further hyperkeratosis and thus onycholysis (Fig. 3.50). Ultimately the underside of the nail is involved, which results in a

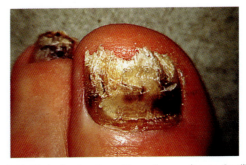

Figure 3.49 Black discoloration of toenail secondary to *Scytilidium dimidiatum*.

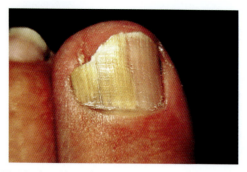

**Figure 3.50** Distal and lateral subungual onychomycosis (DLSO) showing spread to the proximal nail fold.

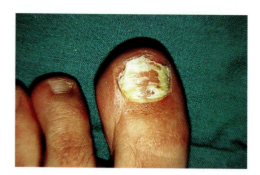

**Figure 3.51** Superficial white onychomycosis (SWO) secondary to *Trichophyton mentagrophytes*.

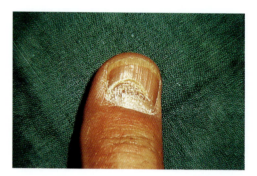

**Figure 3.52** Proximal subungual onychomycosis (PSO) secondary to *Trichophyton rubrum*.

thickening of the nail, which sometimes becomes friable and crumbles away. Sometimes the fungus proliferates in the space between the nail plate and nail bed, and this is known as a dermatophytoma. Such lesions are either round or linear and are important in that such an appearance is the most common cause of treatment failure.

*Scytilidium dimidiatum* produces a similar appearance, although there is a notable black discoloration of the nail in this infection and it is seen only in patients from the tropics or, occasionally, travellers to the tropics. Scopulariopsis brevicaulis and some *Aspergillus* species are occasionally isolated but they are probably secondary pathogens to previously damaged nail in that they are saprophytic moulds that will thrive in dead material but not produce proteases capable of invading the nail themselves. Most non-dermatophyte moulds are resistant to antifungal drugs, and nail removal is usually necessary as treatment.

## CASE STUDY 3.11 **SKIN DERMATOPHYTE INFECTION**

A 19-year-old paraplegic girl presents in the clinic with severe maceration of her toe clefts, which are notably soggy and white looking. She has both sensory and motor loss affecting her feet and is therefore asymptomatic. She uses a hydrotherapy pool for physiotherapy purposes on a regular basis.

It is likely that she has a primary dermatophyte infection, with a secondary infection consisting of both yeasts and bacteria.

Topical Terbinafine should take care of both dermatophytes and yeasts, and in addition Betadine ointment should be used for any bacterial overlay. Potassium permanganate (Condy's crystals) footbaths for 10 minutes each day are always helpful in such cases.

A laboratory specimen for both fungi and bacteria should be submitted before continuing treatment.

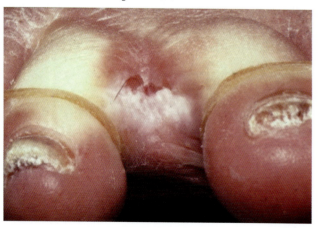

## Superficial white onychomycosis (SWO)

This is a less common variety and is usually the result of a *T. mentagrophytes* infection. However, some moulds, such as *Acremonium* and *Fusarium*, may also be causal, and this is the only type of onychomycosis that affects the dorsal surface of the nail (Fig. 3.51) and thus sometimes responds to topical treatment.

An especially dense, white appearance occurs in patients with AIDS. Although this is not a true SWO, in that the whole thickness of the nail plate is involved, it is certainly white in appearance and is appropriately classified here for the sake of clinical convenience.

## Proximal subungual onychomycosis (PSO)

Yeast infection is the commonest cause of a proximal nail infection, but this is dealt with under the heading of candidal onychomycosis (see below). *T. rubrum* occasionally causes PSO where the disease begins at the proximal end of the nail (Fig. 3.52). This is often seen in patients with intercurrent disease such as AIDS and peripheral vascular disease.

## Total dystrophic onychomycosis (TDO)

All of the above varieties will eventually produce total dystrophy of the nail, which is really a classification for end-stage infection (Fig. 3.53).

## Candidal onychomycosis (CO)

Candidal infection of the nail can exist in four forms. The commonest variety is a proximal infection of the nail secondary to a chronic paronychia. This is generally seen in patients with wet occupations where

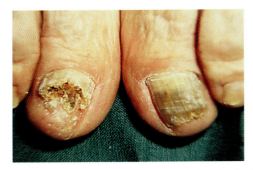

**Figure 3.53** Total dystrophic onychomycosis (TDO) showing both thickening and destruction of the nail plate.

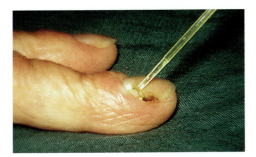

**Figure 3.54** Chronic paronychia showing cuticular detachment.

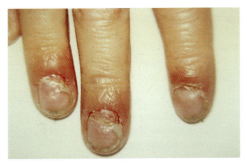

**Figure 3.55** Chronic paronychia with a proximal nail fold dystrophy.

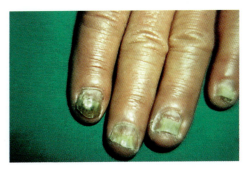

**Figure 3.56** Distal onycholysis in a patient with Raynaud's phenomenon.

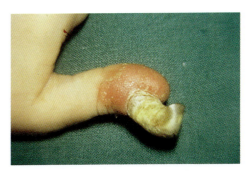

**Figure 3.57** Chronic mucocutaneous candidosis showing gross thickening of the nail plate.

the cuticle becomes detached from the nail plate and infection occurs in the subcuticular space (Fig. 3.54). This is often the result of a mixed infection of yeasts and bacteria, resulting in further swelling of the posterior nail fold, thereby enhancing the cuticular separation. Ultimately, a proximal nail dystrophy will occur because of inflammation in the region of the nail matrix (Fig. 3.55).

Distal infection with yeasts is almost exclusively seen in patients with Raynaud's phenomenon. It is unclear whether the peripheral vasospasm produces onycholysis and a secondary yeast infection, or whether there is a primary yeast infection resulting in onycholysis. The former is logically more likely in that yeasts do not produce proteolytic enzymes capable of dissolving keratin. It is nearly always seen in the fingernails and is not very common (Fig. 3.56). Total candidal nail dystrophy secondary to chronic mucocutaneous candidosis is even less common. Chronic mucocutaneous candidosis is an inborn defect of cell-mediated immunity, of which there are various types that vary with the severity of the immune defect. In the most severe types there is gross thickening and hyperkeratosis of the whole nail, which is packed with yeasts (Fig. 3.57). Such patients are usually

children, who often do not survive into adult life because of the degree of immunodeficiency.

The fourth variety of yeast infection is purely secondary to intercurrent disease, and psoriatic nails are often colonised by yeasts but treatment of the yeast will rarely significantly improve the clinical appearance because psoriasis is the primary defect.

## Tinea incognito

It is appropriate to mention this variety of fungal infection here, although it is a poor name that legitimises misdiagnosed and mistreated infection with topical steroids (Fig. 3.58). When the classic ring-like appearance is seen this disease results in loss of integrity of the ring, a reduction of scaling and the development of nodules, which makes diagnosis even more difficult. It can be seen on the feet and lower legs, when fungal infection is mistaken for a dermatitis reaction and treated with topical steroids. If there is clinical doubt and treatment must be instituted then it is always safer to begin with a topical antifungal, which will do no harm to a dermatitis, whereas a topical steroid will enhance a fungal infection.

## LABORATORY DIAGNOSIS OF DERMATOPHYTE INFECTION

There is no doubt that many cases of fungal foot infection are treated without laboratory confirmation of diagnosis. Many antifungal preparations are now available on an over-the-counter basis and self-treatment is common. Even when patients visit the general practitioner it is rare for the diagnosis to be confirmed by laboratory methods. The clinical appearances of interdigital infection are rela-

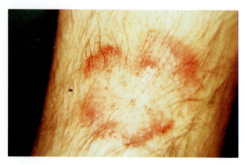

**Figure 3.58** 'Tinea incognito'. Tinea corporis of the lower leg inappropriately treated with topical steroids.

tively typical and this is probably fair enough. However, in order for a therapeutic trial of this sort to be effective it is necessary to use the most effective antifungal preparation. Allylamines are generally much more effective antidermatophyte drugs than azoles, and they are the treatment of choice (see below). It is generally accepted that infections of the sole, and certainly of the nails, should be treated systemically, and in such cases it is always wise to confirm the diagnosis by sending a specimen to a laboratory with expertise in the diagnosis of fungal infections.

In cases of skin infection a skin scraping should be taken from the edge of the lesion, which can either be done dry or following dampening of the area with saline. A blunt scalpel blade can then be used to scrape away the scales, or the slurry when saline is used, and the specimen placed on black paper. The advantages of using the saline method are that it stops skin scales flying around, which makes the specimen difficult to obtain and there is a theoretical risk of inhaling fungal spores thus producing allergy in medical and podiatric practitioners. One should not take the view that this risk is very great, but it is a theoretical one. Because nail infection is primarily a disease of the nail bed rather than the nail plate, collection of hyperkeratotic material from beneath the nail is always best and, of course, a specimen from the most proximal part of the infection contains the most active fungus. A small probe is ideal for removing this material from beneath the nail. Nail clippings are less likely to yield fungus and are more difficult to handle in a laboratory. Scrapings from the nail surface are of no use at all in cases other than SWO.

When the specimens arrive at the laboratory they are cleared with 20% potassium hydroxide and examined directly microscopically. It requires some expertise to differentiate fungal elements from cell walls, and such microscopy should only be carried out by an experienced technician who will usually be able to differentiate a dermatophyte from a non-dermatophyte mould and certainly from a yeast. Culture is carried out in Sabaraud's dextrose agar and a properly taken specimen will usually grow in culture. However, about 30% of nail specimens that are positive on microscopy fail to grow in culture simply because the specimen is taken from an area where the infection is old and the fungus is dead. However, direct microscopy is entirely adequate for diagnosis of infection and institution of treatment because dermatophytes are not commensal organisms and when the fungus is seen microscopically it is indicative of active disease. In a clinical-trial situation, of course, positive microscopy and culture is demanded and greater care should be taken in the collection of specimens.

It is certainly mandatory to confirm the diagnosis of infection in nail disease. Although modern antifungal drugs do produce cure rates in the region of 80% they have to be given for 3 months and thereafter the nail is left to grow out normally. In the case of toenails this takes at least 12 months before the result of the therapeutic trial is known, and this is quite unacceptable where the drugs are costly and possibly even toxic. Although fungal nail infection is the commonest cause of nail dystrophy it still accounts for only 50% of all cases of dystrophic nails that present, and this confirms the need for accurate laboratory diagnosis. If the disease is strongly suspected on clinical grounds and the laboratory test is negative in microscopy and culture, the test should be repeated at least once, and possibly twice, before fungal infection is excluded simply because nails are difficult specimens for the laboratory to handle and no blame can be attached to even the best laboratory if an infection is missed at first pass, especially if the specimen is taken from the wrong area.

## TREATMENT OF FUNGAL FOOT AND NAIL INFECTIONS

Interdigital tinea pedis, the commonest variety of fungal infection, is best treated topically. An antifungal cream should always be used rather than antifungal powder. Antifungal foot powders are useful prophylactically but have no therapeutic role. There are many proprietary brands of topical antifungal but they mainly fall into two drug groups: the azoles and the allylamines. Both azoles and allylamines inhibit sterol biosynthesis in the fungal cell wall. Azole drugs inhibit a cytochrome P450 enzyme, 14 alpha-demethylase, which results in ergosterol depletion. This causes the cell wall to leak; the cell will stop growing and will eventually die. Azoles are generally considered to be less potent in their mode of action, and when used topically should be given for the time taken for the keratin to turn over, which in the case of skin is 4 weeks. Allylamines act on a non-cytochrome P450 enzyme called squalene epoxidase. This results in ergosterol depletion but also in squalene accumulation, and this double mode of action is fungicidal. Topical allylamines therefore need to be used for only one week, and indeed clinical trials have demonstrated that they are more effective over one week of treatment than are azole drugs used over 4 weeks. Furthermore, relapse rates in 'cured' patients are much lower than in those treated with azoles. More recently, topical terbinafine in a more adherent base has been developed for once-only use on skin and the results are encouraging.

Topical allylamines should, therefore, be considered the treatment of choice in interdigital foot infection, and topical terbinafine is now available over the counter in both regular and once-only formulations. Although it is more costly than topical azoles, its higher cure rates over a shorter treatment duration, together with its lower relapse rates make it a much more attractive option. The problem with 4 weeks' treatment is that symptoms will resolve long before the period ends and compliance with the full course of therapy using azole drugs is much less likely. Their failure rate is thus enhanced even further. Although some studies have shown topical terbinafine to be effective in moccasin tinea pedis, it is likely that systemic treatment will be required in some cases for infection of the palms and soles, where the keratin is much thicker and there may be difficulty in penetration by topical agents. Creams have no part to play in the treatment of nail infection, and nail lacquers are generally ineffective other than in the case of superficial white onychomycosis where the dorsal surface of the nail is affected. There are no topical allylamine preparations designed specifically for nails, and amorolfine nail lacquer (Loceryl) is probably the most effective agent, but again it should only be recommended for superficial white onychomycosis or, possibly, as an adjunct to systemic therapy. There are a small number of studies that show that adjunctive topical and systemic treatment works better than systemic treatment alone in nail infections but this requires confirmation in larger properly blinded series.

## Systemic treatment of foot and nail infections

There are currently five oral agents available for oral use in the treatment of superficial fungal infections:

- griseofulvin
- ketoconazole
- itraconazole
- terbinafine
- fluconazole.

Griseofulvin is the oldest of these drugs and is a weakly fungistatic antidermatophyte agent. It must be given for the whole of the time the skin at the infected site takes to turn over, and this is 4–6 weeks at least in infections of the palms and soles, 6–12 months in fingernails and 12–18 months in toenails. Even then, relapse rates are high and the drug no longer has a place in treating infections of the feet. It remains the only drug licensed for use in children and is still used in scalp infections. Although it can still be used in children with toenail infections, the results are so poor as to make it hardly worthwhile. Ketoconazole is no longer licensed for use in the normal run of skin and nail infections because of hepatotoxicity. It was not in any case very much more effective than griseofulvin in dermatophyte infections. Fluconazole is a useful drug in yeast infections and is the most bioavailable of all oral preparations, but it only has relatively weak antidermatophyte activity. It is unlikely ever to become licensed for use in nail disease and its only value in foot infection would be if other agents are contraindicated for some reason.

Itraconazole and terbinafine are the leading players in the treatment of foot and nail infection and terbinafine is the most potent antidermatophyte agent in that it has the lowest minimal inhibitory concentration (MIC) of all of these drugs against dermatophytes, and furthermore the MIC is equivalent to the minimal fungicidal concentration (MFC), making this a truly fungicidal drug in vitro.

Itraconazole can achieve fungicidal concentrations, but its MFC is about ten times greater than its MIC and about 100 times greater (in μg/ml) than the MFC of terbinafine. These in vitro data would suggest that terbinafine is the most potent antidermatophyte agent in vivo, and this is certainly borne out in clinical studies in nail infection. Itraconazole is given in nail infection in a pulsed fashion where 400 mg/day of the drug is given for one week per month and repeated three or four times. Terbinafine, on the other hand, is given in a dose of 250 mg/day for 6 weeks in fingernails and 3 months in toenails, and a large study comparing continuous terbinafine with pulsed itraconazole has revealed terbinafine to be the superior agent by some significant margin.

Terbinafine is, therefore, the treatment of choice in toenail infection, and a number of studies have shown that treatment courses longer than 3 months are not statistically superior. The nail at that stage is not clear of fungus and remains abnormal but studies show that it should thereafter grow out normally in about 80% of cases. If itraconazole is chosen it should be given in four pulses of 400 mg/day for 1 week each over 4 months and again regrowth awaited. An additional month of treatment in the case of terbinafine or an additional pulse in the case of itraconazole may well enhance cure rates in selected cases. Continuing growth of the fungus in culture at the end of the prescribed treatment period is certainly an indication that treatment should be continued for longer.

The two drugs are much closer in terms of efficacy in skin infection, and terbinafine 250 mg/day for 2 weeks is likely to be equivalent to itraconazole 400 mg/day for 1 week in infections of the palms and soles. This is based on historical data and no direct clinical study of these two regimens has been carried out. More importantly there have been no studies of relapse rate, which is likely to be lower with fungicidal agents.

### Safety

Itraconazole and terbinafine do have some potential side-effects, as do all drugs. However, minor side-effects such as nausea and itch are seen in only about 5% of cases, which is the same as for most commonly used drugs. Terbinafine does cause taste disturbance in about 1 in 400 cases; this is reversible on cessation of therapy but should be recognised and the drug stopped should it occur. This disturbance varies from a vague diminution in taste sensation to almost complete loss of taste. Hepatotoxicity occurs in about 1 in 50 000 cases in terbinafine-treated patients, and this usually is in the form of an idiosyncratic cholestasis, which again is reversible. Itraconazole causes abnormality of liver enzymes somewhat more frequently, but this rarely becomes symptomatic and again should not give rise to any problems providing it is recognised and the drug stopped when this side-effect does occur. Although the incidence of significant side-effects with systemic antifungal agents compares favourably with many other drugs, there is no doubt that there is some resistance on the part of both patients and medical attendants to their prescription in nail infection. Topical agents, which are largely ineffective, continue to maintain a significant market share, and ongoing development of effective topical agents for nail infections remains a priority.

### Prophylaxis

Treatment of systemic infection is relatively expensive and, of course, attention should be paid to prophylactic measures after successful treatment to try to prevent reinfection. Nail infection is secondary to toe-cleft disease, and any evidence of recurrence of toe-cleft infection should be treated enthusiastically. Prevention of toe-cleft infection is possible with antifungal foot powders or the wearing of small plastic socks while swimming. The former is probably a more feasible option, and any antifungal foot powder should be applied after swimming or using communal bathing places. Particular attention must be paid to the toe clefts, and such use of powder has been shown to be useful in preventing reinfection in regular users. The degree of spread via contaminated footwear is unknown but it is theoretically possible, and powder may be applied to the inside of shoes as well.

## REFERENCES

Akasu R, Sugiyama H 1996 Dermatoscopic and videomicroscopic features of melanocytic plantar nevi. American Journal of Dermatopathology 18:10–18.

Baran R, Dawber R, Haneke E, Tosti A 1996 Onychomycosis and its treatment. In: A text atlas of nail disorders. Martin Dunitz, London, pp 155–167.

Bart RS, Andrade R, Kopf AW, Leider M 1968 Acquired digital fibrokeratomas. Archives of Dermatology 97:120–129.

Bedi TR, Pandhi RK, Bhutani LK 1976 Multiple palmoplantar histiocytomas. Archives of Dermatology 112:1001–1003.

Bleehen SS 1998 Textbook of dermatology, 6th edn, vol 2, Ch. 39. Rook Wilkinson, Ebling, pp 1753–1815.

Bolognia JL 1995 Bazex syndrome: acrokeratosis paraneoplastica. Seminars in Dermatology 14(2):84–89.

Bouscarat F, Bouchard C, Bouhour D 1998 Paronychia and pyogenic granuloma of the great toes in patients treated with indinavir. New England Journal of Medicine 338(24):1776–1777.

Boyd AS, Neldner KH 1991 Lichen planus. Journal of the American Academy of Dermatology 25:593–619.

Brownstein MH, Shapiro L 1976 Verrucous carcinoma of skin: epithelioma cuniculatum plantare. Cancer 38(4):1710–1716.

Brehler R, Hildebrand A, Luger TA 1997 Recent developments in the treatment of atopic eczema. Journal of the American Academy of Dermatology 36:983–994.

Burton JL, Holden CA 1998 Pompholyx. In: Textbook of dermatology. Blackwell, Oxford.

Casso EM, Grin-Jorgensen CM, Grant-Kels JM 1992 Spitz nevi. Journal of the American Academy of Dermatology 27:901–913.

Cockayne SE, Shah M, Messenger AG, Gawkrodger DJ 1998 Foot dermatitis in children: causative allergens and follow-up. Contact Dermatitis 38:203.

Cohen HJ, Gibbs RC, Minkin W, Frank SB 1970 Painful piezogenic pedal papules. Archives of Dermatology 101:112.

Dalle S, Depape L, Phan B et al 2007 Squamous cell carcinoma of the nail apparatus: clinicopathological study of 35 cases. British Journal of Dermatology 156:871–874.

Dawber RPR, Sonnex T, Leonard J, Ralfs I 1983 Myxoid cysts of the finger: treatment by liquid nitrogen spray cryosurgery. Clinical and Experimental Dermatology 8:153–157.

Dealey C 2005 The Care of Wounds, 3rd ed. Blackwell Scientific Press, Oxford.

De Berker D, Lawrence CM, Dahl MGC 1994 Outpatient surgery for subungual exostoses. British Journal of Dermatology 131(Suppl 44):44.

DeDavid M, Orlow SJ, Provost N 1997 A study of large congenital melanocytic nevi and associated malignant melanomas: review of cases in the New York University Registry and the world literature. Journal of the American Academy of Dermatology 36:409–416.

Demirkesen C, Hoede N, Moll R 1995 Epithelial markers and differentiation adnexal neoplasms of the skin: an immunohistochemical study including individual cytokeratins. Journal of Cutaneous Pathology 22:518–535.

Deschamps P, Leroy D, Pedailles S Mandard JC 1986 Keratoderma climactericum (Haxthausen's disease): clinical signs, laboratory findings and etretinate treatment in 10 patients. Dermatologica 172(5):258–262.

Diaz-Cascajo C, Bastida-Inarrea J, Borrego L, Carretero-Hernández G 1995 Comparison of p53 expression in dermatofibrosarcoma protuberans and dermatofibroma: lack of correlation with proliferation rate. Journal of Cutaneous Pathology 22:304–309.

Dictor M, Rambech E, Way D 1996 Human herpesvirus 8 (Kaposi's sarcoma-associated herpesvirus) DNA in Kaposi's sarcoma lesions, AIDS Kaposi's sarcoma cell lines, endothelial Kaposi's sarcoma simulators, and the skin of immunosuppressed patients. American Journal of Pathology 148:2009–2016.

Drapé JL, Idy-Peretti I, Goettmann S et al 1996 Standard and high resolution magnetic resonance imaging of glomus tumours of toes and fingertips. Journal of the American Academy of Dermatology 35:550–555.

Duran-McKinster C, Herrera M, Reyes-Mugica M, Ruiz-Maldonado R 1993 Infantile digital fibromatosis: spontaneous regression in three cases. European Journal of Dermatology 3:192–194.

Eichenfield LF, Levy ML, Paller AS, Riccardi VM 1997 Guidelines of care for neurofibromatosis type 1. Journal of the American Academy of Dermatology 37:625–630.

Elmets CA, Ceilley RL 1980 Amelanotic melanoma presenting as a pyogenic granuloma. Cuts 25(2):164–166, 168.

Eriksson M-O, Hagforsen E, Lundin IP, Michaelsson G 1998 Palmoplantar pustulosis: a clinical and immunohistological study. British Journal of Dermatology 138:390–398.

Evans J, Clarke T, Mattacks CA, Pond CM 1989 Dermatofibromas and arthropod bites: is there any evidence to link the two? Lancet 2:36–37.

Exner JH, Dahod S, Pochi PE 1983 Pyogenic granuloma-like zone lesions during isotretinoin therapy. Archives of Dermatology 119:808–818.

Fine J-D, Bauer EA, Briggaman RA 1991 Revised clinical and laboratory criteria for subtypes of inherited epidermolysis bullosa. Journal of the American Academy of Dermatology 24:119–135.

Fisher WC, Helwig EB 1963 Leiomyomas of the skin. Archives of Dermatology 88:510–520.

Fujisawa H, Matsushima Y, Hoshino M et al 1991 Differentiation of the basal cell epithelioma-like changes overlying dermatofibroma. Acta Dermatologica Venereologica (Stockholm) 71:354–357.

Garcia C, Poletti E 2007 Sentinel node biopsy for melanoma is still controversial. Journal of the American Academy of Dermatology 56: 347–348.

Giardina VN, Morton BF, Potter GK et al 1996 Metastic endometrial adenocarcinoma to the skin of a toe. American Journal of Dermatopathology 18(1):94–96.

Gloster HM 1996 Dermatofibrosarcoma protuberans. Journal of the American Academy of Dermatology 35:355–374.

Goettman S, Drapé JL, Idy-Peretti I et al 1994 Magnetic resonance imaging: a new tool in the diagnosis of tumours of the nail apparatus. British Journal of Dermatology 130:701–710.

Goldman L 1978 Laser treatment of multiple progressive glomangiomas. Archives of Dermatology 114:1853–1854.

Goldner R 1970 Eccrine poromatosis. Archives of Dermatology 101:606–608.

Griffiths CE, Barker JN 2007 Pathogenesis and clinical features of psoriasis. Lancet 370:263–271.

Griffiths WAD 1980 Pityriasis rubra pilaris. Clinical and Experimental Dermatology 5:105–112.

Grin-Jorgensen C, Kopf AW, Maize JC 1991 Cutaneous malignant melanoma. Periodic Synopsis 712.

Halpern AC, Guerry DIV, Elder DE et al 1993 Natural history of dysplastic nevi. Journal of the American Academy of Dermatology 29:51–57.

Hare PJ, Smith PA 1969 Acquired (digital) fibrokeratoma. British Journal of Dermatology 81:667–670.

Harvell J, Maibach HJ 1992 Skin disease among musicians. Medical Problems in the Performing Arts 7:114–120.

Herman PS, Datnow B 1974 Acquired (digital) fibrokeratomas. Acta Dermato-Veneriologica (Stockholm) 54:73–76.

Hill BB, Sloan DA, Lee EY et al 1996 Marjolin's ulcer of the foot caused by nonburn trauma. Southern Medical Journal 89(7):707–710.

Hodak E, David M, Feuerman EJ 1986 Palmoplantar keratoderma in association with myxoedema. Acta Dermato-Venereologica 66:243–245.

Hoffman D 1997 Leg ulceration with mixed arterial and venous disease. Journal of Wound Care 6(2):53–55.

Hunt SJ, Santa Cruz DJ, Miller CW 1990 Cholesterotic fibrous histiocytoma. Archives of Dermatology 126:506–508.

Judge MR, McLean WHI, Munro CS. 2004 Disorders of keratinisation. In: Burns T, Breathnach S, Cox N, Griffiths C (eds) Rook's textbook of dermatology, 7th edn. Blackwell, Oxford, pp 34.1–34.111.

Kemény L, Gyulai R, Kiss M et al 1997 Kaposi's sarcoma-associated herpesvirus/human herpesvirus-8: a new virus in human pathology. Journal of the American Academy of Dermatology 37:107–113.

Kemmett D, Colver GB 1994 Myxoid cysts treated by infra-red coagulation. Clinical and Experimental Dermatology 19:118–120.

Kimyai-Asadi A, Kotcher LB, Jih MH 2002 The molecular basis of hereditary palmoplantar keratodermas. Journal of the American Academy of Dermatology 47:327–343.

Kint A, Baran R 1988 Histopathologic study of Koenen tumors. Journal of the American Academy of Dermatology 18:369–372.

Kint A, Baran R, De Keyser H 1985 Acquired (digital) fibrokeratoma. Journal of the American Academy of Dermatology 12:816–821.

Klein MB, Pereira FA, Kantor I 1974 Kaposi sarcoma complicating systemic lupus erythematosus treated with immunosuppression. Archives of Dermatology 100:602–605.

Kolbusz RV, O'Donoghue MN 1991 Pyogenic granuloma following treatment of verruca vulgaris with cryotherapy and Duoplant. Cutis 47(3):204.

Kossard S, Rosen R 1992 Cutaneous Bowen's disease. Journal of the American Academy of Dermatology 27:406–410.

Kukita A, Ishihara K 1989 Clinical features and distribution of malignant melanoma and pigmented nevi on the soles of the feet in Japan. Journal of Investigative Dermatology 92:210S–213S.

Kutzner H 1993 Expression of the human progenitor cell antigen CD34 (HPCA-1) distinguishes dermatofibrosarcoma protuberans from fibrous histiocytoma in formalin-fixed, paraffin-embedded tissue. Journal of the American Academy of Dermatology 28:613–617.

Kwa RE, Campana K, Moy RL 1992 Biology of cutaneous squamous cell carcinoma. Journal of the American Academy of Dermatology 26:1–26.

Langley RGB, Barnhill RL, Mihm MC et al 1999 Fitzpatrick's dermatology in general medicine, 5th edn, vol 1, Ch. 92. McGraw Hill, New York, pp 1080–1116.

La Parola IL, Masini C, Nanni G 1997 Kaposi's sarcoma in renal-transplant recipients: experience at the Catholic University in Rome 1988–1996. Dermatology 194:229–233.

Leffell DJ, Fitzgerald, DA 1999 Fitzpatrick's dermatology in general medicine, 5th edn, vol 1, Ch. 81. McGraw Hill, New York.

Lemlich G, Schwam L, Lebwohl M 1987 Kaposi's sarcoma and acquired immunodeficiency syndrome: Post-mortem findings in twenty four cases. Journal of the American Academy of Dermatology 16:319–325.

Lemont H, Pearl B 1992 Juvenile plantar dermatosis. Journal of the American Podiatric Medical Association 82(3):167–169.

Leung AKC 1998 Pruritis in children. Journal of the Royal Society for Promotion of Health 118(5):280–286.

Lever WF, Schaumberg-Leuer G 1990 Histopathology of the skin, Ch. 30. Lippincott, Philadelphia, p. 696.

Lindelöf B, Sigurgeirsson B, Melander S 1992 Seborrheic keratoses and cancer. Journal of the American Academy of Dermatology 26:947–950.

Lookingbill DP, Spangler N, Sexton FM 1990 Skin involvement as the presenting sign of internal carcinoma. Journal of the American Academy of Dermatology 22:19–26.

Lospalluti M, Mastrolonardo M, Loconsole F et al 1995 Classical Kaposi's sarcoma: a survey of 163 cases observed in Bari, South Italy. Dermatology 191:104–108.

Lund HZ, Greensboro NC 1965 How often does squamous cell carcinoma of the skin metastasise? Archives of Dermatology 92:635–637.

McKee PH 1994 Pathology of the skin with clinical correlations. Mosby-Wolfe, London, pp 15.50–15.51.

MacKie RM 1998 Textbook of dermatology, 6th edn, vol 2, Ch. 38. Rook Wilkinson, Ebling, pp 1717–1752.

McLean DI, Gallagher FP 1995 'Sunburn' freckles, café au lait macules, and other pigmented lesions of schoolchildren: the Vancouver mole study. Journal of the American Academy of Dermatology 32:565–570.

Mann PR 1970 Leiomyoma cutis: an electron microscope study. British Journal of Dermatology 82:463–469.

Mautner VF, Lindenau M, Baser ME 1997 Skin abnormalities in neurofibromatosis 2. Archives of Dermatology 133:1539–1543.

Mellerio JE 1999 Molecular pathology of the cutaneous basement zone. Clinical and Experimental Dermatology 24:25–32.

Mikhail GR 1985 Subungual basal cell carcinoma. Journal of Dermatologic Surgery & Oncology 11(12):1222–1223.

Moeller CA, Welch RH, Kaplan DL 1987 An enlarging tumor of the foot. Archives of Dermatology 123(5):653–654.

Monckton Copeman PW, Jones EW 1965 Pigmented hairy epidermal nevus (Becker's nevus). Archives of Dermatology 92:249–251.

Morris J, Wood MG, Samitz MH 1968 Eccrine poroma. Archives of Dermatology 98:162–165.

Ogino A 1976 Linear eccrine poroma. Archives of Dermatology 112:841–844.

Ortonne JP 1999 Recent developments in the understanding of the pathogenesis of psoriasis. British Journal of Dermatology 140:1–7.

Ozedmir HM, Yildiz Y, Yilmaz C, Saglik Y 1997 Tumors of the foot and ankle: analysis of 196 cases. Journal Foot and Ankle Surgery 36(6):403–408.

Patrice SJ, Wiss K, Mullien JB 1991 Pyogenic granuloma (lobular capillary hemangioma): a clinicopathologic study of 178 cases. Paediatric Dermatology 8(4):267–276.

Pernia LR, Guzman-Stein G, Miller HL 1993 Surgical treatment of an aggressive metastasized Eccrine poroma. Annals of Plastic Surgery 30:257–259.

Pinkus H, Mehregan AH 1963 Epidermotropic eccrine carcinoma. Archives of Dermatology 88:597–606.

Pinkus H, Rogin JR, Goldman P 1956 Eccrine poroma: tumors exhibiting features of the epidermal sweat duct unit. Archives of Dermatology 74:511–521.

Pulimood GS, Jacob M 1997 Pain in multiple leiomyomas alleviated by nifedipine. Pain 73:101–102.

Requena L, Baran R 1993 Digital angioleiomyoma: an uncommon neoplasm. Journal of the American Academy of Dermatology 29:1043–1044.

Requena L, Sangueza OP 1997 Cutaneous vascular proliferations. Part II: hyperplasias and benign neoplasms. Journal of the American Academy of Dermatology 37:887–920.

Requena L, Farina C, Fuente C et al 1994 Giant dermatofibroma: a little known clinical variant of dermatofibroma. Journal of the American Academy of Dermatology 30:714–718.

Rhodes AR 1999 Fitzpatrick's dermatology in general medicine, 5th edn, vol 1, Ch. 90. McGraw Hill, New York, pp 1018–1059.

Rivers JK, MacLennan R, Kelly JW 1995 The eastern Australian childhood nevus study: prevalence of atypical nevi, congenital nevus-like nevi, and other pigmented lesions. Journal of the American Academy of Dermatology 32:957–963.

Roth MJ, Stern JB, Haupt HM et al 1995 Basal cell carcinoma of the sole. Journal of Cutaneous Pathology 22(4): 349–353.

Sagebiel RW 1989 The dysplastic melanocytic nevus. Journal of the American Academy of Dermatology 20:496–501.

Salasche S, Dinehart SM, Pollack SV, Skouge JW 1993 Guidelines of care for cutaneous squamous cell carcinoma. Journal of the American Academy of Dermatology 23:628–631.

Sandilands A, Smith FJ, Irvine AD, McLean WH 2007 Filaggrin's fuller figure: a glimpse into the genetic architecture of atopic dermatitis. Journal of Investigative Dermatology 127:1282–1284.

Sasaoka R, Morimura T, Mihara M et al 1996 Detection of human papillomavirus type 16 DNA in two cases of verrucous carcinoma of the foot. British Journal of Dermatology 134:983–984.

Sau P, McMarlin SL, Sperling LC, Katz R 1994 Bowen's diseases of the nail bed and periungual area: a clinicopathologic analysis of seven cases. Archives of Dermatology 130:204–209.

Schwartz RA 1995 Cutaneous metastatic disease. Journal of the American Academy of Dermatology 33:161–182.

Schwartz RA 1996 Kaposi's sarcoma: advances and perspectives. Journal of the American Academy of Dermatology 34: 804–814.

Seehafer JR, Rahman D, Soderstrom CW 1979 Epithelioma cuniculatum: verrucous carcinoma of the foot. Cutis 23:287–290.

Shaw M, McKee PH, Lowe D, Black MM 1982 Malignant eccrine poroma: a study of twenty seven cases. British Journal of Dermatology 107:675–680.

Slade J, Marghoob AA, Salopek TG et al 1995 Atypical mole syndrome: risk factor for cutaneous malignant melanoma and implications for management. Journal of the American Academy of Dermatology 32:479–494.

Smith CH, Anstey AV, Barker JN et al 2005 British Association of Dermatologists guidelines for use of biological interventions in psoriasis. British Journal of Dermatology 153:486–497.

Steel HH 1965 Garlic clove fibroma. Journal of the American Medical Association 191:1082–1083.

Stewart DM, Altman J, Mehregan AH 1978 Speckled lentiginous nevus. Journal of the American Academy of Dermatology 114:895.

Strohal R, Gillitzer R, Sinzits E, Stingl G 1991 Localised vs generalised pyogenic granuloma. A clinicopathologic study. Archives of Dermatology 127(6):856–861.

Tappero JW, Conant MA, Wolfe SF, Berger TG 1993 Kaposi's sarcoma. Journal of the American Academy of Dermatology 28:371–395.

Tateyama H, Eimoto T, Tada T 1995 p53 protein and proliferating cell nuclear antigen in eccrine poroma and porocarcinoma: an immunohistochemical study. American Journal of Dermatopathology 17:457–464.

Tosti A, Baran R, Piraccini BM et al 1996 Nail matrix nevi: a clinical and histopathologic study of twenty two patients. Journal of the American Academy of Dermatology 34:765–771.

Toyama K, Hashimoto-Kumasaka K, Tagami H 1995 Acantholytic squamous cell carcinoma involving the dorsum of the foot of elderly Japanese: clinical and light microscopic observations in five patients. British Journal of Dermatology 133:141–142.

Venencie PY, Puissant A, Boffa GA et al 1982 Multiple cutaneous leiomyomata and erythrocytosis with demonstration of erythropoietic activity in the cutaneous leiomyomata. British Journal of Dermatology 107:483–486.

Verallo VVM 1968 Acquired digital fibrokeratomas. British Journal of Dermatology 80:730–736.

Verma KC, Chawdhry SD, Rathi KS 1973 Cutaneous leiomyomata in two brothers. British Journal of Dermatology 90:351–353.

Vincent CY 1999 Fitzpatrick's dermatology in general medicine, 5th edn, vol 1, Ch. 83. McGraw Hill, New York, pp 873–881.

Warren RB, Griffiths CE. 2008 Systemic therapies for psoriasis: methotrexate, retinoids, and cyclosporine. Clinics in Dermatology 26:438–447.

Wolkenstein P, Freche B, Zeller J 1996 Usefulness of screening investigations in neurofibromatosis type 1: a study of 152 patients. Archives of Dermatology 132:1333–1336.

Zimmerman EH 1997 Subungual exostosis. Cutis 19:185–188.

Zvulunov A, Esterly NB 1995 Neurocutaneous syndromes associated with pigmentary skin lesions. Journal of the American Academy of Dermatology 32:915–935.

# Chapter 4

# Adult foot disorders

*Jean Mooney and Robert Campbell*

## KEYWORDS

Achilles tendonitis
Adductor forefoot
Ankylosing spondylitis
Asymmetrical bowing
Atavistic foot
Bursae
Calcaneonavicular fusion
Capsulitis
Chondromalacia
Clinical biomechanical analysis
Compensated forefoot varus
Crushing apophysitis
Deep retrocalcaneal bursitis
Everted or valgus forefoot
Flat foot
Focal hyperkeratoses
Foot flat
Forefoot supinatus
Forefoot varus
Forefoot valgus
Freiberg's disease
Freiberg's infraction
Functional hallux limitus
Functional metatarsalgia
Gait cycle
Ganglia/ganglionic cyst
Genu valga/valgum (knock knees)
Genu vara/varum (bow leg)
Gouty tophus
Haglund's deformity
Hallux abducto valgus
Hallux limitus/rigidus flexus
Heel lift
Heel pain syndrome
Heel strike
Hypermobile medial column/first ray
Iselin's disease
Joint motion
Kohler's disease
Leg length discrepancy (LLD)
March fracture
Metatarsalgia
Metatarsus primus elevatus
Midstance
Mobile adaptor
Morton's neuroma
Myalgia
Neoplastic disease
Neutral position of the joints
Non-functional metatarsalgia
Osteoarthritis and osteoarthrosis
Osteochondritis dissicans
Osteochondrosis
Osteomyelitis

Painful neuropathy
Paraesthesia
Pes cavus/mobile pes cavus
Pes plano valgus/pes valgus
Pes planus
Plantar fasciitis
Plantar fibromatosis
Plantar-flexed fifth metatarsal
Plantar heel pain
Plantar plate rupture
Policeman's heel
Principle of compensation
Rearfoot varus/valgus
Rheumatological diseases
Ruptured Achilles tendon
Sagittal plane blockade/valgus
Sever's disease
Stance phase
Stress fractures
Subcalcaneal bursitis
Superficial retrocalcaneal bursitis
Tarsal arthritis
Tarsal coalition
Tarsal tunnel syndrome
Tibia vara (bowleg)
Tibialis posterior tendon dysfunction
Toe-off
Traction (or distraction) apophysitis
Uncompensated forefoot valgus varus
Uncompensated rearfoot varus

## CLINICAL BIOMECHANICS

Clinical biomechanical analysis of foot and leg function is essentially qualitative and an exercise in observation and examination:

- observation and quantification of the position of the joints and functional segments of the body
- examination of the quality, range and direction of motion of the joints and functional segments of the limb
- observation, quantification and examination of the functioning limb in gait and movement.

The technological advances that have allowed greater quantitative analysis of gait and movement and decreased subjectivity in biomechanical examination have impacted on therapy, prescription, provision and evaluation. Thus, the practitioner must be fully conversant with biomechanical terminology and have a good knowledge of lower-limb and foot anatomy.

### The neutral or reference position

The neutral position of the joints of the lower limb is used as a reference point from which the clinician can describe and observe variations from the norm and also facilitate anthropometric measurement. They were defined and described by Root et al (1971, 1977), and reviewed by Brown and Yavorsky (1987) as equating to the position adopted by the foot and lower limb in the normal subject when standing in the normal angle and base of gait (Seibel 1988).

The *hip joint* is in the neutral position when the leg is in line with the trunk in the sagittal plane, the femoral condyles lie in the frontal plane and the legs are parallel to one another with the feet slightly apart and abducted. From this position the hip joint can flex, extend, adduct, abduct, internally and externally rotate and circumduct.

The *knee* is in the neutral position when the joint is fully extended and the thigh and lower leg are in line. From this position, the knee joint can flex only.

The *ankle joint* is in the neutral position when the foot lies on a flat horizontal weight-bearing surface and the leg is perpendicular. From this position, the ankle joint may dorsiflex and plantar flex.

The *subtalar joint* is reputed to be in, or near to, its hypothetical neutral position when the posterior aspect of the calcaneum is perpendicular to the weight-bearing surface. From this position the subtalar joint may supinate and pronate.

The *midtarsal joint complex* is in its neutral position when all metatarsal heads lie on the horizontal weight-bearing surface and the joint is maximally pronated. From this position, the midtarsal joint complex can supinate only.

The *first metatarsophalangeal joint (MTPJ)* is in its neutral position when the plantar aspect of the hallux is in ground contact and the hallux is neither adducted nor abducted. From this position, the first MTPJ may dorsiflex, plantar flex, adduct, abduct and circumduct.

The *first ray* is in its neutral position when the first metatarsal head is in line with the lesser metatarsal heads and all the metatarsal heads lie parallel to the ground. From this position, the first ray can dorsiflex and invert, and also plantar flex and evert.

The *lesser rays (2, 3 and 4)* tend to function as a single unit. They are in a neutral position when they are at their most dorsiflexed and lying parallel to the weight-bearing surface. From this position, the lesser rays can plantar flex only.

The *fifth ray* is in neutral when lying parallel to the weight-bearing surface (i.e. on the transverse plane) with the fifth metatarsal head in line with the other metatarsal heads. From this position, the fifth ray can dorsiflex and invert, and also plantar flex and evert.

## The principle of compensation

The principle of compensation simply means that, if a joint or body segment functions in an abnormal manner, then an adjacent joint or body segment may alter its function in an attempt to normalise the function of the body as a whole (Root et al 1977).

Joint motion may be classed as abnormal if the total range of motion of the joint is too great, too little, in the wrong direction or of poor quality (e.g. a knee joint capable of hyperextension, or a subtalar joint that exhibits supination from neutral but no pronation). Joint position may be abnormal if the adjacent bones and body segments are malformed, damaged due to trauma or disease, or are misaligned.

For example, a subject with a dropped foot will, during gait, compensate for this abnormality by increasing knee and hip flexion. Therefore, the knee joint and the hip joint have compensated for the abnormal motion at the foot. Consequently, the hip or knee may, in the long term, exhibit pathologies that have originated from malfunction of the foot.

During locomotion, if all the criteria for normalcy are met there is no need for compensatory mechanisms to occur. The limb will function, in normal activity, with no undue stress, except perhaps in the case of overuse. However, if there are deviations from the norm, then abnormal motion or stress may result. This, in turn, may lead to stress-type injuries in the short term or permanent deformity in the longer term.

There are a number of abnormalities or variations from the norm that may result in abnormal foot and leg function and culminate in foot and leg pathology.

## The gait or walking cycle

The gait cycle describes the sequence of events that occur during normal walking on a flat and level surface. It identifies, describes, analyses and evaluates all aspects of gait. The gait cycle lists sequential events that occur in one limb during one complete stride (i.e. from the initial heel contact (heel strike) of one foot, to the initial heel contact of the same foot at the start of the next stride). It is divided into the stance phase (when the foot or part of the foot is in contact with the walking surface) and the swing phase (when the foot is swinging from one episode of ground contact to the next).

The stance phase is further subdivided into three periods: the contact period, the midstance period and the propulsive period. Simplistically, the foot and limb should be unlocked and mobile to cope with the impact of ground contact during the contact period, be a rigid and stable lever for propulsion during the propulsive period, and be converting from one state to the other during the midstance period.

The contact period of the stance phase of gait occurs from heel strike (i.e. the instant the posterior lateral aspect of the heel contacts the walking surface) to foot flat – (i.e. the instant the weight-bearing surface of the foot begins contact with the walking surface). During this period the foot comes into contact with the ground, the foot and lower limb decelerate rapidly and are subject to high impact forces, which are typically 115% of body weight. The foot and limb at this point should be unlocked and relatively mobile to allow instantaneous adaptation to variations in the walking surface and to allow attenuation of the high ground contact impact forces – this is termed shock absorption or attenuation. The foot and limb are often described as a 'mobile adaptor' during the contact period of the stance phase of gait.

The midstance period of the stance phase of gait occurs from foot flat to heel lift. It describes the period in time when the total weight-bearing surface of the plantar aspect of the foot is in ground contact.

The propulsive period of the stance phase of gait occurs from heel lift to toe-off (i.e. the instant the toes lift off the weight-bearing surface). During the propulsive period, the foot and limb undergo acceleration and propel the body weight forward, on to the contralateral leg. The foot should be locked and rigid to form a stable base for propulsion and to be able to deal efficiently with the propulsive forces, which are typically 112% of body weight. The foot and limb are often described as a 'rigid lever' during the propulsive period of the stance phase of gait.

## Activity of the muscles and joints of the limb in gait

To comprehend lower limb function during gait and activity the practitioner should be aware of the action of all joints, muscles and other soft tissue structures of the limb, and be able to extrapolate the effects that abnormal activity or abnormal musculoskeletal function may have on the overall health of the limb. Functional anatomy of the lower limb is described in Chapters 14 and 15. In particular the practitioner should consider:

- the axes of motion of the major joint complexes of the lower limb, during walking and running.
- the phasic activity of the muscles of the lower limb, during walking and running.
- the effects that the environment (footwear, surfaces) has on lower limb function.

## LOWER LIMB AND FOOT ANOMALIES

Functions of the elements of the lower limb and foot may be described in terms of their relationship to the cardinal planes. Similarly, dysfunction of the limb and foot segments may be categorised in relation to positional deviations from and malalignments along body planes. The functional anomalies and positional variants within the lower limb and foot described in the next section of this chapter are categorised in terms of deviations from the cardinal body planes (i.e. deviations from the frontal, sagittal and transverse body planes).

## FRONTAL PLANE ANOMALIES OF THE LOWER LIMB AND FOOT

### Leg-length discrepancy

The effect of leg-length discrepancy (LLD) on foot and leg function has been, and still is, controversial. It is generally accepted that a significant LLD will affect pain-free normal function of the lumbar spine, the limb and the foot. However, there is considerable disagreement as to what constitutes a 'significant' discrepancy. The obvious difficulty in the precise assessment of the true limb length difference adds to the debate.

### Incidence of LLD

A number of studies have been carried out on the epidemiology of LLD. Most agree that a minor degree of difference in limb length of 1–2 cm is extremely common and occurs in around 90% of the population, and is of little clinical significance (Blustein & D'Amico 1985).

### Causes of LLD

Blustein and D'Amico (1985) attributed LLDs to idiopathic unequal development (53%), unilateral coxa vara (3%), pelvic abnormalities (3%), fractures with shortening (11%), fractures with lengthening (7%), postsurgical shortening (3%) and unilateral subtalar joint pronation (1%). The remaining 19% result from a number of diseases and abnormalities, including neurological disorders (e.g. polio, cerebral palsy), rickets, osteomyelitis, slipped capital femoral epiphysis, irradiation-therapy effects and sciatic nerve injury.

### Effects of LLD

LLDs are associated with a variety of types of musculoskeletal imbalance, including altered gait patterns, equinus contracture at the ankle and increased energy expenditure in gait (Gurney 2002). However, there is no consistent pattern common to all individuals. LLD alters the magnitude of forces acting through joints and also changes the area of force distribution by altering the area of the joint surface that is subject to load. Runners with LLD tend to present with increased vertebral disc and low-back symptoms, and increased incidence of tibial stress fractures, knee pain, shin splints, painful heel syndrome, symptomatic hallux valgus, and sciatica (Fig. 4.1).

The effects of LLD include:

- An increase in activity of the lumbar spine musculature to control the associated spinal scoliosis (Vink & Kamphuisen 1989). Initially the scoliosis involves only the soft tissues, but it has been suggested that, over time, the scoliosis may become osseous and permanent. The pain in the lumbar spine causes a change in the vertebral joint congruency and changes the

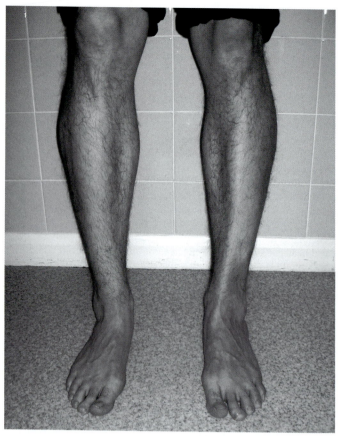

**Figure 4.1** Leg-length discrepancy: 3 cm limb-length discrepancy in a 28-year-old man. The patient was unable to give the cause of his limb-length difference, other than he had spent several months in hospital when 12 years old because his 'left leg was not growing properly'. The patient habitually toe walks on the left foot, and pronates excessively on the right. Examination showed normal sensation and tendon jerks in both legs and no loss of muscle power, although there was a reduction of the muscle bulk on the left side. The forced supination of the left foot is marked by the contraction of the tibialis anterior muscle. He is treated with orthotic therapy to redress the difference in limb length and to control the excessive right foot pronation.

pattern of mechanical stresses within the joints of the lumbar spine. Tensile stress is increased at the short-leg side of the joint (or joints) and compressive stress is increased on the long-leg side. Consequently, the strain on the ligamentous and muscular structures of the spine is asymmetrical and the intravertebral disc becomes wedge shaped. There is also a tendency for body weight to be shifted to the longer leg (Hansen 1993), which often results in lowering of the shoulder on the long-leg side.

- A high correlation (97%) between asymmetrical pronation and LLD (Manello 1992). The subtalar joint of the longer leg undergoes pronation, with supination of the subtalar joint in the shorter leg. Unilateral subtalar joint pronation can be a cause or an effect of LLD. Unilateral pronation can cause anterior knee pain (Chambers 1983).

- An LLD of more than 2 cm can predispose the patient to both early heel lift/ankle equinus on the shorter leg and increased pelvic tilt. These result in reduced or absent heel strike (Menelaus 1991).

- The patient is likely to show an asymmetrical pelvic rotation and uneven arm swing. The hand will be lower on the side of the longer leg, and the shoulders uneven. The shorter leg has to cover the same distance in the same time in an attempt to achieve gait symmetry. Consequently, the shorter leg travels faster, and in effect goes further (proportionally to the length of the leg). The contralateral arm, on the long side, swings further and faster to counterbalance this.

- The patient presents with a shoulder tilt, reciprocating the increased pelvic tilt and the spinal scoliosis.
- Scoliosis of the spine – as a result of the increased pelvic tilt.
- Increased mechanical stress on the hip joint of the longer limb, often resulting in a unilateral osteoarthritis.
- Knee pathologies, due to the failure of the knee on the long side to achieve full extension prior to heel contact. As the flexed knee is not locked, it can cause ligamentous strain and weakness of vastus medialis muscle.
- In 80% of cases of LLD presenting symptoms are worse in the longer limb. This may be due to increased stresses in the longer limb secondary to excessive foot pronation, increased stance time, and internal rotation and incomplete extension of the knee. However, the remaining 20% of cases of LLD have symptoms affecting the shorter limb, and no satisfactory hypotheses have yet been offered to explain this inequality.

## Symptoms of LLD

Symptoms of LLD include arthritis of the knee, psoasitis, anterior knee pain, shin splints, metatarsalgia, sacroiliitis, Achilles tendonitis, quadriceps strain, pes anserinus bursitis, groin (adductor) strain, peroneal tendonitis, neck pain, intermetatarsal neuroma, osteitis pubis, sesamoiditis and sinus tarsi syndrome.

## Significance of the degree of LLD

The literature on the degree to which LLD is likely to produce pathological symptoms is contradictory. The view propounded by Subotnick (1981) suggests that the significance of LLD is relative to the patient's activity levels:

> Minor LLD which would cause significant symptoms in the active athlete … tend to be 3 times more significant when running rather than when walking … the 1/4 inch LLD is therefore as significant in the athlete as the 3/4 inch LLD is in the non-athletic person.

However, even asymptomatic LLD should always be regarded as significant in patients who have lower limb and lower back pathologies.

## Assessment and measurement of LLD

There are two presentations of LLD: true LLD and apparent LLD. It is not always straightforward to determine whether the patient has a true or an apparent LLD. True LLD is noted when the patient presents with a difference in the lengths of the tibiae, femurs or both. An apparent LLD will occur when there is pelvic asymmetry, such as a scoliosis and resultant pelvic tilt, or foot asymmetry such as unilateral subtalar joint excessive pronation or supination.

Measurements, made using a standard tape measure with the patient lying supine, include:

- anterior superior iliac spine to medial malleolus
- greater trochanter to lateral malleolus and sternum to medial malleolus.

The subject can also be assessed in the normal angle and base of gait, and the symmetry of the following may be assessed or measured:

- Equity within the pectoral girdle: shoulder line; hand fall.
- Equity within the pelvic girdle: anterior superior iliac spines, iliac crests, posterior superior iliac spines, gluteal folds, popliteal creases.
- Limb equity: patellae height; height of the tibial tubercles from the floor.

## Management of LLD

LLD is managed by applying height correction to the short limb, and the use of orthoses to control problems in the long limb associated with excessive foot pronation.

- A simple heel lift has been shown to be very effective in controlling symptoms such as low back pain, sciatica and hip pathologies (Freiberg 1983).
- The heel lift can be incorporated in a functional foot orthosis with inbuilt heel lift when the foot and limb pathology warrants such intervention.
- Where the LLD is greater than 2 cm, the use of heel lift is contraindicated. A full-length sole lift, with or without an in-shoe orthosis, should be used to ensure that the patient does not overload the forefoot on the short limb.

### CASE STUDY 4.1 LEG-LENGTH DISCREPANCY

A 27-year-old male recreational runner presented with unilateral, right-side patellofemoral pain, which was induced by exercise and relieved by rest. He had been involved in a road traffic accident 12 years previously, requiring open reduction of lower shaft fractures of the left tibia and fibula. Relaxed calcaneal stance evaluation revealed a right-sided tibial varum, with an excessively pronated foot and internally rotated limb, as noted on patellar squinting. The left leg was within normal limits. The pelvis and knees were symmetrical in the frontal plane.

Neutral calcaneal stance evaluation corrected the alignment of the right limb and foot but created a frontal plane asymmetry in that the knee and pelvis were higher on the right side. It was assumed that his previous surgery may have reduced a congenital tibia vara on the left side and also resulted in slight shortening of the left lower leg. A casted orthosis, posted for rearfoot varus, was fitted to the right shoe and a heel raise fitted in the left. The subject returned to his past level of running with no further problems reported.

## The inverted or varus rearfoot

### Coxa valgum, genu vara, tibia vara (bowleg)

*Coxa valgum* is a frontal plane malalignment of the hip, where the angulation between the femoral neck and the shaft of the femur is greater than 135°. It usually occurs as the outcome of slipped epiphysis of the femoral head. It creates an LLD with relative lengthening of the affected leg. It may induce a limp, together with compensatory pronation within the leg, such as external femoral rotation, internal tibial torsion and pes planus. Cases with coxa valgum usually show genu vara (Hammer 1999).

*Genu vara* and *tibia vara* are frontal plane malalignments of the lower limb, which affect foot and limb function in the same way as a rearfoot varus. In genu vara and tibia vara, the anterior aspect of the subject's thigh will be in a valgus position and the lower leg will be in a varus position when the patient stands in relaxed calcaneal stance. The condition is characterised by 'bowing' of the legs and a noticeable gap between the knees when the patient stands erect.

*Distal tibia vara* is a condition where the lower third of the tibia adopts an inverted (varus) position. When the subject stands erect, the legs will be straight from the hip to the lower third of the tibia, but the lower third of the tibia bows in a varus position. Tibia vara of 5°–10° is normal in the infant and anything up to 5° is probably of little significance in the adult, except perhaps in the overuse situation. Infantile tibia vara usually corrects with maturity. However, not all paediatric or developmental bowlegs will resolve. Pointers for the diagnosis of non-correcting bowlegs are:

- marked local bowing of the leg
- asymmetrical bowing.

## Rearfoot varus

Rearfoot varus is defined as a congenital structural abnormality of the rearfoot, where the rearfoot is inverted relative to the weight-bearing surface, when the subtalar joint is in its neutral position and the midtarsal joint is maximally pronated around both axes. A functional rearfoot varus occurs as a result of a varus attitude of the leg (Pickard 1983, Sgarlatto 1971).

### Causes of rearfoot varus

This frontal-plane deformity most commonly arises as a result of a congenital varus abnormality of the leg or foot. Occasionally fractures or other severe trauma, particularly to growing bones, may result in a unilateral abnormality. Rearfoot varus arises as a result of subjects displaying genu vara (bow legs), tibia vara (bowing of the lower third of the tibia) and tibial epiphyseal vara (varus abnormality of the tibial epiphysis). In the foot, a varus deformity arises as a horizontal plane anomaly of the talus (talar vara), the calcaneus (calcaneal vara) or the subtalar joint (subtalar vara).

Rearfoot varus is present in a significant proportion of the population (Hopper et al 1994, Powers et al 1995). As rearfoot varus of less than 4° is present in 98% of the population (McPoil et al 1988) it could be considered as a normal structural variant, which is congenital in the sense that the subject either is born with the variant or has inherited the trait to develop the variant as they grow. These abnormalities are often very mild and may be quite subtle. However, even mild abnormality may result in foot and leg pathologies if coupled with high levels of physical activity. The sequelae of rearfoot varus can become increasingly apparent with age.

### Classifications of rearfoot varus

Rearfoot varus is traditionally classified according to the ability of the subtalar joint to compensate for the abnormality.

- *Uncompensated rearfoot varus* occurs when there is no additional (abnormal) compensatory pronation of the subtalar joint available to rotate the heel toward the support surface. The foot remains inverted during stance.
- *Fully compensated rearfoot varus* is said to occur when there is sufficient subtalar joint pronation to allow the plantar aspect of the heel to contact the ground fully, allowing ground reaction forces to be fairly evenly distributed across the heel and, therefore, the foot.
- *Partially compensated rearfoot varus* occurs when there is some pronation available to compensate in part for the abnormality but insufficient to allow full and effective weight bearing of the rearfoot (Pickard 1983, Sgarlatto 1971).

### Compensatory mechanisms in rearfoot varus

The normal foot will present to the ground (at initial contact) in a slightly inverted position. Ground reaction force on the lateral infe-rior–posterior aspect of the heel induces rearfoot pronation, as the foot will rotate the foot around the axis of the subtalar joint until the entire plantar aspect of the heel contacts the weight-bearing surface (Perry 1992, Root et al 1977). In rearfoot varus the foot is in a more inverted position at the start of the contact period, and therefore a greater degree of subtalar joint pronation is required to rotate the foot to allow the plantar aspect to contact the weight-bearing surface. The additional subtalar joint pronation is termed 'compensation', and compensatory subtalar joint pronation is abnormal and excessive.

Excessive pronation at the subtalar joint increases the range of motion of the forefoot on the rearfoot at the midtarsal joint, and tends to load the medial side of the foot during the midstance period. Ground reaction force acting on the medial side of the forefoot causes supination of the midtarsal joint, so that the foot remains unlocked and hypermobile during the latter half of the stance phase of gait, when it should be locked and stable for propulsion. However, as it is the abnormally inverted position of the rearfoot that is the cause of the excessive pronation, the foot may rapidly supinate and recover some or all of its stability before toe-off once the heel is raised off the ground at the end of the midstance period. Consequently, rearfoot varus abnormalities tend to be less destructive to foot function than do forefoot abnormalities. Nevertheless, the hypermobility and reduction in osseous stability of the foot, which are characteristic of rearfoot varus, may result in progressive ligamentous laxity and resultant greater pronation than is required to compensate for the inverted rearfoot (Pickard 1983, Root et al 1977, Subotnick 1975).

### Other compensatory mechanisms in rearfoot varus

In addition to an increased amount of pronation at the subtalar joint, rearfoot varus may be compensated by plantar flexion of the distal part of the first metatarsal and by gait modification.

- *Plantar flexion of the first ray*. In some instances, where there is insufficient subtalar joint pronation to compensate for the abnormality, the first metatarsal head may move plantarwards and enable ground contact of the medial side of the forefoot. It is thought that this is brought about by the contraction of the peroneus (fibularis) longus muscle causing plantar flexion of the first metatarsal.
- *Gait modification*. The subject may abduct the foot using the lateral side of the forefoot as a pivot (abductory twist). The abductory twist is visualised as the heel rapidly moving medially after heel lift. This allows the subject to load the medial side of the forefoot after the midpoint of midstance.

### Uncompensated rearfoot varus

This condition will occur where there is no additional subtalar joint pronation available to compensate for the inverted or supinated rearfoot. The calcaneus will remain inverted to the ground during stance, and the medial side of the heel does not bear weight effectively. A true uncompensated rearfoot varus, where there is no compensatory subtalar joint pronation, is an uncommon idiopathic congenital abnormality. It may also arise as the result of earlier limb or foot trauma, after surgical fusion of the rearfoot, subtalar arthritis and neurological pathologies.

In theory, only the lateral side of the foot will bear weight effectively; the midtarsal joint is normal and will be maximally pronated and locked by the ground reaction force acting on the lateral side of the forefoot. As the midtarsal joint cannot pronate further and bring the medial border of the forefoot on the ground, only the lateral side of the forefoot will bear weight. (By definition, this is a rearfoot abnormality. The relationship between the forefoot and the rearfoot is normal.)

### Signs and symptoms of an uncompensated rearfoot varus

These include:

- Superficial hyperkeratotic skin lesions along the lateral border of the foot, including the styloid process.
- Tailor's bunion deformity due to excessive weight bearing on the lateral forefoot, causing abduction of the fifth metatarsal which results in pressure and shear between the fifth metatarsal head and footwear.
- There may be pressure symptoms and lesions under the first metatarsal head if a plantar-flexed first ray is present.
- Lateral (inversion) ankle sprains may occur. This foot type functions in a more inverted position than normal. Uneven walking surfaces or activities requiring rapid changes in direction, such as football and racquet sports, can precipitate forceful inversion of the foot.
- Symptoms that result from disordered shock attenuation. Lack of subtalar joint pronation during the contact period of gait interferes with the normal shock-attenuation process of the leg. This may result in shin, knee and lower spine pathologies.
- Symptoms as a result of disordered transverse-plane motion of the limb. The lack of subtalar joint pronation may result in a reduction in the normal internal rotation of the leg during contact, resulting in knee and shin pathologies.

### Fully compensated rearfoot varus

This condition is characterised by sufficient subtalar joint pronation to allow the plantar aspect of the heel to contact the ground fully, so that ground reaction forces are fairly evenly distributed across the heel and, therefore, the foot.

### Signs and symptoms of fully compensated rearfoot varus

These include:

- Significant lowering of medial 'arch' height on weight bearing.
- Lateral border lesions are less likely, as this foot is plantigrade. However, there are often signs of excessive lateral shoe wear.
- Varying degrees of Haglund's deformity (see rearfoot disorders, below) may be present due to irritation of the lateral–posterior–superior border of the calcaneus, lateral to the insertion of the Achilles tendon. The irritation is brought about by rapid and excessive contact-phase pronation. The heel linings of footwear, particularly sports shoes, often wear through at the corresponding point, due to the excessive movement of the foot within the shoe (Fig. 4.2).

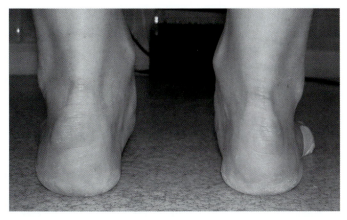

**Figure 4.2** Haglund's deformity. Superficial bursitis and some exostosis formation, particularly on the left heel.

- Reduced first MTPJ motion is common, even in the younger subject with no joint pathology (see Stage 1 functional hallux limitus, in the section on hallux limitus/rigidus, below). The excessively pronated foot restricts the ability of the first metatarsal to plantar flex and move backwards to facilitate dorsiflexion of the hallux after heel lift. This causes restriction to passive and/or active dorsiflexion of the MTPJ, and eventually may cause permanent damage to the dorsal surface of the joint, and structural hallux limitus.
- Tailor's bunion deformity due to forefoot hypermobility is common, as a result of the excessive pronation of the subtalar joint, coupled with excessive lateral loading of the foot during the contact period.
- The re-supinator muscles may become fatigued and traumatised as they attempt to supinate the foot rapidly after heel lift. This often presents clinically as anterior or posterior 'shin splints'.
- Low back pain is also associated with rearfoot varus. The causal mechanism is not well documented but has been hypothesised by Dananberg (1996).
- As in uncompensated rearfoot varus, lateral (inversion) ankle sprains are common, especially in the physically active.

### Partially compensated rearfoot varus

This rearfoot condition is characterised by some available subtalar joint pronation to compensate in part for the abnormality but insufficient subtalar joint pronation to allow full and effective weight bearing of the rearfoot.

### Signs and symptoms of partially compensated rearfoot varus

The signs and symptoms of partially compensated rearfoot varus vary in accordance with the amount of compensation available at the subtalar joint, and reflect aspects of the clinical picture of both compensated and non-compensated rearfoot varus.

### Treatment of rearfoot varus

- *Compensated rearfoot varus.* In the short term, symptomatic treatment using clinical padding, strapping and physical therapies is appropriate. However, the long-term aim is to negate the need for compensatory pronation of the subtalar joint. This is usually achieved by functional foot orthoses with intrinsic or extrinsic medial posting. In cases where high levels of physical activity compound the symptoms, full-length orthoses may be required (Fig. 4.3).
- *Uncompensated rearfoot varus.* Feet with uncompensated rearfoot varus lack mobility and thus are less amenable to functional orthoses. Accommodative orthoses, which off-load and protect, with appropriate shoe advice and local treatment strategies are appropriate.

## Varus rearfoot

Distinction must be drawn between a rearfoot varus (a primary abnormality) and a foot that adopts or functions in a varus position secondary to a malalignment elsewhere in the limb or secondary to another pathology.

The rearfoot may adopt a varus attitude when the subject is standing in a relaxed posture (relaxed calcaneal stance), or the foot may function during gait in a greater degree of varus than is the accepted norm. This may be due to an uncompensated rearfoot varus abnormality, but equally may be due to compensatory movement of the rearfoot as a result of a forefoot valgus or other abnormality that results in compensatory supination of the foot. A varus rearfoot may also be a feature of a neurological pathology.

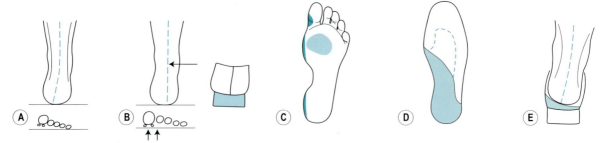

**Figure 4.3** Rearfoot varus. (A) uncompensated rearfoot varus; (B) compensated rearfoot varus; (C) pattern of hyperkeratotic lesions in the compensated foot; (D and E) orthotic therapy and shoe modification to control compensation.

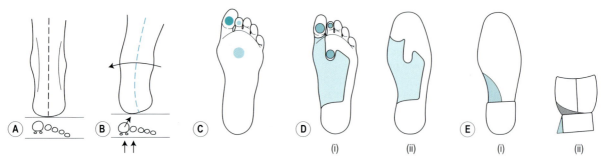

**Figure 4.4** Forefoot varus. (A) normal contact in midstance; (B) pronating after midstance; (C) site of hyperkeratotic lesions; (D) (i) adhesive deflective/protective padding on the foot; (D) (ii) the same padding applied in the shoe on an insole; (E) (i) extended heel on sole of shoe (Thomas heel); (E) (ii) medial heel wedging in the shoe and flare (buttress) on the medial side of the heel of the shoe.

## The inverted or varus forefoot

### Forefoot varus

Forefoot varus is a congenital osseous structural deformity in which the plantar plane of the forefoot is inverted relative to the plantar plane of the rearfoot when the subtalar joint is in its neutral position and the midtarsal joint is maximally pronated around both its axes (Bowden 1983, Hlavlac 1971). A true osseous forefoot varus is probably fairly rare, especially in adults, as years of walking in an overpronated manner on a consequently hypermobile foot is likely to result in soft tissue adaptation (Fig. 4.4).

### Causes of forefoot varus

Forefoot varus is assumed to be an inherited structural condition where there is reduction in the normal developmental valgus rotation of the head and neck of the talus. This theory is not well supported in the literature. This normal developmental, rotational, process is thought to be complete by the age of 6 years. However, there is some evidence that, in some cases, this process takes longer (O'Donnell 1988). Therefore, a forefoot varus is not uncommon in infants under 6 years of age, but by this age (or a little older) developmental valgus rotation of the head and neck of the talus should have brought the forefoot and the rearfoot parallel to one another and parallel to the weight-bearing surface.

### Classifications of forefoot varus

Forefoot varus is traditionally classified according to the amount of available compensatory subtalar joint pronation. Therefore, a forefoot varus is fully compensated when there is sufficient abnormal excessive subtalar joint pronation to compensate for the forefoot abnormality, uncompensated when there is no available compensatory subtalar joint pronation, and partially compensated when there is some avail-

able subtalar joint pronation but insufficient to allow full forefoot compensation.

### Compensatory mechanisms in forefoot varus

In the normal foot, at the midpoint of midstance, the calcaneus is vertical (or possibly slightly inverted), the subtalar joint is near its neutral position, the midtarsal joint is maximally pronated about both its axes, and the plantar planes of the forefoot, and rearfoot are parallel to one another and parallel to the ground.

- In an *uncompensated forefoot varus*, at the midpoint of midstance, theoretically the plantar plane of the forefoot is inverted relative to the plantar plane of the rearfoot and inverted relative to the ground, the calcaneum is vertical, the subtalar joint is in its neutral position and the midtarsal joint is maximally pronated about both its axes. The uncompensated forefoot varus foot weight bears as normal until the fifth metatarsal head comes into ground contact, after which excess rearfoot and/or midtarsal joint pronation would be required to allow the medial plantar forefoot to make ground contact. As the midtarsal joint is already maximally pronated and no further compensatory pronation is available at the subtalar joint, at the midpoint of stance the patient must externally rotate the lower limb. The foot pivots about the fifth metatarsophalangeal head, abducting the whole foot and loading the medial plantar forefoot (i.e. the patient undergoes abductory twist, see above).

- In a *fully compensated forefoot varus*, foot contact is normal until the midpoint of midstance (Fig. 4.4A), when the foot continues pronating to allow the medial side of the foot to bear weight (Fig. 4.4B). The calcaneum therefore becomes everted, as the subtalar joint is abnormally and excessively pronated. Because the midtarsal joint is maximally pronated, the forefoot will only bear weight if the subtalar joint abnormally and excessively pronates. The plantar plane of the forefoot is still inverted relative to the plantar plane of the rearfoot, but it is weight bearing and is therefore parallel to the ground. This excessive compensatory subtalar joint pronation increases the range of motion of the midtarsal joint. The midtarsal joint is therefore unlocked; the forefoot is hypermobile and will distort under load.

- A *partially compensated forefoot varus* is one in which there is some compensatory pronation available at the subtalar joint but insufficient to allow the forefoot to evert completely on to the weight-bearing surface.

### Fully compensated forefoot varus

This occurs in a foot with sufficient available subtalar joint pronation to compensate for the inversion of the forefoot. To allow the medial side of the plantar surface to come into ground contact the foot must pronate excessively at the subtalar joint (the midtarsal joint is already pronated maximally). This excessive pronation of the subtalar joint increases the range of motion of the midtarsal joint, so that the midtarsal joint and the forefoot become hypermobile (i.e. the forefoot is more mobile than it should be, particularly during the propulsive period of the stance phase of gait).

### Signs and symptoms of fully compensated forefoot varus

These include:

- Calcaneal eversion in static stance and during gait from midstance to toe-off.
- Abduction of the forefoot on the rearfoot as a result of the excessive abnormal subtalar joint pronation.
- Excessive lowering of the medial border on weight bearing due to abnormal and excessive pronation of the subtalar joint.
- Forefoot deformity, as a result of forefoot hypermobility, during the propulsive period of the stance phase of gait, including hallux abducto valgus, lesser toe deformities and associated skin lesions.
- Plantar fasciitis, plantar digital neuritis, non-specific 'arch' strains and ankle tendonopathies are now associated with forefoot varus and excessive pronation of the subtalar joint.
- Thigh, groin, shin and knee problems related to excessive pronation of the subtalar joint and associated excessive internal rotation of the limb.
- Low back pain (as a result of disruption to the shock-absorbing mechanism, and functional hallux limitus).

### Uncompensated forefoot varus

A foot shows uncompensated forefoot varus when there is no available additional subtalar joint pronation to compensate for an inverted forefoot. This type of foot is characteristically relatively immobile and has poor shock-absorption qualities. It is often seen in conjunction with a rearfoot varus where all the available subtalar joint pronation has been used up to facilitate heel contact. Severe and marked uncompensated forefoot varus is characteristic of talipes equinovarus.

### Signs and symptoms of uncompensated forefoot varus

- The calcaneus remains vertical (or slightly inverted) at the end of the contact period and there is excessive lateral weight bearing during stance.
- An abductory twist of the foot occurs as the heel lifts after midstance, and the heel is seen to adduct towards the midline of the body. This facilitates medial forefoot contact in the late stance phase and may result in lesions over the interphalangeal joint of the hallux.
- Gross forefoot disruption is unusual, as the forefoot is locked and rigid during propulsion.
- Knee problems are possible due to abductory twist and abnormal leg rotation.
- In some cases, compensatory plantar flexion of the first metatarsal may occur.

### Partially compensated forefoot varus

A foot with partially compensated forefoot varus is characterised by some available compensatory subtalar joint pronation, but insufficient to allow the forefoot to evert completely or to fully contact the weight-bearing surface.

### Signs and symptoms of partially compensated forefoot varus

Partially compensated forefoot varus shows a mix of the features of fully and uncompensated forefoot varus, depending on the degree of compensation and where this takes place.

### Treatment of forefoot varus

In fully compensated forefoot varus, orthoses designed to reduce the compensatory excessive pronation of the subtalar joint, and consequently reduce the hypermobility of the forefoot, are appropriate. Uncompensated forefoot varus requires an orthosis that will accommodate for the abnormality.

## Forefoot supinatus

Forefoot supinatus is an acquired soft tissue deformity of the longitudinal axis of the midtarsal joint, where the forefoot is inverted relative to the rearfoot when the subtalar joint is in the neutral position and the midtarsal joint is maximally pronated around both its axes. The condition arises secondary to long-term (>15 years) excessive pronation at the subtalar joint, where eversion of the calcaneum ultimately results in compensatory forced inversion of the forefoot. Initially the foot can recover its normal position when off-loaded, but with time the local soft tissues become stretched and lose their ability to correct the forefoot back to its normal position (Davis' law), so that the forefoot adopts an abnormal compensatory position (Redmond 2009).

### Causes of forefoot supinatus

Any abnormality or condition that results in excessive pronation of the subtalar joint with resultant eversion of the calcaneum, including forefoot varus, ankle equinus and abnormal limb positions will predispose to the development of forefoot supinatus.

### Clinical recognition of forefoot supinatus

The foot with forefoot supinatus will appear as a foot with forefoot varus. The two conditions are differentiated by the application of a pronatory force to the dorsum of the foot at the talonavicular joint (Hubscher manoeuvre):

- in a forefoot supinatus, spongy resistance to this pronatory force is felt and the forefoot inversion will reduce
- in a forefoot varus, firm resistance to the pronatory force is felt and the forefoot inversion will only reduce if the subtalar joint is allowed to evert (Beeson 2002).

### Treatment of forefoot supinatus

Forefoot supinatus is treated by controlling abnormal calcaneal eversion. A forefoot supinatus should not be supported by an orthosis, as this tends to exacerbate the condition. Instead, the soft tissue supinatus contracture of the forefoot should be totally or partially reduced when taking the plaster impression of the forefoot, and the orthosis manufactured to reflect this degree of control of calcaneal eversion, which may result in long-term reduction of the supinatus.

---

### CASE STUDY 4.2 **TARSAL COALITION**

A 13-year-old boy was brought to the clinic by his mother, as she was concerned about his 'flat feet and clumsy gait'. The patient was extremely tall for his age and of slim build. He experienced no pain or discomfort in his feet or legs under normal circumstances, but remarked that his feet sometimes ached after PE at school. He also admitted to disliking running or sports, partly because he was not particularly good at these activities but mainly because his classmates teased him about his running style, saying he 'ran like a duck'.

Examination revealed severe valgus flat feet and an apropulsive gait. Subtalar joint range of movement was extremely limited, with insufficient inversion to reach neutral. There was no pain on palpation, or movement of the foot. Radiographic examination revealed a bilateral talonavicular bar. The boy was diagnosed as having fixed flatfoot, secondary to tarsal coalition. His foot was initially managed by the use of ankle–foot orthoses, after referral to an orthopaedic consultant. It was anticipated that he would require rearfoot surgery after his bones had fully ossified.

---

## The everted or valgus rearfoot

### Coxa vara and genu valga/valgum (knock knees)

Coxa vara is a frontal plane malalignment of the hip, where the angulation between the femoral neck and the shaft of the femur is less than 120°. It may occur as the result of trauma or bone disease, or as a congenital abnormality. It causes a limb-length discrepancy, with relative shortening of the affected leg. It usually induces a limp and compensatory supination within the limb, such as internal femoral rotation, external tibial torsion, ankle equinus and pes cavus. Cases with coxa vara usually show genu valgum.

Genu valgum is a frontal plane malalignment of the lower limb, in which the anterior aspect of the subject's thigh will be in a varus position and the lower leg will be in a valgus position when the patient stands in relaxed calcaneal stance. The condition is characterised by the knees touching or 'knocking' on their medial aspects (knock knees) and a noticeable gap between the feet, measured at the medial malleoli, when the patient stands erect. It is a normal developmental feature in many children, showing most commonly from 2–4 years until 6–8 years, and from 11–12 years until 14–15 years. Genu valgum in adults may result in compensatory excessive pronation of the subtalar joint, especially in the overweight or obese patient. During stance and gait, the centre of mass of the body acts medial to the foot, causing the foot to adopt a pronated position.

### True rearfoot valgus

A true rearfoot valgus is an exceptionally rare primary congenital osseous abnormality. It is defined as a congenital, structural abnormality of the rearfoot, where the rearfoot is everted relative to the weight-bearing surface, when the subtalar joint is in its neutral position and the midtarsal joint is maximally pronated around both axes. However, it is common for the rearfoot to adopt a valgus attitude in relaxed calcaneal stance, due to a number of conditions that are compensated for by excessive pronation of the subtalar joint.

## The valgus rearfoot

A valgus rearfoot, as observed during gait or in relaxed calcaneal stance, is usually a secondary abnormality and appears mostly as a compensation for a primary abnormality elsewhere in the limb or foot, such as forefoot varus, forefoot supinatus, mobile forefoot valgus and genu valgum. A valgus rearfoot can also arise as the result of trauma such as a Pott's or bi-malleolar fracture, agenesis of the distal aspect of the fibula, congenital absence of a fibula, rupture of tibialis posterior tendon, rheumatoid disease, tarsal coalition, Charcot neuroarthropathy and footballer's ankle (Zhang et al 2002).

## The everted or valgus forefoot

### Forefoot valgus

Forefoot valgus is a congenital osseous deformity where the plantar plane of the forefoot is everted relative to the plantar plane of the rearfoot when the subtalar joint is in the neutral position and the midtarsal joint is maximally pronated around both its axes.

#### Causes of forefoot valgus

The head and neck of the talus normally undergoes a valgus rotation on the body of the talus during normal development. In the normal foot, this rotation ceases when the plantar aspect of the forefoot becomes parallel to the plantar aspect of the rearfoot. In forefoot valgus, an excessive amount of developmental valgus rotation can result in the plantar plane of the forefoot being everted in relation to that of the hindfoot. However, a forefoot valgus can also occur if the first metatarsal head lies in on a lower plane than the lesser (two to five) metatarsal heads. This condition is termed a 'plantar-flexed first ray', or 'partial forefoot valgus' (see below).

#### Classification of forefoot valgus

Traditionally, forefoot valgus has been classified as total forefoot valgus or a partial forefoot valgus, due to plantar flexion of the fist ray. Regardless of whether the valgus position of the forefoot is total or due to a plantar flexed first ray, the foot will function in a similar manner.

- In *total forefoot valgus*, the entire plantar plane of the forefoot is everted relative to the plantar plane of the rearfoot. The metatarsal heads are all in line, one with the other, but are everted relative to the rearfoot.
- In *partial forefoot valgus*, the first ray is plantar flexed in relation to the lesser metatarsal heads, which usually lie on the same plane as the rearfoot.

In addition, each type of forefoot valgus, total or partial, is further subdivided into a *mobile* and a *rigid* type. Because of the differences in function of the two types, forefoot valgus tends to present with either of two distinct clinical patterns, that of a rigid-type forefoot valgus or a mobile-type forefoot valgus.

#### Rigid-type forefoot valgus

A foot with rigid forefoot valgus is characteristically rigid and does not tend to adapt under load. The rearfoot is in a normal relationship to the lower leg, so heel contact in stance is normal. Due to the everted forefoot, the first metatarsal head will contact the ground before the fifth, so the forefoot will load from medial to lateral (rather than from the fifth through to the first MTPJ loading as in the normal foot).

Ground reaction force acting at the plantar aspect of the head of the first metatarsal attempts to supinate the forefoot about the longitudinal axis of the midtarsal joint, but as this foot-type is characteristically rigid there will be little or no supination available at the midtarsal joint. Where the midtarsal joint cannot compensate adequately for the forefoot eversion, additional compensatory supination may be required at the subtalar joint. Thus contact-period pronation is reduced, or prevented, by the compensatory supination. The leg is forced into external rotation, with resultant lateral instability at the ankle–subtalar joint complex and the knees.

### Signs and symptoms of rigid forefoot valgus

The foot with rigid forefoot valgus shows a high-arched, 'pes cavus' type foot and calcaneal inversion, both when weight bearing or non-weight bearing. There may be a lateral 'rock' during gait, as normal subtalar pronation abruptly stops and the subtalar joint undergoes early re-supination. This is known as a 'supinatory rock', and may lead to lateral instability and shock-induced pathologies in the shin, knee, hip and lower back, due to the loss of shock attenuation that is part of normal subtalar joint pronation.

The midtarsal joint shows reduced mobility and the lesser toes may be retracted or clawed in an attempt to stabilise the forefoot. There may be hyperkeratotic pressure lesions on the skin overlying the plantar aspects of the first and fifth metatarsal heads and also posterior–lateral calcaneal irritation. Subjects may express difficulty in obtaining suitable footwear because of the high arch and the deformed lesser toes. They may also comment on excessive lateral shoe sole wear.

### Mobile type forefoot valgus

In mobile forefoot valgus heel contact is normal, but the forefoot accepts load under the MTPJs in the order first to fifth (not fifth to first as in the normal foot). The foot is characteristically mobile and distorts under load. The first ray dorsiflexes and the midtarsal joint supinates. There is seldom a need for the subtalar joint to undergo compensatory supination. The net result is forefoot supination, with unlocking of the midtarsal joint and resultant forefoot hypermobility (Fig. 4.5).

### Signs and symptoms of mobile forefoot valgus

The forefoot instability that characterises mobile forefoot valgus (Fig. 4.5A) results in a high incidence of hallux abducto valgus, lesser toe deformities, plantar hyperkeratosis under the central metatarsal heads, fifth toe corns and a tendency to splayed forefoot and tailor's bunion. Plantar fasciitis, plantar digital neuritis, medial sesamoiditis and first metatarsal–cuneiform joint exostosis may also occur. There is a low incidence of postural lesions as rearfoot function tends to be relatively normal. However, in cases where the calcaneum everts (Fig. 4.5B), postural symptoms may occur, including medial knee pain, shin pain and lower back pain.

### Treatment of forefoot valgus

All presentations of forefoot valgus respond to orthotic therapy. Orthoses that accommodate the everted position of the forefoot, or in the case of a plantar flexed first ray accommodate the plantar flexed position of the first metatarsal head, are indicated. Ideally, these orthoses should project distal to the metatarsal heads, although this may not be practicable, as in rigid forefoot valgus this will negate the need for compensatory subtalar supination. In cases of mobile forefoot valgus, orthoses should be designed to reduce the need for first ray dorsiflexion and midtarsal joint supination.

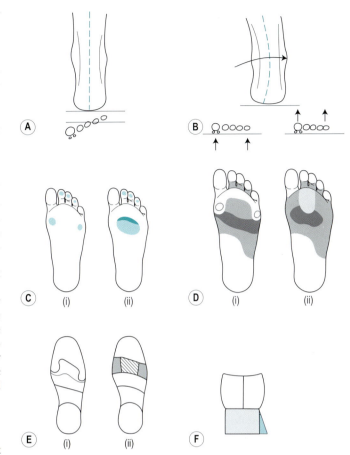

**Figure 4.5** Pes cavus. (A) forefoot valgus, plantar-flexed first ray; (B) hindfoot varus; (C) (i) and (ii) sites for the hyperkeratotic lesions; (D) (i) and (ii) clinical padding to deflect pressure; (E) (i) and (ii) in-shoe or insole padding; (F) buttressed heel on shoe.

## SAGITTAL PLANE ANOMALIES OF THE LOWER LIMB AND FOOT

### Pelvic nutation

Pelvic nutation describes the increase in the angulation of the pelvis in relation to the frontal plane, where the anterior upper poles of the pelvis are oriented more anterior to the frontal plane of the body. This positional variant imposes change within the lower back, such as increased lumbar lordosis, and changes within the lower limb and foot, resulting in excessive foot pronation.

### Genu recurvatum

Genu recurvatum is a common, acquired sagittal plane lower limb anomaly characterised by hyperextension of the knee joint, so that the central part of the lower limb does not lie along the frontal plane. Skeletal deviation is also characterised by soft-tissue laxity at the posterior, posteromedial or posterolateral area of the knee joint throughout weight-bearing gait, with resultant gait effects, including decreased step and stride length, decreased velocity and reduced cadence. Genu recurvatum is noted in association with spasticity of the triceps surae, quadriceps weakness, limb-length discrepancy, hip extensor weakness, generalised joint hypermobility syndromes, ankle equinus and rearfoot varus.

## Ankle equinus

Ankle equinus is a congenital or acquired functional deficiency of sagittal plane motion at the ankle joint, where there is limited dorsiflexion of the ankle (talocrural) joint (Lang 1984) when the subtalar joint is in the neutral position. A minimum of 10° of dorsiflexion is required at the ankle joint to allow normal walking (Rome 1996). Ankle joint dorsiflexion begins just after the midpoint of midstance, allowing forward progression of the trunk over the weight-bearing limb as the knee extends and before the heel lifts off the ground. At this point in the gait cycle, the subtalar joint is in, or near, its neutral position.

### Aetiology and presentations of ankle equinus

A range of foot and limb conditions are characterised by ankle equinus. These include:

- Congenital or acquired contraction of the Achilles tendon complex. Constriction or tightness of the posterior muscle group of the lower leg tends to restrict normal dorsiflexion at the ankle joint. Soft tissue ankle equinus is revealed by testing the range of ankle joint dorsiflexion with the knee extended and the knee flexed. Soft tissue equinus, due to tightness in the gastrocnemius or soleus or both, is noted where the ankle equinus can be reduced by flexing the knee. Where the loss of ankle dorsiflexion is due to a bone anomaly within the ankle joint, the equinus deformity cannot be reduced by flexing the knee. The end feel of the range of the ankle joint movement will be abrupt and hard, as opposed to a soft end feel in soft tissue limitations.
- An apparent or pseudo-ankle equinus can occur in cases where there is a plantar-flexed or equinus forefoot. In this type of foot, a considerable amount of ankle joint dorsiflexion is required to allow the plantar aspect of the forefoot to lie on the same transverse plane as the rearfoot during midstance. There may be an insufficient residual range of dorsiflexion at the ankle joint to allow forward progression of the tibia to reach an angle of 80° with the frontal plane after the midpoint of midstance and before the heel leaves the ground. In this case, the foot functions as an ankle equinus, even though the abnormality is located at the midfoot, not the ankle.
- An equinus gait, also known as 'toe walking' in children, may be due to talipes, spasticity or other neurological disorder. However, a number of small children who are free of pathology habitually toe walk. The problem resolves naturally as the child grows and develops (Tax 1985).
- A unilateral equinus deformity may arise as a compensation for leg-length inequality, with the subject plantar flexing the foot of the shorter leg to improve postural symmetry.
- Excessive use of high-heeled footwear can lead to a bilateral soft tissue equinus, through soft tissue adaptation under the principles of Davis' law (Lang 1984, Rome 1996).

Compensatory dorsiflexion for ankle equinus takes place at the subtalar joint (Fig. 4.6). As the subtalar joint shows trip-planar motion, compensatory dorsiflexion is accompanied by eversion and abduction of the foot. Thus a foot with insufficient ankle dorsiflexion may compensate for the abnormality by forced and excessive pronation of the subtalar joint. This may be observed during barefoot walking by rapid and increased pronation of the subtalar joint, and a loss of height at the medial longitudinal arch as the support limb passes over the stance foot.

### Classification of ankle equinus

Ankle equinus, like other functional abnormalities of the foot, is classified by the degree of effective compensation.

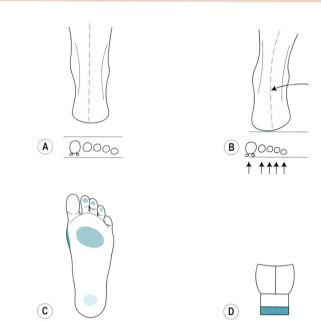

**Figure 4.6** Ankle equinus, short or tight Achilles tendon group. (A) Showing relationship between rearfoot and forefoot; (B) the compensation movements that occur; (C) sites for hyperkeratosis; (D) footwear with extra top piece on heel.

- *Fully compensated ankle equinus* occurs if the foot achieves 10° dorsiflexion, and allows the lower leg to incline to 80° from the transverse plane (10° from the frontal plane) as the body passes over the plantigrade foot. In a normal foot, the ankle joint is able to achieve a minimum of 10° dorsiflexion. With ankle equinus, the ankle joint does not achieve 10° dorsiflexion, and the shortfall is made up from pronation at the subtalar and, if necessary, the midtarsal joints. This compensatory motion at the subtalar and midtarsal joints results in an excessively pronated and hypermobile foot. Fully compensated ankle equinus is one of the most destructive of foot pathologies (Lang 1984, Rome 1996, Sgarlatto 1971). It can result in a grossly pronated foot and may be responsible for actual or incipient hallux abducto valgus, and related sequelae, in children and adolescents. The manifestations of compensated equinus include postural fatigue and other lower-limb pathologies associated with excessive pronation of the subtalar joint. In the foot hallux abducto valgus, lesser toe deformities, digital neuritis, plantar fasciitis, splayed forefoot, abducto-varus fourth and fifth toes, and other hypermobility-related pathologies could be expected.
- *Uncompensated ankle equinus*, where 10° of dorsiflexion cannot be achieved by the combined motions of the ankle, subtalar and midtarsal joints during the stance phase of gait. In this case, the subject bears weight predominantly on the forefoot, resulting in an unstable and apropulsive gait. There may be pressure lesions across the metatarsal heads and lesions associated with clawing of the toes.
- A *partially compensated ankle equinus* occurs where all available ankle dorsiflexion plus abnormal and excessive subtalar joint pronation is still insufficient to allow normal limb movement during midstance. The symptoms associated will be a mix of those associated with uncompensated and fully compensated equinus, depending on the degree of compensation.

Compensation for reduced dorsiflexion at the ankle joint may occur in the lower leg. The subject may show:

- *Premature heel lift*. This compensatory mechanism allows a normal forward progression of the trunk over the stance foot by transferring the inadequate sagittal plane motion of the rearfoot to the MTPJs.
- *Genu recurvatum*. This may occur in cases where soft tissue ankle equinus was present during childhood. The recurved position of the knee reduces the pull on the Achilles tendon, which further shortens under the principles of Davis' law.
- *Excessive knee flexion*. This also has the effect of reducing the tension in the Achilles tendon, and will increase the range of ankle dorsiflexion in soft tissue equinus.
- *Abductory twist*. The subject may adopt an abductory twist to reduce the need for ankle dorsiflexion after the midpoint of midstance. Abduction at the subtalar and midtarsal joints causes the foot to pronate. The pronated foot does not require 10° of ankle dorsiflexion for walking. The abductory twist is noted during gait as a rapid medial rotation of the rearfoot at heel lift.

## Treatment of ankle equinus

The patient must undergo a full biomechanical evaluation to establish the cause of the equinus deformity, in order that the treatment addresses all aspects of the lower limb and foot problem. Therapies include posterior muscle group stretching regimens where soft tissue equinus is diagnosed, orthoses therapy and footwear advice. But care must be taken to ensure that the true ankle equinus is identified and treated, rather than controlling the compensatory pronation at the subtalar and midtarsal joints. The correct diagnosis and treatment of ankle equinus can, however, prevent gross deformity in the longer term.

## Plantar flexed first metatarsal

Plantar flexed first metatarsal is a sagittal plane anomaly of the forefoot characterised by an increased angle of declination of the first metatarsal, so that the head of the first metatarsal is plantar flexed throughout gait, relative to the heads of the lesser metatarsals. It is characteristic of partial forefoot valgus (see above).

A plantar-flexed first ray is an acquired condition, often resulting from a muscular imbalance. Plantar flexion of the first ray is accomplished by contraction of peroneus longus and is opposed by the combined actions of tibialis anterior and tibialis posterior, as they supinate the foot at the subtalar and midtarsal joints. Any disease processes that result in a weakness of the supinators of the foot may result in plantar flexion of the first ray. Thus, a plantar-flexed first ray is also associated with presentations of neuromuscular disease in the foot.

## Hallux limitus/rigidus

Hallux limitus is a progressive pathology characterised by restriction of dorsiflexion of the hallux and degenerative changes within the first MTPJ. It is associated with hypermobility of the first metatarsal, the first ray and/or the whole foot, leading to lower limb and postural effects in the long term. The patient presents with dull pain in and around the first MTPJ that is increased by activity and in the early stages can be decreased by rest. Dorsiflexion at the first MTPJ is markedly decreased, and a characteristic dorsal exostosis and bursa develop in the area of the first MTPJ. The patient is forced to take compensatory action at the mid- and rearfoot to aid ambulation. Treatment is by deflective padding, orthoses to improve foot function and/or surgery.

Hallux limitus is a first ray pathology characterised by restricted dorsiflexion (reduced sagittal plane motion) at the first MTPJ during the propulsive phase of gait. Hallux rigidus is the total absence of dorsiflexion at the first MTPJ, and develops as the end point of the same range of pathologies that cause hallux limitus. The normal range of dorsiflexion at the first MTPJ is 65–70°. Hallux limitus describes a foot with less than 60° of available dorsiflexion at the first MTPJ, and hallux rigidus has less than 5° available dorsiflexion at the first MTPJ.

Hallux limitus is described as structural hallux limitus or functional hallux limitus, and it is possible for elements of both presentations to be seen in the same foot. In structural hallux limitus there is limitation of dorsiflexion at the first MTPJ at all times, whereas in functional hallux limitus dorsiflexion at the first MTPJ is reduced only when the foot is weight bearing. In the unloaded foot with functional hallux limitus, the range of motion at the first MTPJ appears relatively normal, but such a foot cannot function normally during gait. Thus hallux limitus/rigidus is a forefoot syndrome characterised by a progressive reduction in dorsiflexion and degenerative changes at the first MTPJ, and long-term compromise of dynamic foot function.

## Aetiology of hallux limitus

Hallux limitus is a chronic degenerative condition that develops over time, in association with a range of intrinsic (within the lower limb and foot) and extrinsic (e.g. systemic disease) factors. The intrinsic and extrinsic factors and variants of normal foot anatomy that predispose to hallux abducto valgus may also predispose to hallux limitus.

### Intrinsic factors

- Foot shape: the rectus foot (where the metatarsus adductus angle is <15°) is more prone to develop hallux limitus, whereas the adductus-type foot (characterised by metatarsus primus varus) is more prone to develop hallux abducto valgus (Fig. 4.7).
- Biomechanical factors: these are characterised by excessive pronation at the subtalar or midtarsal joints, where the foot remains in pronation from midstance through to toe-off. The factors include: ankle equinus, flexible or rigid pes plano valgus, rigid or flexible forefoot varus, dorsiflexion of the first ray (metatarsus primus elevatus), an elevated or hypermobile first ray, flexor plate immobility, plantar soft tissue contracture (Durrant and Siepert 1993) and functional hallux limitus (Payne et al 2002).
- Structural anomalies: anomalies within the lower limb that predispose to compensatory excessive foot pronation include external tibial torsion, tibial varum, positional variants of the knee (genu valgum/varum/recurvatum), femoral retroversion, leg-length discrepancy, where the long leg pronates excessively throughout gait, and an abducted angle of gait or wide-based gait.
- Relatively long first toe or long first metatarsal.
- Trauma: such as damage to the articular cartilage at the first MTPJ (e.g. osteochondritis, osteoarthritis), soft tissue tears, and sprains (e.g. 'turf' toe) of the soft tissues around the first MTPJ.

### Extrinsic factors

Extrinsic (systemic) factors that are associated with an increased incidence of hallux limitus include:

- Inflammatory joint disease within the foot: such as rheumatoid arthritis, a history of gout affecting the first MTPJ, psoriatic arthropathy and sesamoid degeneration (Camasta 1996).
- Occupations that require repeated and constant forced dorsiflexion of the hallux at the first MTPJ (e.g. carpet fitting),

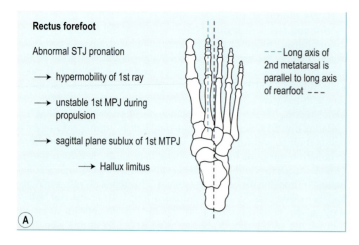

**Rectus forefoot**

Abnormal STJ pronation

→ hypermobility of 1st ray

→ unstable 1st MPJ during propulsion

→ sagittal plane sublux of 1st MTPJ

→ Hallux limitus

- - - Long axis of 2nd metatarsal is parallel to long axis of rearfoot - - -

Ⓐ

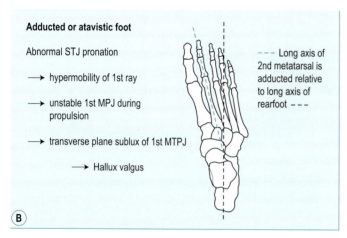

**Adducted or atavistic foot**

Abnormal STJ pronation

→ hypermobility of 1st ray

→ unstable 1st MPJ during propulsion

→ transverse plane sublux of 1st MTPJ

→ Hallux valgus

- - - Long axis of 2nd metatarsal is adducted relative to long axis of rearfoot - - -

Ⓑ

**Figure 4.7** Foot shape: rectus.

sports that require sudden changes in direction of movement or rapid deceleration (e.g. football, tennis, modern dance, basketball, netball), or abnormal weight bearing at the first ray (e.g. ballet dancing en point) all tend to cause repeated/chronic trauma to the first MTPJ, with the probability of developing the degenerative changes at the first MTPJ that characterise hallux limitus or hallux rigidus in later life.

- Pelvic nutation: postural changes may cause sagittal plane pelvic tilt so that the upper poles of the pelvis tilt anteriorly (pelvic nutation) or posteriorly (pelvic antenutation). Pelvic nutation is especially associated with the development of hallux limitus, due to its proximal effects (thoracic kyphosis, lumbar lordosis, internal rotation of the femur at the hip joint, internal rotation of the tibia at the knee joint, and whole foot pronation throughout gait) (Rothbart 2006).
- Shoes do not predispose to hallux limitus unless they are too short for the foot type, but an existing hallux limitus/rigidus may become more symptomatic with certain shoe styles, such as high-heeled shoes, shoes with a thin sole, or a narrow or shallow toe box.

## Pathology of hallux limitus

The primary role of the hallux is to dorsiflex on the first metatarsal head during the propulsive phase of gait. It has been calculated that approximately 70° of dorsiflexion is required at the first MTPJ at toe-off during normal bipedal motion, to allow the body's centre of

mass to progress forward with a smooth transfer of weight from the loaded to the opposite foot. The first MTPJ is a major weight-bearing joint, and at toe-off the full forward momentum of the body mass passes through this joint to be dissipated to the supporting surface.

### Reduction in normal foot function, as the result of first ray anomalies

Any restriction of movement at the first MTPJ predisposes to a range of compensatory changes in foot function, gait disturbance and postural symptoms (Dananberg 1993). Pathology at the first MTPJ affects the normal function of the whole foot, the lower limb and other body areas.

Functional hallux limitus occurs as a result of hypermobility of the first ray, which itself arises secondary to abnormal foot pronation.

- In the normal foot, the midtarsal joint locks from midstance to toe-off: at midstance the midtarsal joint supinates about its longitudinal axis, the first metatarsal stabilises against the support surface, and the first MTPJ dorsiflexes at toe-off. A stable first metatarsal forms a strong lever arm to assist forefoot supination at toe-off. In an excessively pronated foot, the midtarsal joint does not lock/supinate at midstance. The first metatarsal remains mobile and dorsiflexes when loaded at toe-off. The smaller the amount of plantar flexion achieved by the first metatarsal at toe-off, the greater the limitation of dynamic first MTPJ motion.
- To achieve an approximation to normal dorsiflexion of the hallux, compensatory hyperextension occurs at the interphalangeal joint of the hallux. Thus the combined ranges of motion of both the first MTPJ and the hallux interphalangeal joint approximate to 60°, and facilitate a more normal walking pattern. In cases where there is insufficient hyperextension from the combined dorsiflexion of the first MTPJ and hallux interphalangeal joint, the transfer of weight to the opposite foot is facilitated by the patient abducting the foot and toeing off from the medial side of the hallux.

In a structural hallux limitus, immobilisation of the first ray (e.g. due to an excessively long first metatarsal, metatarsus primus elevatus, trauma, sesamoid arthritis or ankylosis, and midtarsal joint arthritis) limits the ability of the hallux to dorsiflex adequately at the first MTPJ.

- Elevation of the first metatarsal, or loss of the arc of plantar flexion of the distal part of the first metatarsal (e.g. due to osteoarthritic changes at the first metatarsal–medial cuneiform joint) predisposes to flexion of the hallux at the first MTPJ to stabilise the forefoot at toe-off. The first MTPJ no longer functions as the primary fulcrum of the foot, and remains unloaded at toe-off. The forward transposition of the main fulcrum of the foot from the first MTPJ to the interphalangeal joint of the hallux allows the foot to supinate at toe-off, but predisposes to hyperextension of the interphalangeal joint of the hallux. Compensatory hyperextension at the hallux interphalangeal joint stretches the tissues of the plantar pulp, with a relative loss of the thickness and loss of cushioning of the plantar pulp of the hallux.
- Forefoot supination without dorsiflexion at the first MTPJ transfers load to the lateral column of the foot.

### Pathophysiological effects of a reduced range of motion at the first metatarsophalangeal joint

In the normal foot, the hallux remains static when under load (i.e. at toe-off), due to hallux purchase (see above). The articular aspect of the base of the proximal phalanx hallux therefore acts as a dynamic buttress to the forward motion of the body, and in effect functions as a 'buffer' to the forward motion of the loaded foot, so that continued onward momentum of the body mass initiates sagittal plane movement at the first MTPJ. There are two components within the sagittal plane movement at the first MTPJ – a hinge movement and a gliding movement – and therefore the first MTPJ is classed as a ginglyomoarthrodial joint (Root et al 1977). The hinge movement occurs as the hallux dorsiflexes at the first MTPJ. The gliding movement (in a plantarwards direction) occurs as the head of the first metatarsal moves down through an arc across the sagittal plane, facilitated by plantar flexion of the first metatarsal at the first metatarsal–medial cuneiform joint. The net result of movement of the first MTPJ is that the first metatarsal moves from a position where is it relatively parallel to the support surface (at midstance), to one where it is almost perpendicular to the supporting surface (at toe-off). As force equals mass/area, the decreased area of foot contact with the support surface at toe-off imposes an increased loading of up to 1.5 times body mass at the first MTPJ. This increased load persists from the latter part of the single support phase of gait until just after the heel strike of the opposite foot, and the weight-bearing limb moves into the swing phase (Dananberg et al 1996).

- When normal first MTPJ motion is reduced, as in hallux limitus, the amount of active dorsiflexion of the hallux at the first MTPJ (the hinge movement) is decreased and its gliding component forms the majority of available first MTPJ motion. The smooth transfer of body weight from the loaded to the opposite foot is compromised. Newton's second law of motion (i.e.: force = mass × acceleration) dictates that, as the patient's body mass remains constant, the force passing through the first MTPJ must increase when the acceleration of the hallux over the head of the first metatarsal is reduced, and forces of forward motion at the head of the first metatarsal and base of the proximal phalanx reciprocally increase.

- In cases where there is reduced movement at the first metatarsal–medial cuneiform joint (e.g. where there is a degree of arthritis at that joint) the plantarwards glide of the first metatarsal head across the sagittal plane is reduced, so that only the dorsiflexion component of the first MTPJ movement is available to facilitate forward momentum of the body from midstance through toe-off (Dananberg et al 1996), with a net restriction of the normal amount of dorsiflexion at the first MTPJ.

- In a normal joint, a feedback mechanism operates to prevent extremes of movement. At the limit of the normal range of movement, nerve endings within the joint secrete substance P and other inflammatory mediators, to initiate the feedback mechanism that prevents the joint moving beyond its normal range. Where the first MTPJ habitually is forced to work at the limits of its (pathologically decreased) range of movement (as outlined above), levels of substance P rise within the joint, triggering a neurogenic inflammation, with pain, swelling, heat, redness and loss of joint function (Light 1996). Thus the feedback mechanism creates and perpetuates the joint pathology, so that inflammation within the first MTPJ leads to even further limitation of joint movement, chronic inflammation, an increasing joint pathology, degenerative changes, the gradual reduction or loss of joint space, osteoarthritis and osteophyte formation, especially at the dorsal aspect of the joint (itself further compromising normal first MTPJ movement) (Fig. 4.8).

## Classification of hallux limitus

The clinical presentation of hallux limitus varies with the stage of the pathology, and thus the progress of the condition can be classified

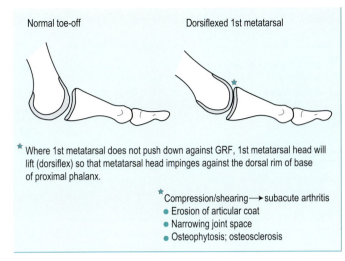

Normal toe-off      Dorsiflexed 1st metatarsal

\* Where 1st metatarsal does not push down against GRF, 1st metatarsal head will lift (dorsiflex) so that metatarsal head impinges against the dorsal rim of base of proximal phalanx.

\* Compression/shearing → subacute arthritis
- Erosion of articular coat
- Narrowing joint space
- Osteophytosis; osteosclerosis

**Figure 4.8** Pathophysiology of hallux limitus. Impingement of the base of the proximal phalanx during gait in a foot with metatarsus primus elevatus and the genesis of hallux limitus.

according to the range of the presenting signs and symptoms (Table 4.1).

## Clinical picture of hallux limitus

The typical patient presenting with hallux limitus is 30–50 years old (Coughlin & Shurnas 2003), with increasing great toe pain and stiffness, especially after walking or exercise involving dorsiflexion at the first MTPJ. There may or may not be a history of minor injury. The first MTPJ area is swollen, tender to touch and painful on passive movement. There may be joint crepitus on movement. The hallux is usually hyperextended (dorsiflexed) at its interphalangeal joint, but in cases where dorsiflexion at the first MTPJ is especially tender and restricted by pain and joint immobility the hallux may be held in slight flexion at the first MTPJ. Gait is modified to accommodate the first MTPJ dysfunction and weight is shifted laterally to the outer border of the foot (Fig. 4.9A and B).

The early clinical signs of functional hallux limitus (Stage 1) are subtle and may go unnoticed: the patient is likely to be free of foot pain, but may show a mildly apropulsive gait and an abductory forefoot twist at toe-off. Patients with Stage 2 mild structural hallux limitus show reduced dorsiflexion at the first MTPJ and reduced heel lift. They tend to compensate for the lack of efficient toe-off by excessively pronating the foot. In Stage 3, severe structural hallux limitus or early hallux rigidus, dorsiflexion at the first MTPJ is much reduced. In Stage 4 the first MTPJ becomes virtually or actually fused/ankylosed. To walk, the patient must pronate, abducting and everting the foot throughout gait, walking in a 'duck-footed' manner. Alternatively, where the ankylosed first MTPJ effectively extends the length of the medial column, it increases the angulation of the line of axis of the MTPJs in relation to the frontal plane, and allows the foot to supinate about the interphalangeal joint of the hallux late into toe-off.

## Gait and posture effects of structural hallux limitus

As walking is modelled as an inverted pendulum system, in which the centre of mass 'vaults' over the rigid stance limb (Lee & Farley 1998), a full range of dorsiflexion at the first MTPJ is an essential component of the normal walking mechanism. During stance, dorsiflexion at the

**Table 4.1** The Classification of hallux limitus/rigidus (after Camasta 1996)

| Stage Criteria | Characteristic features |
| --- | --- |
| Grade 1 (functional hallux limitus)<br>Available dorsiflexion at the first MTPJ ~60 | Functional limitation of dorsiflexion at the first MTPJ:<br>• Hypermobility of the first ray<br>• No marked joint deterioration, but possibly some dorsal osteophyte formation<br>• No sesamoid involvement<br>• First MTPJ dorsiflexion may be near normal in the non-weight-bearing foot<br>• First MTPJ area is usually painful under load |
| Grade 2 (mild structural hallux limitus)<br>Available dorsiflexion at the first MTPJ ~35–55 | Structural limitation of dorsiflexion at first MTPJ:<br>• Joint deterioration shows as broadening and flattening of the head of the first metatarsal and the base of the proximal phalanx<br>• Narrowing of the first MTPJ<br>• Moderate osteophytosis at the first MTPJ area<br>• Osteochondral defect at the first MTPJ (local bone sclerosis)<br>• Structural elevation of the first ray<br>• Sesamoid hypertrophy<br>• Pain in the first MTPJ area on movement and after exercise<br>• Reduced dorsiflexion at the first MTPJ in both the weight-bearing and the non-weight-bearing foot<br>• Possible crepitus at the first MTPJ<br>• Reduced heel lift |
| Grade 3 (moderate structural hallux limitus)<br>Available dorsiflexion at the first MTPJ–15–30 | *Structural loss of dorsiflexion* at the first MTPJ:<br>• Marked joint deterioration, with severe loss of first MTPJ space (near ankylosis)<br>• Extensive dorsal, lateral and medial osteophytosis<br>• Marked osteochondral defects of the first MTPJ complex, with sclerosis, cystic degeneration of subchondral bone, joint 'mice' and extensive hypertrophy of the sesamoids<br>• Structural elevation of the first ray<br>• Reduced height of the medial longitudinal arch<br>• Decrease in calcaneal angulation<br>• Dorsiflexion at the first MTPJ is severely reduced or absent<br>• Crepitus with any movement of the first MTPJ joint<br>• Marked reduction in heel lift |
| Grade 4 (severe hallux rigidus)<br>Available dorsiflexion at the first MTPJ ~<15 | Virtual or actual immobility of the first MTPJ:<br>• Joint obliteration and ankylosis<br>• Increase in depth of the first MTPJ complex due to osteophytosis<br>• Absent heel lift, unless the patient is able to toe-off from the interphalangeal joint of the hallux |

MTPJ, metatarsophalangeal joint.

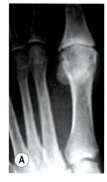
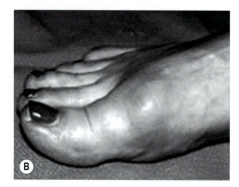

**Figure 4.9** A typical presentation of Stage 3 (moderate) structural hallux limitus. (A) Radiograph showing a reduction of the first MTPJ space and bone sclerosis, degenerative changes of the subchondral bone, hypertrophy of the sesamoids and marginal osteophytosis. (B) Photograph showing the typical clinical presentation of late-stage structural hallux limitus, with hyperextension of the hallux at the interphalangeal joint, elevation of the first metatarsal (metatarsus primus elevatus), the dorsal 'bunion' and an increase in the depth of the foot at the first MTP joint area (reflecting the underlying dorsal osteophytosis).

first MTPJ allows the joint to form the pivot to the 'lever arm' of the leg, allowing the transfer of body mass from the loaded to the opposite foot, whilst maintaining a smooth forward momentum. The loss of normal first MTPJ dorsiflexion in hallux limitus causes marked changes to gait and body posture. The normal response of the first MTPJ is to dorsiflex in direct response to the leverage imposed by heel lift. Where heel lift is reduced secondary to decreased available dorsiflexion at the first MTPJ, the foot is obliged to pronate about the oblique axis of the midtarsal joint, and the patient has to make an abductory twist to assist toe-off. The patient adopts an abnormally abducted angle of gait. Excess pronation imposes changes on limb and skeletal relationships, which include internal tibial torsion, internal rotation and transverse plane motion at the knee, internal rotation at the hips, a forward pelvic tilt (pelvic nutation) due to an increased lumbar lordosis, a thoracic kyphosis and a forward tilt of the cervical spine. Thus the patient with structural hallux limitus or hallux rigidus adopts a short stride length and early knee flexion, shows decreased thigh extension, a hunched back ('bad' posture or thoracic kyphosis), a diminished arm swing (to match the shortened stride length) and tends to either hyperflex the upper cervical spine, in order to face forward, or looks down to the ground whilst walking (Dananberg et al 1996).

## Pain associated with hallux limitus and hallux rigidus

The presenting symptoms of hallux limitus and hallux rigidus vary depending on the stage of the pathology:

- Stage 1: the first MTPJ is often asymptomatic, although the patient may present with one of the several foot pathologies that are associated with excessive foot pronation.
- Stage 2: patients usually complain of pain in and around the first MTPJ. The pain is usually described as a 'deep ache' within the first MTPJ, and is induced by walking or other activities that impose a forced dorsiflexion of the hallux at the first MTPJ (e.g. kneeling or wearing high-heeled shoes), but is relieved by rest.
- Stage 3: the first MTPJ is very painful and often inflamed (due to neurogenic inflammation, see above), both during and after activity. The soft tissues overlying the exostoses at the dorsal joint margins may be traumatised by shoes and be painful. Areas of hyperkeratosis are locally painful.
- Stage 4: the first MTPJ becomes pain free once ankylosis is complete. However, the overall hypertrophy of the first MTPJ complex causes an increased depth of the medial forefoot, and shear forces within the overlying soft tissues cause bursa formation and pain. Focal plantar hyperkeratoses are painful. Hyperextension of the hallux predisposes to local pain and corn and callus formation at the plantar pulp. Toeing-off from the plantar-medial aspect of the hallux is evidenced by a build up of painful callus in this area. The dysfunctional gait of structural hallux limitus or hallux rigidus causes pain in the lower limb (knees and hips) and the lower back.

## Shoe-wear marks

The foot with hallux limitus and hallux rigidus causes characteristic wear marks on the upper and the sole of the shoe. These are more readily visualised in a lace-up shoe, with a leather upper and sole:

- Stage 1: the shoe may show signs of excessive foot pronation, but few or no other characteristic marks.
- Stage 2: there is an increased depth of the upper overlying osteophytosis at the first MTPJ. 'Spin' wear shows on the sole, in relation to the abductory twist.
- Stage 3: in patients with long-standing hallux limitus, a distinct shoe-wear pattern is seen. The sole demonstrates lateral wear, wear beneath the second MTPJ and beneath the hallux interphalangeal joint. The upper shows a diagonal crease, reflecting the angulation of the axis of the hallux interphalangeal joint to the fifth MTPJ line at toe-off.
- Stage 4: in addition to the Stage 3 wear marks noted above, the hallux rigidus foot pronates throughout gait, and thus there is marked wear along the medial area of the sole, with medial 'bulging' of the upper in the area of the throat of the shoe. There may be horizontal creases near the top line of the outer side of the lateral area of the heel counter of the upper, and scratch marks on the outer medial side of the heel. Wear marks can be palpated inside the shoe: the inner surface of the upper will be worn to match the nail of the hyperextended hallux.

## Diagnosis and differential diagnoses

The diagnosis of hallux limitus and hallux rigidus is made from the clinical signs and the patient's symptoms, and confirmed by radiography.

Radiographs (anteroposterior, oblique and lateral views) of a foot with structural hallux limitus show narrowing of the first MTPJ space, with bone sclerosis and formation of dorsal osteophytes (dorsal spur formation). In moderate structural hallux limitus there is progressive enlargement of the sesamoids, increasing osteophytosis and metatarsus primus elevatus. In hallux rigidus, the first MTPJ shows ankylosis and loss of differentiation of the sesamoids, marked metatarsus primus elevatus, decreased inclination of the calcaneum and loss of the cyma line.

The differential diagnoses should rule out inflammatory joint diseases such as rheumatoid arthritis, gout and psoriatic arthropathy, as well as osteochondritis dissicans (in adolescents) and flexor hallucis longus tenosynovitis.

## Treatment of hallux limitus and hallux rigidus

Hallux limitus and hallux rigidus can be treated conservatively, or by surgery, after taking the history and making a full examination and biomechanical evaluation of the patient to determine the extent of the pathomechanical processes associated with the condition. In the past, immobilisation of the first MTPJ was advocated as the principal treatment for hallux limitus and hallux rigidus, in order to unload the joint, promote rest and preserve the remaining joint function (Laing 1995). But Dananberg et al (1996) advocate that the conservative therapy should include manipulative therapy to enhance first MTPJ movement, reduce pain and improve and maintain overall joint function, in order to avoid later gait and postural disturbances.

### Conservative treatments

Conservative treatments include:

- Clinical reduction of plantar hyperkeratoses that form below the second, third, fourth and fifth MTPJs, together with the provision of deflective clinical padding.
- Manipulation: the neurogenic inflammatory response within the joint can be reduced by direct stimulation of mechanoreceptors within the joint through manipulation. The technique involves gentle distraction of the joint surfaces, followed by a rapid thrust of two segments away from each other. For example, the hallux is distracted at the first MTPJ for 15 s, while the thumb of the opposite hand is placed at the base of the first metatarsal. Thrust is simultaneously applied to the hallux, to dorsiflex it, and to the base of the first metatarsal to move it laterally. The calcaneocuboid also benefits from manipulation, in order to maximise the function of the peroneus longus as a stabiliser of the first ray against ground reaction forces (Dananberg et al 1996).
- Shoe style adaptations: the patient should wear a low-heeled shoe that has been properly fitted to the foot. Active dorsiflexion of the hallux at the first MTPJ can be minimised by wearing a shoe with a rigid sole that is curved in the sagittal plane under the forefoot (a rocker sole) (Chapman 1999).
- Functional orthoses for cases of functional hallux limitus help control the abnormal pronatory forces that occur during gait by: maintaining the subtalar joint in the neutral position; stabilising and locking the midtarsal joint, to reduce first metatarsal hypermobility; promoting a normal range of hallux dorsiflexion at the first MTPJ; and encouraging the foot to re-supinate from midstance through to toe-off, and thereby minimise the need for lower limb or postural compensation. Functional orthoses for structural hallux limitus include an accommodation for the first metatarsal head.

Indicative staged conservative treatments include (Dananberg et al 1996):

- Stage 1: Functional hallux limitus. Treatment of stage 1 hallux limitus is essentially prophylactic, as the majority of cases are asymptomatic, and the range of motion at the unloaded first MTPJ is still normal, or near normal. Conservative therapy includes orthoses to stabilise the hypermobile first ray, and manipulation to maintain the normal range of motion at the first MTPJ (Dananberg et al 1996).
- Stage 2: Mild structural hallux limitus. The range of motion of the first ray is reduced, by as much as 50%. If the first MTPJ appears more or less as normal on radiography, Stage 2 structural hallux limitus is treated as the Stage 1 presentation. If any degenerative changes within the first MTPJ are noted, the patient may require a short course of non-steroidal anti-inflammatory drugs (NSAIDs) to reduce joint inflammation and pain (e.g. a 5- to 10-day course of ibuprofen 400 mg q.d.s.) with prescription orthoses to stabilise rear-foot and midfoot function.
- Stage 3: moderate structural hallux limitus. The range of motion at the first MTPJ is reduced by up to 75%, and dorsiflexion of the hallux is very limited; marked degenerative changes within the joint are noted on radiography. Conservative treatment should be attempted, but may not be wholly successful. Manipulative therapy should be carried out daily, preceded by the application of heat (e.g. a foot bath) and followed by the application of an ice pack, to reduce inflammation, and strapping to the joint (fan strapping) (see Ch. 16). A course of ultrasound therapy or iontophoresis may be of benefit. The painful joint should be rested, by means of a rocker-soled shoe (Chapman 1999) and/or the foot should be immobilised by the use of Low Dye® strapping. The patient may need to take painkillers, such as NSAIDs, regularly. Once the signs of joint inflammation have subsided, the patient should be encouraged to continue the manipulative therapy, to regain joint movement, together with the use of antipronatory, in-shoe orthoses.
- Stage 4: severe structural hallux limitus/rigidus, where there is no or very little movement at the first MTPJ, and radiography shows marked osteophytosis at the first MTPJ and the loss of the normal bony architecture within the joint. Any residual movement will be painful, and thus the first MTPJ should be immobilised by means of an orthotic device with a medial forefoot wedge, extended distally as far as the interphalangeal joint of the hallux, in a rocker-soled shoe.

### Surgical treatment of hallux limitus and hallux rigidus

Corrective surgery for structural hallux limitus is recommended when conservative therapies have failed to reduce pain and improve foot function. Surgery includes:

- Procedures to allow a greater range of movement at the first MTPJ whilst essentially preserving joint anatomy, such as the removal of the dorsal exostoses (cheilectomy) together with reducing the pressure within the joint by shortening the first metatarsal (decompression osteotomy, or Valenti procedure). These procedures are indicated in cases of mild–moderate joint damage.
- Procedures that are first MTPJ destructive, such as removal of one aspect of the joint, usually the base of the proximal phalanx (athroplasty) and/or the insertion of a prosthetic joint replacement. These procedures are indicated in cases with intractable pain, with marked joint damage, and in the older patient. Sylastic joint prostheses have an unacceptably high failure rate (Granberry et al 1991).

- Procedures to realign the first metatarsal, to reduce metatarsus primus elevatus (plantar basal closing wedge osteotomy) and to improve overall foot function.
- Surgical fusion of the first MTPJ (arthrodesis) is recommended when the arthritic process has destroyed the articular surface and the patient has intolerable pain. The joint must be fixed (by pins or screws) to allow full fusion of the first MTPJ with the hallux set at a predetermined angle of dorsiflexion. The patient is left with no movement at all at the first MTPJ, and thus will always have to wear shoes of a heel height that reflects the degree of fixed hallux dorsiflexion.

## Hallux flexus (acute hallux limitus)

Whereas in the typical presentation of hallux limitus the patient is middle aged, with a chronic first MTPJ problem an acute presentation of hallux limitus (acute hallux limitus) can occur, usually in a younger person, as the result of sudden local trauma to the first MTPJ. With appropriate treatment, the acute hallux limitus or hallux flexus condition will resolve completely.

### Pathology of hallux flexus

The typical acute hallux flexus patient is a young person who presents with a recent history of trauma to the foot, usually as the result of an accident such as stubbing the toe against a kerb or tripping over a heavy or immovable object. The sudden deceleration of the body mass due to the impact imposes an excessively high load at the articular surfaces of the first MTPJ, resulting in an acute inflammatory response in and around the joint. It is a very painful condition, in which the flexor hallucis brevis muscle goes into spasm as a protective mechanism, creating a metatarsus primus elevatus and excess pain on attempted movement of the first MTPJ. The hallux is held in plantar flexion until the pain, inflammation and muscle spasm subside. Repeated episodes of hallux flexus can predispose to developing structural hallux limitus in later life.

### Diagnosis of hallux flexus

The diagnosis is made from the clinical signs together with the patient history. Radiography will exclude any concomitant fractures caused at the time of the original trauma to the foot.

### Treatment of hallux flexus

Treatment involves pain control, rest, ice, compression and elevation (PRICE):

- Pain control: this can be achieved by rest and limb elevation, together with reduction of inflammation (using ice) and a short course of NSAIDs (e.g.: 5-day course of ibuprofen 400 mg q.d.s.).
- Rest: the patient should be advised not to bear weight on the affected foot until all symptoms subside. Immobilisation (i.e. total rest) can be achieved by use of: a shoe with a stiff/non-bending or rocker sole (see above); strapping the first MTPJ to prevent movement (e.g. fan strapping); soft splintage of the first MTPJ; together with clinical padding of the medial midfoot and forefoot, using an extended valgus filler pad made from semi-compressed felt to support the elevated first metatarsal and prevent weight bearing at the first MTPJ, with or without crutches, to assist ambulation.
- Ice: the patient is advised to use ice in the first 48–72 hours following the initial injury, when the inflammation is most acute. Ice (in the form of a packet of frozen peas or the like

wrapped in a cotton cloth) is applied to the inflamed area at least twice a day. After 72 hours, the application of gentle heat is indicated. Heat can be applied by immersion in a water bath at 45°C for 10 minutes twice daily, or by the use of an infrared lamp or a hot water bottle.

- Compression: compression bandaging (e.g. Coban™ or crepe bandage) is applied to the swollen and inflamed tissues as a 'figure of eight' foot bandage from just above the ankle to just distal to the MTPJs.
- Elevation: this is achieved by sitting with the limb fully supported along its length on a sofa or bed, so that the heel is higher than the buttocks.

## Functional hallux limitus

Functional hallux limitus is noted in a foot with apparent sufficient dorsiflexion of the hallux at the first MTPJ, when tested in the non-weight-bearing foot, but insufficient dorsiflexion of the hallux at the first MTPJ to allow normal gait (i.e. when weight bearing). In a foot with excessive pronation at the subtalar joint, or a foot with a forefoot valgus, the ground reaction force will tend to elevate the head of the first metatarsal and prevent plantarwards movement of the first metatarsal, when under load, at toe-off. This reduces the normal range of dorsiflexion of the hallux at the first MTPJ, resulting in a functional hallux limitus.

Functional hallux limitus is best observed with the patient standing in the relaxed calcaneal stance position, and by carrying out Jack's test. In the normal foot, when the subject is standing in the normal angle and base of gait, the clinician should be able to passively dorsiflex the hallux to 15° at the first MTPJ, without inducing movement elsewhere in the foot. In functional hallux limitus, the great toe is 'locked' to the supporting surface, and forced dorsiflexion of the hallux at the first MTPJ will raise the medial side of the foot away from the ground (see also hallux rigidus/limitus, above).

## Sagittal plane blockade

A foot with functional hallux limitus shows blockade of the sagittal plane motion of the hallux at the first MTPJ until the positional abnormality that caused the limitation no longer influences the movement of the hallux. For example, if the foot is overpronated during the midstance period of gait, normal hallux dorsiflexion will not occur until the foot supinates and allows downwards movement of the first metatarsal, which in turn allows dorsiflexion of the hallux. The normal function of the hallux will be temporarily blocked, showing sagittal plane blockade. This condition has been related to postural problems, and there is growing evidence that chronic low back pain may be a consequence of functional hallux limitus and the associated sagittal plane blockade.

## Hypermobile medial column/first ray

A hypermobile first ray is defined as a foot where the medial column (the first ray) is less stable than in the normal foot. First ray hypermobility may be related to generalised hypermobility, as assessed by the Beighton Score, but there are many cases where the apparent hypermobility is isolated to the medial column of the foot.

## Metatarsus primus elevatus

Metatarsus primus elevatus is defined as a foot in which the transverse plane of the head of the first metatarsal is in a dorsiflexed position compared with that of the second and fifth metatarsals. This may be known as a 'dorsiflexed first ray' or a 'partial forefoot varus'. This foot type functions as a forefoot varus.

## Plantar-flexed fifth metatarsal

A plantar-flexed fifth metatarsal is defined as a foot in which the transverse plane of the fifth metatarsal is in a plantar-flexed position compared with that of the first and fourth metatarsals. This foot type will function as a forefoot varus.

## ABNORMALITIES OF ARCH HEIGHT

There are two terms that are routinely used to describe feet that have an apparent sagittal plane abnormality in the height of the medial longitudinal arch: pes planus and pes cavus. They are both descriptive terms that refer to the appearance of the foot, either with an unusually low or an unusually high medial longitudinal arch, respectively.

- Pes planus describes a foot with a low medial profile. This might be due to overpronation at the subtalar joint, with a resultant lowering of the arch, or instep, on weight bearing. Alternatively, pes planus might be due to a hyperflexible foot that is unable to maintain its normal profile on weight bearing, or a congenitally malformed foot, or a foot damaged by trauma or disease, or a combination thereof.
- Pes cavus describes a foot that has an abnormally high medial profile. This may be due to abnormal development, neurological disease, congenital foot abnormality or trauma.

Although it is very difficult, if not impossible, to provide a definition of normal arch height, the experienced practitioner will always recognise a planus or cavus foot type on sight. Some authors have used navicular height (the distance of the inferior aspect of the navicular tuberosity from the support surface in the weight-bearing foot) and/or navicular drop (the difference in the distance of the navicular tuberosity from the plantar plane of the non-weight-bearing foot compared to its distance from the support surface in the weight-bearing foot) as a measure of the passive and dynamic heights of the instep. However, the reliability and validity of these measures have not been confirmed.

## Pes planus

Pes planus, pes plano valgus and flat foot are all descriptive terms that cover a multitude of conditions that vary in aetiology, pathology, prognosis and management, but all of which are characterised by a foot with a low medial arch profile. These terms are not precise, although some practitioners argue the exact meanings of such terms, and their subtle differences. However, there is no consensus within the literature. Pes planus can be subdivided into a number of categories, depending on its aetiology. It is often subclassified into rigid and flexible pes planus, as either state causes a significant effect on foot and limb function, and each requires a different range of management strategies.

## Classification of pes planus

Pes planus may be classified according to its aetiology; that is, whether it is of functional, congenital, acquired or neurological origin:

- Functional pes planus is characterised by overpronation of the subtalar joint, resulting in a flexible flat foot, although not all overpronated feet will exhibit a low instep, or appear 'flat' during stance (Box 4.1).

Excessive pronation, and resultant functional pes planus, is a feature of the following:
- Compensated forefoot varus
- Mobile forefoot valgus
- Compensated rearfoot varus
- Compensated ankle equinus
- Hypermobile medial column
- Short first metatarsal
- Leg-length inequality, compensated by unilateral pronation of the foot on the longer limb side
- Obesity
- Genu valga
- Genu vara/tibia vara
- Metatarsus adductus
- Internal rotations/torsions of the limb
- Posterior tibial dysfunction (with or without accessory navicular)
- Ligamentous laxity (familial, Downs, Ehler–Danlos, Marfan's etc.)

- Congenital rigid flat foot, such as occurs with congenital convex pes valgus or tarsal coalition (also known as peroneal spastic flat foot – see the section on tarsal coalition later in this chapter).
- Congenital flexible flat foot, such as talipes calcaneo valgus, and hypoplasia of the sustentaculum tali.
- Acquired rigid flat foot, arising in conjunction with tarsal coalition, inflammatory arthritis or traumatic arthritis, or secondary to trauma.
- Neurological causes of both rigid and flexible flat foot as sequelae to, for example poliomyelitis, cerebral palsy, peripheral nerve injuries and muscular dystrophy.

## Consequences of pes planus

Flexible flat foot causes, or is associated with, many foot and lower limb pathologies, including:

- postural symptoms involving the lower limb, pelvis and spine
- apropulsive gait
- forefoot disruption, including hallux abducto valgus (see hallux abducto valgus below) and other digital deformities
- foot pathologies such as metatarsalgia (see functional metatarsalgia), plantar digital neuritis (see functional metatarsalgia), medial arch strains (see plantar fasciitis), hallux limitus (see hallux rigidus/limitus) and abnormal plantar weight distribution.

## Treatment of pes planus

Flexible flat foot is often amenable to treatment, provided the underlying cause has been diagnosed and is addressed by the management strategy. However, some cases of very severe flat feet, particularly those involving late-stage tibialis posterior dysfunction (see plantar heel pain), especially in the elderly, and flat foot of congenital or traumatic origin, are less amenable to conservative treatments. These cases should be referred for an orthopaedic or podiatric surgery opinion. The reader is referred to the wide range of texts (and the considerable debate) available in the literature on surgery for the flat foot.

The rigid flat foot causes a range of symptoms, which will be related in general to the underlying pathology and consequent gait difficulties. Treatment is mostly palliative, but can maximise the function that is available. Referral for surgery may be the option of choice.

## Pes cavus

The term 'pes cavus' describes a foot with a high medial longitudinal arch.

### Aetiology of pes cavus

Pes cavus is often related to neuromuscular dysfunction, congenital abnormality or familial predisposition. For example:

- Neuromuscular dysfunction that results in spasm of the peroneus longus or tibialis posterior, or weakness of the peroneus longus and brevis. This presentation is associated with poliomyelitis, cerebral palsy, spina bifida, hereditary motor and sensory neuropathies, Friedreich's ataxia and spinal cord tumours.
- Severe metatarsus adductus.
- Talipes equinovarus deformities.

However, in a significant number of cases no clear aetiology can be identified, and these cases are classed as being of idiopathic cause. Idiopathic presentations of highly arched feet that do not arise in association with neuromuscular dysfunction, congenital abnormality or familial predisposition are often associated with functional abnormalities and malalignments, which include:

- rigid plantar-flexed first ray
- rigid forefoot valgus
- uncompensated or partially compensated rearfoot varus
- limb-length inequality, where the foot of the shorter leg supinates
- pseudo ankle equinus.

*Mobile pes cavus* is a term used to describe a foot in which, in the non-weight-bearing state, the medial arch appears excessively high but flattens to a more normal profile when the patient stands. This type of pes cavus is mostly associated with a mobile forefoot valgus foot type. The constant adaptive changes in the foot shape between weight-bearing (stance) and non-weight-bearing (swing) result in excessive movements occurring in the foot joints proximal to the first metatarsal. Over time, and as the patient ages, the tarsal joints undergo degeneration, leading to reduced tarsal joint mobility, loss of the weight-bearing adaptation and increased weight-bearing arch height (see tarsal arthritis).

### Treatment of pes cavus

The treatment of pes-cavus-type feet will depend on the presenting symptoms, the resultant gait dysfunction, and the degree of foot-joint mobility. The rigid-type pes cavus foot requires orthoses that cushion and increase shock absorption. The mobile-type pes cavus foot requires dynamic orthoses that maximise foot function and minimise joint deformity. The increase in height of the midfoot means that it can be difficult to obtain footwear that is a good fit and does not traumatise the foot. There are a number of surgical procedures that are indicated to reduce some of the deformity of rigid pes cavus, or to correct the secondary pathologies that characterise mobile pes cavus. The reader is referred to the abundance of literature on this topic.

## TRANSVERSE PLANE ANOMALIES OF THE LOWER LIMB AND FOOT

### Hallux abducto valgus

Hallux abducto valgus is a forefoot pathology, the most obvious sign of which is the lateral deviation of the hallux at the first MTPJ across the transverse plane, with the formation of an exostosis and bursa, or 'bunion' at the medial aspect of the head of the first metatarsal. The lateral drift of the hallux causes the second toe to assume a hammer deformity and/or dislocate at the second MTPJ, the first MTPJ to undergo degenerative changes, and generalised disruption of forefoot function. The incidence of hallux abducto valgus has a strong familial predisposition, but is not inherited per se. Intrinsic causes include a range of biomechanical anomalies that predispose to excessive foot pronation, especially in the period of stance from midstance to toe-off. Extrinsic causes include inflammatory arthropathy. The patient presents with pain on movement and decreased function of the first MTPJ, lesser toe deformities and other forefoot pathologies that are linked to decreased first ray function. Patients are often unable to find a shoe style that does not traumatise the bunion. Treatment includes conservative therapies to treat the associated forefoot soft tissue pathologies, orthoses to address the limb and foot biomechanical anomalies, and surgery to reduce deformity and improve first ray function.

Hallux abducto valgus is defined as a complex, progressive and permanent triplanar forefoot deformity that is most obviously characterised by the lateral deviation of the hallux at the first MTPJ. The clinical picture of hallux abducto valgus includes:

- fibular deviation of the great toe at the first MTPJ
- tibial deviation of the first metatarsal at its distal end (this feature is termed 'metatarsus primus varus')
- progressive loss of or reduction in the normal articular relationships at the first MTPJ, including loss of the normal sesamoid articulation
- instability of the first ray
- structural and soft tissue pathologies at and around the first MTPJ
- other soft tissue and osseous pathologies of the forefoot, secondary to the changes within the first ray and the first MTPJ, and to the development of lesser toe deformities, with resultant disruption of normal foot function.

The features that typify hallux abducto valgus relate to a number of factors, which include variants of normal anatomy as well as pathological changes. To understand the pathology of HAV, one must appreciate the normal anatomy and function of the first MTPJ.

## Normal anatomy of the first ray

The first ray is formed by the medial column of the mid- and forefoot; that is, by the medial cuneiform, the first metatarsal, and the proximal and distal phalanges of the hallux, and their interposed joints i.e. the first metatarsal–cuneiform joint, the first MTPJ and the interphalangeal joint of the hallux.

The first metatarsal–cuneiform joint is a synovial joint that forms the articulation between the base of the first metatarsal and the medial cuneiform bone. The axis of the first metatarsal–cuneiform joint is oriented from proximal–medial–plantar to distal–lateral–dorsal.

- As the first ray supinates at toe-off, the head of the first metatarsal moves into adduction and plantar flexion relative to its base. The first ray tends to evert or rotate about the longitudinal axis of the first metatarsal (Klaue et al 1994).
- In the normal foot the tendency of the first ray to evert is restricted by the orientation of the sesamoid complex and the architecture of the plantar aspect of the head of the first metatarsal (see below), the longitudinal orientation of the pull of the long extensor and flexor tendons (flexor hallucis longus and extensor hallucis longus tendons), the action of the abductor hallucis muscle, and the inelastic and fibrous nature of the capsule of the first MTPJ, especially at its plantar aspect.

The first MTPJ is a synovial joint that forms the articulation between the head of the first metatarsal and the base of the proximal phalanx of the hallux, and of the plantar aspect of the head of the first metatarsal and the sesamoid bones that are embedded within the tendon of the flexor hallucis brevis muscle.

- The axes of motion of the first MTPJ allow sagittal plane movement (dorsiflexion and plantar flexion) and transverse plane movement (adduction and abduction) of the hallux. There is very little active frontal plane movement of the hallux (inversion and eversion) in the normal foot (Fig. 4.10A).
- The capital articular cartilage extends onto the dorsal, plantar, medial and lateral aspects of the first metatarsal head (Fig. 4.10B).
- The sesamoids are two small bones that reinforce the tendon of the flexor hallucis brevis muscle at the point where it crosses the plantar aspect of the first MTPJ. The deep aspects of the sesamoids articulate with the grooves at the plantar aspect of the head of the first metatarsal. The sesamoids have a number of ligamentous attachments to adjacent structures:
  - the medial (tibial) sesamoid ligament inserts into the medial collateral ligament of the first MTPJ and the lateral (fibular) sesamoid ligament inserts into the lateral collateral ligament of the first MTPJ (Fig. 4.10C);
  - the sesamoids have strong fibrous attachments with the deep transverse ligament (Fig. 4.10D);
  - the sesamoids have a number of functions that are essential to normal walking and weight bearing. They increase the strength and prevent wear and tear of the flexor hallucis brevis tendon, provide a groove through which the flexor hallucis longus tendon passes as it crosses the plantar aspect of the first MTPJ, increase the functional depth of the head of the first metatarsal, increase the relative length of the lever arm of the foot and lower limb and, most importantly, provide an articular surface against which the head of the first metatarsal can plantar flex at toe-off. When the sesamoids are compressed into the grooves of the plantar aspect of the first metatarsal head, the first MTPJ is stabilised and abduction of the hallux at the first MTPJ is restricted (Phillips 1994).

The sesamoid complex helps maintain the integrity of the first MTPJ and its associated soft tissue structures:

- The medial and lateral margins of the sesamoids act as points of origin for ligaments that insert into and blend with the fibres of the medial and lateral collateral ligaments of the first MTPJ capsule.
- The sesamoids, embedded within the tendon of flexor hallucis brevis muscle, together with the plantar aspect of the first MTPJ capsule, form a tough structure (the plantar plate). The plantar plate is firmly attached to the plantar aspect of the base of the proximal phalanx of the hallux, but has no firm proximal fixing.
- The medial and lateral collateral ligaments of the first MTPJ are thickened fibrous bands within the medial and lateral aspects of the joint capsule. Their articular cartilage articulates with the capital cartilage at the medial and lateral aspects of the head of the first metatarsal, and effectively form a 'socket' to reciprocate the 'ball' formed by the head of the first metatarsal.
- The medial and lateral collateral ligaments originate at the medial and lateral plantar epicondyles of the first metatarsal head, and insert into the medial and lateral sides of the proximal phalanx of the hallux.
- The structures at the medial part of the capsule of the first MTPJ (the medial collateral ligament, the medial sesamoid ligament and the medial joint capsule) maintain the alignment of the

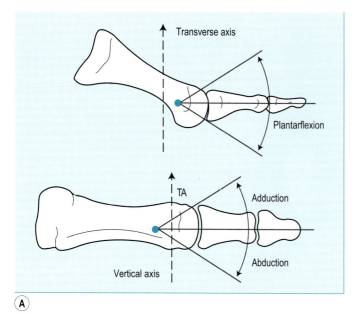

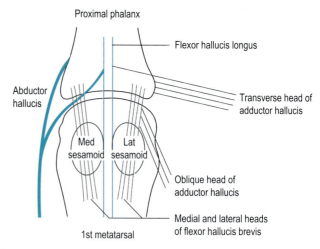

Figure 4.11 Proximal phalanx of the hallux.

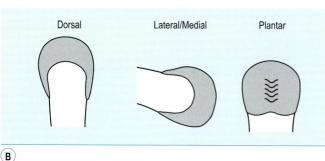

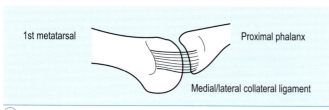

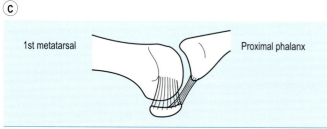

Figure 4.10 The first metatarsal head: functional anatomy. (A) Sagittal plane motion of the hallux (dorsiflexion/plantar flexion) occurs about the transverse axis of the first MTRJ. Transverse plane motion of the hallux (abduction/adduction) occurs about the vertical axis of the first MTPJ. (B) The articular cartilage at the head of the first metatarsal covers the dorsal, medial/lateral and plantar elements. (C) The joint capsule is thickened at the medial and lateral aspects to form the medial and lateral collateral ligaments of the first MTPJ. (D) The sesamoid bones that lie within the paired tendons of the flexor hallucis brevis have ligamentous attachments to the medial and lateral collateral ligaments of the first MTPJ and the base of the proximal phalanx.

first MTPJ on the sesamoid platform. No muscle, tendons or ligaments insert into the head of the first metatarsal.

- There is no direct ligamentous connection between the first and second metatarsal heads. The plantar plate of the first MTPJ attaches to the plantar plate of the second MTPJ by means of the deep transverse ligament.

- All other structures around the first MTPJ are attached to the proximal phalanx of the hallux, or its associated soft tissue structures, and not to the head of the first metatarsal. Thus, when the hallux deviates laterally, the immediately proximal local structures also move laterally (Fig. 4.11).

Tendons crossing the first MTPJ insert into the proximal phalanx and the sesamoids complex:

- Fibres of abductor hallucis tendon blend with the fibres of flexor hallucis longus tendon, and thus the abductor hallucis can act as an auxiliary flexor of the hallux, especially if there is any degree of frontal plane rotation of the hallux.

- Fibres of the tendon of the medial head of flexor hallucis brevis blend with the fibres of the plantar plate, the medial sesamoid ligament and the transverse head of adductor hallucis, as well as inserting into the medial plantar aspect of the proximal phalanx of the hallux.

- Fibres of the tendon of the lateral head of the flexor hallucis brevis blend with the fibres of the oblique head of adductor hallucis at its insertion and the lateral sesamoid ligament, as well as inserting into the lateral plantar aspect of the proximal phalanx of the hallux.

- Fibres of the tendon of the transverse head of adductor hallucis blend with the fibrous tunnel through which the flexor hallucis longus tendon passes onto the plantar aspect of the first MTPJ, as well as inserting into the lateral plantar aspect of the proximal phalanx of the hallux.

- Fibres of the medial slip of the plantar aponeurosis insert into the medial sesamoid, the tendons of the abductor hallucis and the flexor hallucis brevis, as well as into the plantar aspect of the proximal phalanx.

- Fibres of the tendon of the extensor hallucis longus insert into the hood apparatus at the dorsum of the first MTPJ. The hood apparatus is a tough, fibrous structure that cloaks the dorsum of the first MTPJ and inserts into the dorsal periosteum of the proximal phalanx, the plantar plate of the first MTPJ and the fibrous tunnel surrounding the flexor hallucis longus tendon (Fig. 4.12).

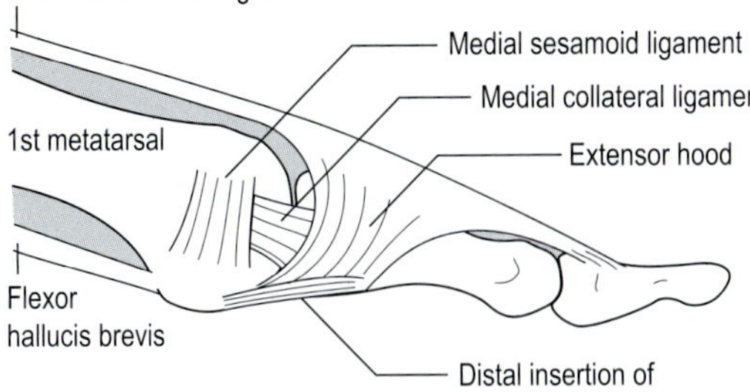

Extensor hallucis longus

Medial sesamoid ligament

Medial collateral ligament

1st metatarsal

Extensor hood

Flexor hallucis brevis

Distal insertion of flexor hallucis longus

**Figure 4.12** Fibrous attachments of the sesamoid complex and the proximal phalanx (ligamentous structures around the first MTPJ).

## Planar movements at the normal first metatarsophalangeal joint

Active weight-bearing movement at the normal first MTPJ includes:

- sagittal plane movement (dorsiflexion and plantar flexion of the hallux on the head of the first metatarsal, and some plantar flexion of the distal part of the first metatarsal relative to the base of the proximal phalanx of the hallux)
- transverse plane movement (potential or slight adduction and abduction of both the hallux and the distal end of the first metatarsal)
- in the normal foot, there is *no* active frontal plane movement, and thus the normal hallux does not invert or evert – static inversion or eversion of the hallux is an indication of foot pathology.

## Incidence of hallux abducto valgus

Hallux abducto valgus affects approximately 1% of all adults. It occurs more often in females, with a male/female ratio of incidence of 1 to 4 (Ferrari et al 2004). There is an age-related increase in incidence, such that 16% (approximately 1 in 6) of people aged over 60 years have a degree of hallux abducto valgus (Gould 1988). There appears to be a genetic predisposition to the development of hallux abducto valgus, although congenital hallux abducto valgus (i.e. hallux abducto valgus noted at birth) is rare.

## Aetiology of hallux abducto valgus

There is no one single cause of hallux abducto valgus, rather the condition develops over time, in association with a range of intrinsic (within the lower limb and foot) and extrinsic (e.g. systemic disease) factors. Variants of normal foot anatomy can also predispose to the development of hallux abducto valgus (Ferrari & Malone-Lee 2002). Contrary to popular lay opinion, shoes, such as high-heeled shoes with a small toe box, or tight-fitting shoes, do not *cause* hallux abducto valgus. However, high-heeled and tight, narrow shoes exacerbate the signs and symptoms of an existing hallux abducto valgus and its associated soft tissue pathologies, and facilitate intrinsic features within normal foot anatomy and function that predispose to the development of hallux abducto valgus.

## Factors that predispose to the development of hallux abducto valgus

Factors that predispose to the development of hallux abducto valgus include intrinsic features of the lower limb and foot, extrinsic features related to systemic pathology, and certain variants of normal foot anatomy.

### *Intrinsic factors*

Intrinsic (within the foot and/or within the lower limb) factors that predispose to the development of hallux abducto valgus include:

- Biomechanical factors, characterised by excessive and compensatory pronation at the subtalar joint or midtarsal joint, where the foot remains in pronation from midstance through to toe-off. These include ankle equinus, flexible or rigid pes plano valgus, rigid or flexible forefoot varus, dorsiflexion of the first ray (known as metatarsus primus elevatus), an overlong second metatarsal, a relatively short first metatarsal, and functional hallux limitus (Payne et al 2002).
- Structural anomalies within the lower limb that also predispose to compensatory excessive foot pronation include external tibial torsion, tibial varum, positional variants of the knee (genu valgum/varum/recurvatum), femoral retroversion, abducted angle of gait or a wide-based gait, and leg-length discrepancy (where the long leg pronates excessively throughout gait).
- Trauma, such as: intra-articular damage within the first MTPJ; soft tissue tears and first MTPJ sprains such as 'turf' toe (see Ch. 13); and dislocation or amputation of the second toe at the second MTPJ.

### *Extrinsic factors*

Extrinsic (systemic) factors that are associated with an increased incidence of hallux abducto valgus include:

- inflammatory joint disease such as rheumatoid arthritis, gout and psoriatic arthropathy
- connective tissue disorders and systemic pathologies characterised by generalised ligamentous laxity, such as generalised hypermobility, Ehlers–Danlos syndrome, Marfan's syndrome and Down's syndrome
- neuromuscular diseases that are characterised by the development of pes cavus and pes plano valgus, such as multiple sclerosis, hereditary sensorimotor neuropathy (also known as Charcot–Marie–Tooth disease or peroneal muscular atrophy), cerebral palsy and poliomyelitis.

### *Variants of normal foot anatomy*

A number of normal anatomical variants may exacerbate a tendency towards developing hallux abducto valgus. These include an adductus or atavistic foot, the relative length of the first metatarsal, unequal muscle function, and idiopathic features.

### *Metatarsus primus varus*

- An adductus or atavistic foot (i.e. a foot with marked metatarsus primus varus) is more likely to develop hallux abducto valgus than a rectus foot (i.e. a foot with a straight medial border). The first ray of an adductus foot tends to function more like that of the hand, with a tendency to frontal plane rotation (eversion) at the medial cuneiform–metatarsal joint and the first MTPJ.
- Excessive foot pronation, of whatever origin, causes adduction at the distal part of the first metatarsal, so that the first metatarsal tends to a varus position (metatarsus primus varus).
- Metatarsus primus varus is accentuated where the angulation of the first metatarsal–cuneiform joint is increased, relative to the longitudinal axis of the foot (Ferrari & Malone-Lee 2002).
- Peroneus (fibularis) longus tendon inserts into the base of the 1st metatarsal. Contraction of peroneus longus muscle causes adduction (toward the mid-line of the body) of the distal part of the first metatarsal, and exacerbates any tendency to metatarsus primus varus.
- The tendency to metatarsus primus varus is increased in a foot with an accessory bone, or os intermetatarsale, at the proximal part of the first intermetatarsal space (Renton 1991).

### Relative length of the first metatarsal

- In a foot with a relatively short first metatarsal, where the first metatarsal is shorter than the fourth metatarsal, the foot must abduct to allow the first MTPJ to function as the major fulcrum of gait. Toe-off occurs at the medial side of the hallux, with abduction of the hallux at the first MTPJ.
- In a foot with a relatively long first metatarsal, where the first metatarsal is longer than the fourth metatarsal, the major fulcrum of the foot (i.e. the first MTPJ) is relatively more distal and thus is loaded later in the gait cycle. As a result, the lateral pull of intrinsic muscles, such as the transverse head of adductor hallucis, is prolonged, and the action of abductor hallucis is not strong enough to overcome the resultant adduction of the hallux at the first MTPJ.

### Decreased muscular function

The tendon of the peroneus longus inserts into the plantar aspect of the base of the first metatarsal. The tendon lies along a vector, the forces of which can be resolved into longitudinal and transverse components. The longitudinal component is relatively larger in a foot that is pronated at toe-off, so that the foot rotates about the longitudinal axis of the midtarsal joint, with resultant pronation, loading of the medial aspect of the hallux at toe-off, and a tendency to hallux abduction.

### Iatrogenic or idiopathic features

- The loss of function of the second toe, due to amputation, traumatic dislocation or congenital hammer deformity, reduces its effect as a lateral buttress to the hallux, allowing the hallux to drift into a valgus subluxation at the first MTPJ.
- Excision of the medial (tibial) sesamoid causes instability of the first MTPJ, as it compromises the insertions of abductor hallucis tendon, the medial band of the plantar aponeurosis and the medial head of the flexor hallucis brevis. There is resultant unequal pull on the base of the proximal phalanx, so that the hallux deviates laterally.

## Pathology of hallux abducto valgus

There are a number of pathomechanical factors that contribute to the pathology of hallux abducto valgus. These include:

- the forefoot effects of excessive, prolonged or compensatory pronation at the rearfoot and midtarsal joints (i.e. the foot that is pronated at toe-off)
- the essential difference in the direction of the axis of motion of the first ray compared with all other axes of motion within the foot
- the orientation of the skeletal and soft tissue components that make up the first ray
- sesamoid dysfunction
- the effects of hallux abducto valgus-induced changes to the function of soft tissue structures within the foot.

### Excessive or prolonged foot pronation

This originates from compensation at the subtalar and midtarsal joints in response to a foot or lower limb anomaly – pronation at the subtalar and midtarsal joints is a normal feature of the midstance phase of gait, and allows the foot to function as a mobile reactor in response to ground reaction forces. The effects of excessive rear- and midfoot pronation include an increase in midfoot mobility, decreased stability of the forefoot joints, and loss of effective forefoot supination at toe-off.

- Propulsive forces of forward motion on an abducted or pronated forefoot load the medial aspect of the forefoot and exacerbate the development of hallux abducto valgus.

- Load at the medial aspect of the forefoot at toe-off causes a loss of or reduction in the midstance locking mechanism at the midtarsal joint. The locking mechanism is triggered in the normal foot by the influence of ground reaction forces at the lateral aspect of the mid- and forefoot. The loss of this mechanism means that the foot remains flexible/mobile in the later stages of stance.
- The flexible foot fails to become a rigid lever at toe-off, with resultant effects on gait efficiency – the patient develops an apropulsive gait.
- Medial forefoot loading results in a loss of or reduction in whole-foot supination at toe-off. Ground reaction forces are focused about the distal–medial area of the first ray, rather than at the plantar area of the MTPJs and the plantar pulp of the hallux, with the result that the hallux is pushed into abduction at toe-off.

### Pronation and supination in the first ray

The axes of motion of all the joints within the foot are angled in relation to the cardinal planes of the body, showing a greater or lesser degree of triplanar movement (supination and pronation). In general, supination is characterised by a combination of inversion, plantar flexion and adduction (towards the midline of the body). Pronation is characterised by a combination of eversion, dorsiflexion and abduction (away from the midline of the body). The axes of motion of all joints within the foot, with the exception of the axis of motion of the first ray, are directed from lateral–plantar–proximal to medial–dorsal–distal. In contrast, the axis of motion of the first ray is oriented in the direction medial–plantar–proximal to lateral–dorsal–distal.

- In a foot where there is a degree of metatarsus primus varus, the tendency to eversion of the first metatarsal at toe-off is maximised.
- The normal resistance to eversion of the first metatarsal is reduced, and the medial sesamoid becomes weight bearing at its medial border.
- The force of the altered pattern of weight bearing and longitudinal pull of the flexor hallucis brevis tendon at the medial sesamoid predisposes to erosion of the crista.
- The apparent transposition of the medial sesamoid to the lateral sesamoid groove is facilitated.

### Change in the orientation of the skeletal and soft tissue components that make up the first ray

In the normal foot, the 65–70° of dorsiflexion at the first MTPJ at toe-off is achieved by a combination of dorsiflexion of the hallux and plantar flexion at the distal end of the first metatarsal within the first MTPJ. Contraction of the extensor hallucis longus contributes only 20–30° of the available dorsiflexion at the first MTPJ at toe-off. Contraction of the peroneus longus muscle, via the insertion of its tendon into the plantar base of the first metatarsal, causes the head of the first metatarsal to move into 40° of plantar flexion at toe-off (Frank et al 2004). Due to its point of insertion, the peroneus longus also tends to exert an adductory pull at the base of the first metatarsal. The contraction of the peroneus longus, occurring just before toe-off, converts the foot from a mobile adaptor to a rigid lever, and increases the tendency to metatarsus primus varus.

- The efficiency of the action of the peroneus longus tendon as a plantar flexor of the first metatarsal is compromised in a pronated foot, so that the degree of whole-foot supination at toe-off is reduced. The peroneus longus tendon operates on a vector that is oriented more towards the longitudinal axis of the foot than the transverse axis, and its supinatory action at the first ray is diminished.

- The loss of peroneus-longus-mediated first metatarsal plantar flexion (as part of supination) at toe-off means that active dorsiflexion at the first MTPJ is reduced by almost two-thirds. As active dorsiflexion at the first MTPJ is then achieved primarily through the action of the extensor hallucis longus, heel lift and the effects of ground reaction forces, the first MTPJ becomes far less stable.
- The reduced efficiency of the peroneus longus also predisposes to dorsiflexion of the first ray. Ground reaction forces at the plantar aspect of the first MTPJ overcome any residual first metatarsal plantar flexion. The first ray moves up into dorsiflexion and the ground reaction forces are transferred to the lesser MTPJs, predisposing to metatarsalgia.
- Dorsiflexion of the first ray reduces the normal (65–70°) dorsiflexion at the first MTPJ. As the same ground reaction and body forces are operating over a shorter distance of movement, the momentum of forward motion at the articular surfaces of the first MTPJ subjects the joint to abnormally high forces, predisposing to joint degeneration.
- The reduced amount of available dorsiflexion at the first MTPJ is both compensated for, and exacerbated by, an increase in abduction of the forefoot (as part of excessive pronation of the subtalar and midtarsal joints). Abduction of the forefoot causes loading of the plantar–medial aspect of the hallux at toe-off, and forces the great toe into an increasing valgus deformity at the first MTPJ.
- The axes of motion of the first metatarsophalangeal and first metatarsal–cuneiform joints may contribute to the development of hallux abducto valgus. Transverse plane motion of the hallux at the first MTPJ (i.e. hallux abduction) is facilitated where the head of the first metatarsal is rounded, rather than of a flatter profile (Ferrari & Malone-Lee 2002). The movement of the first metatarsal into varus is facilitated in an adductus-type foot, where the angulation of the axis of the first metatarsal–cuneiform joint is increased, relative to the frontal and sagittal plane.

## The influence of the position of the sesamoid complex (Fig 4.13)

Sesamoid function is severely compromised by the deformities and foot dysfunction that characterise hallux abducto valgus, and sesamoid dysfunction exacerbates hallux abducto valgus. When the relationship of the sesamoids within the first MTPJ complex is altered, as in hallux abducto valgus, joint stability is decreased and the ability of the hallux and first ray to further resist deforming forces is greatly reduced.

- A tendency to first metatarsal eversion at toe-off, as in metatarsus primus varus, imposes an unequal loading on the sesamoid complex at the plantar aspect of the first MTPJ, so that the medial (tibial) sesamoid receives a greater proportion of ground reaction forces than the lateral sesamoid.
- In an adductus foot, the distal (head) end of the first metatarsal moves medially at toe-off. Tension is created within the plantar joint capsule, generating pressure between the lateral (fibular) side of the medial sesamoid and the medial aspect of crista (the ridge of bone that separates the medial and lateral sesamoid grooves on the plantar aspect of the metatarsal head). The crista tends to undergo resorption, allowing the sesamoids to maintain their normal orientation within the flexor hallucis brevis tendon but becoming disarticulated from their normal position on the plantar aspect of the head of the first metatarsal. There is an apparent lateral drift of the sesamoids.
- The location of the medial sesamoid into the lateral sesamoid groove and the lateral sesamoid to the space between the first

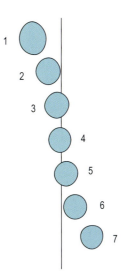

**Figure 4.13** The position of the medial sesamoid in relation to the midline (crista) on the plantar aspect of the head of the first metatarsal (Palladino 1991). Positions 1–3 allow the medial sesamoid to articulate with the medial plantar groove on the plantar aspect of the head of the first metatarsal and maintain the stability of the first MTPJ. A medial sesamoid in position 4–7 cannot locate to the medial groove. The crista becomes eroded and the medial sesamoid 'drifts' laterally. The stability of the first MTPJ is lost and, together with the 'bow string' effect of contraction of the extensor hallucis longus and flexor hallucis longus muscles, there is little to oppose further abduction of the hallux.

and second metatarsals effectively decreases the dorsiplantar dimension of the medial part of the head of the first metatarsal, so that an even greater degree of foot pronation will occur at toe-off.
- The lateral deviation of the hallux on the head of the first metatarsal is characterised by disuse atrophy of the articular cartilage, erosion of the subchondral bone, medial bone proliferation at the head of the first metatarsal, and thus increasing compromise of joint function.
- Adduction of the head of the first metatarsal, as in metatarsus primus varus, causes tension in the medial part of the capsule of the first MTPJ, in the medial collateral ligament and in the medial sesamoid ligament. The structures within the medial capsule stretch and allow the head end of the first metatarsal to adduct further.
- Under the principles of Davis' law, soft tissue structures at the lateral side of the first MTPJ contract and shrink, and thus maintain the abducted position of the hallux.

## Dysfunction of soft tissue structures in hallux abducto valgus

- There are no tendons that insert into the head of the first metatarsal. The integrity of the first MTPJ is maintained by the joint architecture and the correct orientation of the soft tissue structures that pass across it and insert into structures local to it. Orientation on the sagittal plane is maintained by the pull of the long flexor and extensor tendons (flexor and extensor hallucis longus) as they cross the first MTPJ, enhanced by the relationship of the sesamoid complex with the plantar aspect of the first MTPJ, and the contraction of the oblique head of the adductor hallucis muscle. Transverse plane stability is provided by the antagonism of the actions of the abductor hallucis muscle and the transverse head of the adductor hallucis muscle.

- The adductus foot with metatarsus primus varus is characterised by medial deviation of the distal part of the first metatarsal and loss of transverse plane stability (Hockenbury 1999). As the tendons of flexor and extensor hallucis longus pass across the first MTPJ to insert into the phalanges of the hallux, medial deviation of the head end of the first metatarsal (and lateral deviation of the hallux) is exaggerated by the 'bow string' effect of the flexor and extensor hallucis longus tendons as their muscles contract. This effect is maximal at toe-off, increasing the hallux valgus angle (i.e. the transverse and sagittal planes angulation between the base of the proximal phalanx and the longitudinal axis of the first metatarsal), with the result that both the flexor and the extensor hallucis longus act as auxiliary abductors of the hallux.
- The apparent 'lateral shift' of the sesamoids facilitates the bow-string effect of the flexor hallucis longus tendon, as its path is determined by the position of the twin tendons of the flexor hallucis brevis in relation to the plantar aspect of the first MTPJ.
- The greater the lateral displacement of the hallux at the first MTPJ, the greater is the mechanical advantage of the tendons to accentuate the first MTPJ deformity, and the more the medial aspect of the first MTPJ capsule is placed under tension, and the lateral aspect under compression. Davis' law dictates that the medial aspect of the capsule of the first MTPJ stretches, and the lateral aspect contracts and shrinks, so that the joint deformation is perpetuated by soft tissue adaptation.
- Tension within the medial collateral ligament further compromises transverse and sagittal plane stability at the first MTPJ (Kura et al 1998). Lateral drift of the hallux allows the medial area of the capital cartilage of the first metatarsal head to be exposed, so that it no longer articulates with the base of the phalanx. The exposed cartilage undergoes degeneration, and the underlying bone proliferates to form the medial bony eminence that is so characteristic of hallux abducto valgus.
- The tendon of abductor hallucis muscle inserts into the medial aspect of the base of the proximal phalanx of the hallux. Where the hallux has undergone a degree of axial rotation, frontal plane stability of the first MTPJ is compromised. Abductor hallucis insertion becomes oriented more towards the plantar aspect of the foot, and the muscle acts as an auxiliary plantar flexor of the hallux. It is no longer able to apply an efficient transverse plane force to the medial side of the hallux. The adductory force of the transverse head of the adductor hallucis muscle is unopposed, and the hallux pulled further into a valgus (abducted) position.

## Clinical picture in hallux abducto valgus

The patient presents with pain in and around the first MTPJ area. Pain is exacerbated by activity, aggravated by tight or high-heeled shoes, and relieved to some extent by rest or a change of shoe style. The patient is usually concerned about the unsightly appearance of the medial 'bunion', the lesser toe deformities and associated nail pathologies characteristic of the foot with hallux abducto valgus, and the difficulty of obtaining shoes to accommodate the increased width of the forefoot. In addition to the symptoms that the patient reports, the clinician notes: metatarsus primus varus and hallux abducto valgus; a medial eminence at the head of the first metatarsal, which is often overlain with a large bursa; a reduced range of dorsiflexion at the first MTPJ, with pain and/or crepitus on passive movement of the hallux; palpable marginal osteophytes at the first MTPJ; second-toe hammer deformity with associated subluxation of the second toe at the second MTPJ; clawing and/or varus rotation (supination) of the third/fourth/fifth toes; rearfoot and/or forefoot varus; a range of nail

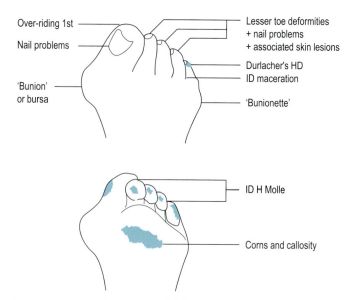

**Figure 4.14** The typical pattern of deformity and forefoot lesions with hallux abducto valgus.

pathologies; and hyperkeratotic lesions on the toes and plantar forefoot (Fig. 4.14).

## Clinical examination in hallux adducto valgus

The underlying, principal cause of the hallux abducto valgus deformity must be determined. This is achieved from the patient history, from a physical examination of the foot and limb (both weight bearing and non-weight bearing) and a biomechanical evaluation of lower limb and foot function.

In the relatively healthy patient, the development of hallux abducto valgus is usually associated with biomechanical and intrinsic factors. Extrinsic factors associated with hallux abducto valgus will either predispose the patient to develop the condition as a direct result of the systemic disease process, or exacerbate any natural tendency to hallux abducto valgus due to inherent intrinsic factors. For example, patients with rheumatoid disease tend to develop marked eversion of the rearfoot, due to the effects of inflammatory arthritis within the subtalar joint. The resultant excessive whole-foot pronation, together with the generalised connective tissue inflammation that characterises the disease (e.g. vasculitis, synovitis, capsulitis, tendonitis, bursitis), predisposes to instability at all forefoot joints, with severe hallux abducto valgus and marked lesser toe deformities.

The biomechanical evaluation should include examination of the lower limb and foot to note:

- Lower limb relationships: hip (internal/external) rotation, knee position (varum/valgum/recurvatum), the presence of external tibial torsion and/or tibial varum.
- Relationships within the foot: the range of available ankle dorsiflexion, the ranges of motion at the subtalar and midtarsal joints, the neutral relaxed calcaneal stance position, the relationship of the calcaneum to the lower leg at the neutral subtalar joint, the relationship of the forefoot and rearfoot at the neutral subtalar joint, the ranges of motion of the first ray and the first MTPJ, and the metatarsal formula.

### Non-weight-bearing examination

With the patient in a non-weight-bearing position, the following should be assessed:

- The position of the hallux on the horizontal plane, in relation to the second toe.
  - Lateral deviation of the hallux may result from subluxation of the hallux at the first MTPJ, or relate to structural changes within the hallux, such as hallux interphalangeus valgus.
  - The hallux may override, underride, abut, or not contact the second toe.
  - Where the extensor hallucis longus has a greater pull than the flexor hallucis longus, the hallux tends to hyperextend and rotate in relation to the frontal plane, so that the medial (tibial) nail wall becomes weight bearing, and the plantar aspect of the pulp of the hallux tends to override the dorsum of the second toe, causing the second toe to adopt a hammer position.
  - Where the flexor hallucis longus has a greater pull than the extensor hallucis longus, the hallux tends to underride the second toe, and the second toe tends to dislocate at the second MTPJ.
- The medial eminence: this is formed by the hypertrophy of the medial and dorsomedial aspects of the head of the first metatarsal. Its junction with the dorsomedial aspect of the head of the first metatarsal is marked by a 'sagittal groove'.
  - The medial eminence is usually associated with the formation of an adventitious bursa within the overlying soft tissues.
  - The bursa may become very large and fluctuant and be subject to inflammation (bursitis), chilling, tissue breakdown and infection. It is often termed a 'bunion'.
- The available range of motion at the first MTPJ: the first MTPJ complex should be taken through its full range of movement (dorsiflexion and plantar flexion, adduction and abduction, inversion and eversion, clockwise and anti-clockwise circumduction) to identify pain, crepitus, restriction or excess movement.
  - The normal non-weight-bearing range of motion at the first MTPJ is 65–70° of dorsiflexion and 15–20° of plantar flexion. The range of dorsiflexion is usually decreased in hallux abducto valgus.
  - The quality of the motion at the first MTPJ should be noted, especially the presence of pain and/or crepitus, which indicates damage to the intra-articular cartilage. Pain on movement without crepitus is indicative of synovitis at the first MTPJ.
  - The degree of abduction of the hallux at the first MTPJ is examined to determine whether the abduction deformity can be corrected passively. An abducted hallux that cannot be passively placed into a corrected (rectus) position indicates contracture and shrinkage of soft tissues at the lateral aspect of the first MTPJ.
- The range of motion at the first ray: the normal range of motion of the first ray at the level of the first MTPJ is 5 mm dorsiflexion and 5 mm plantar flexion (10 mm overall). The resting position of the first ray with the foot in subtalar joint neutral should be assessed by comparison to the position of the second ray, and both should lie in the same plane, and parallel to the ground surface.
  - With hallux abducto valgus, the first ray may be plantar or dorsiflexed relative to the second ray.
  - Transverse motion at the first metatarsal–cuneiform joint and the first MTPJ should be assessed: in a normal foot there is little to no transverse motion available in the medial column, but transverse plane motion is usually noted with hallux abducto valgus.
- The prominence of extensor hallucis longus tendon, and the path taken by the tendon should be noted.

- The path of the extensor hallucis longus tendon on the dorsum of the first MTPJ reflects the path of the flexor hallucis longus tendon at the plantar aspect of the joint, and thus shows the degree of 'bow-stringing' of the extrinsic muscle tendons occurring in association with hallux abducto valgus.
- A prominent extensor hallucis longus tendon indicates soft tissue contracture, hyperextension of the hallux at the first MTPJ, and/or hyperextension of the hallucal interphalangeal joint. It characterises a long-standing hallux abducto valgus deformity.
- The presence of plantar keratoses.
  - Hyperkeratosis in the plantar first MTPJ area indicates excessive plantar pressure at that site secondary to ankle equinus, rigid forefoot valgus, non-mobile pes cavus, a non-reducible plantar-flexed first metatarsal, prominent sesamoids, and/or atrophy of the plantar fat pad below the first MTPJ.
  - Focal plantar hyperkeratosis at the second metatarsal head can indicate a short first metatarsal (bradymetatarsal), a relatively long second metatarsal, a dorsiflexed first metatarsal (metatarsus primus elevatus), hypermobility of the first metatarsal and first ray, and retrograde pressure at the second metatarsal head secondary to deformity of the second toe (a hammered, clawed or retracted second toe).
  - Plantar hyperkeratosis in the second, third, fourth and fifth MTPJs area is associated with lesser toe deformities, where imbalance between the pull exerted by the extensor digitorum longus and the flexor digitorum longus muscles allows the toes to retract, claw or hammer, with resultant dorsiflexion of the proximal phalanges at the MTPJ. The base of the proximal phalanx exerts a plantarwards piston-like action at the dorsal aspect of the head of the metatarsal, and the metatarsal is forced into plantar flexion at toe-off, causing an increase in ground reaction forces at the overlying plantar skin and distal drift of the plantar fibrofatty padding.
  - Diffuse plantar hyperkeratosis in the second/third/fourth MTPJs area is associated with hypermobility of the foot, where the foot fails to supinate fully at toe-off. The height of the medial longitudinal arch is decreased in a pronated foot, and there is a relative lengthening of the foot at midstance that persists into toe-off. Shear forces at the plantar skin overlying the second/third/fourth MTPJs promote the formation of diffuse callosity.
- The presence of digital keratoses.
  - Hyperkeratosis at the medial–plantar aspect of the interphalangeal joint of the hallux indicates excessive foot pronation at toe-off.
  - Hyperkeratosis at the lateral (fibular) aspect of the hallux interphalangeal joint/medial (tibial) aspect of the proximal interphalangeal joint of the second toe indicates abduction of the hallux at toe-off.
  - The lesser toe deformities that characterise a foot with hallux abducto valgus predispose to apical, dorsal and interdigital callosity and corn formation. A deep helloma molle may form at the depth of the fourth/fifth interdigital sulcus, especially in association with sagittal hypermobility of the fifth ray.
- The presence of paraesthesia or reduced sensation at the medial and dorsomedial quadrant of the hallux.
  - Some patients note paraesthesia, pain or reduced sensation in the distribution of the cutaneous nerve, which serves the dorsomedial quadrant of the hallux. The nerve can be chronically irritated by exostoses at the medial/dorsal area of the first MTPJ (Camasta 1996).

- The presence of pain and/or onychophosis and/or onychocryptosis at the hallux nail.
  - Pain in the medial or lateral nail sulcus arises in conjunction with axial rotation of the hallux, where the medial sulcus becomes weight bearing and/or the lateral sulcus is compressed against the medioplantar aspect of the second toe.
  - Subungual pain or a subungual corn indicates that the hallux is in a hyperextended position at toe-off.
- The presence of other forefoot deformities that form the classic clinical presentation of hallux abducto valgus include:
  - lesser toe deformities, such as hammered second and third toes; clawing of the third, fourth and fifth toes; axial rotation or supination of the third, fourth and fifth toes; and associated dorsal, interdigital and apical hyperkeratoses
  - tailor's bunion formation, a similar but more minor deformity than hallux abducto valgus, affecting the fifth ray at the fifth MTPJ
  - a 'diamond'-shaped forefoot due to first ray (metatarsus primus varus and hallux valgus) and fifth ray (metatarsus quinque valgus and digiti minimi varus) deformities, and flat foot (Fig. 4.14).

### Standing examination

A standing examination illustrates how all features of the hallux abducto valgus deformity are increased by weight bearing, and deformities are more exaggerated when the patient stands on tiptoe.

- Both the transverse plane (hallux abduction) and the frontal plane (hallux eversion) moments of the hallux at the first MTPJ are increased on weight bearing.
- The angulation of the first metatarsal (the metatarsus primus varus angle) is increased and the medial prominence at the head of the first metatarsal is more obvious than in the non-weight-bearing foot, with a resultant increase in the tension, stretch and shear within the deep transverse ligament between the plantar plates of the first and second metatarsal heads, and the soft tissues at the medial aspect of the first MTPJ.
- The contracture of the extensor hallucis longus tendon is more obvious, so that any hyperextension (dorsiflexion) of the hallux at the interphalangeal joint or at the first MTPJ is exaggerated.
- *Hallux purchase* reflects the ability of the hallux to stabilise in response to ground reaction forces at toe-off. It can be assessed by the examiner attempting to pull on a piece of paper that is placed under the pulp of the great toe when the patient is standing in their normal angle and base of gait. Hallux purchase is classified as good (when the paper cannot be pulled out from under the toe), fair (when the paper under the hallux tends to move a little when pulled), poor (when the paper can be pulled from under the toe with very little effort) or absent (when the hallux is not in ground contact) (Frank et al 2004).

## Diagnosis of hallux abducto valgus

The diagnosis of hallux abducto valgus is based on the clinical observation of the typical forefoot deformities, and associated hyperkeratotic skin lesions, together with reported pain in and around the first MTPJ, metatarsalgia and the presence of characteristic lesser toe deformities. The differential diagnoses should exclude inflammatory joint disease and other extrinsic factors that predispose to hallux abducto valgus.

Weight-bearing plain radiographs are taken to determine the extent of joint pathology and forefoot deformity prior to carrying out corrective surgery. Views include anteroposterior, lateral oblique, lateral and axial projections.

- Anteroposterior and axial (skyline) views, taken in the angle and base of gait are used to visualise the quality of the sesamoids, the sesamoid–metatarsal joint space, the relationship of the sesamoids to the head of the first metatarsal, any lateral subluxation of the sesamoids from their respective grooves on the plantar aspect of the head of the first metatarsal, and erosion of the crista.
- An anteroposterior view is used to visualise specific relationships between the parts of the forefoot skeleton (Table 4.2), the relative lengths of the first and second metatarsals, the position of the sesamoids in relation to the head of the first metatarsal (Palladino 1991), the condition of the articular surfaces of the first MTPJ, the joint space at the first MTPJ, the quality of the bone stock, the angulation of the first metatarsal–cuneiform joint, the degree of rotation of the hallux, the size of the medial eminence of the first metatarsal head, and the degree of soft tissue pathology (e.g. swelling, chronic inflammation, calcification of intermetatarsal arteries).
- A lateral projection is used to determine the position of the first metatarsal in the sagittal plane (metatarsus primus elevatus) or to visualise the degree of plantar flexion of the first metatarsal

**Table 4.2** First ray relationships (from an anteroposterior view radiograph)

| Angle | Location | Value in a normal foot |
|---|---|---|
| Intermetatarsal angle | The angle subtended by the longitudinal axes of the first and second metatarsals | 8–12° |
| Metatarsus adductus angle (first metatarsophalangeal angle) | The angle subtended by the longitudinal axis of the lesser metatarsals and the first metatarsal | <15° |
| Hallux abductus angle | The angle between the longitudinal axis of the hallux and that of the first metatarsal | <20° |
| Proximal articular set angle (PASA) | The comparison of the plane of the articular surface of the head of the first metatarsal and that of the base of the proximal phalanx of the hallux | <7.5° |
| Distal articular set angle (DASA) | The comparison of the plane of the articular surface of the head of the proximal phalanx and that of the base of the distal phalanx of the hallux | <7.5° |
| Hallux valgus interphalangeus angle | The angle between the longitudinal axis of the proximal phalanx of the hallux and that of the distal phalanx | <10° |
| Sesamoid position | The position of the sesamoids in relation to the head of the first metatarsal | Positions 1–3 |

(normally in the range 15–30°), and to visualise a dorsal exostosis or osteophytes within the first MTPJ.

- The lateral oblique projection is useful in the evaluation of bone stock, to visualise the tarsometatarsal joints and to determine the dimensions of a dorsomedial exostosis.

## Treatment of hallux abducto valgus

Treatment of hallux abducto valgus includes the conservative and symptomatic management of the soft tissue and nail pathologies that are associated with the forefoot deformities, orthotic therapy to address the biomechanical dysfunction that predisposes to the development of the condition, and surgical correction of the deformity.

### Conservative and symptomatic management of nail and soft tissue pathologies

- Reduction of onychauxic nails and sharp debridement of onychophosis that forms in relation to the chronic trauma due to digital deformity.
- Regular sharp debridement of the areas of corn and hyperkeratosis that develop in relation to forefoot deformity, in association with the use of deflective and cushioning digital padding:
  - helloma molle at the interdigital aspects of the proximal and distal interphalangeal joints of adjacent toes and in the depth of the interdigital web spaces
  - digital helloma durum at the dorsum of the proximal interphalangeal joint in a hammer toe, the dorsum of the distal interphalangeal joint in mallet toe, or the apex in clawed toe
  - Durlacher corn at the lateral nail sulcus area in varus toe
  - plantar helloma durum at the MTPJ area of a toe with an associated fixed hammer deformity
  - diffuse plantar callosity at the lesser MTPJ areas.
- Anti-shear measures to reduce trauma to bony prominences:
  - clinical padding/strapping to reduce shear stress to the bursa at the medial aspect of the first MTPJ (see Ch. 16)
  - the use of an appropriate shoe style, such as flat shoes with a wide, deep toe box and positive fixing (laces) to accommodate the breadth of the forefoot, any clinical padding and in-shoe orthoses.
- The provision of bespoke or semi-bespoke shoes that will accommodate both the deformity and an orthotic, and/or shoe adaptations to the first MTPJ area:
  - stretch of the shoe upper to accommodate the medial eminence and lesser toe deformities
  - provision of a false bursa or balloon patch to accommodate the medial eminence and lesser toe deformities.

### Orthotic therapy

- Palliative devices to correct non-fixed digital deformity, and to cushion and deflect plantar pressure, such as:
  - silicone orthodigita
  - moulded cushioned insoles to compensate for loss of the plantar forefoot fibrofatty pad
  - deflective plantar pads to support the medial longitudinal arch and reduce pressure on isolated plantar lesions.
- Dynamic orthoses to stabilise the rearfoot and midfoot and reduce excessive foot pronation. These are not indicated for patients with fixed rearfoot deformity or inflammatory arthritis.

### Surgical correction of the forefoot deformity

There are more than a hundred types of surgical procedure to address the pain and deformity of hallux abducto valgus. Surgery for hallux

**Table 4.3** A range of surgical options for the treatment of hallux abducto valgus

| Patient | Assessment of deformity | Procedure(s) |
|---|---|---|
| Adolescent Young adult | Mild deformity Stable joint HV angle 20–30° IM angle <15° | Distal varus osteotomy (e.g. Mygurd–Thomason) |
| Adolescent Adult <45 years | Moderate deformity No joint degeneration HV angle 30–40° IM angle <15° | Distal displacement osteotomy (e.g. Mitchell or Wilson) |
| Adolescent Adult <45 years | Moderate deformity No joint degeneration HV angle 30–40° IM angle <15° Flat foot | Proximal valgus osteotomy (e.g. Shaft), displacement osteotomy (e.g. Scarfe–Akin) |
| Adult | Moderate deformity Joint degeneration HV angle 30–40° IM angle <15° | Silastic replacement (e.g. Helal or Swanson) |
| Adult | Severe deformity Joint degeneration HV angle >40° IM angle >20° | Basal closing wedge osteotomy (e.g. Allum and Higginson) Screw arthrodesis |
| Adult | Recurrent cases Cases with severe preoperative metatarsalgia | Screw arthrodesis at first MTPJ |
| Adult Elderly | Failed silastic implant Moderate deformity Joint degeneration HV angle 30–40° IM angle <20° Osteophytosis ++ | Excision arthroplasty + wire distraction if IM angle >15° (e.g. Keller) |

IM = Inter-metatarsal; HV = Hallux Valgus; ++ marked.

abducto valgus follows three principles: soft tissue surgery, first-MTPJ-preserving surgery, and first-MTPJ-destructive surgery. Joint-preserving surgery is always indicated for younger patients, and joint-destructive procedures ought to be reserved for older subjects. Where hallux abducto valgus is problematic in a child (i.e. before the bones have fully ossified), soft tissue procedures together with orthotic therapy are indicated. The surgical procedure of choice is the one that will give the best outcome for the presenting array of forefoot pathologies for that particular patient (Table 4.3).

- Soft tissue procedures include tendon division and transfer, and resection of bursae.
- Reduction of the medial bony eminence (cheilectomy or bumpectomy).
- The hallux deformity may be corrected by means of arthroplasty or arthrodesis at the first MTPJ and realignment of the hallux, such as a Scarf–Akin procedure.
- Lesser toe deformities can often be corrected by arthrodesis or arthroplasty at the interphalangeal joint(s) with soft tissue release at the relevant MTPJ.

- Metatarsus primus varus is corrected by first metatarsal shaft realignment, together with removal of the medial exostosis, such as a Scarfe or an Austin procedure, or by arthrodesis of the first metatarsal–medial cuneiform joint.
- An overlong or short first metatarsal can be effectively shortened or lengthened by the use of an appropriate osteotomy technique.
- Midfoot surgery: an unstable first ray may be stabilised by a Lapidus procedure (i.e. fusion of the first metatarsal–medial cuneiform joint).

## OTHER FOOT DISORDERS

## Osteochondrosis/osteochondritis

Osteochondrosis is the generic term used to describe a group of syndromes that share the common pathology of idiopathic bone disease (Ekman & Carlson 1998). The pathogenesis of osteochondritis is unclear, but all presentations are characterised by an interruption of normal enchondral ossification, together with a greater or lesser degree of focal death of the local trabeculated bone (Caselli et al 1998). A number of examples of osteochondritis affecting specific bone sites are named eponymously to the physician who first reported the disease. The onset of osteochondritis generally occurs during childhood, especially during times of rapid growth, but the full effects of the resultant joint and bone damage may not become apparent, and problematic, until adulthood. Osteochondritis may give rise to focal bone deformation during the healing phase of the disease, where the forces imposed by body mass impinge on the areas of abnormal ossification or diseased bone, causing a change in the local bone architecture. The altered shape of the involved bone sites may give rise to pathologies later in life.

## Classification

Osteochondritis may be classified in relation to the anatomical location of the enchondral ossification defect (Griffin 1994):

- osteochondritis of the *primary articular epiphysis* – e.g. Freiberg's disease (of the metatarsal head) and Kohler's disease (of the navicular)
- osteochondritis of the *secondary articular epiphysis* – e.g. osteochondritis dissicans of the talus
- osteochondritis of the *non-articular epiphysis* – e.g. Sever's disease (of the tibial tuberosity) and Iselin's disease (of the base of the fifth metatarsal/styloid process).

Alternatively, osteochondritis may be classified by the effects brought about by local forces on the area of diseased enchondral bone:

- *Crushing apophysitis*, such as Freiberg's disease of the metatarsal head, where the retrograde force applied to the affected metatarsal head by the base of the phalanx, especially at toe-off, induces an eggshell fracture of the cortical bone overlying the area of necrosis, with resultant flattening of the metatarsal head.
- *Traction (or distraction) apophysitis*, such as Sever's disease, which affects the posterior leaflet of the calcaneus. Force due to contraction of the muscles in the posterior compartment of the lower leg is transmitted through the Achilles tendon to its principal site of insertion at the middle posterior facet of the calcaneum, causing the posterior ossification centre to detach from the body of the calcaneus. A similar pathology characterises Iselin's disease, where traction forces imposed by

the peroneus (fibularis) brevis muscle at its tendinous insertion into the styloid process at the base of the fifth metatarsal cause distraction of that secondary ossification centre. Thus Sever's and Iselin's diseases are more correctly termed 'apophyseal injuries'. Apophyses are accessory or secondary ossification centres that develop with bone maturation. They normally overlie a growth plate and are subject to traction forces from ligaments or tendons inserting into that area of the bone (Kaeding & Whitehead 1998). At times of rapid growth, the tension at the tendon insertion, in conjunction with normal action of the muscle, causes a local irritation and micro trauma, resulting in an apophysitis.

- *Fragmentation osteochondritis (osteochondritis dissicans)*: cortical bone overlying an enchondral defect fractures, forming a loose fragment of bone within the joint or at the tendon insertion site. Articular osteochondritides, such as Freiberg's and Kohler's diseases, as well as osteochondritis dissicans, may be characterised by a degree of bone fragmentation. The disease process may arise as the result of minor trauma, or occur as the result of the structural collapse of healthy bone overlying an area of avascular necrosis within the enchondral bone (Griffin 1994, Kaeding & Whitehead 1998). The bone fragment may persist as a 'flap'. Alternatively, it may fully detach to form an intra-articular loose body, which is either later reabsorbed, or enlarges by a process of enchondral ossification.

### Aetiology

The true aetiology of the various presentations of osteochondritis is unknown, but they have been linked to hereditary factors, local trauma, nutritional factors and local ischaemia within the affected area of bone (Ekman & Carlson 1998, Walsh & Dorgan 1988).

### Diagnosis

Plain radiographs are usually used to diagnose osteochondritis, but minor or early-stage lesions may be overlooked as they are difficult to visualise on a plain radiograph. Lesions are identified readily using bone scan, computerised axial tomography scan and magnetic resonance imaging (Bohndorf 1998).

### Differential diagnosis

The differential diagnosis for all the osteochondritides can include osteomyelitis, bone tumours and fractures (Caselli et al 1998).

### Treatment

The treatment of all presentations of osteochondritis focuses on rest and immobilisation to allow the affected bone to heal with no or only minimal distortion, together with the use of painkillers (such as NSAIDs), as necessary, during the acute or early presentations of the disease.

Rest and immobilisation of the affected bone is essential:

- to reduce local pain and swelling
- to promote bone healing
- to prevent or reduce the incidence of unwanted forces at the area of diseased bone, so that the normal bone architecture is preserved and local disruption and distortion minimised.

Early initiation of treatment is especially important where the involved osteochondritic bone forms part of a joint, in order to reduce the likelihood of later osteoarthritic changes, pain and dysfunction of the affected joint.

The format, intensity and duration of the regimen of rest is tailored to the presenting problem, and can be achieved by a variety of means, such as rigid splinting, soft splinting and strapping, and other means to reduce weight bearing, and traction and compressive forces on the involved bone.

- Prolonged or imposed rest will always require a follow-up period of rehabilitation and programmed exercise to assist return to normal muscular function, and overcome disuse atrophy of limb muscles. For example, a patient who is prescribed a below-knee plaster cast as part of the management of Sever's disease may develop ankle equinus as the foot is held in a plantar-flexed position during healing in order to rest the area by minimising the pull of the Achilles tendon on the posterior heel area. The patient is likely to remain in the cast for at least 6 weeks to allow the calcaneum to heal, during which time the Achilles tendon will tend to shorten, under the principles of Davis' law, and the bulk of the muscles of the posterior compartment of the lower leg (gastrocnemius and soleus) will reduce due to disuse atrophy. The rehabilitation programme should ensure that the exercise regimen encourages normal function of the posterior muscle group in order to prevent the subsequent development of a permanent ankle equinus with a resultant alteration to gait, such as an early heel lift and premature loading of the forefoot.
- Where the architecture of the affected bone has become permanently distorted as the result of the disease process, such as in cases of Freiberg's disease, an in-shoe orthosis may be needed to reduce weight bearing at the affected MTPJ.
- A fragment of bone, also known as a loose body or sequestrum, within the joint capsule, formed as the result of osteochondritis dissicans, may later resorb. Alternatively, it may need to be excised as a surgical or arthroscopic procedure. If the fragment of bone has enlarged, it may be reattached by means of an internal fixation procedure.

---

### CASE STUDY 4.3 OSTEOCHONDRITIS DISSICANS: PRESENTATION IN AN ADULT

A 54-year-old woman presented with a 10-month history of pain in the right foot. She worked as a radiography assistant in a local hospital. She recalled that on 16 December of the previous year, whilst walking along a corridor from the x-ray department to one of the wards to deliver a patient's radiograph, she experienced a sudden and severe shooting pain in the right forefoot. The pain located to the base of the second toe, and continued throughout that day, and she was unable to walk without limping heavily on the right foot. That night, she applied ice to the foot, and self-medicated with ibuprofen. By the next day, the pain had not reduced at all. There was some mild local swelling in the area of the right second metatarsophalangeal joint (MTPJ). The patient reported that a radiograph, taken within 24 hours of the incident, failed to show any bone lesion. It was assumed by the GP that she had suffered some form of foot strain. The swelling cleared within 3 weeks, and the severe pain gradually subsided over the next 3 months, although the right second toe continued to be very painful on movement at the second MTPJ.

She was referred to the podiatrist in September of the following year. On examination, it was noted that her feet showed the typical forefoot deformities of moderate hallux limitus, with 45° of available passive dorsiflexion at the first MTPJ. Passive sagittal plane movement of the right second toe was much reduced, with crepitus and pain at the right second MTPJ. There was a palpable dorsiplantar thickening of the right forefoot in the area of the second MTPJ. Plain

radiographs showed marked degenerative changes at the head of the right second metatarsal and the base of the associated proximal phalanx, with flattening of the metatarsal dome, osteophytosis at the head of the right second metatarsal and base of the associated proximal phalanx, and local bone sclerosis.

On the basis of the history and the September radiograph the patient was diagnosed as showing arthritic degeneration of the right second MTPJ. It was presumed that the patient may have suffered an osteochondritis dissicans the previous December, secondary to an overload phenomenon imposed by the loss of movement at the first MTPJ, and possibly in association with a degree of age-related osteoporosis. The bone lesion at the second metatarsal head did not show up on the radiograph taken within 24 hours of the original incident, as the radiograph was taken at too early a stage in the pathology for it to be visible on plain radiography. Subsequent degenerative changes had developed over the ensuing months, causing osteoarthritis at the right second MTPJ.

The right forefoot problem was treated by conservative therapy, initially with defective clinical plantar padding, then with a bespoke cushioned orthotic and the use of a rocker-soled shoe. This reduced her forefoot pain to what the patient felt was an acceptable level. As the patient did not wish to contemplate forefoot surgery, she was not referred to an orthopaedic or podiatric surgeon.

---

## Freiberg's disease (Freiberg's infraction)

This form of osteochondritis affects the metatarsal head(s). In four out of five cases the patient is a girl aged between 12 and 15 years (Griffin 1994, Manusov et al 1996b).

### Pathology

Freiberg's disease may present uni- or bilaterally, as a focus of ischaemia and bone necrosis within the head of a metatarsal, leading to collapse of both the articular surface and the underlying area of subchrondral bone – the so-called eggshell fracture. The head of the second metatarsal is affected in almost 70% of cases, and the third metatarsal head in almost 30% of cases, but any of the metatarsal heads may be subject to infraction (Griffin 1994). The predominance of osteochondritis affecting the second metatarsal head is thought to be due to the greater length of the second metatarsal in relation to the first and third metatarsals, and its resultant susceptibility to local trauma during the gait cycle, especially at toe-off. It is thought that the blood supply to the epiphyseal plate is interrupted by repeated microtraumata, causing an area of avascular necrosis within the metatarsal head (Manusov et al 1996b).

### Clinical picture

The patient presents with increasing pain and associated swelling, and possible bruising on the dorsum of the foot, overlying the affected metatarsal head. Gait is affected and the patient may limp (Caselli et al 1998). The pain worsens on weight bearing and with activity. The range of motion at the affected MTPJ is decreased, particularly when active and/or weight-bearing dorsiflexion of the toes is attempted. Pain and crepitus is likely to be elicited on passive movement of the affected joint.

### Diagnosis and differential diagnosis

In the early stages of the disease plain radiographs may show little apparent bone involvement. In the later stages, as healing progresses, new bone growth in the affected area can be seen. The classical radiographic presentation in the adult who has undergone an episode of Freiberg's infraction as a teenager, or an untreated Freiberg's disease

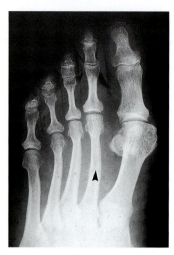

**Figure 4.15** Freiberg's disease: radiograph of the foot on initial presentation appears normal.

in a younger person, is of a flattened metatarsal head, with associated signs of osteoarthritic changes, such as bone sclerosis and osteophyte formation, occurring at the metatarsal head (Fig. 4.15). The base of the associated proximal phalanx may also show degenerative changes. The differential diagnoses of an acute presentation in a young person should exclude a march fracture, rheumatoid arthritis, intermetatarsal bursitis and other overuse injuries that may arise in relation to sports or dancing.

## Treatment

The principal focus of the treatment of Freiberg's disease is to reduce or eliminate weight-bearing forces to the affected bone area during the 6 weeks of the acute phase of the disease. This is achieved by imposing a regimen of non-weight bearing on the affected foot, with rest and painkillers as necessary. Non-weight bearing during the acute phase of the disease is necessary to ensure that retrograde pressure from the base of the proximal phalanx on the affected metatarsal head at toe-off is minimised, allowing bone healing to proceed without loss of the normal architecture of the affected metatarsal head. Non-weight bearing on the affected foot is achieved by the use of crutches, together with soft splintage of the foot, or rigid splintage of the lower limb and foot.

- Soft splintage includes the use of clinical semicompressed felt pads, such as a U-shaped metatarsal pad, a metatarsal shaft pad, or a valgus filler extended as a shaft to support the affected metatarsal, together with supportive bandaging, such as a figure-of-eight bandage to the ankle and foot, or the application of elasticised tubular bandage (e.g. Tubigrip®) from toe to knee. The patient should wear a roomy shoe with a thick firm outer sole and cushioned insole.
- Immobilisation of the foot, ankle and lower leg in a rigid splint, such as a below-knee plaster of Paris cast, or an Aircast® boot may be preferred.
- Painkillers may be used as necessary. NSAIDs may be used to relieve pain, reduce local swelling and inflammation, and thereby promote healing. Aspirin is contraindicated in children below 12 years of age, and is not usually recommended for

children aged between 13 and 16 years. Paracetamol (Calpol™) is not a true NSAID, and may be used to control pain and reduce temperature in children under 16 years old.

Freiberg's disease may cause permanent alteration to or loss of the normal dome shape of the affected metatarsal head, even in cases where the disease has been identified in its early stages. The long-term treatment of these cases includes:

- The provision of an accommodative or functional orthotic, after the acute phase has passed.
- Surgery may be indicated to repair the bone defect. If the joint is pain-free on passive movement, a simple osteotomy will allow the affected metatarsal head to elevate to a non-weight-bearing position. In cases where the head of the affected metatarsal has become very flattened, or the involved MTPJ is painful, normal movement is restricted and has developed osteoarthritis, the affected MTPJ may be replaced by a prosthetic titanium joint or silicon elastomer implant. Alternatively, the affected metatarsal head may be remodelled using autologous or donor bone graft. If the affected metatarsal head is resected, adjacent toes may be syndactylised to prevent shortening of the associated toe as a result of the excision of the metatarsal head. The base of the proximal phalanx is not usually excised, although it too may be surgically remodelled. Excision of the metatarsal head can induce transfer pressure lesions in the skin overlying the adjacent MTPJs, and these metatarsals may also require later corrective surgery, such as an osteotomy.

---

### CASE STUDY 4.4 FREIBERG'S INFRACTION: ADOLESCENT PRESENTATION

A 12-year-old girl presented with a history of recent pain in her left forefoot. She related the onset of her symptoms to a sponsored walk that she had completed 3 weeks previously. She was otherwise in good health, with no marked foot deformity or swelling. She had not experienced any similar event in the past.

On examination the focus of pain was located to the second metatarsophalangeal joint (MTPJ) and the pain was exacerbated by both passive and active extension of the second toe, although there was no crepitus on movement of the second MTPJ. She was unable to stand on tiptoe on the left foot. The differential diagnosis included Freiberg's infraction of the head of the second metatarsal or stress fracture of the second metatarsal. Plain radiographs of the left foot excluded a stress fracture (as there was no indication of bone callous formation, which should have showed 3 weeks after the onset of symptoms) but the radiograph did not point to a definite diagnosis of Freiberg's disease.

The patient was treated symptomatically with orthoses designed to reduce plantar pressures at the painful second MTPJ area. These reduced her pain to a tolerable level. She was advised to rest the foot, and to wear stiff-soled shoes, to reduce movement at the MTPJs. Her condition was monitored. At 6 months after her initial visit a second radiographic examination was requested. The second radiograph showed pathological changes at the left second metatarsal head. The normal domed shape had been lost, and the head of the second metatarsal was flattened and 'squared off', and local bone sclerosis was noted.

After 18 months of palliative care the patient's symptoms subsided. There is an increased risk of this patient developing premature osteoarthritis at the left second MTPJ in later life.

# Kohler's disease

This form of osteochondritis affects the ossification centre of the navicular bone. Classically, Kohler's disease of the navicular affects young boys aged between 2 and 9 years. There is a male/female ratio of 4 : 1.

## Pathology

It is thought that repetitive minor trauma to the navicular bone causes patchy ossification (Manusov et al 1996b).

## Clinical picture

The patient presents with, or the parent notes, pain and possibly swelling in the medial–plantar area of the instep, with focal tenderness in the area of the navicular. Small children may become reluctant to run around or play as normal.

## Diagnosis and differential diagnosis

Initially, little shows on radiography, but radiographs from patients who have had Kohler's disease of the navicular in earlier childhood typically show anteroposterior narrowing (wafering) of the navicular, with increased bone density and loss of normal trabeculation in later life. In this age group, there are few other disease processes that give rise to these presenting features.

## Treatment

Some cases of Kohler's disease are self-resolving. Others require the use of soft splintage, such as semicompressed felt valgus filler pads, or supportive orthoses and appropriate footwear to maintain the architecture of the longitudinal arch of the foot during healing. Paracetamol (e.g. Calpol™) may be used to control pain in young children. Surgery is not usually indicated.

# Osteochondritis dissicans of the talus

Osteochondritis dissicans of the talus more commonly affects the talar head, although it may also affect the trochlear surface. The incidence is reported as 1 in 5000 (Griffin 1994), and it is more common amongst sports people such as skaters, runners and gymnasts (Manusov et al 1996a). There is often a history of recent trauma or severe inversion ankle sprain (Kaeding & Whitehead 1998), or the patient may recall only a relatively minor injury, such as slipping or stumbling.

## Pathology

The bone lesion is classified in four stages of presentation:

- Stage I – a small area of trabeculated subchrondral bone becomes compressed and relatively ischaemic.
- Stage II – the unsupported cortical bone begins to separate from the body of the bone, forming a bone 'flap'.
- Stage III – The cortical fragment dislodges, resulting in a bone crater.
- Stage IV – the detached fragment moves around within the joint cavity, distant to its site of origin, forming a loose body within the joint.

## Clinical picture

The patient presents with a painful, swollen ankle. The location of the pain and the swelling can aid the diagnosis of the exact site of the bone lesion. For example, osteochondritis dissicans of the talar head gives rise to focal pain and swelling in the medial area of the midtarsal joint, whereas osteochondritis dissicans of the trochlear surface of the talus will cause pain and swelling that relates to the anterior aspect of the ankle. However, if a loose body has formed within the ankle or talonavicular joints, the site of the pain and swelling is far less constant, and the patient describes episodes of acute focal pain and swelling that change location from day to day as the fragment of bone moves around within the joint cavity. Patients often report that the ankle 'locks' or 'catches', and that the ankle and subtalar joint area is unstable on weight bearing.

## Diagnosis and differential diagnosis

Radiographs may not identify the damaged area, especially in the early stages. Special views may need to be requested to visualise all aspects of the affected bone. Computerised tomography scans and magnetic resonance imaging are much more sensitive than radiography in the early diagnosis of osteochondritis dissicans of the ankle–subtalar–midtarsal joint complex.

## Treatment

The treatment of stages I and II includes rest and immobilisation for 6 weeks. This is achieved by the use of a below-knee plaster of Paris cast, an Aircast® boot, or an ankle–foot orthosis, together with the use of crutches to aid in walking. As healing progresses, the use of a firm walking boot, rather than a normal shoe, is of benefit, as it restricts movement of the rearfoot complex, yet allows relatively normal ambulation.

Stages III and IV may require surgical removal of the loose bone fragment, via arthroscopy, or internal fixation to reattach the detached bone fragment.

# Sever's disease

Sever's disease is perhaps the most common cause of heel pain in children, aged between 7 and 12 years (Griffin 1994, Manusov et al 1996a).

## Pathology

Heel pain in Sever's disease occurs as the result of an overuse syndrome, and is not a true avascular necrosis. Although it is commonly referred to as an osteochondritis, it is more accurately classified as a traction apophysitis.

The calcaneus has two centres of ossification: the primary centre, which is within the body of the calcaneum; and the secondary centre, which is within the posterior area of the bone. These centres of ossification unite when the bone attains maturity (becomes fully ossified) at about 12 years of age. Traction forces from the Achilles tendon on immature bone can induce epiphyseal distraction, (between the body and the posterior leaflet of the calcaneus) due to its insertion onto the middle third of the posterior surface of the calcaneum. Repetitive contractions of the muscles of the posterior compartment (gastrocnemius and soleus) may also predispose to microfractures at the calcaneal epiphyseal plate. A similar pathology is noted at the insertion of the patellar tendon into the tibial tubercle in Osgood Schlatter's disease (Madden & Mellion 1996).

## Clinical picture

The condition may be unilateral or bilateral. The patient presents with pain and tenderness that localises to the posterior aspect of the calcaneus. Pain is maximal after vigorous or impact exercise, such as running or gymnastics. There may be an associated warmth and oedema at the posterior heel area, and wearing shoes with a close heel counter aggravates symptoms. It affects boys more often than girls, and onset may link with growth spurts, especially in physically active or overweight children (Madden & Mellion 1996). Many patients will also show biomechanical compensation for structural foot anomalies that tend to reduce shock absorption at heel strike and expose the heel to abnormal ground reaction forces (Madden & Mellion 1996).

## Diagnosis and differential diagnoses

Diagnosis in the early stages of the disease is based on the history and the presenting symptoms. Diagnostic signs include: increased pain on passive dorsiflexion of the foot at the ankle, and exacerbation of symptoms when standing on tiptoe (a positive Sever's sign) (Madden & Mellion 1996). Radiographs of the calcaneus appear normal in the early stages of the disease process. As the disorder progresses, the apophyseal area shows sclerosis and fragmentation, although this finding is not necessarily diagnostic as this picture can also been seen in asymptomatic patients (Kaeding & Whitehead 1998).

The differential diagnosis should exclude a duck-bill fracture of the posterior leaflet of the calcaneum, Achilles tendon pathologies and deep retrocalcaneal bursitis.

## Treatment

Many authors believe Sever's disease to be self-limiting, as it tends to resolve spontaneously when calcaneal ossification is completed, usually at about 12 years of age. However, the use of physical therapies such as PRICE (pain control, rest, ice, compression and elevation) is beneficial in the acute phase of the disease. When symptoms are severe, a non-weight-bearing regimen, such as a below-knee cast for 6 weeks, or an Aircast® boot, and crutches, together with a course of NSAIDs is indicated. When the presenting symptoms are mild, the use of a figure-of-eight bandage to the affected rearfoot with a heel raise in the shoe is useful.

A heel raise should continue to be used after the acute phase has passed, in order to reduce the pull of the Achilles tendon on the posterior surface of the calcaneum. This will also minimise further trauma to the epiphyseal plate during the healing phase. Night splints, such as those used for the treatment of plantar fasciitis (Powell et al 1998) are also of benefit. After healing is complete, a regimen of rehabilitation exercises to stretch the Achilles tendon will be needed to prevent or reduce a tendency to ankle equinus, and a programme of stretching exercises and ice massage should continue to be used after strenuous activity. The patient should undergo a full biomechanical evaluation, and orthoses should be prescribed to correct any noted faults. The routine use of well-fitting trainers with good shock absorption should be recommended.

## Iselin's disease

Iselin's disease is a traction apophysitis that affects the base of the fifth metatarsal, at the insertion of peroneus brevis tendon (Lehman et al 1986). The proximal apophysis of the fifth metatarsal usually does not ossify fully until approximately 16 years of age. Overuse of the peroneus brevis tendon prior to full ossification causes inflammation, swelling and tenderness, bruising and pain at the dorsolateral area at the base of the fifth metatarsal (the styloid process). Diagnosis is confirmed by the presenting symptoms, together with increased local pain when the foot is everted against resistance. The differential diagnosis should exclude a stress fracture of the styloid process, a Jones fracture or an avulsion fracture of the styloid process. Symptoms usually respond to a short period of rest (Griffin 1994). In less responsive cases, the foot should be strapped into eversion, to minimise the pull of the peroneus brevis tendon, until the symptoms subside.

# REARFOOT DISORDERS

The distal ends of the tibia and fibular (forming the medial and lateral malleoli, respectively), the talus and the calcaneus, their interposed joints (the ankle joint and the subtalar joint) and the associated and overlying soft tissues (tendons, ligaments, retinaculae, adventitious and congenital bursae, deep and superficial fascia, the skin and subcuticular structures) form the rearfoot. Pathology and pain in the rearfoot may arise from problems with any of these structures. Thus rearfoot pathology can be classified by the tissue type involved in the pathological process (bone, joint, soft tissues), in conjunction with the location of the pathology (plantar, medial, lateral, or posterior).

## Posterior heel pain

Posterior heel pain may be caused by a number of soft tissue pathologies (e.g.: blister formation, infalmmation of the deep or superficial retrocalcaneal bursae, inflammation or rupture I partial rupture of the Achilles tendon), bone pathology (e.g.: Haglund's deformity, posterior heel spur, Sever's disease, 'duck-bill' fracture) or local trauma.

## Superficial retrocalcaneal bursitis

### Pathology

The Achilles tendon inserts into the middle third of the posterior facet of the calcaneus. A bursa readily forms within the soft tissues superficial to the insertion of the Achilles tendon, in response to stress at the central–lateral area of the posterior surface of the heel. This adventitious bursa is known as the superficial retrocalcaneal bursa. Inflammation of the adventitious bursa (superficial retrocalcaneal bursitis) is associated with rearfoot motion in association with compensated rearfoot varus, mobile pes cavus, or in cases where there is an increase in the angle of inclination of the calcaneus. Eversion of the calcaneus (frontal plane motion) occurs during compensation for these pathologies, and the foot rotates about the longitudinal axis of the midtarsal joint. The frontal plane rotation allows the calcaneus to evert, but imposes shear stresses within the soft tissues overlying central–lateral area of the posterior aspect of the heel, as these tissues move relative to the inner surface of the shoe. The continuous compensatory eversion of the heel predisposes to inflammation of the bursa. If the condition is of long standing, there may also be local hypertrophy of the underlying area of the posterior aspect of the calcaneus. The bony prominence thus formed is known as Haglund's deformity, or a 'pump bump'. The shear stresses affecting the overlying soft tissues increase in direct proportion to the size of the bony prominence, and the bursitis can become chronic. If the overlying skin is breached, such as in a broken chilblain or a ruptured blister, the bursa may become infected.

## Clinical features

The condition usually affects adolescent females, who present with pain in the posterior aspect of the heel, especially when wearing, or having worn a particular pair of shoes, such as high heels or a style with a marked heel counter. The patient may report seasonal fluctuations, as the problem may flare up if there is local perniosis (chilblain) affecting this area of the heel, when it is termed 'winter heel'. On examination, there will be an inflamed, fluctuant and very tender area at the central–lateral aspect of the posterior surface of the heel, with a palpable hypertrophy of the superficial fascia, and underlying bone in long-standing cases. The patient is often unable to wear a normal shoe, and the pain of the condition causes her to walk with a limp.

## Diagnosis and differential diagnosis

The diagnosis is usually made by reference to the presenting signs and symptoms. Oblique-lateral radiographs of the rearfoot will also demonstrate any additional bone formation at the central–lateral heel area. The differential diagnosis should exclude other causes of local soft tissue inflammation, such as chilblain or blisters.

## Treatment

Initially, a conservative approach is indicated:

- The patient is advised on appropriate accommodative footwear.
- Cooling lotions, such as witch hazel, or ice can be applied to the skin to reduce an acute inflammation, or rubefacients, such as warm water soaks, or iodine-based ointments are indicated to reduce chronic inflammation.
- If the skin is broken, the area should be treated as an open wound.
- Clinical padding may be used to reduce local stress to the inflamed area. This includes materials such as two-way stretch fleecy web oval to the posterior heel area to minimise shear stress, foam to cushion the area, together with an oval cavity pad fabricated from semicompressed felt to redistribute pressure. These pads can be applied either to the foot or to the inner aspect of the heel of the shoe.
- A heel cup, made of heat-moulded thermoplastic, such as soft density Plastazote™, can be manufactured to be worn within the shoe, or against the foot within the sock or stocking. Alternatively, a heel cup made to a cast of the foot can incorporate a 'doughnut' pad of closed cell padding material.
- Footwear can be modified – the heel stiffening overlying the bump can be removed. New shoes may be problematic, and may require modification before they are worn.

Surgery may be required to reduce the underlying bony prominence. A more laterally placed bony prominence can be reduced, but this becomes more difficult if the area of bone hypertrophy involves the attachment of the Achilles tendon. In those cases, a closing wedge osteotomy may be used to reduce the angle of inclination of the calcaneum.

## Deep retrocalcaneal bursitis

### Pathology

The deep retrocalcaneal bursa is a true anatomical bursa. It is located within the soft tissues at the posterior aspect of the heel, lying between the upper third of the posterior aspect of the calcaneus and the inner aspect of the Achilles tendon, immediately superior to its insertion into the middle third of the posterior aspect of the calcaneus. The bursa is a horseshoe-shaped structure, and in the adult is approximately 2 cm long, 1 cm wide and 0.5 cm deep (Frey et al 1992). Its inferior surface lies on the Achilles fat pad at the posterosuperior aspect of the proximal calcaneus, its anterior surface at the upper third of the posterior surface of the calcaneus, and its posterior surface against the deep aspect of the Achilles tendon.

Pathological changes (deep retrocalcaneal bursitis) can occur in response to local mechanical irritation, such as where the upper edge of a shoe with a marked heel counter traumatises the soft tissues at the superior area of the posterior surface of the heel. The inflamed bursa shows marked thickening and oedema of its walls. The volume of the contained synovial fluid increases, but its viscosity decreases. Deep retrocalcaneal bursitis may also be a feature of inflammatory joint disease, such as rheumatoid disease and seronegative arthropathies. In these cases the area of the calcaneus that receives the insertion of the Achilles tendon may show bone erosions.

## Clinical feature

The patient presents with diffuse pain that locates to the posterior aspect of the heel. The pain is exacerbated by active dorsiflexion of the foot, such as when walking upstairs as the inflamed bursa is compressed further, between the overlying Achilles tendon and the underlying calcaneus. The visible signs of inflammation are not obvious, although there may be some local warmth and swelling. The inflamed bursa is usually palpable as a tender, bi-lobed, fluctuant area of soft tissue, to either side of the Achilles tendon at a point just superior to its insertion into the posterior surface of the calcaneus. Palpation of the inflamed tissue may show a fluid 'thrill'.

## Diagnosis and differential diagnoses

The diagnosis is made from the presenting signs and symptoms. The bursa can be identified by bursography (the injection of a radio-opaque dye into the swollen bursa).

The differential diagnosis should exclude:

- Achilles tendonitis, affecting the Achilles tendon, at a point 2–5 cm superior to its insertion into the calcaneus.
- Superficial retrocalcaneal bursitis, in which there is usually an area of focal pain and inflammation at the central–lateral area of the heel.
- Rheumatoid or seronegative arthritides, which may be excluded by blood assay, and radiographs to seek for evidence of bone erosion.
- Sever's disease: this primarily affects children up to 12 years old, and the area of pain locates to the central area of the posterior aspect of the heel. In Sever's disease, standing on tiptoe, during active plantar flexion induces pain.

## Treatment

The underlying cause of the bursitis must be established, and in cases where there is evidence of underlying inflammatory joint disease the patient should be referred to a rheumatologist. Conservative therapy focuses on resting the traumatised area. This includes a review of the footwear. The use of a trainer, manufactured with a cut-out at the upper margin of the heel counter is very useful. A simple heel raise, such as a 7 mm semicompressed felt plantar heel pad, placed inside the shoe will prevent or reduce trauma from the upper edge of the heel counter and allow the bursal inflammation to subside. Severe cases may require aspiration of the bursa, and injection of a corticosteroid.

# Achilles tendonitis

Achilles tendonitis is a painful and sometimes debilitating inflammation of the Achilles tendon occurring at a point just superior to its insertion into the calcaneum. It is thought to affect up to 20% of runners, and is especially common in athletes who are poorly conditioned, or in recreational joggers who have not trained properly. Participation in activities that involve sudden stops and starts and repetitive jumping (e.g. squash, basketball, netball, football, tennis, fencing and dancing) also increases the risk of developing the condition. The condition is aggravated by the use of high-heel-tab trainers, or by wearing high-heeled shoes with a marked heel counter.

## Pathology

Microtears within the distal part of the Achilles tendon (or heel cord) and resultant local inflammation may be precipitated by a sudden increase in activity levels, training on poor surfaces, or using inappropriate footwear. Achilles peritendonitis may be precipitated by a single incident, or can develop gradually as a general overuse phenomenon. It may also affect women who adopt flat-heeled shoes after habitually wearing high heels, and, much more rarely, may present as a later complication of congenital pes valgus. In both these examples, the undue pull on the Achilles tendon causes a reflex spasm of the posterior calf muscles, with increased tension and the development of microtears within the heel cord.

There are three presentations associated with inflammation of the Achilles tendon: peritendonitis (also known as paratendinitis), tendinosis and peritendonitis with tendinosis.

- Peritendinitis (Paratendinitis) characterised by localised pain in the tendon during or following activity. The pain is primarily felt at a point along the tendon, approximately 5 cm superior to its site of insertion into the calcaneum. As the condition progresses, the pain develops at an increasingly early stage of activity, and may even occur at rest.
- Tendinosis is a degenerative condition of the Achilles tendon that usually does not produce painful symptoms during activity, but is characterised by swelling or a hard knot of tissue (nodule) approximately 5cm superior to the insertion of the tendon into the calcaneus.
- Peritendinitis with tendinosis is characterised by local pain and swelling along the distal Achilles tendon that increases with activity. The presentation of Achilles peritendonitis may progress to partial or complete rupture of the tendon.

## Clinical picture

The patient presents with pain in the distal part of the Achilles tendon that localises to a point approximately 5 cm superior to the point of insertion at the calcaneum. Characteristically the pain develops during strenuous activity and eases with rest. In the later stages of the problem, the pain may be severe and unrelenting even at rest, and prevent normal walking. The soft tissues overlying the affected area may be hot and swollen. If the patient has associated tendinosis, there will be a palpable and tender fusiform thickening along the tendon, or nodule formation at a point approximately 2–5 cm superior to the insertion of the tendon into the calcaneus. Generally the condition has a gradual onset, with mild pain that worsens with continued activity. Patients may also complain of pain on first weight bearing after a period of rest, such as when they first stand up in the morning. Repeated activity in cases of Achilles tendonitis causes an increase in local inflammation and can result in later partial or complete rupture of the tendon. Patients who are prone to this condition often show

excessive compensatory pronation, as pronation tends to reduce Achilles tendon traction.

## Diagnosis and differential diagnosis

The characteristic pain of Achilles tendonitis can be induced by plantar flexion of the ankle against resistance. This effect occurs as the patient begins to stand up from a sitting position, or by going up on tiptoe. In severe cases the patient will be unable to take the full body weight when asked to stand on the affected leg. These results, together with the presenting symptoms and case history facilitate the diagnosis. Severe cases will show inflammation and even tears with the tendon on magnetic resonance imaging. Radiographs of the tendon (a tenogram) will show local inflammation and deterioration of the tendon quality.

The differential diagnosis should exclude Haglund's deformity, deep retrocalcaneal bursitis, inflammatory arthritides and partial or total rupture of the Achilles tendon. Patients with marked fatty nodules along the length of the Achilles tendon should undergo blood tests to exclude raised blood cholesterol levels (Citkowitz 2004).

## Treatment

People, especially those in middle age, who intend to embark on a jogging or running programme should be reviewed for appropriate orthotic therapy, and undergo a programme of stretching exercises *before* carrying out sporting activity in order to reduce the likelihood of developing Achilles tendonitis. In the earliest stages of presentation, a simple heel raise to minimise the pull on the Achilles tendon, together with advice on training and prestretching may be sufficient to resolve an incipient Achilles tendonitis. Of course, it will be necessary to rest from strenuous sports activity until all symptoms have cleared, and to undergo a programme of gradual rehabilitation when sports are resumed. Attention should be paid to the footwear, in particular the shape of the heel counter, to reduce the likelihood of further trauma. More advanced cases, where there is a degree of tendon degeneration, require more active intervention. Steroid injections are contraindicated because of the danger of causing further tendon deterioration, and subsequent rupture. Physical therapies such as the use of pain control, rest, ice and strapping (PRICE) in the acute stages, and a course of twice-weekly ultrasound and contrast footbaths to reduce inflammation are beneficial. Heavy-load, eccentric calf muscle training is very effective (Alfredson et al 1998), but immobilisation in a below-knee cast or Aircast® may be necessary to allow tendon healing, followed by a rehabilitation programme of intensive stretching and exercises, as an essential adjunct to treatment to allow the patient to get back to full weight bearing. After the acute injury has resolved the patient should undergo biomechanical evaluation and any identified faults should be corrected by the prescription of functional orthoses.

# Rupture and partial rupture of the Achilles tendon

The Achilles tendon is prone to rupture at a point 2–5 cm superior to its point of insertion on the posterior surface of the calcaneus.

## Pathology

The Achilles tendon may rupture as the result of an isolated severe traumatic event, or as the culmination of repeated episodes of peritendonitis. The tendon rupture in either case may be partial or total.

## Clinical picture

Patients with either acute or chronic Achilles tendon rupture present ultimately with a similar set of clinical signs. These include a palpable painful swelling overlying and surrounding the distal part of the tendon, a discontinuity along the length of the tendon just superior to its insertion (Fig. 4.16), and inability to stand on tiptoe or plantar flex the foot against resistance, or bear weight normally on the affected foot. In an acute presentation of Achilles tendon rupture, the patient gives a characteristic history of a severe pain and a sudden sensation of something 'snapping' at the back of the heel, usually occurring during an episode of strenuous or sports activity. They experience severe localised pain, usually fall over, and are unable to use that foot to walk normally, as they will have lost the ability to plantar flex the foot against ground resistance. Sometimes they think that someone must have kicked them in the back of their heel. In a chronic presentation, the onset of symptoms is more gradual, as an increasingly severe Achilles tendonitis, leading to eventual partial or total rupture.

## Treatment

In cases of partial Achilles tendon rupture the affected limb must be immobilised in a below-knee cast or Aircast® boot for several weeks to allow the tendon to heal. The patient will need to follow a programme of rehabilitation once the cast is removed and tendon repair is complete in order to regain full strength in the posterior calf muscles, reduce the chance of re-rupture, and prevent the development of ankle equinus due to any contraction of the posterior soft tissue structures that may have occurred during the healing period. More severe cases of partial rupture are corrected surgically.

Cases of full rupture of the Achilles tendon may be corrected surgically. The tendon ends are resutured together, sometimes including the additional use of donor tendon, such as a plantaris tendon graft. The foot is immobilised in a cast for 6–8 weeks, in a plantar-flexed position, and the patient not allowed to weight bear until tendon healing is complete. Wound healing in Achilles tendon repairs can be prolonged. In cases of total Achilles tendon rupture, immobilisation without surgery, even for several months, is not usually successful, and the risk of re-rupture is high in those few cases that do achieve a degree of repair solely by immobilisation.

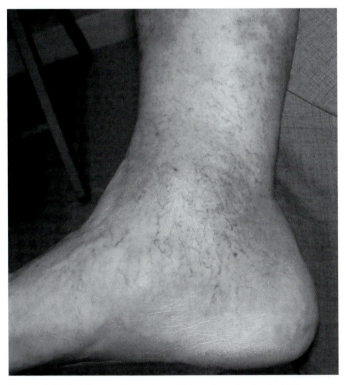

**Figure 4.16** Achilles tendon rupture. This male patient, aged 74 years, developed a rupture of the Achilles tendon several months after experiencing pain at the posterior area of his right heel/lower leg. He was diagnosed as having type 2 diabetes mellitus at age 68 years, with associated chronic hypertension, hypercholesterolaemia, peripheral sensory neuropathy, chronic venous insufficiency and mild obesity. In view of his overall medical condition, the vascular status of the lower limb, and the chronicity of the Achilles tendon injury, the orthopaedic surgeon recommended that surgical repair of the tendon was not in the patient's best interest. The case was managed initially by the use of an Aircast™ walking boot for 6 weeks, followed by prescription orthoses worn in walking boots.

### CASE STUDY 4.5 RUPTURE OF THE ACHILLES TENDON SUBSEQUENT TO CHRONIC ACHILLES TENDONITIS

A 38-year-old man was referred for orthotic therapy subsequent to undergoing surgical repair of the Achilles tendon 6 months earlier. He was in good general health, and on no regular medication. He smoked 20 cigarettes a day. He had been employed as a firefighter since he was 20 years old, but was currently on long-term sick leave due to the Achilles tendon problem.

He presented the following history. At age 17 years he had a cartilage injury to his left knee, which was repaired surgically. He had suffered a recurrent problem with his left Achilles tendon since injuring it when he was 21 years old, whilst playing football. He did not take the advice he was given then to rest the injury, and felt that this had caused him to have a nagging problem ever since. Six months ago, he had slipped down a flight of stairs whilst answering a fire call and snapped the left Achilles tendon. The tendon was repaired, using a peroneus (fibularis) brevis tendon graft. The left limb was put in a below-knee cast for 6 weeks, then an Aircast for a further 6 weeks. He followed an extensive programme of rehabilitation and physiotherapy for a further 3 months, at the end of which he was referred to a podiatrist for orthotic therapy.

He reported the following symptoms: a constant dull ache in his left knee, a painful nodule in the lateral area of the left calf, lower back (lumbar/sacral) discomfort, and a tendency for his left foot to slip when walking on uneven surfaces.

On examination it was noted that the patient had bilateral pes cavus. There was marked contracture of the left Achilles tendon and inversion of the left heel. There was a surgical scar along the lateral aspect of the left foot from the base of the fifth metatarsal to the heel, and another surgical scar along the posterior aspect of the lower left leg extending from the posterior aspect of the heel to the inferior lateral–posterior calf area, with a tender nodule at its proximal end (the stump of the harvested peroneus brevis tendon). There were areas of marked plantar and lateral hyperkeratosis at the left fifth metatarsophalangeal joint area. There was no loss of continuity of the Achilles tendon, but there was some local thickening 3–5 cm superior to its attachment into the calcaneus. The left leg was 1 cm shorter than the right, and the left calf 3 cm narrower than the right. His gait was laboured. The left foot showed an early heel lift and remained inverted throughout gait. He was unable to stand fully on tiptoe on his left foot, and unable to maintain what toe stance he could demonstrate for longer than a few seconds. Muscle power (eversion and plantar flexion) of the left foot was markedly reduced.

His presenting problems related to the injuries he had suffered: the shortening of the left Achilles tendon, as the result of the surgery, caused the early heel lift during gait, and reduced active plantar flexion. The harvesting of the peroneus brevis had reduced his ability to evert the foot. His left foot, therefore, remained inverted throughout gait, causing him to feel unsteady on uneven ground. The loss of shock absorption, due to the loss of midstance pronation, was the cause of his left knee and lower back pain. Casts were made of both feet, to which intrinsically posted orthoses were made. He has now returned to work as a firefighter.

## Plantar heel pain

Pain of the plantar aspect of the heel may be caused by a number of pathologies, which include: heel pain syndrome, plantar fascia rupture, fat-pad atrophy, stress fractures of the calcaneus, proximal plantar fasciitis, distal plantar fasciitis, plantar fibromatosis, tendonitis of the flexor hallucis longus tendon, tumour of the calcaneum, and nerve entrapment or injury (Pfeffer et al 1999).

### CASE STUDY 4.6 RUPTURE OF THE PLANTAR FASCIA FOLLOWING HYDROCORTISONE INJECTION

A 35-year-old woman in good general health presented with severe, chronic plantar heel pain syndrome of the left foot, for which she had been prescribed functional orthoses. The heel pain was debilitating, and although the orthoses did not fully eradicate the pain their regular use reduced the pain to a tolerable level. Her foot pain affected her quality of life, and she was frequently depressed by its unremitting nature. At the same time as having podiatric treatment, the patient underwent a course of hydrocortisone injections into the left heel. The injections were administered by the patient's GP. As she was stepping up a kerbstone shortly after the third injection, she experienced severe pain and a sensation as if something in the sole of her left foot had snapped. The pain subsided over the next few days, but the patient was aware that she was no longer able to walk in her normal brisk manner.

The next time she attended for podiatric treatment it was noted that the longitudinal profile of the left foot was visibly flatter than that of the right. She was unable to go up onto tiptoe on her left foot. The plantar fascia did not tighten, and there was no alteration in the profile of the medial longitudinal arch when the hallux was dorsiflexed passively at the first metatarsophalangeal joint. The patient was diagnosed as having suffered a rupture of the plantar fascia. Her foot pain did not return, although the function of her left foot was altered. Rupture of the plantar fascia following corticosteroid injection has been reported in the literature (Acevedo & Beskin 1998, Rolf et al 1997, Sellman 1994).

## Heel pain syndrome

The most common cause of plantar heel pain is inflammation of the proximal portion of the plantar fascia. It is a common condition that may occur at any time of life, although it tends predominantly to present in the age range 40–60 years, affecting males and females equally. Both feet are affected in 15% of patients. Heel pain can be considered as an overuse syndrome, as there is no single clear aetiology of the condition. Common predisposing factors include a history of increased activity, prolonged standing, excess foot pronation, and recent weight gain or obesity (a body mass index >25) (Aquino & Payne 2001, Hill 1989).

The soft tissues that comprise the plantar aspect of the heel are made up of the glabrous skin that overlies the fibrofatty heel pad, deep to which lies the plantar fascia. The skin and fat pad of the heel are highly specialised to accommodate friction and shock. The plantar heel pad is formed as a honeycombed, interattached meshwork of fibroelastic septa that enclose subcutaneous fat. The deepest parts of the septa merge with the deep fibrous structures that overlie the plantar aspect of the heel. The superficial area of the septa blends with the superficial fascia. This construction allows the absorption of ground reaction forces up to twice body weight, such as occur at heel strike (Singh et al 1997). The heel pad is approximately 18 mm thick in the adult, but often slightly thicker in males (Prichasuk 1994), and tends to atrophy with age, peripheral arterial disease and in cases of rheumatoid disease.

The plantar fascia is also known as the plantar aponeurosis, and is a tough, multilayered inelastic fibrous sheet made up of type I collagen. It is triangular in shape (Fig. 4.17) with the apex directed proximally. The apex originates from the medial calcaneal tuberosity where its deeper fibres merge with the calcaneal periosteum. The more superficial fibres of the plantar fascia merge with the distal Achilles tendon, the fibres of which extend distally to cover the inferior aspect of the proximal calcaneus (Fig. 4.17A) and (Fig. 4.17B). From its point of origin, the plantar aponeurosis fans out distally, becoming gradually broader and thinner, and inserts into the plantar plate on the plantar aspect of the metatarsal heads.

In the area of the MTPJs the plantar fascia separates into five distinct tissue bands. Each of the five bands further subdivides into superficial and deep parts:

- The superficial parts course vertically to attach into the deeper layers of the dermis of the plantar skin that overlies the metatarsophalangeal area of the foot. This mechanism anchors the overlying plantar skin and absorbs shearing forces.
- The deepest layer of each of the five bands splits into medial and lateral portions, which surround the sheaths of the digital flexor tendons and insert into the dorsal periosteum at the base of the proximal phalanges (Kwong et al 1998). Through this mechanism, the plantar fascia is placed under tension whenever the toes are extended or (dorsiflexed) at the MTPJs, storing potential energy and contributing to the 'windlass mechanism' (Hicks 1954) that occurs during the latter stage of stance: as the centre of gravity of the body moves forward through the weight-bearing foot, the foot begins to resupinate and the MTPJs start to extend. The increasing tension in the non-elastic plantar fascia draws the plantar aspect of the heads of the metatarsal and the inferior–proximal angle of the calcaneum towards one another, increasing the height of the medial longitudinal arch and converting the foot from a mobile adaptor to a rigid lever (Fig. 4.18).

## Pathology

Prolonged and continuing traction on the plantar fascia results in inflammation, swelling and pain, especially at its origin at the medial calcaneal tuberosity.

- Normal pronation is associated with a reduction in the height of the medial longitudinal arch or instep, and a relative lengthening of the foot.
- Excess pronation is a feature of compensated rearfoot varus, mobile pes cavus and lower-limb anomalies. Where pronation is excessive, the plantar fascia is under constant tension throughout stance, with increased traction at the attachments and insertions of the plantar fascia.
- Insufficient pronation occurs in cases of uncompensated rearfoot varus and fixed pes cavus. The lack of normal pronation

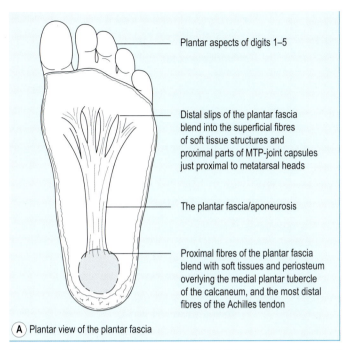

**A** Plantar view of the plantar fascia

Plantar aspects of digits 1–5

Distal slips of the plantar fascia blend into the superficial fibres of soft tissue structures and proximal parts of MTP-joint capsules just proximal to metatarsal heads

The plantar fascia/aponeurosis

Proximal fibres of the plantar fascia blend with soft tissues and periosteum overlying the medial plantar tubercle of the calcaneum, and the most distal fibres of the Achilles tendon

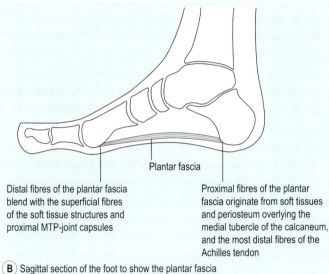

Plantar fascia

Distal fibres of the plantar fascia blend with the superficial fibres of the soft tissue structures and proximal MTP-joint capsules

Proximal fibres of the plantar fascia originate from soft tissues and periosteum overlying the medial tubercle of the calcaneum, and the most distal fibres of the Achilles tendon

**B** Sagittal section of the foot to show the plantar fascia

**Figure 4.17** (A) Plantar view of the plantar fascia; (B) sagittal section of the foot to show the plantar fascia.

at midstance means that the plantar fascia is under constant tension throughout stance, through the windlass mechanism.

- Obesity aggravates any tendency to increased tension at the origin of the plantar fascia, exacerbating the influence of pathomechanical factors and increasing compressive forces on the heel fat pad.
- A reduction in both the thickness (atrophy) and the resilience of the plantar heel pad occurs with advancing age, in peripheral vascular disease, or in association with collagen diseases, such as rheumatoid arthritis. Heel pad reduction predisposes the patient to plantar heel pain, with or without the formation of an associated heel spur or biomechanical anomaly.

It is thought that the repetitive excessive tensile forces created by walking or standing cause microtears in the fascia, leading to acute

and eventual chronic inflammation. If the inflammation affects the entire plantar fascia, it is referred to as a plantar fasciitis; however, if it is isolated to the heel alone, it is called heel pain. Involved tissues undergo changes that typify chronic inflammation. These include collagen necrosis, angiofibroblastic hyperplasia (i.e. overgrowth of local fibrous tissue and blood vessels), chondroid metaplasia (i.e. their transformation into a cartilage-like tissue) and eventual calcification, especially at the origin. In some cases, the first branch of the lateral plantar nerve, known as Baxter's nerve, may become entrapped within the fibrous tissue, causing symptoms of distal sensory neuropathy.

Where the inflammation also affects the periosteum of the medial plantar calcaneal tubercle, an enthesopathy occurs (the insertion of ligamentous or fascial tissues into a bone surface is termed an 'enthesis'). The pull of both the origin of the flexor digitorum brevis muscle and the proximal part of the plantar aponeurosis on the periosteum of the calcaneus acts as a stimulus to new bone formation at their points of insertion, resulting in the formation of a plantar calcaneal or heel spur. A heel spur is usually very painful during its formation, but later may become asymptomatic, as once formed it effectively reduces the tractional forces applied to the medial calcaneal tubercle by the plantar aponeurosis. The presence or absence of a heel spur is not diagnostic of heel pain, as 16% of people with heel spurs do not have heel pain, and 50% of people with heel pain do not have a heel spur (Crawford & Snaith 1996).

## Clinical picture

The patient reports a gradual and increasing pain at the medial–central heel area, which often radiates into the medial longitudinal arch. There is not usually a history of local trauma. The pain, which is usually described as sharp or severe, is worse on weight bearing, especially on first standing in the morning. Typically, the pain subsides gradually after the patient has walked about for a while, but tends to re-establish towards the end of the working day, and recur during the day after periods of rest or non-weight bearing. It is thought that the paradox of pain apparently increased by rest is due to the combined effects of accumulated inflammatory oedema and the sudden traction applied to the inflamed plantar tissues by weight bearing (Wapner & Sharkey 1991). The gradual reduction in the initial pain after walking about is thought to relate to the dispersion of the oedema by the 'massage' effect of walking.

On physical examination, the patient often has tightness of the Achilles tendon, due to the close anatomical relationship of the heel cord with the plantar fascia. Pain is elicited by the examiner applying traction to the plantar fascia by passively extending or dorsiflexing the toes at the MTPJ with one hand whilst palpating along the length of the now tightened medial band of the plantar fascia with the thumb of the other hand from distal to proximal. The examiner's thumb comes to directly palpate the origin of the plantar aponeurosis at the medial plantar calcaneal tubercle (Fig. 4.19). Characteristically, the patient will grimace or verbally indicate pain as the thumb pressure is applied to the point of insertion of the plantar fascia at the medial–plantar heel area, and will also usually describe a sensation of pain as the thumb is moved down the taut plantar fascia.

## Diagnosis and differential diagnosis

The characteristic pattern of pain, tenderness in the medial longitudinal arch and the response to direct compression of the tissues at the origin of the plantar aponeurosis in a sedentary, overweight patient is largely diagnostic. The diagnosis can be confirmed by using ultrasonography and radioisotope bone scans to demonstrate inflammation and early new bone formation at the medial calcaneal tubercle. The presence of a heel spur on plain lateral radiographs is not neces-

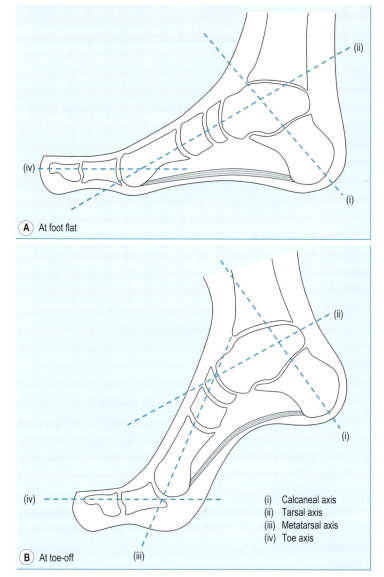

- The longitudinal axis of the tarsus is in line with that of the metatarsals (ii)

- There is only moderate tension in the plantar fascia

**A** At foot flat

- The longitudinal axis of the metatarsals (iii) is plantar-flexed relative to that of the tarsus (ii)

- The angle of inclination of the calcaneus is increased relative to the talus (ii)

- The angle of declination of the talus (ii) is decreased relative to the calcaneum (i)

- The plantar fascia is relatively shorter and under increased tension

- As the heel lifts, the toes dorsiflex at the MTPJs (iv)

- The MTPJs act as a 'windlass drum' around which the distal part of the plantar fascia is 'wound', storing potential energy in the plantar fascia

- As the forefoot leaves the ground the potential energy stored in the plantar fascia converts to kinetic energy, as the tension in the plantar fascia is released, facilitating efficient forward locomotion

(i)   Calcaneal axis
(ii)  Tarsal axis
(iii) Metatarsal axis
(iv)  Toe axis

**B** At toe-off

**Figure 4.18** Windlass mechanism (Hicks 1954).

sarily diagnostic, as asymptomatic heel spur is noted in 10% of people aged over 50 years (Banadda et al 1992) and can be considered as a normal variant when the spur is small and well defined. Large, ill-defined or fluffy heel spurs are seen in conjunction with plantar enthesopathy, especially in cases with seronegative rheumatoid disease (Fig. 4.20).

The differential diagnoses should consider:

- foot strain or plantar fasciitis without heel pain, in which the pain primarily tends to affect the medial band of the plantar fascia in the medial longitudinal arch, rather than the plantar aspect of the heel
- plantar calcaneal bursitis, in which there is marked swelling and inflammation at the central plantar heel area
- calcaneal fracture, where there will be a history of severe trauma and marked swelling, bruising and distortion of the whole heel area
- entrapment neuropathy causing heel pain, where fibres of the first sacral spinal nerve (S1) are traumatised by adjacent vertebrae

- seronegative inflammatory joint disease – Reiter's syndrome, psoriatic arthropathy, ankylosing spondylitis, and Behçet's syndrome are all typified by severe heel pain and the formation of large, ill-defined heel spurs
- seropositive rheumatoid disease – 1 in 50 patients with rheumatoid arthritis shows plantar enthesiopathy and associated heel pain (Renton 1991); these patients should be referred to a rheumatologist for ongoing disease management.

## Other causes of plantar heel pain

### Subcalcaneal bursitis

A subcalcaneal bursitis, also known as policeman's heel, has been described as a cause of plantar heel pain. There is little anatomical evidence of a congenital or acquired bursa in the superficial plantar heel tissues (Lapidus & Guidotti 1965), and it seems likely that the inflammatory symptoms associated with plantar heel pain syndrome (see above) have been confused with the apparent symptoms of an inflamed bursa.

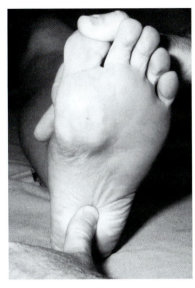

Figure 4.19 To test the exact site of tenderness of plantar heel pain, dorsiflex the great toe, run a thumb from distal to proximal along the plantar fascia until it meets the calcaneum, and apply firm pressure.

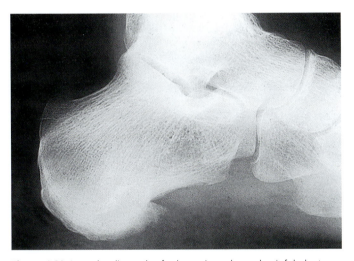

Figure 4.20 Lateral radiograph of a large, irregular and painful plantar heel spur in a patient with psoriatic arthropathy.

### Entrapment neuropathy

Entrapment of the medial calcaneal nerve (Beito et al 1989) or the first branch of the lateral plantar nerve (Schon et al 1993) has been identified as a cause of recalcitrant heel pain. Pain associated with the nerve entrapment is located medially, and is sharp and electrical in nature, and may radiate proximally into the lower leg. Excessive foot pronation is thought to cause repetitive microtraumata, chronic fibrosis of the nerve and resultant paraesthesia. In extreme cases, the nerve may require surgical decompression or excision to achieve pain resolution.

### Radiculopathy of the first sacral spinal nerve (s1 radiculopathy)

Proximal compression of the S1 nerve may cause a referred pain in the distribution of the medial plantar nerve (Schon et al 1993). Referred back pain should be considered in the diagnosis of

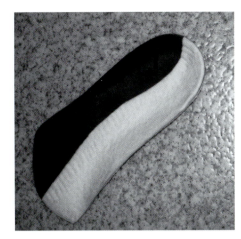

Figure 4.21 Cobra pad.

patients with a history of lower-back problems who present with heel pain.

### Treatment of plantar heel pain

The treatment of plantar heel pain involves isolating the cause of the problem, measures to reduce the painful symptoms, and actions to resolve, where possible, the underlying mechanical or other pathologies. A variety of conservative measures will allow four out of five cases to make a full recovery within 6–9 months of onset of the symptoms, with the podiatric intervention providing palliative care to reduce mechanical stresses on the heel during the painful period. However, the recalcitrant one-fifth of plantar heel pain cases presents a considerable challenge to successfully treatment (Wolgin et al 1994).

*Podiatric palliation* includes the provision of:

- Sponge heel cushions that are made from clinical or orthotic materials, or silicone gel heel pads purchased commercially (Pfeffer et al 1999).
- Ring or doughnut pads that are made from semicompressed felt. The centre of the pad is cut away to match to focus of plantar pain, and thereby reduce compression forces at the site of pain.
- A figure-of-eight crepe ankle bandage or Low-Dye™ taping to invert the calcaneus. The resultant increase in the angle of inclination of the calcaneus will reduce tensile stress along the plantar fascia (Saxelby et al 1997).
- A semicompressed felt tarsal platform, applied over the area of the cuboid, or a distal calcaneal bar applied to the distal calcaneal area will elevate the calcaneocuboid joint, increase the angle of inclination of the calcaneus, and minimise tensile stress in the plantar fascia.
- Temporary antipronatory orthoses, such as a semicompressed felt valgus filler pad extended to a medial heel wedge and a medial forefoot wedge, also known as an adapted cobra pad (Fig. 4.21) tends to limit hindfoot eversion.
- Supportive orthoses, such as soft-moulded orthoses made to a cast of the patient's foot, will support the medial longitudinal arch, especially in patients who have pes cavus.

*Dynamic therapies* include:

- A programme of exercises to stretch the Achilles tendon, together with the use of commercially available prefabricated heel cushions (Pfeffer et al 1999).
- Functional orthoses, such as rigid or semi-rigid prescription orthoses with a deep heel cup, to control rearfoot biomechanical faults (Weil et al 1994).

- Dorsiflexion night splints (Powell et al 1998).
- A course of NSAIDs: a 21-day course of NSAIDs has the maximum anti-inflammatory effect, in patients who are able to tolerate these drugs.
- A weight-loss regimen, in those patients where obesity is an aggravating factor.
- Trigger point acupuncture (Tillu & Gupta 1998).
- Ultra-high-frequency sound diathermy (ultrasound) allows the direction of a localised beam of high frequency sound energy to the painful plantar heel area, to trigger an acute inflammatory response and initiate healing. However, although some patients with heel pain find ultrasound therapy of benefit, it has been shown that a commonly used regimen (0.5 W/cm, 3 Mz pulsed 1 : 4, applied for 8 minutes twice weekly for 4 weeks) was no more effective than placebo in the treatment of plantar heel pain syndrome (Crawford & Snaith 1996).
- Injected hydrocortisone: 1 ml of 25 mg hydrocortisone is injected directly through the plantar tissues, or via a medial heel approach, to deliver the drug to the site of origin of the plantar fascia (i.e. the point of maximum tenderness). This technique has not been proven to be of greater benefit than less invasive therapies (Crawford & Thomson 2003), but can provide symptomatic relief in the short term (Crawford et al 1999). A maximum of two injections is recommended, with the repeat injection administered after an interval of 1 month (see Case Study 4.6). Practitioners are advised to administer the hydrocortisone injection under ultrasound guidance (Tsai 2006). It has recently been reported that 'dry needling' under ultrasound guidance plus a single hydrocortisone injection was very effective in the treatment of plantar heel pain (Kerr 2008). In the UK it is not permissible for podiatrists to mix local anaesthetic and hydrocortisone for injection within the same syringe.
- Surgery: a plantar fasciotomy, to divide the plantar fascia at its point of origin, together with excision of any bone spur is advocated. These techniques can be carried out as 'keyhole' arthroscopic procedures under local anaesthesia. However, such a procedure can affect the biomechanics of the foot, and the patient should be followed up with orthotic therapy (Daly et al 1992).

## Tarsal tunnel syndrome

Tarsal tunnel syndrome is a relatively uncommon entrapment neuropathy affecting the posterior tibial nerve at the point where it passes behind and below the medial malleolus, between the distal end of the tibia and the flexor retinaculum, so that the tibial nerve is entrapped within the fibro-osseous tunnel formed by the calcaneus and the lancinate ligament. The condition is analogous to carpal tunnel syndrome in the hand, and is often associated with inflammatory arthropathies, such as rheumatoid arthritis.

### Pathology

Synovitis of the tibialis posterior tendon, often in association with underlying rheumatoid disease, causes a local chronic inflammation and swelling of the synovial sheath of the tendon as it passes beneath the sustentaculum tali. The resultant local fibrosis causes the tibial nerve to become tethered within the fibro-osseous tunnel formed by the flexor retinaculum of the ankle and the medial malleolus (Cimino 1990). Either direct pressure on the nerve from the fibrous swelling and/or the indirect pressure of rearfoot pronation causes a relative local neuroischaemia, and resultant neural dysfunction, such as

sensory neuropathy. The affected area of nerve shows fibrous thickening (Hadjari Hollis et al 2008).

### Clinical features

The patient experiences a burning pain and paraesthesia in the sole of the foot and toes in the distribution of the distal part of the tibial nerve. The patient often reports paraesthesia affecting the whole of the plantar surface, with maximal symptoms at the medial longitudinal arch and the metatarsal heads area. Alternatively, the patient may describe paraesthesia, including tingling, pins and needles, and cramp-like feelings in the medial longitudinal arch area. Symptoms are exacerbated by weight bearing, and are often worse at night. Percussion over the inferior–medial aspect of the heel at the site of the entrapment, or sustained direct digital pressure to the nerve in the area of the medial malleolus will reproduce the symptoms (a positive Tinel's sign). Long-standing cases may also show frank plantar and digital sensory neuropathy with weakness of intrinsic muscles subserved by the affected nerve.

### Treatment

Treatment of tarsal tunnel syndrome focuses on therapies that reduce the unpleasant and painful symptoms. Clinical padding, such as valgus filler pads or medial heel wedges either affixed to the foot or an insole, helps reduce nerve compression or stretching. Excess rearfoot pronation should be controlled as far as possible by the use of moulded cushioned orthoses, housed within appropriate bespoke shoes, to minimise local pressure at the medial aspect of the heel. The inflammation occurring as the result of the rheumatoid process should be controlled by the relevant drug therapies, including NSAIDs together with disease-modifying antirheumatic drugs (DMARDs) as prescribed by the general practitioner or rheumatologist, but many patients with rheumatoid or other inflammatory arthropathies who develop tarsal tunnel syndrome are already on high doses of NSAIDs, to control other aspects of their disease. Surgical treatment including the decompression of the nerve by freeing it from the surrounding fibrotic tissues, with excision of local fibrous tissue, is indicated in cases that do not respond to conservative measures (Takakura et al 1991).

## Tibialis posterior tendon dysfunction

Tibialis posterior tendon dysfunction is a cause of medial heel pathology that is often overlooked and misdiagnosed, especially in the early stages of its presentation (Wassef & Mikhail 2008). It is a disabling condition, arising as the direct result of the loss of function of the posterior tibial tendon. Chronic inflammation leads to degeneration and elongation of the tendon, with the formation of interstitial tears, attenuation and eventual tendon rupture. The condition, if left untreated, leads to increased misalignment of the rearfoot and midfoot, with calcaneal eversion, plantar flexion of the talus, subluxation of the talonavicular joint and unilateral flat foot.

The tibialis posterior muscle is active during the stance phase of gait: it fires shortly after heel strike and ceases to contract shortly after heel lift. Its belly originates deep within the posterior compartment of the lower limb. Its tendon courses down the lower limb to the posterior aspect of the medial malleolus, where it lies anterior to the tendon of the flexor digitorum longus, the posterior tibial neurovascular bundle (containing the posterior tibial artery, vein and nerve) and the tendon of the flexor hallucis longus. All these structures are restrained by the overlying flexor retinaculum at the medial malleolus. The tibialis posterior tendon runs in a groove behind and below the medial malleolus to split into three slips at the medial aspect of the tarsus. The anterior slip inserts into the tuberosity of the navicular bone; the middle slip continues into the plantar tarsal area to insert into the plantar aspects of the cuneiforms, the cuboid and the bases of the second, third, and fourth metatarsals; and the posterior slip has a band-like insertion into the anterior aspect of the inferior calcaneonavicular (spring) ligament. The vector followed by the tibialis posterior tendon at its point of entry to the foot is changed as it passes behind the medial malleolus which thus acts as a pulley block. This, in conjunction with the position of its points of insertion, allows supination of the rearfoot and midfoot during weight bearing, whilst stabilising the arched construction of the midfoot.

The primary actions of the tibialis posterior muscle are to bring about supination of the subtalar joint, and adduction of the forefoot about the oblique axis of the midtarsal joint:

- during the early stance phase of gait, the tibialis posterior muscle contracts eccentrically to decelerate pronation that occurs at both the subtalar joint and during internal rotation of the tibia
- in the midstance phase of gait, the muscle contracts concentrically, to promote midtarsal joint stability in preparation for propulsion
- at heel lift it provides plantar-flexory torque to allow the heel to leave the ground.

Thus the tibialis posterior muscle acts as a prime stabiliser against rearfoot valgus and forefoot abduction, and is antagonistic to the action of the peroneal muscles, especially to the action of the peroneus brevis.

## Aetiology

The cause of tibialis posterior dysfunction is unclear, but a number of factors are associated with the development of the condition. These include:

- obesity
- excessive foot pronation, which predisposes to compression and reduced vascularity of the tendon as it curves around the medial malleolus deep to the flexor retinaculum
- structural and anatomical anomalies, such as an accessory navicular (os navicularis), rigid or flexible flat foot, osteophytic proliferation in the medial malleolar groove, shallowness of the malleolar grove and ankle equinus
- inflammatory joint diseases, such as rheumatoid arthritis and seronegative arthritides
- collagen vascular disease
- direct trauma, such as tendon laceration due to a medial malleolar fracture
- indirect trauma, such as ankle fracture, eversion ankle sprain, acute avulsion injury of the navicular and tibialis posterior tendon dislocation
- iatrogenic events, such as steroid injections into the area.

## Pathology

The presentation of tibialis posterior dysfunction may be classified into four stages:

- Stage 1 – the asymptomatic stage. Assessment of the patient may show an underlying fault predisposing to the development of the condition, such as fully compensated rearfoot varus or obesity.
- Stage 2 – the initial symptomatic stage. This is characterised by tibialis posterior tendonitis (inflammation of the tendon sheath in the area of the flexor retinaculum). Any associated weakening of the muscles of the tibialis posterior is mild.

- Stage 3 – marked dysfunction stage. This is characterised by a rupture within the tibialis posterior tendon, or by longitudinal tears with elongation, but not rupture, of the tendon, or even by avulsion of the tendon from its insertion onto the navicular tuberosity. Patients present with marked midfoot pronation and forefoot abduction.
- Stage 4 – marked loss of foot function. This is characterised by a rapid progression through Stages 1–3, together with pain, rigid pronation of the affected foot, severely restricted midtarsal joint movement, and pain that locates to the inferior lateral ankle area.

Alternatively, the pathology of tibialis posterior dysfunction may be classified by the duration and severity of the presenting signs and symptoms:

- The acute phase, lasting for the first 2 weeks after onset, during which time the tendon pathology may go undiagnosed. Typically, the patient presents with some diffuse oedema and tenderness over the medial aspect of the ankle. There may or may not be associated aching and muscle fatigue in the lower leg.
- The subacute phase, lasting from 2 weeks to 6 months after onset, during which time the patient presents with pain and oedema along the course of tibialis posterior tendon, extending from the posterior aspect of the medial malleolus into the medial longitudinal arch. There may also be signs of tarsal tunnel syndrome, due to compression of local nerves (see tarsal tunnel syndrome, above). Passive movement of the subtalar and midtarsal joints does not usually cause pain, but walking is affected, with the patient characteristically showing an apropulsive gait, forefoot abduction, and lack of foot supination at heel strike and toe off.
- The chronic phase occurs approximately 6 months after onset, when the patient presents with a unilateral, rigid flat foot. In advanced cases, the pain may transfer from the medial to the lateral area of the sinus tarsi. The lateral pain is caused by the progressive valgus deformity of the rearfoot, which leads to calcaneofibular abutment, periosteal inflammation, peroneal tendonitis and subtalar tendonitis.

## Clinical picture

Approximately 50% of cases present with a history of local trauma, such as a forced eversion of the rearfoot. The typical sufferer of tibialis posterior dysfunction is a female aged over 40 years, although the condition may also affect younger athletes.

- Patients often do not seek help in the earliest stages of the disease, that is in Stage 1 or the acute phase, as their symptoms are slight and do not prompt the patient to seek help.
- Patients typically present at Stage 2, the subacute phase, with diffuse swelling, tenderness and warmth at the medial aspect of the ankle and along the course of the tendon. The patient will experience difficulty or show instability when asked to perform a single heel raise test on the affected side, and the calcaneus fails to supinate and invert as the heel lifts off the supporting surface.
- In Stage 3, the chronic phase, the patient notes a gradual loss of the height of the medial longitudinal arch, with development of unilateral flat foot and reported lower leg fatigue on the affected side when walking. When viewed from the rear, excessive abduction of the fore foot is noted, showing the 'too many toes' sign. The more severe the condition, the greater is the loss of height of the medial longitudinal arch, the abduction of the forefoot on the rearfoot, and the eversion of the calcaneum. Patients generally show excessive medial heel wear of the shoes.

## Diagnosis and differential diagnosis

The integrity of the tibialis posterior tendon can be assessed by palpating the tendon whilst the patient actively plantar flexes and adducts the foot and the examiner applies an abductory force to the forefoot. It is important to determine the exact site of the injury within the tendon, and it is important to compare the problematic foot to the asymptomatic foot. Direct pressure along the course of the tendon will elicit pain, and active inversion of the foot against resistance will show reduced tibialis posterior muscle power. If a partial tendon rupture has occurred, a distinct defect along the integrity of the tendon can be palpated. If the tendon has fully ruptured, the tendon cannot be palpated along its normal course, and the patient is unable to invert the foot against resistance. A partial or complete rupture of the tendon, secondary to trauma, is accompanied by distinct pain at the navicular tuberosity. Overuse injuries and tendon degeneration present with pain just distal to the medial malleolus.

Magnetic resonance imaging is the most useful method of imaging tendons around the ankle, and it is highly sensitive and specific for the detection of a tendon rupture. Other diagnostic tests include bone scans and injection of radio-opaque material into the tendon/tendon sheath. The early diagnosis is not enhanced by a plain radiograph, although views of the foot will show the extent of structural changes in Stage 3 presentations. A standard weight-bearing anterior–posterior view shows an increase in the angle between the longitudinal axis of the talus and the longitudinal axis of the calcaneus, with an anterior break in the cyma line, abduction of the forefoot and displacement of the second metatarsal. The long axis of the forefoot no longer bisects the rearfoot angle. The normal linear relationship of the talus, navicular, medial cuneiform and the first metatarsal is seen to be lost when the foot is viewed on a lateral radiograph. As the condition progresses, osteoarthritic changes may become evident at the first MTPJ, secondary to the development of hallux limitus.

The differential diagnoses should exclude bone anomalies such as os naviculare (os tibiale externum) syndrome, os trigonum syndrome, navicular avulsion, stress fracture of the navicular; osteochondritis or avascular necrosis of the head of the talus or the navicular, fracture of the medial malleolus, subtalar tarsal coalition and medial sinus tarsitis. Soft tissue anomalies such as strain of the deltoid ligament, medial ankle capsulitis and synovitis, tarsal tunnel syndrome, strain of the flexor hallucis longus or flexor digitorum longus, and retrocalcaneal bursitis should be excluded. Other causes of unilateral flat foot, such as true or apparent leg-length inequality and tarsal coalition, should also be considered in the differential diagnosis.

## Treatment

The most appropriate treatment for tibialis posterior dysfunction is dependent on the stage or phase of the pathology, the presenting symptoms and the severity of the pain reported by the patient. Treatment should always be implemented rapidly and aggressively to prevent further deterioration of the tendon. If the patient is seen in the early stages, conservative methods that focus on reduction of inflammation, joint stabilisation and pain control are indicated for up to 8 weeks. In advanced cases or recalcitrant mild cases, surgical repair of the tendon together with joint fixation may be the options of choice.

### Conservative therapies

Conservative therapies of the condition include a course of NSAIDs for cases where the presenting pain is associated with tendon inflam-

mation (tenosynovitis), a course of ultrasound therapy, together with strapping or taping of the rearfoot into inversion to reduce tension on the tibialis posterior tendon. Soft temporary orthoses, such as valgus filler pads or whole-foot medial padding ('cobra pad', Fig. 4.21), are used to invert the rearfoot. Bespoke rigid antipronatory orthoses are prescribed to allow the tibialis posterior muscle to function more effectively by addressing an underlying pathomechanical defect, controlling subtalar joint movement (using a medial heel skive), reducing strain on the tendon, and controlling forefoot abduction (using a lateral flange). A programme of remedial exercises is indicated to strengthen the tibialis posterior muscle. More severe cases may require immobilisation of the foot in an inverted position in a below knee-cast for several weeks. Steroid injections are not recommended as they tend to increase the likelihood of rupture in the already weakened tendon.

### Surgical procedures

Surgical treatments are indicated for Stage 2, or subacute phase, presentations that do not respond to 8 weeks of conservative therapies, or for Stages 3 and 4, or chronic phase, presentations. Procedures for recalcitrant cases with mild tenosynovitis but without overt damage/fraying of the tendon include peritendinous release, synovectomy and tendon debridement. Synovectomy, insertion reattachment or transfer of the flexor digitorum longus is indicated for more severe cases that are characterised by tendon lengthening. Severe cases, with full rupture and fibrosis of the tibialis posterior tendon are treated by transfer of the flexor digitorum longus, shortening of the spring ligament and the talonavicular capsule, and surgical enlargement of the osseous groove below the medial malleolus. Late-stage cases with pain in the lateral rearfoot can be treated by arthrodesis of the rearfoot joints, such as calcaneotalar fusion, subtalar arthrodesis, talonavicular fusion, or combined talonavicular–calcaneocuboid arthrodesis.

The outcome of corrective surgery for tibialis posterior dysfunction is not always straightforward. The procedure requires a long period of recovery and recuperation, with a regimen of postoperative rehabilitation and exercise. The degree of postoperative correction of the planovalgus deformity is difficult to predict with precision, although the patient can expect an increase in stability during stance. Rearfoot degenerative joint disease is likely in the long term due to the loss of normal joint alignment caused by the arthrodeses, and a reconstructed tendon may undergo further attenuation after corrective surgery, with recurrence of the preoperative symptoms.

## Tarsal coalition

Tarsal coalition is an autosomal-dominant, congenital condition, in which two or more bones in the midfoot and/or hindfoot are conjoined due to a failure of development of the intervening joint (Wang et al 2008). Symptomatic tarsal coalition has an incidence of approximately 1% within the general population, but as it is estimated that up to 75% of cases of tarsal coalition are asymptomatic, the true incidence of tarsal coalition may be nearer to 4% (Leonard 1974).

## Pathology

The most common presentations of tarsal coalitions include fusion of the calcaneus with another rearfoot or midfoot bone. These include coalition of the calcaneus and the talus (talocalcaneal coalition), the cuboid (calcaneocuboid coalition) or the navicular (calcaneonavicular coalition) (Fig. 4.22). The condition is normally asymptomatic in early childhood. It becomes symptomatic later in childhood or during adolescence, when the cartilaginous anlage

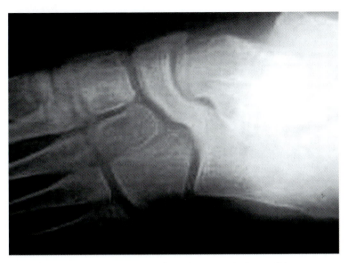

**Figure 4.22** Oblique radiograph of a calcaneonavicular coalition.

undergoes ossification, and the flexibility between the conjoined bones is lost. Presentations of tarsal coalition in adulthood have been reported.

The normal motion of the subtalar joint during weight bearing involves both rotation and gliding. During the stance phase of gait, the axis of the subtalar joint rotates from a position of 4° external valgus to 6° internal varus to compensate for the internal rotation of the tibia. The loss of or reduction in internal rotation at the subtalar joint causes loss of the height of the medial longitudinal arch, flattening of the foot and fixed calcaneal eversion (a valgus heel). The plantar aspects of the midtarsal joints widen, and their dorsal aspects narrow. The navicular tends to override the head of the talus when the foot is in a position of maximum dorsiflexion, causing traction and elongation of both the deep midtarsal and spring ligaments and the talonavicular joint capsule. The overall flattening of the longitudinal profile of the foot leads to adaptive shortening of the peroneal tendons, with reactive spasm of the peroneal muscles – the so-called 'peroneal spastic flatfoot'. Prolonged subtalar joint restriction of motion may lead to long-term degeneration of the posterior facet or arthrosis of the subtalar joint.

## Clinical presentation

The patient with a tarsal coalition presents with a flat foot and marked restriction of available hind- and midfoot eversion. There is associated pain in the foot and lateral compartment of the leg that is usually relieved by rest and aggravated by activity. The patient may also complain of recurrent eversion ankle sprains.

The varying forms of tarsal coalitions ossify at different ages, and thus the age of onset of symptoms is an indicator of the site of the coalition. For example: talonavicular coalitions begin to ossify, and thus become symptomatic, in children aged 3–5 years; calcaneonavicular coalitions begin to ossify in children aged 8–12 years; and talocalcaneal unions become symptomatic during adolescence, most commonly between the ages of 12 and 16 years. The loss of subtalar joint motion and the increasing valgus position of the hindfoot become more apparent as ossification progresses, leading to the development of pes planus. Coalitions involving the middle facet of the subtalar joint are associated with the greatest loss of midtarsal joint motion and are the most likely to cause marked valgus deformity of the foot.

### CASE STUDY 4.7 ADULT PRESENTATION OF CALCANEONAVICULAR FUSION

A 21-year-old female university student was referred for advice on the management of a swollen right heel. She was in excellent health, and had just completed the final examinations for an honours degree.

She reported that the medial area of her right ankle/heel became swollen 3 months ago, after running a half marathon. She did not recall noticing this before, and was concerned that she kept traumatising the swollen inner ankle area of the right foot, causing small local grazes.

On examination, it was noted that the right foot was markedly pronated, with a pronounced medial tarsal 'bulge'. Movement was normal at both ankle joints, but there was no available inversion or eversion at the right subtalar joint, and that on the left was reduced. Pain could not be elicited by palpation, or by passive or active movement of the rearfoot complex. There were no signs of tibialis posterior dysfunction. Plain radiographs demonstrated calcaneonavicular fusions of both feet, that on the right being more marked than that on the left.

This was an unusually late presentation of tarsal coalition, and atypical in that, although both feet showed abnormal bone formation, only that of the right foot was symptomatic, although not painful. It was presumed that the local skin trauma was caused by the inner border of the overpronated right foot being scraped by the left shoe during the swing phase when walking and running.

## Diagnosis and differential diagnoses

Tarsal coalitions are most readily identified by computerised axial tomography or magnetic resonance imaging scans. Plain radiographs require special views to visualise tarsal coalitions. Calcaneonavicular coalition is suggested by the presence of an elongated anterior calcaneal process, and a talocalcaneal coalition is best visualised on a Harris–Beath (also known as an axial or 'ski-jump') view of the hindfoot.

The examiner can evaluate a loss of subtalar joint movement: In the normal weight-bearing foot the tibia and patella externally rotate and the foot supinates when the medial border is raised, the lateral border maintained in contact with the floor, and the heel maintained in the neutral position. When this examination technique is carried out on patients with limited or decreased subtalar joint motion, the amount of available external rotation of the tibia is decreased and the patella does not rotate externally. A loss of subtalar joint motion can also be demonstrated by the absence of or reduction in normal hindfoot inversion and a lack of increase in the height of the medial longitudinal arch when the patient attempts to stand on tiptoe on the affected foot.

The differential diagnoses should exclude bone tumours, rheumatological disease and fractures about the subtalar joint. Tarsal coalitions have been shown to be a feature of other foot deformities, such as talipes equinovarus, and are associated with fibular hemimelia (a congenital abnormality characterised by total or partial absence of the distal half of the limb), Nievergelt–Pearlman syndrome (a rare, autosomal-dominant, inherited bone disease that affects males more than females, characterised by upper limb and hand deformities, symmetric dysplasia of the lower limbs, with genu valgum, clubfoot and deformed great toes, and crura rhomboidei) and Apert's syndrome (acrocephalosyndactylia – a rare developmental condition with characteristic craniofacial and limb anomalies including craniosynostosis (premature fusion of the skull bones), midface underdevelopment, and gross syndacylisation of the fingers and toes).

## Treatment

The early treatment of a non-ossified tarsal coalition includes immobilisation of the foot in rearfoot neutral by the use of an ankle–foot orthosis or ankle callipers to restrict movement of the affected joints and minimise pain. Surgery is indicated after full ossification of the coalition is complete. The procedure of choice is determined by the degree and location of the coalition, and includes resection of the bone bar, or fixation and arthrodesis of the affected degenerate and painful joints.

# MIDFOOT DISORDERS

Midfoot pain may arise in conjunction with a pathology that affects the proximal plantar area or as a distinct entity.

## Plantar fibromatosis

Plantar fibromatosis describes a condition in which the patient tends to develop fibromae or fibrous nodules within the plantar fascia. Males tend to be more commonly affected than females, and the condition presents most frequently in the fifth and sixth decades.

### Pathology

The true pathology of plantar fibromatosis is unclear. Adherent fibrous nodules or fibromae develop, usually within the superficial parts of the plantar fascia, and the associated fascial tissues undergo a degree of contraction. The condition follows a similar pathology to Dupuytren's contracture of the palmar aspect of the hand. Plantar fibromatosis is less common, and generally less disabling than Dupuytren's contracture, as weight-bearing forces prevent the plantar tissues from undergoing the same degree of contraction as the palmar tissues.

### Clinical features

Patients present with single or multiple, painful or asymptomatic nodules, or discrete firm, fluctuant swellings within the soft tissues overlying the plantar aspect of one or both feet.

### Diagnosis and differential diagnosis

The diagnosis is made from the clinical signs and symptoms. Patients presenting with plantar fibromatosis may also have a history of Dupuytren's contracture affecting the hands, and there is a weak association with alcohol abuse.

### Treatment

Asymptomatic cases do not require treatment. Painful presentations may be treated with accommodative orthoses to reduce pressure over the tender nodules. More problematic cases can be treated by an injection of hydrocortisone into the nodule. Surgery may be indicated to excise multiple painful or large nodules, but fibromata tend to recur.

## Tarsal arthritis

Osteoarthritic changes may occur at the joints of the midfoot, leading to local pain and the formation of exostoses.

### Pathology

Degenerative changes occur at the first metatarsal–medial cuneiform and the cuneionavicular joints in feet with pes cavus and pes valgus:

- In mobile pes cavus, subtalar joint movement, as compensation for rearfoot varus, leads to excessive foot pronation in midstance and at toe-off, with dorsiflexion of the first metatarsal and retrograde pressure on the first metatarsal–medial cuneiform joint. In the long term, degenerative changes occur at that joint.
- In rigid pes cavus, the increased angle of inclination of the calcaneum and decreased angle of declination of the talus is compensated by an increased angle of declination of the first ray, so that the distal part of the first ray plantar flexes. The resultant incongruency of the cuneionavicular joint predisposes to degenerative changes at that joint in the long term.
- In pes valgus, the foot is in a position of excessive pronation throughout stance. The resultant dorsiflexion of the first ray and retrograde pressure on the first metatarsal–medial cuneiform joint predisposes to degenerative changes at that joint in the long term.

### Clinical picture

The patient presents with a pain in the dorsal midfoot area that radiates to the plantar aspect of the medial longitudinal arch. There is a palpable thickening of the bony architecture of the first metatarsal–medial cuneiform joint and the cuneionavicular joint, with the development of exostoses at the joint margins (Fig. 4.23). There is a loss of or reduction in the normal gliding movement within the joint, and possible crepitus. The overlying dorsal tissues may become inflamed,

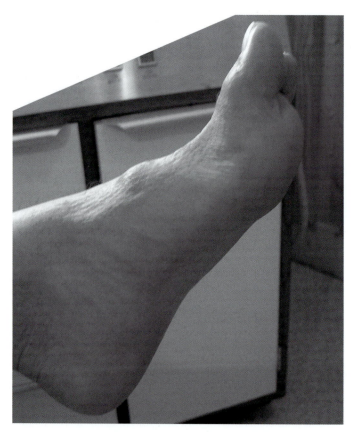

**Figure 4.23** Osteoarthritic changes at the first metatarsal–medial cuneiform joint.

and a dorsal adventitious bursa may develop over these joints due to shoe pressure. In extreme cases, the bursa may even perforate through the overlying dorsal skin. In cases of pes valgus or mobile pes cavus the area of plantar skin overlying the exostoses may develop hyperkeratosis, or even ulcerate, especially in patients with sensory neuropathy or those on parenteral steroid therapy.

### Diagnosis and differential diagnoses

The condition can be confirmed, and the extent of the exostoses and joint degeneration visualised, by plain lateral radiographs of the foot.

The differential diagnosis should exclude midtarsal Charcot arthropathy, such as the neuroarthropathy that arises with diabetes mellitus, other causes of distal sensory neuropathy and midfoot fractures.

### Treatment

Clinical pads may be used to reduce pressure on painful areas. These include cavitied or holed semicompressed felt ovals applied to the dorsal or plantar areas of the midfoot, and fleece ovals, which are used to reduce sheer stress to a dorsal bursa. Shoe-style advice is essential, as the patient should obtain a style that will both accommodate the altered foot shape and reduce trauma to the painful area. Temporary or permanent orthoses can be made to control or reduce the effects of the underlying biomechanical anomaly. The exostoses can be excised surgically, with or without fixation of the affected arthritic joint.

## Plantar fasciitis

Plantar fasciitis (foot strain) is a relatively common foot problem that causes mild to moderate, or moderate to severe pain in the plantar area of the medial longitudinal arch.

### Pathology

The pathology of plantar fasciitis resembles that of heel-pain syndrome. Biomechanical anomalies that predispose to excess tension along the medial column of the foot, together with obesity and prolonged standing predispose to chronic inflammation within the medial band of the plantar fascia.

### Clinical picture

The patient presents with a history of a gradual increase in discomfort or pain radiating along the medial band of the plantar fascia. The pain is worse on first weight bearing in the morning, or after periods of prolonged sitting or rest, and may radiate proximally to the central area of the heel, or distally to the MTPJs. The pain may become intractable and constant, especially by the end of the day. Pain can be induced by asking the patient to stand on tiptoe, or by the examiner palpating the medial band of the plantar fascia with the thumb whilst dorsiflexing the hallux at the first MTPJs. The medial band of the plantar fascia can be easily palpated as a tight, tender cord. Inflammation is not usually obvious. One or both feet may be affected, and sufferers may become quite debilitated, depressed and disabled by the chronic and intractable nature of their foot pain.

### Diagnosis and differential diagnosis

The diagnosis is made on the basis of the presenting signs and symptoms.

The differential diagnosis should exclude heel-pain syndrome, plantar fibromatosis, march fracture and tibialis posterior dysfunction.

### Treatment

Treatment of chronic foot strain is not straightforward, as the patient may have had the condition for several months before seeking treatment. The patient should be advised that they have a chronic soft tissue injury that has probably been present for some considerable time, and is caused by the movements and tensions that occur within the foot during standing and walking. Absolute rest of the foot is impossible to achieve in an ambulant patient, and thus there is no one 'quick fix' treatment for their problem. The recovery period may be protracted, and may not necessarily follow a smooth path to resolution. Thus the patient is likely to have 'good' and 'bad' days. The practitioner is advised to encourage the patient to use combinations of the therapeutic measures listed below, rather than to rely on one type of therapy alone, and to keep on with the treatment for as long as it takes to resolve the symptoms. Empirically, it appears that most cases will respond to a multitherapy approach and the condition will become tolerable within 1–2 months and fully resolve in 6–9 months.

- Biomechanical faults should be identified by a full assessment, and corrected, where possible, with functional permanent orthoses or antipronatory padding, such as a semicompressed felt, whole-foot medial wedge ('cobra' pad, Fig. 4.21), valgus filler pad, or a medial heel wedge applied directly to the foot or affixed to a temporary insole.
- In the obese, weight loss is an essential part of the treatment of plantar fasciitis.
- Any underlying systemic condition (e.g. hypothyroidism) must be diagnosed and managed effectively.
- A course of ultrasound therapy, administered two or three times a week for up to 6 weeks, may be of benefit for some cases.
- A daily regimen of 'triple therapy' is an effective form of home physical therapy, especially when used in conjunction with antipronatory insoles. The 'triple therapy' is used at least once a day and consists of:
  - The use of contrast foot baths (i.e. alternating immersion in warm water at 45°C for 5 minutes, and very cold water at 5°C for 1 minute) for a total of 30 minutes.
  - This is followed by a 5-minute period of toe 'scrunching' exercises, where the patient attempts to gather a tea towel under the foot using only the toes. The towel is laid out on the floor and the toes repeatedly plantar flexed at the MTPJs so that the towel is gradually drawn under the plantar surface of the foot.
  - Finally, the patient rolls the medial longitudinal arch area back and forth for 5 minutes across a cold cylinder (e.g. a bottle of water or a can of cola that has been kept cool in the refrigerator).
- Static daily exercises to impose a lengthening pull on the Achilles tendon are also recommended.
- Night splints, such as a rigid, casted ankle–foot orthosis manufactured to hold the ankle in 10° of dorsiflexion, worn whilst in bed will maintain continued traction on the Achilles tendon overnight (Powell et al 1998).
- A course of NSAIDs to control pain and reduce inflammation, in conjunction with other conservative and mechanical therapies, may be of benefit for those patients who can tolerate these drugs.

## FOREFOOT DISORDERS: METATARSALGIA

'Metatarsalgia' is a generic term used to denote dorsal or plantar, deep or superficial pain in the area of the metatarsals, and thus is a symptom that is associated with a number of forefoot pathologies. Metatarsalgia arises with pathological changes in any forefoot tissues (bones and joints, ligaments, tendons, fascia, the skin and subcuticular tissues, the vasculature, and also in nerve tissue), either as a local problem or as a referred pain from more proximal sites. Other factors that may contribute to metatarsalgia are associated with excessive forefoot forces during weight bearing, and include obesity, pregnancy or occupational factors. Unsuitable or ill-fitting footwear that impedes foot function is implicated as a predisposing or aggravating factor of metatarsalgia. Thus, too short or narrow shoes, shoes with high heels, overlarge shoes, shoes with an incorrect heel-to-ball length, thin-soled and worn-out shoes all contribute to the development of metatarsalgia. Old age or the systemic illnesses that predispose to atrophy or distal displacement of the plantar fat pad also predispose to forefoot pain.

The nature of the underlying problem that has resulted in metatarsalgia must be established in order to fully diagnose and treat the forefoot pain. The diagnosis of metatarsalgia is dependent on gaining a full history of the presenting complaint, together with the examination of the patient, which is itself backed up by the results of diagnostic tests.

- The clinician should question the patient about the presenting problem, exploring areas such as the nature and duration of the pain, and whether it is new, or the recurrence of a previous similar problem. The clinician should establish what induces the forefoot pain, what relieves it, and the sequence of events that lead to its onset. The presence of forefoot swelling or inflammation or bruising, as well as changes in local skin texture or sensation should be noted.
- The examination should include an objective assessment of not just the painful area, but also the complete lower limb and foot, and include details of systemic disease, changes of occupation, exercise levels, and current and previous medications. As a minimum, the examiner should:
  - Palpate the painful area.
  - Look for abnormalities in joints, soft tissues, skin and movement.
  - Assess skin sensation and explore the neurological status of the foot.
  - Assess the skin temperature and explore the vascular status of the foot.
  - Make a static and a dynamic biomechanical assessment of the foot and lower limb. This should include examination of all segments and biomechanical relationships within the lower limb and foot: hip inversion and eversion; patellar position; knee position (genu varum, valgum or recurvatum); tibia varum; tibial torsion; the amount of available dorsiflexion at the ankle (i.e. >10°); the position of the rearfoot in relation to the lower limb (i.e. varus/valgus); the forefoot to rearfoot relationship (supinatus/varus/valgus); the position of the first metatarsal (varus, plantar flexed, dorsiflexed); the range of sagittal plane motion at the first and fifth rays; and the range of movement at the first MTPJ.
  - Check the shoes for wear marks, their fit and their suitability for orthoses.
  - Establish what other treatments have already been used to treat the metatarsalgia, and how effective these were.

From the presenting symptoms and the patient examination, the clinician will be able to reach a working diagnosis. This hypothesis should be confirmed, where possible, by diagnostic tests, including radiographs or other forms of diagnostic investigations such as magnetic resonance imaging or computerised axial tomography scans, bone scan, ultrasound scan and blood tests. The combination of the history, the examination and the results of the diagnostic tests will allow the clinician to form the final diagnosis, and allow him or her to formulate a management plan, so that the presenting problem is treated in the most appropriate manner.

## Classification of metatarsalgia

'Greater metatarsalgia' is a term that may be used to describe pain that relates to first-ray pathology, and 'lesser metatarsalgia' for pain relating to pathology in the area of the second to fifth rays. Alternatively, metatarsalgia may be classified as functional or non-functional.

## Functional metatarsalgia

Functional metatarsalgia is the term used to describe the forefoot pain that arises from the pathomechanical stresses, such as compression, shearing and tensile stress arising within the lower limb, the whole foot, the rearfoot or the forefoot, during both stance and gait. Pathologies associated with metatarsalgia are often ascribed to one particular form of abnormal stress, but which, in reality, develop as the result of combined stresses. For example, concurrent abnormal compression and shearing induces the formation of hyperkeratotic plantar lesions: the patient with a fixed plantar-flexed metatarsal may present with diffuse, asymptomatic, shear-stress-related plantar callosity overlying a compression-related deep painful corn.

Functional metatarsalgia may arise due to anomalies of the forefoot bone structure, such as the relative length of the metatarsals, a localised metatarsal equinus or iatrogenic structural change.

- The normal *metatarsal formula*, that is the frontal plane relationship of the metatarsal heads across the metatarsal parabola, is $2 > 3 = 1 > 4 > 5$, or $2 > 1 > 3 > 4 > 5$. A relatively long metatarsal is prone to overload at its head, and a relatively short metatarsal predisposes to overload of the metatarsal head adjacent to it. If a second or third metatarsal is relatively long, its head will lie in a plantar-flexed position in relation to the adjacent metatarsal heads, predisposing to the formation of associated plantar hyperkeratosis, joint capsulitis and digital deformity. A previous episode of Freiberg's disease at the second metatarsal head may cause apparent shortening of the metatarsal due to loss of the dome of the head, and the development of transfer metatarsalgia at the adjacent MTPJs. A relatively short fourth metatarsal is a congenital condition that arises due to premature closure of the epiphyseal plate and is associated with an apparently short and retracted fourth toe (Fig. 4.24). A similar situation is noted with a very rare inherited condition, pseudo-pseudohypoparathyroidism, where subjects show abnormally short fourth metacarpals and metatarsals, amongst other skeletal dysplasias.
- A *localised metatarsal equinus*, that is relative plantar flexion of the head of an individual metatarsal, tends to give rise to metatarsalgia, due to an associated capsulitis at the affected metatarsal joint.
- *Iatrogenic structural changes* may arise as the result of a previous surgical intervention to the metatarsal area, and require further surgery to correct the problem.

### Pathology

Persistent intermittent abnormal compression of the plantar tissues results in contusion and inflammation of soft tissues, and predisposes to the formation of focal, nucleated plantar keratoses. Abnormal compression forces at the plantar fibrofatty pad of the forefoot are associated with:

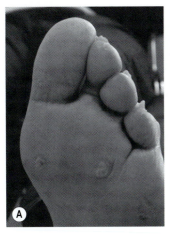 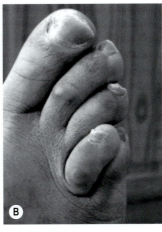

**Figure 4.24** Congentially short 4th metatarsal in male aged 38 years (A), and the resultant plantar hyperkeratotic transfer lesions (B), affecting the skin over the head of the 3rd and 5th metatarsals.

- Inflexibility of the foot, such as in rigid pes cavus, uncompensated ankle equinus and forefoot equinus; loss of subtalar joint movement, due to tarsal coalition, an old foot injury, or the glycation of ligamentous protein that occurs in long-term diabetes mellitus.
- Fixation of one or more metatarsals or MTPJs, such as occurs with the fixed plantar flexion of the first and/or fifth rays, noted with rigid pes cavus.
- Fixed toe deformity, including non-reducible triggering, retraction or clawing of the toes, fixed hammer or mallet toe formation and associated plantar flexion of the associated metatarsal.
- Subluxation or dislocation of any of the MTPJs. For example, the second toe tends to adopt a hammer position in cases with hallux abducto valgus, so that the toe is subluxed at the second MTPJ.

## Clinical presentation

Persistent abnormal shear stress predisposes to the development of plaques of diffuse plantar hyperkeratosis of skin overlying the MTPJs, and formation of adventitious bursae especially beneath the -first MTPJ. Abnormal shear stress primarily arises as the result of hypermobility. The hypermobility may affect the whole foot, such as is seen in generalised whole-body hypermobility. But it is also associated with biomechanical anomalies such as mobile pes cavus and fully compensated rearfoot varus. Associated excessive compensatory pronation at the subtalar and midtarsal joints causes a reduction in the height of the medial longitudinal arch, with a resultant relative lengthening of the foot on weight bearing and abnormal shear stress of plantar soft tissues. The forefoot is stabilised, in part, by the transverse metatarsal ligament and the tone of the transverse head of the adductor hallucis muscle, which together control the transverse spread of the metatarsal heads when under load. The first and fifth metatarsals are unable to resist metatarsal splaying in the hypermobile foot, with the development of metatarsus primus varus and metatarsus qinque valgus, a resultant increase in the width of the forefoot and associated hallux abducto valgus and digitus quintus varus deformities. In these cases the medial aspect of the first MTPJ and the lateral aspect of the fifth MTPJ are subjected to shoe-related shear stress, with resultant bursa formation at these sites. Over-large or slip-on shoes also predispose to shear stresses at the skin surface, with resultant development of painful diffuse plantar keratoses at the forefoot.

Abnormal tensile stresses occur as the result of chronic strain on fascial tissues. Examples of metatarsalgia associated with abnormal tensile foot stresses include chronic foot strain, and strain on the transverse intermetatarsal ligaments with associated fatigue of intrinsic musculature due to splaying of the metatarsals, such as is seen in pes cavus and hallux abducto valgus.

## Management

The successful management of functional metatarsalgia depends on the identification and elimination, or mitigation, of the underlying pathomechanical cause of pain. In cases where metatarsalgia is symptomatic of a forefoot (rather than hindfoot) malfunction, the management focuses on the promotion of maximum function of the lesser toes and their MTPJs, by the use of clinical padding, the use of correctly fitting shoes, the use of functional orthoses and surgery.

- The function of non-fixed retracted and clawed toes is increased by the use of orthodigital splints. These devices improve both the alignment of the interphalangeal joints and their associated MTPJs, and promote better toe function.
- Toe function can be increased by the use of plantar metatarsal padding or orthoses designed to reduce both plantar flexion of the metatarsal and excessive dorsiflexion of the proximal phalanx at the MTPJ.
- Anomalies of foot function that predispose to metatarsalgia, such as compensated, or part-compensated, or non-compensated rearfoot–lower limb and forefoot–rearfoot malalignments should be identified through biomechanical assessment and corrected, where possible, by the use of functional in-shoe orthoses.
- Exercise regimens, such as those recommended for the resolution of foot strain (above), and physical therapies (see Ch. 16) will help improve function of the intrinsic musculature.
- Palliative metatarsal in-shoe or orthosis-based cushioning is indicated for cases where the plantar fibrofatty pad has atrophied or has become distally displaced.
- Surgery may be indicated for those cases of metatarsalgia that relate to overload or prominence of a single metatarsal head, or where the symptoms cannot be relieved by conservative measures. Procedures include metatarsal osteotomy to realign the head of the affected metatarsal within the metatarsal parabola. Plantar skin transfer lesions or hyperkeratosis may develop over the adjacent MTPJ area subsequent to metatarsal surgery, but the secondary lesions tend to be far less painful than the original problem.

## Non-functional metatarsalgia

This is a term used to describe painful forefoot conditions that do not primarily relate to biomechanical problems within the lower limb and foot. Examples would include Freiberg's disease and Morton's neuroma. However, as the foot is a dynamic, weight-bearing structure, it is very difficult to isolate presentations of non-functional metatarsalgia from the influence of biomechanical and weight-bearing factors. Thus the remainder of this review of metatarsalgia groups the presentations of forefoot pain in relation to the tissues involved.

### Categorisation of non-functional metatarsalgia

Metatarsalgia can be considered within three broad causative categories:

- metatarsalgia relating to soft tissue pathology
- metatarsalgia relating to bone and joint pathology
- metatarsalgia relating to systemic pathology.

## Focal hyperkeratoses

### Metatarsalgia relating to soft tissue pathologies

Focal hyperkeratoses (also known as intractable plantar keratoses [IPK]), tyloma, helloma vasculare and helloma neurovasculare) are deep-seated fibrous corns that form within the skin overlying the plantar aspects of the lesser metatarsal heads. They may incorporate a vascular or neurological element and are frequently underlain by fibrous tissue formation. They are difficult to remove in a pain-free manner without the use of local analgesia.

### Pathology

Focal hyperkeratoses are noted in association with:

- relative depression of a metatarsal head, itself associated with fixed hammer-toe deformity or rigid pes cavus
- a dorsally displaced or elevated first metatarsal, where the corn forms within the plantar skin overlying the second MTPJ, and often occurs in association with hallux rigidus and hallux abducto valgus (see below)
- idiosyncratic skin types
- plantar skin scars.

### Clinical picture

The patient presents with a persistent painful hyperkeratotic lesion that usually locates within skin overlying a specific metatarsal head. The lesion requires frequent reduction to control the localised pain it causes, but tends to reform within a very short time after apparent full removal. Total enucleation of the central keratin plug is not always possible, as the patient may be unwilling or unable to accept local anaesthesia or tolerate the pain caused by debridement, especially in cases where a neural or vascular element is included at the deepest part of the hyperkeratotic plug. The long-standing nature of the lesion is characterised by chronic inflammation, which leads to the gradual replacement of that area of the normal fat pad with tough fibrous tissue, deep to the lesion. The resulting replacement of an area of the softer fibrofatty plantar pad with tough fibrous tissue reduces local tissue resilience and exacerbates the problem. Plantar cushioning is further reduced if the lesion is associated with a hammer-toe deformity within the same ray, or clawing or retraction of the lesser toes, which causes the plantar fibrofatty pad to be drawn distally away from the MTPJs and towards the plantar webbing area, as soft tissues are more firmly attached to the plantar basal area of the proximal phalanx than to the metatarsals. The volume and function of the tissues overlying the plantar aspects of the MTPJs is reduced, so that the plantar aspects of the metatarsal heads appear to be prominent and are easily palpated. The residual plantar fibrofatty pad is of reduced thickness, and unable to resist the compression imposed by the combination of body weight and ground reaction forces. Atrophy of the plantar fibrofatty pad is a feature of the elderly or rheumatoid foot, and is noted in patients with peripheral vascular disease.

### Diagnosis

The association with prominence of a particular metatarsal head can be established on an anteroposterior radiograph of the forefoot, where the location of the skin lesion is marked by affixing small metal marker, such as a small circle or wire, to the skin over the hyperkeratotic focus.

### Treatment

The conservative treatment of focal plantar hyperkeratosis does not always lead to resolution, and all approaches are indicated to ensure best results. Treatment options include:

- Meticulous reduction of all overlying plantar callosity, and enucleation of the plug of keratin. The enucleation may require administration of a local anaesthetic, such as a tibial nerve block, or the use of self-administered transcutaneous electrical nerve stimulation (TENS) during the enucleation. Astringent chemicals, such as 75–95% silver nitrate, or caustic chemicals such as 20% wheat germ oil and 20% pyrogallol ointment, may be applied after enucleation to discourage lesion reformation. Strong astringents and caustics are contraindicated in patients with neuropathy or peripheral vascular disease, and some patients are unable to tolerate the pain that can occur for a short time after the application of these chemicals.
- The use of the Podospray™ drill, which is reputed to cause less pain during lesion enucleation.
- The application of clinical padding or the provision of accommodative insoles to deflect compressive forces away from the painful plantar area.
- The manufacture of orthoses that are prescribed to correct any underlying biomechanical abnormality in the younger foot.
- Electrosurgery, under tibial block local anaesthesia, to excise the lesion.
- Ray surgery to correct an associated lesser toe deformity, with or without osteotomy to improve metatarsal alignment.

## Metatarsalgia due to synovial tissue pathologies

### Ganglia/ganglionic cysts

Weakness in the wall of a synovial tendon sheath or a joint capsule predisposes to the formation of a local fluctuant swelling, often at the dorsum of the foot, especially at the point where the tendon sheath emerges from the overlying retinaculae.

### Pathology

The tendon sheath or joint capsule herniates, to form a thin-walled, cyst-like structure that lies within subcuticular structures. The cyst is continuous with the lining of the tendon sheath or joint capsule, and is filled with synovial fluid. The cyst may present as forefoot pain, due to the tension within the cyst, or due to local pressure from footwear. Where the cyst forms as a herniation of the distal interphalangeal joint, it can cause mucoid cyst formation with distortion of the local nail matrix, with resultant deformation of the visible nail plate.

### Clinical picture

The ganglion shows translumination when the beam from a bright torch is shone through it. The swelling usually has an easily palpable margin, delineating the limits of the lesion. The examiner can detect a 'fluid thrill' within the lesion. The examiner places two fingers on the ganglion and applies pressure with the tip of one of the fingers. The second finger detects the change in fluid pressure as the ganglion fluid moves in response to the applied pressure.

### Treatment

The most appropriate treatment is determined by the severity of the presenting problem, and can range from no active treatment through to lesion excision or bone surgery. The range of treatments include:

- Direct pressure to the lesion, using a compression dressing, such as Coban®. In days gone by, ganglia were traditionally dispersed with sudden pressure, from a large book.
- The application of deflective or cushioning clinical padding to reduce local pressure from shoes.
- Aspiration of the cystic fluid under local anaesthesia, using a wide-bore needle; however, the lesion tends to reform over time.

- Surgical excision of the ganglion, with cauterisation of the basal sinus to prevent reformation. Cysts formed by herniation of an interphalangeal joint may require partial joint excision (hemiphalangectomy) to prevent recurrence.

## Capsulitis

Capsulitis is the term used to describe inflammation of a joint capsule. Capsulitis frequently arises secondary to osteoarthritis and rheumatoid arthritis, or as the result of ongoing, low-grade joint trauma.

### Pathology

The articular synovium associated with joint ligaments and local tendon sheaths becomes engorged, swollen and softened by the inflammatory process. Where capsulitis is associated with rheumatoid arthritis, the toes may sublux at the MTPJs. Where the process is induced by trauma, such as stubbing the great toe leading to capsulitis of the first MTPJ, the clinical picture is one of acute hallux flexus (see below).

### Treatment

The condition can be treated by:

- Physical therapies, such as gentle heat at the subacute or chronic stage of inflammation, or the use of PRICE (pain control, rest, ice, compression and elevation) in the first 24–48 hours of an acute presentation.
- The use of NSAIDs to control associated pain and reduce inflammation.
- Referral for treatment of any underlying rheumatoid condition with disease-modifying antirheumatic drugs (DMARDs).
- Reduction of local trauma to allow the area to rest, and to minimise inflammation, promote healing and prevent joint distortion.

## Gouty tophus

Gout is a crystal deposition disease that predisposes to arthropathy in susceptible subjects.

### Pathology

Insoluble uric acid in blood is converted by enzymic action into soluble urea. Raised uric acid levels predispose to the deposition of crystalline sodium urate in peripheral and cooler soft tissues, causing severe local pain and inflammation. The long-term accumulations of sodium urate within soft and joint tissues form gouty tophi (singular: tophus). Gout has a predilection to affect the first MTPJ, although tophi may arise in any area of superficial soft tissue, including the nail bed and the outer margin of the pinna of the ear. The disease tends to affect males, over 30 years of age, but postmenopausal women are also predisposed to gout.

### Clinical picture

Urate crystal deposition within soft tissues acts as a mediator of acute inflammation. Typically, the patient wakes in the middle of the night with severe pain in the first MTPJ. The affected area shows severe acute inflammation: it is very swollen and shiny, very red and hot, and far too tender to touch. Gradually, over the subsequent days, the inflammation gradually subsides, and the area becomes much less swollen, red and painful, and the involved area of skin may peel, reflecting the severity of the earlier acute inflammatory process. The inflammation may totally subside or may persist as a chronic condition. Repeated episodes of gout or prolonged chronic inflammation predispose to ongoing osteoarthritic and degenerative changes within the affected joint. The skin overlying the tophus may perforate or ulcerate and reveal an accumulation of bright, white urate crystals within the affected soft tissues. Where gouty tophi form in subungual tissues, the nail shows onycholysis and subungual breakdown. The nail matrix may be distorted by the long-term inflammation leading to dystrophy and thickening (onychauxis) of the nail plate.

### Diagnosis

The classic presentation of gout arthropathy and tophus formation is almost self-diagnostic. Radiographs of affected joints show characteristic 'punched out' erosions at the joint margins. In the acute phase of the disease, blood urate levels and the erythrocyte sedimentation rate will be raised, but these tend to fall to near-normal values between episodes. Polarised-light microscopy of aspirated joint fluid shows birefringent crystals.

### Treatment

The treatment of gout includes the use of drugs to control pain and inflammation, and agents to reduce blood urate levels.

- NSAIDs are the first line of pharmaceutical therapy. They are used to reduce joint inflammation and prevent later arthrosis and degenerative changes in affected joints. They are used in conjunction with rest, or non-weight bearing at the painful area.
- Uricosuric agents (i.e. drugs that are specific to the control of blood urate levels) may be required to prevent further episodic flare-up.

## Problematic bursae

Adventitious bursae form over bony prominences in relation to local shear stresses. In the long term they may become fibrous, distended, inflamed, infected or even calcified. The skin overlying the bursa may be prone to chilling. Patients with forefoot deformities, such as hallux abducto valgus, are prone to develop adventitious bursae over the medial exostosis at the first metatarsal head, and patients with rheumatoid arthritis tend to develop very large and distended bursae over the bunion joint and the plantar aspects of the MTPJs (see below).

### Treatment

The treatment of bursae focuses on the reduction of local shear stress together with palliation. The range of treatments includes:

- the application of antishear padding and strapping, such as fleecy web, Moleskin® and Spenco second skin®
- the manufacture of moulded cushioned insoles
- aspiration of bursal fluid, under local anaesthesia, to reduce tissue distension
- The modification of shoe wear, such as the provision of balloon patches and slits cut into the upper to increase the internal dimension of the toe box, and the provision of bespoke or semi-bespoke shoes to accommodate the deformity and reduce shear stresses.

## Rheumatoid nodules and rheumatoid bursae

Patients with rheumatoid arthritis are prone to develop large adventitious bursae within the plantar tissues overlying the MTPJs, and fibrinoid nodules over bony prominences (see Ch. 8).

### Pathology

The autoimmune inflammation that characterises rheumatoid arthritis is associated with bursa and nodule formation. Bilateral symmetrical multilobed, distended, fluid-filled soft tissue swellings form over the plantar aspects of the MTPJs, and fibrinoid deposits arise in areas of low-grade trauma, such as at the posterior aspect of the heel or the outer surface of the elbow.

### Clinical picture

These lesions are prone to flare-up, and become very swollen and acutely tender. The patient with distended plantar bursae describes a sensation of walking on 'hot coals'. The plantar skin overlying the bursae may be covered with thin callus. Both rheumatoid bursae and nodules are subject to tissue breakdown, and secondary infection may occur, due to the decreased tissue viability that is a feature of rheumatoid arthritis, and the range of drugs that are used to control pain and inflammation. Disease modifying anti-rheumatic drug (DMARD) and NSAID regimens both tend to cause thinning of the skin and tissue breakdown.

### Treatment

The aim of treatment is to minimise trauma to the painful area, particularly during a time of flare-up.

- Any area of tissue breakdown should be treated as an open wound, and protected with appropriate sterile dressings and clinical padding until healing is complete.
- Full-length, soft, moulded insoles made from layers of soft- and medium-density Plastazote® are formed to a cast of the patient's foot to cushion the area and reduce local shear stresses.
- Moulded, soft-density Plastazote® heel cups can be used to protect nodules at the posterior heel area.
- Bespoke or semi-bespoke shoes of a type that will accommodate both the casted insole and the foot deformity are essential to minimise soft tissue trauma.

## Plantar plate rupture

The plantar plate is a tough, rectangular, fibrocartilaginous structure that overlies the plantar aspects of the MTPJs. It is formed from the distal part of the plantar aponeurosis and the plantar aspects of the capsules of the MTPJs. It has a weak origin at the plantar aspects of the necks of the metatarsals and a strong insertion into the plantar aspect of the base of the proximal phalanges. Its function is to reduce load at the plantar aspects of the metatarsal heads, stabilise the digit in association with the collateral ligaments and the intrinsic and extrinsic muscles, and guide the line of pull of the tendons that insert into the digits, such as the tendons of the lumbrical and flexor digitorum longus muscles. The plantar plate acts as an attachment for the distal part of the plantar fascia and has a role in the windlass mechanism (Hicks 1954), resisting hyperextension of the MTPJ. The loss of the integrity of the plantar plate is implicated in the genesis of hammer toe. When rupture of the plantar plate occurs at the first MTPJ the condition is termed 'turf toe', and commonly affects young men who engage in vigorous sports (see Ch. 13).

### Pathology

The plantar plate is subject to severe extension forces at toe-off. Any weakness at an origin of the plantar plate predisposes to the development of chronic digital hyperextension at the associated MTPJ, with subsequent attenuation (thinning), or even rupture, of the plantar plate. As a result, the MTPJ becomes unstable, and spontaneous joint dislocation may occur, especially at the second MTPJ. In some cases the rupture presents as a central tear in the joint capsule, allowing synovial fluid to leak out from the joint space into the surrounding tissues, where it acts as a mediator of acute inflammation. In cases where the affected toe deviates laterally, the tear is likely to have occurred in the collateral ligament.

### Clinical picture

Rupture or attenuation of the plantar plate at the second to fifth MTPJs occurs more frequently in women. It is thought that both the increase in the weight-bearing load at the forefoot and the forced hyperextension at the MTPJs imposed by wearing high-heeled shoes predisposes to plantar plate dysfunction. The condition has also been associated with a long second metatarsal, a short first metatarsal, inflammatory arthropathies, diabetes mellitus, age-related degeneration of the joint tissues and biomechanical anomalies. Athletes are also prone to this condition, as repetitive hyperextension of the MTPJ induces elongation and attenuation of the plantar aponeurosis and joint capsule.

The second MTPJ is most commonly affected by plantar plate rupture. Patients commonly present with chronic focal pain underlying the second MTPJ. The patient may report a history of tripping, and complain of an awareness of a 'lump' or a 'bruised feeling' on the plantar aspect of the second MTPJ. There may be associated mild swelling to the plantar and dorsal aspects of the joint. Commonly, patients note gradual sagittal (hammering) and/or transverse plane (lateral drift) deformity of the second toe.

The presentation of a plantar plate rupture may vary from a relatively mild local metatarsalgia to an exuberant and acutely painful inflammation with synovitis of the affected MTPJ and associated flexor tendon, with marked functional disability. More commonly, the patient presents with a progressive subluxation or frank dislocation of the second toe, and idiopathic inflammation about the associated MTPJ. The patient usually reports a history of sudden onset of foot pain whilst walking that locates to the base of the toe and the associated MTPJ. The disruption of the proximal phalanx retaining mechanism allows alteration in the alignment of the pull of the flexor tendons, with subsequent and progressive hammering and transverse deviation of the digit.

### Diagnosis and differential diagnoses

The clinical diagnosis is made from the history and presenting symptoms. A positive vertical stress test allows the affected toe to be elevated in a dorsal direction at the MTPJ, when the associated metatarsal is stabilised. Translocation of the digit by more than 2 mm in relation to the associated metatarsal head is indicative of rupture of the plantar plate. The tear within the plantar plate and the resultant leak of synovial fluid out of the joint space can be visualised on a radiograph when a radio-opaque dye is injected into the affected joint space (arthrography). The lesion shows on a magnetic resonance imaging scan as an increase in signal intensity in and around the plantar plate (Fig. 4.25), with discontinuity of the integrity of the plate, synovitis of the

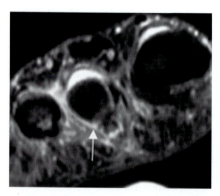

**Figure 4.25** Magnetic resonance image of the second MTPJ, showing loss of integrity of the plantar plate.

MTPJ and flexor tendon sheath, and persistent hyperextension of the proximal phalanx.

The differential diagnosis should exclude synovitis in association with rheumatological disease, traumatic subluxation of the toe, osteochondritis of the metatarsal head (Freiberg's disease), stress fracture and plantar digital neuroma.

### Treatment

The treatment of plantar plate rupture can be approached conservatively or surgically.

Conservative treatments of plantar plate rupture are designed to ease local pain, rest the painful area, and minimise digital deformity whilst inflammation subsides and tissue healing occurs.

- Conservative measures include taping to maintain the correct alignment of the toe at the MTPJ, clinical plantar pads to dorsiflex the metatarsal and plantar flex the toe at the MTPJ, and orthoses to correct any underlying biomechanical faults, realign the digit and reduce pressure at the painful MTPJ.
- It should be noted that pads or orthoses that incorporate a U-shaped cut-out for the affected MTPJ may exacerbate the presenting problem. A reciprocal dorsiflexion of the proximal phalanx of the affected joint can be exacerbated by unrestricted plantar flexion of the distal part of the metatarsal with the result that the interosseous and lumbrical tendons adopt a near-vertical orientation. The digital deformity may worsen and the likelihood of full plantar plate rupture is increased.
- Exercises to strengthen the action of the plantar intrinsic muscles may be of benefit once the acute phase has passed (see foot strain, above)
- Recalcitrant pain may be relieved by a course of NSAIDs and/or intra-articular hydrocortisone injection. It must be noted that hydrocortisone may further weaken the affected tissues.

Surgery is indicated for cases that fail to respond to conservative therapies. Recommended procedures include osseous correction of the deformed digit together with flexor-to-extensor tendon transfer to restore the correct alignment of the toe and MTPJ, with surgical repair of the tear in the plantar plate or collateral ligament.

## Neurological problems

### Sensory problems, paraesthesia and painful neuropathy

Patients with painful neuropathy or hyperalgesia experience radiating burning, sharp or shooting pains in the distribution of the affected nerve. Their symptoms are usually exacerbated by movement. Tinel's sign (i.e. distal tingling and paraesthesia) or Valleix' sign (i.e. proximal tingling and paraesthesia) may be noted when the affected nerve trunk is percussed or palpated. Patients with abnormal sensory function will have altered nerve conduction rates on testing. Painful neuropathy or hyperaesthesia may be a feature of diabetic sensory neuropathy, and often precedes severe loss of peripheral sensation.

### Nerve entrapment/Morton's neuroma

Morton's neuroma, also known as plantar digital neuroma, causes spasmodic neurological pain in the forefoot. It is a common condition, often affecting middle-aged women. Durlacher first described the painful syndrome in 1845, although it is named after TG Morton who wrote on the condition in 1876. In 1883, Hoadley was the first person to identify a nerve lesion at a symptomatic area. Many clinicians have theorised on the true nature and cause of the pain of plantar digital neuroma: some theories are feasible, but others are anatomically incorrect. Plantar digital neuroma affects women more often than men, and the most likely age band of onset is 40–60 years. Sufferers show a tendency to the upper limit of the normal body mass index (BMI). The BMI is calculated as the body weight in kilograms divided by the square of the height in meters. The normal BMI range is 20–25. Patients with plantar digital neuroma tend to the upper levels of the normal BMI (i.e. a BMI of 25 or greater). Neuroma can affect either foot, but bilateral presentation is less common, as is the occurrence of more than one lesion in the same foot. The neuroma lies approximately 5–10 mm deep to the plantar skin, just proximal to the point of division forming the plantar digital nerves proper. Plantar digital neuroma arises as an entrapment pathology affecting an intermetatarsal nerve, causing focal thickening of the nerve at the point where it divides to form the plantar digital nerves. Approximately 90% of cases affect either the second–third or third–fourth web spaces, and only 10% affect the first–second or fourth–fifth interspaces.

### Pathology

Branches of the tibial nerve give rise to the lateral and medial plantar nerves, which subdivide to form paired plantar digital nerves proper. The lateral plantar nerve gives off digital branches that supply both sides of the fifth toe and the lateral side of the fourth toe. The medial plantar nerve gives off digital branches that supply both sides of the first, second and third toes, and the medial side of the fourth toe. There is often a communicating branch of the lateral plantar nerve that anastomoses with the medial plantar nerve, and also supplies the third web space. Other communicating branches anastomose with nerves deeper within the foot, and thereby tether the nerve in the third–fourth web space (Fig. 4.26). The metatarsal heads are separated by bursae, which lie superior (dorsal) to the transverse plantar ligament. The neurovascular bundles and lumbrical muscles lie within

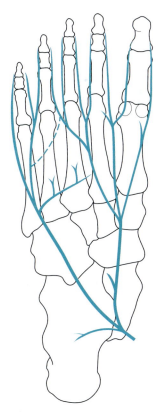

**Figure 4.26** Plantar digital neuritis: the plantar nerves.

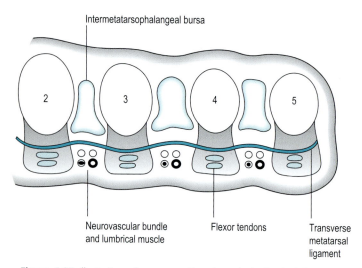

Intermetatarsophalangeal bursa

2    3    4    5

Neurovascular bundle
and lumbrical muscle        Flexor tendons        Transverse
                                                  metatarsal
                                                  ligament

**Figure 4.27** Illustration of a cross-section through the level of the metatarsal necks 2–5.

the intermetatarsal spaces, deep (plantar) to the transverse metatarsal ligament (Fig. 4.27).

Factors that predispose to the development of plantar digital neuroma include nerve compression and tension, especially in the third–fourth interspace, the distal extension of the intermetatarsal bursa at toe-off, transient nerve ischaemia and biomechanical factors.

## Compression and tension of the plantar digital nerves

There are a number of factors that predispose to compression and tension of the plantar digital nerves. These include:

- Nerve thickness: the third common digital nerve is thicker than other common digital nerves, as it is formed of branches from both the medial and lateral plantar nerves.
- Movement between the medial and lateral columns of the foot: the third metatarsal is relatively immobile in comparison to the range of sagittal plane movement available to the fourth metatarsal. Thus, the third common digital nerve is tensioned by sagittal plane movement of the fourth metatarsal relative to the more static third metatarsal.
- Hyperextension of the toes at the MTPJs: for example, shoes with high heels pitch the centre of gravity of the body forward towards the forefoot, and decrease the area of foot–ground contact. They impose hyperextension of the MTPJs, so that the digital nerve is forced upwards against the inflexible transverse intermetatarsal ligament.

## Distal extension of the intermetatarsal bursa

The intermetatarsal bursae lie between adjacent metatarsal heads (Fig. 4.27). The distal margins of the intermetatarsal bursae project just distally to the associated MTPJ and the distal limit of the transverse intermetatarsal ligament, to lie between the bases of the proximal phalanges. At toe-off the bursal fluid tends to move into the more distal parts of the bursae. This effect is implicated in the pathogenesis of plantar digital neuroma:

- hypermobility of the forefoot, associated with abnormal subtalar joint pronation and compounded by lateral compression from constricting footwear, creates shear and friction on the intermetatarsal bursa, inducing inflammation and an increased volume of fluid within the bursa

- the rise in fluid pressure within the bursa causes it to extrude distally and impinge against the neurovascular bundle, leading to an entrapment neuropathy, compression of the local artery and resultant ischaemic pain
- the resultant chronic inflammation leads to perineural fibrosis, where fibrous tissue develops around and compresses the nerve.

### Transient ischaemia

The vasa nervosum (the artery serving the affected nerve) and the digital artery (which lies within the same neurovascular bundle as the affected nerve) are subject to intermittent compression during gait, by the distal distension of the intermetatarsal bursa, causing a local transient ischaemia, and acute ischaemic pain.

### Biomechanical influences

Empirical observation indicates that a majority of cases with plantar digital neuroma present with inversion of the forefoot when the foot is non-weight bearing. This is compensated at toe-off by sagittal plane movement between the second–third or third–fourth metatarsals. That is, the lateral column of the foot moves dorsally, and the medial column moves relatively in a plantar direction when the forefoot comes under load, leading to stretching of the intermetatarsal tissues, chronic inflammation and the development of local fibrosis around the plantar nerve at the point where it divides to form the plantar digital nerves. The fibrous tissue ensheaths the nerve, exacerbating the condition.

The affected plantar digital nerve shows a fusiform thickening of the perineural tissues, and hypertrophy of the plantar digital nerves – a neuroma. The neuroma is white to yellow in colour, and shiny. Microscopically, there is juxtaneural fibrosis of the nerve that is continuous with the intermetatarsal bursa, intraneural fibrosis and collagen deposition, subperineural hyalinised nodules (Renault's bodies), fibrosis of endoneural blood vessels (endarteritis), demyelination of the involved nerve fibres and axonal loss. These pathological changes to the plantar digital nerve confirm the diagnosis of Morton's neuroma, and indicate that the lesion forms as the result of degenerative processes, consistent with an entrapment neuropathy.

### Clinical picture

The patient typically reports a sudden, sharp, shock-like, burning, paroxysmal, spasmodic debilitating pain at the plantar aspect of the second–third or third–fourth intermetatarsal webbing area. The pain is often triggered by prolonged standing, walking or running, and may also occur during rest. The pain may be acute and disabling. Patients often report urgent need to remove the shoe and massage the foot to try to reduce the pain. Pain can be induced or aggravated by wearing tight or narrow shoes, thin-soled shoes or high-heeled shoes. Pain can also occur spontaneously and during the night. The pain often radiates into the toes that lie to either side of the affected web space, to the dorsum of foot and/or into the lower part of the back of the leg. The patient often describes a sensation of walking on a 'lump' or 'pebble' in the vicinity of the focal point of the pain at the plantar webbing, and has disturbed sensation, such as paraesthesia, tingling and numbness in the toes to either side of the affected web space. Sometimes the pain of plantar digital neuroma may present as an isolated apical pain. There may be a palpable thickening and oedema of the affected webbing area, which can be detected by palpating the dorsal–plantar dimension of the webbing tissues and comparing this with the same site on the other foot or the adjacent web space. Local oedema may cause the toes at the affected web space to diverge slightly, especially on weight bearing (the sunray sign).

## CASE STUDY 4.8 **MORTON'S NEUROMA**

The patient was a 47-year-old woman, who was in good general health and worked as a home help. She presented with acute pain at the tip of the left fourth toe. The pain had been present for approximately 6 months, beginning gradually, but recently increasing to almost intolerable levels. She was otherwise in good health, although inclined to asthma and eczema.

On examination, the left fourth and fifth toes were in a marked varus position, with a large Durlacher's corn deep in the lateral sulcus of the left fourth toe. Enucleation of the lesion gave almost instantaneous relief. However, as the pain re-established within 2 months, the outer segment of the left fourth nail was later excised under local anaesthetic, and the exposed pocket of matrix phenolised to prevent nail regrowth. Healing was uneventful, and the left fourth toe was pain free.

However, 1 year later, the patient returned, complaining of exactly the same apical pain in the left fourth toe. The pain was worse when wearing court shoes, and was described as like 'toothache' in its sudden and unpredictable onset. There was no sign of nail regrowth, or hyperkeratotic lesion. However, thumb pressure to the left thirrd/fourth plantar webbing whilst simultaneously applying lateral compression across the forefoot (Mulder's test, Fig. 4.28) triggered the pain spasm. She was diagnosed with plantar digital (Morton's) neuroma.

A temporary insole with a medial heel/instep/forefoot (cobra) pad was made, and this gave some considerable, but short-lived, relief of the symptoms. Finally, the patient underwent day-case surgery, and a large neuroma was excised from the left third/fourth interspace via a web splitting incision. The area healed well, and the patient has been symptom-free in the 10 years since.

This was an unusual presentation of Morton's neuroma, as the typical signs and symptoms were not obvious, and the treatments of the primary lesions gave good, but only temporary, relief. As the pain of the diagnosed neuroma was no different to that of either the Durlacher's corn and nail trauma, it was assumed that the neuroma was the underlying cause of the forefoot pathology.

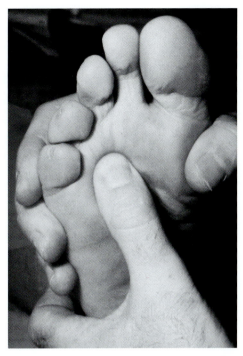

**Figure 4.28** Mulder's test: Apply pressure to the third and fourth web spaces, using the thumb, to elicit pain. The forefoot should simultaneously be compressed laterally to test for a palpable, painful 'Mulder's' click.

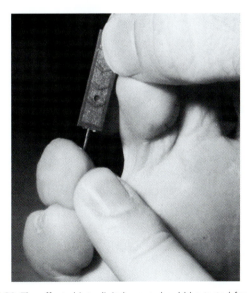

**Figure 4.29** The affected interdigital space should be tested for loss of sensation using a sharp instrument e.g. a neurotip.

### Diagnosis and differential diagnosis

The diagnosis of plantar digital neuroma is generally made on the basis of the highly characteristic presenting symptoms, together with elicitation of the pain by lateral compression of the metatarsal heads whilst simultaneously applying direct pressure in a dorsal–proximal direction with the thumb at the affected web space (Mulder's test) (Fig. 4.28). The patient will also characteristically show a degree of paraesthesia or hypoaesthesia in the associated interdigital cleft, in comparison to the unaffected interdigital areas (Fig. 4.29). Unambiguous loss of sensation at the affected interdigital space and adjacent toes can be taken as strong supportive evidence of a positive diagnosis of plantar digital neuroma. The patient with plantar digital neuroma or neuritis will experience a full reduction of pain, even when the action that normally triggers the pain is undertaken, by the injection of local anaesthetic, such as 2 ml of 1% lignocaine plain solution, into the area of the neuroma via the interdigital space. The nerve lesion is not visible on radiography, unless it is very large, when the adjacent metatarsal heads may show divergence. The lesion can be well visualised on magnetic resonance imaging, and high-resolution ultrasound imaging is a very useful indicator of the presence of plantar digital neuroma, showing the lesion as a hypoechoic mass, varying in density from the surrounding tissue and oriented parallel to the long axis of the metatarsals (Fig. 4.30A and B). Nerve conduction tests are not always conclusive in the diagnosis of Morton's neuroma.

The differential diagnosis of Morton's neuroma or plantar digital neuritis should exclude forefoot pain arising as the result of: lumbar radiculopathy, tarsal tunnel syndrome, metatarsal or stress fracture, Freiberg's infraction, peripheral neuritis or neuropathy, intermetatarsal bursitis, arthritides, metatarsal and soft tissue tumours, rupture of the plantar plate and MTPJ capsulitis.

### Treatment

The treatment of plantar digital neuroma should address all aspects of the presenting problem, as well as the associated predisposing factors.

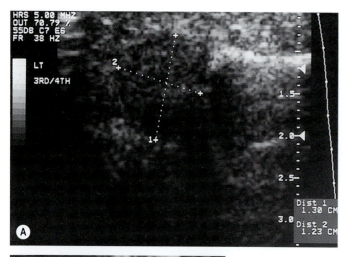

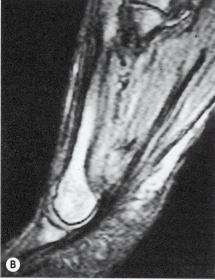

**Figure 4.30** (A) Ultrasound scan of the third–fourth intermetatarsal space revealing a large neuroma. (B) An MRI scan of the same site, however, failed to identify the neuroma. (Photographs printed with kind permission of Miss A. Wilson, The London Foot Hospital.)

- The patient should undergo a full biomechanical assessment, and any anomaly, such as forefoot inversion/rearfoot varus, should be corrected with the provision of a temporary clinical antipronatory orthotic, such as a 'cobra' pad (Fig. 4.21), or the prescription and manufacture of appropriate orthoses made to a cast of the patient's foot. Simple antipronatory clinical orthoses in appropriate accommodative shoes reduce the pain of neuroma to a tolerable level in approximately half of all cases (Mooney et al 1999).
- The patient should be urged to change to an appropriate shoe style, such as a flat, laced style, with a thick cushioned sole and a wide, deep toe box, or a roomy training shoe, and warned that the condition is likely to recur should they resume the use of their former ill-fitting, constrictive shoes.
- A course of NSAIDs may help control foot pain and reduce local inflammation.
- The injection of corticosteroid (e.g.: 1 ml (25 mg)) of hydrocortisone delivered under a local anaesethic cover, and ultrasound guidance can reduce pain and minimise local inflammation. This therapy should be administered a maximum

of two times, approximately one month apart. It is fully effective in approximately one-third of cases, gives some reduction in the overall pain or gives full but only temporary relief in a further one-third of cases, but is ineffective in the remaining one-third of cases.

- Surgical excision of the neuroma, with or without excision of the associated intermetatarsal bursal sac, should be reserved for those cases that have failed to respond to conservative and drug therapy. The neuroma can be excised via a dorsal incision (which will also divide the intermetatarsal ligament), a plantar incision (which causes a possibly problematic plantar scar) or an interdigital or web-splitting incision (which is technically more awkward to perform, but gives a very good cosmetic result). Alternatively, the intermetatarsal ligament may be divided via a dorsal or plantar incision, leaving the neuroma in situ but free of the trauma of compression against the intermetatarsal ligament. Microsurgical techniques are also used to reduce nerve compression: fibrous tissue is dissected away from around the nerve, leaving the nerve intact and in situ, but free of constrictive perineural fibrosis (Fernandez et al 1999).

## Metatarsalgia arising in association with bone pathologies

### Stress fracture

Stress fractures are hairline cracks that develop in bone as the result of the repeated application of low-level forces – such as the forces arising during prolonged exercise, or unaccustomed activity. Stress fracture of a metatarsal is given as an example of this process, and the principles of the recognition and treatment of stress fractures elsewhere in the foot are discussed.

### Pathology

Bone fractures occur either as the result of high-level trauma, such as the sudden major exchange of energy that happens in an impact injury, or bone can develop a fracture as the result of the application of repeated minor trauma. This principle is illustrated by cutting a paper clip or a piece of wire. Considerable force, such as that applied by wire cutters, is needed to cut the wire in a single action, but wire can be easily broken if it is repeatedly bent and straightened with the fingers. The accumulated effect of the repeated movements breaks a paper clip after only four or five bend–straighten actions. If other bone pathologies coexist, such as osteoporosis in conjunction with the menopause or steroid therapy, disuse osteoporosis in conjunction with persistent foot pain or distal ischaemia, local Paget's disease or bone tumour, the likelihood of stress fracture increases. General overall levels of fitness or disease states may also predispose to the development of stress fracture.

### Signs that indicate a stress fracture

- A history of pain that has not resolved together with recent-onset, local soft tissue swelling or bruising.
- Pain in the area after exercise.
- Local tenderness on palpation of the painful area.
- Pain that can be induced by tensioning the soft tissues that cross the affected bone, such as when the local tendons, fascia, ligaments and retinaculae are tightened.
- Local, soft tissue swelling.
- An increase in the temperature of the local tissues.

### Factors that predispose to stress fracture

- Age: stress fractures are more common in people over 40 years of age.

- Menopause-related osteoporosis.
- An excess of unaccustomed activity, especially in the unfit or untrained foot. Examples of unaccustomed activity include long walks, prolonged ladder work, sports and carrying heavy weights.
- Foot surgery or limb immobilisation, where the stress fracture develops due to osteoporosis of disuse.
- Revascularisation of an ischaemic limb.

### Diagnosis

The diagnosis of a stress fracture is made from the history and the presenting signs and symptoms. These include an insidious onset of pain or aching that is increased by activity, together with local swelling with or without bruising. The patient may limp. There may be generalised foot or local oedema. The clinician will be able to palpate an isolated, excessively tender point in relation to the underlying bone. In cases of metatarsal fracture, pressure applied under the forefoot induces pain, as will the use of ultrasound over the fracture site, or attempting to move the opposing sides of the fracture in relation to one another.

Early-stage stress fractures do not usually show on plain radiographs, although a technetium-90 radioisotope bone scan will show an area of increased uptake of contrast medium, or 'hot spot', at the fracture site, early in the case. From weeks 3–4 onwards the fracture shows as a dark line surrounded by an area of diffuse bone callus on plain radiograph (Fig. 4.31). The fracture line may follow an oblique, transverse, longitudinal or spiral course through the bone tissue. Once healing is complete, the bone callus resorbs, but the cortical bone may remain permanently thickened around the site of the earlier fracture.

### Treatment

It is important to follow a regimen of rest and immobilisation from 4–6 weeks to allow bone healing to take place. NSAIDs are indicated to control pain during the early stages of healing.

## March fracture

The typical stress fracture in the foot affects the second, third or fourth metatarsal shaft, and is termed a 'march' fracture. The fault develops

within the shaft of the metatarsal, at the point one-third from the head and two-thirds from the base, but stress fractures of the first and fifth metatarsals tend to affect the more proximal part of the bone shaft. Classically, the lesion develops at the medial aspect of the affected metatarsal. Usually only one metatarsal per foot is affected at any one time. The patient rarely gives a history of an exciting incident or trauma, although he or she may have undergone a period of extra exercise or standing, or have experienced weight gain in the weeks prior to the problem developing.

### Clinical picture

The patient complains of pain and aching in the metatarsal area after, and sometimes during, exercise and when walking or standing, and may have noticed some dorsal swelling and bruising at the time of onset of the pain. Symptoms are often quite mild, so the patient may not seek help at first. The swelling and bruising tend to subside over the subsequent 2–3 weeks, but the pain persists, especially on direct palpation of the fracture site. Wearing certain shoe styles, such as high heels, exacerbates the symptoms, as the increased tension they induce in the plantar fascia causes potential movement in the metatarsal shaft at the fracture site. For the same biomechanical reason, pain is induced when the patient stands on tiptoe – due to the bowing effect of the tightened plantar fascia on the metatarsals.

### Diagnosis and differential diagnosis

The diagnosis is suggested by the history, and the presenting signs and symptoms, such as residual swelling and/or bruising at the dorsum of the foot.

The fracture rarely shows on a plain radiograph in its early stages, but after 3–4 weeks the bone repair subsequent to the fracture shows as an increase in the diameter of the bone shaft where diffuse bone callus is forming (Fig. 4.3). The fracture line shows as a radiolucent (black) area traversing the cortex at one aspect of the shaft. Seldom does a stress fracture cause a full trans-shaft fracture. A stress fractures is visible from its earliest stages on bone scan, due to the increased take up of contrast medium in the acute inflammation that characterises the fracture site.

The differential diagnoses of a march fracture should exclude metatarsal osteochondritis, bone tumour, Charcot neuroarthropathy and bone infection (osteomyelitis).

### Treatment

March fractures, as all bone fracture within the lower limb and foot, require immobilisation and protection from weight bearing and ground reaction forces to promote and allow uncomplicated bone healing.

- If symptoms are severe, rest can be achieved by the use of a below-knee plaster cast or an Aircast® boot for 4–6 weeks, with elbow crutches to reduce the load on the affected foot and aid mobilisation.
- Alternatively, in cases where the acute phase has passed, immobilisation can be achieved by the use of soft splints made from clinical padding materials such as semicompressed felt. These include shaft pads applied over the dorsal and plantar aspects of the affected metatarsal, and a valgus filler pad incorporating a lateral forefoot wedge, to reduce any tendency to metatarsal plantar flexion at toe-off.
- The application of elastic tubular bandage, such as Tubigrip®, from the toes to the knee helps, together with the use of a 'figure-of-eight' crepe bandage applied to the rear- and midfoot (see Ch. 16). Both forms of bandage apply local compression and reduce intrinsic movements within the foot, thereby imposing a degree of immobility at the fracture site.

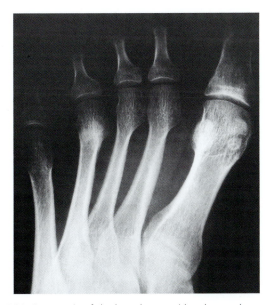

**Figure 4.31** Osteopenia of the lateral sesamoid and avascular necrosis.

- Clinical strapping, such as bow strapping (see Ch. 16) or a false plantar fascia applied from the plantar heel to the distal webbing, in conjunction with a felt valgus filler pad tends to stabilise the foot and reduce intrinsic movements.
- The use of a shoe with a stiff, curved profile, or a rocker sole, allows the foot to be used in a relatively normal manner during walking, whilst preventing both dorsiflexion of the toes and tightening of the plantar fascia through the windlass mechanism (see above). In a similar manner, the use of a walking boot stabilises the ankle and rearfoot, and thereby reduces sagittal plane movement of the metatarsals during gait.

In the majority of cases, healing of a march fracture is uncomplicated, and seldom requires complex interventions, such as internal fixation. However, the predisposing factor(s) that induced the initial bone lesion must be identified and eradicated to ensure good healing and to prevent future recurrence. For example, a 50-year-old woman with a BMI of 29 who is currently employed full time as a traffic warden, but is also working night shifts stacking shelves in a supermarket to earn extra money for a holiday, might develop a march fracture. The problem may be related entirely to her extra workload, but her obesity and age cannot be ignored as contributing factors to the bone pathology. Thus, in addition to the regimen of rest and immobilisation outlined above, the patient should be counselled to seek the advice of her general practitioner about possible menopausal or postmenopausal osteoporosis and help with weight loss. She should also consider whether her increased workload is detrimental to her general health.

## Principles of recognition and treatment of stress fractures elsewhere in the foot

Other bones in the foot may be prone to develop stress fracture.

- Calcaneum: a stress fracture of the calcaneum gives rise to a vague heel pain that eludes diagnosis. As it may be up to 3 months before the fracture shows on radiography, bone scans are indicated as the diagnostic test of choice.
- Sesamoids: stress fractures of the sesamoids that lie within the tendon of flexor hallucis brevis muscle, adjacent to the plantar aspect of the first metatarsal head, may be difficult to differentiate from the presentation of bipartite or enlarged sesamoids. But close inspection of the radiograph shows that the bone cortex is discontinuous with sesamoid fracture and continuous on bipartite sesamoids. Bone scan should be the investigation of choice to avoid ambiguity of diagnosis.
- Styloid process of the fifth metatarsal: dancers, especially ballet dancers, tend to develop stress fractures of the styloid process at the base of the fifth metatarsal. A stress fracture of the styloid process should be distinguished from Iselin's disease, which is a traction apophysitis of the styloid process (see above), as it may require screw fixation to promote bone healing.

## Sesamoid pathologies

Sesamoids are small bones that occur within tendons, especially at points where the tendon crosses a joint. The sesamoid reinforces the tendon, and facilitates its movement across the joint as the deep aspect of the sesamoid is covered with cartilage and articulates with the other bones of the joint complex. Sesamoid bones are classified as constant or variant. Constant sesamoids are found in almost all humans. Examples of constant sesamoids include the patella that forms part of the knee joint complex, and the paired sesamoids that form part of the first MTPJ complex. Variant sesamoids, and bi- or tripartite sesamoids within the foot occur far less often, and their incidence and presentation varies from person to person.

All sesamoids are subject to all bone pathologies. These include subluxation, dislocation, fractures of all types, osteochondritis, chondromalacia, osteoarthritis and osteoarthrosis, osteomyelitis, bone tumour and associated bursitis.

There are paired, constant sesamoids that form part of the first MTPJ. These are each approximately the size of a grapefruit pip and lie within the tendon of the flexor hallucis brevis muscle to articulate at their deep aspects with the medial (tibial) and lateral (fibular) grooves on the plantar aspect of the first metatarsal head. Their function is to form part of the first MTPJ and contribute a channel on the plantar aspect of the first MTPJ through which the tendon of the flexor hallucis longus muscle courses as it passes to its insertion at the plantar aspect of the distal phalanx of the great toe. The sesamoids reinforce the flexor hallucis brevis tendon, increase the relative depth of the first metatarsal head so that tension within the flexor hallucis longus tendon is maintained, even at toe-off, and increase the functional length of the lever arm of the lower limb at the first MTPJ. Thus the paired sesamoids of the first MTPJ stabilise the joint and increase foot function during gait. The medial sesamoid tends to be larger than the lateral one, but either may present in a mono- or multi- (bi-, tri-, or quadri-) partite form. Bipartite sesamoids are encountered twice as often as multipartite sesamoids, and whilst up to one-third of medial sesamoids are noted as bipartite, only 2% of lateral sesamoids show bipartitism.

Metatarsalgia in the area of the plantar aspect of the first MTPJ may relate to sesamoid pathology.

### CASE STUDY 4.9 SESAMOID PATHOLOGY DUE TO OSTEOCHONDRITIS OF THE LATERAL SESAMOID

A 31-year-old woman presented with pain in the first metatarsophalangeal joint of the right foot. The area had been symptomatic for just over 1 year and the pain was becoming progressively worse. The patient was otherwise in good health, and normally a very active individual. She used to play netball for an amateur league team but since the onset of the right forefoot problem had had to give up sport altogether.

The patient presented with fixed pes cavus, with rearfoot inversion and a plantar-flexed first ray. Movement and direct palpation at the right first metatarsophalangeal joint (MTPJ) area was warm, puffy and very painful, with an exquisitely tender point at the lateral plantar aspect of the first MTPJ. A dorsiplantar weight-bearing radiograph showed osteopenia of the lateral sesamoid and a healing stress fracture of the fourth metatarsal.

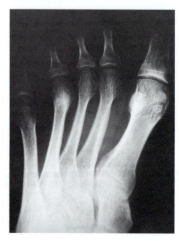

Osteopenia of the lateral sesamoid and avascular necrosis.

A diagnosis of avascular necrosis of the lateral sesamoid was made. It was presumed that the metatarsal fracture had developed as stress fracture due to lateral forefoot overload and the patient's inability to load the medial area of the right forefoot, secondary to the sesamoid problem.

The patient presented with fixed pes cavus, with rearfoot inversion and a plantarflexed first ray (partial forefoot valgus). Movement and direct palpation at the first metatarsophalangeal joint (MTPJ) area was warm, puffy and very painful, with an exquisitely tender point at the lateral plantar aspect of the first MPTJ. A dorsiplantar weight-bearing radiograph showed osteopenia of the lateral sesamoid shown in figure, indicating a continuing pathology. As her pain was so debilitating and unrelenting she was referred to a podiatric surgeon, who excised the lateral sesamoid, to good outcome.

## Relationship of flexor hallucis brevis sesamoids and the first metatarsal head

The normal relationship of the sesamoids to the plantar aspect of the first metatarsal head is lost in hallux valgus (see hallux valgus, above), with the result that the lateral sesamoid comes to lie in the first inter-metatarsal space, and the medial sesamoid articulates with the lateral plantar groove of the first metatarsal head. As a result of this, the relative depth of the first metatarsal head is reduced by approximately 30% and normal first MTPJ function and stability is compromised in hallux abducto valgus. The loss of the normal orientation of the medial sesamoid increases the opportunity of the foot to pronate, rather than supinate, at toe-off, and efficient propulsion at toe-off is compromised by the overall reduction in joint stability.

*Chondromalacia*, or dystrophy of sesamoid articular cartilage (at the deep aspect of the sesamoid), is a relatively common cause of sesamoid pathology. It tends to affect the medial sesamoid more often than the lateral one, especially in cases where the medial sesamoid shows bipartitism. The patient presents with a nagging pain or ache that localises to the plantar aspect of the medial sesamoid, especially on weight bearing or during exercise. The condition can be treated by the application of deflective clinical padding or by the manufacture of orthoses that elevate the distal part of the first metatarsal. Surgical removal of the medial sesamoid, or planing the plantar aspect of the sesamoid whilst leaving the deep cartilaginous articular surface intact is advocated for intractable cases that do not respond to conservative measures (see Ch. 13).

*Sesamoiditis*, or ongoing inflammation and pain around the sesamoid, is a common condition that typically affects physically active young girls, such as dancers and gymnasts. Any activity, even walking, that places constant and repetitive force on the head of the first metatarsal may cause sesamoiditis. Any pathology that damages the sesamoid, such as stress fractures of the medial sesamoid, can also induce sesamoiditis (Kliman et al 1983).

### Clinical picture

The patient complains of aching, tenderness and swelling in the plantar area of the first MTPJ, especially towards the medial–plantar angle of the joint. The pain increases insidiously, but may cause constant throbbing. Alternatively, movement, especially active and forced dorsiflexion of the great toe, may trigger or exacerbate the pathology. The soft tissues surrounding the affected sesamoid become tender and inflamed. The majority of cases do not show bruising or redness, but pain and swelling limits normal dorsiflexion and plantar flexion at the first MTPJ, so that walking is difficult, and the patient may limp.

### Diagnosis and differential diagnosis

The clinical picture of sesamoiditis, which is a history of the gradual onset of and increasing pain at the plantar aspect of the medial–

plantar border of the first MTPJ area, with local swelling and a decreased range of joint movement in a young otherwise healthy and active young person, is indicative of medial sesamoiditis.

### Treatment

Minor presentations of sesamoiditis respond to a regimen of rest. This includes minimal weight bearing, cessation of the provocative activity and the use of deflective clinical padding to reduce pressure at the painful plantar–medial area. 'Fan' strapping (see Ch. 16) or soft splintage of the first MTPJ to restrict joint movement is also of help, as is a course of NSAIDs to help reduce local pain and swelling. More severe cases may require fixed immobilisation in a below-knee walking cast, together with intra-articular injection of corticosteroid. Once symptoms have subsided, the patient should undergo a full biomechanical assessment to determine the underlying cause of sesamoiditis. Predisposing causes include a plantarflexed first metatarsal (partial forefoot valgus), pes cavus and excessive rearfoot or midfoot pronation. Appropriate prescription orthoses should be made to control or minimise the predisposing factors, to prevent recurrence of the pathology.

### Sesamoid fractures

A fracture of one or both sesamoids at the first MTPJ will show symptoms that mimic sesamoiditis, such as pain on the plantar aspect of the first MTPJ and the medial forefoot area, with swelling and limited sagittal plane movement of the first MTPJ. However, the patient with a sesamoid fracture usually presents a history of traumatic injury to the plantar first MTPJ area, such as landing heavily following a fall from a height, with the onset of severe pain that relates to the time of injury. Following the sesamoid fracture, the forefoot becomes very tender, swollen and bruised, with focal pain at the first MTPJ. The fracture is confirmed by a plain radiograph, although a naturally bipartite sesamoid can mimic the appearance of a fractured sesamoid. In these cases, a bone scan is indicated.

The fractured sesamoid is treated by rest and full immobilisation for 6–8 weeks in a below-knee cast to restrict first MTPJ movement. Non-union of the fracture may require the affected sesamoid to be excised, with resultant loss of aspects of normal first MTPJ function.

### Sesamoid osteochondritis

See the section earlier in this chapter on osteochondritides (Fig. 4.32).

## Freiberg's infraction

Freiberg's infraction, or osteochondritis of the metatarsal head, causes metatarsalgia most commonly in the area of the second MTPJ area. It may present as a primary problem in teenagers, or as a secondary degenerative arthrosis in later life. See the section earlier in this chapter on Freiberg's disease.

## Complications following metatarsal surgery

Metatarsalgia may develop as the result of forefoot or metatarsal surgery. Complications arising after metatarsal surgery can include delayed union, malunion, non-union and the development of a pseudoarthrosis, recurrence of the original metatarsal problem, or the development of plantar hyperkeratotic 'transfer' lesions over adjacent MTPJs. Where the integrity of the MTPJ is lost as the result of surgery, such as a Keller's arthroplasty, used to correct hallux abducto valgus, the patient may develop a 'floating' digit. Other postsurgical complications can include the overexuberant formation of bone callus, with loss of the normal bone architecture; displacement of the metatarsal head and loss of MTPJ integrity; aseptic necrosis of the capital fragment of the metatarsal following osteotomy; and osteomyelitis (bone infection).

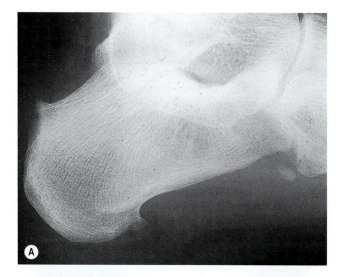

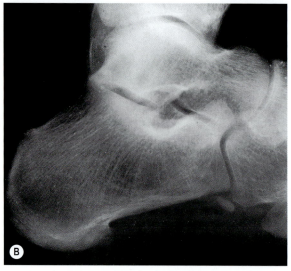

Figure 4.32 (A) Lateral radiograph of plantar and posterior heel spurs. This patient was later diagnosed as having ankylosing spondylitis. (B) subsequent radiograph taken during disease remission shows remodelling of the calcaneum and reduction of the spurs.

## Systemic diseases that may give rise to metatarsalgia

### Rheumatological diseases

Any generalised pathology that affects the locomotor system is likely to give rise to pain in the foot, and thus can be a cause of metatarsalgia. Diseases of the locomotor system fall into two broad categories:

- Arthropathies: diseases that affect joint function.
- Other diseases: conditions that cause back pain, and give rise to a referred pain in the foot; conditions that affect foot and limb function due to pain or muscular imbalance, or soft tissue rheumatism, where the rheumatoid disease process primarily affects muscular, tendinous and ligamentous structures; and miscellaneous causes.

The text in the following section gives only a summary of the main features of these diseases. For greater detail the reader is advised to consult a textbook on general medicine.

### Arthropathies

#### Osteoarthritis

Osteoarthritis (see Ch. 8) causes joint degeneration. It presents more commonly in the older population. Although statistically 1 in 10 people in the UK have osteoarthritis and half of all sufferers are over 60 years old. Osteoarthritis presents as a non-symmetrical monoarthritis, in which cartilage erodes and thins, joint space narrows, and osteophytes form at the margins of the affected joints. Osteoarthritis affects primarily the weight-bearing joints, such as the hip, the knee and the first MTPJ, but it also affects joints that have been damaged by an earlier pathology, such as osteochondritis, or affected by adverse pathomechanical influences such as hallux abducto valgus and metatarsus primus elevatus. Crystal deposition disease, such as gout, predisposes the affected joint to develop later osteoarthritis.

#### Rheumatoid arthritis

Rheumatoid arthritis is caused by an autoimmune-mediated inflammation that results in vasculitis in connective tissues. It characteristically causes hypertrophy of the synovium of the smaller joints of the hands and feet. The rheumatoid arthritis process leads to marked destruction of joint and periarticular tissues, with resultant marked and typical hand and foot deformities. Deformities include lateral deviation and subluxation of digital, and metacarpophalangeal joints and MTPJs, with associated muscle wasting and tendon rupture. Joint effects are noted first and more frequently in the feet, with radiologically evident erosions showing initially at the fifth metatarsal head, with subsequent third, fourth, second then first MTPJ involvement (Renton 1991). Early manifestations of rheumatoid arthritis in the feet include tenderness and swelling of the MTPJs due to synovitis and joint effusions. Characteristically, periarticular swelling causes the toes to diverge – the 'daylight' or 'sunray' sign. Persistent synovial disease leads to joint erosion, destruction and subluxation, with distal displacement of the fibrofatty pad and the formation of large painful plantar bursae that are prone to tissue breakdown and ulceration. Local bone becomes porotic, but joint ankylosis may also occur. Patients may require forefoot surgery to reduce the deformation and achieve pain relief. Procedures include forefoot arthroplasty such as Fowler's procedure.

Extra-articular features of rheumatoid arthritis include the formation of rheumatoid or fibrinoid nodules on the extensor surfaces of the limb, tenosynovitis, and characteristic plantar bursae overlying the plantar aspects of the MTPJs. Subjects may develop neuropathy, such as glove and stocking sensory loss, and motor weakness with a positive Tinel's sign in the affected dermatome of the tibial nerve. Vasculitis of the skin, where acute inflammation of small blood vessels is provoked by the deposition and accumulation of immune complexes, leads to tissue breakdown and ulceration, especially over distorted joints or in association with the plantar bursae. Joint surfaces become eroded and joint spaces widen.

### CASE STUDY 4.10 HEEL SPUR IN ASSOCIATION WITH SERONEGATIVE RHEUMATOID DISEASE

A 27-year-old man, who was referred by his GP, had a 2-year history of lower back and hip pain and increasing heel pain, for which he had been prescribed ibuprofen. The patient reported that he thought he was otherwise in good general health, although he had had to give up playing amateur football each week since the onset of his foot and back problems. He worked as a gemstone polisher, which required him to stand all day long on a concrete floor. He was concerned that he had had to take several episodes of sick leave in the past year, because of the increasing severity of the back and heel pain. In the course of the past month, the heel pain had become severe and prevented him from wearing any shoe other than a trainer with a thick cushioned insole. His feet were now a source of considerable daily pain, no matter which type of shoes or cushioned insoles he wore. He also reported that he was finding it increasingly difficult to bend down to cut his toenails. He was currently on sick leave.

On examination: both feet were of normal shape, but with a generalised marked lack of joint mobility. There were no areas of hyperkeratosis, and all pulses in the feet were easily palpable. There was a gross swelling at the posterior aspect of the calcaneum at the insertion of the Achilles tendon (left worse than right), which was extremely tender to touch, and pain was induced by palpating the central plantar heel pad. Plain lateral radiographs showed marked irregularity of the posterior and inferior areas of the calcanei (see figure). Blood tests showed a raised erythrocyte sedimentation rate (ESR) (a normal ESR is <20; a raised ESR indicates a non-specific generalised inflammation).

The patient was made and issued with moulded cushioned insoles, and an appointment was made for him to receive ongoing nail care by the podiatry assistant. A letter to his GP requested an early referral to a rheumatologist, as his symptoms, gender, age and history suggested that he might have ankylosing spondylitis. This diagnosis was confirmed by the rheumatologist following further blood tests. The ankylosing spondylitis had caused posterior and inferior heel spur formation and sacroiliac enthesiopathy. The patient was prescribed a course of disease-modifying antirheumatic drugs (sulfasalazine), and radiographs taken some months later showed a degree of disease remission and resultant calcaneal remodelling (see figure).

### Ankylosing spondylitis

Ankylosing spondylitis is a rheumatological disease that typically affects young men of the HLA B27 tissue type. It causes progressive stiffening of the spine, with calcification of ligaments and tendons at their insertions into bone. It predisposes to plantar and posterior heel spur formation (Fig. 4.32 and case study 4.10).

### Connective tissue disorders

Connective tissue disorders, such as systemic lupus erythematosus, systemic sclerosis, polymyalgia rheumatica and dermatomyositis, are all characterised by a generalised immune-complex-mediated vasculitis, which can affect all body tissues. Vasculitis at specific body sites causes a range of presenting symptoms. These include rheumatoid-arthritis-like arthropathy, a characteristic facial 'rash' known as a butterfly rash, ischaemia of the finger and toe pulps with apical ulceration, Raynaud's phenomenon and severe chilling, levedo reticularis, calcinosis, skin and epithelial sclerosis, telangectasia, polymyositis and muscular weakness, and sensory and kidney dysfunction. Vasculitis of medium-sized vessels characterises polyarteritis nodosa.

### Infective and reactive arthritis

Arthritic joints, especially in those seen with severe rheumatoid disease, are prone to develop staphylococcal infection. Other generalised infections, such as tuberculosis (which itself is predisposed by alcoholism), diabetes mellitus or other chronic debilitating disease states, gonorrhoea, salmonella, rubella, and Lyme's disease, may all cause transitory arthritis. Joints affected by transitory arthritis may become subject to later osteoarthritis. Reiter's syndrome, which is often triggered by a gastrointestinal infection, affects males of the HLA B27 tissue type. It gives rise to heel and forefoot pain, and is characterised by Achilles tendonitis, plantar fasciitis and heel spur forma-tion. Associated systemic symptoms include eye and urinary tract infections.

### Arthropathy associated with other disease states

Crohn's disease, chronic active hepatitis, Whipple's disease and psoriasis can all cause forefoot pain. Psoriasis causes dactylitis – the isolated acute inflammation and swelling of a toe. Psoriasis may also cause arthritis mutilans, which is a form of seronegative arthritis that resembles the most severe joint effects of rheumatoid arthritis. Arthropathy may be a feature of many other diseases. For example, Charcot neuroarthropathy is a feature of long-standing diabetes mellitus and also of late-stage untreated syphilis. Small-joint arthritis can be a presenting feature of hypothyroidism. Acromegaly and joint pain are features of hyperpituitarism. The formation of large bone spurs within the foot area is a feature of Forrestier's disease (characterised as showing four or more large anterior osteophytes within vertebral disc spaces in the absence of the disc-space narrowing). Avascular necrosis within joints can be associated with sickle-cell disease, thalassaemia and hypercholesterolaemia. Behçet's syndrome can cause rheumatoid-type arthritis. Generalised hypermobility and foot strain is a feature of Ehlers–Danlos syndrome.

## Other causes of metatarsalgia

### Plantar fibromatosis

The development of fibrous nodules on the plantar fascial structures is reviewed in the section on plantar fibromatosis (see earlier in this chapter).

### Altered tissue perfusion and reduced vascular drainage

This can cause forefoot and generalised foot pain.

- *Chronic arterial insufficiency of the whole lower limb.* Poor arterial perfusion, for example due to arteriosclerosis, atherosclerosis, diabetes mellitus, intermittent claudication, rest pain, and other classic signs of reduced tissue perfusion, can all give rise to forefoot ischaemia and metatarsalgia.
- *Chronic venous insufficiency of the whole lower limb.* Impaired venous drainage, characterised by lower-limb oedema, varicosed veins, varicose eczema, hemosiderosis, lipodermatosclerosis and stasis ulcers, can also cause generalised foot and forefoot pain. Impaired venous drainage is more likely in a foot that overpronates throughout stance, as the venous foot pump functions maximally when the foot fully supinates at toe-off.
- *Chronic lymphatic insufficiency of the lower limb.* Reduced or absent lymphatic drainage, such as in Milroy's disease, causes gross, woody, oedema and induration of the lower leg. Patients with chronic heart disease and kidney failure develop a similar clinical picture of generalised lower-limb and foot oedema. These cases are prone to foot pain.

### Generalised muscular pathology

Myalgia or muscle pain of a muscle unit or group is characterised by muscular stiffness and pain on movement. Myalgia may occur as a feature of repetitive movements, intermuscular sensory neuritis (also known as fibrositis, fibromyositis and myositis) tendonitis, muscle strains, traumatic injury and contusions. Symptoms vary from a transient stiffness, to agonising pain, and can be set off by pressure at trigger points within the affected muscle. Acupuncture of the trigger and more proximal pressure points, or trigger point massage, is a useful therapy to reduce the pain of myalgia (Sandberg et al 2004).

## Neoplastic disease

Neoplasm is rare in the foot, accounting for less than 0.05% of foot lesions. There are a number of relatively benign neoplasms that affect the foot and may possibly cause metatarsalgia. These include squamous-cell papilloma, dermatofibroma, naevi, eccrine poroma, angiokeratoma, giant-cell tumour of tendon sheaths, lipoma, benign fibrous histiocytoma, chondroma, leiomyoma, myxoma and lipoblastoma. Primary malignancies within the foot and lower limb are rare. Those that do arise may provoke metatarsalgia, and include synovial sarcoma, melanoma, verrucous carcinoma, squamous-cell carcinoma, basal-cell carcinoma, fibrosarcoma, malignant fibrous histiocytoma, leiomyosarcoma, chondrosarcoma, myosarcoma, lymphangiosarcoma and malignant neurofibroma. Those malignant neoplastic tumours that affect the bones of the foot tend to occur as a secondary tumour to a primary tumour of lung, breast or kidney. However, the possibility of bone tumours in the foot cannot be ignored, as, although bone tumours below the knee are very rare, 25% of those malignancies that do arise in the lower leg affect the bones of the foot.

## Back pain

Lumbar pain can cause pain in the legs and feet, referred within the distribution of the sciatic nerve. Classically, heel pain can be a feature of spinal nerve compression at the S1 level.

## Soft tissue effects of rheumatic disease

Large plantar bursae are a feature of rheumatoid arthritis. Tenosynovitis and plantar enthesiopathies characterise rheumatoid diseases and Reiter's syndrome. Nerve-compression syndromes, such as tarsal tunnel syndrome, can arise as the result of local autoimmune-mediated inflammation and vasculitis of the vasa nervosum.

## Miscellaneous systemic causes of metatarsalgia

Paget's disease, which is characterised by bone pain, enlargement of the medullary cavity and thinning of the cortex of long bones, can predispose to stress fractures. Bone infections, such as osteomyelitis and tuberculosis, are very painful, even in cases with sensory neuropathy, and are difficult to treat, requiring surgery and prolonged courses of antibiotics. Neoplastic disease, muccopolysaccharide disorders, skeletal dysplasia (e.g. achondroplasia, osteomalacia), and hereditary diseases such as osteogenesis imperfecta and osteopetrosis all predispose the patient to fractures that are as likely to affect the bones of the foot as elsewhere in the skeleton.

Obese patients with a BMI of over 30, and/or a waist measurement of more than 1 m may experience foot pain due to chronic tension on the plantar fascia. Foot pain can be a feature of the later stages of pregnancy. Any biomechanical anomalies are exaggerated by the increase in body weight, the change in the centre of gravity of the body due to the gravid uterus, and the generalised ligamentous laxity that characterises late pregnancy. Patients who suffer from alcoholism often develop painful neuropathies that affect the feet and legs.

## REFERENCES

Acevedo JI, Beskin JL 1998 Complications of plantar fascia rupture associated with corticosteroid injection. Foot and Ankle International 19(2):91–97.

Alfredson H, Pietilä T, Jonsson P, Lorentzon R 1998 Heavy-load eccentric calf muscle training for the treatment of chronic Achilles tendinosis. American Journal of Sports Medicine 26:360–366.

Aquino A, Payne CB 2001 Function of the windlass mechanism in excessively pronated feet. Foot and Ankle International 18(11):705–709.

Banadda B, Gona G, Vaz R, Ndlovu D 1992 Calcaneal spurs in a black African population. Foot and Ankle International 13(6):352–354.

Beeson P 2002 Orthopaedic assessment. pp 199–200, In: Merriman LM, Turner W (eds) Assessment of the lower limb, Ch. 8. Churchill Livingstone, Edinburgh.

Beito SB, Krych SM, Harkless LB 1989 Recalcitrant heel pain: traumatic fibrosis versus heel neuroma. Journal of the American Podiatric Medicine Association (79)7:336–339.

Blustein SM, D'Amico JC 1985 Limb length discrepancy. Identification, clinical significance and management. Journal of the American Podiatric Medicine Association 75(4):200–206.

Bohndorf K 1998 Osteochondritis (osteochondrosis) dessicans: a review and new MRI classification. European Radiology 8(1):103–112.

Bowden PD 1983 The pathomechanics of forefoot valgus. The Chiropodist 38(12):445–451.

Brown LP, Yavorsky P 1987 Locomotor biomechanics & pathomechanics, a review. Journal of Orthopaedic and Sports Physical Therapy 9(1):3–10.

Camasta CA 1996 Hallux limitus and hallux rigidus. Clinics in Podiatric Medicine and Surgery 13(3):423–445.

Caselli M, Sobel E, McHale KA 1998 Pedal manifestations of musculoskeletal disease in children. Clinics in Podiatric Medicine and Surgery 15(3):481–497.

Chambers MRC 1983 Running on leg length discrepancy. Athletes World 6:55–58.

Cimino WR 1990 Tarsal tunnel syndrome: review of the literature. Foot and Ankle International 11(1):47–51.

Citkowitz E 2004 Familial hypercholesterolaemia. www.emedicine.com

Chapman C 1999 Rocker soles. Podiatry Archives. Available at: http://www.mailbase.ac.uk/podiatry January 1999.

Coughlin MJ, Shurnas PS 2003 Hallux rigidus: demographics, etiology, and radiographic assessment. Foot and Ankle International 24(10):731–743.

Crawford F, Atkins D, Young P, Edwards J 1999 Steroid injection for heel pain: evidence of short-term effectiveness. A randomized controlled trial. Rheumatology 38:974–977.

Crawford F, Snaith M 1996 How effective is therapeutic ultrasound in the treatment of heel pain? Annals of Rheumatic Diseases 55:265–267.

Crawford F, Thomson CE 2003 Interventions for treating plantar heel pain. Cochrane Database Systematic Review 2003(3): CD000416.

Daly PJ, Kitaoka HB, Chao EYS 1992 Plantar fasciotomy for intractable plantar fasciitis: clinical results and biomechanical evaluation. Foot and Ankle 13:188–195.

Dananberg HJ, Phillips AJ, Blaakman HE 1996 Non-surgical treatment of hallux limitus. Advances in Podiatric Medicine and Surgery 2:67–69.

Dananberg HJ 1993 Gait style as an etiology to chronic postural pain. Part 1–Functional hallux limitus. Journal of the American Podiatric Medicine Association 83(8):432–441.

Durrant MN, Siepert KK 1993 Role of soft tissue structures as an aetiology of hallux limitus. Journal of the American Podiatric Medicine Association 83(40):173–180.

Ekman S, Carlson CS 1998 The pathophysiology of osteochondrosis. Vetinary Clinics of North America 28(1):17–32.

Fernandez E, Pallini R, Lauretti L, et al 1999 Neurosurgery of the peripheral nervous system: entrapment syndromes of the lower extremity. Surgical Neurology 52(5):449–452.

Ferrari J, Malone-Lee JG 2002 Relationship between proximal articular set angle and hallux abducto valgus. Journal of the American Podiatric Medicine Association 92(6):331–335.

Ferrari J, Hopkinson DA, Linney AD 2004 Size and shape differences between male and female foot bones: is the female foot predisposed to hallux abducto-valgus deformity? Journal of the American Podiatric Medicine Association 94(5):434–532.

Frank CJ, Robinson DE, Dalenberg DD 2004 Hallux valgus. Available at: http://www.eMedicine.com.

Freiberg O 1983 Clinical symptoms and biomechanics of lumbar spine and hip joint in leg length inequality. Spine 8(6):643–651.

Frey C, Rosenberg Z, Shereff MJ, Kim H 1992 The retrocalcaneal bursa: anatomy and bursography. Foot and Ankle International 13(4):203–207.

Gould JS 1988 The foot book. Williams and Wilkins, Baltimore, OH.

Granberry WM, Noble PC, Bishop JO, Tullos HS 1991 Use of a hinged silicone prosthesis for replacement arthroplasty of the first metatarsophalangeal joint. Journal of Bone and Joint Surgery 73(10):1453–1459.

Griffin DW 1994 Common sports injuries of the foot and ankle seen in children and adolescents. Orthopaedic Clinics of North America 25(1):83–93.

Gurney B 2002 Leg length discrepancy. Gait and Posture 15(2):192–206.

Hadjari Hollis M, Lemay DE, Jensen RP 2008 Nerve entrapment syndromes of the lower extremity. Available at: http://emedicine.medscape.com/article/1234809-overview.

Hammer WI 1999 Functional soft tissue examination and treatment by manual methods, 2nd edn, Ch. 6. Jones & Bartlett, Sudbury, MA.

Hansen TES 1993 Correlation between leg length inequality and lateral weight distribution. Thesis, Anglo-European College of Chiropractic, Bournemouth.

Hicks JH 1954 The mechanics of the foot, 2. The plantar aponeurosis and the arch. Journal of Anatomy 88:25–31.

Hill JJ, Cutting PJ 1989 Heel and body weight. Foot and ankle international 9(6):254–256.

Hlavac HF 1971 The foot book -advice for athletes. World Publications, California.

Hockenbury RT 1999 Forefoot problems in athletes. Medicine & Science in Sports & Exercise 31(7), 448–457.

Hopper D, Bryant A, Elliott B 1994 Foot types and lower limb injuries in elite netball players. JAPMA 8(7):355–362.

Kaeding CC, Whitehead R 1998 Musculoskeletal injuries in adolescents. Primary Care 25(1):211–223.

Kerr M 2008 Needle punctures plus corticosteroid injection relieve plantar fasciitis symptoms. Presented at 94th Scientific Assembly and Annual Meeting of the Radiological Society of North America, 30 November– 5 December 2008, Chicago, IL.

Klaue K, Hansen ST, Masquelet AC 1994 Clinical, quantitative assessment of first tarso-metatarsal mobility in the sagittal plane and its relationship to hallux valgus deformity. Foot and Ankle 15(1):9–13.

Kliman ME, Gross AE, Pritzker KP, Greyson ND 1983 Osteochondritis of the hallux sesamoid bones. Foot and Ankle 3(4):220–223.

Kura H, Luo Z-P, Kitaoka HB, An K-N 1998 Role of the medial capsule and transverse metatarsal ligament in hallux valgus deformity. Clinical Orthopaedics and Related Research Vol 354 pp235–240 Sept.

Kwong PK, Kay D, Voner VT, White M 1998 Plantar fasciitis: mechanics and pathomechanics of treatment. Clinics in Sports Medicine 7(1):119–126.

Lang L 1984 Ankle equinus. The Chiropodist 39(1):4–7.

Laing P 1995 The painful foot. In: Merriman LM, Tollafield DR (eds) Assessment of the lower limb. Churchill Livingstone, Edinburgh.

Lapidus PW, Guidotti FP 1965 Painful heel: report of 323 patients with 364 painful heels. Clinical Orthopaedics and Related Research 39:178–186.

Lee CR, Farley CT 1998 Determinants of tne center of mass trajectory in human walking and running. J Exp Biol Nov;201(Pt 21): 2935–2944.

Lehman RC, Gregg JR, Torg E 1986 Iselin's disease. American Journal of Sports Medicine 14:494–496.

Leonard MA 1974 The inheritance of tarsal coalition and its relationship to spastic flat foot. Journal of Bone and Joint Surgery – British Volume 56B(3):520–526.

Light MR 1996 Dynamics and function of the first metatarsophalangeal joint. Advances in Podiatric Medicine and Surgery 2:41–48.

McPoil TG, Schuit D, Knecht HG 1988 A comparison of three positions used to evaluate tibial varum. Journal of the American Podiatric Medicine Association. 78(1):22–28.

Madden CC, Mellion MB 1996 Sever's disease and other causes of heel pain in adolescents. American Family Physician 54(6):1995–2000.

Manello DM 1992 Leg length inequality. Journal of Manipulative and Physiological Therapeutics 15(9):576–590.

Manusov EG, Lillegard WA, Raspa RF, Epperly TD 1996a Evaluation of pediatric foot problems: part II. The hindfoot and the ankle. American Family Physician 54(3):1012–1026.

Manusov EG, Lillegard WA, Raspa RF, Epperly TD 1996b Evaluation of pediatric foot problems: part I. The forefoot and the midfoot. American Family Physician 54(2):592–606.

Menelaus MB 1991 The management of limb inequality. Churchill Livingstone, Edinburgh.

Mooney J, Ramsamy H, McCoshim G, et al 1999 The resolution of the pain of plantar digital neuritis after surgical excision of neuroma. British Journal of Podiatry 2(3):93–100.

O'Donnell MM 1988 In: Thomson P (ed.) Introduction to podopaediatrics. Chapter 7 General Medicine; WB Saunders, London.

Palladino SJ 1991 Pre-operative evaluation of the bunion patient: aetiology, biomechanics, clinical and radiographic assessment, In: Gerbert J (ed.) Textbook of bunion surgery, 2nd edn. Futura, New York, pp 1–87.

Payne C, Chuter V, Miller K 2002 Sensitivity and specificity of the functional hallux limitus test to predict foot function. Journal of the American Podiatric Medicine Association 92(5):269–271.

Perry J 1992 Gait analysis, normal & pathological function. Slack, Thorofare, NJ.

Pickard JM 1983 Pathomechanics of rearfoot varus. The Chiropodist 38(10):379–383.

Pfeffer G, Bacchetti P, Deland J, et al 1999 Comparison of custom and prefabricated orthoses in the initial treatment of proximal plantar fasciitis. Foot and Ankle International 20(4):214–223.

Phillips D 1994 Biomechanics. In: Hetherington VJ (ed.) Hallux valgus and forefoot surgery. Churchill Livingstone, Melbourne, pp 39–66.

Powell M, Post WR, Keener J, Wearden S 1998 Effective treatment of chronic plantar fasciitis with dorsiflexion night splints: a cross over prospective randomized outcome study. Foot and Ankle 19(1):10–18.

Powers CM, Maffucci R, Hampton S 1995 Rearfoot posture in subjects with patello-femoral pain. Journal of Orthopaedic & Sports Physical Therapy 22(4):155–160.

Prichasuk S 1994 The heel pad in plantar heel pain. Journal of Bone and Joint Surgery 76B(1):140–142.

Redmond A 2009 In: Merriman LM, Turner W (eds) Assessment of the lower limb, Ch. 10. Churchill Livingstone, Edinburgh.

Renton P 1991 Radiology of the foot. In: Klenerman L (ed.) The foot and its disorders, 3rd edn, Ch. 13. Blackwell Scientific, Edinburgh.

Rolf C, Gunter P, Ericsater J, Turan I 1997 Plantar fascia rupture: diagnosis and treatment. Journal of Foot and Ankle Surgery 36(2):112–114.

Rome K 1996 Ankle joint dorsiflexion measurement studies. A review of the literature. Journal of the American Podiatric Medicine Association 86(5):205–211.

Root ML, Orien WP, Weed JH 1971 Normal and abnormal function of the foot. Clinical biomechanics, Vol. I. Clinical Biomechanics Corp. Los Angeles.

Root ML, Orien WP, Weed JH (1977) Normal and abnormal function of the foot. Clinical biomechanics. Vol. II. Clinical biomechanics Corp., Los Angeles, CA.

Rothbart BA 2006 Relationship of functional leg length discrepancy to abnormal pronation. Journal of the American Podiatric Medicine Association 96(6):499–504.

Sandberg M, Lindberg L-G, Gerdle B 2004 Peripheral effects of needle stimulation (acupuncture) on skin and muscle blood flow in fibromyalgia. European Journal of Pain 8(5):163–171.

Saxelby J, Betts RP, Bygrave CJ 1997 Low-dyetaping on the foot in the management of plantar-fasciitis. The Foot 7:205–209.

Schon L, Glennon T, Baxter D 1993 Heel pain syndrome: electrodiagnostic support for nerve entrapment. Foot and Ankle International 14(3):129–135.

Seibel MO 1988 Foot function: a programmed text, Williams and Wilkins, Baltimore.

Sellman JR 1994. Plantar fascia rupture associated with corticosteroid injection. Foot and Ankle International 15(7):376–381.

Sgarlatto TE 1971 A compendium of podiatric biomechanics. California College of Podiatric Medicine, Oakland, CA.

Singh D, Angel J, Bentley G, Trevino SG 1997 Plantar fasciitis. BMJ 315:172–175.

Subotnick SI 1975 Biomechanics of the subtalar and midtarsal joints. Journal of the American Podiatric Medicine Association 65:756–764.

Subotnick SI 1981 Limb length discrepancies of the lower extremity, (the short leg syndrome). Journal of Orthopaedic & Sports Physical Therapy 3:11–16.

Takakura Y, Kitada C, Sugimoto K, et al 1991 Tarsal tunnel syndrome. Journal of Bone and Joint Surgery 73B:125–128.

Tax HR 1985 Podopaediatrics, 2nd edn. Williams and Wilkins, Baltimore, OH.

Tillu A, Gupta S 1998 Effect of acupuncture treatment of heel pain due to plantar fasciitis. Acupuncture in Medicine 16(2):66–68.

Tsai WC, Hsu CC, Chen CP, Chen MJ, Yu TY, Chen YJ, 2006 Plantar fasciitis treated with local steroid injection: comparison between sonographic and palpation guidance. J Clin Ultrasound 34(1):12–16.

Vink P, Kamphuisen HAC 1989 Leg length inequality, pelvic tilt and lumbar back muscle activity during standing. Clinical Biomechanics 4(2):115–117.

Walsh HP, Dorgan JC 1988 Etiology of Freiberg's disease – trauma? Journal of Foot Surgery 27(3):243–244.

Wang EA, Gentili A, Masih S, Wang MC 2008 Tarsal coalition. Available at: http://emedicine.medscape.com/article/396694-overview.

Wapner KL, Sharkey PF 1991 The use of night splints for treatment of recalcitrant plantar fasciitis. Foot and Ankle International 12:135–137.

Wassef S, Mikhail M 2008 Ankle, tibialis posterior tendon injuries. Available at: http://emedicine.medscape.com/article/386322-overview.

Weil LS, Gowlding PB, Nutbrown NJ 1994 Heel spur syndrome. A retrospective study of 250 patients undergoing a standardised method of treatment. The Foot 4:68–78.

Wolgin M, Cook C, Graham C, Mauldin D 1994 Conservative treatment of plantar heel pain: long term follow up. Foot and Ankle International 15(3):97–102.

Zhang Y, Jun H, Hiroaki I, Katsuya N 2002 Footballer's ankle: a case report. Chinese Medical Journal (English) 115(6):942–943.

# Chapter 5

# Circulatory disorders

*Brian M Ellis*

## KEYWORDS

Acrocyanosis
Ankle–brachial index
Arteriosclerosis
Atherosclerosis
Buerger's test
Capillary refill time
Chronic venous stasis
Deep venous thrombosis (DVT)
Diabetes mellitus
Doppler sounds
Erythema ab igne

Erythromelalgia

Filariasis

Frostbite

Homocysteine

Hypercholesterolaemia

Hypertension

Immersion foot (trench foot)

Intermittent claudication

Lipid disorders

Livedo reticularis

Lymphatic disease

Lymphoedema

Microvascular disease

Mönckeberg's medial sclerosis

Obesity

Peripheral arterial disease (PAD)

Polyarteritis nodosa

Primary lymphoedema (Milroy's disease)

Pulmonary thromboembolism

Raynaud's phenomenon

Rest pain

Rheumatoid vasculitis

Secondary lymphoedema

Thromboangiitis obliterans (Buerger's disease)

Thrombophilia

Thrombosis vasculitis

Vasospastic disorders

Venous filling time

## INTRODUCTION

Circulatory disorders of the lower limb can be broadly classified as arterial (macrovascular) or capillary (microvascular) disease, which results in ischaemia, or as venous or lymphatic disease, which impairs venous drainage of blood and interstitial fluid. Clinically, the most important of these three groups is arterial disease, because of its potential threat to limb viability and the very significant negative impact on the patient's quality of life. The most common form of peripheral arterial disease (PAD) is atheromatous arterial disease.

PAD has been regarded as the 'Cinderella' of cardiovascular disease, secondary to coronary artery disease and cerebrovascular disease. This view is slowly changing as it is recognised that risk modification in people with PAD is beneficial in reducing the incidence of subsequent cardiovascular disease. As a consequence, effective modification of the risk factors for PAD is now regarded as being cardioprotective and this has highlighted the importance of accurate diagnosis and timely management of PAD.

## ARTERIOSCLEROSIS (HARDENING OF THE ARTERIES)

Arteriosclerosis is a term that should be restricted to describing the age-related changes in which the intima and media of the arterial wall become thickened and fibrosed, and there is replacement of the smooth muscle and elastic fibres of the media with collagen. The overall effect of this condition is to increase the rigidity and tortuosity of the vessel and contribute to the age-related increase in blood pressure. In malignant hypertension there is fibrinoid necrosis in the arterioles, and in diabetes mellitus there may be medial calcification (Mönckeberg's medial sclerosis). This definition of arteriosclerosis is not universally accepted, and the name is sometimes used as a generic term to describe the pathological changes associated with arteriosclerosis and atherosclerosis.

## ATHEROSCLEROSIS (MACROVASCULAR DISEASE)

The term atherosclerosis describes thickening of the intima of large and medium-sized arteries, and consequent narrowing of the artery because of lipid and fibrous deposition. Atherosclerosis is a major cause of morbidity and mortality in the western world, due to coronary artery disease, cerebrovascular disease and peripheral vascular disease. It is responsible for about 80% of all deaths in Europe, USA and Japan. This condition causes a progressive narrowing, or occlusion, of the arteries, resulting in ischaemia of the tissues supplied by the diseased vessel. In addition, atheromas serve as sites for thrombus formation, which can result in acute symptoms. The development and rate of progression of the atheroma varies from vessel to vessel (e.g. femoral artery to cerebral artery) and from patient to patient; symptoms usually develop when the arterial obstruction equates to a 50–75% reduction in the diameter of the vessel lumen. Typically, a patient will present with symptoms of ischaemia in one anatomical region (e.g. lower limbs, heart or brain) but as the condition advances symptoms frequently develop in one or both of the other two regions (e.g. patients who present with PAD have a four- to six-fold increased risk of dying from a cardiovascular event).

### Epidemiology

In the UK, 5% of men and 2.5% of women over the age of 50 years have intermittent claudication, which is the commonest manifestation of atheromatous PAD, and about 8–12% of these patients will progress to critical limb ischaemia. The prevalence rate of PAD increases with age, and rises to 8% of the population over the age of 70 years. Approximately 50% of all claudicants will be dead within 5 years from the onset of symptoms.

In the USA, 8 to 12 million people are reported to have PAD, with 20–40% presenting with the symptoms of intermittent claudication.

### Pathology

In western countries atheromatous plaques begin to appear in the second and third decade of life. The formation of the plaque within the intima of the artery is thought to be the end product of a complex process of repair, initiated in response to an injury to the endothelium. The widely accepted mechanism that explains this process is known as the 'response to injury hypothesis'.

Atherosclerosis is a complex inflammatory process in which lipids, smooth muscle cells and macrophages accumulate in the intima to form atheromatous plaques. The vascular endothelium plays a pivotal role in maintaining vascular integrity and homeostasis. There are many possible mechanisms by which the endothelium is injured, including mechanical factors (e.g. hypertension and increase in turbulent flow), biochemical abnormalities (e.g. diabetes mellitus, elevated levels of low-density lipoprotein (LDL) and plasma homocysteine), immunological factors (e.g. elevated levels of free radicals), inflammation induced by infection (e.g. *Helicobacter pylori*) and genetic factors.

The earliest stage of the atheromatous plaque is fatty streaks, which appear microscopically as flat yellow dots or lines on the endothelium. They can be present from childhood onwards, and develop at bifurcations of vessels where turbulent flow may contribute to the damage of the endothelium. The streak develops as circulating monocytes migrate into the intima, taking up oxidised LDL and, because of their histological appearance, these are referred to as foam cells. These cells rupture, releasing their contents and increasing the extracellular pool of lipids. Not all these fatty streaks will evolve into the next stage of development of the atheromatous plaque; many will regress. The next stage of plaque formation is mediated through the release of cytokines, such as platelet-derived growth factor and transforming growth factor-β (TGF-β) by macrophages, monocytes and damaged endothelial cells. These cytokines trigger the accumulation of macrophages, as well as smooth muscle cell migration and proliferation from the media into the intima. Smooth muscle cells produce increased amounts of collagen, which encroaches on the lumen, disrupting laminar flow and reducing blood flow.

The mature fibrolipid plaque is characterised by a core of extracellular lipids, smooth muscle cells and foam cells, which protrude into the lumen of the vessels. The media of vessel beneath the plaque is thinned, and this may contribute to aneurysmal dilatations. The endothelial lining of the plaque is prone to fissure/rupture, resulting in embolus formation and the development of a thrombosis, which may result in acute occlusion of the artery. Thrombosis can arise by two different mechanisms: by superficial endothelial injury, which exposes subendothelial connective tissue, triggering platelet adhesion and resulting in the formation of a thrombus on the surface of the atheromatous plaque; or, in advanced disease, where there is a deep fissure within the plaque, blood from the lumen enters the plaque, resulting in a thrombosis within the plaque, which will distort the vessel and extend into the lumen.

# RISK FACTORS

## Modifiable factors

### Smoking

Cigarette smoking is the single most powerful risk factor for PAD, and it is dose dependent. The relative risk (RR) of developing atherosclerosis if you smoke is up to 10 times higher compared with a matched non-smoker. This risk declines to almost normal after 10 years of abstention. Smoking results in repetitive endothelial injury, and is associated with high levels of carboxyhaemoglobin and low levels of oxygen delivery to tissues. Tissue hypoxia will stimulate the proliferation and migration of arterial smooth muscle cells into the intima, and may diminish the degradation of LDL by smooth muscle cells.

### Lipid disorders

Elevated levels of plasma cholesterol (>5.2 mmol/l) positively correlate with an increase in the incidence rate of atherosclerosis. The excess risk is associated with an increase in the concentration of LDL cholesterol (often referred to as the atherogenic particle) and is inversely related to the plasma high-density lipoprotein (HDL) cholesterol concentration. In addition, there is weak positive correlation between increased plasma triglyceride concentration and athero-

sclerosis. The hypertriglyceridaemia risk factor becomes stronger if LDL cholesterol is raised and HDL cholesterol reduced. Increased concentrations of specific lipoproteins may be primary (i.e. due to hereditary defects in lipoprotein metabolism) or secondary to certain diseases.

### Primary hyperlipidaemias

Two genetic disorders which can cause hypercholesterolaemia are:

- Familial hypercholesterolaemia (FH), an autosomal-dominant condition affecting about 1 in 500 of the population, is due to a defect in the LDL receptor that prevents the uptake of LDL cholesterol into the liver, resulting in an increase in the level of plasma LDL. Homozygotes that have grossly elevated levels of LDL cholesterol (>15 mmol/l) have severe forms of atherosclerosis and die very prematurely from coronary atherosclerosis. Heterozygotes have moderately reduced LDL receptor activity (>9 mmol/l) and frequently present with coronary artery disease in their forties. Both genotypes present with xanthomata – cholesterol deposits that can thicken the Achilles tendon or present as nodules over the patella.
- Familial combined hyperlipidaemia, the genetic origin of which is uncertain, is thought to affect 1 in 250 of the population and predisposes to atherosclerosis.

### Secondary hyperlipidaemias

These may arise in untreated diabetes mellitus, oral oestrogen or thiazide diuretic therapy, hypothyroidism, alcohol abuse, nephritic syndrome and liver disease.

## Diabetes mellitus

Atherosclerosis is much more common in patients with non-insulin-dependent diabetes mellitus (RR 1.5–4.0). This risk is very much related to the background population; for example, European diabetics are much more likely to develop atherosclerosis than are diabetic patients from Japan. The excess risk of amputation of a foot for gangrene is increased 50 times in a diabetic compared with the general population. This increased susceptibility to atherosclerosis is related to: duration of diabetes; increasing age; systolic hypertension; hyperinsulinaemia; hyperlipidaemia, particularly hypertriglyceridaemia; protein urea; and altered vascular reactivity. Other factors are the same as for the general population.

## Hypertension

Hypertension is an important risk factor for atherosclerosis, with the risk increasing incrementally with increasing levels of blood pressure. Raised blood pressure (systolic pressures are more predictive than diastolic pressures) is associated with an increased risk (RR 3) of developing atherosclerosis through endothelial shear injury.

## Obesity

Obesity is an independent risk factor, particularly if it is central or truncal, but it is frequently seen in association with other risk factors such as diabetes mellitus, sedentary lifestyle and hypertension.

## Homocysteine

High levels of this thrombosis-associated amino acid are associated with thromboembolism through the adverse effects on the vascular endothelium. Plasma levels of homocysteine are influenced by a range of genetic and non-genetic factors.

## Haemostatic variables

Increased levels of factor VII, factor VIIIC and serum fibrinogen are associated with an increased risk of atherosclerosis. It is not yet known if a reduction in these factors lowers the incidence rate of ischaemic attacks.

## Sedentary lifestyle

Lack of regular exercise is associated with an increased risk of atherosclerosis. Exercise has a protective and therapeutic effect, which is related to the increase in HDL cholesterol, development of the collateral circulation and a reduction in blood pressure.

## Dietary deficiencies of antioxidant vitamins and polyunsaturated fatty acids

Diets with low levels of vitamin C, vitamin E and other antioxidants may facilitate the production of oxidised LDLs. Diets high in saturated fats are associated with coronary atherosclerosis.

## Type A behaviour pattern (TABP)

This classification describes people who tend to exhibit aggression, ambitiousness, restlessness, time urgency and high anxiety. However, it is the individual trait of aggression that is associated with atherosclerosis, and this may relate to an increased level of circulating catecholamines.

## Fixed factors

### Age and sex

Atherosclerosis in more common in males, but after the menopause the incidence rate increases in women, approaching that of males of the same age.

### Family history

Atherosclerosis does show familial patterns, and this could be due to genetic factors, lifestyle choices or a combination of both. It has been estimated that 40% of the risk of developing ischaemic heart disease is determined by genetic factors and the remaining 60% by lifestyle factors.

An alternative explanation to the response to injury/lifestyle hypothesis was put forward by the epidemiologist David Barker in the 1980s, which postulates that the adverse conditions in utero and during infancy increase the risk of cardiovascular disease in later life (Barker hypothesis or fetal origins hypothesis). This hypothesis was built around longitudinal and retrospective case–control studies, where the early health records of newborn babies and young children were matched with the current health status of these babies who are now adults (>50 years old). The results reported that people who are small at birth or during infancy remain biologically different throughout their lives. They have higher blood pressure, a higher incidence rate of type 2 diabetes mellitus, different pattern of lipids, different bone density, altered stress response, less elastic arteries, thicker ventricular walls, and are more likely to age quicker. A number of subsequent studies have added weight to this hypothesis, but it still remains controversial. Perhaps the risk factors for atherosclerosis cannot be explained by one single hypothesis but are embedded in fetomaternal, environmental, inheritance and life-course risk factors.

## CLINICAL FEATURES

Patients presenting with PAD will frequently have features of atherosclerosis in vessels supplying other organs (e.g. ischaemic heart disease and cerebrovascular disease). The three cardinal features of symptomatic PAD are intermittent claudication, rest pain and gangrene, each of which reflects an increasing degree of ischaemia. Symptoms usually occur when the arterial obstruction reaches 50–70%. Typically, patients initially present with intermittent claudication, and as the pathology advances this may progress to rest pain, and in a small percentage of patients it may result in peripheral gangrene. In many cases the leg ischaemia does not have time to deteriorate to gangrene because the associated coronary atherosclerosis is responsible for a high and premature mortality rate.

## Intermittent claudication

Intermittent claudication typically causes pain in the calf (because the femoropopliteal vessels are the most commonly affected arteries) that is brought on by exercise and relieved by rest. Although the calf is a common site for ischaemic pain, depending on the location of the atheroma pain may also be felt in the buttock, thigh or even on the plantar aspect of the foot. The pain is initially located in one limb, but pathology is usually present in both limbs but to different degrees. The symptoms are described as cramping, tightness or, in the case of the elderly, as a loss of power/movement. All these symptoms will force the patient to stop and rest for a few minutes, during which time there is relief from pain. The symptoms are progressive and start during strenuous exercise, but as the pathology advances pain is eventually felt during mild exercise. Key diagnostic questions must demonstrate that the pain is located in muscle and not in joints. The pain should be exacerbated by an increased level of activity (e.g. walking uphill or into the wind, or climbing stairs) and be relieved by short periods (a few minutes) of rest, but reoccur with exercise. It should be noted that a few patients are able to walk through the claudication; this is probably due to reducing the work rate of muscle.

---

### CASE STUDY 5.1 INTERMITTENT CLAUDICATION

A 50-year-old male patient is referred to you complaining of leg pain on exercise.

#### QUESTION

What three key questions would you ask to confirm a clinical diagnosis of intermittent claudication?

#### ANSWERS

1. Ask the patient to describe the type of pain, onset pattern and how it is relieved – typically pain is described as cramping and is brought on by progressive exercise and is relieved by rest within 2–3 minutes.
2. Ask the patient to point to the location of the pain – they should point to muscle mass (e.g. centre of calf, midthigh, buttock) or the centre of the sole of the foot.
3. Ask the patient whether this pain occurs each time they are walking – pain typically occurs when the patient has walked a certain distance; this may be increased if they are walking slowly or down an incline, and conversely may be shortened if they are walking up a hill or into a strong wind, or are carrying bags.

# Rest pain

Rest pain signifies a more precarious blood supply to the limb than does intermittent claudication, indicating a failure in flow at the microcirculatory level. The pain, which is typically felt at night or when the lower limbs are elevated and warmed, can be excruciating and is described as burning in nature, often located in the forefoot and associated with symptoms of paraesthesia. Patients are wakened from sleep and have to resort to placing their limbs in a dependent position with their feet on cold surfaces to alleviate the pain. In severe cases, patients may not be able to sleep through a complete night because of ischaemic rest pain, and may have to resort to sleeping semi upright with their feet in a dependent position. With progressive ischaemia, rest pain may eventually be continuous despite all attempts to increase blood flow through limb dependency.

Other complaints might include cold feet, which is of a persistent nature and present even in high environmental temperatures. Colour changes may vary, and include: pallor, which is due to diminished blood flow, cyanosis, which is seen when the blood flow is sufficient to prevent blanching; and erythrocyanosis, which is produced by anoxic damage to capillaries and venules, resulting in continued vasodilatation.

Physical signs of PAD will include decreased or absent peripheral pulses below the site of obstruction, premature limb blanching when the limb is elevated from the supine position, the ruddy cyanotic hue that spreads over the lower limbs within 3 minutes when the limb is placed in a dependent position from elevation, and increased capillary filling time (>10 seconds). Congenital absence of peripheral pulses has frequently been reported in the literature (e.g. 10% of people have a congenital absence of the dorsalis pedis), but it is now recognised that this is not as prevalent as the original studies reported. Additional physical signs might include nail changes (e.g. thickening, slow nail plate growth through to loss of the nail plate with scarring), atrophic skin changes (characterised by anhidrosis) and thinning of the skin and loss of subcutaneous tissues.

*Critical limb ischaemia* is a term used to describe an advanced stage of PAD that is regarded as limb-threatening ischaemia. Five to ten percent of patients develop critical leg ischaemia, with pain in the foot, ulceration or gangrene. Chronic critical limb ischaemia is defined in both diabetic and non-diabetic patients by either of the two following criteria:

- persistently recurring ischaemic rest pain requiring regular adequate analgesia for >2 weeks with an ankle systolic pressure of <50 mmHg and/or a toe systolic pressure of <30 mmHg; or
- ulceration/gangrene of the foot/toes, with an ankle systolic pressure of <50 mmHg or a toe systolic pressure of <30 mmHg.

The impact of PAD on the patient cannot be simply measured or assessed in terms of distance walked and the severity of pain experienced. Research shows that patients with PAD:

- are frequently frustrated as a result of the delay in diagnosis and the acquisition of knowledge to assist them to manage their disease
- are limited in their social and role function, which is expressed as an inability to meet the desired and required social demands of life
- are compromised by their ability to function in society in a manner consistent with their beliefs about how they should be able to function
- have a sense of uncertainty and fear, where fear is seen in the context of loss of function and independence, amputation and loss of life

- experience a negative impact on mood that is positively correlated with disease severity.

## DIAGNOSIS

The diagnosis of PAD in primary care is frequently based on the clinical method, which includes:

- *Medical history* – evidence of atherosclerotic disease in other anatomical regions (e.g. ischaemic heart disease or cerebrovascular disease), signs and symptoms of anaemia or other blood disorders, and the presence of risk factors for atherosclerosis (e.g. cigarette smoking and diabetes mellitus).
- *Examination of peripheral pulses* – this should include palpation of the popliteal, posterior tibial and dorsalis pedis arteries for strength and volume. The quality of pulses is noted, with the clinician using a light touch with two fingers over the pulse points. Clinicians with very warm hands should avoid using their index fingers to palpate pulses, as this can give rise to confusion over the pulse they are palpating.
- *Presenting symptoms* – intermittent claudication and/or rest pain (see above for a description of the symptoms).
- *Presenting signs* – a cold limb with a lack of hair, translucent atrophic skin with or without ulceration, infection and gangrene.
- *Ankle–brachial index* – an index <0.9 indicates PAD, with progressively lower values correlating with more marked ischaemia (e.g. with intermittent claudication the index is typically 0.5–0.9, and with critical leg ischaemia the value is <0.5). Values >1.3 are indicative of vessel calcification. The evidence base is such that a degree of variance (0.05–0.1) must be accepted and ankle–brachial index values should not be taken in isolation. Common errors in measurement include incorrect cuff size, rapid deflation of the pressurised cuff, and failure to maximise the Doppler signal by placing the probe at the correct angle of 45° to the direction of flow. Toe-pressure measurements (toe–brachial index) are useful when patients present with medial sclerosis, as there is less calcification in toe vessels.
- *Segmental systolic pressure* – this has been reported to assist in the location of vascular obstructions.
- *Doppler sounds/spectral wave analysis* – the interpretation of Doppler sounds is subject to observer bias. However, triphasic and biphasic sounds are indicative of normal flow, a high-pitched monophasic sound indicates arterial occlusion, and a lowering of the sound pitch indicates distal disease. In addition to the waveform being altered by atherosclerotic disease, decreased cardiac output and aortic valve disease will also have an adverse affect on waveforms.
- *Venous filling time* – this test assesses the time taken for blood to refill the drained lower limb veins. The clinician should identify a prominent foot vein before placing the patient in a supine position with their leg elevated at 45° to the horizontal for a period of 60 seconds. On placing the limb into a dependent position following the period of elevation, the time taken for the selected vein to refill should be noted: 15 seconds is normal; 20–30 seconds is indicative of moderate ischaemia; and >40 seconds indicates severe ischaemia. In the presence of venous incompetence this test is invalid due to venous reflux.

- *Buerger's test* – this is the observation of changes in skin colour in response to limb elevation and dependency. The patient is placed in a supine position, with their lower limb elevated for 60 seconds; the leg is then placed in a dependent position and the time taken for the limb colour to return to the blanched limb is noted. In addition to noting the time taken for the limb colour to return, the consistency of the colour should also be noted; ischaemic limbs are characterised by a patchy dependent rubor. Despite this test being widely used, there is no standard protocol for its use or interpretation.
- *Capillary refill time* – blanching the capillary and subcapillary vessels using light digital pressure and recording the time taken for the colour to return is frequently reported as a valid test for assessing skin blood flow. Although refill times in excess of 5 seconds are used to indicate abnormal flow, research reports that the predictive value of this test remains low.

Specialist vascular laboratory investigations may include:

- *Digital subtraction arteriography* – traditionally the first-line imaging investigation for patients with PAD, it is today still considered the gold standard (despite a number of flaws, e.g. overestimation of the length of occlusions) against which other techniques are measured.
- *Duplex ultrasound* – combines B-mode ultrasound and colour Doppler ultrasound to identify haemodynamically significant lesions.
- *Magnetic resonance angiography* – three-dimensional, contrast-enhanced magnetic resonance angiography has largely replaced two-dimensional techniques. Research reports that this technique is accurate for detecting haemodynamically significant stenoses (>50%) and is cost effective in comparison to digital subtraction angiography.
- *CT angiography* – non–invasive imaging modalities should be employed in the first instance for patients with intermittent claudication who are being considered for intervention.
- *Treadmill exercise testing* – the pre- and postexercise ankle brachial indices are plotted to determine the time to recovery. Maximum walking distance can also be measured objectively using the treadmill; this test is indicated when there is a discrepancy between the history and the clinical signs.

---

### CASE STUDY 5.2 **PERIPHERAL ARTERIAL DISEASE AND SEVERE VASCULAR DISEASE**

Two new patients are referred to you with peripheral arterial disease, and you measure their ankle/brachial pressure index (ABPI) in each patient. In one patient the value is 0.8 and in the other patient it is 0.4.

#### QUESTION

What action would you take and why?

#### ANSWER

Both patients have clinical evidence of peripheral arterial disease. In the patient with an ABPI of 0.8 the severity of the disease is mild, and therefore it is very unlikely that any surgical intervention would be considered at this stage. However, the patient should be assessed for risk factors for arterial disease and these should be modified where possible. An ABPI of 0.4 is indicative of very severe vascular disease (critical limb ischaemia) and this patient should be immediately referred to a vascular clinic.

## ASSESSMENT OF SKIN BLOOD FLOW

Many podiatrists ask if is it is possible to measure skin blood flow because they wish to know whether or not the skin blood flow (volume not quality) is adequate to support wound healing. There are many different methods and instruments used in the assessment of skin blood flow, these including laser Doppler flowmetry and imaging, capillaroscopy, spectrophotometry, thermography, plethysmography and transcutaneous blood gas monitoring. Measuring skin blood flow is complex and difficult, and cannot be undertaken in routine clinic. Skin blood flow is influenced by many physiological and environmental variables (e.g. temperature, respiration and anxiety), and it is compounded by the fact that skin blood flow exhibits both spatial and temporal variations, all of which make it difficult to establish baseline blood flow norms. Nearly all the instruments are used to measure changes in skin blood flow following a vascular challenge (e.g. iontophoresis of an endothelium-dependent (acetylcholine) or endothelium-independent vasodilator (sodium nitroprusside)). These techniques have made important contributions to our understanding of skin blood flow in both health and disease. The description of each of these techniques is outside the scope of this chapter. However, of note is capillaroscopy, which is a relatively unknown technique in the UK. This allows direct visualisation of the morphology of capillaries located in the eponychium, and, more recently, measurement of capillary blood flow. This technique has contributed to our knowledge of the different morphological changes seen in Raynaud's disease and Raynaud's syndrome.

Historically, podiatrists have assessed skin colour, condition and temperature as indicators of the patency of the cutaneous microcirculation. For example, colour and temperature are used as indicators of perfusion and oxygenation:

- pink and warm – adequate flow and oxygen saturation
- red and warm – high flow and oxygenation (e.g. as seen in inflammation or abnormal shunting)
- cyanotic and cold – decrease in flow and oxygen saturation
- red and cold – reduced perfusion
- white – occlusion, either fixed or vasospasm
- black – tissue necrosis.

The technique for assessing skin temperature is to run the back of both hands down both legs simultaneously, noting any significant differences in temperature between the left and right limbs, and the proximal and distal segments. This assessment should be undertaken when the patient has been rested in an environmental temperature of 24°C for 15 minutes. Skin will deteriorate when vascular perfusion and oxygenation is compromised, becoming dry, thin, inelastic, shiny, and hairless, and nail growth will slow or cease. These cutaneous changes take time to develop, and may not always be present at the time of diagnosis of PAD, and are not exclusive to arterial disease.

The classification of PAD can be based on symptoms (e.g. claudication distance, ankle–brachial index, critical limb ischaemia) or on the Fontaine classification. The Fontaine classification consists of four stages:

- Stage I   asymptomatic
- Stage II   intermittent claudication
- Stage III   rest pain/nocturnal pain
- Stage IV   necrosis/gangrene.

## CLINICAL MANAGEMENT

The effective management of PAD must include a reduction in the risk factors as well as effective management of symptoms. Patients with PAD, even in the absence of ischaemic heart disease and ischaemic stroke, have approximately the same relative risk of death from cardiovascular disease as patients with a history of coronary or cerebrovascular disease. Therefore, the focus of management must be on reducing cardiovascular complications, managing pain and improving quality of life. This can only be effectively achieved through a multidisciplinary approach, which places the patient at the centre, ensuring that he or she is informed, engaged and empowered. Patients with suspected PAD should be referred into secondary care when:

- you are not confident about the diagnosis of PAD
- risk factors are not being managed appropriately
- the patient has symptoms that limit lifestyle and has objective signs of arterial disease
- young healthy adults present prematurely with claudication.

## Risk reduction

### Smoking

Although there is a paucity of high-quality research evidence (meta-analyses, systematic reviews of randomised controlled trials) concerning smoking-cessation therapy for patients with PAD, there is clear evidence that smoking is associated with a range of vascular disorders, and as a consequence all PAD patients should be actively discouraged from smoking. The selection of the methodology for smoking cessation should be informed by published guidelines, with podiatrists taking a more prominent role in this aspect of management.

### Elevated cholesterol

There is good-quality evidence of a benefit of lipid-lowering therapy (e.g. statins) for patients with PAD whose cholesterol levels are >3.5 mmol/l.

### Glycaemic control

Research reports that in patients with type 2 diabetes mellitus good glycaemic control reduces the risk of cardiovascular morbidity and mortality (e.g. a 1% reduction in HbA1c is associated with a 14% reduction in risk of myocardial infarction over a 10-year period). Despite the lack of research evidence linking glycaemic control with PAD, good glycaemic control for all patients with diabetes mellitus will reduce the incidence of cardiovascular disease.

### Blood pressure control

Hypertension (>140/90 mmHg) is a recognised risk factor for atherosclerosis, and the literature reports a strong association with cardiovascular and cerebrovascular events, and premature mortality. In the context of patients with hypertension and PAD, treatment for hypertension should adhere to the national guidelines, which are applicable to the general population. Concern has been reported about the adverse effect of peripheral vasoconstriction in PAD patients who are prescribed beta blockers.

### Obesity

Obesity, which is defined as a body mass index (BMI) >30 k associated with a number of cardiovascular risk factors, such as pressure, plasma cholesterol and thrombogenesis. It also walking capacity, and therefore could have a negative impact on treatment/rehabilitation.

### Antiplatelet therapy

All patients with intermittent claudication should be put onto antiplatelet therapy (e.g. 75–150 mg/day aspirin).

### Elevated homocysteine

Elevated levels of plasma homocysteine are reported to be a risk factor for atherosclerotic disease, but there is insufficient evidence to recommend homocysteine-lowering therapy (folic acid and vitamin $B_6$) for patients with PAD.

### Drug therapy

Five drugs are licensed for the symptomatic treatment of intermittent claudication: Cilostazol has antiplatelet and vasodilator effects, and is used in patients with short claudication distances. Naftidrofuryl also has a vasodilator effect and is recommended for use in patients who have tried exercise programmes and report a poor quality of life. Oxpentifylline and Inositol nicotinate are vasodilatatory; however, there is no evidence for their efficacy in the treatment of intermittent claudication. Finally, Cinnarizine, which works antagonistically to a number of vasoconstrictors, also lacks evidence of efficacy.

### Exercise therapy

Exercise programmes are a relatively inexpensive, low-risk option compared with other more invasive therapies for patients with intermittent claudication. A Cochrane Review investigated the effects of exercise programmes on intermittent claudication, particularly in respect to the reduction of symptoms on walking and an improvement in quality of life. Compared with usual care or placebo, exercise significantly improved maximal walking time and distance, with an overall improvement in walking ability of 50–200%. Improvements were seen for up to 2 years. Due to limited data it was not possible to assess the effect of exercise, compared with placebo or usual care, on mortality, amputation or peak exercise calf blood flow. The authors concluded that exercise programmes were of significant benefit, compared with placebo or usual care, in improving walking time and distance in selected patients with leg pain from intermittent claudication. There still remains considerable debate about what constitutes the optimum exercise regimen, and why there is such a variance in patient compliance.

### Alternative therapies

Both *Gingkgo biloba* and vitamin E are reported to be beneficial in the management of PAD. However, the research evidence is not strong enough to draw any definite conclusions about their effectiveness in the treatment of PAD.

### Vascular intervention

Surgical intervention for stable intermittent claudication is rarely required, as the risk to limb viability is low. It is estimated that 6–10%

of patients per year will require a surgical intervention. Surgical treatment falls into two groups: angioplasty and stenting, which is most useful in patients with focal disease; and bypass surgery, for those patients with severe disability impacting negatively on their quality of life, who failed to benefit from exercise therapy, risk-factor reduction and medical treatment.

---

### CASE STUDY 5.3 MILD CLAUDICATION IN THE LEG

A patient with mild claudication in his leg is reluctant to modify his lifestyle, as he believes that once you start to develop vascular disease it cannot be reversed.

#### QUESTION

How might the patient help in the management of his claudication?

#### ANSWER

1. Maintain an optimum body weight
2. Eat a balanced diet with five portions of fruit/vegetables per day
3. Reduce his intake of saturated fats
4. Stop smoking cigarettes
5. If he is unable to stop smoking, then reduce the number of cigarettes smoked
6. Start regular daily walking up to the point of claudication pain

---

## ACUTE ARTERIAL OCCLUSION

This is commonly due to embolism from the heart as a result of mural thrombosis after myocardial infarction or endocarditis. Emboli frequently become lodged in aortic, iliac or popliteal bifurcations, resulting in the limb becoming extremely painful, pale, cold and numb, with an absence of pulses distal to the occlusion, and eventually loss of function. Thrombosis is also a cause of acute occlusion, and this typically occurs in atheromatous arteries. Acute occlusion is a medical emergency that requires pain relief, heparinisation and prompt surgical embolectomy.

## VASCULITIS

The term vasculitis describes a group of mixed conditions that are characterised by local inflammation of the wall of the arteries or arterioles, with the inflammation extending to affect veins and capillaries in some cases. The three most frequently seen inflammatory conditions that affect the lower limb vessels are thromboangiitis obliterans, polyarteritis nodosa and vasculitis seen in association with rheumatoid arthritis.

### Thromboangiitis obliterans (Buerger's disease)

Leo Buerger's original description in 1924 refers to a perivascular inflammation involving distal arteries, veins and nerves, which were frequently agglutinated by fibrous tissue. These segmental lesions, which could develop rapidly, were typically located in distal sections of vessels.

### Epidemiology

The typical age at onset is 20–45 years, with males being affected 7–8 times more frequently than females. This higher prevalence rate in males is changing, probably as a consequence of increasing cigarette smoking in young females. Overall, the prevalence rate of the disease is thought to be falling.

### Aetiology

Although the exact aetiology remains unknown, Buerger's disease is now considered to be an accelerated form of atheroma that affects heavy-smoking, young males. There is a slight genetic predisposition associated with HLA A9 and B5.

### Clinical features

Patients develop superficial migratory thrombophlebitis, cool dysaesthetic feet, claudication or rest pain, and gangrene. The migratory thrombophlebitis is usually present for at least a year prior to the development of arterial symptoms. Arterial disease is present in both the lower and upper limbs, and the features typically include cold feet/hands, paraesthesia, claudication, severe rest pain, and trophic ulceration and gangrene. Claudication, if present, is typically located to intrinsic foot muscles, and this symptom is often misdiagnosed as metatarsalgia of orthopaedic origin. Proximal limb pulses are usually normal, with distal ones being absent or diminished.

### Pathology

The vasculitis affects medium and small arteries and veins. Short segments of the vessel are occluded by thrombus, and there is intense infiltration of the thrombus and the whole thickness of the vessel wall by inflammatory cells, but the wall does not tend to ulcerate. These changes eventually evolve into chronic inflammation and, finally, fibrosis. Different areas of the vessels are affected at different times, with the upper limbs often being the primary site.

### Differential diagnosis

The differential diagnosis is from premature atherosclerosis. Features that assist in differentiating thromboangiitis obliterans from premature atherosclerosis include:

- Early-onset symptoms (before age 45 years)
- evidence of addictive smoking
- inflammation
- evidence of distal disease
- involvement of vein and associated nerve
- upper-limb ischaemia
- exclusion of other risk factors.

### Treatment

- Stopping smoking will arrest the development of the disease.
- Adequate pain relief.
- Acute cases may require hospitalisation for anticoagulant therapy and/or amputation.
- A wide range of drugs have been reported to have beneficial effects.
- Good management of trophic ulcerations.
- Careful attention to foot hygiene.

### Prognosis

Prognosis is poorer for the foot than the hand.

## Polyarteritis nodosa

Polayarteritis nodosa (PAN) is a necrotising vasculitis affecting medium-sized arteries. This rare disorder affects twice as many males as females and, although it can affect any age group, it has a peak incidence in the fourth and fifth decades of life. It is associated with circulating immune complexes containing the hepatitis B surface antigen, and in populations where hepatitis B is common there is a corresponding high incidence of PAN.

### Clinical features

The symptoms and signs of PAN relate to its devastating multisystem inflammatory nature, and vary depending on which organs are predominantly affected. Classical signs include vague systemic illness, muscle pains, mononeuritis multiplex (as a consequence of the involvement of the vas nervorum), abdominal pains, severe hypertension, chest pain, renal impairment, arthritis, claudication, and cutaneous lesions such as palpable purpura, ulceration and gangrene.

### Differential diagnosis

This is mainly from other collagen vascular disorders, which can produce indistinguishable lesions. The diagnosis is based on clinical features; angiography shows multiple aneurysms and smooth narrowing of affected vessels. Immunological studies may assist in excluding other collagen vascular diseases:

- hypersensitivity vasculitis
- Henoch–Schönlein purpura
- cryoglobulinaemia
- vasculitis associated with malignancy.

### Treatment

Antiviral therapy for the hepatitis-B-related variety or immunosuppressive therapy is beneficial in most cases. Mortality is less than 20%, although relapses are common.

## Rheumatoid vasculitis

Vasculitis is seen in approximately 20% of patients with rheumatoid arthritis who present with nodules and are positive for rheumatoid factor. Vasculitis affects small vessels (terminal arterioles and capillaries), resulting in nail-fold infarcts and small areas of tissue ulceration. In other patients, vasculitis affects small arteries and is responsible for larger areas of cutaneous ulceration and digital gangrene. In some patients the usual signs of vaculitis (skin infarction, neuropathy and scleritis) may be absent, and the key features may be rapid weight loss, fever, malaise and a persistently raised erythrocyte sedimentation rate.

## VASOSPASTIC DISORDERS

### Raynaud's phenomenon

In Europe, the broad term Raynaud's phenomenon is used to describe any form of cold-related vasospasm. This broad classification can then be subdivided into Raynaud's disease (RD), when the symptoms are consistent with the original description given by Maurice Raynaud in 1862 and where connective tissue disease is absent both clinically and serologically, and Raynaud's syndrome (RS), where there is an associated disease. This nomenclature allows patients to progress from RP to RS; however, the term Raynaud's phenomenon is used when there is uncertainty.

Raynaud's disease is a common condition, occurring in 5–10% of the population, and it is especially common in women aged 20–40 years. The range of disorders associated with Raynaud's syndrome is wide and includes:

- Immune mediated:
  - systemic sclerosis (affects 95% of patients)
  - systemic lupus erythematosus (affects 10–45% of patients)
  - mixed connective tissue disease (affects 85% of patients)
  - polymyositis/dermatomyositis (affects 20% of patients)
  - Sjögren's syndrome (affects 33% of patients)
  - rheumatoid arthritis (affects 10% of patients)
  - cryoglobulinaemias.
- Drug induced:
  - anti migraine compounds
  - cytotoxic drugs
  - beta blockers (particularly non-selective).
- Occupation-related:
  - vibration exposure (affects up to 50% of workers)
  - cold injury (frozen-food packers)
  - polyvinyl chloride exposure.
- Obstructive vascular disease:
  - atherosclerosis
  - microemboli
  - thromboangiitis obliterans
  - thoracic outlet syndrome.

## Clinical features

On exposure to cold, typically two or three fingers or toes (in up to 50% of cases) go into a prolonged vasospasm, and turn initially white and feel numb with a progressive loss of fine movement. This is followed by cyanosis, which is due to a slow blood flow and desaturation, and finally the fingers or toes become bright red and painful from a reactive hyperaemia.

## Pathology

A number of abnormalities of vascular control have been identified in patients with RD and RS. In RD, increased sympathetic nervous activity is thought to be involved, probably a local vascular hyperreactivity to the sympathetic activity. In addition, calcitonin-gene-related peptide (CGRP), a potent vasodilator, is reduced in patients with RD. The vascular endothelium, a regulator of vascular tone through the production of chemicals such as nitric oxide, endothelin and prostacyclin, has been shown to be involved in the pathogenesis of both RD and RS. Changes in haemostasis, fibrinolysis and haemorrheology have all been reported in patients with RD and RS. Capillaroscopy has demonstrated morphological changes (tortuosity, dilation and drop-out) in nail-fold capillaries in patients with RS.

## Treatment

- Explanation on prevention and self-management (e.g. avoiding cold exposure and the use of heated gloves).
- Vasodilator therapy (e.g. nifedipine).
- In severe cases, prostaglandin analogues.

A patient complains intermittently of three cold toes, which appear white in colour from the proximal interphalangeal joints distally.

**QUESTIONS**

1. What is the most likely diagnosis?
2. What would you base your diagnosis on?
3. How might this condition be managed?

**ANSWERS**

1. Raynaud's phenomenon
2. Clinical presentation – colour changes (white/blue followed by a reactive hyperaemia), evidence of paraesthesia/loss of sensation and/or loss of movement
3. Explanation of the condition, maintain central body temperature, keep feet warm and insulated. If symptoms persist, consider referral for vasodilator therapy (e.g. nifedipine)

## ACROCYANOSIS

This is a benign condition that presents with persistently cyanosed, cold, clammy and puffy skin, and is seen typically in the hands, feet and, rarely, the face. Peripheral pulses are normal and trophic changes are very rare. It is thought to be due to increased vasomotor tone and a dilatation of the capillaries/venules. Seen mainly in young females it is of minimal clinical significance and improves when the patient moves into a warmer atmosphere.

## ERYTHOMELALGIA

This is a rare condition that is characterised by intense paroxysmal hyperaemia, pain and heat. This condition typically affects the hands, feet and face. It is seen in association with a number of disorders, including hypertension, diabetes mellitus, connective tissue disease, spinal cord injury, myeloproliferative disorders and multiple sclerosis.

Treatment is focused on rest, aspirin and treatment of any underlying disorders.

## LIVEDO RETICULARIS

This painless condition is characterised by purple rings with central islands of pallor. The typical location is on exposed limbs – backs of the legs and forearms. This condition can be a primary disorder, and is probably due to an increase in vasomotor tone. In other patients it is secondary, and it is seen in association with PAD.

## ERYTHEMA ABIGNE

Erythema abigne (also known by many other names, such as fireside tartan and granny's tartan) presents initially as multiple circular red rings on the sides of legs exposed to direct heat. In advanced cases, the red colour may be replaced by darker brown rings, which are due to the activation of melanocytes. In heavily sedated or demented patients the condition may advance to ulceration due to repeated or continual exposure of the skin to heat.

## FROSTBITE

Frostbite is the result of severe cold exposure and the combined effects of wind chilling. The affects are variable and depend upon the extent of the pathology, which might include direct damage to skin, prolonged vasoconstriction and sludging in the microcirculation. The typical picture of mild frost bite is one of pain or numbness, and pale waxy skin that typically blisters within 1–2 days of chilling.

## IMMERSION FOOT (TRENCH FOOT)

This condition describes excessive exposure to water. The clinical picture will vary depending on whether the foot is exposed to cold or warm water. Exposure to cold water presents with cold, pulseless, numb, mottled skin, which tends to ulcerate, exposing healthy tissue; exposure to warm water produces painful, tender, macerated tissues that are prone to blistering and bruising.

## MICROVASCULAR DISEASE

Microvascular disease occurs in both insulin-dependent and non-insulin-dependent diabetes mellitus, and its development is linked to the duration of diabetes and the degree of glycaemic control. The term microvascular disease refers to the changes seen in the smallest vessels (capillaries and arterioles). Understanding the nature and pathophysiology of microvascular disease will make significant contributions to our knowledge of cutaneous ulceration and its treatment. The vascular endothelium plays key roles in the regulation of blood flow, vascular remodelling, haemostasis and thrombosis, and in inflammation. Microvascular disease damages endothelial cells, impairs their function and thickens the basement membrane. The resultant effect is decreased blood flow and reduced vasodilatatory capacity. This impairs wound healing, and limits the tissue's ability to respond to traumatic incidents and invasion of microorganisms. In diabetes, microvascular disease is frequently seen in the small vessels of the retina, renal glomeruli and nerve sheaths. Microvascular signs typically develop 10–20 years after the diagnosis of diabetes in young patients, but may present earlier in older patients, possibly due to the period of time for which they have had unrecognised diabetes.

## VENOUS DISEASE

Venous disease encompasses thrombosis and thrombophilia (an inherited or acquired state leading to an increased risk of thromoembolic disease).

In 1856, Virchow proposed that thrombosis (homeostasis in the wrong place) would require two of the following three states (referred to as Virchow's triad):

- Blood stasis:
    - all conditions with immobility
    - impaired limb mobility

- congestive heart failure
- compression of a vein (e.g. pressure from a tumour or abscess).
- Alteration to the vein wall:
  - history of previous thrombosis
  - inflammation/infection around the vein
  - direct vein wall trauma (e.g. cannula or surgical trauma)
  - varicose veins.
- Hypercoagulability states:
  - deficiencies in, for example, antithrombin, protein S and protein C
  - antiphospholipid syndrome
  - hyperhomocysteinaemia
  - surgery (especially lower-limb surgery), trauma and injury
  - childbirth
  - polycythemia
  - neoplastic disease
  - oral contraceptive (oestrogen therapy).

Although Virchow proposed the three broad headings, developments and research in haematology and vascular medicine have added considerable knowledge and understanding of the biochemical pathways of each mechanism. The clinical presentation of venous thromboembolic disease can vary:

- deep venous thrombosis (DVT), typically affecting the calf veins
- pulmonary embolism as a secondary complication of DVT
- recurrent DVT
- atypical thrombosis in the cerebral, axillary and mesenteric veins
- recurrent midtrimester fetal loss.

## Deep venous thrombosis (DVT)

This is a common and important condition that should be recognised early in its development and have the diagnosis confirmed. Failure to diagnose and instigate effective treatment may result in pulmonary embolism, which could be fatal, or permanently damage and impair the lower-limb venous drainage.

In addition to the risk factors for thrombosis and thrombophilia (see above), the profile of the patient is likely to include: increasing age, obesity, pregnancy, history of previous thrombosis and/or surgery (frequently hip and knee surgery), and use of oral contraceptives.

### Clinical diagnosis

The diagnosis is notoriously difficult and there is a proneness to false-positive results when validated against objective tests. Clinical diagnosis (based on signs and symptoms) is reported to be incorrect in up to 70% of cases. Objective tests are based on diagnostic imaging (venography, ultrasound, plethysmography, spiral computerised tomography or magnetic resonance imaging) and haematological assay (usually in patients with a history or family history of DVT) such as for antiphospholipid antibody, homocysteine, factor V Leiden, and protein C and S and antithrombin.

### Clinical features

The most common site is the calf, where it is confined to the sinuses of the soleus muscle and the posterior tibial and peroneal veins. The next most common sites are the femoral vein and iliofemoral vein, which produce the most severe manifestations because of their proximal position.

The following are features of DVT:

- it is silent in up to 50% of cases
- it often starts 3–10 days after surgery
- slight pyrexia
- a mild pain in the calf is made worse by exercise
- swelling distal to the thrombosis
- distension of the superficial veins
- a slight increase in tissue temperature distal to the clot
- a cyanotic colour to the distal tissues
- a positive Homan's sign (pain in the calf on ankle dorsiflexion)
- symptoms of pulmonary embolism.

These symptoms are variable and may be attenuated, depending on the magnitude of the thrombosis, the vessel affected and the state of the collateral circulation. Differential diagnosis should include:

- muscle injury
- Baker's cyst (compressing the popliteal vein)
- contusion of the calf muscle
- cellulitis
- arthritis
- oedema due to other causes.

## Treatment

The aims of treatment are to prevent propagation of the thrombosis, pulmonary embolism and valvular damage, which could lead to long-term impairment of venous drainage. Treatment will include:

- Physical measures:
  - bed rest (limb elevated) for 1 week, as this is the time taken to stabilise the clot
  - elastic stocking, to reduce swelling and protect the superficial veins
  - limitation of prolonged standing for 3–6 months.
- Anticoagulants:
  - This is the mainstay of treatment as it prevents thrombus extension, new thrombus formation and embolisation of the thrombosis, and reduces the complications of developing pulmonary embolism.
  - Heparin is administered either subcutaneously or intravenously for 6–8 days depending on the extent of the thrombosis. In most patients warfarin therapy will commence at the same time, as it take 2–3 days to decrease the concentration of the vitamin-K-dependent clotting factors. Heparin should be continued until the international normalised ratio (INR) is >2.0 for 2 days consecutively.
  - Following a single episode of venous thromboembolism it is the norm to continue with the oral anticoagulant for 3–6months, but this period will be increased if the patient has a thrombophilic condition. It is important to remember that common drugs such as non-steroidal anti-inflammatory drugs (NSAIDs) can affect the action of warfarin, and therefore patients should have their INR checked when starting and stopping additional medication.
- Thrombolysis:
  - Thrombolytic agents are designed to dissolve the thrombus and should only be considered in significant proximal thrombosis where the DVT is considered a significant risk. Haemorrhage is a potential complication of this type of therapy and must be taken into consideration when considering this option.
- Surgical:
  - Vena caval filters are mechanical devices that prevent emboli reaching the lungs, and are used in patients where anticoagulation is contraindicated or has failed to prevent pulmonary embolism.

## PULMONARY THROMBOEMBOLISM

The most common origin of a pulmonary embolism is from a DVT in the legs (80%) followed by thrombosis in the pelvis (15%). In the UK, 30 000 deaths per year are attributable to pulmonary thromboembolism.

The features of pulmonary thromboembolism depend on the magnitude of the thromboembolism:

- Small embolus:
  - dyspnoea on excursion
  - tiredness
  - cardiac arrhythmias (rare).
- Medium-sized embolus:
  - pleuritic pain
  - cough and haemoptysis
  - dyspnoea.
- Massive embolus:
  - chest pain
  - shock
  - tachycardia
  - acute, right-sided cardiac failure
  - death.

## SUPERFICIAL THROMBOPHLEBITIS

This is a common, and often recurring, problem seen in primary care that presents with a local area of skin around a superficial vein being, tender, swollen, warm and red. The vein feels indurated and resistant to light finger compression. The onset of the condition is often sudden, and can be triggered by direct trauma to the vein. Superficial thrombophlebitis does not require anticoagulation. Analgesic NSAIDs are usually sufficient, when combined with correct compression therapy (compression is contraindicated in a patient with PAD and an ankle–brachial plexus index of <0.8) and an exercise walking regimen. Antibiotics should only be used when there is evidence of infection.

## CHRONIC VENOUS STASIS

This common condition, which affects 1% of the adult population, results from either extensive or repeated venous thrombosis and/or valvular incompetence associated with varicose veins or a failure in the venous pump mechanism(s). There is a familial clustering of the condition, and there is thought to be a genetic element to its development.

Following a DVT there is an increase in venous hypertension in the deep, perforating and superficial veins, which results in damage at the microcirculatory level. The nature of this damage has been extensively debated, and theories have included: tissue hypoxia due to stasis of flow; excessive atrioventricular shunting; and a fibrin cuff acting as a barrier to diffusion. All these theories have been challenged and, while there is agreement that there is a failure at the level of the microcirculation, the exact mechanisms are still to be fully elucidated. Recent interest has been focused on the plugging of the microcirculation by activated white blood cells.

### Clinical features

- Pain on standing (often described as a bursting sensation which is relieved by elevation).
- Oedema, which is initially pitting but becomes non-pitting with chronicity.
- Cyanotic appearance.
- Lipodermatosclerosis, due to the leakage of fibrinogen through the vessel wall. This fibrinogen becomes converted and forms the fibrin cuff, which tightens the skin and gives the leg the shape of an inverted bottle of champagne.
- Reduced ankle movement, due to the fibrin cuff.
- Atrophie blanche – white, irregular-shaped areas of tissue with one or two dilated capillaries visible. This is due to slow necrosis of tissue and is the potential site of venous ulceration.
- Telangiectasia – dilated capillaries.
- Ulceration, typically located on the lower third of the leg on the medial and lateral sides.
- Lichenification – the excessive scales are often due to continual bandaging, which interferes with desquamation.
- Dermatitis, which is frequently caused by topical medication.

### Treatment

The treatment of chronic venous stasis remains unsatisfactory. Treatment is directed at reducing venous hypertension by compression therapy, regular exercise walking regimens and, where possible, limb elevation to aid venous drainage. If chronic venous stasis is due to isolated superficial venous incompetence, surgical ligation, stripping and local sclerosing agents may be a long-term cure.

## LYMPHATIC DISEASE

The function of the lymphatic system is to remove macromolecules and excessive fluid from the interstitial spaces and allow transfer of lymphocytes from the lymph nodes to the circulation. Disease of the lymphatic system causes oedema.

## LYMPHOEDEMA

### Primary lymphoedema (Milroy's disease)

This is caused by a failure in the development or an absence of lymphatic vessels in embryonic life. It can be seen in isolation or in association with other congenital anomalies (e.g. Turner's syndrome). The development of the oedema is insidious, and the age at onset will reflect the varying degrees of failure. Lymphograms show varying degrees of hypoplasia, or even aplasia, in the main vessels or, less frequently, there may be gross varicose dilatations and reflux into the skin.

There are three different subtypes:

- *congenital lymphoedema* – appears at or near birth
- *lymphoedema praecox* – appears after birth and before 35 years of age (typically at puberty)
- *lymphoedema tarda* – lymphoedema after the age of 35 years.

### Secondary lymphoedema

Secondary lymphoedema is due to an obstruction of the lymphatic vessels by some known pathological process:

- *Filariasis* – parasitic worms (*Wuchereria bancrofti*) indigenous to West Africa, India and part of South America cause an allergic lymphangitis. Recurrent episodes may lead to lymphatic obstruction and lymphoedema, which may affect the legs, arms, breast and genitalia, and become permanent. This condition is also known as elephantiasis.
- *Malignant disease* – due to infiltration of the vessels and nodes by tumour cells or by compression of the vessels.
- *Radiotherapy* – causes obstruction and fibrosis of the vessels.
- *Trauma.*
- *Chronic infection.*

### Clinical features

The age of onset varies, and in secondary lymphoedema it depends upon the underlying cause. Primary lymphoedema affects both sexes, although 70–80% of cases are female. In only 10% of cases is oedema present at birth; in 80% of cases it is present before the age of 35 years, and the remaining 10% presents after the age of 35 years. In 80% of primary cases the features develop in one lower limb. The oedema is initially of the pitting type, which is reduced with elevation, but eventually it becomes non-pitting and indurated as a result of fibrosis. The epidermis is classically 'warty and hyperkeratotic in appearance' and may predispose to opportunistic infections in 20% of cases.

### Diagnosis

Diagnosis is based on the clinical history and presentation, and exclusion of other cause(s) of oedema. A lymphangiogram is a definitive test to confirm lymphatic obstruction.

### Treatment

- Eliminate the underlying cause, where possible (e.g. treatment of chronic infections).
- Encourage limb elevation, compression therapy and exercise.
- Pneumatic massaging devices (e.g. Flowtron boots).
- Careful attention to skin hygiene.
- Diuretic therapy.
- Microsurgical techniques to improve drainage (these are continuing to be developed).

## FURTHER READING

Belch JJF, Walker F, McCollum P 1996 Colour atlas of peripheral vascular diseases. Mosby-Wolfe, London.

Bergan J 2007 The vein book. Academic Press, Oxford.

Creager M, Dzau V, Loscalzo J 2006 Vascular medicine. A companion to Braunwald's heart disease. Saunders, Philadelphia, PN.

Hands L 2007 Vascular surgery. Oxford University Press, Oxford.

Huether SE, McCrane KL 2007 Understanding pathology, 4th edn. Mosby, Edinburgh.

Loscalzo J, Creager MA, Dzau VJ 1996 Vascular medicine: a textbook of vascular

biology and diseases. Little Brown, Boston, MA.

McCrane KL, Huether SE 2006 Pathophysiology. The biologic basis for disease in adults and children, 5th edn. Mosby, Edinburgh.

Moore WS 2006 Vascular and endovascular surgery. Saunders, Philadelphia, PA.

Myers KA, Clough A 2004 Making sense of vascular ultrasound. A hands-on guide. Arnold, London.

Scottish Intercollegiate Guidelines Network 2006 Diagnosis and management of peripheral arterial disease, 89. Available at: http://www.sign.ac.uk.

Stone J 2007 Rheumatic diseases clinics of North America. WB Saunders, Philadelphia, PA.

Tooke JE, Lowe GDO 1996 Textbook of vascular medicine. Arnold, London.

Watson L, Ellis B, Leng G 2008 Exercise for intermittent claudication. Cochrane Database of Systematic Reviews, Issue 4, Art No. CD000990.

Yates B 2009 Merriman's assessment of the lower limb. Edinburgh Churchill Livingstone, Edinburgh.

# Chapter 6

# Neurological disorders in the lower extremity

*Jacqueline Saxe Buchman*

Roussy–Levy syndrome

Spinal radiculopathies

Spinocerebellar tract

Spinothalamic tracts

Sudek's atrophy

Superficial peroneal nerve

Sural nerve

Sydenham's chorea or St Vitus' dance

Neurological disorders in the lower extremity result from disease processes that involve sensory, motor and autonomic nervous systems. They can result from a hereditary or metabolic process, create progressive or static deformity, and be treatable or refractory. Injury at any level within the central or peripheral nervous system is capable of influencing lower extremity function.

## THE SPINAL CORD PATHWAYS AND CLINICAL EXAMINATION

The spinal cord is made up of many afferent and efferent pathways. Afferent sensory fibres transmit impulses for striated muscles, joints, skin and subcutaneous tissues. Visceral afferent fibres transmit sensory impulses from smooth muscle, cardiac muscle and glands. These sensory fibres enter the spinal cord in two groups of bundles. The larger medial bundle is composed of medium and larger, more heavily myelinated fibres, whereas the lateral bundle is composed of finely myelinated and unmyelinated small fibres.

### Ascending pathways

*The dorsal or posterior columns* are composed of the fasciculus gracilis and fasciculus cuneatus, representing the incoming medial bundles. They enter the cord just dorsomedial to the tip of the posterior grey columns. The fasciculus gracilis carries impulses from the lower extremity and is made up of afferent nerve fibres from the lower thoracic, lumbar and sacral dorsal roots. These nerve fibres are located in a more medial position within the dorsal columns. The fasciculus cuneatus carries impulses from the upper extremities. Conscious proprioception, light touch, vibratory and position sense are carried within this pathway, receiving input from Meissner corpuscles (light touch), Pacinian corpuscles (vibratory sense) and muscle fibres and Golgi tendon organs (position sense).

These ascending sensory fibres enter the spinal cord and ascend on the same side to the level of the brainstem where they decussate and continue on to the thalamus. Some fibres carrying light touch decussate after ascending only one or two vertebral levels beyond their entry. It is because of this small percentage of ipsilateral fibres that light touch sensation will be spared with a unilateral spinal cord lesion.

Clinical evaluation of vibratory sense is the most sensitive indicator of the integrity of the dorsal columns and may be evaluated in several ways (see Ch. 1). The use of a C (128 Hz) tuning fork is quick and easy, but the method lacks the ability to be reliably duplicated or quantified. The fork is placed on the various dermatomes, and the patient, with eyes closed, is asked to evaluate when vibration stops (Fig. 6.1). A biothesiometer, although not as convenient to use as a tuning fork, can quantify findings and is reproducible. The rate of vibration can be varied, with the instrument displaying a scale of 0–50. As the rate of vibration increases, the readings increase. A patient who does not feel vibration at a setting of 25 is considered to

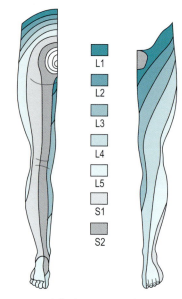

**Figure 6.1** Dermatomes of the lower extremity.

be at risk of neurotrophic injury. Decreased vibratory sense is associated with several disease processes, most notably diabetes mellitus, alcohol abuse, $B_{12}$ vitamin deficiencies and tabes dorsalis. It decreases with the normal ageing process, and patients over the age of 50 years may have a measurable level of decrease in sensation distally. Care should be taken to separate this loss from that of true dorsal column pathology.

Position sense evaluates the integrity of conscious proprioception. It can be assessed simply by asking the patient, with eyes closed, to determine whether the hallux is dorsiflexed or plantar flexed. Light touch can be evaluated by passing a wisp of cotton over the dermatomes of the foot. The patient should not be 'tickled' as this represents evaluation of subliminal pain.

The *spinothalamic tracts* lie within the anterior lateral aspect of the spinal cord and are composed of A-δ and type C nerve fibres. Pain, temperature and crude touch sensations are carried within this pathway. Sensory fibres enter the spinal cord and ascend no more than one or two vertebral levels before decussating into the contralateral side of the cord. From here, they travel on to the thalamus and are relayed to the cerebral motor cortex.

Evaluation of pain sensation is performed by pricking the patient over the various dermatomes of the extremity with a moderately sharp needle. Any area of decreased sensation should be carefully mapped out and compared from distal to proximal and bilaterally. Temperature may be evaluated with an alcohol-saturated swab. The swab is squeezed to trickle a small amount over the foot. The patient is then asked to identify the cold sensation associated with the evaporation of the alcohol.

The *spinocerebellar tract* is an extrapyramidal pathway that carries input regarding unconscious proprioception and stereognosis. It remains ipsilateral, the ascending fibres remaining within the cord on the side of entry. Neurons enter the cerebellum via the superior and inferior peduncles.

A cerebellar lesion results in awkwardness and uncoordination of movement. In the lower extremity, the heel-to-shin test is the most reliable clinical indicator of pathology. The patient is placed in a supine position and asked to place the heel of one foot on the contralateral knee or shin and asked to draw the heel distally along the shin. This test should normally display smooth and even movement.

**Table 6.1** Damage to upper and lower motor lesions

| Upper motor neuron lesion | Lower motor neuron lesion |
| --- | --- |
| Spastic paralysis | Flaccid paralysis |
| Hyper reflexia | Hyporeflexia |
| Babinski sign present | Babinski sign absent |
| No fasciculations or fibrillations | Fasciculations and fibrillations |

Awkwardness or an inability to place the heel on the knee is suggestive of cerebellar disease. Romberg's test may also be used. The patient is asked to stand with the feet close together and with eyes closed. In the presence of cerebellar pathology the patient will sway.

## Descending pathways

The *corticospinal tract* is the primary motor pathway exiting the cerebral cortex and is responsible for voluntary motor control. It descends from the motor cortex to the brainstem, decussating at the junction of the brainstem and spinal cord and providing contralateral motor control. This tract synapses in the anterior motor horn of the spinal cord. Injuries to this tract result in an upper motor neuron lesion, which characteristically exhibits weakness, hyper reflexia and increased tone (see Table 6.1).

Evaluation of the voluntary motor system includes the observation of muscle power, bulk and tone, with note taken of any involuntary movements such as fasciculations or tremors, chorea or athetosis. Movement is assessed for smoothness and coordination. Deep tendon reflex responses are evaluated. The presence of an upper motor neuron lesion may be identified by the presence of a pathological reflex response (Fig. 6.2).

A Babinski sign is virtually pathognomonic for the presence of an upper motor neuron lesion when present beyond the age of 2 years. It is elicited by stroking the lateral aspect of the foot from proximal to distal and then onward across the ball of the foot. If present, the foot will exhibit extension of the great toe with flexion and fanning of the lesser digits. This is a slow response, which occurs over 1–2 seconds, and should not be mistaken for a withdrawal response as seen in a 'ticklish' patient. In the presence of a positive withdrawal response, alternative methods to produce a response include the Chaddock, Oppenheim and Gordon reflexes (Fig. 6.2).

Clonus is associated with increased muscle tone and hyper-reflexia, and reflects the presence of a corticospinal tract lesion. Ankle joint clonus is elicited by a quick, vigorous dorsiflexion of the foot with the knee held in flexion. Greater than three beats suggests nerve injury.

Altered deep tendon reflex responses are often associated with lower or upper motor neuron lesions. They also provide information about an intact reflex arc which represents the integration of five components: an intact afferent sensory nerve, a functional synapse at the spinal cord level, an intact motor nerve, an intact and functional neuromuscular junction, and a competent muscle. Abnormalities must be correlated with other aspects of the neurological examination to identify the level of pathology (Table 6.2).

The symmetry of skeletal muscles should be noted and the muscles evaluated for the presence of spasticity or weakness.

## PERIPHERAL NERVE INJURY

The peripheral nerve comprises axons from the sensory, motor and autonomic nervous systems. These fibres are surrounded by different layers of connective tissue and packaged to form mixed nerves. Each individual axon is surrounded by the endoneurium, a loose connective tissue covering that serves at the blood–nerve barrier. It is made up of a thin inner layer that surrounds the Schwann cells and 'dips' into the nodes of Ranvier. Its outer layer does not dip. These axons are then bundled up into fascicles or funiculi, which are held together by the perineurium. The perineurium comprises many connective tissue layers, with perineural cells held together by tight junctions (Burnett & Zager 2004). These junctions provide the barrier against infectious agents. Groups of fascicles are then packaged together by the epineurium, which is made up of collagen and elastin fibres. It is connected loosely to the surrounding structures and provides the peripheral nerve with flexibility. Peripheral nerves undertake a long journey on their way to the lower extremity and are subject to injury at many levels along their course. The ability of a nerve to recover from injury is dependent on the extent to which the nerve is compromised. Two classification systems exist to help identify nerve injury and predict the probability of nerve repair.

Seddon's (1943) classification is based on the pathophysiological changes that occur within the injured nerve. Neuropraxia represents a transient loss of conductivity. It frequently occurs with mild compression. There is no actual disruption of the neurofibrils. Full recovery is made within a few days to weeks. Axonotmesis represents axonal nerve damage within the structural framework of the peripheral nerve – the nerve sheath remains intact. Axons distal to the nerve injury undergo degeneration, with subsequent regeneration within the intact neural tubes. Recovery is generally at a rate of 1 mm/day and growth can be evaluated using Tinel's sign. Neurotmesis represents disruption of the structural framework of the nerve, involving the nerve sheath and the axons contained within it. Regeneration of the nerve is not possible and may result in a 'stump' neuroma.

Sunderland (1990) developed a classification system based on an ascending order of the severity of the injury. First-degree nerve injury represents a conduction deficit within an intact axon. There may be some demyelination and the patient may experience an 'irritable' stage, with pain, paraesthesias and hyperaesthesias; however, recovery is complete. In second-degree nerve injury, the axon is severed within an intact endoneural sheath. The nerve will regenerate with no residual conduction anomalies. Third-degree nerve injury represents damage to both the axons and fascicles. Degeneration of axons occurs with compromise of the internal structure of the fascicles. Regeneration of the nerve does occur, but healing is unpredictable, with residual motor and/or sensory defects. Pain with this type of nerve injury may be persistent. Fourth-degree nerve injury occurs when the axon, endoneurium and perineurium are disrupted. The nerve trunk becomes a tangled mess of nerve parts. Regeneration is impossible and a neuroma in continuity develops. Complete transaction of the nerve results in fifth-degree injury. Recovery cannot occur without surgical repair (Fig. 6.3).

## PERIPHERAL ENTRAPMENT NEUROPATHIES

The peripheral nerves, as they course to their destiny in the lower extremity, are subject to numerous types of injury. Aetiologies include gradual constriction of anatomical structures about the nerve, chronic compression of the nerve against an unyielding fibrous or skeletal

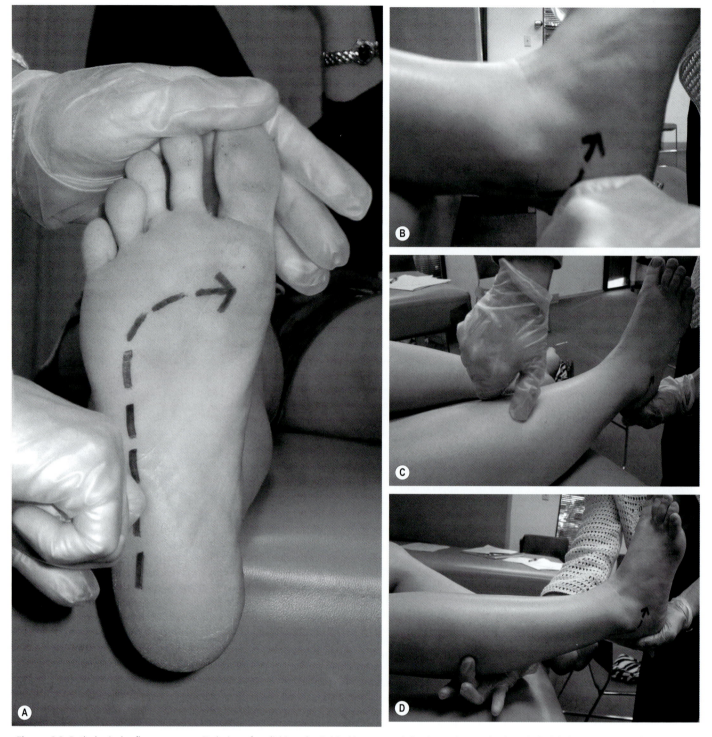

**Figure 6.2** Pathological reflex responses. Technique for eliciting the Babinski response (A). Alternative methods include (B) the Chaddock reflex response elicited by stroking behind the fibular malleolus from proximal to distal; (C) the Oppenheim reflex response elicited by stroking the tibial crest using the fingers as callipers from proximal to distal; and (D) the Gordon reflex response, elicited by squeezing the posterior calf. All the reflex responses, when present, will demonstrate flexing and fanning of the lesser digits.

structure and external trauma resulting in oedema or increased compartmental pressures. Clinically, these injuries present insidiously, with gradual development of sensory and motor changes and pain referred along the distribution of the involved nerve. Electromyography and nerve-conduction studies are helpful in identifying the location of the lesions and aid in the confirmation of the diagnosis.

*Saphenous nerve entrapment* occurs very rarely. Arising from the lumbar plexus, it is the largest and longest sensory branch of the femoral nerve. It supplies sensation to the skin over the medial aspect of the thigh, leg and foot. It courses with the femoral artery in the femoral triangle, and then descends and dives medially under the sartorius muscle. The terminal portion of the nerve courses inferiorly

**Table 6.2** Percussion responses

| Tendon percussed | Spinal nerve roots | Reflex response |
|---|---|---|
| Biceps brachialis | C5–C6 | Flexion of forearm |
| Triceps brachialis | C7–C8 | Extension of forearm |
| Patellar | L3–L4 | Knee joint extension |
| Achilles | S1–S2 | Ankle joint plantar flexion |

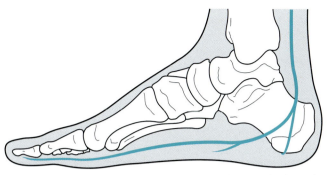

**Figure 6.4** Branches of the posterior tibial nerve. The medial calcaneal, medial plantar and lateral plantar branches of the posterior tibial nerve are illustrated.

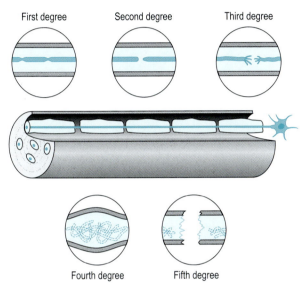

**Figure 6.3** Classification of a nerve injury as described by Sunderland (1990).

with the greater saphenous vein, ending at the level of the first metatarsal head. Entrapment can occur where the nerve exits the subsartorial canal just proximal to the knee joint and exhibits loss of cutaneous sensation along the distribution of the nerve. As there are no motor branches, there is no concomitant muscular weakness or diminished deep tendon reflex responses.

The *posterior tibial nerve* is the anterior division of the sciatic nerve arising from the sacral plexus. It is a mixed nerve providing motor, sensory and autonomic innervation to structures of the superficial and deep posterior compartments of the lower leg. The nerve courses inferiorly, passing underneath the flexor retinaculum, where it bifurcates into the medial and lateral plantar nerve. It also gives off a small medial calcaneal branch at this level. As the medial plantar nerve enters the vault of the foot, it courses with the medial plantar artery to supply motor innervation to only four plantar muscles: the abductor hallucis, flexor hallucis brevis, flexor digitorum brevis and first lumbricale. The lateral plantar nerve, after entering the vault of the foot, courses laterally, working its way over the heel and plantar lateral aspect of the foot. It provides motor innervation to all remaining intrinsic plantar muscles and sensory innervation to the lateral aspect of the fourth and all of the fifth toe (Fig. 6.4).

*Proximal tarsal tunnel syndrome* is a result of entrapment of the posterior tibial nerve or its branches, typically occurring under the flexor retinaculum. Many factors may contribute to the impingement of this nerve. Excessive subtalar joint pronation is the most common underlying aetiology, creating a narrowing of the tarsal canal. With weight bearing, the tarsal tunnel becomes narrowed. Tarsal tunnel syndrome occurs as the nerve becomes impinged or compressed between the osseous architecture of the foot and surrounding soft-tissue structures. Other aetiologies include entanglement of the nerve within the septal attachments of the flexor retinaculum, or compression from an enlarged abductor hallucis muscle belly, enlarged navicular tuberosity or os tibiales externum. Ischaemic injury or vascular insufficiency may compromise the blood flow to the posterior tibial nerve. Varicosities within the tarsal tunnel, when engorged, may produce tarsal tunnel syndrome. Tarsal tunnel syndrome has also been linked with hypothyroidism and diabetes mellitus.

Clinical presentation, regardless of the underlying aetiology, is a symptom complex of tingling, burning and numbness along the plantar aspect of the foot. These symptoms may be reproduced with percussion of the posterior tibial nerve at the level of the flexor retinaculum. The patient typically has a flexible flat foot with concomitant gastrocnemius–soleus equinus. Electrodiagnosis is helpful; however, studies may remain normal, despite the presence of entrapment. Diagnosis is frequently made on clinical findings alone.

*Distal tarsal tunnel syndrome* reflects the isolated entrapment of the medial or lateral plantar nerves. The medial plantar nerve becomes compressed between the navicular tuberosity and the abductor hallucis muscle belly, and may be referred to as 'jogger's foot'. The first branch of the lateral plantar nerve, referred to as Baxter's nerve, may become entrapped as it courses laterally between the abductor hallucis and quadratus plantae muscles on its way to the abductor digiti quinti muscle belly. Baxter's neuritis may present as infracalcaneal heel pain, a history of insidious onset and the persistence of symptoms at rest.

Irritation of a *plantar intermetatarsal nerve* may lead to the development of a neuroma, an enlargement of the nerve at the level of the metatarsal heads. Symptoms may be described as tingling, burning or numbness and radiate distally into the digits. High-heeled or tight-fitting footwear exacerbates the discomfort. Clinically, direct palpation of the nerve or compression of the metatarsals (Mulder's sign) will reproduce the patient's symptoms; the digits innervated by the intermetatarsal nerve may appear separated from each other (Sullivan's sign). Any of the plantar intermetatarsal nerves may be involved, but the third is most common (Table 6.3).

Treatment for an intermetatarsal space neuroma includes patient education regarding the use of proper fitting footwear, mechanical, orthotic control to minimise subtalar joint pronation, and the use of metatarsal 'cookie' pads, which help to spread the metatarsal heads. Injections into the intermetatarsal space of anaesthetic and glucocorticoids or the use of a 4% alcohol sclerosing agent may be of benefit. Surgical resection of the nerve may be indicated when conservative management fails.

**Table 6.3** Results of nerve trunk irritation

| Involved nerve | Nomenclature |
|---|---|
| Medial plantar digital proper | Joplin's neuroma |
| First plantar intermetatarsal nerve | Houser's neuroma |
| Second plantar intermetatarsal nerve | Heuter's neuroma |
| Third plantar intermetatarsal nerve | Morton's neuroma |
| Fourth plantar intermetatarsal nerve | Islen's neuroma |

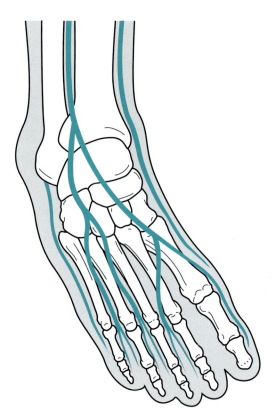

**Figure 6.6** Bifurcation of the superficial peroneal nerve into the medial and intermediate dorsal cutaneous nerves.

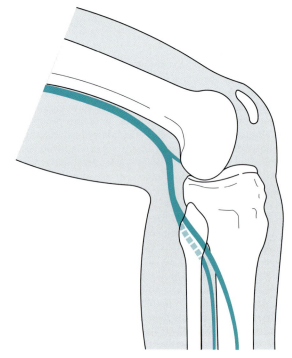

**Figure 6.5** Common peroneal nerve at the level of the head and neck of the fibula.

The *common peroneal nerve* branches laterally from the sciatic nerve trunk within the popliteal fossa. It becomes superficial at this level and winds inferiorly and laterally around the head of the fibula. It then divides into the superficial peroneal nerve within the lateral compartment of the calf and the deep peroneal nerve within the anterior compartment of the calf. The common peroneal nerve is very vulnerable to compression injuries (Fig. 6.5). Neuropraxia can occur simply from crossing one's legs. Iatrogenic injury may occur secondary to positioning on the operating room table or the placement of a below-knee cast where the proximal edge impinges on the nerve with knee joint flexion. Blunt trauma to the area or traction on the nerve from an inversion ankle injury can cause pathology. Clinical findings include muscular weakness of the lateral and anterior compartments, creating a drop foot deformity. Nerve-conduction and electromyographic (EMG) studies help to confirm the diagnosis.

The *superficial peroneal nerve*, also known as the musculocutaneous nerve, courses inferiorly between the peroneal muscles. It becomes superficial, piercing through the fascia, approximately 10 cm superior to the tip of the lateral malleolus. It is at this point that it may become entrapped. Symptoms may be reproduced with dorsiflexion and ever-sion of the ankle joint against resistance and direct percussion of the nerve where it exits the fascia.

The superficial peroneal nerve then continues distally to bifurcate into the intermediate and medial dorsal cutaneous nerves (Fig. 6.6). The *intermediate dorsal cutaneous nerve* provides sensory innervation to the majority of the dorsal aspect of the foot. At the level of the ankle joint it rests approximately 1 cm anterior to the lateral malleolus, just medial to the sinus tarsi. It is extremely susceptible to damage, with inversion ankle injuries and with ankle arthroscopy, by virtue of its proximity to the classic anterolateral portal. The *medial dorsal cutaneous nerve* sends its branches to the medial aspect of the first ray and the second intermetatarsal space. It may be compressed by footwear, often at the level of the first metatarsal cuneiform joint. It is also vulnerable to laceration during surgical procedures addressing the base of the first metatarsal or the first cuneiform.

The *deep peroneal nerve*, also known as the anterior tibial nerve, courses inferiorly within the anterior muscular compartment. At the level of the ankle joint the nerve anatomically flattens and rests between the extensor hallucis longus and extensor digitorum longus tendons, and it is at this location that the nerve becomes damaged. Entrapment of the deep peroneal nerve is known as anterior tarsal syndrome. Aetiological factors include exostoses of the tarsal bones and tight or ill-fitting shoes, particularly ski boots and high-topped shoes, which demonstrate a maximum point of contact at the dorsal talonavicular joint. Patients will present with a complaint of paraesthesias over the dorsal aspect of the foot and numbness within the first intermetatarsal space. Percussion of the nerve at the level of the ankle joint and provocative testing of ankle joint plantar flexion with concomitant dorsiflexion of the digits will reproduce symptoms. There may be motor weakness of the extensor hallucis longus. Nerve-conduction and EMG studies may confirm the diagnosis.

The *sural nerve* arises from branches of both the tibial and common peroneal nerves and originates inferior to the popliteal fossa. It courses inferiorly between the heads of the gastrocnemius muscle bellies to rest posterior to the fibular malleolus, continuing distally along the lateral aspect of the foot. Injury commonly occurs at the level of the ankle joint, iatrogenically with a surgeon's 'slip of the hand' or from fibrosis secondary to an inversion ankle injury.

## HEREDITARY MOTOR AND SENSORY NEUROPATHIES

The hereditary motor and sensory neuropathies represent a slowly progressive degenerative process of the peripheral motor nerves and the spinocerebellar tracts. This genetically transmitted disorder is divided into two major types: the demyelinating form and the neuronal form. The demyelinating form is characterised by degeneration of the posterior columns, loss of anterior horn cells and degeneration of the spinocerebellar tracts. This form demonstrates slowed nerve-conduction velocities and hypertrophic nerve changes. The neuronal form is characterised by axonal degeneration of the peripheral nerve. The prevalence of these disorders is approximately 1 in 2500 individuals.

*Charcot–Marie–Tooth disease type I* is also referred to as peroneal muscular atrophy. It is an autosomal-dominant, inherited disorder that results from a mutation in the gene coding for peripheral myelin protein-22 on chromosome 17. Unstable myelin is synthesised and breaks down, resulting in segmental demyelinisation of the peripheral nerves and conduction deficits. To attempt repair, Schwann cells proliferate and lay down defective myelin, which subsequently breaks down, and a vicious cycle develops, resulting in hypertrophy of the peripheral nerves resembling an 'onion' bulb.

The onset of symptoms usually occurs between the ages of 5 and 15 years with a presenting complaint of difficulty in walking, muscle cramps and paraesthesias in the legs. Signs of classic lower motor neuron disease develop initially in the peroneal and intrinsic muscle groups of the calf and foot. As the motor weakness progresses, the normal agonist–antagonist relationship between the peroneus longus and brevis and the anterior and posterior tibialis muscles is lost, resulting in the development of a high-arched or cavus-appearing foot. Clawed toe deformities develop from the inability of the intrinsic muscles to stabilise the digits against ground reactive force (Figs 6.7, 6.8). Flaccid paralysis develops, frequently with fascicular twitching in the wasting muscles. Deep tendon reflex responses are decreased or completely absent. Lower extremities are observed as slender legs with plump thighs and are often described as 'an inverted champagne bottle' or 'ostrich legs'.

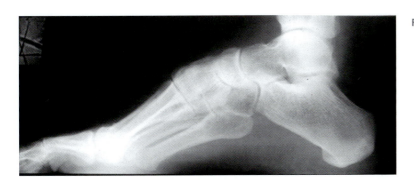

Figure 6.7 Charcot–Marie–Tooth disease.

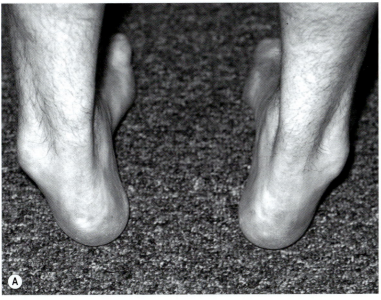
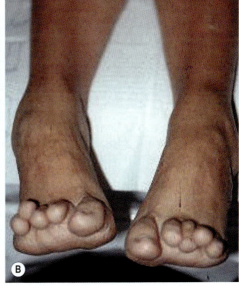

Figure 6.8 Charcot–Marie–Tooth disease. (A) View from rear. (B) View from front.

Diagnosis is suggested by the presence of weakness and atrophy of the peroneal muscle group along with a positive family history. Nerve-conduction studies reveal diffuse and uniform slowing of nerve conduction in both sensory and motor nerves. Nerve biopsy is seldom needed but reveals the typical onion-bulb formation comprising Schwann cells and their processes. There is no effective medical management of this demyelinating process. Early in the disease process, passive stretching and strengthening exercises and splinting of unopposed muscle groups may be somewhat helpful but cannot deter the progression of the disease. Advanced cases require surgical intervention to achieve joint immobilisation.

*Roussy–Levy syndrome* is also known as hereditary areflexic dystasia (Auer-Grumbach et al 1998). Transmitted as an autosomal-dominant trait, symptoms generally develop in early childhood. It is characterised by the presence of an essential tremor and is otherwise very similar clinically to Charcot–Marie–Tooth disease. Patients present with a sensory ataxia or poor judgement of movement, distal muscular atrophy of the peroneal muscles and, frequently, a kyphoscoliosis.

*Dejerine–Sottas disease* is also known as Charcot–Marie–Tooth disease type III or as hypertrophic polyneuritis. It is transmitted via autosomal-recessive inheritance with onset of symptoms occurring in early infancy. The histological picture and clinical course is much more severe than Charcot–Marie–Tooth type I, resulting in delayed motor milestones, poor walking and an inability to run. Additional findings include sensory conduction deficits with paraesthesias and lightning-like pains in the lower extremities. There is slowly progressive distal muscular weakness with peroneal atrophy, resulting in a cavus foot deformity.

*Refsum's disease* is also known as Charcot–Marie–Tooth disease type IV. This extremely rare, autosomal-recessive disorder presents clinically as a triad of retinitis pigmentosa, peripheral neuropathy and cerebellar ataxia. It is the result of a gene mutation that prevents the enzymatic degradation of phytanic acid, an exogenous fatty acid found in chlorophyll, resulting in elevated serum and tissue levels that are associated with neurotoxicity. Onset generally occurs within the first years of life, with lower extremity manifestations of progressive distal neuropathy leading to cavus foot deformity, foot drop and cerebellar ataxia. Dietary control and plasmaphoresis help attenuate the progression of the disorder.

# SPINAL RADICULOPATHIES

Radiculopathy is defined as pathology pertaining to the spinal nerve roots and is secondary to irritation, inflammation or trauma. The fourth and fifth lumbar and the first and second sacral spinal cord nerve roots provide the majority of the innervation to the lower extremity. These nerves exit the spinal column through the vertebral foramina, where they are subject to impingement by bony spurs, tumours and herniated vertebral discs. Radicular pain may present as focal irritation of a nerve root, or 'local', as visceral pain secondary to nerve root irritation, as 'referred' pain, which follows the distribution of the nerve involved, or as 'radicular' pain.

Radicular pain is a common lower extremity complaint frequently involving the fifth lumbar or first sacral nerve distribution – the junction of the flexible spine upon the fixed sacrum. It must be differentiated from peripheral nerve pathology. Symptoms associated with nerve root irritation include a complaint of 'pseudoclaudication'. This discomfort is often unilateral, radiating from the buttock to the thigh or leg, exacerbated by standing or walking and described by the patient as pain, numbness or weakness. Sensory and motor loss occurs

**Table 6.4** Nerve root damage

| Nerve root | Sensory deficit | Motor deficit | Deep tendon reflex response |
|---|---|---|---|
| Fourth lumbar | Medial lower leg<br>Medial malleolus<br>Medial foot | Quadriceps femoris | Diminished patellar<br>Normal Achilles |
| Fifth lumbar | Anterolateral lower leg<br>Dorsal foot | Extensor hallucis longus | Normal patellar<br>Normal Achilles |
| First sacral | Posterolateral lower leg | Triceps surae<br>Plantar foot | Normal patellar<br>Diminished Achilles |

along the distribution of the nerve root. Deep tendon reflex responses are hyporeflexic or absent (Table 6.4).

Elevation of the leg with the hips and knees in full extension should reproduce symptoms; the distribution of these symptoms should identify the involved nerve root. The patient may walk with small steps, keeping knees semi-flexed to prevent stretching the nerve root. The spine should be evaluated for abnormal lumbar lordosis, thoracic kyphosis or scoliosis. Evaluation should include imaging studies to determine the nature of the nerve irritation. Treatment is directed toward the underlying aetiological factor and minimising the inflammation, both pharmacologically and biomechanically. The use of functional orthoses, with or without a heel lift, may benefit patients with a leg-length discrepancy.

# CHARACTERISTICS OF CEREBELLAR LESIONS

In the lower extremity, the cerebellum controls unconscious posture, balance and the coordination of voluntary movements. Anatomically, it is divided into three lobes. The paleocerebellar, or anterior, lobe is responsible for unconscious posture, balance and proprioception. The flocculonodular, or middle, lobe is vestibular, controlling unconscious equilibrium. The neocerebellar, or posterior, lobe receives input from the cerebral motor cortex and coordinates voluntary skilled movements. Afferent input to the cerebellum is received from the cerebral cortex, vestibular tracts and the spinocerebellar tract, an ipsilateral spinal cord pathway relaying input from the lower extremities. Efferent output is then initiated from the cerebellar nuclei, integrated with input from the red nucleus and basal ganglia and relayed to the motor cortex. Any disease process, trauma or physiological insult to the elements regulating cerebellar activity may result in impairment of the coordination of volitional movements.

Clinically, cerebellar pathology in the lower extremity is recognised by classic, uncoordinated ataxic gait. *Dysynergy* is a component of cerebellar disease. Voluntary movements cannot be performed smoothly due to the lack of normal coordination between muscular agonists, antagonists and synergists. This is referred to as *decomposition of movement*. It is recognised by the utilisation of accessory muscles, a wide arc of motion when the patient attempts to reach a goal, easily tired muscles, or asthenia and hyporeflexia.

Other elements of cerebellar ataxic gait include abnormal timing and coupling of movements known as *dysrhythmia* concomitant with the inability to gauge distance, speed, strength and velocity of movement known as *dysmetria*. Patients have a tendency to 'overshoot' a desired point or to stop before it is reached. Excessive rebound and delay in the initiation or cessation of movement results from faulty postural fixation of the limbs. An intention tremor exists, with initiation of voluntary movement recognised by an oscillating frequency that varies and often intensifies as the goal is neared. Finally, speech is dysarthric, sounding slurred, jerky or explosive in nature (i.e. syllabic).

Cerebellar gait is recognised as a wide-based gait with a slow, jerky and irregular cadence. Stride length and foot placement vary from step to step and the patient may frequently lose his or her balance. The foot will contact the ground in two phases – heel strike followed by toe contact. This gait pattern has a characteristic 'double tap' sound. The patient will undergo numerous postural 'adjustments' and may tend to favour one side if the cerebellar lesion is unilateral.

Treatment for cerebellar ataxia is generally palliative. Measures should be taken to increase stability in ambulation. The use of a quad cane or forearm crutch, functional or accommodative orthoses and physical therapy to augment muscular coordination and strength can be very effective.

*Friedreich's ataxia*, also known as hereditary spinocerebellar ataxia, is the most common of the inherited ataxias. It is transmitted by an autosomal-recessive gene defect carried on the pericentric region of chromosome 9. This gene codes for the protein frataxin, which is normally present within the mitochondria of the nervous system, heart and pancreas and required for oxidative phosphorylation and iron homeostasis. The cerebellum, spinocerebellar tract, corticospinal tract and posterior columns are all involved in the evolution of this disease process, which is characterised by the progressive loss of voluntary muscle coordination, obstructive cardiac hypertrophy and the possibility of diabetes mellitus.

Symptoms associated with Friedreich's ataxia generally begin between the ages of 5 and 15 years. Early clinical findings include an early loss of vibratory and position sense, loss of the Achilles and patellar deep tendon reflex responses, and a positive Babinski sign. Patients may have delayed motor milestones and a tendency to stagger and fall. Voluntary coordination progressively deteriorates, resulting in classic ataxic gait with a wide stance, multiple postural corrections and a steppage pattern. Of patients with Friedreich's ataxia, 80–90% will develop a slowly progressive thoracic scoliosis, 50% will develop cardiac disease and 10% will develop diabetes mellitus.

Lower extremity findings reveal distal muscle weakness that is greatest in the peroneal muscle group. This results in the development of a cavus foot type with flexion contracture of the digits. Gait is unsteady, with a wide base. Most patients become non-ambulatory approximately 15 years after the onset of the disease process. Death usually occurs due to cardiac failure. There is no known cure for this disease and medical management is generally palliative.

## CHARACTERISTICS OF BASAL GANGLIA LESIONS

The basal ganglia are a collection of nuclei located deep to the white matter within the brain. Upon receiving input from the premotor cortex regarding a planned movement, efferent output from the basal ganglia will then control this movement. These ganglia, therefore, control intentional movement. Lesions will result in the presence of awkward, unintentional or involuntary movements.

The ganglia that play a role in movement include the caudate, putamen and substantia nigra. The caudate and putamen (which collectively are termed the striatum) receive the majority of their input from the cerebral cortex, sending it on to the globus pallidus. The primary neurotransmitters of the striatum are acetylcholine and γ-aminobutyric acid (GABA). The globus pallidus then 'outputs' this information to the thalamus, exerting an essentially inhibitory effect on the thalamus. Degeneration of the caudate and putamen results in the development of choreic, dance-like movements or athetotic, snake-like movements. The globus pallidus also receives input from the subthalamic nucleus. Injury to this nucleus will result in hemiballismus or flailing movements of an arm and leg.

The substantia nigra, which produces dopamine, an essential neurotransmitter for movement, communicates directly with the caudate and putamen. Deterioration of this nucleus results in the symptoms of parkinsonism.

The effect of the basal ganglia on the thalamus is inhibitory. For example, if one needs to sit still, the basal ganglia will inhibit movements other than those associated with postural reflexes. On the other hand, when one needs to move, the basal ganglia will inhibit unnecessary postural reflexes. Disorders of the basal ganglia are classified as hypokinetic or hyperkinetic dyskinesias.

## Hyperkinetic dyskinesias

### Huntington's chorea

This disorder was first described by George Huntington in 1872. 'Chorea' is literally taken from the Greek word 'to dance'. It is a chronic, progressive, degenerative, central nervous system disease occurring in adulthood. It is transmitted by autosomal-dominant inheritance and is characterised by choreic involuntary movement, progressive dementia, and psychiatric and behavioural disturbances. Nervous system pathology is generally confined to the brain, with advanced cases demonstrating extensive atrophy of the cerebral cortex, basal ganglia and cerebellum. Diagnosis is by the appropriate clinical presentation and the demonstration of caudate atrophy on magnetic resonance imaging.

Huntington's chorea is prevalent throughout the world, occurring in all ethnic and racial groups with an incidence of 5–10 per 100 000. The disease does not typically manifest until after the age of 40 years, although there is a juvenile variant that has an onset at under 25 years of age. Symptoms result from a selective loss of nuclei in the caudate and putamen. Gradual development of choreic movements and mental deterioration are the predominant clinical manifestations, which progressively worsen over 15–20 years and result in death.

There is no specific pharmacological treatment that will attenuate the disease process, so management is directed towards minimising symptomatology. Haloperidol may be effective in minimising the irregular movements in the extremities or facial muscles. Patients may also benefit from the use of antidepressant medications.

### Sydenham's chorea or St Vitus' dance

Sydenham's chorea is the most important form of chorea in childhood. It is one of the five major diagnostic criteria for rheumatic fever as described by Jones. It may occur up to 6 months following tonsillitis or pharyngitis caused by a group A β-haemolytic streptococcal infection. It is thought to be the result of autoantibodies that target certain areas of the basal ganglia.

Sydenham's chorea is more common in girls, with a peak incidence at 8 years of age. The onset of symptoms is generally insidious, and may first be recognised by the presence of facial grimacing slowly progressing to involuntary flinging movements and sudden jerks, which may be more prevalent in the upper extremities. Movements are exacerbated when the patient attempts to control them and disappear while sleeping. Diagnosis is predominantly clinical and from past medical history. Serological testing may reveal elevated acute-phase reactants and the presence of streptococcal antibody titres.

Cerebrospinal fluid will demonstrate increased serum glucose and leukocytosis.

Treatment must initially be directed toward the underlying aetiology (i.e. the streptococcal infection). Penicillin is still considered the drug of choice, with the use of erythromycin in penicillin-allergic individuals, and must be administered for a minimum of 10 days. Management of the chorea is palliative and usually resolves in 3–6 weeks. In rare instances, when the symptoms are severe or become chronic, valproic acid, carbamazepine or haloperidol may be effective.

## Hypokinetic dyskinesias

### Parkinsonism

Parkinsonism was first described by James Parkinson in 1817 as the 'shaking palsy'. It is a distinctive symptom complex characterised by tremor, muscular rigidity, bradykinesia and characteristic alterations of posture and attitude of the extremities, and is sometimes referred to as paralysis agitans. The aetiology is unknown; theories include exposure to unidentified environmental toxins, generation of free radicals and, perhaps, very rarely, inheritance.

Prevalence is roughly 1% of the population in the USA, with a mean age of onset of 55–60 years. Approximately 50 000 new cases are diagnosed each year and this does not appear to be changing with time. The course of the disease is slow, with gradual progression. With appropriate treatment life expectancy will approach the norm.

The major pathological feature is the loss of dopaminergic neurons in the substantia nigra. Via direct and indirect pathways these neurons modulate thalamic input to the cerebral motor cortex. Up to 80% of the neurons are lost before the reduced excitation of the cerebral cortex demonstrates clinical signs of parkinsonism.

Clinical features include the insidious onset of tremor, rigidity, bradykinesia and disturbances in gait and posture. A resting, 'pill-rolling' tremor of 4–6 Hz is a common presenting sign and is the initial complaint in 70–75% of cases. It usually begins unilaterally, affecting one hand or, less often, one foot. Rigidity is demonstrated by the stiffness and slowness of movement. A cog-wheeling phenomenon may be superimposed on the rigidity and is more prominent in the extremities. As the rigidity progresses, the patient acquires a stooped posture, with the head tilted forward and the arms flexed at the wrists and elbows, and walks with a shuffling gait. Bradykinesia is observed as slowness, with muscular fatigue on voluntary movement, and may progress to akinesia, which is recognised as a lack or poverty of movement. Loss of facial expression is noted early in the disease, leading to a monotonous, stuttering, 'deliberate' speech pattern. As the disease process continues, voluntary muscle fatigue leads ultimately to a 'masked facies' and disabling postural difficulties.

Patients with advanced disease present with a classic shuffling gait. Due to the deterioration of postural reflexes patients develop a forward or backward lean. To correct a forward lean, festination occurs. This is a gait pattern characterised by sudden, short, shuffling steps that become progressively shorter and faster. To correct a backward lean, retropulsion occurs. This is characterised by rapid backward steps.

Classic treatment for parkinsonism is pharmacological intervention directed at providing dopamine with levodopa and carbidopa, or the use of dopamine agonists such as pergolide that stimulate the dopamine receptors. Other medications may be used to address individual movement deficits. Surgical management has also become a treatment option, with procedures directed toward destruction of specific sites within the basal ganglia, stimulation of the thalamus and even fetal cell transplants.

Lower extremity management is essentially palliative. The patient should be encouraged to participate in a regular, moderate exercise programme. Physical therapy modalities that address balance compensation may also help improve ambulation.

## CEREBRAL PALSY

Cerebral palsy is a chronic, non-progressive disorder affecting motor dysfunction and, in 60% of patients, mental status. Generally becoming evident in the second year of life, underlying aetiologies are varied and the specific insult is frequently unidentifiable. Prenatal injury is often idiopathic. It may be secondary to hereditary disorders, gestational diabetes, erythroblastosis fetalis, toxaemia and even the presence of more than one fetus in the womb. Natal injury is the most frequent cause, and this encompasses any insult that occurs during birth or within the first week of life. Prematurity, anoxia and respiratory distress are common factors. Postnatal injury includes any insult occurring after the first week of life and up to the second birthday. Aetiologies include infection, poisoning, seizures and trauma. Some form of cerebral palsy occurs in up to 7.5 of every 1000 live births.

Cerebral palsy may involve the pyramidal tracts, extrapyramidal tracts or a mixture of both. Pyramidal tract or spastic cerebral palsy is the most common type, accounting for up to 70% of cases. It represents a lesion within the cerebral cortex demonstrating the characteristics of an upper motor neuron lesion, and may be further categorised by areas of the body affected (Table 6.5).

Early clinical signs of spastic cerebral palsy include a change in muscle tone, asymmetry of movement where there is greater involvement of one side or limb, and delayed motor milestones such as sitting up, crawling and walking. The spastic limbs are usually thinner and smaller, presenting with hyper reflexia and clonus. The Babinski

**Table 6.5** Cerebral palsy

| Type of cerebral palsy | Area of injury | Clinical involvement |
|---|---|---|
| Spastic: 50–70% | Motor cortex lesion | |
| Monoplegia | One limb involved | Spastic movement of arm or leg |
| Diplegia/paraplegia | Two limbs involved | Spastic movements of arms or legs |
| Quadriplegia | Four limbs involved | Spastic movement of all four limbs |
| Hemiplegia | One side affected | Ipsilateral involvement of arm and leg |
| Double hemiplegia | Both sides affected | Spastic movement is not symmetrical |
| Athetoid: 10–20% | Basal ganglia lesion | Uncontrolled, uncoordinated movements |
| Ataxic: 5–10% | Cerebellar lesion | Incoordination of movement or balance |
| Mixed: 10% | Combination of lesions | Spastic/athetoid most common |

sign is usually present in postnatal cases. In the lower extremity, spasticity of the hip flexors and adductors results in internal hip rotation; involvement of the knee flexors and plantar extensors results in toe walking and a cavo varus foot deformity. Arms are held adducted at the shoulders and flexed at the elbows and wrists. Patients demonstrate what is classically described as a 'scissored' gait. Treatment is directed towards physical and occupational therapy. Bracing is of some benefit in preventing adaptive contracture. The use of the exotoxin derived from *Clostridium botulinum* (Botox) may be beneficial. It exerts its effect at the neuromuscular junction, preventing the release of acetylcholine. The result is temporary relaxation of the spastic muscles, creating a transient flaccid paralysis. Within a few months these muscles develop new acetylcholine receptors and paralytic effects are reversed. Surgical intervention may be used to release muscular contractures and restore some normal agonist–antagonist balance between involved muscle groups.

*Athetotic cerebral palsy* is the result of a basal ganglion lesion. It is characterised by slow, uncontrolled, writhing movements, which may be continuous or intermittent. There is a slow, serpentine movement of the arms and legs interposed on postures of flexion with supination and extension with pronation. These limb movements are accompanied by rotatory movements of the neck. Dyskinesia subsides while sleeping. An increased incidence of athetotic cerebral palsy has been linked to postnatal kernicterus.

*Ataxic cerebral palsy* occurs secondary to cerebellar dysfunction. It is characterised by an inability to control the rate, range, direction and force of fine motor movements. Typically, there is a balance disturbance that is compensated for by a wide base of gait. There is an intention tremor with the initiation of intentional movement.

*Mixed cerebral palsy* represents more than one type of motor lesion. Most commonly it is a combination of spastic and athetotic movements. Treatment for the extrapyramidal involvement in cerebral palsy is directed towards the underlying movement disorder.

## AUTONOMIC NERVOUS SYSTEM

The autonomic nervous system is primarily responsible for the regulation of peripheral organ systems. Efferent nerves affect the rate and strength of cardiac, smooth and vascular muscle contraction, endocrine and exocrine secretions of glands, as well as visual accommodation and papillary size. It receives afferent input regarding respiratory and vasomotor reflexes from these various systems. It is under the master control of the hypothalamus, which coordinates the automatic reflexes dictating homeostasis.

The system comprises two divisions:, the sympathetic and parasympathetic nervous systems. Both systems are made up of preganglionic axons that synapse with postganglionic fibres innervating the effected organ system. Preganglionic motor neurons of the sympathetic system arise from the intermediolateral columns of the spinal cord between T1 and L2 (the thoracolumbar region). The fibres then pass into the paravertebral sympathetic ganglia, which are organised into two chains running parallel to and on either side of the spinal cord, where they travel up or down the chain for considerable distances before synapsing. This first synapse is cholinergic. Postganglionic fibres continue on to innervate peripheral organs. The second synapse is adrenergic, with the exception of the sweat glands.

The parasympathetic motor nerves originate in the medulla oblongata. The cell bodies of this system occupy a position in the intermediolateral columns of the spinal cord at levels S2 through S4 and cranial nerves three (pupil and ciliary body constriction), seven (tearing and salivation), nine (salivation) and ten (vagus). This is known as the 'craniocaudal' region. The synapses of the parasympathetic nervous system are typically close to or within the viscera. The majority of both synapses in this system are cholinergic.

## Sympathetic nervous system dysfunction in the lower extremity

Clinical signs of sympathetic nervous system dysfunction in the lower extremity are recognised by visible changes in colour, temperature and hydration of the extremity. Overactivity results in vasoconstriction and hyperhidrosis, resulting in a cyanotic-appearing, cool, clammy extremity. Underactivity or a lack of sympathetic regulation causes vasodilatation and anhidrosis, identified by the presence of bounding pulses, erythema and significant xerosis. With prolonged dysfunction trophic changes persist, muscle bulk is lost and demineralisation of bone may occur.

*Hyperhidrosis* represents increased activity of the sympathetic nervous system. The hands are generally affected to a greater extent than the feet. Patients with hyperhidrosis are more prone towards tinea, cutaneous diphtheroid infections and bromhidrosis. Treatment with astringents such as glutaraldehyde and antiperspirant creams with aluminium salts is generally effective. Anhidrosis results from complete loss of sympathetic input. Spinal cord transaction above the level of T7 will produce total loss of sweating in both the upper and lower extremities.

*Raynaud's disease* represents vasomotor instability mediated by the sympathetic nervous system. It occurs most frequently in women aged between 18 and 40 years. When it is associated with an identifiable underlying aetiology, as with many collagen vascular diseases, it is referred to as Raynaud's phenomenon. Clinically, Raynaud's disease is characterised by a 'triphasic' colour response of pallor, cyanosis and rubor. Pallor occurs initially as a result of constriction of the small cutaneous vessels. Capillaries and venules then dilate, resulting in sluggish slow blood flow resulting in cyanosis. Reflex hyperaemia then occurs, a process that may be quite painful and results in rubor. Patients may complain of pain, paraesthesias and stiffness of the fingers and toes. Symptoms may be exacerbated by cold environs.

Diagnosis is made on the basis of clinical presentation and elimination of any underlying disorder. A complete blood count (CBC) including a differential rheumatoid profile and erythrocyte sedimentation rate may be quite useful. It will identify the presence of a collagen vascular disease and help to rule out a haematological disorder, and lead or arsenic exposure. Patients should be educated regarding potential triggering factors and taught to minimise anxiety and stress that may cause sympathetic nervous system overactivity. Treatment of the vasomotor instability is palliative, directed toward 'insulating' the digit. The use of several pairs of socks or the application of petroleum jelly may prevent heat loss. Nitroglycerine pastes applied to the base of the digits and drug therapy to decrease peripheral vasoconstriction can be effective.

*Acrocyanosis* occurs secondary to an overactive sympathetic nervous system, although the exact aetiology is unknown. It is characterised by patchy cyanosis at the distal portions of the extremities. It is differentiated from Raynaud's disease by the persistence of cyanosis. It has a greater incidence in women during the winter months. Symptoms include swelling, decreased touch, heat, cold and pain perception, paraesthesias and hyperhidrosis. It is managed by patient education and measures directed at minimising cold exposure.

*Familial dysautonomia* is another disorder of autonomic nervous system dysfunction. It is also known as Riley–Day syndrome and is characterised by a complete indifference to pain. It is inherited as an autosomal-recessive trait and occurs in individuals of Mediterranean descent. The most distinctive clinical feature is the absence of tears with emotional crying. A weak suckling response and misdirected swallows lead to feeding difficulties and an increased risk of aspiration pneumonia. Patients may experience a dysautonomic crisis with psychological or physiological stress, experiencing vomiting, tachycardia, hypertension and emotional lability. Classic findings include hyperhidrosis, orthostatic hypotension and an incomplete distribution of indifference to all forms of pain. Mentality is often dulled, and deep tendon reflexes are hyporeflexic or absent. A cavus foot type and the presence of trophic ulcers are frequent findings in the lower extremity. Treatment is palliative. Accommodative footwear should be used to off-load osseous prominences and maintain a normal distribution of the weight-bearing load throughout the gait cycle. Good wound care is essential.

*Reflex sympathetic dystrophy* was renamed 'complex regional pain syndrome type I' in 1993 by the International Association for the Study of Pain. It is believed to occur as a secondary vasomotor instability that is in some way mediated by the sympathetic nervous system. Frequently associated with a minor form of trauma, such as sprains, soft-tissue wounds, fractures of varied severity, surgical procedures and infection, there is no obvious nerve lesion. Causalgia was renamed 'complex regional pain syndrome type II' and is characterised by the same clinical presentation; however, there is an identifiable nerve injury. Sympathetically maintained pain is an additional classification of this type of injury, and is characterised as pain restricted to the distribution of a single nerve. The key finding in all these syndromes is pain out of proportion to the severity of the injury.

The underlying aetiology of complex regional pain syndromes is uncertain and several theories exist to proffer explanation. Doupe in 1944 described a 'short circuit' that occurs between the sympathetic nervous system and the nociceptive efferent pathways that occurs after injury. He postulated that, following an injury, the insulation of the nerve is damaged, resulting in disruption of normal nerve impulses. Nerve impulses are then misdirected, resulting in cross-stimulation of afferent pain fibres. Livingston, in 1943, hypothesised that the internuncial neurons within the spinal cord became overstimulated by the afferent input of an irritative nerve lesion. These internuncial neurons, that act as 'liaisons' between the afferent and efferent stimulus responsible for mediating reflex responses, then in turn influence skeletal and smooth muscle efferent motor nerves in the spinal cord. Hence, a vicious cycle is established, resulting in the observed symptoms of vasomotor instability, hyperalgesia and impairment of motor function.

Complex regional pain syndrome type I is divided into three stages. The acute stage usually lasts 2–3 months. It is recognised by the presence of severe burning pain along with warmth, swelling and joint stiffness distributed not to a single dermatome or myotome but to an entire region. Symptoms may be exacerbated by limb dependency, emotional stress or physical contact (Fig. 6.9). Radiographs may demonstrate early demineralisation of bone. This is then followed by the dystrophic phase, which includes trophic changes of the skin and more advanced demineralisation of bone.

The second or dystrophic stage may last for several months. The warm oedematous phase gives way to a firm, cyanotic, cool extremity. Pain remains the predominant symptom, and this becomes constant, unrelenting and exacerbated by any stimulus. Radiographs demonstrate diffuse osteoporosis, historically heralding the onset of Sudek's atrophy. Flexion contractures of the digits may begin to develop. The disease process is still reversible at this stage.

This process, without successful treatment, progresses into the atrophic phase, which is irreversible. The pain may diminish, be absent or become intractable. Skin and subcutaneous tissues become atrophic and flexion contractures of the foot become irreversible. Radiographically, the osteoporosis advances and the bone has been characterised as having a 'ground-glass appearance'.

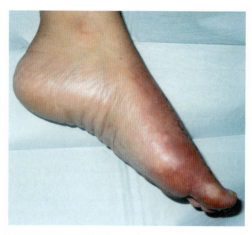

**Figure 6.9** Complex regional pain syndrome. Mottled cyanosis with oedema in a 31-year-old female 3 weeks following surgical correction of a bunion deformity. Symptoms were brought on abruptly by placing the foot in a dependent position.

Incidence is distributed among individuals of all ages, although it is quite uncommon in children under the age of 10 years. Women are up to three times more likely to develop complex regional pain syndrome. Many patients seem to fit a psychological profile – they are overanxious, inquisitive, type A personalities.

Early recognition and treatment of complex regional pain syndrome is critical if there is to be any hope of successful treatment. Diagnosis is generally based on clinical findings along with radiographic changes in the extremity. A triphasic technetium bone scan will demonstrate intense, focal periarticular uptake in the delayed imaging phase. Thermography may also provide diagnostic information. Symptomatic relief in response to a sympathetic nerve block is indicative of sympathetically maintained pain.

Treatment must include aggressive physical therapy in the early phases of the disease process directed towards preventing abnormal joint contractures and muscle wasting. It can include local application of heat, massage, and range of motion and occupational therapy. The extremity should never be immobilised! Sympathetic nerve blocks can be administered on a biweekly basis, directed towards interfering with the aberrant cycling of nerve impulses. Many different classes of medications have been used in the treatment of complex regional pain syndrome; however, none have produced consistent results. The use of non-steroidal anti-inflammatory drugs may be helpful for pain management. The use of narcotic analgesics should be discouraged. Tricyclic antidepressants and anticonvulsants may help with the depression and nerve-mediated pain. Severe cases may require regional anaesthetic blocks or surgical sympathectomy.

## DIABETIC PERIPHERAL NEUROPATHY

Peripheral neuropathy is an all too frequent complication of diabetes, affecting the sensory, motor and autonomic neurons of the peripheral nervous system and the organs that these neurons innervate. Hyperglycaemia and the duration of the disease appear to be the primary factors in its development.

Distal symmetrical polyneuropathy is the most common type of neuropathy in diabetics. It develops insidiously and may affect the small sensorimotor nerve fibres, large sensorimotor nerve fibres, or both. Small, unmyelinated C fibres are composed of autonomic and sensory axons that transmit thermal perception and sympathetic function. These are affected early in the disease process. Patients present with prominent paraesthesias and autonomic nervous system dysfunction recognised by the presence of orthostatic hypotension, resting tachycardia and distal anhidrosis.

Large myelinated axons include both motor and sensory nerves. They conduct proprioception, light touch, vibratory and pain sensations. Symptoms of large-fibre involvement include tingling, burning, numbness, allodynia or deep lancinating pain. Sensory ataxia may occur as a result of diminished vibratory and proprioceptive sense. Sensory changes do not always correlate with nerve-conduction deficits. Deep tendon reflex responses are attenuated or absent and there may be distal motor weakness. The neuropathy develops in a length-dependent fashion, progressing from distal to proximal in a 'stocking and glove' distribution. Progression of nerve injury leads to the loss of protective threshold or the ability to detect small objects or stimuli, resulting ultimately in the neurotrophic or insensate diabetic foot. This is the cause of diabetic ulceration in up to 85% of patients.

The exact pathophysiology of nerve damage in diabetes remains unclear. A number of theories exist, which include the polyol pathway, microcirculation complications secondary to the stimulation of protein kinase, and the non-enzymatic glycosylation of proteins throughout the body.

The polyol pathway has long been implicated. Peripheral nerve tissue does not require insulin for glucose uptake. Hyperglycaemia results in increased cellular glucose levels within nerve tissue, which require an alternative catabolic pathway to be cleared. Via oxidative reactions, glucose is converted to sorbitol, and sorbitol converted to fructose. Initially it was believed that the accumulation of sorbitol and fructose led to osmotic stress, resulting in nerve injury. However, it is now thought that it is the oxidative stress resulting from the breakdown of intraneural glucose that metabolically compromises neurons and leads to nerve damage. Functional loss of axons seems to occur as a length-dependent loss, resulting in an initial distal neuropathy.

Intracellular hyperglycaemia stimulates the activation of protein kinase C. This enzyme facilitates the transfer of phosphate groups from a donor molecule. Although there are many isoenzymes of protein kinase C, the β-2 form has been implicated as the mediator of microvascular damage. These elevated levels of protein kinase C β-2 result in increased basement membrane matrix protein deposition, leucocyte activation, and smooth muscle proliferation and contraction. This process results in decreased endoneural blood flow, resulting in nerve damage.

Exposure of proteins to high levels of glucose initiates a multistep process, resulting in non-enzymatic glycosylation of these proteins – referred to as advanced glycation end-products (AGEs). Proteins, lipids and nucleic acids are all affected, with a resultant change in metabolic function. The large protein complexes may also be difficult for the body to clear, resulting in AGE accumulation in susceptible tissues. Interaction with collagen in endoneural vessel walls thickens the walls, compromising microcirculation to the nerves.

The wide reach of diabetic neuropathy therefore results in many changes in the lower extremity. Sensory involvement results in a loss of protective threshold and the development of a neurotrophic foot. It is recognised early on as a loss of protective threshold and dorsal column involvement characterised by a loss of vibratory and position sense. This is the most prominent factor in the development of foot ulceration and the clinical path to lower extremity amputation.

Motor involvement affects initially the intrinsic musculature of the foot, leading to what is sometimes referred to as an 'intrinsic minus' foot. Atrophy of the intrinsic musculature results in digital contractures, plantar prominence of the metatarsals and abnormal distribution of the normal weight-bearing load with ambulation. In advanced neuropathy a drop foot may develop secondary to anterior compartment muscle wasting in the lower leg. The gastrocsoleus complex,

having lost its antagonistic muscle group, then gains mechanical advantage, resulting in ankle joint equinus. This deformity adds further to the weight-bearing load borne by the forefoot, placing the patient at even greater risk of forefoot ulceration.

Autonomic nervous system involvement in the lower extremity results in a profound vasodilatation of all vessels to the lower extremity and sudomotor changes. The foot will present clinically as warm, erythematous and dry. Increased vascular flow to the foot results in demineralisation of bone; it is literally 'washed away'. This is a major contributing factor to the pathogenesis of Charcot joint disease.

Medical treatment for diabetic peripheral neuropathy must begin with rigid glucose control and patient education regarding the risks and hazards associated with nerve damage. Superficial nerve pain can be managed with capsaicin creams. Deeper nerve pain may be managed with tricyclic antidepressant medications such as amitriptyline or antiseizure medications such as gabapentin. Muscle relaxants may provide relief of deep pain. Disease-modifying drugs that would modulate the pathogenesis of neuropathy are in clinical trials and will open a new frontier in the prevention of neuropathic complications in the diabetic patient.

Treatment in the lower extremity should be directed towards preventing ulceration. Accommodative footwear is indicated in all patients who have lost protective threshold. A laminated plastazote and poron insole provides the ability to offload plantar prominences and provide absorption of abnormal shearing forces. Often an extra-depth shoe will provide ample room for the diabetic foot; however, if severe foot deformities are present, custom-moulded shoes are indicated. Physical therapy is an important adjuvant therapy in the diabetic patient, with treatments directed towards increasing the patient's balance and muscular strength.

## CHARCOT JOINT DISEASE

Charcot joint disease is also referred to as neuropathic osteoarthropathy. There are two forms: atrophic and hypertrophic. It is a destructive process that can occur very rapidly. The atrophic form, or diabetic osteolysis, is much less common and is characterised by severe bone resorption. The hypertrophic form is characterised by severe osseous proliferation followed by bony coalescence or 'healing'. The end result is significant foot deformity.

Atrophic joint disease occurs much less frequently. It may be referred to as diabetic osteolysis and is a form of bone resorption thought to be brought on by hyperaemia. Bones are literally 'washed away' and there is a characteristic pencilling of the metatarsal heads, with a 'sucked-candy' appearance. It is generally localised to the forefoot.

The pathogenesis of hypertrophic Charcot joint disease is most likely multifactorial (Table 6.6); however, two popular theories exist. The 'neurotraumatic' theory attributes the bone destruction to the loss of pain and proprioception coupled with repetitive microtrauma. The sensory neuropathy prevents the patient from recognising joint subluxation or the presence of pain associated with it. The 'neurovascular' theory suggests that, due to autonomic neuropathy, increased blood flow to the bones results in periarticular osteopenia. This decreased mineralisation coupled with trauma results in joint destruction. Pedal pulses will be bounding, the foot erythematous and warm. Motor neuropathy contributes to the development of structural deformity. Abnormal distribution of the weight-bearing load during gait creates pathological stress throughout the osseous architecture of the foot. This may create microstress fractures. Finally, the non-enzymatic glycosylation of collagen decreases the strength of the joint capsules and ligaments, permitting greater joint subluxation.

**Table 6.6** Modified classification system of Eichenholtz

| Stage | Radiographic findings |
|---|---|
| 0 Clinical | Erythema, oedema and increased temperature |
| I Development | Generalised demineralisation<br>Periarticular fragmentation<br>Loose-body formation<br>Joint dislocation |
| II Coalescence | Organisation and early healing of fracture fragments<br>Periosteal new bone formation<br>Resorption of bony debris |
| III Reconstruction or consolidation | Greater definition of bony contours<br>Reconstruction or ankylosis of involved bones |

Hypertrophic Charcot joint disease (Table 6.7) usually occurs at the midfoot, rearfoot or ankle. Incidence is higher in patients who have had diabetes for an average of 12–18 years and which has been poorly controlled. Patients are often in their fifth or sixth decade of life. Males and females are affected equally. During the development phase there are bony changes consistent with an exaggerated form of osteoarthritis. Clinically, pulses will be bounding, the foot is red, hot, swollen and generally, pain free. Radiographically there is generalised demineralisation, cartilaginous fibrillation and loose-body formation (Fig. 6.10). A Charcot foot can, unfortunately, closely mimic osteomyelitis. As these clinical and radiographic findings mimic infection, osseous malignancy or deep venous thrombosis, the importance of accurate diagnosis cannot be overstated.

The coalescence stage is characterised by resorption of osseous debris, with early healing of fracture fragments. During the reconstruction phase the foot becomes stable, resulting in well-defined bony contours and ankylosis of involved joints.

**Table 6.7** Clinical features of hypertrophic Charcot joint disease

| Vascular | Neuropathic | Skeletal | Cutaneous sequelae |
|---|---|---|---|
| Bounding pulses | Diminished or absent | 'Rocker bottom' foot | Hyperkeratosis |
| Erythema | Pain and vibratory sense | Midfoot subluxations | Neurotrophic ulceration |
| Oedema | Proprioception | Digital contractures | Secondary infection |
| Warmth | Deep tendon reflexes | Hypermobility | |

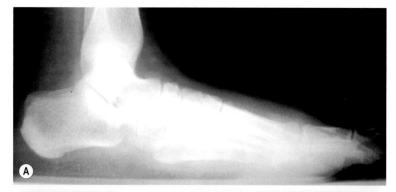

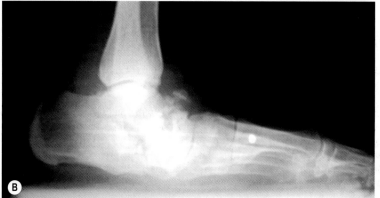

**Figure 6.10** (A) Charcot joint disease in a 58-year-old, non-insulin-dependent female. (B) Following surgical correction of a bunion deformity the patient experienced Charcot-mediated collapse of the subtalar joint.

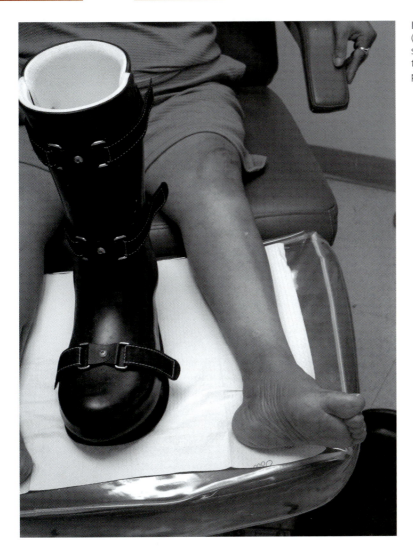

**Figure 6.11** Custom-made Charcot restraint orthotic walker (CROW) boot designed for Charcot joint changes in the subtalar joint. The patient was able to remain weight bearing throughout all clinical stages of the Charcot joint disease process.

Early recognition is critical to avoid significant foot deformity. Early immobilisation with cessation of weight bearing provides the best clinical outcome. A total contact cast or a Charcot restraint orthotic walker (CROW) boot is used once the oedema associated with the development stage has subsided (Fig. 6.11). A bone stimulator may aid in the reconstructive stage. At the conclusion of this disease process, the patient is left with significant foot deformity. Custom-moulded shoes are required and the possibility of surgical intervention to eliminate bony prominences or fuse subluxed joints must be considered.

## DISORDERS OF NEUROMUSCULAR TRANSMISSION

These disorders are associated with weakness and fatigability on exertion. The 'neurological' lesion rests within the generation of a motor end-plate potential, which is unable to trigger a muscle response. Although management of these disorders is primarily medical, it is important to differentiate these neuromuscular junction diseases from myopathic diseases.

*Myasthenia gravis* is an acquired autoimmune disorder, the symptoms of which were first described by Thomas Willis in 1672. The formation of autoantibodies against nicotinic acetylcholine receptors at the neuromuscular junction results in a chronic, progressive weakness of the voluntary skeletal muscles. Involvement may be limited to the external ocular muscles or generalised. The frequency and recognition of myasthenia gravis is increasing, with an annual incidence of 2 per 100 000. The presence of a thymic tumour is a significant predisposing factor, with 30–60% of thymomas associated with myasthenia gravis. Early-onset disease occurs before the age of 40 years, is more common in women and tends to coexist with other autoimmune disorders. Late-onset disease is slightly more common in males, has no thymus enlargement, and has recently shown an increase in frequency. Respiratory failure and aspiration pneumonia are the most severe complications encountered.

The most characteristic feature is painless muscle fatigue exacerbated by exertion. Ptosis and diplopia are the initial presenting symptoms in 50% of patients. These are usually bilateral and asymmetric. Bulbar and facial muscle weakness results in reduced facial expression, with difficulty in swallowing and speaking clearly. Limb weakness is symmetrical, more pronounced proximally and more frequent in the upper extremities. When the lower extremity is affected, the hip flexors, quadriceps and hamstring muscles are affected, the foot plantar flexors and dorsiflexors being less commonly involved. Clinical findings include abnormal fatigability of the limb muscles. Patients may have dyspnoea with only mild to moderate exertion, and experience difficulty climbing stairs, walking or running. Deep tendon reflex responses and sensory findings remain normal throughout the course of the disease.

Diagnostic tests used include the assay of blood serum for the presence of antibodies against the acetylcholine receptors. The presence of these antibodies is diagnostic for the disease, and the degree of elevation of these titres correlates loosely with the severity of the disease. Pharmacological testing may be done with edrophonium, a short-acting acetylcholinesterase inhibitor. Transient improvement of muscle weakness is suggestive of myasthenia gravis. Treatment may include the use of anticholinesterases, prednisolone, plasmapheresis and thymectomy.

*Lambert–Eaton myasthenic syndrome* is also an acquired autoimmune disorder. The defect in this disease process is with the actual numbers of presynaptic acetylcholine quartals released. The postsynaptic response to acetylcholine is normal. The incidence is equal between men and women, and is strongly associated with underlying tumours, particularly small-cell carcinomas of the lung. Patients will demon-strate weakness and fatigability of the proximal limb and thoracic muscles, and have difficulty with chewing, swallowing and speech. The eye muscles are rarely involved. Diagnosis is confirmed by the presence of antibodies in the serum directed against the calcium channels on the presynaptic side of the motor nerve. Electromyographic findings demonstrate an increase in the amplitude of the action potential following voluntary muscular contraction. Treatment may include the anticholinesterases; however, the effect is not as dramatic as with myasthenia gravis. Guanidine increases the actual numbers of acetylcholine quartals released but carries with it serious side-effects. Management of any underlying malignancy is essential.

There are many *congenital myasthenic syndromes*, which must be distinguished from the immune-mediated, acquired disorders. There are presynaptic, synaptic and postsynaptic forms, most of which are inherited through autosomal-recessive transmission. Symptoms usually develop by the age of 2 years. The progression and severity of these processes is dependent on the type of myasthenic syndrome.

## REFERENCES

Auer-Grumbach M, Strasser-Fuchs S, Wagner K 1998 Roussy–Levy syndrome is a phenotypic variant of Charcot–Marie–Tooth syndrome IA associated with a duplication on chromosome 17p11.2. Journal of Neurological Science 154(1):72–75.

Burnett MG, Zager EL 2004 Pathophysiology of peripheral nerve injury: a brief review. Neurosurgery Focus 16(5):E1.

Seddon HJ 1943 Three types of nerve injury. Brain 66:237–288.

Sunderland S 1990 The anatomy and physiology of nerve injury. Muscle and Nerve 13:771–784.

## FURTHER READING

### Peripheral nerve injury

Feinberg JH, Nadler SF, Krivickas LS 1997 Peripheral nerve injuries in the athlete. Sport and Medicine 24(6):385–408.

Ochoa J, Danta G, Fowler TJ 1971 Nature of the nerve lesion caused by a pneumatic tourniquet. Nature 233:265–266.

Ochoa J, Fowler TJ, Gilliatt RW 1972 Anatomical changes in peripheral nerves compressed by a pneumatic tourniquet. Journal of Anatomy 113:433–455.

### Low back pain

Deyo RA, Weinstein JN 2001 Low back pain. New England Journal of Medicine 344(5):363–370.

Deyo RA, Rainville J, Kent DL 1992 What can the history and physical examination tell us about low back pain? JAMA 268:760–765.

Malmivaara A, Häkkinen U, Aro T 1995 The treatment of acute low back pain – bed rest, exercises, or ordinary activity? New England Journal of Medicine 332:351–355.

### Hereditary motor and sensory neuropathies

Dyck PJ, Lambert EH 1968 Lower motor and primary sensory neuron diseases with peroneal muscular atrophy. I. Neurologic, genetic, and electrophysiologic findings in hereditary polyneuropathies. Archives of Neurology 18(6):603–618.

Harding AE, Thomas PK 1980 The clinical features of hereditary motor and sensory neuropathy types I and II. Brain 103(2):259–280.

Jansen GA, Waterham HR, Wanders RJ 2004 Molecular basis of Refsum disease: sequence variations in phytanoyl-CoA hydroxylase (PHYH) and the PTS2 receptor (PEX7). Human Mutation 23(3):209–218.

Keller MP, Chance PF 1999 Inherited peripheral neuropathy. Seminars in Neurology 19(4):353–362.

Krajewski KM, Lewis RA, Fuerst DR et al 2000 Neurological dysfunction and axonal degeneration in Charcot–Marie–Tooth disease type 1A. Brain 123(7):1516–1527.

Njegovan ME, Leonard EI, Joseph FB 1997 Rehabilitation medicine approach to Charcot–Marie–Tooth disease. Clinical Podiatric Medicine and Surgery 14(1):99–116.

Pareyson D 2004 Differential diagnosis of Charcot–Marie–Tooth disease and related neuropathies. Neurological Science 25(2):72–82.

Ouvrier RA, McLeod JG, Conchin TE 1987 The hypertrophic forms of hereditary motor and sensory neuropathy. A study of hypertrophic Charcot–Marie–Tooth disease (HMSN type I) and Dejerine–Sottas disease (HMSN type III) in childhood. Brain 110(1):121–148.

### Entrapment neuropathies

Bailie DS, Kelikian AS 1998 Tarsal tunnel syndrome. Diagnosis, surgical technique, and functional outcome. Foot and Ankle International 19(2):65–78.

Boc SF, Hatef J 1995 Space occupying lesions as a cause of tarsal tunnel syndrome. Journal of the American Podiatric Medical Association 85(11):713–715.

Cimino WR 1990 Tarsal tunnel syndrome: review of the literature. Foot and Ankle 11(1):47–52.

Dyck PJ, Dyck PJ, Grant IA 1996 Ten steps in characterizing and diagnosing patients with peripheral neuropathy. Neurology 47(1):10–17.

Goecker RM, Banks AS 2000 Analysis of release of the first branch of the lateral plantar nerve. Journal of the American Podiatric Association 90(6):281–286.

Hayes DW Jr, Mandracchia VJ, Webb GE 2000 Nerve injury associated with plantarflexion-inversion ankle sprains. Clinical Podiatric Medicine and Surgery 17(2):361–369, vi–vii.

Kanbe K, Kubota H, Shirakura K et al 1995 Entrapment neuropathy of the deep peroneal nerve associated with the extensor hallucis brevis. Journal of Foot and Ankle Surgery 34(6):560–562.

Leach RE, Purnell MB, Saito A 1989 Peroneal nerve entrapment in runners. American journal of Sports Medicine 17(2):287–291.

Lorei MP, Hershman EB 1993 Peripheral nerve injuries in athletes. Treatment and prevention. Sports Medicine 16(2):130–147.

Mahan KT, Rock JJ, Hillstrom HJ 1996 Tarsal tunnel syndrome: a retrospective study. Journal of the American Podiatric Medical Association 86(2):81–91.

McCluskey LF, Webb LB 1999 Compression and entrapment neuropathies of the lower extremity. Clinical Podiatric Medicine and Surgery 16(1):97–125, vii.

McCrory P, Bell S, Bradshaw C 2002 Nerve entrapments of the lower leg, ankle and foot in sport. Sports Medicine 32(6):371–391.

McMinn RM, Hutchings RT, Logan BM 1996 Color atlas of foot and ankle anatomy, 2nd edn. Mosby-Wolfe, Sydney.

Oh SJ, Meyer RD 1999 Entrapment neuropathies of the tibial (posterior tibial) nerve. Neurology Clinics 17(3):593–615, vii.

Poncelet AN 1998 An algorithm for the evaluation of peripheral neuropathy. American Family Physician 15 February:755.

Sammarco GJ, Chalk DE, Feibel JH 1993 Tarsal tunnel syndrome and additional nerve lesions in the same limb. Foot and Ankle 14(2):71–77.

Schon LC, Baxter DE 1990 Neuropathies of the foot and ankle in athletes. Clinical Sports Medicine 9(2):489–509.

## Cerebellar lesions

Bradley JL, Homayoun S, Hart PE et al 2004 Role of oxidative damage in Friedreich's ataxia. Neurochemistry Research 9(3):561–567.

Delatycki MB, Williamson R, Forrest SM 2000 Friedreich's ataxia: an overview. Journal of Medical Genetics 37(1):1–8.

Durr A, Cossee M, Agid Y et al 1996 Clinical and genetic abnormalities in patients with Friedreich's ataxia. New England Journal of Medicine 335(16):1169–1175.

Ponka P 2004 Hereditary causes of disturbed iron homeostasis in the central nervous system. Annals of the New York Academy of Sciences 1012:267–281.

Stolze H, Klebe S, Peterson G et al 2002 Typical features of cerebellar ataxic gait. Journal of Neurology, Neurosurgery and Psychiatry 73:310–312.

## Basal ganglion disease

Cummings JL 1995 Behavioral and psychiatric symptoms associated with Huntington's disease. Advances in Neurology 65:179–186.

Davutoglu V, Kilinc M, Dinckal H et al 2004 Sydenham's chorea-clinical characteristics of nine patients. International Journal of Cardiology 96(3):483–484.

Dajani AS, Ayoub E, Bierman FZ, et al 1993 Special Report: Guidelines for the Diagnosis of Rheumatic Fever: Jones Criteria, Updated 1992: Special Writing Group of the Committee on Rheumatic Fever, Endocarditis, and Kawasaki Disease of the Council on Cardiovascular Disease in the Young. American Heart Association Circulation 87(1):302–307.

Hermanowicz N 2001 Management of Parkinson's disease: strategies, pitfalls, and future directions. Postgraduate Medicine 110(6).

Jones TD 1944 Diagnosis of rheumatic fever. JAMA 126:481–485.

Kirkwood SC, Su JL, Conneally P, Foroud T 2001 Progression of symptoms in the early and middle stages of Huntington disease. Archives of Neurology 58(2):273–278.

Korn-Lubetzki I, Brand A, Steiner I 2004 Recurrence of Sydenham's chorea: implications for pathogenesis. Archives of Neurology 61(8):1261–1264.

Lang AE, Lozano AM 1998a Parkinson's disease. First of two parts. New England Journal of Medicine 339(15):1044–1053.

Lang AE, Lozano AM 1998b Parkinson's disease. Second of two parts. New England Journal of Medicine 339(16):1130–1143.

Martin JB 1999 Molecular basis of the neurodegenerative disorders: New England Journal of Medicine 341(18):1407.

Rosenstein LD 1998 Differential diagnosis of the major progressive dementias and depression in middle and late adulthood: a summary of the literature of the early 1990s. Neuropsychology Reviews 8(3):109–167.

Sapp E, Schwarz C, Chase K et al 1997 Huntingdon localization in brains of normal and Huntington's disease patients. Annals of Neurology 42(4):604–612.

Swedo SE, Leonard HL, Schapiro MB et al 1993 Sydenham's chorea: physical and psychological symptoms of St Vitus dance. Pediatrics 91(4):706–713.

Veasy LG, Wiedmeier SE, Orsmond GS et al 1987 Resurgence of acute rheumatic fever in the intermountain area of the United States. New England Journal of Medicine 316(8):421–427.

## Cerebral palsy

Gordon N 1999 The role of botulinus toxin type A in treatment – with special reference to children. Brain Development 21(3):147–151.

Graham HK, Selber P 2003 Musculoskeletal aspects of cerebral palsy – review article. Journal of Bone and Joint Surgery (British) 85-B:157–166.

Grether JK, Nelson KB, Emery ES, Cummins SK 1996 Prenatal and perinatal factors and cerebral palsy in very low birth weight infants. Journal of Pediatrics 128(3).

Kuban KC, Leviton A 1994 Cerebral palsy. New England Journal of Medicine 330(3):188–195.

Schulman LH, Sala DA, Chu MLY et al 1997 Developmental implications of idiopathic toe walking. Journal of Pediatrics 130(4):541–546.

Torfs CP, van den Berg B, Oechsli FW, Cummins S 1991 Prenatal and perinatal factors in the etiology of cerebral palsy. Journal of Pediatrics 118(1):161.

## Diabetic neuropathy

Arnal JF et al 1999 Endothelium-derived nitric oxide and vascular physiology and pathology. Cell and Molecular Life Science 55:1078–1087.

Albert SW, Koval KJ, Zuckerman JD 1996 Neuropathic arthropathy: review of current knowledge. Journal of the American Academy of Orthopedic Surgeons 4:100–108.

Caputo GM, Ulbrecht J, Cavanagh PR, Juliano P 1998 The Charcot foot in diabetes: six key points. American Family Physician 57(11).

England JD, Asbury AK 2004 Peripheral neuropathy. Lancet 363(9427):2151–2161.

Feldman EL 2003 Oxidative stress and diabetic neuropathy: a new understanding of an old problem. Journal of Clinical Investigation 111(4):431–433.

Moncada S, Higgs A 1993 The L-arginine–nitric oxide pathway. New England Journal of Medicine 329:2002–2012.

Pittenger GL, Malik RA, Burcus N et al 1999 Specific fibre deficits in sensorimotor diabetic polyneuropathy correspond to the cytotoxicity against neuroblastoma cells of sera from patients with diabetes. Diabetes Care 22:1839–1844.

Sommer TC, Lee TH 2001 Charcot foot: the diagnostic dilemma. American Family Physician 64(9).

Sumpio BE 2000 Foot ulcers. New England Journal of Medicine 43(11):787–793.

Vinik AI 2002 Neuropathy: new concepts in evaluation and treatment: Southern Medical Journal 95(1):21–23.

Wautier JL, Guillausseau PJ 2001 Advanced blycation end products, their receptors and diabetic angiopathy. Diabetes Metabolism 27:535–542.

## Complex regional pain syndrome

Anderson DJ, Fallat LM 1999 Complex regional pain syndrome of the lower extremity: a retrospective study of 33 patients. Journal of Foot and Ankle Surgery 38:381–387.

Lee KJH, Kirchner JS 2002 Complex regional pain syndrome and chronic pain management in the lower extremity. Foot and Ankle Clinics of North America 7:409–419.

Maleki J, LeBel AA, Bennet GJ, Schwartzman RT 2000 Patterns of spread in complex regional pain syndrome, type I (reflex sympathetic dystrophy). Pain 88(3):259–266.

Pittman DM, Gelgrade MJ 1997 Complex regional pain syndrome. American Family Physician 56(9).

## Myasathenic syndromes

Drachman DB 1994 Myasthenia gravis. New England Journal of Medicine 30(25):1797–1810.

# Chapter | 7 |

# Podiatry in the management of leprosy and tropical diseases

*Donald L Lorimer*

## KEYWORDS

Anaesthesia
Autonomic impairment
Bacterial
Bites
Complications of ulceration
Cutaneous infections
Drug reactions
Ectoparasites
Epidemiology
Foot in the traveller
Fungal
Hansen's disease
Infection control
Mal perforans
Motor paralysis

## INTRODUCTION

The use of podiatric skills in the management of foot and lower limb conditions has continued to widen and it is now seen as essential to use podiatric interventions in a range of situations where the underlying pathology is not common in temperate climates. The value of such intervention, particularly in the case of leprosy, has been shown to be capable of giving significant improvement to the life of the sufferer. The present-day podiatrist now needs to be aware of an ever-widening range of conditions that present clinically, particularly as international air travel makes it possible for conditions that were previously seen solely in the tropics to be a not too uncommon occurrence in temperate zones.

## LEPROSY

Hansen's disease (HD), or hanseniasis, are preferred terms for leprosy as they do not evoke the connotations that leprosy does. Once an individual has been diagnosed as having leprosy, his or her role in society will lead to an inevitable social death. The patient's experience of the disease is profoundly affected by the social beliefs and expectations of the society of which the individual is a part. Leprosy is not simply a dysfunction of physiological order, it also has psychosocial manifestations that profoundly affect the patient's family and community.

Ironically, the tragedy of leprosy has little to do with the bacillus that causes the disease. The general perception of leprosy within a community is confined to conditions associated with the characteristic secondary deformities. Thus it is possible that, long after Hansen's disease has been cured, the sequelae of the disease, unless controlled, may continue to deform and disable the patient. It is such patients who will then continue to be perceived as having leprosy. Impairment control is a practicable objective, but it demands life-long vigilance. The podiatrist has a specialised approach to chronic pedal disorders. Podiatric training is, therefore, particularly appropriate for the implicit needs of impairment control. The podiatrist is trained to accept the challenge posed by incurable conditions and is uniquely facilitated to develop a provider–receiver relationship that can protect the patient physically and rehabilitate him or her socially.

## Epidemiology

Hansen's disease is essentially a problem in developing countries. Findings published by the World Health Organization in 1998 showed that, globally, there were 804 436 registered cases (WHO 1999). The Indian subcontinent remains the region with the highest prevalence; however, in 1998 prevalence was declining in India, whereas it was increasing in Brazil. Countries with the highest prevalence rates are shown in Table 7.1. There have been problems with the interpretation of the data because case definitions vary between countries.

The prevalence figures only suggest the number of people registered for treatment, and do not give any indication of those who are 'cured' but remain permanently impaired. Figures for the total number of leprosy-affected people are not available, but they could number millions.

After diabetes mellitus, Hansen's disease is the most common cause of sensory neuropathy globally, and is probably the major cause of neuropathy in Asia and Africa, where it affects predominantly the lower socio-economic groups.

The mode of transmission remains a topic of investigation, and the three possible routes are the respiratory tract, the skin and the gastrointestinal tract. Direct skin-to-skin contact is no longer considered the most likely form of transmission, as it appears that *Mycobacterium leprae* is not capable of penetrating the papillary zone of the dermis. However, transmission through skin abrasions has not been excluded (Jopling & McDougal 1988).

Aerosol contamination remains the most likely form of transmission, and there is evidence that demonstrates that infected droplets can be expelled during sneezing, coughing and even talking. Droplets may also be absorbed by dust, and viable *M. leprae* has been identified in desiccated secretions a week after expectorating. The principal theory of transmission is that contaminated droplets are inspired, *M. leprae* enters the capillaries around the alveoli and then continues to target cells via a haematological route. It has also been suggested that damage to the nasal mucosa provides an accessible portal of infection from the same source. The most significant target cell is the Schwann cell, but *M. leprae* is also found in significant numbers in macrophages, endothelium, chondrocytes and melanocytes.

The bacillus is not virulent; infected subjects can host vast numbers without feeling any ill effect, and chemotherapy rapidly compromises the viability of the bacillus. It is therefore from undiagnosed, multibacillary hosts that the threat of infection is greatest.

## Classification

Host resistance to the bacillus will determine the classification of the disease type. The Ridley–Jopling classification is the most widely respected, but more simple classification systems are now used in most field programmes. The Ridley–Jopling classification describes the spectrum of disease from tuberculoid (TT), which demonstrates vigorous resistance and low infection (paucibacillary (PB)), to lepromatous (LL), which demonstrates severely compromised resistance and massive infection (multibacillary (MB)). Borderline (BB) describes resistance that lies between the two polar responses. Further subdivisions are made that represent responses that lie between the principal responses (Jopling & McDougal 1988).

### Neuropathy in tuberculoid leprosy

The most significant changes in tuberculoid leprosy involve the cutaneous and subcutaneous nerves. Nerve damage is an inherent effect of host response and is not related to massive proliferation of bacilli. Infected nerves are invaded and destroyed beyond recognition by epithelioid granulomae. An intense response to infection may lead to necrosis and the development of nerve abscesses. Where a nerve trunk is affected, the sensorimotor deficit will be superimposed, giving rise to the localised mixture of neurological defects characteristic of tuberculoid leprosy. The destruction of dermal nerves explains the localised anaesthetic patches, sometimes the only indication of polar tuberculoid leprosy. Autonomic loss is a feature of tuberculoid lesions, where axon reflex and sweating are found to be absent. Involvement of nerve trunks, being in proximity to skin lesions, is probably secondary to cutaneous nerve involvement. The most frequently affected nerves in the lower limb are the common peroneal and the posterior tibial nerves. The saphenous and the sural nerves are less commonly affected.

### Neuropathy in lepromatous leprosy

Due to depressed cell-mediated immunity in lepromatous leprosy, the haematogenous spread of the bacilli allows the unchecked proliferation of bacilli. Nerve damage is slower to become apparent than in other forms of leprosy. While bacilli continue to multiply within Schwann cells and perineurium, others are dispersed with the destruction of the same. Liberated bacilli are engulfed by histiocytes in which they are not destroyed, and the histiocyte becomes a vehicle that transports multiplying bacilli to other regions of the nerve or other

**Table 7.1** Countries with the highest prevalence rates of Hansen's disease in 1998 (WHO 1999)

| Country | Prevalence | Prevalence per 10 000 | New-case detection rate |
|---|---|---|---|
| India | 527 344 | 5.3 | 53.16 |
| Brazil | 72 953 | 4.33 | 25.86 |
| Indonesia | 29 225 | 1.41 | 7.42 |
| Myanmar | 13 581 | 2.74 | 18.35 |
| Bangladesh | 13 248 | 1.03 | 8.80 |
| Nigeria | 12 878 | 1.06 | 5.89 |
| Nepal | 12 540 | 5.30 | 31.49 |
| Mozambique | 11 072 | 6.24 | 23.64 |
| Madagascar | 11 005 | 6.78 | 71.23 |
| Philippines | 8 749 | 1.22 | 6.89 |

tissues. It is these cells that are known as lepra cells, carrying masses of bacilli collectively called globi.

Symmetrical and bilateral sensory loss of lepromatous leprosy is explained by the massive and widespread distribution of bacilli. The sites of nerve lesions appear to be related to body temperature. Sabin and Swift (1984) presented repeated patterns of surface temperature obtained by thermographic scanning of normal subjects. By comparing gradients between different body temperatures and the evolution of neurological deficit, a clear relationship between the usual distribution of surface temperatures and sensory loss was demonstrated.

## Neuropathy in borderline (dimorphous) leprosy

While nerve damage in borderline leprosy is essentially limited to the same sites as those common in lepromatous leprosy, the potential for uncharacteristic neurological defects is greater. Cases of borderline leprosy demonstrate the greatest potential for catastrophic peripheral nerve damage. This is explained by a dual effect. An inadequate host response ensures that an initial haematogenous spread of disease is not prevented. However, unlike lepromatous leprosy, there is a degree of resistance, resulting in a prompt and radical response when bacilli are detected. As a result, widespread, tuberculoid-type nerve damage is demonstrated early in the disease.

Where a borderline case demonstrates a tendency to fall closer to the tuberculoid pole (BT), paralysis and sensory loss are always asymmetrical. Where borderline cases lie at the midpoint of the spectrum (BB), involvement is asymmetrical and indicates intracutaneous nerve dysfunction because the borders of insensitivity do not conform to dermatomes. In a low-resistance borderline case (BL) there will be numerous lesions, symmetrically distributed. Areas of insensitivity may exceed the borders of lesions, and temperature-linked patterns of sensory loss become apparent. However, the spread of involvement is less diffuse than in lepromatous leprosy and is not as symmetrical (Sabin & Swift 1984).

## The lower limb in Hansen's disease

### Anaesthesia

The integrity of the foot is dependent on safety information relating to current conditions of the substratum. The high density of Vater–Pacini corpuscles in the subcutaneous fat chambers provides an acute sense of deep pressure and vibration. These modalities are associated with high-frequency shock and tissue displacement, whereas it is postulated that the Meissener's corpuscles register low-frequency shock. The dual effect of these modalities is that the foot's movement against the ground and the character of the weight-bearing surface may be perceived. The ability to register pressure coupled with withdrawal and postural reflexes is essential for self-protection (Jorgensen & Bosjen-Moller 1991). The major factor compromising the foot in Hansen's disease is anaesthesia. Denied the benefits of sensory feedback, the undesirable effects of pathomechanical forces are undetected. Tissue may be strained by mechanical stress beyond its threshold of competence, in which case it breaks down.

### Factors associated with plantar ulceration

- Motor paralysis.
- Pre-existing pathomechanical foot function.
- Tarsal disintegration.
- Absorption and pathological fractures.
- Autonomic impairment.
- Social and behavioural variables.

### Motor paralysis

It has been suggested that only 6% of ulcerated feet display anaesthesia alone; when the foot was further compromised by intrinsic muscular paralysis, this figure was increased ten-fold (Brand 1991). It is probable that paralysis of the intrinsic muscles increases the vulnerability of the foot by creating instability during propulsion. The extent to which pre-existing functional abnormalities could exacerbate this condition has not been widely considered.

### Claw toes

Claw toe deformity is a common feature of the neuropathic foot in Hansen's disease and is generally considered to indicate intrinsic muscle paralysis. (The development of the deformity should not be taken as a qualification for muscle paralysis per se, as muscle imbalance due to other mechanical factors is also a cause of claw toe deformity (Root et al 1977).) The extension of the proximal phalanges results in the plantar flexion of the metatarsal heads and anterior drifting of the fibrofatty pad. Compromised by the loss of digital stabilisation, the metatarsal heads are exposed to abnormally directed, excessive forces, focused on a reduced area of loading. Extreme peak pressure readings have been reported under the ulcerated metatarsal heads of leprosy-impaired subjects (Bauman et al 1963).

### Extrinsic muscle paralysis

*M. leprae* appears to have a predilection for cooler sites, such as the peroneal nerve as it winds around the fibular neck. This site is particularly vulnerable to infiltration, Peroneal and anterior compartment paralysis is not uncommon. The resulting foot drop deformity can severely compromise an affected person. Excessive lateral and forefoot loading predisposes the patient to ulceration, particularly under the fifth metatarsal head. The plantar flexors and posterior tibialis have not been found to be affected by neuropathy in Hansen's disease.

### Pre-existing pathomechanical foot function

Factors of a congenital and/or developmental origin affecting foot function are probably implicated in the development of plantar ulceration. It has been reported that 85% of plantar ulcers occur in the forefoot, with the remaining 15% occurring in the heel (10%) and lateral border (5%) (Brand 1991). The predilection for forefoot ulceration suggests that standing pressure and injury are less likely to be causative factors than is walking.

Of initial ulcers that occur on the forefoot, the most common sites are:

- on the plantar aspect of the proximal phalanx of the hallux
- the second metatarsal head
- the area between the first metatarsal head and the proximal phalanx of the hallux.

The frequency of occurrence at these sites suggests an association with excessive or abnormal loading, which is generally associated with compensatory subtalar pronation for rearfoot or extrinsic abnormalities.

### Tarsal disintegration

In late lepromatous leprosy, a complication may be the massive infiltration of bacilli into the bones of the foot. Such infiltration may cause rarefaction of cancellous bone and some loss of trabeculae. Mechanical stress, during phases of acute infiltration, can result in fracture and disintegration of tarsal bones. In most cases of this nature, the acute phase is followed by a period of recalcification. During this period, the skeleton either returns to normal, if undamaged, or is reorganised following disintegration or fracture. Tarsal disintegration as a direct consequence of infiltration is unusual (about 1% of all cases of leprosy).

A more common cause of disintegration and absorption is a perio-steal osteoclastic action, which occurs as a consequence of hyperaemia following ulceration (Kulkarni & Mehta 1983). It is, however, the combination of neuropathy and pathomechanical foot function that most disadvantages the patient with Hansen's disease. Talonavicular and calcaneocuboid instabilities have been implicated as major compromising features, as tarsal disintegration most commonly begins from either of these joints. Excessive calcaneal eversion, with subtalar pronation, may result in the impingement of the lateral process of the talus into the crucial angle of the calcaneus. A splitting of the calcaneus at this location is also a common early feature of tarsal disintegration.

### Absorption and pathological fractures

Brand (1991) recorded that just over 33.3% of patients with Hansen's disease show distinct radiological changes in the bones and joints of the feet. These changes are caused either by infiltration of *M. leprae* (4%) or by secondary changes, including periostitis, osteoporosis, and sequestration with associated pathological fractures and disintegration of bone. *M. leprae* has been described as a specific pathogen with a predilection for infecting bone (in multibacillary disease). However, the more common invasive and destructive nature of non-specific osteomyelitis is attributed to secondary infection. Active secondary infection of ulceration may lead to periostitis and osteomyelitis, which commonly leads to sequestration.

Hyperaemia, associated with chronic plantar ulceration, and active infection of bone can also cause osteoporosis. The osteoporotic state of bone predisposes it to pathological fractures, particularly when pain sensation in the joints is lost. Fracture and infection may lead to absorption of bone, giving rise to short foot or tarsal disintegration. The gross organisation of such feet predisposes them to further ulceration due to the vulnerability of the tissue beneath bony prominences.

### Autonomic impairment

The impairment of dermal sympathetic nerve function may result in the loss of sweat and axon reflexes. Dehydration of the epidermis results in the loss of keratin flexibility and elasticity. The integrity of the skin is therefore compromised and tensile stress causes fatigue and breakdown. Apart from being a contributory factor affecting ulceration, anhidrosis very commonly causes fissures, which are a potentially serious complication for patients as they provide a portal for infection (Fig. 7.1).

### Social and behavioural variables

Hansen's disease is predominantly a problem among lower socio-economic groups. Patients are constrained to continue working to avoid dependence on family members and loss of dignity. Very often the employment opportunities available to sufferers are limited to manual labour and agricultural occupations, where patients are compelled to submit their feet to excessive demands and are unable to rest (Fig. 7.2). Poverty dictates that such patients are unable to purchase suitable footwear, if indeed they can purchase any at all. Podiatry has mainly focused therapeutic developments around the interaction between the foot and footwear. Treating underprivileged, unshod populations is a daunting challenge.

## Complications of ulceration

### Secondary infection

Common causative organisms implicated are *Staphylococcus aureus*, *Streptococcus haemolyticus*, *Pseudomonas aeruginosa*, *Proteus mirabilis* and

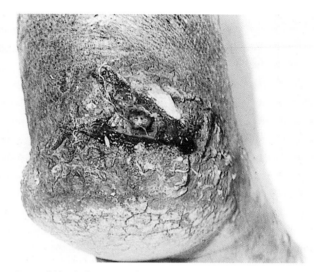

**Figure 7.1** Anhidrotic fissure on the posterior aspect of the heel extending to the calcaneus.

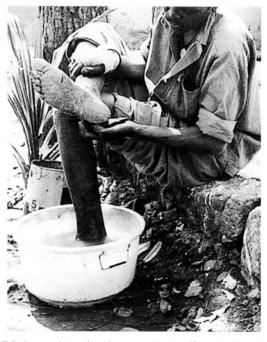

**Figure 7.2** Appropriate education to motivate self-care is the mainstay of impairment control for Hansen's disease patients. A midday break provides a good opportunity for this man to wash his feet in soapy water and rub away hardened skin with a stone. Such diligence is rare.

*Escherichia coli*. Aggravated by continuous mechanical forces in the absence of pain, infection spreads rapidly along tendon sheaths and into synovial joint spaces. Infective arthritis and osteomyelitis are common sequelae found in a 'complicated ulcer'.

### Squamous-cell carcinoma

The chronic irritation of regenerating epithelium around an ulcer and osteomyelitis with chronic discharging sinuses are two of the predisposing factors thought to influence the development of squamous-cell carcinoma. Hyperplasia, influenced by chronic irritation, initiates the regeneration of cells, which manifest as papillomatoses adapted to irritation. Continued irritation leads to dysplasia with decreasing cell differentiation and, ultimately, carcinoma (Sane & Mehta 1988).

## Treatment of pedal pathologies

When treating Hansen's-disease-related foot problems in developing countries, the availability of materials and medications will dictate management options. A sound understanding of therapeutic principles, a pragmatic philosophy and imaginative resourcefulness will be the key attributes of the successful clinician in such circumstances.

### Ulceration

The treatment of neuropathic ulceration should aim to enhance the normal response to trauma. The physiological response to wound healing follows a recognised sequential pattern. The biochemical and cellular responses, demonstrated as inflammation, proliferation and maturation, demonstrate a continuous process that aims to restore continuity and tissue strength. Where the overlapping phases of inflammation, epithelialisation, contraction and connective tissue formation are continuously disrupted, the process of resolution or organisation is confounded by the effects of chronic inflammation. Chronic inflammation is perpetuated by foreign-body irritation and repeated microtrauma. A prolonged inflammatory response is associated with a delay in tissue regeneration and consequent retarded development of tissue tensile strength.

The normal physiological response to ulceration demonstrates three phases:

1. the active phase
2. the proliferative phase
3. the maturation, or remodelling, phase.

### The active phase of ulceration

The leucocytic migration to a traumatised location results in the active debridement and solubilisation of devitalised tissue. Complementing phagocytic activity is the monocytic production of collagenase and proteoglycan-degrading enzymes. Associated with the increased migration of macrophages and plasma proteins is the accumulation of transudate. The normally clear, straw-coloured serous exudate displays discoloration and odour, reflecting its altered status as a cellular aggregate. The viscous and purulent aggregate of cells and debris that drains from an opened wound is a sterile exudation. Within a week, the cells and plasma constituents of the exudate cease to function and become incorporated into a necrotic coagulum. Necrotic tissue (slough) may remain relatively fluid or dehydrates to become a hardened eschar. In the active phase of ulceration, discharge is copious. The volume of exudate inhibits the consolidation of materials to form an eschar. Oedema and infection can contribute considerably to the amount of exudate expressed.

Unresolved disruptive forces perpetuate haemostatic mechanisms. The occlusion of microcirculation serves to exacerbate the anoxic necrosis of tissue. Where pressure is implicated as a precipitating factor, endothelial cells lining the microcirculation become separated. The resultant separation of junctional complexes allows contact between procoagulants of the blood and subendothelial tissues, notably collagen, causing an aggregation of platelets. Platelet aggregation leads to vascular occlusion and further tissue necrosis (Barton 1976, Cruickshank 1976).

The pathological process during the destructive phase of ulceration causes the lesion to spread inwards, thereby destroying subcutaneous tissue faster than the overlying skin. The undermined edges of active

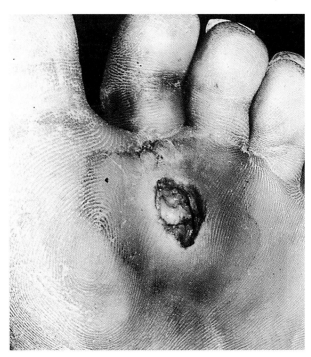

**Figure 7.3** The undermined edges of active ulcers are a characteristic feature. The second metatarsal head is a common site for the first ulcer.

ulcers are a characteristic feature (Fig. 7.3). Recently formed and active ulcers have been described as exhibiting a mobile relationship with deeper tissues. The organisation of fibrous tissue associated with chronicity results in the lesion being tied to deeper structures, thereby reducing its mobility. The indurated and punched-out edges of chronic ulceration are the manifestation of the accumulation of collagen (Kloth & Miller 1990).

### The proliferative phase of ulceration

*Granulation.* A primary indication of ulcer resolution is the appearance of granulation tissue at the base of an ulcer. Granulation tissue is a vascular and lymphatic system in a gel-like matrix, contained within a fibrous collagen network. The matrix is composed of hyaluronic acid and fibronectin, with other salts and colloidal materials. The vascular network carries nutrients to macrophages and fibroblasts, while the lymphatics prevent oedema. Granulation tissue is produced until the wound cavity is filled, reducing the depth of the ulcer almost to the level of the surrounding skin (Thomas 1990).

*Re-epithelialisation.* The spread of granulation to the level of the skin stimulates the activation of the epithelium, which begins to proliferate over the wound (Thomas 1990). It has been suggested that wounded tissue does not produce chalones, and therefore that the separated surfaces at a free edge would not be subject to the inhibitory effect of chalone on biological events. This hypothesis may explain the common occurrence of hyperkeratinisation around the periphery of ulcers (Daly 1990).

*Factors influencing healing during the active and proliferative phases.* Vitamin C and oxygen are fundamental factors influencing the hydroxylation of proline and lysine. When there is a deficit of these factors there follows an inhibition of collagen synthesis. Vitamin A deficiency has been recorded as delaying re-epithelialisation. Protein deficiency results in an amino acid deficit, causing a consequent lack of availability of material to structure granulation tissue. Protein deficiency may have an inhibiting effect on host defence against infection. Deficiency of trace elements, particularly zinc and copper, has been implicated as a cause of delayed healing (Daly 1990, Westaby 1982, Zederfeldt et al 1986).

Other factors recorded as inhibiting wound healing include systemic and topical steroids, antineoplastic drugs, haemostatic agents, non-steroidal anti-inflammatory drugs, nicotine and many systemic antibiotics. Local conditions may be compromised by the effects of antimicrobial toxicity, while dressings may adversely affect healing by creating an unsuitable environment for this process (Daly 1990, Westaby 1982).

### The maturation or remodelling phase of ulceration

An outline of events characterising this phase includes the decline in concentration of fibroblasts and the complex reorientation of collagen fibres. The result is eventual consolidation of scar tissue, which displays a maximum strength of 20% less than that of intact skin. The realignment of collagen fibres is thought to be a response to pressure. When pressure is applied, collagen releases piezoelectric substances. It is postulated that these stress-generated voltages are responsible for the realignment and general maintenance of collagen (Price 1990).

### Mal perforans

Complicated ulcers (Fig. 7.4) extend to involve tendons, synovial sheaths, joint capsules and bone. Pyogenic infection of bone may result from the localisation of infection via a haematogenous route or from abscesses. Infection may lead to chronic osteomyelitis with multiple sinus formation. A more common causative factor contributing to involvement of deeper tissue is secondary infection of an uncomplicated ulcer. Sequestration, remodelling of bone and copious periosteal reaction are associated with pyogenic infection. In such cases,

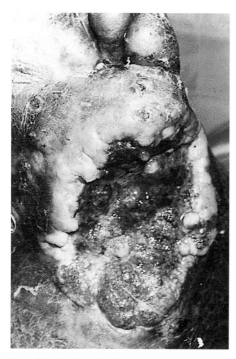

**Figure 7.4** Complicated ulcer. The hypergranulating surface suggests the involvement of necrotic bone.

restoration of tissue stability is dependent on overcoming infection and the removal of necrotic bone and soft tissue. In the absence of compromising factors, complicated ulcers proceed to heal by secondary intention.

### Enhancing the healing process

Factors that should be taken into account include:

- infection control
- maintaining an optimal wound environment
- rest.

### Infection control

Hansen's disease is not associated with generally compromised immunological defences. Where other variables are addressed, healing is usually faster than diabetic ulceration, because Hansen's disease is not complicated by vascular disease. The immune system may, however, be suppressed by systemic and topical steroid therapy, malnutrition and nicotine. These factors should be considered when planning infection control. The choice of antiseptic medicaments should be balanced between the perceived threat of infection and the cytotoxicity of available medicaments.

### Maintaining an optimal wound environment

The general principles of ulcer management are that the lesion should be kept clean and clear of slough, avascular or necrotic soft tissue (see Ch. 10). Overlying callus and epidermis should be excised to reduce stress and encourage healing by secondary intention. Excessively discharging complicated lesions or hypergranulating lesions indicate investigation for sequestrae or other foreign bodies, which must be removed.

The lesion should be kept moist at all times. During the active phase, dressings capable of absorbing exudate are indicated. During the proliferative and remodelling phases there is greater danger from the wound becoming too dry; the choice of dressings should be considered accordingly.

An ideal wound environment can be maintained where the following are ensured:

- thermal stability (exposure to cold or heat will impede healing)
- unimpeded gaseous exchange
- inaccessibility to microorganisms, arthropods and foreign bodies (including fibres from dressings)
- avoidance of strike-through of gauze-type dressings (strike-through can provide access to the lesion for microorganisms)
- careful removal of adherent dressings (delicate granulation and/or epithelium are easily traumatised)
- avoidance of inappropriate dressings (incorrect dressings can counteract the healing process by compromising the wound environment).

### Rest

Wherever possible, patients with acute ulceration should be treated with bed rest and medication. Where this is possible, after a week the oedema and discharge will have diminished and a walking plaster can be applied. Plaster casting is contraindicated for profusely discharging ulcers. If, after a week, the ulcer continues to discharge copiously, involvement of bony tissue should be considered. Swelling subsides rapidly when the foot is immobilised, and unless the plaster is removed after the first week, the cast may become loose and problematic. Further plaster casts can be applied and changed depending on the rate of discharge from the ulcer, looseness of cast and the extent of wear. Although ulcers have been known to heal within 3 weeks, the patient should be advised not to expect healing before 6 weeks. Attention to plaster-casting technique cannot be overemphasised. Well-applied plaster, appropriately placed padding, and either a rubber heel or wooden rocker will immobilise the foot and distribute forces over the foot and up the leg.

Debate continues about the efficacy of window casting. The advantage is that direct access is given to the ulcer for dressing and assessment. The major disadvantage is that oedema can result in the protrusion of the ulcer into the window. In such cases healing is delayed and the ulcer is vulnerable to further trauma.

## Orthotic options

Simple ulcers of 1 cm diameter have been shown to heal using appropriate appliance therapy (Cross et al 1995, 1996). Appliance therapy is also particularly useful for the preservation of the foot after healing by plaster casting. The recurrence of ulceration after cast removal is a common problem.

Resource availability will dictate orthotic prescription and manufacture. There is no substitute for a thorough grounding in functional anatomy, biomechanics and the therapeutic rationale supporting appliance therapy.

*Note.* Functional orthoses should not be supplied unless the patient can be monitored diligently.

Orthotic prescription is based on:

- footwear
- availability of the patient for monitoring
- biomechanical examination of the foot
- gait analysis.

Detailed screening and examination may indicate patients at risk of ulceration or tarsal disintegration. Timely orthotic intervention may be a valuable adjunct to other disability-prevention measures (ILEP Medical Commission 1993, Watson 1986).

## Case studies

*The context.* Case studies 7.1 and 7.2 were recorded at the Lalgadh Leprosy Services Centre, Nepal. The centre serves a rural community in an area of high endemicity for leprosy (18 per 10 000). The region in which the hospital is situated is underdeveloped, and as a consequence the catchment area is extensive. People may walk for 2 days to avail themselves of services; however, for most a visit to the Outpatient Department constitutes a full day away from home and employment. Cultural factors dictate that women (apart from the destitute) may not travel unaccompanied. Very few people are able to visit more frequently than once a month, and for many even this is not an option due to economic pressures.

### CASE STUDY 7.1 **IMPAIRMENT CONTROL**

*History.* A 14-year-old boy presented at the Outpatient Department. The patient's father had become suspicious of the hypopigmented patches on the boy's face and legs and had brought his son for further investigations. Neither the patient or his father were certain of the time since the appearance of the patches. However, it was approximately a year since the patient's peers had noticed the patches and had begun to persecute him.

There was no previous history of Hansen's disease in the family.

## ON EXAMINATION

*Skin examination.* The anaesthetic macules demonstrated a morphology typical of borderline tuberculoid leprosy.

*Nerve function assessment.* Sensory testing was conducted using Semmes–Weinstein monofilaments (Brandsma 1994) and the boy was found to present with sensory loss affecting the plantar aspects of both feet. The development of anhidrotic fissures was evidence of possible autonomic palsy. There was no loss of muscle function affecting the lower limb, but a weakness of fifth finger function (right hand) suggested impairment of the ulnar nerve. Following careful questioning it was ascertained that the posterior tibial nerve function impairment was of approximately 4 months duration and that the ulnar nerve impairment was of approximately 2 months duration.

*Biomechanical assessment.* On weight-bearing examination the boy presented with excessively pronated subtalar joints in the relaxed calcaneal stance position. This was considered to be a compensation for marked genu varum. The neutral calcaneal stance position demonstrated that when the subtalar joint was neutral the calcaneums were aligned at 10° inversion.

On non-weight-bearing examination of the feet no forefoot abnormalities were found.

Gait analysis revealed that aphasic subtalar pronation extended throughout the gait cycle.

## TREATMENT

The boy and his father were counselled carefully to enable them to accept that the boy did have Hansen's disease and that he required treatment with multidrug therapy for 1 year.

He was supplied with abendazole for the treatment of intestinal infestation prior to receiving an initial supply of steroids. A course of prednisolone, tapering after 2 weeks from an initial dose of 45 mg, was prescribed for the restoration of nerve function. (Steroid therapy is indicated where nerve function impairment is of less than 6 months duration.)

He was supplied with sandals supporting microcellular rubber soles. The sandals incorporated appliances, which have become known among leprosy organisations of the Indian subcontinent as 'hatti pads'. The function of the appliance is essentially to limit the extent of pronation and to support the arch to facilitate better first-ray function. The hatti pad incorporates a heel meniscus where the medial aspect is broader than the lateral aspect and is angled to limit the extent to which the heel may otherwise evert. It extends to include an arch support. The arch support is carefully designed and manufactured to give maximum support beneath the navicular. It slopes anteriorly to end immediately proximal to all the metatarsal heads (except the fifth) and laterally to the lateral tread line. It thus conforms closely to the architecture of the arch.

The boy and his father were offered places in the Self-care Training Centre to assist the boy in his orientation to the disease and its treatment. The Self-care Training Centre offers a 14-day programme that aims to enable people affected by leprosy to learn how to adopt safe practices for the prevention of further impairment and possible disability. A further objective is that on completion of the course people affected by leprosy will be better able to cope with possible psychosocial effects of the disease.

## FOLLOW-UP

The boy returned monthly for monitoring and supply of drugs, footwear and foot appliances. He did recover function in the ulnar nerve but sensory function was not restored to the plantar surfaces of his feet. Up to the time of reporting this study he has avoided plantar ulceration and has managed to maintain his plantar skin in reasonably good order. He has adjusted well to the disease and receives strong family and community support.

## CASE STUDY 7.2 IMPAIRMENT MANAGEMENT, DISABILITY LIMITATION AND SOCIAL EMPOWERMENT

### HISTORY

A woman of uncertain age (between 25 and 35 years) presented at the Outpatient Department with a foul-smelling plantar ulcer on her left foot.

The patient's file catalogued a complex history over the previous 6 years. Four years earlier she had completed treatment for lepromatous leprosy, complicated by recurrent episodes of type 2 reaction and iritis. Since cure from the disease she had presented on numerous occasions and had been treated for ulceration of her hands and feet.

The patient had extensive impairments, including an anaesthetic clawed right hand, an anaesthetic left hand with loss of index and ring fingers and clawing and shortening of other fingers. Both feet were anaesthetic. The patient's right foot had undergone extensive damage, resulting in short foot deformity, while her left foot had lost all toes. The patient's nasal septum had collapsed.

The records related that the patient had lost two children and that her husband had evicted her from their home. Until recently, she had been living in a neighbour's buffalo shed where her husband and others had from time to time sent her food.

### ON EXAMINATION

An ulcer issuing copious foul-smelling exudate was found beneath the first metatarsal head. The distal aspect of the lower left leg was hot, and on palpation the left groin lymph node was found to be swollen and very tender.

Further examination using a probe revealed that the metatarsal head was fragmenting. Some maggots were extricated from recesses in the wound.

The patient was found to be detached and unresponsive to questioning.

### DIAGNOSIS

The patient's primary presenting problem was an acute infected complicated ulcer with osteomyelitis of the first metatarsal head. Secondary effects were cellulitis and lymphadenectasis.

There were indications that the patient was depressed.

### TREATMENT

The patient was admitted for treatment of an acute septic condition.

As an inpatient, immediate bed rest with elevation of the limb was ordered. Following consultation, the physician prescribed amoxicillin, gentamicin and intravenous infusion of Ringer's lactate.

Necrotic soft tissue was excised, sequestrae were removed and the distal end of the metatarsal shaft was resurfaced. Further examination revealed that the infection had begun to track along the sheath of flexor hallucis longus. An incision was made proximally to expose the tendon and 2 cm of infected tendon was excised. Betadine packing with a secondary gauze dressing was applied and the wound was bandaged. Following examination the next day secondary sutures were applied.

Betadine dressings were applied until the removal of sutures. Following the removal of sutures saline dressings were applied for a further week, after which a walking plaster was applied for 4 weeks. On removal of the plaster the wound had resolved to the extent that it had become a simple ulcer. At this stage the patient began self-care of the ulcer.

During conversations with the patient it became apparent that she was unable to wear protective footwear in her village due to the censure of the community. Simple self-care procedures (soaking and oiling of plantar and palmar skin) also drew strong negative reactions. It was also apparent that the attitude of the community had seriously eroded the patient's self-esteem, making it unlikely that she would be motivated to take any appropriate precautionary measures. A further stage of the treatment, therefore, was to address the social pathology. A visit was made to the village where discussion with village leaders and the patient's neighbours gave an opportunity to educate the community concerning the true nature of the problem. Having the benefit of understanding, the community agreed to take positive action to help the patient. It was also agreed that Lalgadh Leprosy Services would establish means by which she would become less dependent on the community for economic assistance (in this instance breeding goats were supplied for the patient).

During the remainder of her period of admission a biomechanical assessment was undertaken. The patient's right foot had been reduced to little more than an apropulsive prop. It was essential, therefore, to locate areas that would be vulnerable to the effects of high pressure and to manufacture an appropriate 'moulded' insole to palliate the foot.

The patient's left foot presented with a pronated subtalar joint during weight bearing. On non-weight-bearing examination the loss of the first metatarsal head resulted in a superior displacement of the medial aspect of the forefoot. The potential for high shearing stress injury resulting from late and excessive subtalar pronation to compensate for the iatrogenic forefoot varus was considered a high risk. The medial aspect of the foot was also extremely vulnerable due to the recent episode of ulceration. For this foot a tarsal cradle constructed from microcellular rubber was prescribed.

Both appliances were manufactured and placed into custom-made microcellular rubber sandals. These were supplied with Velcro fittings for ease of wear with deformed hands.

### FOLLOW-UP

The patient continued to return on an occasional basis for repeat footwear/appliance supply. The patient's social conditions had improved, as had her attitude. However, she did continue to present with simple ulcers on the plantar aspect of her right 'short foot'. The episodes were much less frequent and the injuries very much less severe on presentation.

## TROPICAL DISEASES

Skin infection and tropical diseases presenting on the foot may represent a primary condition or a secondary manifestation of illness elsewhere in the body. Cutaneous larva migrans, madura foot and localised cutaneous simple leishmaniasis are examples of the former, whereas the latter can be exemplified by systemic conditions such as leprosy, disseminated leishmaniasis and coccidioidomycosis.

When approaching a patient with a tropical skin disease on the feet the podiatrist should carry out a thorough exercise in history taking. This must include detailed information on previous skin disease, travel history, occupation, duration of signs and symptoms, evolution of clinical signs, and a fast practical assessment of the patient's immune status. The identification of extracutaneous signs such as fever, enlarged lymph nodes and general malaise indicate systemic illness, and these findings should prompt immediate action for an appropriate referral. Particular epidemiological settings determine exposure and attack rates of specific diseases, and hence an understanding of the global geographical pathology and living conditions of the overseas population is required.

The prevalence of skin diseases in the tropics is similar to that found in developed countries. The main differences found in tropical settings are a higher incidence of endemic infectious diseases, a lower frequency of skin malignancy, and a lack of or decreased availability of podiatric and dermatological services. Moreover, poor living conditions, overcrowding and malnutrition account for a variety of cutaneous signs and symptoms related to poverty. A vast number of tropical diseases manifest on one or both feet, and this chapter contains up-to-date information on this field of podiatry. The following sections are organised to present the most relevant conditions grouped by aetiological agents, and the main emphasis is on clinical findings and diagnosis as a practical guide to everyday work in podiatry. Pathogenesis of disease and management of conditions are also included.

# Bacterial infections

## Pyogenic infections

### Aetiology and pathogenesis

Common bacterial infections of the skin are caused by *Staphylococcus* and *Streptococcus* species. These infectious agents are ubiquitous in both urban and rural environments, and are capable of causing disease in individuals of all age groups. Healthy and immunocompromised hosts develop pyogenic infections of the foot following direct inoculation of bacteria. Less often, haematogenous dissemination to the lower limb, and even a septicaemic state, may develop as a result of a minor injury on the foot. The port of entry for these pathogenic organisms is often unnoticed by both the patient and doctor, but minor injuries, insect bites, friction blisters or superficial fungal infection are the commonest means of entry found in clinical practice. Other clinical circumstances, such as burns, use of indwelling catheters in children and surgical procedures, also play a role as risk factors for these infections.

Pyogenic bacteria cause damage in the infected tissue by the pathogenic action of proteases, haemolysins, lipoteichoic acid and coagulases. Erythrogenic toxins are responsible for the erythema commonly observed on feet infected by *Streptococcus* species (Bisno & Stevens 1996).

### Clinical findings and diagnosis

The clinical spectrum of pyogenic infections of the foot includes folliculitis, furuncle and carbuncle formation on areas with hair follicles. Plaques of impetigo and infiltrated thickened dermis can affect any region of the foot, and are caused by *Staphylococcus* and *Streptococcus* species, respectively. Abscess formation, cellulitis, and necrotic ulceration represent the more severe end of the spectrum.

The perimalleolar regions are far more commonly affected than other areas of the foot, as they are exposed to mechanical trauma. The dorsum, toes and heels follow in frequency.

Common clinical signs of pyogenic infections include a variety of manifestations such as erythema, inflammation, pus discharge, abscess formation, ulceration, blistering, necrotising lesions and gangrene (Figs 7.5–7.8). Most pyogenic skin infections are painful.

The diagnosis of pyogenic infection of the foot is based on the clinical history and findings. Bacteriological investigations and sensitivity profile to antibiotics must be carried out if possible. Disseminated, chronic or severe infections require an immediate referral to a dermatologist or an infectious disease specialist.

### Management and treatment

Mild infections are successfully treated by bathing or soaking the affected foot in potassium permanganate solution (1 : 10 000 dilution in water) for 15 minutes daily. Other mild superficial infections, such as isolated plaques of impetigo or impetiginised eczema, respond well to antiseptic or antimicrobial creams and ointments containing cetrimide, chlorhexidine, fucidic acid or mupirocin. Acute or chronic

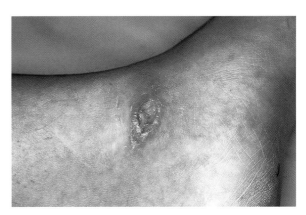

Figure 7.5 Pyogenic ulcer on the medial malleolus.

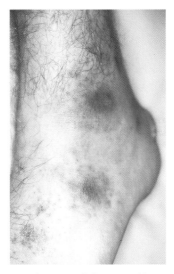

Figure 7.6 Purpuric patches and cellulitis caused by *Streptococcus* species.

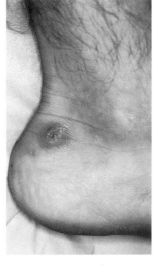

Figure 7.7 Seaborne pyogenic verrucous lesion surrounded by erythema.

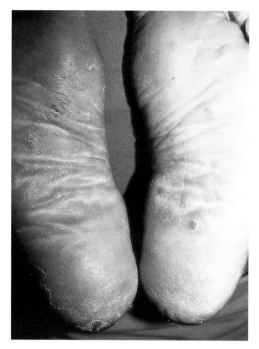

**Figure 7.8** Syphilis. Asymptomatic bilateral papules and scaling.

foot eczema requires treatment with potent topical steroids in order to eliminate risk factors for infection. Infections with multiple lesions, or those involving larger areas of the foot, require a complete course of systemic β-lactam or macrolide antibiotics in addition to the above topical treatments. Recurrent episodes of cellulitis require longer courses of these antibiotics, and hospitalisation followed by surgical debridement is mandatory in necrotic lesions, gangrenous plaques and deeper infections with severe fasciitis. Superficial infections of the foot skin complicated by deeper involvement with necrosis of soft tissues carry a high mortality rate (up to 25%) (Elliot et al 1996).

## Treponemal infections

Cosmopolitan treponemal diseases such as secondary *syphilis* present with an asymptomatic, symmetrical papular eruption and scaling of plantar regions (Fig. 7.8). Other clinical features, such as concurrent palmar involvement, the history of a primary chancre and the characteristic trunkal rash, confirm the clinical suspicion. A definitive diagnosis can be established by specific tests such as a positive darkfield microscopy from early skin lesions, as well as from highly sensitive treponemal serology (Young 1992). Despite the fact that syphilis is not strictly a tropical disease, it represents a significant problem for the returning traveller involved in high-risk sexual activities while in the tropics (WHO 1986). The treatment of choice is penicillin, but allergic individuals respond to erythromycin or tetracyclines.

*Yaws* is a treponemal tropical disease manifesting on the feet and periorificial skin on the face. This condition affects mainly the male rural population in South America, Sub-Saharan Africa and South East Asia. This disease is associated with poverty in the humid tropics (Sehgal et al 1994) and one of the characteristic clinical presentations is that of plantar hyperkeratosis. Late tertiary infection results in asymptomatic palmoplantar keratoderma that develops nodular hyperkeratotic lesions leading to painful disability; hence the characteristic walk known as 'crab yaws'. The clinical picture can be difficult to differentiate from that of other types of infectious and non-infectious plantar keratodermas. Tests for diagnosis include dark-field microscopy of early lesions and treponemal serology. The treatment of choice is penicillin but *Treponema pallidum pertenue* also responds to tetracyclines and macrolides.

## Other bacterial infections manifesting on the foot

Tropical *seaborne infections* by halophilic *Vibrio vulnificus* can produce localised or systemic disease manifested by acute and painful erythema, purpura, oedema and necrosis on one or both feet. The infection is acquired by direct traumatic inoculation in estuaries and seawater, or by ingestion of raw seafood, particularly oysters. Male individuals with a history of liver disease and iron-overload states are the group at highest risk of this infection (Serrano-Jaen & Vega-López 2000). Severe cases require immediate referral to a specialist hospital physician, as intravenous antibiotics and early surgical debridement represent the treatment of choice.

Exfoliation of the plantar skin is part of the complex and severe picture in cosmopolitan cases with *staphylococcal scalded skin syndrome* (SSSS) (Cribier et al 1994), whereas necrotic ulceration of the foot can result from tropical *cutaneous diphtheria* caused by *Corynebacterium diphtheriae* (Belsey & LeBlanc 1975). Cutaneous diphtheria commonly manifests as a non-healing single ulcerated lesion on the toe or toe cleft lasting between 4 and 12 weeks.

## Mycobacterial infections

### Aetiology and pathogenesis

Several mycobacterial species can cause primary or secondary infection of the foot. The 'swimming' or 'fish-tank granuloma' is an infection caused by *Mycobacterium marinum*. Other common chronic mycobacterial tropical infections include leprosy, tuberculosis and Buruli ulcer. These are caused by *Mycobacterium leprae*, *Mycobacterium tuberculosis* and *Mycobacterium ulcerans*, respectively. Mycobacterial skin diseases can be acquired by direct skin contact with a patient, by direct accidental or occupational inoculation, and by inhalation of the infective organisms. Particular clinical forms of cutaneous tuberculosis result following haematogenous dissemination from a primary infection elsewhere. The respiratory route is particularly important for leprosy and diverse forms of pulmonary tuberculosis. In the case of Buruli ulcer it has recently been suggested that contact with infected water in rural areas of Africa may represent the main source of infection. A toxin called mycolactone seems to be responsible for the severe tissue destruction and ulceration seen in patients with Buruli ulcer (Thangaraj et al 1999). In general, however, it is accepted that agents causing mycobacterial skin diseases have a low pathogenic potential, as most infected individuals in endemic regions do not develop clinical mycobacterial diseases.

Mycobacteria are very complex organisms; most of them are ubiquitous in nature as saprophytes, but a number of species cause disease in other animals. A very thick wall surrounds the cytoplasmic membrane of mycobacteria and contains virulence factors such as proteins and glycolipids. Mycobacteria can inhibit an efficient phagocytosis and intracellular killing by macrophages and can also interact with the host's immune cells. This interaction results in chronic inflammation, tissue damage, and immunopathology, all of which account for the signs and symptoms observed in the wide range of mycobacterial diseases.

### Clinical findings and diagnosis

#### Fish-tank granuloma

This affects more commonly the fingers or hand dorsum but it has also been described on the foot. *M. marinum* frequently infects freshwater fish, and hence individuals handling fish tanks represent the main population at risk (Gray et al 1990). Direct inoculation into the foot presents with similar clinical findings to those found in infections of the upper limb. The disease manifests as a localised progressing swelling with variable pain, and the appearance, within a few weeks, of nodular or verrucous skin lesions on the affected area. These lesions can show ulceration and bleeding from the disease process itself but also from mechanical trauma. The nodular lesions, measuring from a few millimetres up to 2–3 cm, may resolve spontaneously after a few months, but they can also disseminate proximally by haematogenous or lymphatic spread. The dorsal aspects of the foot and the malleolar regions are exposed to trauma, and therefore direct inoculation commonly takes place on these regions. Once the condition is suspected, microbiological and histopathological investigations represent the most sensitive tests to confirm the clinical diagnosis.

## Leprosy

Advanced disease manifests with skin atrophy, pigmentary changes and, in severe cases, chronic ulceration leading to disability (Fig. 7.9). Mutilating lesions of the toes result from bone resorption, mechanical trauma, and secondary bacterial infection.

The clinical diagnosis of leprosy can be easily established in most cases that occur in endemic regions of the world (Bryceson & Pfaltzgraff 1990). Epidemiological, clinical, histopathological, bacteriological and immunological criteria have been used for many years to diagnose and classify the cases of leprosy within a disease spectrum. This spectrum considers two polar groups or forms, called tuberculoid and lepromatous, as well as intermediate forms of the disease defined as borderline. Early disease may not present characteristics of any of the above groups and such cases are called indeterminate. Patients with early disease, and particularly those presenting to the podiatrist in countries non-endemic for leprosy, often pose diagnostic difficulties. The delay in establishing an accurate diagnosis and treatment inevitably results in irreversible nerve damage and chronic complications with variable degrees of disability.

## Skin tuberculosis

This affects individuals of all ages and both sexes, who present with a wide variety of clinical pictures that frequently affect the lower limbs and particularly one or both feet (Chopra & Vega-López 1999). However, lupus vulgaris and papulonecrotic tuberculide are more common in females, whereas tuberculosis verrucosa cutis is rare in children. By far the main clinical presentation of cutaneous tuberculosis affecting the adult foot is called tuberculosis verrucosa cutis. The tuberculous bacilli cause disease following direct inoculation into the skin but clinical disease can also result from haematogenous dissemination. Unilateral involvement is the rule in almost all cases. Commonly observed asymptomatic lesions include dry patches of atrophic skin, pigmentary changes, nodules and plaques of verrucous lesions. The total plaque of tuberculosis can measure 2–12 cm in diameter, but chronic and larger lesions can involve most of the foot dorsum and lateral aspects. The course of cutaneous tuberculosis is indolent and chronic, but determines skin atrophy and variable degrees of scarring with a consequent degree of local skin insufficiency. The clinical diagnosis can be confirmed by histopathology, bacteriology and polymerase chain reaction (PCR) investigations.

## Buruli ulcer

This affects mainly young individuals in rural Africa – and particularly in West Africa where an increase in incidence has been reported (Thangaraj et al 1999). More than two-thirds of the cases present in children below the age of 15 years. The initial lesions present as papules or small nodules that slowly increase in size to the point of causing an area of inflammation and subsequently ulceration of the skin. The ulcer characteristically presents with undermined edges and manifests active indolent phagedenism, often involving large areas of the affected limb. A single ulcer, or smaller coalescing ulcers, present more frequently on the lower leg above the ankles, but other regions of the foot can be involved as well. Oedematous forms may progress rapidly and cause a panniculitis with destruction of underlying tissues such as fascia and bone. In cases where a large ulceration is followed by healing, contractures of the affected limb result from scarring. Severe scarring and contractures have been identified as a high morbidity factor for disability and up to 10% require amputation of the deformed limb (Josse et al 1994).

## Management and treatment of mycobacterial infections

All mycobacterial diseases require highly specialised diagnostic investigations that, in many cases, can be carried out only in a tertiary hospital setting. Most mycobacterial diseases affecting the skin represent public health priorities, not only in the endemic countries where they occur but also at an international level as established by the WHO. Following the diagnosis of individual cases, a long-term multidrug therapeutic regimen can be prescribed only by specialised physicians. Mycobacteria are known to develop resistance to antibiotics, and it is imperative that all cases be treated with combinations of at least two drugs. The main drugs with antimycobacterial activity are rifampin, ethambutol, pirazinamide, clofazimine, sulfone, isoniazide, macrolide antibiotics, tetracyclines and quinolones. The management of all mycobacterial diseases must consider not only the medical treatment but also a full range of educational initiatives aimed at the patient, the community and the health personnel. Early lesions of fish-tank granuloma, skin tuberculosis, and particularly those caused by Buruli ulcer require surgical excision.

## Bacterial mycetoma

### Aetiology and pathogenesis

*Nocardia*, *Actinomadura* and *Streptomyces* species are the common aetiological agents of 'madura foot' or actinomycetoma. This form of

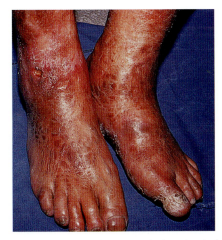

**Figure 7.9** Atrophy, pigmentary changes and ulceration in leprosy.

bacterial mycetoma occurs in tropical countries, and the main case series have been reported from Sudan, Senegal, Nigeria, Saudi Arabia, India and Mexico. The infection is acquired by direct inoculation of bacteria into the skin. Young male individuals living in endemic regions and dedicated to agricultural activities have been reported to have the highest incidence of actinomycetoma (López-Martínez et al 1992). Bacteria causing actinomycetoma have a thick wall surrounding the cytoplasmic membrane that is rich in lipid and carbohydrate compounds. Some of these compounds, such as lipoarabinomannan and mycolic acids, have been identified as virulence factors. These bacteria are capable of blocking the adequate killing mechanisms by the cells of the infected host; however, it is considered that they have a low pathogenic potential and most of them live as saprophytes in the soil.

### Clinical findings and diagnosis

The clinical disease is characterised by a chronic course, with inflammation, formation of sinus tracts discharging 'grains' and progressive deformity of the affected foot (Fig. 7.10). Healing of discharging sinus tracts over the years determines scarring, with atrophic skin plaques and secondary pigmentary changes. Asymptomatic nodular or verrucous lesions can also be found, and in a few cases a variable range of symptoms is present. These include pain that often results from superimposed pyogenic infection, acute inflammation and bone involvement. The chronic infection with deformity of the foot determines periosteal involvement and subsequently osteomyelitis. Variable but often severe degrees of disability complete the chronic course of actinomycetoma.

The clinical picture manifested on one foot is highly suggestive of the diagnosis. The main differential diagnosis includes mycetoma caused by fungi (see the section on eumycetoma, below) but other forms of 'cold' abscess formation, histoplasmosis, chromoblastomycosis, cutaneous tuberculosis and sarcoidosis are the other main conditions to consider. Direct microscopy to disclose the 'grains' discharged from sinus tracts confirms the diagnosis, and the culture of this material also provides a definite diagnosis of actinomycetoma.

### Management and treatment

Effective drugs against the agents of bacterial mycetoma include streptomycin, dapsone and trimethoprim/sulfamethoxasol (Welsh 1991). Recently, a report revealed efficacy with a combination of trimethoprim/sulfamethoxasol, amikacin and immunomodulators (Serrano-Jaén, personal communication, 1999). The treatment has to be administered for several months and the therapeutic response is variable. Early cases of mycetoma presenting with small lesions can be

cured by surgical excision. In contrast, advanced cases with periosteal involvement and those with osteomyelitis do not respond to medical treatment, and radical surgery of the foot represents the only therapeutic option.

## Parasitic diseases, ectoparasite infestations and bites

### Cutaneous larva migrans

#### Aetiology and pathogenesis

This dermatosis results from the accidental penetration of the human skin by parasitic larvae from domestic canine and feline hosts. Cats and dogs pass ova of these helminths within the stools and larval stages develop in the soil or beach sand. Close contact with human skin allows the infective larvae to burrow into the epidermis and cause clinical disease. The main aetiological agents are *Ancylostoma brasiliensae*, *A. caninum*, *A. ceylanicum* and *A. stenocephalae* but other species affecting ruminants and pigs can also cause human disease. Following penetration into the skin, the larvae are incapable of crossing the human epidermodermal barrier, and stay in the epidermis creeping across spongiotic vesicles until they die a few days or weeks later. Multiple infections can, however, last for several months.

#### Clinical findings and diagnosis

The plantar regions of one or both feet represent the main anatomical site affected by cutaneous larva migrans, but any part of the body in contact with infested soil or sand can be involved. Individuals of all age groups and both sexes can be affected, and the disease is a common problem for tourists on beach holidays where they walk bare foot or lie on the infested sand. A report of 50 cases presenting in returning travellers attending a specialised clinic in London revealed that 70% of the lesions were located on one foot (Blackwell & Vega-López 2000). The initial lesion is a pruriginous papule at the site of penetration that appears within a day following the infestation. An erythematous, raised, larval track measuring 1–3 mm in width and height starts progressing in a curved or looped fashion (Fig. 7.11). New segments of larval track reveal that the organism can advance at a speed of 2–5 cm/day. Commonly, the larval track measures between a few millimetres up to several centimetres in the region adjacent to the penetration site, but uncommon cases may present long larval tracks surrounding large areas of the foot with a well-defined

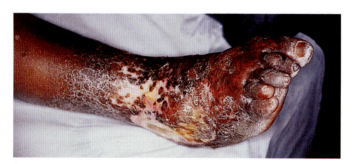

**Figure 7.10** Actinomycetoma with deformity, multiple sinus tract formation and scarring.

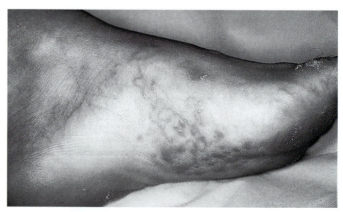

**Figure 7.11** Tracks and inflammatory reaction in cutaneous larva migrans.

perimalleolar distribution. Localised clinical presentations on the toes may present with only papular lesions, but other presentations include blisters and urticarial wheals. Secondary complications to the presence of the parasite in the epidermis include an inflammatory reaction, eczematisation, impetiginised tracks or papules, and even deeper pyogenic infections. Variable in severity, but most commonly intense, pruritus and burning sensation are the main symptoms.

The diagnosis is based on the clinical history and physical findings on the affected skin. The histopathological investigation has little, if any, value in the diagnosis of cutaneous larva migrans. The study of 332 cases in central Mexico over 10 years in the 1980s (Orozco, personal communication, 1993) revealed that haematoxylin–eosin (HE) preparations of affected skin show a spongiotic acute or subacute dermatitis with a variable presence of larval structures. A mild perivascular lymphocytic infiltrate was frequently observed in the dermis, and a low proportion of cases may develop peripheral eosinophilia, but this is not a constant finding.

### Management and treatment

The treatment of choice is the systemic administration of albendazol for 3 days. Topical options include a 10% thiabendazol cream applied several times daily for 10 days, and one or more sessions of cryotherapy with liquid nitrogen. Resistant cases may respond to a single dose of systemic ivermectin (Caumes et al 1992).

## Leishmaniasis

### Aetiology and pathogenesis

*Leishmania* species parasites are protozoan organisms transmitted to humans and other vertebrates by the bite of female sandflies of the genera *Phlebotomus* or *Lutzomya*. Most *Leishmania* species can cause skin or mucocutaneous disease, but a few of them affect internal organs as well. It is estimated that 15 million individuals are infected by *Leishmania* in 88 countries. The main endemic foci are found in Asia, the Middle East, Africa, Southern Europe and Latin America. Hot and humid environments such as those found in rain forest jungles provide adequate habitats for the vectors in Latin America. In contrast, desert conditions favour breeding sites for the vectors in the Middle Eastern and North African endemic regions (WHO 1990).

Following the bite from a *Leishmania*-infected sandfly, humans can either heal spontaneously or develop localised or disseminated skin disease. Sandfly and *Leishmania* species causing skin disease in humans have been classified in geographical terms as Old World and New World cutaneous leishmaniasis. Both can affect the skin of one foot, but multiple infective bites or disseminated forms may present with lesions on both feet. The bite of the sandfly commonly targets exposed areas such as the external ankles during walking or the medial regions of the foot when the host is at rest. Depending on the area left uncovered by light footwear, the foot dorsum, heel, toes, lateral aspect and plantar region can also be affected by bites.

*Leishmania* parasites can resist phagocytosis and damage by complement proteins from the host by the action of lipophosphoglycan and glycoprotein antigens. Following phagocytosis, the intracellular forms of *Leishmania* parasites induce a delayed-type hypersensitive granulomatous reaction, which adds to the tissue damage.

### Clinical findings and diagnosis

The clinical picture of cutaneous leishmaniasis was recently reviewed by Chopra and Vega-López (1999). The bite of a sandfly may induce an inflammatory papular or nodular lesion of prurigo, but in some cases it may go unnoticed for several weeks. The incubation period can be as short as 15 days but commonly it is estimated at about 4–6 weeks. Certain forms may take longer to develop clinically. A non-

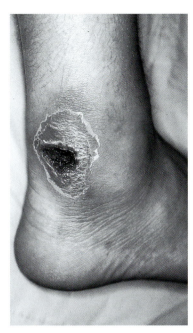

**Figure 7.12** *Leishmania brasiliensis* infection. Ulceration and severe inflammatory reaction.

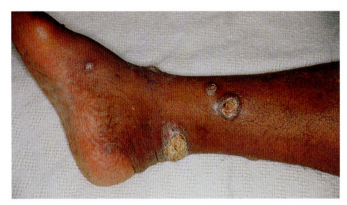

**Figure 7.13** *Leishmania tropica* infection. Multiple nodular ulcers with crust formation.

healing papule with surrounding erythema and pain may also indicate superimposed bacterial infection that subsequently develops ulceration (Fig. 7.12). On average, 6–8 weeks after the sandfly bite a violaceous nodule, with or without nodular borders, starts to enlarge and ulcerate. The ulcer is partially or completely covered by a thick crust (Fig. 7.13) that, following curettage, reveals a haemorrhagic and vegetating bed. Cutaneous leishmaniasis on the foot can manifest clinically as nodules covered with crust, ulceration with a raised inflamed solid border, tissue necrosis and lymphangitic forms. Advanced late forms present with scarring, skin atrophy and pigmentary changes. The plantar regions may be affected by pigmented and hyperkeratotic lesions in a clinical form called 'post-kala-azar dermal leishmaniasis', which presents after an episode of visceral leishmaniasis.

The clinical picture of leishmaniasis on the foot and the history of exposure in an endemic region of the world strongly suggest the diagnosis. Complementary tests include histology of a skin specimen, slit skin smears stained with Giemsa for direct microscopy, and tissue samples for culture and for genetic analysis by PCR techniques.

## Management and treatment

The general public and health personnel easily establish the diagnosis of cutaneous leishmaniasis in endemic areas of the world. Following referral to a physician, one or more treatment options are available. However, in non-endemic regions, and particularly in non-tropical countries, the patient requires attention by a doctor experienced in tropical medicine, infectious diseases or dermatology. Several drugs are effective against *Leishmania* parasites and these include pentavalent antimonials, amphotericin B, triazole and alylamine antifungal compounds. However, the only treatment of choice for a number of species is the intravenous administration of antimonials carefully monitored in hospital and administered only by experienced personnel. A number of patients require long-term follow-up as leishmaniasis may relapse in some cases.

## Gnathostomiasis

### Aetiology and pathogenesis

A number of *Gnathostoma* species live as adult worms in the intestine of domestic cats. Humans can acquire the disease by eating contaminated fish that have ingested small crustaceans acting as intermediary hosts in this condition. The larval stages do not reach maturation in the human body and can cause disease in several internal organs as well as in the skin. The disease is prevalent in South East Asia, China, Japan, Indonesia and Mexico.

### Clinical findings and diagnosis

Episodes of migrating, intermittent, subcutaneous oedema with pruritus constitute the main clinical picture, and cases can adopt a chronic protracted course for years. The episodes of oedema can be quite inflammatory and painful, and the larvae can erupt out from the affected skin. The feet are not commonly affected.

### Management and treatment

The surgical extraction of the larva from the skin represents the curative therapeutic approach (Taniguchi et al 1992).

## Tungiasis

### Aetiology and pathogenesis

Tungiasis is a localised skin disease commonly affecting one foot and caused by the burrowing flea *Tunga penetrans*. This is also known as chigoe infestation, jigger, sandflea, chigoe and puce chique (in France). It has been reported that this flea originated in Central and South America (Ibanez-Bernal & Velasco-Castrejón 1996) and was subsequently distributed in Africa, Madagascar, India and Pakistan. It is a very small organism (~1 mm long) that lives in the soil near pigsties and cattle sheds. Fecundated females require blood, and their head and mouthparts penetrate the epidermis to reach the blood and other nutrients from the superficial dermis. After nourishment over several days, eggs are laid to the exterior and the flea dies.

### Clinical findings and diagnosis

These fleas commonly affect one foot, penetrating the soft skin on the toe web spaces, but other areas of the toes and the plantar aspects of the foot can be affected (Douglas-Jones et al 1995). The initial burrow and the flea body can be evident in early lesions, but within 3–4 weeks a crateriform single nodule develops with a central haemorrhagic point. Superimposed bacterial infections may be responsible for impetigo, ecthyma, cellulitis and gangrenous lesions.

The diagnosis is clinical, but skin specimens for direct microscopy and histopathology with HE stain reveal structures of the flea and eggs.

## Management and treatment

Curettage, cryotherapy, surgical excision or other careful removal of the flea and eggs are the curative therapeutic choices. Early treatment and avoidance of secondary infection are of the utmost importance in all infested hosts, and particularly in individuals with diabetes mellitus, leprosy or other debilitating conditions of the feet. A haemorrhagic nodule due to *Tunga penetrans* may be difficult to discern from an inflamed common wart or a malignant melanoma, but the short duration of the lesion and the history of exposure indicate the acute nature of this parasitic disease.

## Myasis

### Aetiology and pathogenesis

A number of diptera species in larval stages (maggots) may colonise the human skin. The infestation mechanisms include direct deposition of eggs, contamination by soil or dirty clothes, other insects acting as vectors, or actual penetration into the skin by larvae. Species of *Dermatobia* and *Cordylobia* are the commonest found in the tropics, in the Americas and Africa, respectively, whereas European cases originate from *Hypoderma* species (Lui & Buck 1992). A local inflammatory reaction to the larvae with secondary infection is responsible for the signs and symptoms of disease.

### Clinical findings and diagnosis

Elderly and debilitated individuals of both sexes with exposed chronic wounds or ulcers are at a higher risk of suffering from this infestation. Furunculoid and subcutaneous forms may affect any part of the body, but in children the scalp is a commonly affected site. Chronic ulcers of the lower legs and feet represent a predisposing factor, and myasis often complicates severe infections by bacteria or fungi (see e.g. Fig. 7.18). Larvae feed on tissue debris and may not cause discomfort or any symptoms at all. Cases are observed throughout the year in tropical regions where the standards of hygiene, nutrition and general health are poor. The diagnosis is based on clinical suspicion and physical findings.

### Management and treatment

The treatment of choice is the mechanical removal or surgical excision of the larvae (Lui & Buck 1992). Single furunculoid lesions can be covered by thick Vaseline or paste to suffocate the larvae that, following death, can be subsequently extracted. Superficial infestations respond to repeated topical soaks or baths in potassium permanganate solution over a few days.

## Scabies

### Aetiology and pathogenesis

Scabies is a cosmopolitan problem, but individuals in poor tropical countries with low standards of hygiene and, particularly, overcrowding suffer from cyclical outbreaks of severe and chronic forms. The human scabies mite *Sarcoptes scabiei* commonly affects the skin of both feet of infants and children. Adults rarely manifest scabies on the lower limbs below the knees (Hebra lines), but exceptional cases of crusted or Norwegian scabies may present with lesions on both feet. The scabies mite burrows a tunnel of up to 4 mm into the superficial layer of the epidermis, where eggs are laid. The eggs hatch and reach the stage of nymph, and subsequently become an adult male or female mite. Female individuals live for up to 6 weeks and lay up to 50 eggs. A new generation of fecundated females penetrates the skin in regions adjacent to the nesting burrow, but the mite infestation can

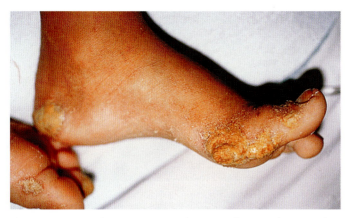

**Figure 7.14** Crusted or Norwegian scabies. Hyperkeratotic lesions with erythema and scaling.

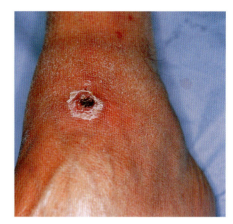

**Figure 7.15** Tick bite. Eschar with central necrosis surrounded by scaling and erythema.

also be perpetuated by clothes, or by reinfestation from another host in the family.

### Clinical findings and diagnosis

Papules, with or without excoriation, and S-shaped burrows are the elementary classic lesions of scabies. Infants and young children present with papular, vesicular and/or nodular lesions on both plantar regions, but other parts of the feet can be affected. Children rarely have access to a consultation with a podiatrist, but adults with chronic crusted scabies may present with eczematisation, impetiginised plaques and hyperkeratosis similar to those observed in the paediatric case shown in Figure 7.14. Large crusts covering inflammatory papular lesions contain a high number of parasites, and careful examination is required to prevent the health personnel from acquiring the infestation.

The clinical findings and intense pruritus support the diagnosis. Confirmation is obtained by direct microscopy of skin scrapings from a burrow revealing the structures of the mite.

### Management and treatment

Topical treatment overnight with benzyl benzoate, malathion, lindane or permethrine, lotion or cream, is usually effective. A second course is recommended 10 days after the original application, and all the affected members of a household require treatment at the same time to prevent cyclical reinfestations. Severe cases, or individuals in particular community settings such as those living in homes for the elderly, orphans, prisons or psychiatric wards, require oral treatment with a single dose of ivermectin as originally described by Macotela in 1991 (personal communication). This drug can be prescribed only by a qualified physician. Other therapeutic measures are directed at controlling the symptoms, inflammation and infection. Clothes and bed linen require washing at high temperature to kill all young fecundated females, but a number of authors have demonstrated that this is not necessary. In the right epidemiological context scabies may represent a venereal disease. Pruritus may last for several weeks after cure.

### Ticks

### Aetiology and pathogenesis

Ticks are cosmopolitan ectoparasites capable of transmitting severe viral, rickettsial, bacterial and parasitic diseases. The transmission of infectious agents takes place at the time of taking a blood meal from a human host that becomes infested accidentally. Soft ticks of the

Argasidae family are more prevalent in the tropics and subtropical regions of the world and transmit agents of tick-borne relapsing fever.

### Clinical findings and diagnosis

The bite of a tick is painful and the patient is aware of this episode. The bite produces a local inflammatory reaction, suggesting initially an ordinary papular insect bite, that subsequently causes localised superficial vascular damage with necrosis. The characteristic clinical picture manifests as an eschar that can be easily recognised on careful physical examination (Fig. 7.15). An area of circular scaling of the skin surrounding the original haemorrhagic bite can be seen after 7–10 days. Residual chronic lesions may leave hyperpigmented patches with a central induration.

### Management and treatment

Careful removal of the tick can be carried out by applying a tight dressing or cloth impregnated with chloroform, petrol or ether on the tick body. The organism is carefully removed a few minutes later, avoiding the rupture of head and mouth parts, which can be left behind in the skin. A careful follow-up and self-surveillance is indicated as systemic illness may start a few days or weeks following the tick bite. Symptoms such as fever, skin rash, lymph node enlargement, fatigue and night sweats indicate systemic disease, and the patient requires referral to a hospital physician or a specialist in tropical medicine.

## Fleas

### Aetiology and pathogenesis

The common human flea *Pulex irritans* is cosmopolitan but a number of other species, such as the tropical rat flea *Xenopsylla cheopis*, show preference for tropical climates. Fleas bite humans in order to get a blood meal, and in so doing produce a localised inflammatory reaction. History of exposure can reveal that an individual host or family member recently moved house or acquired a second-hand piece of wooden furniture, where fleas can live for months without taking blood meals.

### Clinical findings and diagnosis

A clinical picture of prurigo with papules, vesicles or small nodules on both feet and lower legs is characteristic, and the lesions are often found in clusters (Fig. 7.16). The papular discrete lesions may reveal a central haemorrhagic punctum, and the lesions in clusters often show a remarkable asymmetry. Modification of the initial pruriginous

**191**

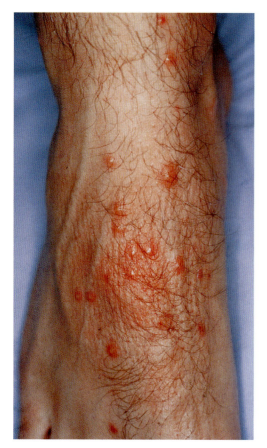

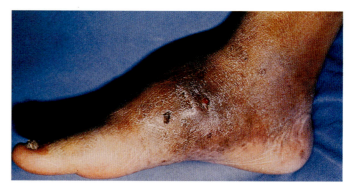

**Figure 7.17** Eumycetoma caused by *Madurella mycetomatis*. Deformity, sinus tract formation, pigmentary changes and scarring. (Courtesy of Dr Rubén López, Mexico City.)

**Figure 7.16** Flea bites. Numerous pruriginous papules in clusters.

lesions may result from intense scratching and superimposed secondary bacterial infection.

### Management and treatment

Fumigation can be successfully achieved by using common insecticide products approved for domestic use. Severe reactions of prurigo require a topical steroid cream, and impetiginised cases require topical or systemic antibiotics. Antihistamine lotions or tablets may provide symptomatic relief. Severe cases are treated with a single dose or short course of systemic corticosteroids.

## Fungal conditions

### Eumycetoma

#### Aetiology and pathogenesis

*Madurella mycetomatis, Pseudoallescheria boydii* and *Leptosphaeria senegalensis* are the main aetiological agents of true fungal mycetoma, also known as eumycetoma. A generic term, 'Madura foot' is currently used to describe all forms of bacterial and fungal mycetoma (see section on bacterial mycetoma, above). Eumycetoma occurs in Sudan, Senegal and Saudi Arabia, particularly in arid or semi-arid regions (Abbott 1956). Cases also occur in India and Central and South America. Infective organisms penetrate the skin of the foot by direct traumatic inoculation, and once in the host's tissue the agents multiply and infect adjacent structures. Changes in the fungus cell wall and melanin production are the main virulent factors involved in local pathogenesis.

### Clinical findings and diagnosis

Eumycetoma affects predominantly young male individuals between 20 and 50 years of age. It has been estimated that more than 70% of cases of eumycetoma manifest on one foot. The perimalleolar region and the dorsum are the most commonly affected sites, but any region of the foot can suffer the direct inoculation of infective organisms (Fig. 7.17). The characteristic clinical signs include a nodule or irregular swelling followed by sinus tract formation and discharge of purulent material containing the characteristic grains. Pigmentary changes of the skin and scarring result from the chronic inflammatory process that persists over months or years. Periosteal involvement is the starting point of bone resorption, osteolysis and irreversible osteomyelitis.

The epidemiological context and characteristic clinical picture are diagnostic. This is confirmed by direct microscopy of pale or black grains that measure 0.5–1 mm and contain fungal structures measuring 2–4 μm. This material grows in agar containing glucose and peptone, and the histological sections of deep skin specimens reveal the characteristic, and in many cases pathognomonic, grains of particular fungal species. Radiological investigation of the affected foot discloses periosteal involvement, cortical resorption and osteolysis.

### Management and treatment

Early nodular lesions or small papular forms called 'micromycetoma' can be treated by complete surgical excision. However, the delay in diagnosis results in advanced cases that respond poorly to medical treatment. Systemic antibiotics in combination, such as streptomycin, cotrimoxazol, amikacin, dapsone and rifampin, are the drugs of choice and require long-term administration. Nearly two-thirds of cases caused by *M. mycetomatis* respond to ketoconazole (Mahgoub & Gumaa 1984). Severe cases with bone involvement can be cured only by radical surgery.

## Chromoblastomycosis

### Aetiology and pathogenesis

This is a chronic infection caused by fungi of the genera *Fonsecaea, Cladosporium* and *Phialophora*. The disease is widely distributed in the tropics and affects predominantly agricultural workers who acquire the infection through direct inoculation into the skin. Numerous cases have been reported from Costa Rica, Cuba, Brazil, Mexico, Indonesia and Madagascar.

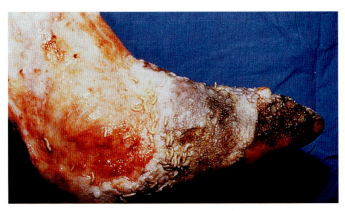

**Figure 7.18** Chromoblastomycosis with verrucous lesions, chronic ulceration and complicated by myasis.

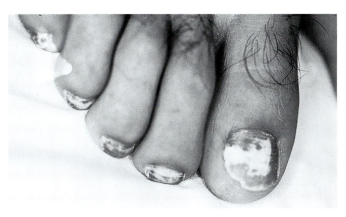

**Figure 7.19** Subungual white onychomycosis by Trychophyton rubrum.

## Clinical findings and diagnosis

The initial lesion starts as a papular or nodular inflammatory reaction that subsequently develops a warty appearance. Over time, this lesion slowly enlarges and becomes a characteristically large verrucous asymptomatic plaque. The commonest site affected in sporadic infections is the foot, and the chronic verrucous plaque appears on the dorsum or the perimalleolar region. The plaque may become very thick over several years and may cause gross deformity of the affected foot (Fig. 7.18). Varying degrees of disability and recurrent secondary infections and/or infestations are a common problem for the foot with chromoblastomycosis.

The diagnosis is made on clinical grounds and confirmed by direct microscopy and mycological culture in glucose–peptone agar. The histopathology of skin specimens is characteristic, showing acanthosis with a granuloma formation and the presence of typical fungal structures known as 'fumagoid' cells.

## Management and treatment

Flucytosine and thiabendazol have been used in combination without a consistent efficacy. Triazole compounds such as itraconazol have resulted in cure but, in general, it is accepted that chromoblastomycosis is not easy to treat medically, and patients require long-term treatment. Localised and early cases respond successfully to complete surgical excision of the lesion, and thermosurgery has also been reported to be of benefit. All patients affected by chromoblastomycosis require attention and follow-up by specialists in mycology, infectious diseases and/or dermatology.

## Dermatophytes

### Aetiology and pathogenesis

Superficial fungal infections by dermatophytes are cosmopolitan and affect one or both feet. These fungi are transmitted to humans by direct skin contact from their habitat in the soil, vegetation or other individuals. Local conditions on the skin, such as a moist and hot environment, are predisposing factors. Dermatophyte infections are highly prevalent in tropical climates, as this represents an ideal environment for these organisms, and numerous case series and epidemiological studies from Latin America have been reported to the literature in Spanish and Portuguese. The main genera involved in human infections are *Trychophyton*, *Epidermophyton* and *Microsporum*, but infections of the foot, including the toenails, are particularly caused by *Trychophyton rubrum*, *Trychophyton mentagrophytes* and *Epidermophyton floccosum*. Dermatophytes are keratinophilic organ-

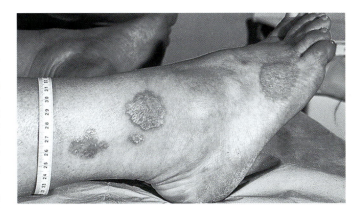

**Figure 7.20** Granuloma anulare in the differential diagnosis of *tinea pedis*.

isms and exert their pathogenesis through attachment to the skin, nail or hair surfaces (see Ch. 3).

### Clinical findings and diagnosis

Individuals of both sexes and all age groups are affected by dermatophytes; however, children under the age of 10 years rarely present with *tinea pedis*. The main clinical pictures are those of localised *tinea pedis*, interdigital, plantar hyperkeratosis and onychomycosis. Common names for these conditions include ringworm and athlete's foot. Dermatophyte infections can manifest as localised single or multiple circinate plaques, with erythema and variable degrees of scaling on the foot dorsum or perimalleolar regions. Toe web involvement is commonly bilateral, presenting with erythema, burning sensation, pruritus and scaling – particularly of the fourth interdigital toe web space. Chronic plantar lesions develop asymptomatic large hyperkeratotic plaques, and a particular form of toenail infection by *T. rubrum* manifests clinically as a subungual white onychomycosis (Fig. 7.19). Severe acute forms present with painful erythema and blistering in a pattern similar to that found in cases of acute eczema or pompholyx. Varying degrees of temporary disability may result from severe infections.

Discrete plaques of granuloma anulare (Fig. 7.20) have to be considered in the differential diagnosis of localised ringworm, whereas thickened plaques of plantar psoriasis (Fig. 7.21) may pose diagnostic difficulties with chronic hyperkeratotic infections by dermatophytes. Other superficial skin and nail infections of the foot, such as those caused by *Candida* and *Scytalidium* species, may also represent a diagnostic difficulty.

**193**

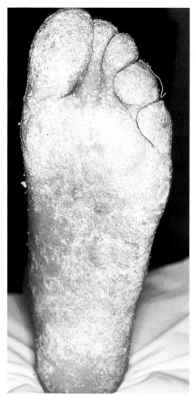

Figure 7.21 Plantar psoriasis in the differential diagnosis of hyperkeratotic dermatophyte infection.

The diagnosis of dermatophyte infection on the foot is made on clinical grounds. Additional diagnostic measures include direct microscopy of skin scrapings in 10–12% potassium hydroxide solution, and the identification by culture of the causative organism in Sabouraud's medium.

### Management and treatment

The therapy of choice includes the use of topical and/or systemic azole or alylamine antifungal compounds. Localised infections require topical therapy for 3–4 weeks but interdigital athlete's foot may require 6–8 weeks. Topical steroids are often required to control the inflammatory picture, but are administered only when effective antifungal treatment is already in place. Systemic therapy with antifungals is indicated in severe skin infections and onychomycosis of the toenails. Other therapeutic measures address the control of symptoms, secondary eczematisation and superimposed bacterial infection. Measures of general hygiene and appropriate footwear are useful to prevent re-infection, which is a common problem.

## Systemic mycosis manifesting on the feet

Infections by *Coccidioides immitis* and *Paracoccidioides brasiliensis* commonly manifest with disease of the lungs, but haematogenous dissemination results in the appearance of skin lesions on both feet.

Patients with foot involvement from systemic fungal disease require immediate referral to an experienced hospital physician or specialists in mycology, infectious diseases or dermatology.

### Coccidioidomycosis

This is acquired through inhalation of infective spores in tropical, but also subtropical, desert regions of the world, particularly in the

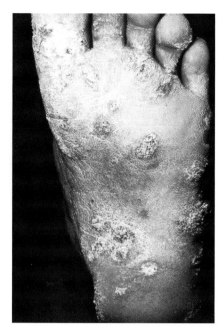

Figure 7.22 Coccidioidomycosis with isolated and confluent verrucous plaques. (Courtesy of Dr Sergio González, Monterrey, Mexico.)

American continent. The skin of one or both feet is involved, and lesions manifest as erythematous verrucous or scaling nodules on the plantar surface or any other part of the foot (Fig. 7.22). A history of exposure in endemic regions as well as the cutaneous and extracutaneous clinical picture support the diagnostic possibility. Other investigations such as serology, chest radiographs and culture for the isolation of the organism confirm the diagnosis. Culture of agents causing systemic mycoses should be carried out only in specialised laboratories, as they represent a serious biological hazard. Systemic therapeutic options for coccidioidomycosis include amphotericin B and triazole compounds.

### Paracoccidioidomycosis

This occurs in Mexico and Central and South America, and predominantly affects males. Actual evidence of the mode of transmission is incomplete, but the respiratory route seems to be common in acquiring the infection. Following a chronic picture of lung involvement, weight loss and fatigue, the skin of one or both feet can be affected. Painful nodular, haemorrhagic, ulcerated and verrucous lesions can be observed, covered by a thick crust (Fig. 7.23), and severe disability results in advanced forms of the disease. The diagnosis is based on the history of exposure in an endemic region and the clinical picture, supported by investigations to reveal the presence of the typical large, budding yeast cells. These can be observed on direct microscopy, and preparations for histology and are easily identified in culture. Effective systemic treatment has been reported with triazole compounds and amphotericin B.

## Viral infections

Most common viral skin diseases presenting on the foot are cosmopolitan, but the onset may coincide with a trip to the tropics and pose problems in the differential diagnosis of the returning traveller. Viral infections with foot involvement that are prevalent in the tropics include plantar warts, Kaposi's sarcoma (Figs 7.24, 7.25), and severe blistering forms caused by varicella (Fig. 7.26). Severe cases require a full diagnostic protocol, with specimens for culture, electron micros-

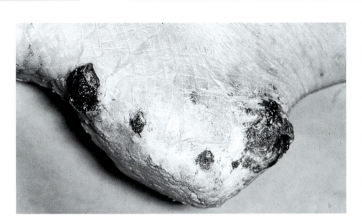

**Figure 7.23** Hyperkeratotic and verrucous haemorrhagic lesions in chronic infection by *Paracoccidioides brasiliensis*.

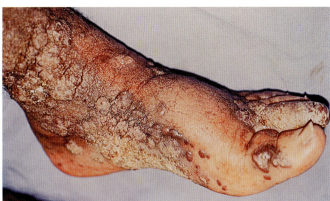

**Figure 7.25** Verrucous lymphangiomatous lesions in Kaposi's sarcoma.

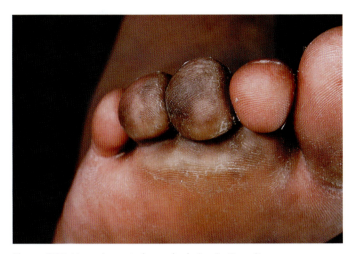

**Figure 7.24** Hyperpigmented vascular lesion in Kaposi's sarcoma.

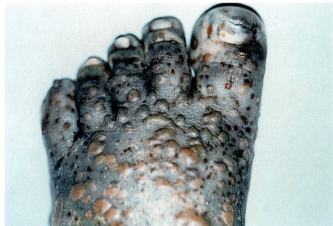

**Figure 7.26** Blistering and oedema in varicella herpes infection.

copy, serology and histopathology, followed by specialised treatment in tertiary medical centres.

## Miscellaneous conditions

### Ainhum

This uncommon condition affecting the fifth toe of adults in tropical Africa is also called spontaneous dactylolysis. A painful constricting band of fibrotic tissue results in spontaneous amputation of the toe. A number of contributing factors have been identified, including familial occurrence, decreased blood supply locally, mechanical trauma from walking barefoot, and chronic diseases with neuropathy such as leprosy and diabetes mellitus. General hygiene measures, avoidance of infection and surgical amputation, if required in advanced cases, are the therapeutic interventions of choice (Browne 1976).

### Pellagra

Pellagra is caused by a nutritional deficiency of niacin and classically manifests with the triad of dermatitis, diarrhoea and dementia. Clinically, it manifests as a remarkable photosensitive rash that may show an eczematoid pattern with hyperpigmentation. Most lesions affect the face and neck, and both lower limbs present with signs similar to those found in stasis dermatitis. Eczematoid changes,

xerosis and hyperpigmented patches are present symmetrically on both feet (Stratigos & Katsambas 1977). Oral treatment with niacin amide is indicated, and podiatric care includes general hygiene, moisturising and avoidance of infectious or mechanical trauma.

### Drug reactions, chronic dermatitis and other skin conditions

Drug reactions occur worldwide but may coincide with a trip to the tropics and in some cases result from sun exposure. A variety of medicines induce moderate to severe reactions, and the patient's history often identifies the use of antibiotics, carbamazepine, sulfamides, diuretics or beta blockers. More than three-quarters of all patients with drug reactions manifest with erythema (rash) and/or urticaria. Other severe forms of drug reaction commonly manifesting on both feet include erythema multiforme and toxicodermias. The finding of vasculitis presenting with purpura (Fig. 7.27) or severe exfoliation with hyperpigmented lesions and epidermal detachment (Fig. 7.28) indicates systemic illness due to a drug reaction. Specialised management in hospital is required for all severe cases, as mortality can be high for toxic epidermal necrolysis (Brocq–Lyell syndrome) and Stevens–Johnson's syndrome.

Finally, a number of chronic skin conditions that are eczematous in nature result in bilateral and remarkably symmetrical hyperpigmented skin patches (Fig. 7.29). A symmetrical rash suggests contact

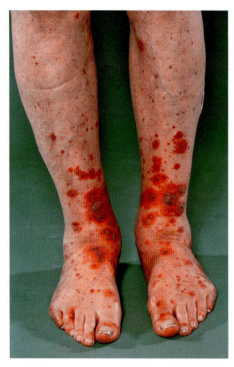

**Figure 7.27** Bilateral purpura and vasculitis by drug reaction.

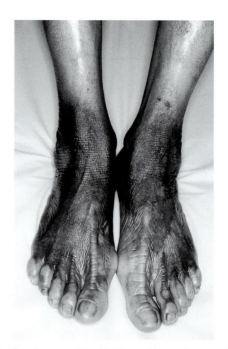

**Figure 7.29** Chronic dermatitis with bilateral hyperpigmentation.

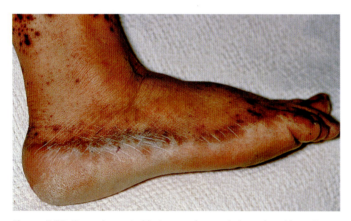

**Figure 7.28** Hyperpigmented lesions and necrosis in toxic epidermal necrolysis.

dermatitis, but complex cases involve a vascular deficit secondary to venous hypertension. Psoriasis may also present with a chronic recurrent eczematous picture, affecting the heel and medial plantar aspects on both feet.

## Seaborne conditions

Holiday-makers who have been in tropical seawater present to local podiatrists following contact or traumatic skin injury from jellyfish, coral, anemones, sea-urchins and venomous fish. A variety of acute clinical pictures manifest as contact eczema, stings, burns and penetrating injuries, whereas vasoactive phenomena represent the common pathogenic mechanism in direct skin poisoning. The returning traveller commonly manifests postinflammatory lesions characterised by hyperpigmentation and scarring. Chronic eczematous reactions and secondary bacterial infections require specific treatment.

## REFERENCES

Abbott PH 1956 Mycetoma in the Sudan. Transactions of the Royal Society of Tropical Medicine and Hygiene 50:11–24.

Barton AA 1976 The pathogenesis of skin wounds due to pressure. In: Kenedi RM, Cowden JM (eds) Bed sore biomechanics. Macmillan, London.

Bauman JH, Girling JP, Brand PW 1963 Plantar pressures and trophic ulceration. Journal of Bone and Joint Surgery 45B:652.

Belsey MA, LeBlanc DR 1975 Skin infections and the epidemiology of diphtheria: acquisition and persistence of *C. diphtheriae* infections. American Journal of Epidemiology 102:179–184.

Bisno AL, Stevens DL 1996 Streptococcal infections of skin and soft tissues. New England Journal of Medicine 334:240.

Blackwell V, Vega-López F 2000 Two years of cutaneous larva migrans in London. British Journal of Dermatology 143: 53–54.

Brand P 1991 The insensitive foot (including leprosy). In: Jahss MH (ed.) Disorders of the foot and ankle. WB Saunders, Philadelphia, PA.

Brandsma JW 1994 Terminology in leprosy rehabilitation and guidelines for nerve function assessment. Tropical and Geographical Medicine 46:88–92.

Browne SG 1976 Ainhum. International Journal of Dermatology 15:348–350.

Bryceson A, Pfaltzgraff RE 1990 Symptoms and Signs. In: Leprosy, 3rd edn. Churchill Livingstone, Edinburgh, pp 25–55.

Caumes E, Datry A, Paris L 1992 Efficacy of ivermectin in the therapy of cutaneous larva migrans. Archives of Dermatology 128:995–996.

Chopra S, Vega-López F 1999 Skin granulomas in clinical practice. In: James DG, Zumla A (eds). The granulomatous disorders. Cambridge University Press, Cambridge, pp 507–510, 513–517.

Cribier B, Piemont Y, Grosshans E 1994 Staphylococcal scalded skin syndrome in adults. Journal of the American Academy of Dermatology 30:319–324.

Cross H, Sane S, Dey A, Kulkarni VN 1995 The efficacy of podiatric orthoses as an adjunct to the treatment of plantar ulceration in leprosy. Leprosy Review 66:144–157.

Cross H, Dey A, Kulkarni VN, Rendall G 1996 Plantar ulceration in patients with leprosy. Journal of Wound Care 5(9):406–411.

Cruickshank CND 1976 The micro anatomy of the epidermis in relation to tissue trauma. In: Kenedi RM, Cowden JM (eds) Bed sore biomechanics. Macmillan, London.

Daly MD 1990 The repair phase of wound healing – re-epithelialisation and contraction. In: Kloth LC, McCulloch JM, Feedar JA (eds) Wound healing: alternatives in management. FA Davis, London.

Douglas-Jones AG, Llewelyn MB, Mills CM 1995 Cutaneous infection with *Tunga penetrans*. British Journal of Dermatology 133:125–127.

Elliot DC, Kufera JA, Myers RA 1996 Necrotizing soft tissue infections. Risk factors for mortality and strategies for management. Annals of Surgery 224:672–683.

Gray SF, Smith RS, Reynolds NJ 1990 Fish tank granuloma. British Medical Journal 300:1069–1070.

Ibanez-Bernal S, Velasco-Castrejón O 1996 New records of human tungiasis in Mexico (Siphonaptera: Tungidae). Journal of Medical Entomology 33:988–999.

ILEP Medical Commission 1993 Guidelines for leprosy control programmes. ILEP, London.

Jopling WH, McDougal AC 1988 Handbook of leprosy, 4th edn. Heinemann, Oxford.

Jorgensen U, Bosjen-Moller F 1991 The plantar soft tissues: functional anatomy and clinical applications. In: Jahss MH (ed.) Disorders of the foot, Vol. 1. WB Saunders, Philadelphia, PA.

Josse R, Guedenon A, Aguiar J et al 1994 Buruli's ulcer, a pathology little known in Benin. Apropos of 227 cases. Bulletin de la Société de Pathologie Exotique 87:170–175.

Kloth L, Miller K 1990 The inflammatory response to wounding. In: Kloth LC, McCulloch JM, Feedar JA (eds) Wound healing: alternatives in management. FA Davis, London.

Kulkarni VN, Mehta JM 1983 Tarsal disintegration (TD) in leprosy. Leprosy in India 55(2):338–370.

López-Martínez R, Méndez-Tovar LJ, Lavalle P, et al 1992 Epidemiología del micetoma en México: Estudio de 2105 casos. Gaceta Médica de México 128:477–481.

Lui H, Buck W 1992 Cutaneous myasis: a simple and effective technique for extraction of *Dermatobia hominis* larvae. International Journal of Dermatology 31:657–659.

Mahgoub ES, Gumaa SA 1984 Ketoconazole in the treatment of eumycetoma due to *Madurella mycetomi*. Transactions of the Royal Society of Tropical Medicine and Hygiene 78:376–379.

Price H 1990 Connective tissue in wound healing. In: Kloth LC, McCulloch JM, Feedar JA (eds) Wound healing: alternatives in management. FA Davis, London.

Root ML, Orien WP, Weed JH 1977 Normal and abnormal function of the foot. In: Clinical Biomechanics, Vol. 11. Clinical Biomechanics Corporation, Los Angeles, CA.

Sabin TD, Swift TC 1984 Leprosy. In: Dyck PJ, Thomas PK, Lambert EH, Bunge R (eds) Peripheral neuropathy, Vol. 2. WB Saunders, Philadelphia, PA.

Sane SB, Mehta J 1988 Malignant transformation in trophic ulcers in leprosy: a study of 12 cases. Indian Journal of Leprosy 60:93–99.

Sehgal VN, Jain S, Bhattacharya SN, Thappa DM 1994 Yaws control and eradication. International Journal of Dermatology 33:16–20.

Serrano-Jaén L, Vega-López F 2000 Fulminating septicaemia caused by *Vibrio vulnificus*. British Journal of Dermatology 142:386–387.

Stratigos JD, Katsambas A 1977 Pellagra: a still existing disease. British Journal of Dermatology 96:99–106.

Taniguchi Y, Ando K, Isoda K 1992 Human gnathostomiasis: successful removal of *Gnathostoma hispidum*. International Journal of Dermatology 31:175–177.

Thangaraj HS, Evans MRW, Wansbrough-Jones MH 1999 *Mycobacterium ulcerans* disease; Buruli ulcer. Transactions of the Royal Society of Tropical Medicine and Hygiene 93:337–340.

Thomas S 1990 Wound management and dressings. Pharmaceutical Press, London.

Watson J 1986 Disability prevention in leprosy patients. Leprosy Mission International, London.

Welsh O 1991 Mycetoma. Current concepts in treatment. International Journal of Dermatology 30:387–398.

Westaby S 1982 Wound care No. 8 – Wound infection: causes and prevention. Nursing Times 16(Suppl):29–32.

WHO 1986 Expert Committee on Venereal Diseases and Treponematoses. Sixth Report. Technical Report Series, No 736. World Health Organization, Geneva.

WHO 1990 Control of leishmaniasis. Report of a WHO Expert Committee. Technical Report Series, No 793. World Health Organization, Geneva.

WHO 1999 Global leprosy situation in 1998. Available at: http://www.who.int/lep/12htm.

Young H 1992 Syphilis: new diagnostic directions. International Journal of Sexually Transmitted Diseases and AIDS 3:391–413.

Zederfeldt B, Jacobsson S, Ahonen J 1986 Wounds and wound healing. Wolfe Medical, London.

## Further reading

Brand P 1991 The insensitive foot (including leprosy). In: Jahss MH (ed.) Disorders of the foot and ankle. WB Saunders, Philadelphia, PA.

Brandsma JW, Heerkens YF, Lakerveld-Heyl K, Mischner-Van Ravensberg CD 1992 The international classification of impairments, disabilities and handicaps in leprosy control projects. Leprosy Review 63:337–343.

First T 1996 Don't treat me like I have leprosy! ILEP, London.

Hastings RC (ed.) 1985 Leprosy. Churchill Livingstone, New York.

Summers A 1993 Leprosy for field staff. Leprosy Mission, London.

Srinivasan H 1993 Prevention of disabilities in patients with leprosy. A practical guide. WHO, Geneva.

Van Brakel WH, Anderson AM 1997 Impairment and disability in leprosy: in search of the missing link. Indian Journal of Leprosy 69(4):361–373.

Watson JM 1991 Essential action to minimise disability in leprosy patients. The Leprosy Mission, London.

Weis MG, Doongaji DR, Siddharatha S et al 1992 The explanatory model interview catalogue. Contribution to cross cultural research methods: from a study of leprosy and mental health. British Journal of Psychiatry 160:819–830.

# Chapter | 8 |

# Musculoskeletal disorders

*Anthony Redmond and Phillip Helliwell*

## KEYWORDS

Ankylosing spondylitis
Behçet's syndrome
Beighton score
Benign familial joint hypermobility syndrome
Crohn's disease
Crystal arthropathies
Disease-modifying antirheumatic drugs (DMARDs)
Ehlers–Danlos syndrome
Fibromyalgia
Gout
Immune-mediated inflammatory diseases
Infective arthritis
Juvenile idiopathic arthritis
Lisfranc's joint
Marfan syndrome
Osteoarthritis
Osteogenesis imperfecta
Polymyalgia rheumatica (PMR)
Pseudogout
Psoriatic arthritis
Reactive arthritis
Regional examination of the musculoskeletal system (REMS)
Reiter's syndrome
Retrocalcaneal bursitis
Rheumatoid arthritis
Rigid/semi-rigid, functional orthoses
Seropositive inflammatory arthritis
Scleroderma
Sjögren's syndrome
Systemic lupus erythematosus (SLE)
Vasculitis
Whipple's disease

## INTRODUCTION

This chapter is intended to provide an introduction for readers either potentially or actually involved in the care of the foot in

**199**

patients with rheumatic conditions. An overview of the medical management is provided because foot pathologies do not normally present in isolation in these patients and so the systemic context is important. However, the chapter is about the foot and so focuses mainly on the foot conditions, the processes underlying them and the treatment options available. The evidence supporting many of the therapies for disorders of the foot in rheumatology is often weaker than would be desirable. This chapter represents, therefore, a digest of available literature, combined with the authors' experience of clinical practice and research within an academic multidisciplinary rheumatology team supported by a comprehensive foot health service.

## DEFINING RHEUMATOLOGY AND THE MUSCULOSKELETAL DISEASES

Rheumatology practice covers a heterogeneous range of more than 200 disorders with varied aetiologies, and which affect joints, bones, muscles and soft tissues (Linaker et al 1999, Symmons et al 2002). The rheumatic disorders have a variety of systemic features, but their common feature is their effect on the musculoskeletal system. Those working with foot problems are probably familiar with disorders arising from purely biomechanical and local factors, and these disorders are dealt with elsewhere in this book. This chapter focuses on the broader rheumatic diseases affecting the feet and their associated systemic or extended local disease processes. Many of the disorders seen in rheumatology practice are the consequence of a disordered immune response, and are therefore sometimes referred to as immune-mediated inflammatory diseases. Typical examples of immune-mediated inflammatory diseases are RA, the spondyloarthropathies, and the connective tissue diseases such as lupus and scleroderma (described later). Other systemic presentations include diseases caused by disordered metabolism, such as gout and osteoporosis; and complex, multifactorial disorders such as OA.

## GENERAL EPIDEMIOLOGY OF RHEUMATIC CONDITIONS

Approximately 1 in 7 adults in the UK has ongoing musculoskeletal symptoms, with some 1 in 20 people suffering moderate to severe disability secondary to a musculoskeletal disorder (Symmons et al 2002). The prevalence of musculoskeletal disease increases steadily with age, and by the age of 75 years can be as high as one person in three (Urwin et al 1998, Symmons et al 2002). Musculoskeletal pain also presents in multiple sites, and only one-third of people report their musculoskeletal pain to be confined to a single joint (Urwin et al 1998). Unsurprisingly, the degree of impact on quality of life increases as the number of affected sites increases (Urwin et al 1998).

The disability pathway from the underpinning local joint inflammation through to the impact on quality of life is well described for arthritis, and is summarised in Figure 8.1. Controlling symptoms and the effects of disease on quality of life are the focus of much of the therapeutic process. It should be remembered, however, that the disability pathway is influenced not only by disease factors, and that approximately one-quarter of disability is predicted by a range of modifying factors such as age, gender, lifestyle, work demands and psychological status (Escalante & Del Rincon 1999, 2002).

## BURDEN OF DISEASE

The burden of musculoskeletal disability to the health system is significant, with musculoskeletal conditions accounting for about one in five of all GP consultations, a proportion that continues to increase (Arthritis Research Campaign 2002, Symmons et al 2002). The musculoskeletal diseases are to some degree a social problem, because the prevalence is significantly higher in more deprived socio-economic groups and in workers engaged in more physical activities (Arthritis Research Campaign 2002, Urwin et al 1998).

The direct cost to the UK health service is approximately £5.5 billion each year, but indirect costs (such as the 206 million days a year lost to work, reduced incomes, social security and mortality) raise the total cost to the UK economy to £18 billion per year (Arthritis Research Campaign 2002).

## THE EPIDEMIOLOGY OF FOOT PROBLEMS GENERALLY AND IN RHEUMATOLOGY

Nearly one-quarter of all people aged over 55 years report ongoing foot pain, which in the majority of cases leads to impairment to daily activities (Benvenuti et al 1995, Chen et al 2003, Gorter et al 2001, Leveille et al 1998, Thomas et al 2004). Some 20–24% of all adults have had foot pain in the past month and some 60% have had foot pain in the past 6 months, with the foot pain causing measurable disability in half of these cases (Garrow et al 2004). Musculoskeletal disorders account for more than three-quarters of all foot pain (Gorter et al 2000) or, in other words, for foot pain in up to 7% of the total population (Cunningham & Kelsey 1984).

The incidence of foot problems is known to increase with age, and to be as much as five times higher in females than males (Benvenuti et al 1995, Black & Hale 1987, Dunn et al 2004, Garrow et al 2004, Leveille et al 1998, Munro & Steele 1998). Foot pathology often also coexists with other musculoskeletal morbidity such as knee or hip pain (Gorter et al 2000, Leveille et al 1998, Munro & Steele 1998, Odding et al 1995), and this should be considered in assessment and treatment planning. As well as the musculoskeletal manifestations themselves, plantar hyperkeratoses have been found in 66% of people with musculoskeletal or connective tissue disease, digital lesions in 24% and ulcerations in as many as 17% (Port et al 1980).

## A BRIEF OVERVIEW OF DEVELOPMENTS IN MEDICAL RHEUMATOLOGY

In many rheumatic diseases, the classical approach of slowly escalating drug therapy has been superseded by a new paradigm of early and aggressive treatment, and combination therapies using disease-modifying antirheumatic drugs (DMARDs). This change in approach has been further enhanced in recent years by the development of a new range of pharmaceuticals, the so-called 'biological' immunotherapies, which provide a highly effective treatment option for patients who do not respond adequately to conventional therapies. The significant medical advances are also reflected in the management of rheumatology patients by allied health professionals, as the emphasis moves from compassionate management of physical decline to more dynamic and proactive approaches.

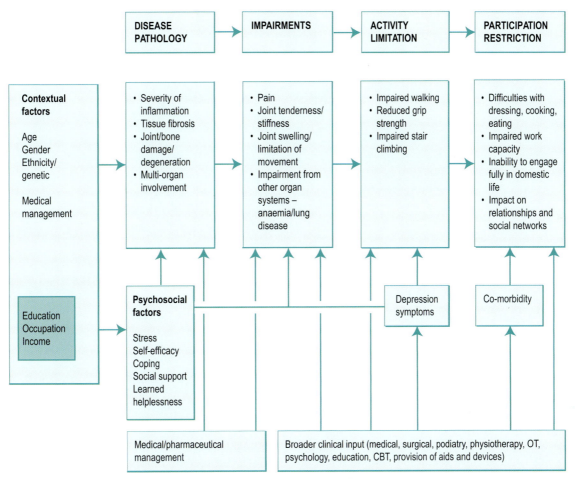

**Figure 8.1** Factors affecting the disability pathway in inflammatory arthritis. From the original concept proposed by Nagi (1965) and modified by Escalante (Escalante & Del Rincon 2002), adapted to incorporate WHO ICG definitions.

## MEDICAL MANAGEMENT IN RHEUMATOLOGY – OVERVIEW ACROSS DISEASES

Medical management in rheumatology has undergone nothing short of a revolution in recent years. While the non-inflammatory conditions such as OA continue to be managed according to fairly traditional principles, treatment of immune-mediated inflammatory diseases has been, quite literally, turned on its head.

Between the 1950s and the mid-1990s, patients with inflammatory arthritis would be managed according to the severity of presenting symptoms, using what was described as a 'treatment pyramid', where drug therapy was escalated slowly and incrementally in response to treatment failure (Cannella & O'Dell 2003, Fries et al 1996, Pincus et al 1999). High doses of non-steroidal anti-inflammatory drugs (NSAIDs) would be used, with doses increasing until patients were no longer able to tolerate therapy. When disease control was inadequate using NSAIDS, other disease-modifying drugs such as the antimalarials, gold, penicillamine and sulfasalazine would be introduced sequentially to try to suppress the inflammation as far as practicable. These second-line DMARDs were often not introduced until 5–10 years of disease duration had passed and, as we now know, damage had already accrued (Wolfe et al 2001). In the 1990s, methotrexate came to prominence such that it became the recommended DMARD

to be given early in the course of the disease, with rapidly escalating doses if response was suboptimal.

Furthermore, better understanding of the pathological processes involved, the discovery of the role of cytokines in the early 1980s, and the development of anti cytokine drugs in the past 10 years (Feldmann 2002) have led to a total paradigm shift. The new paradigm is known as the 'inverted pyramid' or 'step-down bridge' approach (Fries et al 1996, Pincus et al 1999) (Figure 8.2).

In the step-down approach early management is aggressive and combinations of DMARDs are used to suppress inflammation nearer to disease onset, so limiting irreversible joint damage (O'Dell 2004). There is compelling evidence that the new approach improves outcomes substantially in a range of immune-mediated arthropathies (Cannella & O'Dell 2003, Rao & Hootman 2004) and that the earlier that treatment is instigated the better (Bukhari et al 2003, Hazes 2003, Lard et al 2001, Puolakka et al 2004). The Arthritis and Musculoskeletal Alliance (ARMA) national standards of care for rheumatoid arthritis (RA) require that all patients with suspected inflammatory arthritis are seen by a rheumatology specialist within 12 weeks of first presentation, and preferably within 6 weeks (Arthritis and Musculoskeletal Alliance 2004a).

In inflammatory arthritis, the goal at first presentation is to establish and maintain disease remission, and this can often be achieved with standard (i.e. traditional non-biological) therapies (Bukhari et al 2003). Patients are started on NSAIDs (ibuprofen, diclofenac, indometacin or cyclo-oxygenase-2 (cox-2) inhibitors, according to

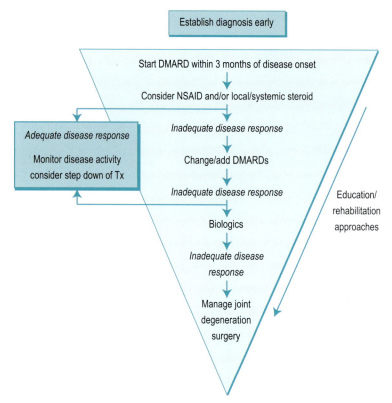

**Figure 8.2** An abridged schema for the medical management of RA (adapted from ACR guidelines 2002).

risk factors), which provide immediate reduction in pain and stiffness (O'Dell 2004). NSAIDs are not used in isolation, however, as they do not prevent erosions and joint damage and so do not alter long-term prognosis (Aletaha & Smolen 2002, American College of Rheumatology Subcommittee on Rheumatoid Arthritis 2002, Choy et al 2002, Fries et al 1996). Much has been made of the potential benefits offered by the new cox-2 selective NSAIDS, although the objective evidence suggests that the effectiveness of the cox-2 inhibitors is no greater than traditional (and cheaper) NSAIDs such as ibuprofen, naproxen and diclofenac, with benefits confined to slightly better tolerance (Garner et al 2004a,b). Importantly, new data emerging have indicated a potential for increasing the risk of cardiovascular events with cox-2 drugs, and one of this new class of NSAIDs (rofecoxib) has already been withdrawn from the market (Juni et al 2004). Prescribers are therefore advised to be cautious and to avoid these drugs in anyone with a high risk, or history, of cardiovascular disease (Fitzgerald 2004). Furthermore, it is now becoming clear that even traditional NSAIDs carry an increased risk of vascular disease. These developments have led to an aversion by physicians to prescribing NSAIDs – if they are prescribed the recommendation is for the smallest possible dose for the shortest possible time.

There is good evidence that instigation of DMARD therapy within 3 months of disease onset is highly effective in controlling immune-mediated inflammatory diseases (American College of Rheumatology Subcommittee on Rheumatoid Arthritis 2002, O'Dell 2004), and so patients are normally started on a suitable DMARD immediately. The most commonly used DMARDs at present are methotrexate and hydroxychloroquine, with sulfasalazine becoming increasingly marginalised. Leflunomide is a new DMARD with good tolerability, which can be used in conjunction with methotrexate or as a fallback when patients cannot use methotrexate (American College of Rheumatology Subcommittee on Rheumatoid Arthritis 2002, Olsen & Stein 2004; Osiri et al 2004). Methotrexate is usually the DMARD of first choice because of its significant therapeutic effects when used in isolation,

and because of its adjunctive effects when used in combination with other DMARDs (O'Dell 2004, Verstappen et al 2003a,b). Methotrexate is the best tolerated DMARD for long-term therapy, and many patients use methotrexate for many years (O'Dell 1997, Rau et al 1997, Verstappen et al 2003). Used in this way, methotrexate is often referred to as an 'anchor drug' (Pincus et al 1999).

There is some controversy on the use of oral corticosteroids as a first-line treatment because of their wide ranging systemic side-effects. Recent high-profile studies on intensive treatment regimens have used oral steroids (BeST and TICORA) but their use is not widespread in the UK. Oral steroids are useful in early disease as a 'bridging therapy' before the DMARDs take effect, and, given systemically, for short-term suppression of disease flares (O'Dell 2004). Low-dose systemic steroid therapy may be required on an ongoing basis in some patients but the dose is kept to a minimum (American College of Rheumatology Subcommittee on Rheumatoid Arthritis 2002).

The new, biological DMARDs inhibit cytokine activity high up in the inflammatory pathway and can be highly effective even in patients who have failed on conventional DMARD therapy (O'Dell 2004, Olsen & Stein 2004). The most common 'biologicals' are the agents active against tumour necrosis factor α (TNFα) (etanercept (Enbrel), infliximab (Remicade) and adalimumab (Humira)), although new ones are now appearing (Olsen & Stein 2004). The effect of anti-TNF therapy is often striking, with some patients showing a positive response within days or even hours. Biological DMARDs are expensive, however, costing £8,000 to £10,000 for a year of treatment, and so their publicly funded use is restricted to those patients with active disease who have already failed on conventional DMARDs. Because they demonstrate better efficacy than conventional DMARDS, a case is being made for their use in early disease (Emery & Seto 2003, Breedveld et al 2004), where it is contended that the significant reduction in (work-related) disability associated with biological therapy makes these therapies cost effective when viewed in the context of savings to the country from lost work days (9.4 million days, equiva-

### Box 8.2 The preferred protocol for assessing the foot in rheumatology at the authors' centre

**History**

Clerking information

Demographics

General medical history – including (as appropriate) duration of disease, medications, disease activity markers

Presenting complaint – history and documentation, including pain maps and patient-completed baseline health outcome measures (MFPDQ, FFI, LFIS – see the section on assessing outcomes in rheumatic disease later in this chapter)

**Observation (non-weight bearing)**

Musculoskeletal system/disease state:

  Limb alignment

  Joint/soft tissue swellings

  Dermal signs

Presenting complaint:

  Visible lesions measured and dimensions recorded

  Recording of tender and swollen joints counts on a Ritchie-type chart

  Footwear assessment – suitability, wear patterns, distortion of uppers

**Observation (weight bearing)**

Limb alignment – large joint and limb segment alignment, foot posture in quiet standing (supplemented with photographic images as appropriate)

Comparison of weight-bearing observations with non-weight-bearing ones

Observation of gait

**Examination**

Provocation/reproduction of pain/symptoms – palpation, active motion, passive motion

Systematic palpation and movement of structures moving from proximal to distal – bony structures, joints, soft tissues

---

lent to £833 million a year for RA alone) (Arthritis Research Campaign 2002) and decreased dependence on the state benefits system.

Another family of therapies are drugs aimed at reducing the activity and number of B-cells, which are important mediators of the immune-mediated inflammatory response. Rituximab is now well established as a therapy for RA and connective tissue diseases, and good results are reported up to 30 weeks after initial injection without short-term immunocompromise (Edwards et al 2004, Tsokos 2004). Other biological therapies are emerging every year. Currently, the T-cell costimulation blocker abatacept is licensed for use in RA and the anti-interleukin-6 (anti-IL6) compound toclizumab newly available. It is likely that all these therapies will be restricted to those people who have failed on conventional (and cheaper) DMARDs but, common to all, there is an increased risk of infection and practitioners must keep this in mind when caring for patients on these drugs. We still do not know whether drugs such as those in the anti-TNF class will cause an increased tumour incidence with long-term therapy, but the initial indications are good (see box 8.1).

Medical management is usually combined with other approaches such as physical and occupational therapies. Exercise programmes have been found to improve outcomes in a range of rheumatological conditions, including low back pain, lupus, fibromyalgia and ankylosing spondylitis (Rao & Hootman 2004). Other physical therapies in widespread use are heat and cold therapies (baths, thermal packs etc.), therapeutic ultrasound, transcutaneous electrical nerve stimulation (TENS), mobilisation and massage.

Patients with rheumatological disorders often have to live with chronic pain. It is important to recognise the limitations of medical management, and to ensure that the standard approaches are supplemented with specific strategies directed towards living with chronic pain or disability (Rao & Hootman 2004). Cognitive–behavioural strategies are important in enabling patients to understand the condition, and moderate their beliefs and behaviours (Rao & Hootman 2004).

## THE FOOT IN RHEUMATOLOGY – OVERVIEW ACROSS DISEASES

### Assessing the foot

There is no validated, standardised assessment for the foot in musculoskeletal conditions. A number of validated assessments that include the foot are used in medical practice, but podiatrists tend to use more individualised assessments.

The GALS (gait, arms, legs, spine) screen is now considered a minimum standard for all musculoskeletal assessments in medical rheumatology, and this includes at least an observational assessment of the feet. Where lower-limb involvement is suspected, this may be followed up using a new validated assessment, the REMS (regional examination of the musculoskeletal system) assessment, which is being introduced to the rheumatology community (Coady et al 2004). REMS includes a fairly detailed assessment of the feet, although it must be remembered that the GALS and REMS approaches are intended to be part of a general medical work-up and are inadequate for detailed assessment of the foot.

In the absence of a standardised foot assessment, we have developed a preferred protocol for foot assessment at the Leeds centre, which is based on a history–observation–examination (or look–feel–move) model (Box 8.2).

This assessment protocol provides most of the information required to inform a diagnosis and management plan. However, it is sometimes helpful to supplement this assessment with objective data from more 'high-tech' investigations, and patients may also be referred for objective, dynamic functional assessments, such as plantar pressure evaluations, or for radiographic imaging. Gait laboratory assessments are not mainstream outside of teaching centres and are not detailed here, but radiographic imaging is central to rheumatology practice and will be accessed widely by foot practitioners.

The plain radiograph is usually still the imaging modality of first choice, although it is increasingly being supplemented by a range of alternatives. Plain films will differentiate gross radiographic features, such as joint-space narrowing, osteophyte formation or periarticular erosion, but the images are limited to two dimensions. Menz et al (2007) have produced a useful atlas of radiographic classification of joint disease in the foot which may help to standardise interpretation. Plain films are limited in the new paradigm of early and aggressive intervention, however, because they are not sensitive to many of the changes that often occur early in the disease process (Devauchelle-Pensec et al 2002, Ostergaard & Szkudlarek 2003). To image more subtle pathologies of the musculoskeletal system, other modalities are coming to prominence. Magnetic resonance imaging (MRI) allows good visualisation of soft-tissue structures such as ligaments, tendons and synovium. Methods such as T1- and T2-weighted sequences and STIR, particularly if enhanced with a contrast agent such as gadolinium-DTPA, allow for good differentiation of healthy and inflamed soft tissues, and identification of bony oedema and erosions (Bouysset et al 1995, Ostergaard & Szkudlarek 2003). Advances in imaging technology allow for sophisticated three-dimensional reconstructions that can be used to provide valuable visual and quantitative data on the severity of disease activity locally (Woodburn et al 2002a,c). MRI is expensive and time consuming, however, and cannot be considered a first resort. For high-resolution imaging of bony structures, computed tomography (CT) remains the modality of choice. However, CT requires exposure to ionising radiation and is unsuitable for screening or repeated use.

High-resolution ultrasound (HRUS) is becoming increasingly popular as a 'bedside' modality in rheumatology, as it is low risk, differentiates soft tissues structures well and involves no exposure to ionising radiation (Ostergaard & Szkudlarek 2003, Wakefield et al 2000). It is possible using HRUS, to reliably differentiate between inflamed and healthy soft tissues, identify erosions that are undetectable on a plain radiograph and also to investigate structures dynamically (Olivieri et al 1998, Ostergaard & Szkudlarek 2003, Szkudlarek et al 2003, Wakefield et al 2000). There are some limits to HRUS imaging where features of interest, such as those within larger joints such as the ankle, lie too deep to the surface to be imaged, or lie in the ultrasound shadow of structures that form a barrier to the imaging signal. More validation studies are needed, but HRUS imaging is an area of rapid development in musculoskeletal radiology and is proving of considerable clinical use (Riente et al 2006).

## Management principles

In a dedicated rheumatology foot health service, callus reduction, footwear advice and provision, and orthosis prescription are mainstays of management. In a Bradford multidisciplinary rheumatology clinic, some 76% of patients required foot orthoses and 43% required replacement footwear (Helliwell 2003), while in a Rochdale audit the requirement (not the provision) for orthoses and footwear was estimated to be 60% and 10%, respectively. An audit of our Leeds clinic indicates that just over one-quarter of our patients are referred on for footwear intervention, with another quarter receiving orthoses. General foot care (nails, corns and callus) also accounts for one-third of our caseload, a figure lying between those reported separately by Williams & Bowden (2002) and Helliwell (2003), and illustrating the variability in caseloads between services.

Injectable steroid is useful in many cases for controlling local areas of inflammatory activity such as articular synovitis or tenosynovitis.

Injection of corticosteroid has been shown to be effective in relieving plantar heel pain in the short term (Mulherin & Price 2009) and is used widely to control local sites of inflammation associated with inflammatory arthritis (Cardone & Tallia 2002, Crawford et al 1999). Local injection of corticosteroid now falls within the extended scope of practice of a number of allied health professionals and can be a valuable adjunct to traditional conservative therapies for pain in the foot. It is generally recommended that steroid injections are used sparingly because of the degenerative effects on tissues following repeated injection. Patients also need to rest the body part for 24–48 hours after injection because of the risk of local tissue damage while there are high concentrations of steroid present in the tissues and to limit dispersion of the agent (Cardone & Tallia 2002).

Traditionally, most injections of local corticosteroid have been administered 'blind', that is without the aid of radiographic imaging to direct the needle accurately to the desired point of deposition. Recently, the wider availability of ultrasound imaging in musculoskeletal practice has led to a move towards using 'guided' injections, where the agent can be delivered more accurately to the required site.

## Provision of foot health services – current provision, multidisciplinary involvement, surgery

There is a clear gap between the need for foot health services generally and the provision of these services in the UK. Approximately 1 in 10 people with foot pain have nothing at all done about it, and a further 40% self-manage their painful foot problems (Gorter et al 2001). However, the fact that foot problems are substantially underreported (Gorter et al 2000, Munro & Steele 1998) makes services planning and evaluation difficult.

Only one-quarter of those needing foot health services have adequate access provided by NHS services (White & Mulley 1989) and 30–40% of people needing access to foot care services simply do not have services available to them from any source (Garrow et al 2004, Harvey et al 1997). The discrepancy is greater still in the rheumatology population, with a recent survey of 139 patients attending rheumatology outpatients at a North of England hospital finding that 89% of patients had foot problems. Sixty per cent of these patients had no access to foot care services on clinical examination (Williams & Bowden 2002). The inequity in foot health provision to patients with rheumatic disorders has been noted by rheumatologists and podiatrists alike (Helliwell 2003, Michelson et al 1994, Otter 2004).

Multidisciplinary care is important in managing rheumatology patients, and there are two sides to this. On the one hand, rheumatology patients are often complex medically, and it is essential that the practitioner managing the foot problems has a dialogue with, and good back up from, the patient's rheumatology physician. Conversely, expertise in dealing with foot problems is often limited among rheumatologists, and a strong case can be made for better integration of foot health services into rheumatology (Korda & Balint 2004).

While multidisciplinary care is well established and of proven benefit in other disciplines such as diabetology, provision of multidisciplinary foot health services in rheumatology is highly variable. Multidisciplinary clinics will often cover the medical basics, education and coping strategies, but it is less common to find podiatry included as a core part of the team despite the level of need in this patient group nearing 80% (Prier et al 1997). We surveyed rheumatology departments in the UK and established that, while 85% of rheumatology departments include rheumatology specialist nurses in the team and 44% include physiotherapy, only 27.1% include podiatry (Redmond & Helliwell 2005). The provision of foot health services also varies widely geographically, ranging from 65% in Yorkshire and the North East; to 50% in London and the South East, to 25% and 33% in Scotland and Wales, respectively.

Only half the rheumatology departments in our survey reported having access to foot heath services for important functions such as nail care and corn/callus reduction. We have criticised the lack of coordination of foot services in rheumatology previously, noting the problems that are created with patient dissatisfaction, and impediment to the development of the service within the medical teams (Helliwell 2003). We have suggested, from local experience, that a multidisciplinary foot team should consist of at least a rheumatologist, a podiatrist and an orthotist, and it would be quite appropriate to extend team membership to orthopaedics and physiotherapy as resources permit. The Arthritis and Musculoskeletal Alliance (ARMA) and Podiatry Rheumatic Care Association (PRCA) Standards of Care (2008) provide a useful mechanism for evaluating musculoskeletal foot health services and planning strategically to best integrate medical and foot health teams. Succession planning is imperative, as small teams such as these can be highly dependent on individual people for their success, and it is all too easy for a successful service to run into problems if one of the team leaves and his or her replacement is unable to participate at the same level. To ensure a level of professional development appropriate to a specialist team it is advisable that arrangements are made for continuing professional development, and for update courses to be undertaken jointly with the rest of the rheumatology team (Otter 2004).

A good multidisciplinary rheumatology foot health service is likely to tap into considerable unmet need for foot health services (Prier et al 1997) and it is our and others' experience that the service will expand rapidly and attract referrals for a range of conditions (Helliwell 2003, Prier et al 1997). A robust business plan should be devised prior to initiating a service in order to pre-empt these potential problems and to ensure the long-term success of such a venture. The initial business plan should also be supplemented with careful documentation of patient outcomes (Prier et al 1997) so that the merits of the service can be quantified and the cost effectiveness evaluated in the long term.

Within a rheumatology multidisciplinary team, rheumatology specialist nurses play an increasingly central role, responsible for administering, monitoring and modifying patients' medication, education, and a valuable psychosocial support role (NICE 2009). The therapy professions, specifically physiotherapy and occupational therapy, are also important in the overall management of the symptoms associated with inflammatory arthritis, and NICE (2008, 2009) has produced explicit guidance on these roles in rheumatology. The main roles for rehabilitation therapies are to help people limit disability through skills training, exercise training, pain management, joint protection programmes, and provision of splints and orthoses (Steultjens et al 2004). The merit of providing splints as part of a regimen of occupational therapy has been demonstrated, and echoes the data for foot orthoses provided as part of podiatric management (Budiman-Mak et al 1995, Steultjens et al 2004, Woodburn et al 2002a).

## Service provision

The foot health services that should be provided as part of a multidisciplinary foot health team in rheumatology fall into five categories.

1. Education and self-management advice, including footwear advice.
2. Provision of, or assistance with, finding orthoses and footwear.
3. General foot care, nail cutting, corn and callus reduction, provision of padding.
4. High-risk management of the vasculitic or ulcerative foot.
5. Extended scope practice and surgery.

### Education and self-management advice

In an era of increased patient empowerment, education programmes have become more commonplace. Self-management is known to result in improved health status (Rao & Hootman 2004), but there is conflicting evidence over the merit of formal education programmes for patients with rheumatic disorders. Education is the mainstay of management in non-systemic conditions such as chronic mechanical low back pain, and provides demonstrable benefits over traditional medical management of this condition (Rao & Hootman 2004). In the inflammatory diseases the picture is less clear, however, and the measurable benefits are probably confined to short-term effects on the psychological factors and impact of disability (Riemsma et al 2004). Education in RA provides measurable improvement in knowledge but only small and non-significant changes in objective and health-related quality of life measures (Helliwell et al 1999). In OA, a small reduction in the use of healthcare services was reported after individualised education, but again no changes in patient outcomes have been found (Riemsma et al 2004, Ward 2000). Rheumatology patients can be overwhelmed with information at diagnosis, however, and it may be best to introduce education selectively, focusing on issues of particular relevance at any given time. This is equally true for foot health advice, and clear guidance on the provision of information has been provided in the ARMA/PRCA Standards of Care (2008).

### General foot care, nail cutting, corn and callus reduction, provision of padding

Patients with musculoskeletal conditions have an increased need for a range of basic foot care services. Deformities of the foot associated with joint changes and soft-tissue lesions create areas of pressure that result in callus and corn formation. Arthritis in the hands may make foot care and hygiene tasks difficult, and spinal involvement can make bending to attend to basic foot care tasks impossible.

It is well accepted anecdotally and in simple cohort studies (Redmond et al 1999, Woodburn et al 2000) that debridement of symptomatic callosities and removal of cornified nuclei reduces pain in the short term. One randomised trial has provided contradictory evidence, however, suggesting that callus debridement was no better than placebo at reducing pain scores in patients with RA (Davys et al 2004). The study authors do not recommend abandoning callus debridement because the anecdotal evidence and patient demand is so overwhelming, but it is clear that more research is needed into this important area of podiatric practice. Offloading strategies are essential for managing the deformed rheumatic foot, and podiatrists can be useful in providing orthoses and/ or footwear (Korda & Balint 2004).

### High-risk management of the vasculitic or ulcerative foot

This is a sometimes neglected aspect of rheumatology practice. Risk of ulceration is raised in a number of musculoskeletal diseases, such as RA, in which the point prevalence is about 3% (Firth et al 2008). Management of the high-risk foot accounts for approximately one-quarter of the Leeds foot health appointments, and in one report of the case profile of multisystem wound care service rheumatology patients made up 6% of the total caseload (Steed et al 1993). Prevention and management of the high-risk foot is an important part of the foot health service in rheumatology (Korda & Balint 2004) (Figure 8.3).

### Extended scope practice and surgery

The advent of the extended scope practitioner (ESP) has created the opportunity for foot health services to be more responsive to patients' needs. The new ESPs are able to access enhanced investigations and can intervene more proactively, making amendments to patients'

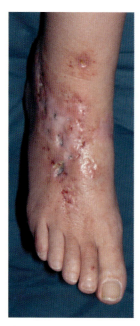

**Figure 8.3** A high-risk foot with localised rheumatoid vasculitis.

pharmacological management and using injectable steroids. More sophisticated surgical techniques and better integration of surgeons into the early management have also improved the surgical management of the foot in rheumatology.

## SPECIFIC DISEASES

## Seropositive inflammatory arthritis

### Rheumatoid arthritis

#### Definition

RA is a chronic, immune-mediated inflammatory disease with polyarthritis as its main feature. Chronic inflammation leads to joint damage and functional impairment (van Gestel et al 1996). Rheumatoid factors are detectable by serological testing in a large proportion of cases.

#### Epidemiology

The prevalence of RA in the population is approximately 7.7 per 1000 (0.8%), a risk that is doubled for relatives of confirmed cases (Hawker 1997). Approximately two-thirds of new cases arise in females, and mostly in the fourth and fifth decades of life, although there is wide variation and some suggestion that the age of onset is increasing. In one large UK cohort reported recently, the average age at onset was 55 years (Young et al 2000).

#### Diagnosis

Diagnosis is made according to diagnostic criteria defined by the American College of Rheumatology (Box 8.3). Key serological markers for the systemic inflammatory response are a raised erythrocyte sedimentation rate and C-reactive protein. Testing for rheumatoid factor aids in diagnosis and estimating the prognosis (American College of Rheumatology Subcommittee on Rheumatoid Arthritis 2002). Rheumatoid factor is present in 65–80% of patients with RA, and those who are rheumatoid factor positive are predisposed to more severe disease. Radiographic changes are often not present in early disease or on plain film. Radiography may not help with diagnosis, although it does provide a useful baseline for future assessment (American College of Rheumatology Subcommittee on Rheumatoid Arthritis 2002). Enhanced visualisation of inflamed synovium is possible with modern HRUS, and this modality may be helpful in early cases.

There is an important role for primary care practitioners in aiding with the early recognition of as yet undiagnosed inflammatory arthritis (American College of Rheumatology Subcommittee on Rheumatoid Arthritis 2002). The foot is the first site of involvement in about 1 in 8 cases of RA, and some 20% of patients report foot pain before any other manifestation of the disease (O'Brien et al 1997).

A consensus-based referral recommendation for primary care practitioners (Emery et al 2002) states that inflammatory (rheumatoid) arthritis should be considered, and patients referred rapidly for a rheumatology opinion if they demonstrate:

- three or more swollen joints
- pain on lateral compression of the metacarpo- or metatarsophalangeal joints (a positive squeeze test)
- Morning stiffness of ≥30 minutes duration.

#### Pathology

The underlying histopathology is of an immune-mediated synovitis caused by a faulty autoimmune response to proteins such as immunoglobulin G. The synovial membrane of the affected joint becomes hyperplastic, and infiltrated with inflammatory cells that promote secretion of proinflammatory cytokines (including TNFα) (Feldman & Maini 2008). The synovial membrane proliferates further, forming a pannus, which increasingly intrudes into the joint space (Choy & Panayi 2001). Cells in the pannus release enzymes that degrade cartilage and the connective tissue matrix (Choy & Panayi 2001). Erosion is more extensive around the margins of joints, because the articular cartilage affords some initial protection to the subchondral bone (Gold et al 1988).

#### Clinical course

The disability pathway for inflammatory arthritis and the specific factors affecting the clinical course in RA are summarised in Figure 8.1. Modifiers include endogenous factors that affect the underlying pathology, biopsychosocial factors and exogenous factors.

The presence of rheumatoid factor is a key marker for subsequent disease severity and is found in about 60% of new cases (American College of Rheumatology Subcommittee on Rheumatoid Arthritis 2002, Young et al 2000). Modern antibody testing, including for anti-CCP antibodies, has further improved diagnostic specificity and prognostic prediction (van Venrooij et al 2008). Other important prognostic factors include HAQ score, delay in instigating therapy, smoking, and the presence of certain immunogenetic markers (Sanmarti et al 2003, Young et al 2000).

There appears to be some shortening of the lifespan because of the disease course itself and also because of the risks associated with therapies such as oral steroids and DMARDs (Hawker 1997). RA is associated with decreased ability to undertake both paid work, and unpaid work such as domestic duties (Backman et al 2004), and everyday activities of work and leisure take longer to perform (March & Lapsley 2001). Work disability increases with disease duration. Approximately 20% of people with RA report significant work disability within a year of diagnosis, one-third by 2 years and up to 60% within 10 years of onset (Barrett et al 2000). A third of people with RA will leave the workforce permanently within 3 years of diagnosis (Barrett et al 2000).

The clinical course of the disease improved markedly with improvements in DMARD therapy in the 1980s and 1990s, and more recently with the advent of biological immunotherapy. Patients treated with conventional DMARDs will typically do moderately well, with some 13% going into long-term remission, and just under one-half following a moderated disease course with episodes of remission and relapse (Young et al 2000). Patients following this disease course will do better than those untreated or on NSAIDs only, but joint degeneration does accrue in the long term (>10 years) and disability remains a factor in established RA (Gordon et al 2001). Joint-space narrowing occurs early in RA, and is initially symmetrical and uniform, although it becomes less regular as the joint degenerates (Kumar & Madewell 1987). Some ongoing joint degeneration will occur in all but the mildest or best-controlled cases, and joint replacement remains a mainstay of management in end-stage disease. Currently, some 1 in 10 people will require at least one joint replacement within 5 years of diagnosis (Young et al 2000), although it might be expected that this number will fall as early DMARD therapy starts to improve prognosis.

## Medical management

The outline of medical management in rheumatology described in the earlier section of this chapter is derived primarily from the principles of management of RA and needs no repetition here. There are clear guidelines provided by the American College of Rheumatology Subcommittee on Rheumatoid Arthritis (2002) and in the UK by the National Institute for Clinical Excellence (NICE 2009). An abridged schema adapted from the American College of Rheumatology guidelines for the medical management of RA can be seen in Figure 8.2.

It should be noted that while this schema represents an ideal clinical pathway, complete remission is still unusual (American College of Rheumatology Subcommittee on Rheumatoid Arthritis 2002), and some patients respond particularly poorly to specific DMARDs, even to new biological agents (Feldmann 2002). Where full remission is not achieved, the management goals become symptom relief and maximisation of quality of life (American College of Rheumatology Subcommittee on Rheumatoid Arthritis 2002). Medical treatment should thus be undertaken within a multidisciplinary setting, with other disciplines providing valuable input to the chronic disease process (NICE 2009).

## The foot in rheumatoid arthritis

The prevalence and impact of foot problems is strongly related to disease duration (Michelson et al 1994) and the foot is eventually affected in nearly all people with RA, usually in a symmetrical pattern. Joint pain and stiffness is the most common initial presentation, but a range of other features may also be found, including tenosynovitis,

nodule formation and tarsal tunnel syndrome, reflecting the widespread soft-tissue involvement. Foot-related impact is a consequence of a combination of factors, including pain, inflammation and mechanics (Turner et al 2008), with involvement of the feet both contributing to (van der Leeden et al 2008a) and representing a marker for impaired mobility and functional capacity in RA (Wickman et al 2004). In about three-quarters of people with RA, the foot contributes to difficulty with walking, and the foot is the main or only cause of walking impairment in one-quarter (Kerry et al 1994).

Some 20–25% of all surgical operations for RA relate to manifestations of the disease in the feet (Hamalainen & Raunio 1997). Despite this high demand, the success of surgical interventions is only moderate. Fewer than 50% of patients undergoing forefoot surgery for RA report 'very good' or 'excellent' outcomes. Indeed, 13% of patients undergoing foot surgery for inflammatory arthropathy require subsequent reoperation because of poor outcomes (Hamalainen & Raunio 1997).

### Hindfoot

Retrocalcaneal bursitis is common in RA, and often coexists with inflammation of the Achilles tendon and long flexor and extensor tendon sheaths (Stiskal et al 1997). This in turn leads to the development of longitudinal tendon tears and structural degeneration, which in the long term can occasionally lead to complete rupture of the tendon, especially in high-load tendons such as the tendon of tibialis posterior (Bouysset et al 1995, Kumar & Madewell 1987). Tendinopathy is best imaged using HRUS or gadolinium-enhanced MRI (see earlier), which will show a greater frequency of involvement than the clinical examination (Bouysset et al 1995). Lesions were found in the posterior tibial tendons of 53/67 patients in one recent study (Bouysset et al 2003), but complete rupture of the tendon is uncommon, even in severely deformed feet (Jernberg et al 1999, Masterton et al 1995). Spurs can be found on the plantar surface of the calcaneus in about one-third of established RA cases, with a similar prevalence of posterior spurs at the insertion of the Achilles tendon, although posterior spurs tend to be smaller and are often asymptomatic (Bouysset et al 1989). The degree of soft-tissue involvement is largely dependent on the systemic disease activity, but local areas of severe inflammation may respond to infiltration of steroid into joints or soft tissues (McGuire 2003).

Ankle (talocrural) joint degeneration occurs relatively rarely in RA, and is confined to severe and late-stage disease (1 in 10 patients after 20 years). Ankle-joint change is almost always preceded by subtalar joint involvement (Belt et al 2001), and may therefore be a consequence of altered hindfoot alignment (Cimino & O'Malley 1999). Subtalar joint disease is suggested where there is pain on walking over uneven ground and swelling posterior to the medial malleolus or in the sinus tarsi (Bouysset et al 1995). The subtalar joint is affected in about a quarter of long-standing RA patients (Bouysset et al 1987) but rarely in early disease.

In the longer term, synovitis in the hindfoot joints leads to systematic changes in hindfoot structure and function (Woodburn et al 2002). The altered function, combined with the effect of load bearing and increased soft-tissue laxity, lead the hindfoot to function in a progressively more pronated position, with the heel becoming more inclined into valgus and the tibia more internally rotated (Bouysset et al 1987, Keenan et al 1991, Woodburn et al 2002b) (Figure 8.4).

Initially, the deformities are largely reducible, and the elastic response of the soft tissues allows for correction. Rigid functional orthoses have been shown to restore normal function at this early stage, and to slow the progression of fixed deformity (Woodburn et al 1999). If uncorrected, bony adaptation and disease-related changes in soft-tissue histology will lead to irreducible structural changes.

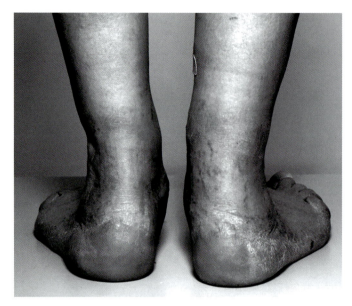

**Figure 8.4** Valgus hindfoot deformity in RA.

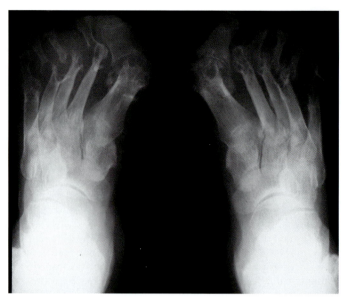

**Figure 8.5** Plain radiograph of severe forefoot deformity in RA.

Varus deformities of the hindfoot occur in fewer than 1 in 30 people with RA (Kerry et al 1994, Vidigal et al 1975), and usually as a direct consequence of compensation strategies such as inversion of the forefoot to offload painful medial metatarsophalangeal joints (MTPJs).

It is important to note that health-related quality of life is better related to rearfoot pain than rearfoot deformity (Platto et al 1991), and so interventions should be provided on the basis of patient reports of impairment rather than reserved for those with the appearance of worse foot deformity.

In the valgus rheumatoid foot, synovitis and compression of tissues on the medial aspect of the hindfoot can lead to tarsal tunnel syndrome (Jernberg et al 1999). This manifests as a paraesthesia or as a burning sensation over the distribution of the tibial nerve on the plantar surface of the foot. Tarsal tunnel syndrome may respond to local injection of corticosteroid, but may require surgical decompression.

Surgical procedures most commonly performed on the rheumatoid hindfoot include tarsal tunnel decompression, and ankle, subtalar or talonavicular arthrodesis (McGuire 2003). There have been calls for surgical interventions to be considered earlier, as it is proposed that an early correction may improve local mechanics and minimise subsequent degeneration in neighbouring joints (Cimino & O'Malley 1999, Cracchiolo 1993). At present, however, most surgical interventions in the rheumatoid hindfoot are performed on feet in the late stages of disease.

Subtalar arthrodesis is often indicated following rupture of the tendon of tibialis posterior, where tendon repair is often not possible because of the degenerate nature of the tissue. In the absence of repair, the continued lack of medial stability leads to a poor prognosis unless the joint is fused surgically (Bouysset et al 1995). The salvage procedure for severe cases of hindfoot structural change is triple arthrodesis following corrective wedge osteotomies to restore better alignment (Cimino & O'Malley 1999). Ankle and hindfoot arthroplasty in RA is directed toward addressing the degenerative joint changes, and so these procedures are discussed more fully in the later section on OA.

In the presence of significant deformity, adaptive footwear might be necessary. The addition of external flanges to the heel, along with reinforcement of the heel counter and medial arch of the upper of the shoes can aid with hindfoot stability. Extra-depth shoes allow for an orthosis to be better accommodated.

## Midfoot

The joints of the midfoot are affected widely, with the talonavicular joint and Lisfranc's joints affected in 15–30% of cases (Bouysset et al 1987). Diffuse joint degeneration may occur, although the characteristic erosions seen in the forefoot (Figure 8.5) are generally less common in the rheumatoid midfoot.

## Forefoot

The MTPJs are the joints most commonly affected in RA (Weinfeld & Schon 1998), and MTPJ involvement often precedes that of any other joints, again with a symmetrical distribution (Pensec et al 2004, Priolo et al 1997). Early synovitis can lead to swelling of the digits (Kumar & Madewell 1987), and MTPJ synovitis, which is noted clinically as a warm boggy feeling to the joint on palpation, can lead to separation of neighbouring toes (the so-called 'daylight sign').

In the longer term, the acute phase will reduce (van der Leeden et al 2008b) and the rheumatoid forefoot will develop a typical marked hallux-valgus-type presentation and hammer toe deformities of the lesser toes (Figure 8.6). The hallux valgus deformity of RA is severe, with a large medial eminence, and it often results in first MTPJ subluxation (Weinfeld & Schon 1998). The second, third and fourth toes will typically exhibit lateral drift in addition to the hammer toe deformity, while the fifth toe will often be directed toward the midline, coming to lie over or under the fourth toe. It is common for the lesser digits to cease weight bearing entirely, and in combination with anterior displacement and atrophy of the plantar fat pads this leads to significantly increased pressure under the MTPJs (Turner & Helliwel 2003), which in turn is associated with greater impairment (Schmiegel et al 2008). Prominent adventitious bursae develop under the metatarsal heads, and these are frequently overlaid with callus (Figure 8.7). Bursitis at this site will be painful, and localised areas of skin ulceration are not uncommon (Figure 8.8). Plantar pressure data show the areas of increased pressure to be highly localised, and patients often describe a feeling of 'walking on pebbles'.

The pain from the forefoot, and to a lesser extent the midfoot and hindfoot joints leads to characteristic changes in the gait of people with RA. Gait velocity decreases, as both the cadence and stride length are reduced. The double-support period extends to minimise the forces applied to the foot, and a reluctance to load the forefoot leads

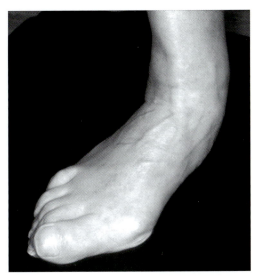

**Figure 8.6** The clinical appearance of the forefoot deformity typical of RA.

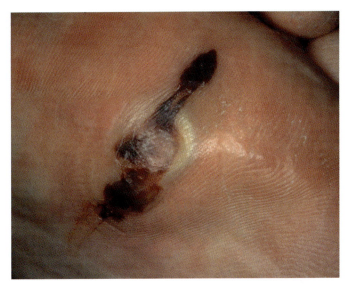

**Figure 8.8** Ulceration of the skin overlying plantar bursae.

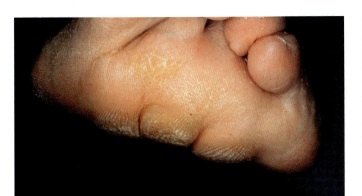

**Figure 8.7** Prominent plantar bursae in established RA.

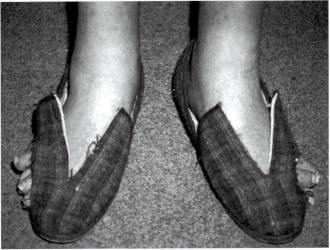

**Figure 8.9** Self-help by a patient with RA who requires non-standard footwear.

to delay in loading and a change in the velocity of centre-of-pressure profile (Hamilton et al 2001, Keenan et al 1991, O'Connell et al 1998, Turner & Helliwel 2003).

The severity of the changes that occur in the rheumatoid forefoot can often lead to a requirement for non-standard footwear (Figure 8.9). Traditionally, prescription footwear was bespoke (i.e. shoes were made to an individual cast or model) and were intended to account for specific individual features. Long-standing dissatisfaction with this approach, due to the high costs and unacceptable levels of patient (and practitioner) satisfaction (Williams et al 2007) has seen a change in approach in more recent years (Herold & Palmer 1992, Lord & Foulston 1989). One recent Dutch study indicated that about one-third of RA patients had been provided with orthopaedic footwear and, in an encouraging trend, 80% of this was in daily use (de Boer et al 2009).

Accommodative footwear can be provided off-the-shelf if the requirement is simply for extra depth or soft uppers in the toe box. The patient's own shoes may be adapted in some cases, or bespoke shoes may still be made. Off-the-shelf shoes have been shown to provide significant improvements in pain, quality of life and gait parameters (Fransen & Edmonds 1997, Williams et al 2007), and are especially effective when combined with semi-rigid orthoses (Egan et al 2003). There is evidence for similar levels of satisfaction with bespoke and off-the-shelf shoes for people with RA (Kerry et al 1994).

Prescription footwear is usually provided in the NHS by orthotists working to a consultant prescription, but commercial alternatives provide other avenues that are increasingly available. Patient compliance is often problematic, and there is increasing evidence for benefits associated with better consideration of patient choice in the design and provision of bespoke footwear (Williams et al 2007).

Soft, flexible uppers made of soft leathers or stretchable textile can be very helpful in reducing the pressure on deformed digits (Figure 8.10), and in accommodating the increased width of the rheumatoid forefoot. The material characteristics and the presence of seams also warrant extra consideration where there is a risk of ulceration secondary to impaired arterial supply or vasculitis. The increased pressure found under the rheumatoid forefoot is aided by the addition of cushioning, and this can be provided separately or incorporated into prescription footwear (Egan et al 2003, Hodge et al 1999).

Rigid or semi-rigid, functional orthoses are known to be effective in limiting the rate of hindfoot and forefoot deformity, and in redis-

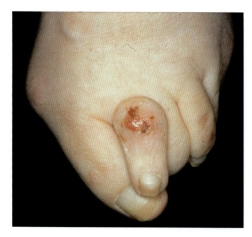

**Figure 8.10** Digital deformity and ulceration in a patient with RA.

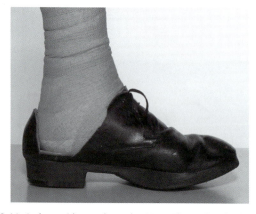

**Figure 8.11** A shoe with a rocker sole. *Note:* The patient had cut the heel counter of the shoe away herself to reduce pressure and discomfort.

tributing load away from the forefoot (Budiman-Mak et al 1995, Redmond et al 2004, Woodburn et al 2003), and contrary to past anecdotal opinion are well tolerated by people with RA (Woodburn et al 2002a). This approach, combined with forefoot cushioning, is effective at reducing pressure and pain in the painful forefoot (Chalmers et al 2000, Hodge et al 1999, Redmond et al 2004) and improving basic gait parameters (Kavlak et al 2003).

When joint pain is severe, the demand for painful motion in the forefoot joints during walking can be reduced by the provision of shoes with a rocker sole (Figure 8.11). A rocker sole is a straightforward adaptation little used in podiatry generally, but which can be quite effective in patients with RA.

Patients with RA affecting their back and/or hands may experience difficulties with shoe fastenings. Advice can be given when people are purchasing shoes to minimise this problem. Standard laces can be changed for elastic laces in existing shoes, removing the need for the wearer to bend and tie them. Alternative fastenings such as Velcro or elastic should be considered when choosing or prescribing orthopaedic footwear.

Many people with forefoot involvement require surgery and, because the forefoot is more affected by RA, forefoot procedures are generally performed before the hindfoot is operated on. However, if there is severe concomitant hindfoot involvement, stabilisation of the hindfoot does take precedence (Cracchiolo 1993).

The surgical approach to the forefoot joints is normally via dorsal incisions, as scarring on the weight-bearing plantar surface of the foot can lead to painful callus formation later. Plantar incisions are used when the skin quality on the dorsum of the foot might lead to problems with healing. Because of the severity of the joint degeneration in RA, excision arthroplasty is a part of most procedures, and the metatarsal heads, the base of the phalanges, or both are usually excised. Different procedures are used for the first MTPJ and lesser MTPJs. First MTPJ procedures, such as Keller's excision arthroplasty, joint arthrodesis and replacement arthrodeses, are described elsewhere and will not be detailed here. For a severe lesser toe deformity, such as seen in RA, there are many procedures available, with those described by authors such as Clayton, Kates and Fowler forming the mainstay of rheumatoid foot surgery through the latter half of the 20th century. All lesser MTPJs are usually operated on simultaneously, because more conservative approaches involving surgery on only one of the most affected joints tend to have poorer long-term results in people with RA (Hughes et al 1991). Metatarsal head resection provides significant reduction in pain and forefoot pressure (Bitzan et al 1997, Rosenberg et al 2000), although the postoperative function cannot be considered normal and results tend to worsen in the longer term (Toolan & Hansen 1998). Modern variations, including techniques involving interposition of the plantar plate and preservation of the metatarsal head, are gradually supplanting the more traditional approaches (Cracchiolo 1993).

### Subcutaneous lesions

Subcutaneous rheumatoid nodules are thought to arise in about one-quarter of patients with RA, usually those who are rheumatoid-factor positive and who have more severe disease (Gilkes 1987). The fibrotic nodules are associated with subcutaneous vasculitis and subsequent fibrosis, and arise at points of high stress, such as the extensor surfaces of elbows or knees. One study detected histological signs of rheumatoid necrosis (nodules) in the forefeet of 65% of a sample of people with RA, although most were subclinical (Berger et al 2004). Clinically evident nodules are not common in the feet, but affected sites include the posterior aspect of the heel and the dorsum of the forefoot. Rarely, nodules may break down or cause ulceration of overlying skin. If rheumatoid nodules are causing problems with shoe fitting or weight bearing, they may require surgical excision.

### Skin and nails

Patients with RA of long disease duration will develop significant skin atrophy, with the skin taking on a pale, translucent quality (Gilkes 1987). The nails may be thickened and ridged, but are not usually symptomatic. The involvement of the hand, and difficulties with bending over for people with RA, mean that many patients need help with general foot health tasks such as nail cutting and maintenance of foot hygiene.

### Vasculitis

Although better disease control appears to be reducing the prevalence of RA-related vasculitis (Turesson & Matteson 2009), it is not uncommon for vasculitis and ulceration to affect the rheumatoid foot, especially in patients who are rheumatoid-factor positive or have other signs of severe disease such as rheumatoid nodules (Cawley 1987). Usually, the pedal pulses are unaffected and the vasculitis is localised, affecting only part of the foot. The most common vasculitis in RA is endarteritis obliterans, in which inflammation of the intimal layer of the small blood vessels leads to occlusion of blood flow (Cawley 1987). The clinical features of endarteritis obliterans are infarcts in the nail beds and/or toe pulps. These are initially red and uncomfortable, but often turn black and painless within a few days, although in some cases the infarct progresses to form an ulcer. A second form, necrotising vasculitis, is caused by vessel-wall destruction (Genta et al 2006). If necrotising vasculitis

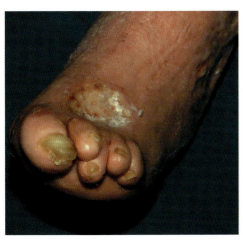

**Figure 8.12** Necrotising vasculitis leading to a large ulcer on the dorsum of the foot.

affects the venules, it leads to local exsanguinations under the skin (palpable purpura). Necrotising vasculitis affecting arterioles leads to larger areas of ulceration, usually on the dorsum of the foot and toes (Cawley 1987) (Figure 8.12). Vasculitis can affect the vasa nervorum, leading to peripheral sensory neuropathy in some people with RA.

The foot is at high risk of ulceration in people with RA (Genta et al 2006). The risk is elevated because of the tendency to vasculitis and the thinning of the skin, and also because of the deformity accompanying the disease, which leads to the development of areas of high pressure, both on the dorsal and on the plantar aspects of the foot (Firth et al 2008). These risk factors are also present in addition to the usual cardiovascular risk factors present in an older population. In the Leeds rheumatology foot health clinic some 15% of the patients have vascular/high-risk presentations, and they account for over a quarter of appointment slots.

The site of the ulcer will give clues as to the important underlying pathology; breakdown over obvious pressure sites, such as the dorsum of deformed interphalangeal joints, might be expected to respond well to offloading of pressure. Breakdowns on the dorsum of the foot and lower leg are more likely to be of predominantly vasculitic origin (Cawley 1987) and need multidisciplinary management, including review of antirheumatic medication and possible supplementary therapy with agents such as Iloprost (Kay & Nancarrow 1984). The vasculitis associated with RA is also reported to respond well to anti-TNF therapy (Olsen & Stein 2004).

The increased susceptibility of many rheumatology patients to infection has been discussed previously, and must be considered in the care of this group.

## Juvenile idiopathic arthritis

### Definition

Juvenile idiopathic arthritis is a heterogeneous group of inflammatory arthropathies indicated by the presence of an inflammatory arthropathy, with an onset at less than 16 years of age, affecting one or more joints for longer than 6 weeks.

### Epidemiology

Around 12 000 children in the UK have juvenile idiopathic arthritis, and girls are almost three times more likely to be affected than boys (Arthritis Research Campaign 2002).

### Classification

Juvenile idiopathic arthritis has undergone a number of different classifications in the last 20 years. Each new classification is based on emerging knowledge of the taxonomy, natural history and immunopathology of the condition. The latest classification was decided upon in Durban in 2000 and suggests seven classes for children with juvenile idiopathic arthritis: systemic arthritis, oligoarthritis, polyarthritis (two classes depending on rheumatoid factor status), psoriatic arthritis, enthesitis-related arthritis and 'undifferentiated' (Petty et al 1991). Better information on treatment and prognosis will be forthcoming as further studies of these groups are published.

### Diagnosis

The diagnosis of juvenile idiopathic arthritis is based on the exclusion of other provisional diagnoses, such as infection and trauma. The history is usually of a chronic idiopathic synovitis, with onset in a single joint, typically the knee, ankle, hip or wrist (oligoarticular onset). Blood tests are less helpful in diagnosis than in adult-onset arthritis, but can help the clinician to decide to which subgroup the patient belongs.

### Pathology

The pathophysiology is specific to the subgroup, but is essentially that of a chronic immune-mediated inflammatory synovitis. The enthesis, however, is the primary site of inflammation in enthesitis-related arthritis and psoriatic arthritis (see the section on adult seronegative arthropathy later in this chapter). The inflammatory pathways are similar in children and adults, and so the driving cytokine in many of the groups is TNFα.

### Clinical course

Onset is often before 4 years of age, and the clinical course is variable and dependent on the clinical subgroup. In a good proportion of cases of oligoarticular disease, the disease may remit spontaneously with no long-term joint damage. In the majority of cases of polyarticular arthritis, the disease will continue for many years, sometimes without remission throughout the lifespan. Many cases positive for rheumatoid factor go on to a clinical course similar to RA.

### Medical management

The general principle is of support rather than cure, and management is aimed at limiting symptoms, maintaining function and minimising permanent changes. NSAIDs will be the initial intervention. Intra-articular steroids are often used in severe monoarticular or oligoarticular forms. Disease-modifying drugs are used in cases with a poor prognosis, which will include those in the polyarticular group, the juvenile RA group and the systemic onset group.

The principal drugs used are methotrexate, corticosteroids and biological drugs such as anti-TNFα (Olsen & Stein 2004).

The local management of the foot and legs in these children will complement these therapies, as in the adult. It is, however, important to note the differences between children and adults with arthritis. Children are naturally stoic and will get on with their life as long as the symptoms are tolerable. Consequently, they are also more prone to loading inflamed joints and have little sense of joint protection.

### The foot in juvenile idiopathic arthritis

#### Polyarticular type

The foot, especially the hindfoot and ankle, is involved in some two-thirds of polyarticular cases (Hendry et al 2008). Involvement of centres of ossification can lead to alterations in the shape of the growing bones and may cause deformity and brachydactyly (Moll

1987). Pes planus or pes cavus deformities may develop, as can the hallux-valgus-type picture seen in adult RA (Chen 1996).

### Enthesitis-related arthritis and psoriatic arthritis

As noted previously, this presentation mirrors that of the adult seronegative arthropathies. The joints most affected in the foot are the hindfoot and interphalangeal joints, and entheseal inflammation at the insertion of the Achilles tendon and plantar fascia is common. Spinal involvement is common as the disease progresses. Inflammation in the mid- and hindfoot joints may lead to subsequent ankylosis, a not infrequent end point in this subgroup.

Particular attention should be given to the feet in juvenile idiopathic arthritis, as deformity will occur quickly. Better therapies have improved prognosis generally, but foot involvement remains common (Hendry et al 2008). Children are usually very accepting of in-shoe orthoses, but these must be reviewed annually, and more frequently during growth spurts. Joint inflammation may cause overgrowth or undergrowth of the adjacent long bones, so a careful watch for limb-length discrepancy should be maintained.

## Seronegative inflammatory arthritis:

### Introduction – common features

The seronegative arthritides are again a diverse group of conditions with a number of common features. There is a known association with the human leucocyte antigen (HLA) B27, and some 90% of patients with seronegative arthropathy of various types test positive for this antigen. Clinically, there is frequent involvement of the spine (axial involvement) in the seronegative arthritides, and many will first present as back pain before differentiating later. The inflammatory process in the seronegative arthropathies is also associated with enthesopathy – inflammation at the insertion of ligaments or tendons (Olivieri et al 1998). The most common sites for enthesopathy in the foot are the posterior calcaneus at the insertion of the Achilles tendon, the plantar calcaneus (the plantar fascia and the short flexor muscles), the base of the fifth metatarsal and the forefoot (McGonagle et al 2002, Olivieri et al 1998). There may be localised swelling at superficial insertions such as that of the Achilles tendon (Figure 8.13), and swellings can be especially pronounced when the enthesopathy extends to involve local bursae. In the fingers and toes the enthesitis and synovitis can present with marked dactylitis or 'sausage digits' (Figure 8.14). More widespread inflammation can lead to noticeable general swelling in the foot.

On radiography there may be periarticular proliferation of periosteum and bone, usually whiskery or fluffy in character, which contrasts with the bony erosions seen in RA. New bone formation may also be seen at the entheses as a consequence of the inflammatory process. It is uncommon for the foot in the seronegative arthropathies to be associated with vasculitis (Cawley 1987).

## Ankylosing spondylitis (inflammatory back pain)

### Definition

Ankylosing spondylitis is a progressive seronegative spondyloarthropathy that affects the axial skeleton (the spine and surrounding structures) predominantly, but which also has peripheral features that can involve the foot.

### Epidemiology

The incidence of AS is approximately 1%, with men affected by AS three times as frequently as women (Braun & Sieper 2007). The ankle is affected in one-quarter of people with AS, and the forefoot in about 10% (Moll 1987). The inflammatory spondyloarthropathies cause 1.4 million working days to be lost each year, costing the UK economy some £122 million.

### Diagnosis

Diagnosis is based on the modified New York criteria of the presence of one of:

- inflammatory back pain of >3 months duration
- limited spinal mobility in two planes
- limited chest expansion, plus evidence of sacroiliitis on the plain radiograph.

However, these criteria have been criticised for having limited sensitivity (van der Heijde 2004).

### Pathology

The pathology is not well understood overall, but appears to be driven by enthesitis. The sacroiliac joints are the worst affected, and initial inflammation can give way to ossification of the joints. TNF appears important in the pathological process, and overexpression of TNF precipitates an ankylosing-spondylitis-type presentation in transgenic mice. Preliminary findings from treatment studies suggest that TNF blockade appears even more beneficial in people with ankylosing spondylitis than in those with RA (Marzo-Ortega et al 2001).

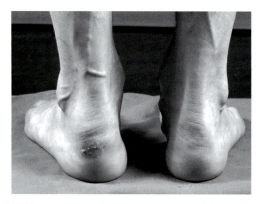

**Figure 8.13** Heel enthesopathy in seronegative arthritis (psoriatic arthritis).

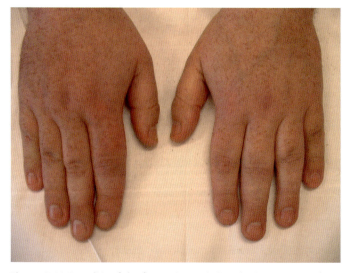

**Figure 8.14** Dactylitis of the fingers in psoriatic arthritis.

### Clinical course

Ankylosing spondylitis tends to manifest itself initially as low back or buttock pain because of sacroiliitis. Peripheral symptoms (including those in the foot) occur early in the disease but become less problematic over time, leaving the spondyloarthropathy as the main feature of long-standing disease. Spinal curvature increases over time as the long-standing inflammatory process leads to ankylosis and bone formation. The clinical course is generally less severe than in RA, and some cases will remit spontaneously. One notable feature of ankylosing spondylitis is the presence of fatigue as a significant factor for patients (van der Heijde 2004).

### Medical management

NSAIDs are the mainstay of medical management in ankylosing spondylitis, although DMARDs, such as sulfasalazine, are also beneficial for the peripheral arthritis (DeJesus & Tsuchiya 1999, Olivieri et al 1998). Anti-TNF drugs are now established as major symptom-modifying drugs in ankylosing spondylitis. In one study of patients who had already failed to respond to conventional DMARD therapy, TNFα blockade caused complete resolution of 86% of entheseal lesions and led to substantial improvement in pain and quality of life (Marzo-Ortega et al 2001). Even supposedly end-stage 'fixed' spinal kyphoses can show some restoration of function once the inflammatory process has been suppressed. The Assessment in Ankylosing Spondylitis (ASAS) group have defined response criteria similar to those used for RA, which have allowed for better evaluation of therapies (Lukas et al 2009).

### The foot in ankylosing spondylitis

About 20% of patients with ankylosing spondylitis will have enthesitis in the feet, although any involvement of the foot in ankylosing spondylitis is usually transient and tends not to progress to severe degenerative joint disease (Kumar & Madewell 1987, Olivieri et al 1998). Involvement of the enthesis of the plantar fascia is accompanied by soft-tissue oedema in most cases and also by bone oedema in many (McGonagle et al 2002). Retrocalcaneal bursitis occurs fairly frequently in ankylosing spondylitis (Moll 1987).

If the foot is involved more extensively, the presentation has much in common with the other seronegative arthropathies, and erosions, periosteal proliferation and, characteristically, joint ankylosis are all seen. Affected joints will be swollen and tender, and radiographic investigation reveals that initial periarticular erosion is followed by bony proliferation and bone spur formation (Kumar & Madewell 1987).

The management of ankylosing spondylitis in the foot centres on systemic disease control supplemented by local measures. Where isolated sites in the foot are symptomatic, local injection of corticosteroid may reduce inflammation, and padding or orthoses may provide mechanical relief. Achilles tendon insertional enthesitis in seronegative spondyloarthropathy can, unfortunately, be intractable, although there is promise of effective therapy with anti-TNF drugs (Olivieri et al 2007).

## Psoriatic arthritis

### Definition

The diagnosis of psoriatic arthritis is usually used to refer to an inflammatory arthropathy occurring in the presence of psoriasis and in the absence of rheumatoid factor. In practice, it is not always possible to be so precise about the definition, as the joint involvement may be variable, and in some cases may even pre-date the development of skin lesions. Spinal involvement is characteristic, but peripheral joint involvement may range from the widespread and severe arthritis seen

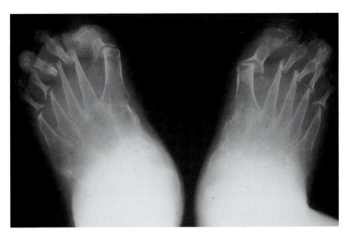

**Figure 8.15** Arthritis mutilans of the forefoot associated with psoriatic arthritis.

in the form arthritis mutilans (Figure 8.15), to a relatively mild monoarthritis. One form of psoriatic arthritis follows a disease course almost indistinguishable from that of RA.

### Epidemiology

Psoriasis of the skin or nails affects 2–3% of the population, with approximately 12% of dermatological cases developing arthritis. There is no association between joint involvement and type of psoriatic presentation in the skin. Psoriatic arthritis is the second most common inflammatory arthropathy after RA (Veale & FitzGerald 2002).

### Diagnosis

There are no widely agreed diagnostic criteria for psoriatic arthritis, and so diagnosis is based on clinical features and the often difficult exclusion of other inflammatory arthritides such as RA and ankylosing spondylitis (Brockbank & Gladman 2002). Serology is not as useful as in RA, because the association between inflammatory markers and disease activity is less clear (Brockbank & Gladman 2002). Recently, new classification criteria for psoriatic arthritis have been developed by a large international group, and it appears that these criteria may also function well as diagnostic criteria (Taylor et al 2006).

### Pathology

The immunogenetics of skin psoriasis and psoriatic arthritis are complex, and at present seem only marginally interrelated, although the cellular features of inflammatory cell infiltration and membrane hyperplasia show some similarities (Veale & FitzGerald 2002). The precise pathological pathway leading to psoriatic arthritis is not well understood, although it is known that the process relates to enthesitis as well as the synovitis seen in RA. TNFα is expressed at higher levels than normal, but the relative proportions of other cytokines in psoriatic synovium are different to those seen in RA (Veale & FitzGerald 2002).

### Clinical course

The textbook presentation is of a unilateral dactylitis (a 'sausage digit'), although in reality the initial presentations are diverse. Early axial involvement is found in 40% of people with psoriatic arthritis. Case reports have suggested a temporal association between the onset of psoriatic arthritis and joint trauma in some cases, mimicking the Köebner phenomenon seen in psoriatic skin (Veale & FitzGerald

2002). Distal interphalangeal joint involvement is characteristic, contrasting with the proximal interphalangeal joint presentation seen in RA (Brockbank & Gladman 2002). Metacarpal or metatarsal joints can be affected, and again it is most common for the early presentation to be asymmetrical (Gold et al 1988).

The presence of arthritis in four or more joints is a significant predictor of a worse prognosis (Brockbank & Gladman 2002).

If the disease follows the arthritis mutilans course, the digital deformities tend to occur in haphazard directions, contrasting with the classic lateral drift seen in RA (Gold et al 1988). Ankylosis of affected joints is common and results in rigid deformity. Alternatively, where erosions predominate, flail digits may develop (Brockbank & Gladman 2002).

### Medical management

Medical management of psoriatic arthritis is often similar to that of RA, with methotrexate and other DMARDs proving effective in combination with NSAIDs and exercise (Brockbank & Gladman 2002, DeJesus & Tsuchiya 1999). Psoriatic arthritis has proven highly responsive to anti-TNFα therapy in recent trials (Olsen & Stein 2004), and etanercept and infliximab suppress both the joint disease and the skin presentations (Leonardi et al 2003). Local corticosteroid injection into affected joints or tendon sheaths may be helpful (Brockbank & Gladman 2002). Treatment recommendations have recently been published by the Group for Research and Assessment of Psoriasis and Psoriatic Arthritis, which provides guidance on effective treatments for the different disease manifestations (Ritchlin et al 2009).

### The foot in psoriatic arthritis

The foot may show the changes typical of psoriatic skin disease, with erythematous patches on the extensor surfaces, or plantar hyperkeratosis or pustule formation on the plantar surfaces. Pitting, discoloration, hyperkeratosis and lysis of the nails may occur, and splinter haemorrhages may be found around the apices of the toes.

Psoriatic arthritis will often present initially in the interphalangeal and then the metatarsophalangeal joints of the feet or hands (Gold et al 1988), although other joints may be affected, sometimes in a single ray pattern (Brockbank & Gladman 2002, Kumar & Madewell 1987).

Inflammation at the entheses results in bony erosions, and on radiographic investigation non-marginal erosions are evident early, with subchondral bone involved soon afterwards (Kumar & Madewell 1987). Reactive new bone formation around affected joints is characteristic, leading to a fuzzy appearance on the radiograph. Endosteal sclerosis will occasionally lead to a substantial increase in density of the shaft, the so-called 'ivory phalanx'. The highly erosive pathology leads to a whittling of the joint margins and an unusual 'pencil in cup' appearance in advanced cases, where the distal end of the affected phalanx is cupped within an excessively concave surface at the proximal end of the more distal phalanx (Gold et al 1988, Kumar & Madewell 1987). Conversely, bony ankylosis can occur instead. Resorption of the distal phalanx occurs in about 5% of patients, resulting in a characteristic, pointed toe pulp (Gold et al 1988, Moll 1987).

Hindfoot involvement mimics that of other seronegative arthropathies. Clinical involvement of the Achilles tendon and plantar fasciitis occurs in about one-third of people with psoriatic arthritis, although pathological signs are observable on ultrasonography in more than three-quarters of patients (Galluzzo et al 2000, Olivieri et al 1998). Bony proliferation of the entheses and exuberant spur formation may be seen on radiography (Gold et al 1988, Kumar & Madewell 1987) (Figure 8.16).

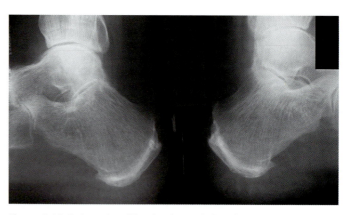

**Figure 8.16** Entheseal proliferation in psoriatic arthritis.

## Reactive arthritis

### Definition

Reactive arthritis can occur in conjunction with urethritis and conjunctivitis (and other features). Reactive arthritis is an acute inflammatory arthritis arising after a local or systemic infection, typically sexually acquired or postdysenteric. The disease usually affects younger males and is associated with the HLA B27 antigen in more than 90% of cases. The initial presentation is usually in the knee or foot, but spondyloarthropathy is a universal feature as the disease progresses. The disease course is of flares and remissions, which will self-limit in time. A small proportion of cases will persist, but the disease tends to be milder than other inflammatory arthropathies (Kumar & Madewell 1987).

### Diagnosis

Reactive arthritis should be suspected where there is an inflammatory arthritis presenting predominantly in the lower limb, especially where the arthritis is accompanied by bony proliferation (Jacobson et al 2008). Multiple joints may be affected, but usually asymmetrically (Moll 1987). The most commonly affected regions in the foot are the metatarsophalangeal joints, the Achilles tendon and its insertion, and the origin of the plantar fascia (Moll 1987).

Keratoderma blenorrhagica can occur in conjunction with the arthritis (Figure 8.17), and it can be difficult to differentiate the skin lesions seen in reactive arthritis from those of psoriasis, leading to confusion over the diagnosis (Kumar & Madewell 1987, Moll 1987).

### Medical management

NSAIDs are the first-line treatment, reducing pain and subduing the inflammatory process to some degree (DeJesus & Tsuchiya 1999). Often a course of DMARDs is all that is necessary. DMARDs (typically sulfasalazine and methotrexate) are used for persistent cases. The use of anti-TNF has also been proposed as an approach in reactive arthritis, because early suppression of this relatively short-lived arthritis may result in preservation of maximum joint integrity once the inflammatory stage has passed.

### The foot in reactive arthritis

The involvement in the foot largely mirrors that of other seronegative arthropathies, focusing on the hindfoot and, to a lesser extent, the forefoot, but largely sparing the midfoot (Kumar & Madewell 1987). In the hindfoot, the radiological findings of reactive arthritis are similar to those of psoriatic arthritis, with whiskery spurs resulting from enthesopathy at the insertion of the Achilles tendon and

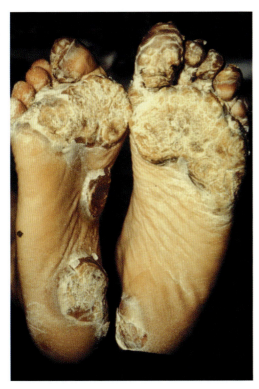

**Figure 8.17** Keratoderma blenorrhagica associated with reactive arthritis.

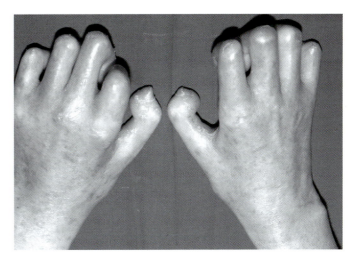

**Figure 8.18** Fibrosis and contracture in the hands of a patient with scleroderma.

plantar fascia. Nodular thickenings may also be found in the tendons (Gerster et al 1977). There is greater differentiation from psoriatic arthritis in the forefoot, however, and reactive arthritis shows less predilection for the lesser interphalangeal joints, with involvement usually confined to the interphalangeal joint of the hallux (Gold et al 1988, Kumar & Madewell 1987). Local corticosteroid injection has been reported to provide symptom relief (Gerster et al 1977).

## Connective tissue diseases – scleroderma and lupus

The connective tissue diseases are a mixed group of conditions sharing some clinical features but with differing pathophysiologies. The two most common discrete forms are scleroderma and systemic lupus erythematosus (commonly known as lupus), although there are forms with less clear differentiation (the so-called mixed connective tissue diseases). Scleroderma and lupus are dealt with as separate entities in this chapter for simplicity, but the interested reader is directed to a dedicated rheumatology text for more detail on this complex group of conditions.

## Scleroderma

### Definition

Scleroderma comes in several forms, including progressive systemic sclerosis, and localised or limited sclerosis. It is an immune-mediated disorder characterised by inflammatory and fibrotic soft-tissue changes. In the systemic form, vascular lesions are also characteristic, affecting the skin and internal structures such as the gastrointestinal system, heart, lungs and kidneys.

### Epidemiology

There are around 1500 diagnosed cases of scleroderma in the UK, with a male/female gender split of 1:4 (Arthritis Research Campaign 2002).

### Diagnosis

There are long-standing American College of Rheumatology criteria for the classification of systemic sclerosis, which have been updated recently but not well validated (Walker et al 2007). Antinuclear antibodies are usually present in the blood, and extractable nuclear antibodies to SCL-70, centromere and RNP may be found, as may rheumatoid factor. The precise pathology is unknown, although it is well accepted that the underlying aetiology is immune mediated.

### Clinical course

The initial presentation of systemic sclerosis may simply be with Raynaud's phenomenon accompanied by oedema of the hands or feet. The skin in the extremities thickens and tightens, leading to the typical presentation of sclerodactyly. The affected fingers and toes develop flexion contractures that cause limited mobility (Figure 8.18). Fibrosis and resorption of the soft tissue and underlying bony substance of the digital apices can lead to a classical atrophic appearance to the ends of the digits. Changes in the face lead to a mask-like appearance, with puckering of the skin around the mouth. Altered pigmentation is common.

One variant of scleroderma is the CREST syndrome, named after the features Calcinosis, Raynaud's phenomenon, (o)Esophagitis, Sclerodactyly, and Telangectiasis. In CREST the scleroderma is usually limited to the hands and forearms. The calcinosis may manifest as small subcutaneous nodules on the hands and feet – these resemble gouty tophi clinically but clearly show themselves as containing calcium on plain radiographs. CREST is not a benign condition, having a relatively high prevalence of lung and heart involvement. Indeed, in systemic sclerosis, pulmonary, cardiac and renal involvement leads to shortening of the lifespan (Gold et al 1988), although better modern medical management has improved the prognosis considerably.

Synovitis may be present, but tends to affect large joints rather than the feet (Gold et al 1988). Calcification of peripheral soft tissues may occur in long-standing cases, and calcinosis of the skin may be seen.

## Medical management

Much of the literature relating to scleroderma focuses on the management of the vascular complications, such as Raynaud's phenomenon, and the effects on internal organs. There is little high-quality evidence for most of the current approaches to medical management. The underlying pathology remains poorly understood, and while DMARDs have been shown to be effective in reducing the skin thickening (Lin et al 2003), their effectiveness overall is unclear. Nevertheless, improved medical management of the renal and pulmonary aspects of the disease has led to increased life expectancy in recent years.

## The foot in scleroderma

The foot will be involved during the course of the disease in about 90% of patients with systemic sclerosis, but involvement is less common and less severe than in the hands (La Montagna et al 2002). Disorders of the skin and vascular system are the most common (see box 8.4), but the skeletal structures of the foot are involved in three-quarters of patients with progressive systemic sclerosis. Musculoskeletal pain occurs in about one-third of sufferers, even in the absence of arthritis. Radiographic foot involvement is associated with a generally poorer prognosis (La Montagna et al 2002, Ueda et al 1991).

Raynaud's syndrome is almost universal in the hands, and occurs in the feet of about 90% of sufferers, the incidence increasing with longer disease duration (La Montagna et al 2002). Localised vasculitic lesions and ulceration, typically of the dorsum of the forefoot and the apices of the toes, are also seen in these patients, with a prevalence of 30% and 20–25%, respectively. There is growing evidence for large-vessel involvement in some cases also (La Montagna et al 2002, Sari-Kouzel et al 2001). Subcutaneous calcinosis can be problematic later in the disease, although it occurs in fewer than 20% of feet and less frequently than in the hands. Ulcerative skin lesions are often very painful in patients with connective tissue disease, contrasting with the neuropathic ulceration seen in diabetes. The healing process is typically protracted because of the vasculitis, and when healing does occur it is often through necrosis and fibrosis rather than the granulation and re-epithelialisation process that occurs during the resolution of many other forms of ulceration.

The combination of skin and subcutaneous fibrosis, along with the changes in the underlying skeletal structures lead to difficulties with shoe fitting (Sari-Kouzel et al 2001), and these patients may require assistance with sourcing adequate footwear. It is desirable that all patients with systemic sclerosis undergo regular checks of their foot health and have ready access to foot health services where follow-up is needed.

# Lupus

## Definition

Systemic lupus erythematosus (SLE) is an immune-mediated connective tissue disease affecting many organ systems and with a variable course and prognosis. In addition to the musculoskeletal effects, renal and cardiopulmonary disease are common features (Maddison 2002). Discoid lupus is a localised form affecting only the skin.

## Epidemiology

Estimates of the prevalence of SLE range from 15 per 100 000 to 68 per 100 000 (Bongu et al 2002). SLE is between two and eight times more common in women than in men (McAlindon 2000), and there is a marked variation according to ethnicity (McAlindon 2000) and age (Bongu et al 2002). People of South-Asian or Afro-Caribbean origin are prone to more severe presentations. About two-thirds of patients with SLE will have non-erosive arthritic manifestations, often in the ankle or metatarsophalangeal joints (Gilkes 1987).

## Diagnosis

Classically depicted by the characteristic malar 'butterfly' rash on the cheeks, the diagnosis of SLE is made on the basis of the 1982 American Rheumatology Association criteria, an 11-item set of criteria including physical characteristics and laboratory investigations such as HLA typing, detection of antinuclear antibodies (McAlindon 2000, Maddison 2002) and antibodies to double-stranded DNA (Maddison 2002). Where the diagnosis is unclear, patients are considered to have 'undifferentiated connective tissue disease' (McAlindon 2000). It is common for patients to remain undifferentiated for years before the progress of the disease leads to a clinical picture meeting the criteria for frank SLE.

## Pathology

In people with an innate susceptibility, an external trigger is thought to be required to precipitate cases. Infection is a widely noted precipitating factor, with seropositivity for the Epstein-Barr virus associated with a 50-fold increase in risk of developing lupus. Lupus is also thought to be precipitated by exogenous factors in some cases, and a variety of environmental agents such as drugs (antihypertensives, antiarrhythmics) and household chemicals, such as those found in cosmetics and domestic spray cans, have been implicated (McAlindon 2000).

## Clinical course

The early clinical course is fairly predictable across the range of lupus-type disorders, with the disease tending to differentiate into one of the more specific forms later (Maddison 2002). The systemic effects result in shortening of the lifespan, and survival rates after 20 years of disease are only 70%, mainly as a consequence of renal disease or increased susceptibility to infection (Bongu et al 2002). There also is increasing evidence of accelerated arthrosclerosis in patients with lupus (Theodoridou et al 2003).

Most patients with SLE will have some musculoskeletal symptoms, and about one-third will develop a non-erosive but rheumatoid-like arthritis (Bongu et al 2002, Reilly et al 1990).

## Medical management

There is good recent evidence that early and aggressive treatment improves outcomes for people with lupus (Rao & Hootman 2004). NSAID therapy is used sparingly because of an increased risk of renal dysfunction (Solsky & Wallace 2002). Antimalarial drugs are effective for mild SLE, but the mainstays of therapy are steroids and immunosuppressive drugs.

## The foot in lupus

Vascular signs occur in 90% of people with SLE, Raynaud's disease, with telangectasia and purpura affecting the feet widely. Vasculitis and ulceration are relatively common in this group of patients, affecting between 10% and 20%, often in the lower extremity (Cawley 1987). In addition to the small-vessel vasculitis seen in RA, people with SLE can also develop large-vessel vasculitis (Gladstein et al 1979) and accelerated atherosclerosis (Theodoridou et al 2003), leading to frank gangrene and risk of amputation. Ankle–brachial pressure indices are abnormal in many SLE sufferers and should be used to detect large-vessel disease early in this group (Theodoridou et al 2003).

Patients with SLE may have RA-type presentations in the feet (Mizutani & Quismorio 1984), although there is less joint destruction and erosions are not seen. Tendinopathy can be seen, especially in the Achilles tendon (Bongu et al 2002).

Patients can present with onycholysis and pitting of the nails, similar to that seen in psoriasis. Splinter haemorrhages may also be seen in the nail beds, reflecting the vascular involvement. Skin lesions are common, with discoid or annular erythematous lesions occurring on the legs and feet exacerbated by exposure to sunlight (Callen 2002).

## Osteoarthritis

### Definition

Osteoarthritis (OA) is characterised by progressive loss of articular cartilage, and remodelling of and change in the structure of subchondral bone.

### Epidemiology

OA is the most common form of arthritis and affects between 12% and 35% of the population (Felson et al 2000). The figures vary because of differences in definition, and because of sampling effects as the prevalence rises with age. Osteoarthritic changes based on radiological definitions are very common and lead to higher estimates of prevalence, while prevalence data based on clinical presentations (symptoms/pain) yield lower prevalence rates. The prevalence of OA is known to be higher in women (Arthritis Research Campaign 2002, Hawker 1997) and the most common sites are the hands (1%), hips (0.9%), knees (2.4%) and feet (Hawker 1997). Joint pain is common in the feet of older adults but, importantly, presents most commonly in combination with pain in other joints such as the knees, back, hands and hips (Keenan et al 2006). Subclinical signs are often reported at higher incidence, especially in older patients, with one study of 100 cadaveric lower limbs reporting moderate or severe degeneration in 24% of older hips, 66% of knees and 47% of first metatarsophalangeal joints (Muehleman et al 1997). Apart from the first metatarsophalangeal joint, the joints of the foot and ankle appear fairly resistant to primary OA, and so most cases are secondary to earlier trauma (Thomas & Daniels 2003).

OA leads to the loss of 36 million working days a year, costing the UK economy over £3 billion.

### Diagnosis

Diagnostic criteria have been proposed by the American College of Rheumatology and others, although the clinical diagnostic criteria are usually joint specific and therefore too numerous to be listed here. Menz et al (2007) have developed a useful classification system for foot joint OA, based on an atlas of plain film radiographic images. The clinical signs are general stiffness and an aching pain in the affected joint, and there may be tenderness at the joint margins on palpation (Demetriades et al 1998). Crepitus may be felt on passive movement of the body part.

Confirmation of the clinical signs requires radiographic investigation. Radiographic signs featured in the Menz system include narrowing of the joint space on a plain radiograph, bony proliferation around joint margins (osteophyte formation), and sclerosis and cyst formation in the subchondral bone. Periarticular erosions are not seen in OA.

### Pathology

OA can be primary (i.e. occurring spontaneously) or may be secondary to trauma or other insult to the joint. OA is no longer considered a simple 'wear and tear' arthritis, as it is clear that the process involves elements of repair as well as inflammation and degeneration (Felson et al 2000). Subtle differences in the presentation and local pathology at different sites have led to suggestions that the balance between the biological and mechanical factors is variable, and that OA at such different sites as weight-bearing hip joints and non-weight-bearing finger joints could even be considered separate entities (Felson et al 2000).

Risk factors for OA include inherent factors such as age, ethnicity and gender, combined with acquired factors such as local mechanics, obesity, trauma and deformity (Felson et al 2000).

The pathology involves the whole of the affected joint, as well as focal changes at specific sites. Primary OA can start with a significant inflammatory element, and can cause significant pain, especially early in the disease process. Osteophytes develop at the margins of the articular surfaces near the attachments of the capsule, ligaments or tendons. Endochondral ossification follows, spreading to involve neighbouring soft-tissue structures. In both primary and secondary presentations the cartilage reduces in thickness as the matrix degenerates, especially in regions of higher stresses (Marijnissen et al 2003). Chondrocyte biochemistry leads to a self-promoting degenerative cascade, hastening the process of deterioration (Marijnissen et al 2003). The subchondral bone becomes sclerotic and cysts become evident, again in areas of high stress. The soft-tissue structures such as the synovium and ligaments can be involved, but not to the extent seen in the inflammatory arthritides (Felson et al 2000).

### Clinical course

Initial soreness may be accompanied by soft-tissue swelling in primary OA; alternatively, the onset may be quite insidious. Osteophytes form early and are often readily palpable. The initial pain of primary OA may ease as the disease progresses.

Osteoarthritic changes in the hands (Figure 8.19) have been noted to be more severe in those with more physically demanding jobs but OA is not clearly associated with limb dominance (Bergenudd et al 1989). Obesity has been linked to the prevalence of OA in both non-weight-bearing and weight-bearing joints (Hawker 1997). Degenerative joint disease can be superimposed on other forms of arthropathy, and is cumulative and currently irreversible.

### Medical management

As noted at the start of this chapter, the medical management of OA still relies on the traditional pyramid approach, in contrast to the paradigm shift for treating immune-mediated inflammatory diseases. In recent years there has been increased emphasis on patient empowerment, and so education and self-management have been adopted as central features of the Arthritis and Musculoskeletal Alliance (ARMA) national standards of care for OA (Arthritis and Musculoskeletal Alliance 2004b). NICE (2008) recommend exercise as the core treatment for early OA, and this can be self-directed. Simple analgesia is NICE's recommended first line of pharmaceutical therapy, with NSAIDs used if pain persists. Some NSAIDs may themselves be harmful to cartilage and, although there is no strong evidence, the new cox-2 inhibitors have been suggested to be moderately chondroprotective (Marijnissen et al 2003).

As more is known about the cellular and cytokine mechanisms involved in OA, new targeted biological drugs will emerge. Already there are early trials on drugs that modify enzymes involved in the degradation of cartilage. It is possible that future therapies for OA will

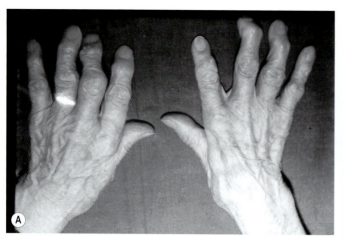 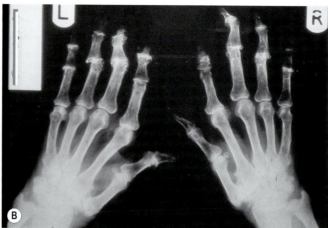

Figure 8.19 Osteoarthritis in the hands: (A) the clinical appearance and (B) the radiographic appearance.

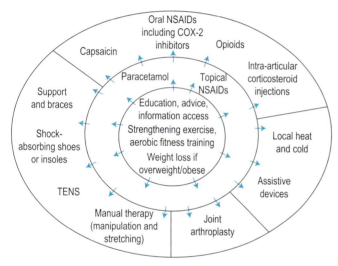

Figure 8.20 A schema for the management of osteoarthritis.

be just as effective (and costly) as the biological drugs in the inflammatory immune-mediated diseases.

Moderate exercise is known to be effective in reducing pain and the impact of OA on quality of life, and exercise programmes should supplement all medical and podiatric management.

The ideal management of OA is to reverse the degenerative process, although to date there has been very little success with this approach medically. While techniques such as autologous chondrocyte implantation have been used to stimulate small amounts of cartilage regeneration, the technique remains useful only for isolated cartilage defects. Chondrocyte supplementation with mesenchymal stem cells is an avenue receiving some considerable attention in medical research, but any clinical applications remain some way off. The success of replacement arthroplasty is highly joint specific, and implants for foot joints have not been especially successful. A schema for the medical management of OA is presented in Figure 8.20, describing the relationships between the treatments recommended by NICE.

### The foot in osteoarthritis

The foot and ankle area has not generally been considered an important anatomical region for OA. Indeed the ankle is notable for being a weight-bearing joint that is particularly resistant to OA (Buckwalter & Saltzman 1999). However, osteoarthritic changes are observable in radiographs of the foot joints in approximately half of people (Lemont & Gibley 1982), and clinical changes are evident in 16% of those aged 55 years and over (Bergenudd et al 1989). The first metatarsophalangeal joint has been proposed to be a highly prevalent site for joint degeneration, second only to the knee (Muehleman et al 1997). Other joints in the foot are affected more sporadically, most often following trauma (Chen 1996). Proximal foot joints in the tarsus and tarsometatarsal region showed degeneration in between 10% and 36% of a cohort of older cadaveric specimens (mean age 76 years).

In one study (Greisberg et al 2003), midfoot OA (Figure 8.21) was considerably more prevalent in patients with severe pes planus than in a control group, but the severity was not related to the degree of deformity.

The most common presentations of OA in the foot are as hallux limitus, hallux rigidus or in association with hallux valgus. In these presentations, degenerative changes at the first metatarsophalangeal joint lead to functional limitation. Pain and stiffness are felt in the affected joint, especially in maximal dorsiflexion, and this may interfere with normal walking (Weinfeld & Schon 1998). Periarticular

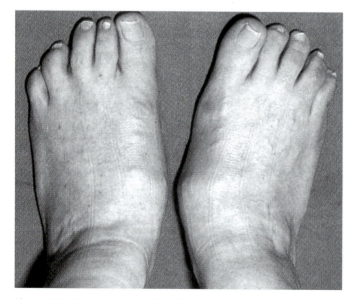

Figure 8.21 Severe osteoarthritis in the midtarsal joints.

osteophyte formation leads to thickening of the first metatarsophalangeal joint, and sometimes the formation of an adventitious bursa. The osteophytic change will be evident on the radiograph, as will joint-space narrowing. The limitation of the joint range of movement may be progressive, with decreasing range associated with increasing impairment (Weinfeld & Schon 1998).

OA in the foot is a significant factor in predicting utilisation of healthcare services, and the presence of foot OA doubles the risk of dependence on health support services (Gorter et al 2001). Treatments for OA of the foot vary in their success. NSAIDs have been shown to be beneficial in OA of the foot and may be advised by podiatrists (Jennings 1994), and paracetamol has shown a systematic, if limited, effect on the pain associated with OA generally (Towheed et al 2004). However, long-term oral analgesic or NSAID use should only be undertaken under medical supervision. Weight loss and low-impact exercise are of known benefit, and some effort should be directed towards exercise counselling during the clinical consultation (Rao & Hootman 2004, Thomas & Daniels 2003).

Over-the-counter remedies for osteoarthritic symptoms include a range of pharmaceutical topical agents, and more recently a growing number of alternative treatments, which are used by up to one-third of people with OA (Arthritis Research Campaign 2002). Alternative therapies include fish oil (which is high in omega-3 fatty acids), glucosamine and chondroitin sulfate. Glucosamine has been reported to provide benefit in OA (Matheson & Perry 2003), but NICE (2008) concluded that the evidence was not strong enough to recommend this approach.

Local therapies can be geared toward ameliorating abnormal mechanics or addressing the symptoms, and the following are recommended by NICE. Contoured foot orthoses, provided either to a neutral cast or off the shelf, are effective at reducing foot joint motions and offloading the forefoot and heel regions, and so may help some patients. Similarly, shock-absorbing insoles or footwear can provide symptom relief, and accommodative padding may reduce pressure over prominences resulting from osteoarthritic changes. Footwear adaptations such as rocker-bottom shoes limit the need for movement of degenerate joints while facilitating sagittal plane motion (Thomas & Daniels 2003).

Intra-articular injection of steroid may provide symptom relief for up to 8 weeks (Thomas & Daniels 2003), although in practice the effect rarely lasts longer than 2–4 weeks. Hyaluronate injections have produced moderate benefits in large joints such as the knee, but their use in small joints such as those of the foot is experimental only.

NICE recommended the use of thermal therapies (i.e. application of local heat or cold), and a range of approaches have been described, including direct application of heat, ultrasound and low-level laser therapy. A Cochrane Review of the latter approach concluded that the evidence was equivocal (Brosseau et al 2004), and so 'low-tech' solutions are more justifiable.

Surgical intervention is usually definitive, with arthrodesis, or replacement or excision arthroplasty reducing pain significantly. Surgery to the first metatarsophalangeal joint is discussed in detail elsewhere and so is not discussed further here. Less commonly, surgery is required for the subtalar joint, ankle joint and midfoot, where joint degeneration is usually secondary to trauma.

Ankle joint surgeries include arthroscopic and open approaches and are varied. Unless there is advanced degeneration and deformity, arthrodesis of the ankle is considered a salvage procedure, because the significant physical demands on this joint (Marijnissen et al 2003) and the high risk of perioperative infection make this a difficult procedure, with variable intermediate and long-term results (Mann & Chou 1995, Van Eygen et al 1999). More wide-ranging arthrodeses of the ankle and hindfoot, such as the pantalar and triple arthrodeses, are similarly regarded as salvage procedures only (Acosta et al 2000).

Intermediate OA of the ankle may respond positively to a low tibial osteotomy, which redistributes loading stress within the joint (Chen 1996). Surgical joint distraction using external Ilizarov fixation is another experimental technique being used to promote cartilage regeneration, and this has produced some encouraging early results in severe arthritis of the ankle (Marijnissen et al 2003).

Where degenerative changes in the midfoot, hindfoot or ankle joint are severe, arthrodesis is currently the preferred surgical approach. Functionally, neighbouring joints are usually able to accommodate the loss of motion in the fused joint reasonably well, at least initially (Demetriades et al 1998), although ankle arthrodesis leads to premature degeneration in the neighbouring foot joints in the long term (Coester et al 2001). Excision arthroplasty can result in instability, and so the use of this technique is confined to the metatarsophalangeal joints and digits. Joint replacements have a chequered history in the foot because the combination of large forces and small amounts of bone stock leads to prosthetic loosening and tissue reaction to wear debris (Weinfeld & Schon 1998). The proportion of failures associated with foot joint replacement is higher than would be acceptable for larger joints such as the knee and hip. Some success was reported in the early days of total ankle replacement arthroplasty, but follow-up results were poor and the technique fell from favour (Demetriades et al 1998). Several generations of refinement have led to some resurgence in interest, and modern ankle replacements with mobile bearings appear to have better functional outcomes and lower failure rates (Wood et al 2008). Nevertheless, the lifespan of these replacements still falls short of that seen in large-joint implantation (Thomas & Daniels 2003).

## Crystal arthropathies (gout and pseudogout)

### Definition

The crystal arthropathies, gout and pseudogout, are the clinical manifestations of an inflammatory response to crystal deposition in synovial joints.

### Epidemiology

Gout occurs in around 1% of men and 0.3–0.6% of women (Harris et al 1999, McGuire 2003) and the incidence increases with age, being rare in adults under 30 years old. Pseudogout is much less common and is predominantly a disease of the elderly.

### Diagnosis

The definitive diagnosis of crystal arthritis is usually simple, and there are long-standing diagnostic criteria (Box 8.5). Crystals may be viewed directly within joint aspirate under polarised light microscopy. The clinical picture in true gout is usually obvious, and microscopy is often only confirmatory, although joint aspiration should always be performed to exclude septic arthritis or coincidental degenerative or inflammatory arthritis (Harris et al 1999). Recent advances in imaging, such as dual-energy computerised tomography, offer a potentially improved method for quantifying the extent of joint and soft-tissue involvement (Choi et al 2008), but these techniques are not yet in widespread use.

### Pathology

The underlying pathology of gout is of crystal deposition into the joint space as a result of elevated levels of monosodium urate in the blood stream. Pseudogout occurs when calcium pyrophosphate dihydrate, a normal component of articular cartilage, enters the joint space and is taken up by white cells. A less common form is caused by deposition of calcium hydroxapatite.

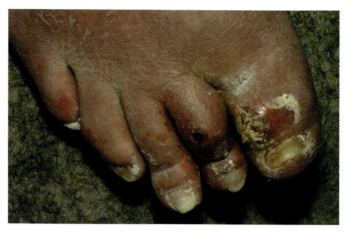

**Figure 8.23** Chronic tophaceous gout.

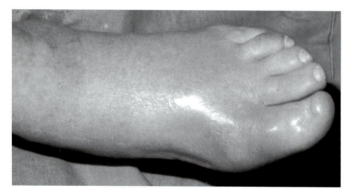

**Figure 8.22** Classic acute gout in a first metatarsophalangeal joint.

The local pathology within the affected joint is of crystal deposition leading to severe synovitis. Synovial proliferation occurs and the inflammatory cascade is instigated and modulated by leucocytes, monocytes and lymphocytes. Tophi are the consequence of phagocytosis of crystals, and are composed of high concentrations of crystals and the detritus of deceased polymorphs.

### Clinical course

There are four phases of gout: (1) asymptomatic hyperuricaemia, (2) acute gouty arthritis, (3) intercritical gout and (4) chronic tophaceous gout (Harris et al 1999).

The initial presentation is typically a severe and acute monoarthritis lasting a few days (Figure 8.22). Preceding an acute attack there may be a history of precipitating factors, such as dietary change, an alcohol binge or minor trauma to the joint (Weinfeld & Schon 1998). Onset is often overnight, with a rapid development of a severe monoarthritis manifest as heat, redness and marked swelling. More diffuse swelling can result if more than one joint is involved (Chen & Schumacher 2003). If untreated, episodes may become more frequent and longer in duration. Medical management of the acute phase for all crystal arthropathies is with high therapeutic doses of NSAID. Other therapies, such as oral steroid, are available for patients unable to tolerate high doses of NSAIDs, but are not preferred. Colchicine is only appropriate in the earliest stages of an acute episode of gout. Oral or injected steroid may be of assistance where single or few accessible joints are

involved (Harris et al 1999). Local therapies such as the application of ice may be helpful.

The length of the intercritical periods can vary, but will tend to shorten in poorly controlled gout. Three-quarters of patients suffer a second attack within 2 years of the first (Harris et al 1999). Recurrences of acute gouty attacks occur more frequently over time and involve other joints, often symmetrically.

Tophaceous deposits may form in the longer term, initially in joints and tendon sheaths, but as time progresses more extensively in soft tissues (Harris et al 1999, Kerman et al 1993). On plain film radiography joint spaces will be initially preserved, but later marked periarticular erosions will form (Kerr 1998). The tophaceous deposits may be fairly large and, in the foot, can result in problems with shoe fitting (Figure 8.23). Occasionally, large tophi will ulcerate (Weinfeld & Schon 1998).

Preventive regimens of drugs, such as low-dose colchicine, uric clearance promoters, such as Probenecid, and the xanthine oxidase inhibitor allopurinol, can be effective in reducing the frequency of subsequent attacks when combined with dietary modification (Chen & Schumacher 2003, Kerr 1998). For some time patients who were allergic to Allopurinol had no alternatives, but a new inhibitor of xanthine oxidase, Febuxostat, has been developed. Febuxostat is as good as or better than allopurinol in reducing the concentration of uric acid in the blood, and has now been approved by NICE for those people who cannot take allopurinol (Becker et al 2005).

### The foot in crystal arthropathies

True gout will onset in the first metatarsophalangeal joint in about half of all cases, although it also has a predilection for other sites in the foot such as the other metatarsophalangeal joints, the first interphalangeal joint, midfoot joints, the subtalar joint and the ankle (Egan et al 1987, Kerr 1998). Pseudogout presents with a less severe synovitis and affects larger joints such as the ankle and knee (Kerr 1998). At onset, crystal arthropathies are characterised by a hyperacute monoarthritis, accompanied by severe swelling erythema and pain. The joint will typically be too painful to move or to touch.

In the chronically gouty joint, there will be considerable joint damage, which in the later stages may require excision or replacement to resolve symptoms (McGuire 2003). Periarticular erosions may have characteristic punched-out or overhanging edges (Egan et al 1987). Two separate case reports have highlighted tophaceous gout affecting the hallucal sesamoids and mimicking tumour or fracture (Reber et al 1997, Liu et al 2003). Other unusual intraosseous presentations reported in the foot include involvement of the navicular and the third metatarsal bone (Surprenant et al 1996, Thomas et al 1998). Tophi may arise extensively in the soft tissues such as tendons, including the Achilles (Kerman et al 1993), and subcutaneous tophi may extrude through the skin (Egan et al 1987).

## Infective arthritis

Infective (septic) arthritis arises as a direct response to the presence of infective organisms (usually bacteria) in the joint, and so usually presents as an acute monoarthritis, often with an accompanying systemic presentation of fever. It is uncommon in the foot joints, preferring larger joints such as the knee (Kerr 1998). Infective arthritis is more common in children than adults.

### The foot in infective arthritis

Although the foot is rarely affected, infective arthritis can occur secondary to ulceration or following a penetrating injury (Kerr 1998), and so is more prevalent in people with sensory neuropathy (Weinfeld & Schon 1998). Infective arthritis should be considered in the case of an acute monoarthritis in the foot after surgery (Weinfeld & Schon 1998). Infective arthritis requires aspiration of joint fluids and long-term antibiotic therapy, but will usually resolve completely (Kerr 1998).

## Other rheumatological conditions

### Fibromyalgia

#### Definition

Fibromyalgia (FM) is a label given to a presentation of chronic, widespread pain in both muscles and joints. It is diagnosed according to criteria published by the American College of Rheumatologists on the basis of 11 or more tender points at specific sites in the body. Prevalence is estimated at 1–2%, the majority of cases arising in females (Linaker et al 1999). It is known that fibromyalgia is associated with higher scores on anxiety and depression scales, and its prevalence increases with age (Linaker et al 1999). Patients report chronic musculoskeletal fatigue and pain, often severe enough to interfere with their ability to work and participate in leisure activities. The clinical course is variable but fairly poor, and fewer than 50% of sufferers are in remission by 10 years. The medical management is directed towards management of chronic pain and its attendant psychological effects. Pain relief is required, usually using analgesics or NSAIDs, although these may not be effective alone. Managing the psychological aspects of fibromyalgia may be helpful, and selective serotonin reuptake inhibitors (SSRIs) or tricyclic antidepressants such as amitriptyline are often prescribed, and may be combined with non-pharmaceutical approaches such as exercise and cognitive–behavioural therapy.

Exercise has been demonstrated to improve outcomes in patients with fibromyalgia in a number of studies (Rao & Hootman 2004). The foot is not an especially common site for involvement in fibromyalgia, but many patients with fibromyalgia will have incidental foot pain, and the general prevalence of foot problems in this group will be at least as high as in the general population. These complex patients will be seen often in foot health clinics.

### Polymyalgia rheumatica

Polymyalgia rheumatica is a musculoskeletal pain syndrome usually seen in females over 65 years old. It affects about 7 people per 1000. Musculoskeletal symptoms occur mainly around the upper (in the shoulders and neck) and lower (buttocks and upper thighs) limb girdles. The onset of symptoms may be dramatic over a few days and can lead to severe disability. Systemic symptoms such as fever and night sweats may occur, as may weight loss. The pathology is unknown, although there is a link with giant-cell arteritis, which has provided some clues. This link is vital, however, as new-onset temporal headache with polymyalgic symptoms may herald acute and permanent loss of vision. The clinical course is of diffuse musculoskeletal pain early, and because of its dramatic course patients usually present early. Treatment with NSAIDs may help but low-dose oral steroids have an equally dramatic benefit on the symptoms, this response being part of the criteria for diagnosis. Polymyalgia rheumatica does not affect the feet directly but patients with difficulty bending and with reduced grip strength due to polymyalgia rheumatica may need assistance with basic foot care.

## Sjögren's syndrome

Sjögren's syndrome is a connective tissue disorder that mainly affects the salivary and tear glands. It is relatively rare and may occur as a primary form (i.e. in the absence of any other disease) or in a secondary form associated with other rheumatic diseases such as RA or lupus. Its main effects are to cause dryness of the mucous membranes, especially the eyes and mouth. The skin can be affected also, and anhidrosis is the most common manifestation in the foot. Patients can benefit from education about the importance of an emollient regimen, including footbaths and creams.

Sjögren's syndrome can be associated with vasculitis, and the toes can be involved. Management is the same as for the other forms of vasculitis in the rheumatology clinic (Cawley 1987).

## Joint hypermobility syndromes

### Definition

There are several conditions that are associated with a generalised hypermobility of joints. The most common are the benign familial joint hypermobility syndrome (BFJHS), the nine basic classifications of Ehlers–Danlos syndrome (EDS), Marfan syndrome and osteogenesis imperfecta.

BFJHS and EDS type III are essentially the same condition (Grahame 2000), and in these two presentations the signs are largely confined to joint laxity and skin hyperextensibility. The other disorders present with other systemic effects to a greater or lesser extent. The systemic complications are not detailed in this chapter, and we focus on the musculoskeletal manifestations using BFJHS/EDS type III by way of example.

### Epidemiology

The prevalence of hypermobility and related symptoms varies considerably with ethnicity. Inheritance patterns are specific to the disorder (e.g. the EDS classification), with recessive, dominant and X-linked forms all reported. Benign familial joint hypermobility nominally follows an autosomal-dominant pattern of inheritance, although penetrance is variable (Beighton & Horan 1970). The prevalence of hypermobility in Caucasians is reported to be around 5%, while in some racial groups, such as those from the Middle East and the Indian subcontinent, the prevalence is reported to be as a high as 38% (Al-Rawi et al 1985, Biro et al 1983, Larsson et al 1993, Wordsworth et al 1987). BFJHS is more common in women than men (Hudson et al 1995) and joint hypermobility declines with age (Larsson et al 1993). The association between underlying joint hypermobility and symptoms is incomplete, but BFJHS accounts for a large proportion of rheumatology referrals (far more than ankylosing spondylitis or psoriatic arthritis), and so the symptoms apparently have a significant

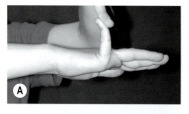
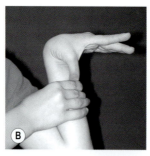
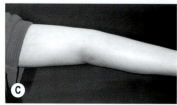
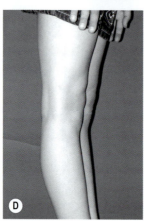
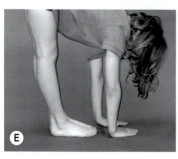

**Figure 8.24** The Beighton–Carter–Wilkinson scale for assessing joint hypermobility. (A) Hyperextension of the fingers past 90°. (B) Touch the thumb to the volar aspect of the forearm. (C) Elbow hyperextension >10°. (D) Knee hyperextension >10°. (E) Being able to place the palms flat on the floor with knees extended. One point is given to each positive sign (one point for each positive limb for signs A–D) to yield a score out of 9.

---

**Box 8.6 Revised Brighton (1998) Criteria for the diagnosis of benign familial joint hypermobility syndrome (BFJHS)**

BFJHS is diagnosed in the presence of two major criteria, or one major and two minor criteria, or four minor criteria. Two minor criteria will suffice where there is an unequivocally affected first-degree relative.

BFJHS is excluded by presence of Marfan or Ehlers-Danlos syndrome (other than Ehlers-Danlos syndrome type III).

**Major criteria**

1. A Beighton score of 4/9 or greater (either currently or historically)
2. Arthralgia for longer than 3 months in 4 or more joints

**Minor criteria**

1. A Beighton score of 1, 2 or 3/9 (0, 1, 2 or 3 if aged ≥50 years)
2. Arthralgia (≥3 months) in 1–3 joints, or back pain (≥3 months), spondylosis, spondylolysis/spondylolisthesis
3. Dislocation/subluxation in more than one joint, or in one joint on more than one occasion
4. Soft-tissue rheumatism ≥3 lesions (e.g. epicondylitis, tenosynovitis, bursitis)
5. Marfanoid habitus (tall, slim, span:height ratio >1.3, upper:lower segment ratio <0.89, arachnodactyly (+Steinberg/wrist signs))
6. Abnormal skin: striae, hyperextensibility, thin skin, papyraceous scarring
7. Eye signs: drooping eyelids or myopia or anti-mongoloid slant
8. Varicose veins or hernia or uterine/rectal prolapse

---

observations and are specific to benign familial hypermobility syndrome (Box 8.6).

### Pathology

The pathology of hypermobility syndrome derives from disordered structure of type I and III collagen (Grahame 2000). Gradation in bundle size is lost, and type I:type III ratios are deranged, leading to decreased tensile strength of connective tissues in the skin and articular structures.

### Clinical course

In people with BFJHS and EDS type III the collagen disorder manifests in a tendency to easy bruising and papyraceous scars from impaired healing. Old scars are usually observed readily on the knees of people with BFJHS/EDS type III. More profound manifestations are suggestive of EDS type I. Musculoskeletal symptoms in the hypermobility syndromes are often intermittent, at least at first, and other than long-term and low-grade mechanical joint damage the clinical course is stable. The majority of patients with BFJHS have multiple intermittent joint and soft-tissue pain, with pain in the back, hands, wrists and shoulders being at least as common as lower limb problems (Ainsworth & Aulicino 1993, Gazit et al 2001, Hudson et al 1995, Sacheti et al 1997). Dislocations are common and, while they usually reduce spontaneously, they are painful in the short term and often recur repeatedly, leading to a worsening of the joint stability (Ainsworth & Aulicino 1993).

The clinical rule of thumb is that people with joint hyperlaxity develop similar sorts of overuse-type symptoms as the rest of the population (tenosynovitis, arthralgia etc.) but do so more frequently and more severely.

---

impact in adults (Grahame 1993, Guma et al 2001, Hudson et al 1995, Sacheti et al 1997).

### Diagnosis

Diagnosis can be difficult and, because of debate over the definition and importance of hypermobility, the condition is often ignored entirely, especially in mild to moderate cases (Grahame & Bird 2001). Many patients express frustration at the delay in obtaining a diagnosis and a lack of understanding from clinical staff (Gazit et al 2001, Gurley-Green 2001).

The diagnosis of hypermobility as a generic physical presentation has long been made on the basis of the well-known Beighton score (Beighton & Horan 1969), a five-item, nine-point scale recording the physical features associated with systemic joint laxity (Figure 8.24). The physical tests used in the Beighton scoring system are among a number of joint features that patients often use as 'party tricks'. It is worth noting that repeated performance of these actions can be detrimental to joints, and clinicians should request their demonstration sparingly, and patients should be discouraged from performing them ad hoc (Gurley-Green 2001).

There may be some variation in the anatomical distribution of joint hyperextensibility even within individuals. While overall quantifications are useful, the clinician should pay careful attention to individual joints of interest.

A more specific set of diagnostic criteria was introduced in 2000 to differentiate BFJHS from other sources of hypermobility and idiopathic musculoskeletal pain (Grahame et al 2000). The Revised Brighton Criteria include a number of physical features and historical

The link between joint hypermobility and subsequent OA has long been noted (Beighton & Horan 1969, Grahame 2000), although at least one recent study has suggested that generalised joint hypermobility might reduce the risk of arthritis in hand joints (Kraus et al 2004).

Marfan syndrome is associated with joint hypermobility but also with a range of cardiovascular pathologies, and in osteogenesis imperfecta the bony fragility is the primary feature. In both of these conditions the joint laxity is considered a secondary feature and may be of less consequence than the systemic effects.

### Medical management

There is little that can be done medically that will directly affect joint mobility. Treatment is aimed at symptom relief, so the mainstays of the management of patients with hypermobility are NSAIDs and selective local corticosteroid in the short term, combined with physical and occupational therapy. Physical therapies must be tailored to the specific needs of patients with joint hypermobility because standard approaches can increase the severity of problems (Gurley-Green 2001). Exercises to strengthen and stabilise affected joints have been demonstrated to reduce joint pain, but the exercise regimens must be continued indefinitely to maintain their effect (Barton & Bird 1996). BFJHS is also noted to be associated with poor proprioception (Grahame 2000), and in our clinic rehabilitation strategies, including proprioception training, are prescribed for hypermobile patients.

Patients with joint hypermobility may develop a chronic pain state, which may be helped by psychological intervention and antidepressant therapy (Grahame 2000, Sacheti et al 1997). There is also a link between BFJHS and fibromyalgia, a recognised chronic pain syndrome (Hudson et al 1995; Karaaslan et al 2002).

### The foot in hypermobility syndrome

Hypermobility of large joints in the lower limb is common and leads to musculoskeletal symptoms and reduced quality of life (Redmond et al 2006b). Repeated dislocations can occur, causing altered gait. Ankle and foot hypermobility has been reported to affect as many as 60–94% of adults with hypermobility syndrome (Bulbena et al 1992, Riano et al 2001), but our experience of a large cohort currently enrolled in a clinical trial suggests that, while the prevalence of pes planus in BFJHS is higher than is found in the general population, it might not be as high as others have suggested (Redmond et al 2006a). Certain forms (such as EDS type I) may be more closely associated with pes planus than others.

Where the generalised joint laxity in our BFJHS patients is reflected in the foot, instability appears to be more manifest in the joints of the midfoot than the hindfoot complex (Figure 8.25). It is notable in some of these patients that the instability of the foot joints is more apparent during walking than quiet standing (Redmond et al 2006a), and we consider a dynamic evaluation to be an essential part of the examination of the hypermobile patient.

Joint hypermobility can be associated with some unusual presentations in the feet, including a 'skewfoot'-type presentation often seen in Marfan syndrome, and talipes-equinovarus-type features (Agnew 1997).

Musculoskeletal pain is common in the feet of people with BFJHS (Redmond et al 2006b), and ankle instability is often troublesome also (Finsterbush & Pogrund 1982).

It can be difficult to achieve satisfactory local analgesia in patients with hypermobility syndrome as the agent diffuses rapidly, preventing adequate nerve blockade (Grahame 2000). Tissue fragility leads to problems with wound closure during surgery, and also contributes to a tendency to wound dehiscence postoperatively. It is common for scar formation following surgery or trauma to be hypertrophic (Tompkins & Bellacosa 1997).

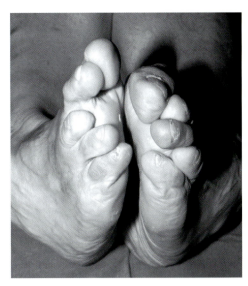

**Figure 8.25** Benign familial joint hypermobility in the foot.

## Miscellaneous other conditions

The foot can be involved in a number of other rheumatic conditions. In ulcerative colitis, synovitis occurs in the metatarsophalangeal joints of 2% of sufferers, with ankle involvement in 5–7% (Moll 1987). In Crohn's disease, the ankle joint is affected in one-third of patients, a similar prevalence to that seen in Whipple's disease (Moll 1987). Behcet (with cidilla) syndrome usually presents as ulceration in the mouth or genitalia, but can present with ankle synovitis and pustule formation on the feet.

## ASSESSING OUTCOMES IN RHEUMATIC DISEASE

Rheumatology as a discipline has been proactive in establishing inventive measures of disease progress and outcome. Outcome measures range from general measures of the impact of musculoskeletal impairment, to particular measures of disease activity and disease-specific impact scales.

For example, the *American College of Rheumatology* diagnostic criteria for RA have been supplemented by explicit criteria for defining and quantifying improvement or remission (Felson et al 1993, van Gestel et al 1998). This enables clear therapeutic guidelines to be drawn up and has removed much of the ambiguity that hampers other areas of practice. These outcome measures are valuable for evaluating the effect of therapies in clinical trials and in day-to-day clinical practice. Outcomes data can be quick to collect, and provide useful objective information on the merits of a clinical service, as well as helping practitioners reflect on their own practice. We recommend that all practitioners involved in the provision of foot health services in rheumatology include some basic outcome-assessment tools in their standard assessment protocol.

Health outcomes tools can be objective, such as the acute-phase inflammatory markers erythrocyte sedimentation rate (ESR) and C-reactive protein (CRP) measured in assessing underlying rheumatoid disease activity, through to more subjective measures, such as pain or impact on quality of life. Some objective measures of function, including basic gait parameters (gait speed, cadence, stride length), are highly correlated with more subjective measures of the impact of disease, such as the Sickness Impact Profile (O'Connell et al 1998). The basic gait parameters are easily and quickly measured without expensive equipment, and are valid and responsive measures of therapeutic change (Fransen & Edmonds 1999, Hamilton et al 2001).

Pain, health status and quality-of-life measures – the easiest way to evaluate the patient-oriented outcomes associated with existing foot health services – can be generic, or disease- or anatomy-specific. Generic measures, such as the Sickness Impact Profile (Bergner et al 1976), SF-36 (Ware et al 1993) and EQ-5D (The Euroqol Group 1990) health assessment questionnaires, measure overall health status and are comparable across diseases.

Disease-specific tools, such as the ASQoL (Doward et al 2003) or the RAQoL (Whalley et al 1997), quality-of-life measures for ankylosing spondylitis and RA, respectively, are intended to pick up features more directly associated with the specific conditions and can be more sensitive.

There are several foot-specific outcomes measures available, the most commonly used being the Foot Function Index (Budiman-Mak et al 1991), the Foot Health Status Questionnaire (Bennett et al 1998) and the Manchester Foot Pain and Disability Questionnaire (Garrow et al 2000), the last of which has recently been revised by Cook et al (2007). These measures are useful, but all have documented shortcomings.

We have developed and validated a foot-specific measure, the Leeds Foot Impact Scale, that is also specific to patients with RA (Helliwell et al 2005). This scale has high validity for foot problems in people with RA, and is the preferred tool for this group. In other rheumatology populations we use the Manchester Foot Pain and Disability Questionnaire and the pain subscale of the Foot Function Index, although in the authors' opinion some improvements could be made in both these measures, and they need to be used with due consideration of their weaknesses. This is an area where the methodologies informing the development of new instruments is maturing rapidly, and further new tools will doubtless be developed in coming years.

## SUMMARY

The foot is often affected in people with rheumatic disorders. The provision of foot health services for this patient group is patchy at best, and frankly inadequate at worst. Foot-related musculoskeletal conditions often coexist with other morbidity, and may even be secondary to impairments associated with systemic effects. Practitioners involved in caring for this group of patients should be aware of current trends in medical management, and should seek to integrate with the rheumatology team. All clinicians engaged in the care of foot-related conditions should remember the high degree of association between the foot and systemic rheumatic disorders, and be mindful of their role in identifying systemic disease if it first presents in the foot.

This is an exciting and developing area of practice in its own right, and more so now that the foot is receiving the recognition is deserves from the rheumatology community.

## ACKNOWLEDGEMENTS

We are indebted to Professor Jim Woodburn and Dr Deborah Turner, both of Glasgow Caledonian University, and former members of the FASTER group, and to Heidi Siddle and all the staff in the Academic Unit of Musculoskeletal Disease for their assistance. We would also like to acknowledge the National Institute of Health Research and the Arthritis Research Campaign for funding the programme of foot research in rheumatology at the authors' institution.

## REFERENCES

Acosta R, Ushiba J, Cracchiolo A 2000 The results of a primary and staged pantalar arthrodesis and tibiotalocalcaneal arthrodesis in adult patients. Foot & Ankle International 21(3):182–194.

Agnew P 1997 Evaluation of the child with ligamentous laxity. Clinics in Podiatric Medicine & Surgery 14(1):117–130.

Ainsworth SR, Aulicino PL 1993 A survey of patients with Ehlers–Danlos syndrome. Clinical Orthopaedics & Related Research 286:250–256.

Aletaha D, Smolen JS 2002 Advances in anti-inflammatory therapy. Acta Medica Austriaca 29(1):1–6.

Al-Rawi ZS, Al-Aszawi AJ, Al-Chalabi T 1985 Joint mobility among university students in Iraq. British Journal of Rheumatology 24(4):326–331.

American College of Rheumatology Subcommittee on Rheumatoid Arthritis 2002 Guidelines for the management of rheumatoid arthritis 2002 Update. Arthritis & Rheumatism 46(2):328–346.

Arthritis and Musculoskeletal Alliance: 2004a Standards of care for people with musculoskeletal conditions – inflammatory arthritis. London.

Arthritis and Musculoskeletal Alliance: 2004b Standards of care for people with musculoskeletal conditions – osteoarthritis. London.

Arthritis and Musculoskeletal Alliance and Podiatry Rheumatic Care Association 2008 Standards of care for people with musculoskeletal foot health problems. London.

Arthritis Research Campaign 2002 Arthritis: the big picture. Chesterfield.

Backman CL, Kennedy SM, Chalmers A, Singer J 2004 Participation in paid and unpaid work by adults with rheumatoid arthritis. Journal of Rheumatology. 31(1):47–56.

Barrett EM, Scott DG, Wiles NJ, Symmons DP 2000 The impact of rheumatoid arthritis on employment status in the early years of disease: a UK community-based study. Rheumatology 39(12):1403–1409.

Barton LM, Bird HA 1996 Improving pain by the stabilization of hyperlax joints. Journal of Orthopaedic Rheumatology 9(1):46–51.

Becker MA, Schumacher HR Jr, Wortmann RL, et al 2005 Febuxostat compared with allopurinol in patients with hyperuricemia and gout. New England Journal of Medicine 353(23):2450–2461.

Beighton P, Horan F 1969 Orthopaedic aspects of the Ehlers–Danlos syndrome. Journal of Bone & Joint Surgery – British Volume 51(3):444–453.

Beighton PH, Horan FT 1970 Dominant inheritance in familial generalised articular hypermobility. Journal of Bone & Joint Surgery – British Volume 52(1):145–147.

Belt EA, Kaarela K, Maenpaa H, et al 2001 Relationship of ankle joint involvement with subtalar destruction in patients with rheumatoid arthritis. A 20-year follow-up study. Joint, Bone, Spine: Revue du Rhumatisme 68(2):154–157.

Bennett PJ, Patterson C, Wearing S, Baglioni T 1998 Development and validation of a questionnaire designed to measure foot-health status. Journal of the American Podiatric Medical Association 88(9):419–428.

Benvenuti F, Ferrucci L, Guralnik JM, et al 1995 Foot pain and disability in older persons: an epidemiologic survey. Journal of the American Geriatrics Society 43(5):479–484.

Bergenudd H, Lindgarde F, Nilsson B 1989 Prevalence and coincidence of degenerative changes of the hands and feet in middle age and their relationship to occupational work load, intelligence, and social background. Clinical Orthopaedics & Related Research 239:306–310.

Berger I, Martens K, Meyer-Scholten C 2004 Rheumatoid necroses in the forefoot. Foot & Ankle International 25(5):336–339.

Bergner M, Bobbitt RA, Pollard WE, et al 1976 The Sickness Impact Profile: validation of a health status measure. Medical Care 19(1):57–67.

Biro F, Gewanter HL, Baum J 1983 The hypermobility syndrome. Pediatrics 72(5):701–706.

Bitzan P, Giurea A, Wanivenhaus A 1997 Plantar pressure distribution after resection of the metatarsal heads in rheumatoid arthritis. Foot & Ankle International 18(7):391–397.

Black JR, Hale WE 1987 Prevalence of foot complaints in the elderly. Journal of the American Podiatric Medical Association 77(6):308–311.

Bongu A, Chang E, Ramsey-Goldman R 2002 Can morbidity and mortality of SLE be improved. Clinical Rheumatology 16(2):313–332.

Bouysset M, Bonvoisin B, Lejeune E, Bouvier M 1987 Flattening of the rheumatoid foot in tarsal arthritis on X-ray. Scandinavian Journal of Rheumatology 16(2):127–133.

Bouysset M, Tebib J, Weil G, et al 1989 The rheumatoid heel: its relationship to other disorders in the rheumatoid foot. Clinical Rheumatology 8(2):208–214.

Bouysset M, Tavernier T, Tebib J, et al 1995 CT and MRI evaluation of tenosynovitis of the rheumatoid hindfoot. Clinical Rheumatology 14(3):303–307.

Bouysset M, Tebib J, Tavernier T, et al 2003 Posterior tibial tendon and subtalar joint complex in rheumatoid arthritis: magnetic resonance imaging study. Journal of Rheumatology 30(9):1951–1194.

Braun J, Sieper J 2007 Ankylosing spondylitis. The Lancet 369(9570):1379–1390.

Breedveld FC, Emery P, Keystone E, et al 2004 Infliximab in active early rheumatoid arthritis. Annals of the Rheumatic Diseases 63(2):149–155.

Brockbank J, Gladman D 2002 Diagnosis and management of psoriatic arthritis. Drugs. 62(17):2447–2457.

Brosseau L, Welch V, Wells G, et al 2004 Low level laser therapy (classes I, II and III) for treating rheumatoid arthritis. Cochrane Database of Systematic Reviews 2:2.

Buckwalter JA, Saltzman CL 1999 Ankle osteoarthritis: distinctive characteristics. Instructional Course Lectures 48:233–241.

Budiman-Mak E, Conrad KJ, Roach KE, et al 1991 The Foot Function Index: a measure of foot pain and disability. Journal of Clinical Epidemiology 44(6):561–570.

Budiman-Mak E, Conrad KJ, Roach KE, et al 1995 Can foot orthoses prevent hallux valgus deformity in rheumatoid arthritis? A randomized clinical trial. Journal of Clinical Rheumatology 1(6):313–321.

Bukhari MA, Wiles NJ, Lunt M, et al 2003 Influence of disease-modifying therapy on radiographic outcome in inflammatory polyarthritis at five years: results from a large observational inception study. Arthritis & Rheumatism 48(1):46–53.

Bulbena A, Duro JC, Porta M, et al 1992 Clinical assessment of hypermobility of joints: assembling criteria. Journal of Rheumatology 19(1):115–122.

Callen JP 2002 Management of skin disease in patients with lupus erythematosus. Clinical Rheumatology 16(2):245–264.

Cannella AC, O'Dell JR 2003 Is there still a role for traditional disease-modifying antirheumatic drugs (DMARDs) in rheumatoid arthritis? Current Opinion in Rheumatology 15(3):185–192.

Cardone DA, Tallia AF 2002 Joint and soft tissue injection. American Family Physician 66(2):283–288.

Cawley MI 1987 Vasculitis and ulceration in rheumatic diseases of the foot. Baillière's Clinical Rheumatology 1(2):315–333.

Chalmers AC, Busby C, Goyert J, et al 2000 Metatarsalgia and rheumatoid arthritis – a randomized, single blind, sequential trial comparing 2 types of foot orthoses and supportive shoes. Journal of Rheumatology 27(7):1643–1647.

Chen BX 1996 Arthritis of the foot and ankle. Current Opinion in Orthopedics 7(3):87–91.

Chen J, Devine A, Dick IM, et al 2003 Prevalence of lower extremity pain and its association with functionality and quality of life in elderly women in Australia. Journal of Rheumatology 30(12):2689–2693.

Chen LX, Schumacher HR 2003 Gout and gout mimickers: 20 clinical pearls: a bigger diagnostic and management challenge than it may seem. Journal of Musculoskeletal Medicine 20(5):254–258.

Choi HK, Al-Arfaj A, Eftekhari A, et al 2008 Dual energy computed tomography in tophaceous gout. Annals of the Rheumatic Diseases ard.2008.099713 (Epub).

Choy EH, Panayi GS 2001 Cytokine pathways and joint inflammation in rheumatoid arthritis. New England Journal of Medicine 344(12):907–916.

Choy EHS, Scott DL, Kingsley GH, et al 2002 Treating rheumatoid arthritis early with disease modifying drugs reduces joint damage: a randomised double blind trial of sulphasalazine vs diclofenac sodium. Clinical & Experimental Rheumatology 20(3):351–358.

Cimino WG, O'Malley MJ 1999 Rheumatoid arthritis of the ankle and the hindfoot.

Clinics in Podiatric Medicine & Surgery 16(2):373–389.

Coady D, Walker D, Kay L 2004 Regional Examination of the Musculoskeletal System (REMS): a core set of clinical skills for medical students. Rheumatology 43(5):633–639.

Coester LM, Saltzman CL, Leupold J, Pontarelli W 2001 Long-term results following ankle arthrodesis for post-traumatic arthritis. Journal of Bone & Joint Surgery American 83(2):219–228.

Cook CE, Cleland J, Pietrobon R, et al 2007 Calibration of an item pool for assessing the disability associated with foot pain: an application of item response theory to the Manchester Foot Pain and Disability Index. Physiotherapy 93(2):89–95.

Cracchiolo IA 1993 The rheumatoid foot and ankle: pathology and treatment. Foot 3(3):126–134.

Crawford F, Atkins D, Young P, Edwards J 1999 Steroid injection for heel pain: evidence of short-term effectiveness. A randomized controlled trial. Rheumatology 38(10):974–977.

Cunningham LS, Kelsey JL 1984 Epidemiology of musculoskeletal impairments and associated disability. American Journal of Public Health 74(6):574–579.

Davys H, Turner D, Emery P, Woodburn J 2004 A comparison of scalpel debridement versus sham procedure for painful forefoot callosities in rheumatoid arthritis. Annals of the Rheumatic Diseases 63(Suppl 1): 427.

de Boer IG, Peeters AJ, Ronday HK, et al 2009 Assistive devices: usage in patients with rheumatoid arthritis. Clinical Rheumatology 28(2):119–128.

DeJesus JM, Tsuchiya C 1999 Pharmacologic management of the arthritic foot and ankle. Clinics in Podiatric Medicine & Surgery 16(2):271–284.

Demetriades L, Strauss E, Gallina J 1998 Osteoarthritis of the ankle. Clinical Orthopaedics & Related Research 349: 28–42.

Devauchelle-Pensec V, Saraux A, Alapetite S, et al 2002 Diagnostic value of radiographs of the hands and feet in early rheumatoid arthritis. Joint Bone Spine 69(5):434–441.

Doward LC, Spoorenberg A, Cook SA, et al 2003 Development of the ASQoL: a quality of life instrument specific to ankylosing spondylitis. Annals of the Rheumatic Diseases 62(1):20–26.

Dunn JE, Link CL, Felson DT, et al 2004 Prevalence of foot and ankle conditions in a multiethnic community sample of older adults. American Journal of Epidemiology 159(5):491–498.

Edwards JCW, Szczepanski L, Szechinski J et al 2004 Efficacy of B-cell-targeted therapy with Rituximab in patients with rheumatoid arthritis. New England Journal of Medicine 350:2572–2581.

Egan M, Brosseau L, Farmer M, et al 2003 Splints/orthoses in the treatment of rheumatoid arthritis. Cochrane Database of Systematic Reviews 1:CD004018.

Egan R, Sartoris J, Dresnick D, et al 1987 Radiographic features of gout in the foot. Journal of Foot Surgery 26(5):434–439.

Emery P, Breedveld FC, Dougados D, et al 2002 Early referral recommendation for newly diagnosed rheumatoid arthritis: evidence based development of a clinical guide. Annals of the Rheumatic Diseases 61(4):290–297.

Emery P, Seto Y 2003 Role of biologics in early arthritis. Clinical & Experimental Rheumatology 21(5 Suppl 31):S191–S194.

Escalante A, Del Rincon I 1999 How much disability in rheumatoid arthritis is explained by rheumatoid arthritis? Arthritis & Rheumatism 42(8):1712–1721.

Escalante A, Del Rincon I 2002 The disablement process in rheumatoid arthritis. Arthritis & Rheumatism 47(3):333–342.

Feldmann M 2002 Development of anti-TNF therapy for rheumatoid arthritis. Nature Reviews. Immunology 2(5):364–371.

Feldmann M, Maini R 2008 Role of cytokines in rheumatoid arthritis: an education in pathophysiology and therapeutics. Immunological Reviews 223(1):7–19.

Felson DT, Anderson JJ, Boers M, et al 1993 The American College of Rheumatology preliminary core set of disease activity measures for rheumatoid arthritis clinical trials. The Committee on Outcome Measures in Rheumatoid Arthritis Clinical Trials. Arthritis & Rheumatism 36(6):729–740.

Felson DT, Lawrence RC, Dieppe PA et al 2000 Osteoarthritis: new insights. Part 1: The disease and its risk factors. Annals of Internal Medicine 133(8):635–646.

Finsterbush A, Pogrund H 1982 The hypermobility syndrome. Musculoskeletal complaints in 100 consecutive cases of generalized joint hypermobility. Clinical Orthopaedics & Related Research 168:124–127.

Firth J, Hale C, et al 2008 The prevalence of foot ulceration in patients with rheumatoid arthritis. Arthritis & Rheumatism (Arthritis Care and Research) 59(2):200–205.

Fitzgerald GA 2004 Coxibs and cardiovascular disease. New England Journal of Medicine 351:1709–1711.

Fransen M, Edmonds J 1997 Off-the-shelf orthopedic footwear for people with rheumatoid arthritis. Arthritis Care & Research 10(4):250–256.

Fransen M, Edmonds J 1999 Gait variables: appropriate objective outcome measures in rheumatoid arthritis. Rheumatology 38(7):663–667.

Fries JF, Williams CA, Morfeld D, et al 1996 Reduction in long-term disability in patients with rheumatoid arthritis by disease-modifying antirheumatic drug-based treatment strategies. Arthritis & Rheumatism 39(4):616–622.

Galluzzo E, Lischi D, Taglione E, et al 2000 Sonographic analysis of the ankle in patients with psoriatic arthritis. Scandinavian Journal of Rheumatology 29(1):52–55.

Garner S, Fidan D, Frankish R, et al 2004a Rofecoxib for rheumatoid arthritis. Cochrane Database of Systematic Reviews 2:2.

Garner S, Fidan D, Frankish R, et al 2004b Celecoxib for rheumatoid arthritis. Cochrane Database of Systematic Reviews 2:2.

Garrow AP, Papageorgiou AC, Silman AJ, et al 2000 Development and validation of a questionnaire to assess disabling foot pain. Pain 85(1–2):107–113.

Garrow AP, Silman AJ, Macfarlane GJ 2004 The Cheshire Foot Pain and Disability Survey: a population survey assessing prevalence and associations. Pain 110(1–2):378–384.

Gazit Y, Nahir AM 2001 Hypermobility syndrome – a disease or not a disease? Annals of the Rheumatic Diseases 60(Suppl 1).

Genta MS, Genta RM, Gabay C 2006 systemic rheumatoid vasculitis: a review. Seminars in Arthritis and Rheumatism 36(2):88–98.

Gerster JC, Vischer TL, Bennani A, Fallet GH 1977 The painful heel. Comparative study in rheumatoid arthritis, ankylosing spondylitis, Reiter's syndrome, and generalized osteoarthrosis. Annals of the Rheumatic Diseases 36(4):343–348.

Gilkes JJ 1987 Skin and nail changes in the arthritic foot. Baillière's Clinical Rheumatology 1(2):335–354.

Gladstein GS, Rynes RI, Parhami M, Bartholomew LE 1979 Gangrene of a foot secondary to systemic lupus erythematosus with large vessel vasculitis. Journal of Rheumatology 6(5):549–553.

Gold RH, Bassett LW, Seeger LL 1988 The other arthritides. Roentgenologic features of osteoarthritis, erosive osteoarthritis, ankylosing spondylitis, psoriatic arthritis, Reiter's disease, multicentric reticulohistiocytosis, and progressive systemic sclerosis. Radiologic Clinics of North America 26(6):1195–1212.

Gordon P, West J, Jones H, Gibson T 2001 A 10 year prospective followup of patients with rheumatoid arthritis: 1986–96. Journal of Rheumatology 28(11):2409–2415.

Gorter K, Kuyvenhoven M, de Melker R 2001 Health care utilisation by older people with non-traumatic foot complaints. What makes the difference? Scandinavian Journal of Primary Health Care 19(3):191–193.

Gorter KJ, Kuyvenhoven MM, de Melker RA 2000 Nontraumatic foot complaints in older people. A population-based survey of risk factors, mobility, and well-being. Journal of the American Podiatric Medical Association 90(8):397–402.

Grahame R 1993 Topical reviews: hypermobility syndrome. ARC Reports on Rheumatic Diseases Series 2(25).

Grahame R 2000 Pain, distress and joint hyperlaxity. Joint, Bone, Spine: Revue du Rhumatisme 67(3):157–163.

Grahame R, Bird H 2001 British consultant rheumatologists perceptions about the hypermobility syndrome: a national survey. Rheumatology 40(5):559–562.

Grahame R, Bird HA, Child A 2000 The revised (Brighton: 1998) criteria for the diagnosis of benign joint hypermobility syndrome (BJHS). Journal of Rheumatology 27(7):1777–1779.

Greisberg J, Hansen ST Jr, Sangeorzan B 2003 Deformity and degeneration in the hindfoot and midfoot joints of the adult acquired flatfoot. Foot & Ankle International 24(7):530–534.

Guma M, Roca J, Holgado S, et al 2001 An estimation of the prevalence of hypermobility. Annals of the Rheumatic Diseases 60(Suppl 1):Thu: 0220.

Gurley-Green S 2001 Living with the hypermobility syndrome. Rheumatology 40(5):487–489.

Hamalainen M, Raunio P 1997 Long term followup of rheumatoid forefoot surgery. Clinical Orthopaedics & Related Research 340:34–38.

Hamilton J, Brydson G, Fraser G, Grant M 2001 Walking ability as a measure of treatment effect in early rheumatoid arthritis. Clinical Rehabilitation 15(2):142–147.

Harris MD, Siegel LB, Alloway JA 1999 Gout hyperuricemia. American Family Physician 59(4):925–934.

Harvey I, Frankel S, Marks R, et al 1997 Foot morbidity and exposure to chiropody: population based study. BMJ 315(7115):1054–1055.

Hawker G 1997 Update on the epidemiology of the rheumatic diseases. Current Opinion in Rheumatology 9(2):90–94.

Hazes JM 2003 Determinants of physical function in rheumatoid arthritis: association with the disease process. Rheumatology 42(Suppl 2):ii17–ii21.

Helliwell PS 2003 Lessons to be learned: review of a multidisciplinary foot clinic in rheumatology. Rheumatology 42(11):1426–1427.

Helliwell PS, Allen N, Gilworth G, et al 2005 Development of a foot impact scale for rheumatoid arthritis. Rheumatology 47:ii27–ii28.

Helliwell PS, O'Hara M, Holdsworth J, et al 1999 A 12-month randomized controlled trial of patient education on radiographic changes and quality of life in early rheumatoid arthritis. Rheumatology 38(4):303–308.

Hendry G, Gardner-Medwin J, Watt GF, Woodburn J 2008 A survey of foot problems in juvenile idiopathic arthritis. Musculoskeletal Care 6:221–232.

Herold DC, Palmer RG 1992 Questionnaire study of the use of surgical shoes prescribed in a rheumatology outpatient clinic. Journal of Rheumatology 19(10):1542–1544.

Hodge MC, Bach TM, Carter GM, et al 1999 Novel Award First Prize Paper. Orthotic management of plantar pressure and pain in rheumatoid arthritis. Clinical Biomechanics 14(8):567–575.

Hudson N, Starr MR, Esdaile JM, Fitzcharles MA 1995 Diagnostic associations with hypermobility in rheumatology patients. British Journal of Rheumatology 34(12):1157–1161.

Hughes J, Grace D, Clark P, Klenerman L 1991 Metatarsal head excision for rheumatoid arthritis. 4-year follow-up of 68 feet with and without hallux fusion. Acta Orthopaedica Scandinavica 62(1):63–66.

Jacobson JA, Girish G, Jiang Y, Resnick D 2008 Radiographic evaluation of arthritis: inflammatory conditions. Radiology 248(2):378–389.

Jennings MB 1994 Comparison of piroxicam and naproxen in osteoarthritis of the foot. Journal of the American Podiatric Medical Association 84(7):348–354.

Jernberg ET, Simkin P, Kravette M, et al 1999 The posterior tibial tendon and the tarsal sinus in rheumatoid flat foot: magnetic resonance imaging of 40 feet. Journal of Rheumatology 26(2):289–293.

Juni P, Nartey L, Reichenbaum S, et al 2004 Risk of cardiovascular events and rofecoxib: cumulative meta-analysis. Lancet 364:2021–2029.

Karaaslan Y, Haznedaroglu S, Ozturk M 2002 Joint hypermobility and primary fibromyalgia: a clinical enigma. Journal of Rheumatology 27(7):1774–1776.

Kavlak Y, Uygur F, Korkmaz C, Bek N 2003 Outcome of orthoses intervention in the rheumatoid foot. Foot & Ankle International 24(6):494–499.

Kay S, Nancarrow JD 1984 Spontaneous healing and relief of pain in a patient with intractable vasculitic ulceration of the lower limb following an intravenous infusion of prostacyclin: a case report. British Journal of Plastic Surgery 37(2):175–178.

Keenan MA, Peabody TD, Gronley JK, Perry J 1991 Valgus deformities of the feet and characteristics of gait in patients who have rheumatoid arthritis. Journal of Bone & Joint Surgery 73(2):237–247.

Keenan A-M, Tennant A, Fear J, Emery P, Conaghan PG 2006 Impact of multiple joint problems on daily living tasks in people in the community over age fifty-five. Arthritis and Rheumatism 55:757–764.

Kerman BL, Mack G, Moshirfar MM 1993 Tophaceous gout of the foot: an unusual presentation of severe chronic gout in an undiagnosed patient. Journal of Foot & Ankle Surgery 32(2):167–170.

Kerr LD 1998 Arthritis of the forefoot. A review from a rheumatologic and medical perspective. Clinical Orthopaedics & Related Research (349):20–27.

Kerry RM, Holt GM, Stockley I 1994 The foot in chronic rheumatoid arthritis: a continuing problem. Foot 4(4):201–203.

Korda J, Balint GP 2004 When to consult the podiatrist. Best Practice & Research in Clinical Rheumatology 18(4):587–611.

Kraus VB, Li, YJ, Martin ER, et al 2004 Articular hypermobility is a protective factor for hand osteoarthritis. Arthritis & Rheumatism 50(7):2178–2183.

Kumar R, Madewell JE 1987 Rheumatoid and seronegative arthropathies of the foot. Radiologic Clinics of North America 25(6):1263–1288.

La Montagna G, Baruffo A, Tirri R, et al 2002 Foot involvement in systemic sclerosis: a longitudinal study of 100 patients. Seminars in Arthritis & Rheumatism 31(4):248–255.

Lard LR, Visser H, Speyer I, et al 2001 Early versus delayed treatment in patients with recent-onset rheumatoid arthritis: comparison of two cohorts who received different treatment strategies. American Journal of Medicine 111(6):446–451.

Larsson LG, Baum J, Mudholkar GS, Srivastava DK 1993 Hypermobility: prevalence and features in a Swedish population. British Journal of Rheumatology 32(2):116–119.

Lemont H, Gibley CW Jr 1982 Prevalence of osteoarthritis of the foot. Journal of the American Podiatry Association 72(5):214–216.

Leonardi CL, Powers JL, Matheson RT, et al 2003 Etanercept as monotherapy in patients with psoriasis. New England Journal of Medicine 349(21):2014–2022.

Leveille SG, Guralnik JM, Ferrucci L, et al 1998 Foot pain and disability in older women. American Journal of Epidemiology 148(7):657–665.

Lin AT, Clements PJ, Furst DE 2003 Update on disease-modifying antirheumatic drugs in the treatment of systemic sclerosis. Rheumatic Diseases Clinics of North America 29(2):409–426.

Linaker CH, Walker-Bone K, Palmer K, Cooper C 1999 Frequency and impact of regional musculoskeletal disorders. Baillière's Clinical Rheumatology 13(2):197–215.

Liu SZ, Yeh LR, Chou YJ, et al 2003 Isolated intraosseous gout in hallux sesamoid mimicking a bone tumor in a teenaged patient. Skeletal Radiology 32(11):647–650.

Lord M, Foulston J 1989 Surgical footwear: a survey of prescribing consultants. BMJ 299(6700):9.

Lukas C, Landewe R, Sieper J, et al 2009 Development of an ASAS-endorsed disease activity score (ASDAS) in patients with ankylosing spondylitis. Annals of the Rheumatic Diseases 68(1):18–24.

Maddison PJ 2002 Is it SLE? Clinical Rheumatology 16(2):167–180.

Mann RA, Chou LB 1995 Tibiocalcaneal arthrodesis. Foot & Ankle International 16(7):401–405.

March L, Lapsley H 2001 What are the costs to society and the potential benefits from the effective management of early rheumatoid arthritis? Best Practice & Research in Clinical Rheumatology 15(1):171–185.

Marijnissen AC, van Roermund PM, van Melkebeek J, Lafeber FP 2003 Clinical benefit of joint distraction in the treatment of ankle osteoarthritis. Foot & Ankle Clinics 8(2):335–346.

Marzo-Ortega H, McGonagle D, O'Connor P, Emery P 2001 Efficacy of etanercept in the treatment of the entheseal pathology in resistant spondylarthropathy: a clinical and magnetic resonance imaging study. Arthritis & Rheumatism 44(9):2112–2117.

Masterton E, Mulcahy DMC, Elwain J, McInerney D 1995 The plano valgus rheumatoid foot – is tibialis posterior tendon rupture a factor? British Journal of Rheumatology 34(7):645–646.

Matheson AJ, Perry CM 2003 Glucosamine: a review of its use in the management of osteoarthritis. Drugs & Aging 20(14):1041–1060.

McAlindon T 2000 Update on the epidemiology of systemic lupus erythematosus: new spins on old ideas. Current Opinion in Rheumatology 12(2):104–112.

McGonagle D, Marzo-Ortega H, O'Connor P, et al 2002 The role of biomechanical factors and HLA-B27 in magnetic resonance imaging-determined bone changes in plantar fascia enthesopathy. Arthritis & Rheumatism 46(2):489–493.

McGuire JB 2003 Arthritis and related diseases of the foot and ankle: rehabilitation and biomechanical considerations. Clinics in Podiatric Medicine & Surgery 20(3):469–485, ix.

Menz HB, Munteanu SE, Landorf KB, et al 2007 Radiographic classification of osteoarthritis in commonly affected joints of the foot. Osteoarthritis and Cartilage 15(11):1333–1338.

Michelson J, Easley M, Wigley FM, Hellmann D 1994 Foot and ankle problems in rheumatoid arthritis. Foot & Ankle International 15(11):608–613.

Mizutani W, Quismorio FP Jr 1984 Lupus foot: deforming arthropathy of the feet in systemic lupus erythematosus. Journal of Rheumatology 11(1):80–82.

Moll JMH 1987 Seronegative arthropathies in the foot. Baillière's Clinical Rheumatology 1(2):289–314.

Muehleman C, Bareither D, Huch K, et al 1997 Prevalence of degenerative morphological changes in the joints of the lower extremity. Osteoarthritis & Cartilage 5(1):23–37.

Mulherin D, Price M 2009 Efficacy of tibial nerve block, local steroid injection or both in the treatment of plantar heel pain syndrome. The Foot 19(2):98–100.

Munro BJ, Steele JR 1998 Foot-care awareness. A survey of persons aged 65 years and older. Journal of the American Podiatric Medical Association 88(5):242–248.

NICE 2002 Guidance on the use of etanercept and inflixmab for the treatment of rheumatoid arthritis. Technology Appraisal Guidance No. 36. National Institute for Clinical Excellence, London.

NICE 2008 Clinical Guideline CG 59: The care and management of osteoarthritis in adults. NICE Clinical Guidelines. National Institute for Health and Clinical Excellence, London.

NICE 2009 Clinical Guideline CG 79: The care and management of rheumatoid arthritis in adults. NICE Clinical Guidelines. National Institute for Health and Clinical Excellence, London.

O'Brien TS, Hart, TS, Gould JS 1997 Extraosseous manifestations of rheumatoid arthritis in the foot and ankle. Clinical Orthopaedics & Related Research 340:26–33.

O'Connell PG, Lohmann Siegel K, Kepple TM, et al 1998 Forefoot deformity, pain, and mobility in rheumatoid and nonarthritic subjects. Journal of Rheumatology 25(9):1681–1686.

O'Dell JR 1997 The therapeutic pyramid: a work in progress. Journal of Rheumatology 24(6):1028–1030.

O'Dell JR 2004 Therapeutic strategies for rheumatoid arthritis. New England Journal of Medicine 350:2591–2602.

Odding E, Valkenburg HA, Algra D, et al 1995 Association of locomotor complaints and disability in the Rotterdam study. Annals of the Rheumatic Diseases 54(9):721–725.

Olivieri I, Barozzi L, Padula A 1998 Enthesiopathy: clinical manifestations, imaging and treatment. Baillière's Clinical Rheumatology 12(4):665–681.

Olivieri I, Scarano E, Padula A, et al 2007 Switching tumor necrosis factor alpha inhibitors in HLA-B27-associated severe heel enthesitis. Arthritis & Rheumatism 57(8):1572–1574.

Olsen N, Stein M 2004 New drugs for rheumatoid arthritis. New England Journal of Medicine 350:2567–2579.

Osiri M, Shea B, Robinson V, et al 2004 Leflunomide for treating rheumatoid arthritis. Cochrane Database of Systematic Reviews 2:2.

Ostergaard M, Szkudlarek M 2003 Imaging in rheumatoid arthritis – why MRI and ultrasonography can no longer be ignored. Scandinavian Journal of Rheumatology 32(2):63–73.

Otter SY, Cryer A 2004 Biologic agents used to treat rheumatoid arthritis and their relevance to podiatrists: a practice update. Musculoskeletal Care 2(1):51–59.

Pensec VD, Saraux A, Berthelot JM, et al 2004 Ability of foot radiographs to predict rheumatoid arthritis in patients with early arthritis. Journal of Rheumatology 31(1):66–70.

Petty RE, Southwood TR, Baum J, et al 1991 Revision of the proposed classification criteria for juvenile idiopathic arthritis: Durban, 1997. Journal of Rheumatology 25(10):1991–1994.

Pincus T, O'Dell JR, Kremer JM 1999 Combination therapy with multiple disease-modifying antirheumatic drugs in rheumatoid arthritis: a preventive strategy.

Annals of Internal Medicine 131(10):768–774.

Platto MJ, O'Connell PG, Hicks JE, Gerber LH 1991 The relationship of pain and deformity of the rheumatoid foot to gait and an index of functional ambulation. Journal of Rheumatology 18(1):38–43.

Port M, McCarthy DJ, Chu S 1980 The foot and systemic disease in the Veterans Administration: a quantitation of the relationship between systemic disease and pedal problems. Journal of the American Podiatry Association 70(8):397–404.

Prier A, Berenbaum F, Karneff A, et al 1997 Multidisciplinary day hospital treatment of rheumatoid arthritis patients. Evaluation after two years. Revue du Rhumatisme (English Edition) 64(7–9):443–450.

Priolo F, Bacarini L, Cannista M, et al 1997 Radiographic changes in the feet of patients with early rheumatoid arthritis. Journal of Rheumatology 24(11):2113–2118.

Puolakka K, Kautiainen H, Mottonen T, et al 2004 Impact of initial aggressive drug treatment with a combination of disease-modifying antirheumatic drugs on the development of work disability in early rheumatoid arthritis: a five-year randomized followup trial. Arthritis & Rheumatism 50(1):55–62.

Rao JK, Hootman JM 2004 Prevention research and rheumatic disease. Current Opinion in Rheumatology 16(2):119–124.

Rau R, Schleusser B, Herborn G, Karger T 1997 Long-term treatment of destructive rheumatoid arthritis with methotrexate. Journal of Rheumatology 24(10):1881–1889.

Reber PU, Patel AG, Noesberger B 1997 Gout: rare cause of hallucal sesamoid pain: a case report. Foot & Ankle International 18(12):818–820.

Redmond A, Allen N, Vernon W 1999 Effect of scalpel debridement on the pain associated with plantar hyperkeratosis. Journal of the American Podiatric Medical Association 89(10):515–519.

Redmond AC, Helliwell PS 2005 A national survey of foot health services in UK rheumatology practice. Unpublished.

Redmond AC, Keenan A, Landorf KB, Emery P 2004 Off-the-shelf contoured orthoses demonstrate comparable mechanical properties to custom-made foot orthoses at less cost. Rheumatology 43(4):ii149.

Redmond AC, Hain J, Bird HA, et al 2006a The distribution and prevalence of symptoms associated with hypermobility syndrome. Annals of the Rheumatic Diseases 65(Suppl II):241.

Redmond AC, Helliwell PS, Bird HA, et al 2006b Pain and health status in people with hypermobility syndrome are associated with overall joint mobility and selected local mechanical factors. Rheumatology 45(1):108.

Reilly PA, Evison G, McHugh NJ, Maddison PJ 1990 Arthropathy of hands and feet in

systemic lupus erythematosus. Journal of Rheumatology 17(6):777–784.

Riano F, Sanchez O, Pena NZT 2001 Joint hypermobility syndrome: a prospective study of articular and non-rheumatic manifestation in a Venezuelan population. Annals of the Rheumatic Diseases 60(Suppl 1):Thu: 0217.

Riemsma RP, Kirwan JR, Taal E, Rasker JJ 2004 Patient education for adults with rheumatoid arthritis. Cochrane Database of Systematic Reviews 2:2.

Riente L, Delle Sedie A, Iagnocco A, et al 2006 Ultrasound imaging for the rheumatologist. V. Ultrasonography of the ankle and foot. Clinical and Experimental Rheumatology 24:493–498.

Ritchlin CT, Kavanaugh A, Gladman DD, et al 2009 Treatment recommendations for psoriatic arthritis. Annals of the Rheumatic Diseases 68:1387–1394.

Rosenberg WWJ, De Waal Malefijt MC, Laan RFJM, Go SL 2000 Forefoot reconstruction with combined first metatarsus osteotomy, metatarsophalangeal fusion and resection of the lesser metatarsal heads in rheumatoid patients. Foot & Ankle Surgery 6(2):99–104.

Sacheti A, Szemere J, Bernstein B, et al 1997 Chronic pain is a manifestation of the Ehlers–Danlos syndrome. Journal of Pain & Symptom Management 14(2):88–93.

Sanmarti R, Gomez A, Ercilla G, et al 2003 Radiological progression in early rheumatoid arthritis after DMARDS: a one-year follow-up study in a clinical setting. Rheumatology 42(9):1044–1049.

Sari-Kouzel H, Hutchinson CE, Middleton A, et al 2001 Foot problems in patients with systemic sclerosis. Rheumatology 40(4):410–413.

Schmiegel A, Rosenbaum D, Schorat A, et al 2008 Assessment of foot impairment in rheumatoid arthritis patients by dynamic pedobarography. Gait & Posture 27(1):110–114.

Solsky MA, Wallace DJ 2002 New therapies in systemic lupus erythematosus. Clinical Rheumatology 16(2):293–312.

Steed DL, Edington H, Moosa HH, Webster MW 1993 Organization and development of a university multidisciplinary wound care clinic. Surgery 114(4):775–778; discussion 778–779.

Steultjens EMJ, Dekker J, Bouter LM, et al 2004 Occupational therapy for rheumatoid arthritis. Cochrane Database of Systematic Reviews 2:2.

Stiskal M, Szolar DH, Stenzel I, et al 1997 Magnetic resonance imaging of Achilles tendon in patients with rheumatoid arthritis. Investigative Radiology 32(10):602–608.

Surprenant MS, Levy AI, Hanfit JR 1996 Intraosseous gout of the foot: an unusual case report. Journal of Foot & Ankle Surgery 35(3):237–243.

Symmons D, Asten P, McNally R, Webb R 2002 Healthcare needs assessment for musculoskeletal diseases: the first step – Estimating the number of incidents and prevalent cases. arc Epidemiology Unit, University of Manchester, Manchester.

Szkudlarek M, Court-Payen M, Jacobsen S, et al 2003 Interobserver agreement in ultrasonography of the finger and toe joints in rheumatoid arthritis. Arthritis & Rheumatism 48(4):955–962.

Taylor W, Gladman D, Helliwell P, et al 2006 Classification criteria for psoriatic arthritis: development of new criteria from a large international study. Arthritis and Rheumatism 54:2665–2673.

The Euroqol Group 1990 EuroQol: a new facility for the measurement of health related quality of life. Health Policy 16(3): 199–208.

Theodoridou A, Bento L, D'Cruz DP, et al 2003 Prevalence and associations of an abnormal ankle–brachial index in systemic lupus erythematosus: a pilot study. Annals of the Rheumatic Diseases 62:1199–1203.

Thomas E, Olive P, Canovas F, et al 1998 Tophaceous gout of the navicular bone as a cause of medial inflammatory tumor of the foot. Foot & Ankle International 19(1):48–51.

Thomas E, Peat G, Harris L, et al 2004 The prevalence of pain and pain interference in a general population of older adults: cross-sectional findings from the North Staffordshire Osteoarthritis Project (NorStOP). Pain 110:361–368.

Thomas RH, Daniels TR 2003 Current concepts review. Ankle arthritis. Journal of Bone & Joint Surgery – American Volume 85A(5):923–936.

Tompkins MH, Bellacosa RA 1997 Podiatric surgical considerations in the Ehlers–Danlos patient. Journal of Foot & Ankle Surgery 36(5):381–387.

Toolan BC, Hansen ST Jr 1998 Surgery of the rheumatoid foot and ankle. Current Opinion in Rheumatology 10(2):116–119.

Towheed TE, Judd MJ, Hochberg MC, Wells G 2004 Acetaminophen for osteoarthritis. Cochrane Database of Systematic Reviews 2:2.

Tsokos G 2004 B-Cells be gone – B-cell depletion in the treatment of rheumatoid arthritis. New England Journal of Medicine 350:2546–2548.

Turesson C, Matteson EL 2009 Vasculitis in rheumatoid arthritis. Current Opinion in Rheumatology 21(1):35–40.

Turner DW, Helliwell P 2003 Pes plano valgus in RA: a descriptive and analytical study of foot function determined by gait analysis. Musculoskeletal Care 1(1):23–33.

Turner DE, Helliwell PS, Lohmann Siegel K, Woodburn J 2008 Biomechanics of the foot in rheumatoid arthritis: identifying abnormal function and the factors associated with localised disease impact. Clinical Biomechanics 23(1):93–100.

Ueda H, Akahoshi T, Kashiwazaki S 1991 Radiological changes in feet of patients with progressive systemic sclerosis. Japanese Journal of Rheumatology 3(1):73–78.

Urwin M, Symmons D, Allison T, et al 1998 Estimating the burden of musculoskeletal disorders in the community: the comparative prevalence of symptoms at different anatomical sites, and the relation to social deprivation. Annals of the Rheumatic Diseases 57(11):649–655.

van der Heijde D 2004 New directions in classification and outcome assessment in ankylosing spondylitis. Current Rheumatology Reports 6(2):98–101.

van der Leeden M, Steultjens M, Dekker JHM, et al 2008a Is disease duration related to foot function, pain and disability in rheumatoid arthritis patients with foot complaints? Clinical Biomechanics 23(5):693–693.

van der Leeden M, Steultjens MPM, et al 2008b Prevalence and course of forefoot impairments and walking disability in the first eight years of rheumatoid arthritis. Arthritis & Rheumatism (Arthritis Care and Research) 59(11):1596–1602.

Van Eygen P, Dereymaeker G, Driesen R, De Ferm A 1999 Long-term follow-up of open ankle arthrodesis. Foot & Ankle Surgery 5(4):271–275.

van Gestel AM, Prevoo ML, van't Hof MA, et al 1996 Development and validation of the European League Against Rheumatism response criteria for rheumatoid arthritis. Comparison with the preliminary American College of Rheumatology and the World Health Organization/International League Against Rheumatism Criteria. Arthritis & Rheumatism 39(1):34–40.

van Gestel AM, Haagsma CJ, van Riel PL 1998 Validation of rheumatoid arthritis improvement criteria that include simplified joint counts. Arthritis & Rheumatism 41(10):1845–1850.

van Venrooij WJ, van Beers JJBC, Pruijn GJM 2008 Anti-CCP antibody, a marker for the early detection of rheumatoid arthritis. The Year in Immunology 1143:268–285.

Veale DJ, FitzGerald O 2002 Psoriatic arthritis – pathogenesis and epidemiology. Clinical & Experimental Rheumatology 20(6 Suppl 28):S27–S33.

Verstappen SM, Jacobs JW, Bijlsma JW, et al 2003a Five-year followup of rheumatoid arthritis patients after early treatment with disease-modifying antirheumatic drugs versus treatment according to the pyramid approach in the first year. Arthritis & Rheumatism 48(7):1797–1807.

Verstappen SMM, Jacobs JWG, Bijlsma JWJ, et al 2003b The Utrecht experience with different treatment strategies in early rheumatoid arthritis. Clinical & Experimental Rheumatology 21(5 Suppl 31):S165–S168.

Vidigal E, Jacoby RK, Dixon AS, et al 1975 The foot in chronic rheumatoid arthritis. Annals of the Rheumatic Diseases 34(4):292–297.

Wakefield RJ, Gibbon WW, Conaghan PG, et al 2000 The value of sonography in the detection of bone erosions in patients with rheumatoid arthritis: A comparison with conventional radiography. Arthritis & Rheumatism 43(12):2762–2770.

Ward MM 2000 Health services in rheumatology. Current Opinion in Rheumatology 12(2):99–103.

Walker JG, Pope J, Baron M, et al 2007 The development of systemic sclerosis classification criteria. Clinical Rheumatology 26(9):1401–1409.

Ware J, Snow KK, Kosinski M, Gandek B 1993 SF-36 Health Survey. Manual and interpretation guide. Boston Health Institute, New England Medical Center, Boston, MA.

Weinfeld SB, Schon LC 1998 Hallux metatarsophalangeal arthritis. Clinical Orthopaedics & Related Research 349: 9–19.

Whalley D, McKenna SP, de Jong Z, van der Heijde D 1997 Quality of life in rheumatoid arthritis. British Journal of Rheumatology 36(8):884–888.

White EG, Mulley GP 1989 Footcare for very elderly people: a community survey. Age & Ageing 18(4):276–278.

Wickman AM, Pinzur MS, Kadanoff R, Juknelis D 2004 Health-related quality of life for patients with rheumatoid arthritis foot involvement. Foot & Ankle International 25(1):19–26.

Williams A, Bowden A 2002 An audit of foot problems in rheumatic disease. Society of Chiropodists and Podiatrists National Conference, Nottingham.

Williams AE, Rome K, et al 2007 A clinical trial of specialist footwear for patients with rheumatoid arthritis. Rheumatology 46(2):302–307.

Wolfe F, Rehman Q, Lane NE, Kremer J 2001 Starting a disease modifying antirheumatic drug or a biologic agent in rheumatoid arthritis: standards of practice for RA treatment. Journal of Rheumatology 28(7):1704–1711.

Wood PLR, Clough TM, Smith R 2008 The present state of ankle arthroplasty. Foot and Ankle Surgery 14(3):115–119.

Woodburn J, Turner DE, Helliwell PS, Barker S 1999 A preliminary study determining the feasibility of electromagnetic tracking for kinematics at the ankle joint complex. Rheumatology 38(12):1260–1268.

Woodburn J, Stableford Z, Helliwell PS 2000 Preliminary investigation of debridement of plantar callosities in rheumatoid arthritis. Rheumatology 39(6):652–654.

Woodburn J, Barker S, Helliwell PS 2002a A randomized controlled trial of foot orthoses in rheumatoid arthritis. Journal of Rheumatology 29(7):1377–1383.

Woodburn J, Helliwell PS, Barker S 2002b Three-dimensional kinematics at the ankle joint complex in rheumatoid arthritis patients with painful valgus deformity of the rearfoot. Rheumatology 41(12):1406–1412.

Woodburn J, Helliwell PS, Barker S 2003 Changes in 3D joint kinematics support the continuous use of orthoses in the management of painful rearfoot deformity in rheumatoid arthritis. Journal of Rheumatology 30(11):2356–2364.

Woodburn J, Udupa JK, Hirsch BE, et al 2002c The geometric architecture of the subtalar and midtarsal joints in rheumatoid arthritis based on magnetic resonance imaging. Arthritis & Rheumatism 46(12):3168–3177.

Wordsworth P, Ogilvie D, Smith R, Sykes B 1987 Joint mobility with particular reference to racial variation and inherited connective tissue disorders. British Journal of Rheumatology 26(1):9–12.

Young A, Dixey J, Cox N, et al 2000 How does functional disability in early rheumatoid arthritis (RA) affect patients and their lives? Results of 5 years of follow-up in 732 patients from the Early RA Study (ERAS). Rheumatology 39(6):603–611.

# Chapter | 9 |

# Metabolic disorders

*Michael E Edmonds*

Metabolic disorders have a considerable importance with regard to public health and may result in significant disease to the foot. They include diabetes, obesity and metabolic bone disorders.

## DIABETES MELLITUS

The manifestations of diabetes result from a persistently raised blood glucose level as a consequence of reduced production and/or impaired effectiveness of insulin.

Diabetes mellitus can be divided into two main groups: type 1 diabetes mellitus and type 2 diabetes mellitus. In addition, there is a small group with secondary diabetes.

## Type 1 diabetes

Type 1 diabetes indicates that there is an almost complete lack of effective insulin, and in the absence of insulin treatment these patients will usually progress to diabetic ketoacidosis. Most of these patients are children and young people under 30 years of age, although it is important to note that type 1 diabetes can present in middle age and in the elderly.

Type 1 diabetes results from damage to the pancreatic beta cells, and genetic, immunological and, probably, environmental (e.g. viral) factors are involved, which lead eventually to total destruction of the beta cell. Type 1 diabetes is a polygenic disease, indicating that many different genes contribute to its expression. The important genetic risk factor for the development of type 1 diabetes is the major histocompatibility complex (MHC) antigens/human leucocyte antigens (HLA). Ninety per cent of people with diabetes in the UK have either HLA-DR3 or HLA-DR4, or both. This leads to the beta cell demonstrating improper antigens to T cells, and eventually results in the production of antibodies that attack the beta cell. Lymphocytes infiltrate the islets of Langerhans, and antibodies against islet cells are present in the sera of 80% of type 1 diabetic patients. There may be certain trigger events, such as viral infections, which precipitate this series of reactions. An increased prevalence of newly diagnosed type 1 diabetes has been found in children aged 4–6 and 11–14 years. These age groups coincide with entry to primary and secondary school.

## Type 2 diabetes

In type 2 diabetes there is a relative, but not an absolute, lack of insulin. Peripheral tissue becomes insulin-resistant; that is, less sensitive to the effects of insulin. There is also a strong inheritable genetic association in type 2 diabetes: having relatives (especially first-degree relatives) with type 2 diabetes increases the risk of developing type 2 diabetes very considerably. In 25% of cases a first-degree relative has type 2 diabetes, and virtually all identical twins of patients with type 2 diabetes develop the disease, even if brought up in different environments.

Type 2 diabetes is the most common type of diabetes. Patients are usually older than 40 years at diagnosis but may be younger, and are often obese. Although considered a disease of adults, type 2 diabetes is increasingly diagnosed in children in association with rising obesity rates. Patients with type 2 diabetes may have relatively few symptoms and do not usually develop ketoacidosis. These patients have normal or increased levels of insulin but this is associated with relative ineffectiveness of insulin at the cellular level. Type 2 patients may, nevertheless, receive insulin therapy and, indeed, up to 25% of patients do so simply to control their blood glucose. They do not need insulin for survival; however, in certain stressful reactions, such as infection and coronary thrombosis, patients with type 2 diabetes patients may also require insulin therapy.

## Secondary diabetes

Secondary diabetes occurs when there is direct damage, removal or impairment of action of the mass of beta cells. This type of diabetes is uncommon but causes of a beta-cell deficit include:

- genetic defects in beta-cell function, genetic defects in insulin action
- pancreatic destruction – carcinoma of the pancreas, pancreatitis, cystic fibrosis, haemochromatosis, pancreatectomy
- antagonism to the action of insulin – Cushing's disease, acromegaly, phaeochromocytoma
- drug- or chemical-induced – such as in the treatment of acquired immunodeficiency syndrome (AIDS) or after organ transplantation, thiazide diuretics, steroid therapy.

Gestational diabetes is impaired glucose tolerance that occurs in pregnancy.

## Diagnosis

Diabetes is diagnosed on finding a random blood glucose level of more than 11.1 mmol/l and symptoms of hyperglycaemia. The standard oral glucose tolerance test is rarely required to establish the diagnosis, although the accepted values of capillary blood glucose of a 75 g glucose load to diagnose diabetes is ≥7.0 mmol/l fasting and ≥11.1 mmol/l at 2 hours.

## Clinical features

The classic symptoms are thirst, polyuria and weight loss, combined with pruritus vulvae or balanitis. The intensity of symptoms varies greatly; they tend to be more severe or more acute in type 1 than type 2 diabetes. The lack of insulin leads initially to hyperglycaemia, and when the glucose concentration in the blood reaches a level of 10 mmol/l the glucose exceeds the tubular reabsorptive capacity and glycosuria results.

In states of severe insulin deficiency, glucose has to be obtained by metabolising amino acids from the breakdown of proteins in a process called gluconeogenesis. Increased breakdown of fat also occurs with the formation of ketone bodies, including acetone, which leads to severe metabolic acidosis, so-called ketoacidotic coma.

The duration of symptoms in type 1 diabetes is usually a few weeks. This can lead to wasting and physical weakness and eventually to vomiting and dehydration. Insulin is needed urgently and, if not given, ketoacidosis will develop, presenting as drowsiness, dehydration and overbreathing (together with acetone in the breath). These are the clinical features of ketoacidosis, which requires urgent admission to hospital and insulin therapy. Occasionally, patients with type 1 diabetes may have a late onset and a slow but persistent progression of the disease.

The presentation of type 2 diabetes is generally less acute. Patients sometimes complain of only one of the classic symptoms. Symptoms develop over variable periods, frequently over several weeks or months. An increasing number of patients are found to have diabetes at routine screening examinations of either urine or blood. Some older patients with type 2 diabetes present for the first time because of diabetic complications. Foot sepsis or ulceration presenting as an emergency almost always indicates a diagnosis of diabetes.

## Treatment

### Treatment of type 1 diabetes mellitus

Type 1 diabetes results from the complete absence of insulin, and this can be treated effectively by the replacement of that insulin. Human insulin, commonly prepared by genetic manipulation of yeast, is now widely used. There are also insulin analogues that contain a slightly different structure to that of human insulin.

Types of insulin can be divided into very rapid-acting analogues, fast-acting, intermediate-acting and long-acting human insulin and extended long-acting analogues. Pre-mixed insulins containing a fixed ratio of rapid- or fast-acting insulin to intermediate-acting insulin are also available. Many insulins are now available in cartridges to fit the several available pen injection devices. To achieve glycaemic targets people with type 1 diabetes need multiple daily injections (3 or 4 per day) or to have a continuous subcutaneous insulin infusion (CSII) via an insulin pump; the latter should be considered as part of an intensive diabetes management programme.

Regular amounts of carbohydrate at fixed times are important in insulin treatment to reduce the swings of blood glucose and, in particular, to avoid hypoglycaemia. Thus, the importance of snacks mid-morning, mid-afternoon and before bedtime should be emphasised. During infection or illness the blood glucose tends to increase. Insulin needs to be increased at these times, particularly when patients stop eating or are vomiting, because hepatic production of glucose in itself often leads to significant hyperglycaemia.

Stress-related 'resistance' to insulin and the consequent increase in the hepatic release of glucose explains why the insulin requirements in the sick patient will be the same or even greater than normal, even if the patient is not eating. An adequate fluid and calorie intake with appropriate insulin must be maintained, all monitored by regular blood glucose measurements.

## Treatment of type 2 diabetes mellitus

Diet is the cornerstone of treatment, and elimination of simple rapidly absorbed sugars is the minimum necessary requirement. Furthermore, for overweight patients, energy supply must be restricted in order to reduce to ideal weight; 50% of the calorie intake should be from carbohydrates and not more than 35% from fats.

Treatment of type 2 diabetes consists of lowering the insulin requirements, together with the use of agents such as sulfonylureas that can increase beta-cell production of insulin, biguanides to modify glucose output, and acarbose to reduce the rates of glucose absorption. Recently introduced are the thioglitazones, pioglitazone and rosiglitazone, which can improve sensitivity to insulin, and in particular increase peripheral glucose utilisation. These drugs should not be used in patients with heart failure, as there is an increased risk of fracture in females. New therapies for type 2 diabetes have recently become available that are based on incretins, which are intestinal hormones that increase insulin from the pancreas and inhibit glucagon release. They are released after the contact of food with the gut. The main incretin of therapeutic use is glucagon-like peptide-1 (GLP-1), which improves beta-cell responsiveness to glucose, inhibits gastric emptying and has a central nervous system effect, resulting in reduced food intake. Endogenous incretin peptides are short-lived due to their degradation by the enzyme dipeptidyl-peptidase-IV (DPP-IV). The recruitment of the incretin–DPP-IV pathways into diabetes management has led to the development of GLP-1 analogues that are resistant to the actions of DPP-IV and DPP-IV inhibitors, which protect the natural incretin hormones from deactivation. Exenatide (Byetta) is the first GLP-1 analogue available in the UK, and it is licensed for use in addition to oral antihyperglycaemic agents. Sitagliptin and vildaglipti are oral DPP-IV inhibitors that can be used to treat type 2 diabetes, either as monotherapy or added to other therapies such as sulfonylurea, metformin or glitazones (DeFronzo et al 2005).

When drug and dietary therapy fails, insulin must be prescribed.

## Hypoglycaemia

In the diabetic patient, a fall in glucose to symptomatic levels represents a temporary mismatch of insulin level to intestinal glucose uptake – a meal may have been missed or delayed, a dose of insulin mismeasured, or unusual exertion undertaken. Symptoms vary from patient to patient, but remain fairly consistent within the individual.

Patients may experience symptoms of hypoglycaemia when the blood glucose is <3 mmol/l, although some who have lost their warning symptoms may pass below this threshold. Others who have suffered previously poor control may be aware of hypoglycaemia at slightly higher levels. With increasing age and duration of diabetes, especially in those who keep their diabetes tightly controlled, there is an increasing tendency towards loss or warning hypoglycaemia.

Symptoms fall into two groups: sympathetic symptoms from activation of the sympathetic nervous system in response to hypoglycaemia; and neuroglycopaenic symptoms, which result from a reduction of glucose supply to the brain.

Early warning sympathetic symptoms are shaking, trembling, sweating and pins and needles in the tongue and lips.

Mild neuroglycopaenic symptoms are double vision, difficulty in concentrating and slurring of speech. Moderate symptoms are confusion, change in behaviour and truculence, and late symptoms are epileptic fits, especially in children, hemiplegia in the elderly and unconsciousness.

Treatment can be as simple as persuading the diabetic patient to take sugar in some form. If the patient is conscious then oral glucose as a drink, tablet or gel can be used. The following items contain 10 g of carbohydrate: Lucozade 60 ml, Ribena 15 ml, Coke (not diet) 80 ml. To prevent relapse of hypoglycaemia, this should be followed by more slowly absorbed carbohydrate such as biscuits or sandwiches. The unconscious patient should be placed in the recovery position with the airway maintained and should be treated with intravenous glucose, usually 20–50 ml of 50% glucose. If the response is not immediate a further dose should be given after 5 minutes, followed by an infusion of 10% glucose.

If intravenous access cannot be obtained, intramuscular glucagon (1 mg) can be given. When oral hypoglycaemics are the cause of hypoglycaemia, the patient should be admitted to hospital, as these agents can continue to cause hypoglycaemia for up to 48 hours.

## Complications and control of diabetes

Diabetic patients may develop a variety of complications, which include microvascular disease (retinopathy and nephropathy), nervous system abnormalities and macrovascular disease (coronary, peripheral vascular and cerebral vascular disease). It is now known that sustained optimal diabetic control in young insulin-dependent diabetic patients delays the onset and retards the progress of diabetic complications.

Retinopathy, nephropathy and neuropathy are reduced by 35–70%, as demonstrated in the Diabetic Control and Complications Trial (DCCT) (Diabetic Control and Complications Trial Research Group 1993) in the USA, which compared the effects of tight control with conventional control in 1441 patients. However, hypoglycaemia was three times more common in the tight-control group compared with conventional treatments. In type 2 diabetes, the UK Prospective Diabetes Study (UKPD) demonstrated significant reductions in microvascular and neuropathic complications with intensive therapy. (UK Prospective Diabetes Study (UKPDS) Group 1998).

With regard to macrovascular disease there is no definite evidence that controlling diabetes can alter the course of the disease. In the DCCT there was a trend toward a lower risk of cardiovascular disease events with intensive control (risk reduction 41%, 95% CI 10–68%) but the number of events was small. The UKPDS observed a 16% reduction in cardiovascular complications (combined fatal or non-fatal myocardial infarction and sudden death) in the intensive glycaemic control group, although this difference was not statistically significant ($p = 0.052$) and there was no suggestion of benefit on other cardiovascular disease outcomes such as stroke in type 2 diabetes.

The microvascular and neurological complications of type 1 diabetes are rarely seen before 5–7 years' disease duration, and occur most commonly after 10–20 years. However, in patients with type 2 diabetes 20% have evidence of complications at diagnosis.

## Eye disease

Diabetes is the most common cause of blindness under the age of 65 years in the UK. Ten per cent of diabetic patients who have had retinopathy for 40 years or more become blind, while many more have impaired vision. Eye complications include:

- cataracts, which occur earlier and with increased frequency, probably related to repeated osmotic damage of the lens. Cataracts have an increased prevalence in adult diabetics with a three- to four-fold increased risk in the age range 50–64 years, with excess risk decreasing in later years.
- there are transient refractive changes, with blurring of vision, which occur when blood glucose levels are altered rapidly.
- retinopathy is a consequence of the microvascular damage, which is partly ischaemic. This can be divided into background and proliferative retinopathy.

## Background retinopathy

There is increased capillary permeability. Dilatation of retinal veins is the earliest recognisable sign. First, microaneurysms appear; these look like red dots and then develop over the retina and may involve the macula. Haemorrhages, which are large and more irregular in shape than microaneurysms, then occur. Large haemorrhages may extend into the vitreous humour. Hard exudates are yellow-white discrete particles of lipid that can occur in rings around leaking capillaries. They can cause blindness when they develop on the macula and are more common in type 2 diabetes.

## Proliferative retinopathy

Proliferative retinopathy reflects capillary non-perfusion. There is new vessel formation, often near the disc, with venous irregularity, cluster haemorrhages and cotton-wool spots. Haemorrhages into the vitreous cause sudden blindness, and are followed by fibrosis, leading to retinal detachment. New vessels are treated with laser photocoagulation.

## Kidney disease

Diabetic nephropathy is now the leading cause of end-stage renal failure. While type 1 diabetes is responsible for the majority of cases in those under 50 years of age, there are now more patients with type 2 diabetes in end-stage renal failure, especially in the non-white populations. The development of proteinuria, which is indicative of nephropathy, is a serious prognostic factor, anticipating not only a decline in renal function but also an increase in cardiovascular disease.

The clinical hallmark of diabetic nephropathy is persistent proteinuria, which is defined as a 24-hour urinary excretion of ≥500 mg of protein on at least three occasions over at least 6 months. An earlier stage, microalbuminuria or incipient nephropathy, is associated with lower levels of albumin excretion. Eighty per cent of these patients progress to overt proteinuria. Regular measurement of blood pressure in these patients is crucial, and effectively tracks progression of renal damage. Renal support treatment is now well established for diabetic patients, comprising dialysis – usually chronic ambulatory peritoneal dialysis (CAPD) and haemodialysis and renal transplantation.

## Neuropathy

Peripheral nerves are prone to several different types of damage in diabetes and there are thus highly distinctive syndromes. These include:

- the common symmetrical sensory neuropathy associated with autonomic neuropathy, which progresses slowly

---

> **Box 9.1 Classification of diabetic neuropathies**
>
> **Progressive**
> Symmetrical sensory polyneuropathy and autonomic neuropathy
>
> **Reversible**
> Acute painful neuropathies, radiculopathies and mononeuropathies (including proximal motor neuropathy/femoral neuropathy and diabetic amyotrophy)
>
> **Pressure palsies**
> Carpal tunnel syndrome
> Ulnar nerve depression
> Foot drop

- acutely painful neuropathies and mononeuropathies, which have a relatively acute presentation and normally recover
- pressure palsies (especially carpal tunnel syndrome, ulnar nerve compression and lateral popliteal nerve palsy).

A classification of diabetic neuropathies is summarised in Box 9.1.

## Symmetrical sensory and autonomic neuropathy

This is a very common condition affecting 11–50% of diabetic patients, depending on the criteria used or the population selected. Neuropathy is always diffuse and symmetrical (stocking distribution), probably starting with involvement of the smallest fibres (pain, temperature, autonomic) and sometimes, but not always, progressing to involve all types of nerve fibre.

Small, non-medullated nerve fibres are the first to be affected and this gives rise to some of the characteristic features of diabetic neuropathy. This small-fibre degeneration leads to loss of pain- and temperature-sensing modalities, with associated autonomic features, and in these early stages other sensory modalities can remain intact, notably light touch sensation. Early neuropathy is frequently not detected in the clinic because temperature and pain sensation are difficult to assess. Sympathetic failure causes loss of sweating and denervation of peripheral vessels, leading to vascular rigidity and calcification, with a very high peripheral blood flow, chiefly from opening of arteriovenous anastomoses. These blood flow changes can occur quite early in the course of diabetes but need sophisticated techniques for their detection.

Small-fibre neuropathies sometimes progress as a selective entity in some patients, leading to symptomatic autonomic neuropathy (causing diarrhoea, gastroparesis, orthostatic hypotension, impotence, neurogenic bladder, gustatory sweating and other problems), often associated with Charcot joints (Winkler et al 2000). These patients sometimes develop iritis as well, and there is some evidence that immune mechanisms may be involved. On the other hand, in some patients neuropathy progresses to involve all types of nerve fibre, and in the worst cases the feet and lower legs become anaesthetic. Major motor involvement is surprisingly uncommon, even in the severest cases.

The evolution of sensory and autonomic diabetic neuropathy is extremely slow and very variable, occurring over many years, with the increasing age of the patient and duration of diabetes. It never remits. Study is further complicated by the differential rate of progression of the different types of fibre, and there are only a few observations over periods of 5–10 years.

## Neuropathies that recover, mononeuropathies, radiculopathies and acute painful neuropathies

Painful neuropathies in diabetes have highly characteristic features, which include constant 'burning', paraesthesia and shooting pains, together with exquisite contact discomfort caused by clothes and bedclothes. The pains are continuous day and night and cause severe insomnia. They are accompanied by profound weight loss. They occur either in a symmetrical sensory stocking distribution affecting both feet, or they may be confined to a single or adjacent group of nerve roots affecting the feet and/or legs, or to one or both thighs, often but not always accompanied by wasting and sometimes debilitating weakness, causing falls. The latter syndrome is known as proximal motor neuropathy or diabetic amyotrophy and is due to either radiculopathy or femoral neuropathy. All these conditions normally recover in 6–18 months.

Neurological examination of the feet in cases of symmetrical painful neuropathy can be confusing, because abnormalities range from severe sensory neuropathy with major deficits in all modalities (the 'painless painful foot') to an almost complete lack of neurological abnormalities. This makes assessment and diagnosis of this condition very complex.

## Pressure palsies

Median nerve compression in the carpal tunnel syndrome (usually bilateral) may occur in up to 10% of patients. Diagnosis may be difficult in diabetic patients with severe polyneuropathy involving the hands. Electromyographic studies are necessary to measure conduction in the median nerves. Treatment is by surgical decompression. Ulnar nerve compression is less frequent, but again should be investigated by means of conduction studies. Patients should be advised not to lean on their elbows.

## Symptomatic autonomic neuropathy

Autonomic function declines with age in the same way that peripheral nerve conduction progressively slows through life. Deterioration of neurological function is accelerated in diabetes, although this decline is not uniform. In some patients it is scarcely different from normal, while in others it is accelerated to the point of severe symptomatic autonomic neuropathy, which is associated with an increased mortality. Symptomatic autonomic neuropathy is surprisingly uncommon compared to the extremely common finding of abnormal autonomic function tests, which can be demonstrated in any diabetic population (Edmonds 2004).

### Symptoms

Numerous symptoms can be ascribed to diabetic autonomic neuropathy. Dysfunction may be present in the cardiovascular system, causing postural hypotension, and in the gastrointestinal system, causing severe uncontrollable diarrhoea. In the genitourinary system, difficulty with micturition and impotence are important symptoms. A classic symptom of autonomic neuropathy is gustatory sweating (i.e. sweating in the upper third of the body provoked by eating cheese or spicy food).

The presence of autonomic neuropathy may be confirmed by abnormalities in standard autonomic function tests.

### Diagnosis

Loss of heart-rate variability during deep breathing is the most reliable and simplest test of autonomic neuropathy. It is best assessed using a cardiotachograph during deep respirations (6 breaths/min), taking average readings over six breaths; it can be performed using an ordinary electrocardiograph during a single deep breath (5 seconds in, 5 seconds out). The heart-rate difference (maximum rate during inspiration minus minimum rate during expiration) in those aged under 55 years is always >10. The increase in heart rate on standing up should be >12 at 15 seconds and there should normally be an overshoot as well. The Valsalva manoeuvre can be included in the tests; a mercury sphygmomanometer is used, the patient blowing hard through the empty barrel of a 20-ml syringe to maintain the mercury column at 40 mm for 10 seconds. Maximum heart rate during blowing, followed by minimum heart rate after cessation are recorded. There should be a bradycardia after cessation of blowing. The ratio of maximum to minimum heart rate is normally >1.21 and is clearly abnormal when <1.10.

## Vascular disease

Major arterial disease that affects the coronary circulation and cerebral arteries and causes peripheral vascular disease of the feet and legs may represent the most serious of the problems. The prevalence is higher in a diabetic than in a non-diabetic population but it is much greater in those patients who develop proteinuria from diabetic nephropathy. Three-quarters of diabetic patients diagnosed over 60 years of age die from cardiovascular disease, chiefly from myocardial infarction. The proportion is even higher among those with nephropathy. Other risk factors are well known, namely smoking, hypertension, hyperlipidaemia and obesity.

The clinical features of major arterial disease are very similar to those in non-diabetic patients but the following differences should be noted:

- atheromatous arterial disease has a tendency to a more peripheral distribution in diabetes, especially in the legs but probably in the coronary vessels as well. Distal lesions are not always amenable to manipulation by angioplasty or arterial surgery but, nonetheless, proximal lesions are still common and often treatable. Diabetic patients should be offered these treatments using exactly the same criteria as those used for non-diabetic patients.
- medial arterial calcification (Monckeberg's sclerosis) of distal arteries is a feature of diabetes and becomes much commoner in those with severe neuropathy. This may result from a medial degeneration in sympathetically denervated vessels. Calcification is further increased and more distal in its distribution in patients with nephropathy. Calcified vessels become more rigid than normal, although the effects on blood flow are uncertain.
- symptomless myocardial infarction is more common in a diabetic population. The presence of autonomic neuropathy is thought to be responsible for the absence of chest pain but the evidence is conflicting. Mortality in acute myocardial infarction is doubled in diabetic patients.

## The diabetic foot

The foot in diabetes can be affected by neuropathies and circulatory changes with or without additional problems from trauma and infection, causing potentially serious foot problems (Edmonds & Foster 2005). The clinical abnormalities affecting the lower limb are thus diverse, ranging from permanent abnormalities and symptoms in the feet to the crippling but reversible disorders due to mononeuropathy (proximal motor neuropathy), causing a painful wasting disease of the thigh. A summary of potential disorders affecting the leg is shown in Table 9.1.

The feet are the target of peripheral neuropathy, leading chiefly to sensory deficit and autonomic dysfunction. Ischaemia results from

**Table 9.1** Leg abnormalities in diabetes

|  | Neuropathy | Ischaemia |
|---|---|---|
| Symptoms | None | None |
|  | Paraesthesiae | Claudication |
|  | Pain | Rest pain |
|  | Oedema |  |
|  | Painful wasted thigh |  |
|  | Foot drop |  |
| Structural damage | Ulcer | Ulcer |
|  | Sepsis | Sepsis |
|  | Abscess | Gangrene |
|  | Osteomyelitis |  |
|  | Digital gangrene |  |
|  | Charcot joints |  |

atherosclerosis of the leg vessels which, in the diabetic, is often bilateral, multisegmental and distal, involving arteries below the knee. Infection is rarely a sole factor but often complicates neuropathy and ischaemia. Nevertheless, it is responsible for considerable tissue necrosis in the diabetic foot.

For practical purposes the diabetic foot can be divided into two entities: the neuropathic foot, in which neuropathy predominates and there is a good circulation, and the neuroischaemic foot, where there is both neuropathy and the absence of foot pulses. The purely ischaemic foot, with no concomitant neuropathy, is rarely seen in diabetic patients, and its management is the same as for the neuroischaemic foot.

The neuropathic foot results in a warm, numb, dry and usually painless foot in which the pulses are palpable. It leads to three complications: the neuropathic ulcer, which is found mainly on the sole of the foot; the neuropathic (Charcot) foot; and, rarely, neuropathic oedema. In contrast, the neuroischaemic foot is cool and the pulses are absent. It is complicated by rest pain, ulceration on the margins of the foot from localised pressure necrosis and gangrene.

## The neuropathic foot

### Neuropathic ulcer

Neuropathic ulcers result from noxious stimuli, unperceived by the patient because of loss of pain sensation, causing mechanical, thermal and chemical injuries. This characteristically occurs at sites of high mechanical pressure on the plantar surface of the foot. The presence of neuropathy (even in its earliest stage, with relatively mild sensory defects) may itself disturb the posture of the foot and so predispose to local increases in pressure, which are also commonly caused by deformities such as claw or hammer toes, pes cavus, Charcot joints and previous ray amputations. The high vertical and shear forces under the plantar surface of the metatarsal heads and toes lead to the formation of callosities of which the patient is often unaware. Repetitive mechanical forces lead to inflammatory autolysis and subkeratotic haematomas, which eventually break through to the skin surface, forming an ulcer. Direct mechanical injuries to the plantar surface result from treading on nails and other sharp objects. However,

the most frequent cause of ulceration brought about by mechanical factors is the neglected callosity.

### Complications of ulceration

Ulcers can become infected by staphylococci, streptococci, coliforms and anaerobic bacteria. If untreated, cellulitis can develop, with tracking of infection to involve underlying tendons, bones and joints. Staphylococci and streptococci act synergistically when they are present together: streptococci produce hyaluronidase, which facilitates spread of necrotising toxins from the staphylococci.

In the deep tissues of the foot, aerobic organisms act synergistically with microaerophilic or anaerobic organisms, leading to necrotising infection, the production of subcutaneous gas and, finally, gangrene.

### Management of ulceration

Excess callous tissue should be reduced with a scalpel by the podiatrist to expose the floor of the ulcer and allow efficient drainage of the lesion. The broken skin increases the great risk of infection to the patient because there is a clear portal of entry for invading bacteria to enter the foot. In addition, in the presence of neuropathy and ischaemia, the inflammatory response is impaired. The patient lacks protective pain sensation, which would otherwise automatically force him or her to detect the problem and rest the foot.

Bacterial growth in ulcers impedes the wound-healing rate. Quantitative microbiology has shown that wound healing slows with increased bacterial load. There is a complex host–bacteria relationship. Many wounds are colonised with a stable bacterial population. If the bacterial burden increases there will be bacterial imbalance, which may show itself as increased exudate before frank infection develops. The crucial problem is when to intervene with antibiotics.

It is important to look for early signs of infection, and the next step is to take a bacteriological swab from the floor of the ulcer and, according to the organisms isolated, prescribe the appropriate oral antibiotics until the ulcer has healed (e.g. amoxicillin 500 mg t.d.s. for streptococcal infections; flucloxacillin 500 mg q.d.s. for staphylococcal sepsis; metronidazole 400 mg t.d.s. for anaerobic infections; and ciprofloxacin 500 mg b.d. for Gram-negative infections). If the ulcer is superficial and there is no cellulitis, treatment can take place on an outpatient basis.

Redistribution of weight-bearing forces on vulnerable parts of the foot should be attempted using special footwear, such as moulded insoles with energy-absorbing properties (e.g. plastozote and microcellular rubber). Special shoes may be needed to accommodate the shape of the foot. In cases of severe deformity it is necessary to construct shoes individually for the patient. However, in most patients, extra-depth 'stock' shoes will usually suffice (Chantelau & Leisch 1994).

In the case of large indolent ulcers, total contact plaster casts may be used that conform to all the contours of the foot, thereby reducing shear forces on the plantar surface (Mueller et al 1989). Various casts are available and their use is governed by local experience and expertise. Techniques include:

- total-contact cast
- Scotchcast boot
- Aircast (walking brace).

Great care must be taken, especially with the fitting of plasters, to prevent chafing and subsequent ulcer formation elsewhere on the foot or ankle. Alternatively, a removable cast walker may be used.

If cellulitis or skin discoloration is present, the limb is threatened and urgent hospital admission should be arranged. After samples for blood cultures have been taken, intravenous antibiotics are administered to treat possible infection with staphylococci, streptococci, Gram-negative bacteria and anaerobes (flucloxacillin 500 mg i.v. 6-hourly; amoxicillin 500 mg i.v. 8-hourly; ceftazidine 1 g i.v. 8-hourly; and metronidazole 500 m.g. i.v. 8-hourly). This antibiotic regimen may need revision after the results of bacterial cultures are available. If the toe complicated by ulceration becomes necrotic, then the patient should undergo digital or ray amputation (which includes the metatarsal head). Such wounds usually heal extremely well in the neuropathic foot (see Ch. 10).

## Neuropathic (Charcot) joint

The precipitating event for a neuropathic joint is usually a minor traumatic episode, such as tripping, which results in a swollen, erythematous, hot and sometimes painful foot. Initially, radiographs are likely to be normal, but subsequently serial radiographs show evidence of bony fracture, osteolysis, fragmentation, new bone formation, subluxation and joint disorganisation.

This destructive process often takes place over only a few months and can lead to considerable deformity of the foot. The metatarsal–tarsal joints are most commonly involved (Sanders & Frykberg 2008).

Early diagnosis is essential. The initial presentation of unilateral warmth and swelling in a neuropathic foot is extremely suggestive of a developing Charcot joint. Bone scans are more sensitive indicators of new bone formation than is radiography and should be used to confirm the diagnosis.

### Management

This comprises immobilisation of the injured part, which can be achieved by non-weight bearing, using crutches or a total contact plaster cast. The immobilisation is continued until the oedema and local warmth have resolved. The foot should then be gradually mobilised using a moulded insole in a special shoe. Recently, bisphosphonates have been used to inhibit osteoclastic activity, leading to a reduction in foot temperature and resolution of symptoms.

## Neuropathic oedema

Neuropathic oedema consists of swelling of the feet and lower legs associated with severe peripheral neuropathy; it is extremely uncommon. Ephedrine (30 mg t.d.s.) has been shown to be useful in reducing the peripheral blood flow and increasing the renal excretion of sodium.

## The neuroischaemic foot

### Pathogenesis

The neuroischaemic foot results from atherosclerosis of the vessels of the leg with neuropathy predisposing it to minor trauma. In diabetic patients atherosclerosis is multisegmental, bilateral and distal, often involving the popliteal, the tibial and the peroneal arteries.

### Presentation

The clinical features of ischaemia are intermittent claudication, rest pain, ulceration and gangrene. However, the most frequent symptom is ulceration. The ulcers present as areas of necrosis often surrounded by a rim of erythema. In contrast to ulceration in the neuropathic foot, callous tissue is usually absent. Furthermore, ulceration in the ischaemic foot is often painful, although this varies from patient to patient according to the coexistence of a peripheral neuropathy. In the ischaemic foot the most frequent sites of ulceration are the tips of the toes, the medial surface of the head of the first metatarsal, the lateral surface of the fifth metatarsal head and the heel.

### Management

Medical management is indicated if the ulcer is small and shallow and is of recent onset (i.e. within the previous month). Ischaemic ulcers may be painful and it may be necessary to prescribe opiates. It is the role of the podiatrist to remove necrotic tissue from the ulcers and, in the case of subungual ulcers, to cut back the nail to allow drainage of the ulcer. Ulcer swabs are taken as with the neuropathic foot, and the ulcers are cleaned with normal saline and dressed with a sterile non-adherent dressing. It is important to eradicate infection with prompt and specific antibiotic therapy after consultation with a microbiologist. However, severe sepsis in the ischaemic foot is an indication for emergency admission: first, to control sepsis by intravenous antibiotics and surgical debridement; and, secondly, to assess the possibility of revascularisation by either angioplasty or reconstruction. Footwear should be supplied to accommodate the foot, and in most cases an extra-depth ready-made shoe to protect the borders of the foot is adequate, unless there is severe deformity, when bespoke shoes will be needed. If any lesion, however small and trivial, in the pulseless foot has not responded to conservative treatment within 4 weeks, the patient should be considered for arteriography and revascularisations.

One of the most important advances in the last 20 years has been the development of new techniques of revascularisation of the diabetic foot. Patients with relatively localised disease (e.g. stenosis or short (<10 cm) occlusions) often do well with angioplasty, particularly in the iliac, superficial femoral and popliteal arteries. However, diabetic patients often have lesions in the calf arteries, but recent advances in catheter techniques and imaging have made it possible to perform angioplasty. Such endovascular procedures have been shown to be feasible and successful in the tibial and peroneal arteries of the diabetic patient (Faglia et al 2005). More recently, subintimal angioplasty has been used to recanalise long arterial occlusions in the tibial arteries (Lazaris et al 2004). Given the same lesion, a diabetic patient will do as well as a non-diabetic patient following femoral popliteal angioplasty, assuming equality of other factors such as inflow and outflow.

Angioplasty must be applied when tissue loss is not extensive and when arterial stenoses and occlusions are still suitable for this procedure. Angioplasty has become an important part of the management of the ischaemic foot that has become infected. Diabetes is not a contraindication to arterial bypass in the leg, and distal bypass to either the tibial or peroneal vessels is often necessary to restore pulsatile blood flow to the diabetic foot, which is vital in cases of severe sepsis and necrosis.

There is a different approach to dry digital necrosis or gangrene in the ischaemic foot compared with the neuropathic foot. If it is possible to improve the circulation by arterial reconstruction then digital amputation can be performed in the ischaemic foot. However, if it is not feasible to improve the circulation, amputation of a necrotic toe should not be performed as the stump is unlikely to heal. Recently, the use of a vacuum assisted closure (VAC) pump has improved healing in postoperative wounds in the ischaemic foot, allowing digital amputation in the ischaemic foot even though it may not have been revascularised. Successful autoamputation, in which the necrotic digit drops off to reveal a healed stump, can occur as long as infection is controlled and there is regular debridement by the podiatrist along the demarcation line.

# OBESITY

Excess of body fat can be measured only indirectly, and the commonest assessment is weight in relation to height and age. The body mass index (BMI) is commonly used and equals weight (in kg) over height (in metres); the normal range is up to 25. Genetic, environmental and socio-economic factors are important in the aetiology of obesity. Rarely, endocrine diseases such as hypothyroidism and Cushing's syndrome may be a direct cause of obesity.

Obesity in the human species is a disorder of intake. Excess energy intake or decreased energy expenditure are the major determinants of obesity in genetically susceptible individuals. In animal studies, a defect in thermogenesis has been identified in brown fat cells which limits the ability of these animals to burn off calories, although these findings have not been confirmed in humans. Obese subjects have disturbed regulation of appetite and energy expenditure. They often have a reduced perception of their calorie intake.

Major long-term health hazards of obesity are type 2 diabetes and the effects on the cardiovascular system, including hypertension and coronary artery disease. Osteoarthritis is a very common condition in obese individuals. Excess weight imposes a severe burden on individuals with respiratory disease, and in simple obesity one of the most frequent complaints is breathlessness on mild exertion. Back ache is also common and is induced by ligamentous strain. Obesity protects against osteoporosis.

An increase in body fat is associated with an increased morbidity and mortality, and associated risk factors such as hyperlipidaemia, hyperglycaemia, hypertension, hyperuricaemia and lack of exercise play a major role.

Specific disorders associated with obesity, such as myxoedema and Cushing's syndrome, should be searched for and treated. The cornerstone of treatment is to reduce the calorie intake to below energy expenditure, with a supervised diet and exercise and behaviour modification.

Crash diets may induce severe metabolic disturbances and even cardiac arrest, but their effects are not permanent. The aim of treatment is to achieve a healthy and enjoyable pattern of eating with the patient in control of his or her weight reduction. Rapport also is important to improve compliance, and initially weight-reduction targets should be modest.

Medical treatments to decrease appetite have a limited role. Currently available are sibutramine, a serotonin and non-adrenergic reuptake inhibitor and appetite suppressant, and orlistat, an intestinal lipase inhibitor.

There are more radical approaches, such as bariatric surgery, which can be divided into malabsorptive surgery to shorten the length of the gut by gastric bypass, and restrictive surgery to induce early satiety (e.g. gastric stapling, gastric balloon). Wiring of the jaws, prolonged behavioural courses and surgical removal of excess adipose tissue have also been used. However, these approaches are not without dangers.

## METABOLIC BONE DISEASE

A brief account of bone metabolism is given here, and the clinical features of hyper- and hypocalcaemia are described, followed by short accounts of osteomalacia and rickets, hyperparathyroidism, renal osteodystrophy and Paget's disease.

### Bone and calcium metabolism

The connective tissue matrix of bone, the osteoid, consists of collagen fibres in a polysaccharide ground substance. The osteoid is made rigid by the deposition of mineral, mainly of crystalline bone salts of calcium phosphate and carbonate. The mineralisation of osteoid is dependent partly on the chemical concentration at the tissue surface of calcium, phosphate and hydrogen ions, and of the enzyme alkaline phosphatase, and partly on the activity of osteoclasts and osteoblasts. Parathormone (PTH) and calcitonin strongly affect the osteoclasts and osteoblasts, and vitamin D acts especially on the chemical environment.

### Hormonal physiology

PTH is synthesised in the parathyroid glands and is the main factor in calcium homeostasis. Its secretion increases when calcium levels fall, stimulating calcium release from bone and calcium reabsorption by the kidney. Calcitonin is secreted by parafollicular cells (C-cells) of the thyroid gland. When infused at high levels, it diminishes plasma calcium by reducing the rate of osteoclastic resorption of bone and increasing urinary excretion. Vitamin D, in its active form, influences calcium and phosphate flux in bone, kidney and intestine. Over 90% of the parent hormone is synthesised in the skin, and the level of the critical highly active form $1,25(OH)_2D_3$ is directly influenced by the concentration of calcium ion and PTH.

### Hypercalcaemia

The commonest causes of hypercalcaemia are malignancy and hyperparathyroidism. Any tendency to hypercalcaemia can be aggravated by dehydration, impaired renal function, or circumstances stimulating bone demineralisation, such as immobilisation or fracture.

Hypercalcaemia interferes with reabsorption of water by the renal tubules, producing polyuria and causing thirst, eventually producing renal stones. There is decreased neuromuscular excitability, which may lead to general muscle weakness. Decreased excitability also affects smooth muscle, causing constipation. Anorexia and vomiting are also common. Patients with hypercalcaemia may feel generally ill and depressed, and may be diagnosed as having some psychological disorder. Calcium deposits may occur at the junction of the cornea and sclera. The deposits have a granular gritty appearance and are associated with increased vascularity. If bone is affected by the primary disease there may be pain and weakness, perhaps with fractures. Severe hypercalcaemia produces confusion, coma, anuria and death, sometimes through cardiac arrest.

If possible, a specific diagnosis of the cause of hypercalcaemia should be made, but other general measures are useful as temporary expedients or to achieve symptomatic relief. Rehydration is essential and diuresis may be further encouraged by the combination of generous intravenous fluid infusion with normal saline and loop diuretics such as furosemide. Steroids (hydrocortisone 400 mg/day i.v. intravenously infusion or prednisolone 40–60 mg/day orally) can be effective, especially in malignancy.

### Hypocalcaemia

Calcium is an ion of considerable importance in numerous cell systems, but the acute clinical effects of hypocalcaemia are mainly those of increased neuromuscular excitability, while the long-term effects are mainly ectodermal.

In hypocalcaemia and tetany, there may be peripheral paraesthesia, muscle cramps, epileptic fits, laryngeal spasm in children, occasionally acute hypertension, or psychosis, and the important physical signs, Chvostek's and Trousseau's.

Chvostek's sign is elicited by tapping over the facial nerve as it emerges from the parotid gland beneath the zygoma. A hemifacial twitch constitutes a positive response. Trousseau's sign is elicited by the application of a cuff to the arm and raising the pressure to above the patient's systolic blood pressure for 3 minutes, by which time the hands should have adopted the classic 'main d'accoucher' position (wrist and metacarpophalangeal joints flexed and fingers extended).

The signs of long-standing hypocalcaemia may also include: a dry, scaly skin; loss of eyelashes, thin eyebrows, patchy alopecia and scanty axillary and pubic hair; brittleness of nails; (in children) hypoplasia or aplasia of teeth; cataracts; calcification in the basal ganglia; rarely, papilloedema; susceptibility to moniliasis, probably due to immune deficiency; and cardiomegaly, with a prolonged QT interval on the electrocardiogram.

In emergencies, a slow intravenous injection of 10–20 ml of 10% calcium gluconate solution (diluted in 100–200 ml of 0.9% saline) should be instituted until symptoms are relieved or total plasma calcium reaches 1.9 mmol/l.

In the long term, dietary calcium can be supplemented and a vitamin D preparation administered carefully. To avoid overdose, levels of calcium and phosphate should be monitored frequently at first and then at intervals not exceeding 6 months, even when the situation is apparently stable. 1-$\alpha$-hydroxylated derivatives of vitamin D are preferred for their shorter half-life. Usual daily maintenance doses are 1 $\mu$g for 1-$\alpha$-(OH)D$_3$ (alfacalcidol) and 1,25(OH)$_2$D$_3$ (calcitriol).

# Osteoporosis

By definition, osteoporosis is the state of less bone being present than is normal for the patient's age and sex. It is associated with loss of structural integrity of the internal architecture of bone. Osteoporosis becomes clinically important only after fracture, but treatment of the disorder after the onset of fractures is less than satisfactory, with prevention being a more effective approach.

Although osteoporosis does occur commonly in the foot and ankle after injury, often to a severe degree, the two forms encountered most often are the senile and the related postmenopausal osteoporosis. Osteoporosis is related to an inequality between the rates of osteoblastic accretion of new bone and osteoclastic removal of old bone. Although the spine and proximal femur are the sites of the most significant fractures in osteoporosis, the foot and ankle are frequent sites for fractures in an osteoporotic patient. Toe and metatarsal fractures are very common. However, a bone with osteoporosis is not deficient in its response to fracture repair, and usually a very active osteoblastic response leads to adequate fracture callus.

A patient with osteoporosis may present for the first time with an injury to the foot without a prior diagnosis of osteoporosis having been reached. Usually, osteoporosis is a diagnosis of exclusion, and osteomalacia, renal pathology and hyperparathyroidism should be excluded by screening for serum calcium, phosphorus and alkaline phosphatase, although the last of these may be slightly increased following fracture (especially of long bones).

The aim of therapy is to reduce the rate of bone loss by adequate calcium intake, female hormone-replacement therapy (which prevents menopausal bone loss), regular physical exercise and a diet with a daily intake of 1–1.5 g/day calcium (one pint of milk contains approximately 750 mg of calcium). In severe cases, drug therapy may be used, including bisphosphonates, raloxifene and parathyroid hormone.

# Osteomalacia and rickets

Osteomalacia and rickets are conditions in which there is defective mineralisation of the matrix of bone. In rickets, the defect is present in infancy and childhood. Osteomalacia is the adult counterpart of rickets. In children, rickets is rarely seen until the patient is over 1 year old, when he or she presents with abnormal patterns of bone modelling, epiphyseal growth and dentition. Rickets is rarely seen in children today because of the addition of vitamin D to milk.

There are many causes of osteomalacia (and rickets), some of which are very rare. They may be divided into three main groups: nutritional, malabsorptive and renal. Nutritional causes follow from lack of vitamin D, either due to deficient synthesis in the skin or low dietary intake. Malabsorption of vitamin D occurs in coeliac disease, gastric surgery, bowel resection and biliary cirrhosis. With regard to the kidney, osteomalacia and rickets can follow from renal glomerular failure as well as renal tubular failure. The effects of renal glomerular failure on the skeleton are complex and are termed 'renal osteodystrophy', with excessive bone resorption, defective bone mineralisation and, in some cases, osteoporosis (see below). Many renal tubular disorders also lead to osteomalacia.

In the adult, osteomalacia may produce bone and muscle tenderness, often due to subclinical fractures. In the leg, the presenting symptom may be aching pain adjacent to an affected portion of the tibia. An increased blood flow is indicated by the increased warmth in the anterior leg. Deformity results from weight bearing and the gastrocneminus pulling forces on the tibia when the disease is in its lytic and weakened phase. Patients who have developed bowing of the femurs and tibias can then develop degenerative arthritis of both the ankle and knee joints due to the abnormal wear on the articular surfaces secondary to the bone deformity.

Rickets is not seen until after the patient is 1 year old, when swelling of the ankles and wrists may be an early physical finding. The earliest clinical symptoms are tiredness and muscular weakness. There is bone pain and pain on movement. Dentition is delayed and the teeth may be deformed and quickly become carious. Swelling and tenderness of the distal ends of the radius and ulna are common, as is the rickety rosary (costochondral swellings). Frontal and parietal bossing of the skull occurs and occipitoparietal flattening may result from the softness of the skull (craniotabes). If the child can stand or walk, bowing of the legs may result from weight bearing and kyphoscoliosis may appear. Radiographs show widening and decreased density of the line of calcification next to the metaphysis, with irregularity and concavity of the metaphysis itself. In severe cases, there may be rarefaction with deformities in the shaft of the bone.

Rickets and osteomalacia can always be cured by administering vitamin D or one of its potent derivatives – alfacalcidol or calcitriol. Patients will need a long-term maintenance dosage of one of these derivatives. Surgical correction of deformity is occasionally required.

# Hyperparathyroidism

The majority of patients are asymptomatic, but hyperparathyroidism may present as a form of osteoporosis with a fracture. Very occasionally, the giant-cell tumour seen in association with severe hyperparathyroidism may present as a mass in the tibia. The radiological abnormalities are due to bone resorption by osteoclasts and subperiosteal resorption of the cortices of phalanges in the feet, as well as the hands, is the early bony abnormality.

# Renal osteodystrophy

The skeletal disorders found in chronic renal failure are collectively called renal osteodystrophy and may occur singly or in various combinations. The condition may develop early in the course of chronic renal disease and may persist after renal transplantation. The main bone changes that occur are osteomalacia, caused by the deficiency of active metabolites of vitamin D, and secondary hypoparathyroidism, which is associated with increased retention of phosphate by the kidneys. Retention of phosphate, with resulting hypocalcaemia, stimulates the parathyroid glands to secrete parathormone, which leads to mobilisation of calcium from bone by osteoclastic resorption. Bony pathology includes hyperparathyroidism with osteitis fibrosa, osteomalacia, and decreased availability of vitamin D, calcium and phosphates, osteoporosis, ostenonecrosis, osteosclerosis and periosteal new bone formation (a radiographic finding) and extraskeletal calcification.

A further abnormality seen in the steroid-treated renal patient is a vascular necrosis of the talus, often in association with a renal transplant.

Management of renal osteodystrophy is according to the mechanisms involved in the pathogenesis of the disease. Treatment with phosphate-binding agents or a low-phosphate diet decreases phosphate retention and prevents progressive secondary hyperparathyroidism and soft-tissue calcification. Vitamin D therapy is indicated in hypoparathyroidism and in osteomalacia due to vitamin D deficiency. Parathyroidectomy is indicated in patients with severe forms of secondary hyperparathyroidism.

## Paget's disease

Paget's disease is a focal disorder of bone remodelling characterised by excessive osteoclastic resorption. Patients with Paget's disease are usually aged over 40 years but the prevalence essentially doubles with every decade over the age of 50 years.

The majority of patients are asymptomatic. In patients with symptoms the most notable feature is bone pain, which is probably a result of combined increased vascularity and new bone formation, which stretches the periosteum. Degenerative joint disease leads to distortion of the articular surface. The abnormal bone texture allows long bones to bend, and fractures commonly develop on the convex margin. Neurological symptoms may result from involvement of the spine, leading to paraplegia. Neuropathies of the cranial and peripheral nerves may occur secondary to entrapment.

The earliest radiological abnormality in a long bone is resorption of a previously normal cortex. Microscopically, osteoclasts are noted within resorption cavities and this is associated with increased osteoblastic activity with the formation of new osteotrabeculae adjacent to the site of bone resorption.

Serum alkaline phosphatase is a marker for bone formation and provides a simple method of evaluating a patient over the course of time. Indeed, the detection of Paget's disease may be due to the elevated alkaline phosphatase levels obtained during screening examinations. The urinary excretion of hydroxyproline indicates collagen breakdown, and this level is markedly raised in many patients with Paget's disease, often in association with the degree of elevation of the alkaline phosphatase activity.

The biochemical changes are similar in rickets and osteomalacia. The plasma calcium is usually a little low and occasionally considerably reduced. The plasma phosphate level is low but the alkaline phosphatase is frequently increased.

The treatment of Paget's disease is by drugs that inhibit bone resorption. This is reflected by an early fall in urinary hydroxyproline and then serum alkaline phosphatase. Bisphosphonates act directly on osteoclasts to inhibit resorption of bone. Calcitonin appears to be equally effective but must be administered by injection and is not now generally used.

## METABOLIC DISORDERS AND PODIATRIC MANAGEMENT

Metabolic disorders are complex, some producing unique challenges for the podiatrist in formulating patient management plans. Metabolic diseases, in particular those affecting bone, will provide problems for podiatric management.

Diabetes mellitus is the commonest metabolic disorder seen by podiatrists. The management of podiatric complications of diabetes is discussed in Chapter 10 and elsewhere in this chapter.

The podiatrist must be familiar with metabolic disorders for two major reasons. First, signs and symptoms presenting in the feet and lower limbs enable the practitioner to make the primary diagnosis of a metabolic disorder. The second reason is that established metabolic disease will have implications for patient risk categorisation and provision of podiatric care.

Many metabolic disorders involve bone; the podiatric implications of metabolic bone disease will be discussed. Osteoporosis may be idiopathic or secondary to other conditions such as renal disease or steroid therapy. Localised osteoporosis occurs after limb immobilisation. Podiatric complications associated with osteoporosis include fractures, including 'minimal trauma' stress fractures (march fracture). Following fractures of the femur the gait may be altered, with consequent effects on the feet.

Abnormal neurological signs and symptoms are often detected in the feet following nerve root irritation and damage associated with vertebral-body osteoporosis. In rare cases, damaged vertebrae may compress the spinal cord.

Fractures affecting the upper limb (e.g. a Colles' fracture associated with a fall onto an outstretched hand) are associated with osteoporosis. The immediate and possibly longer term restriction of mobility at the wrist will compromise a patient's ability to care for his or her feet.

It must be remembered that if osteoporosis is secondary to another disorder or pathology the underlying cause can itself have adverse effects on the feet. Abnormal mechanical forces applied to osteoporotic bone increase the likelihood of fractures. This can occur in a limb affected by poliomyelitis, when the bones may be osteoporotic from disuse but may also be subjected to abnormal stresses. Osteoporosis is a secondary complication in people receiving steroid therapy; the other iatrogenic effects from the drug can compromise tissue viability in the feet. Rheumatoid arthritis is complicated by localised osteoporosis where, again, the primary disease has profound effects on the feet and lower limb (see Ch. 8).

In the adult the podiatric effects of osteomalacia are relatively non-specific, but include bone pain and tenderness that can restrict mobility. Hypotonia of muscles and proximal muscle weakness can produce a waddling gait. Fractures and pseudofractures (Looser's zones) may be seen on radiographs. There may be signs and symptoms of hypocalcaemia, which may cause peripheral paraesthesia and even tetany.

In children the condition is known as rickets; the resultant bone softening leads to skeletal deformity. Rickets results in impaired growth at the epiphyses leading to skeletal abnormalities such as bowing of the tibia, fibula and femur, with concomitant alterations in gait. Gait can also be adversely affected because of kyphosis and lordosis of the spine, associated hypotonia of muscles, and muscle weakness may compound the problem. Pathological fractures can also occur.

The feet may be affected by Paget's disease of the bone. This localised disorder of bone remodelling leads to abnormal organisation of woven and lamellar bone. The effects of Paget's disease on the foot and lower limb include pain, particularly affecting the pelvis, lumbar spine and femur. 'Sabre tibia', describes the appearance of the tibia when it becomes bowed in the sagittal plane; this will alter biomechanical stresses within the leg and alter the direction of mechanical stress to the foot and ankle. Stress fractures can occur, particularly in weight-bearing bones such as the metatarsals and fibula. Osteoarthroses eventually occur at joints where mechanical forces have altered congruity. Neurological effects may be detected in the foot, secondary to nerve compression at a local or at spinal-cord level. Osteosarcoma, a rare complication of Paget's disease, occurs in 0.2% of patients, and often involves the pelvis or femur. The disease can alter the bone structure of the skull and cause enlargement. Auditory nerve compression may ensue and cause deafness; this will have implications for effective communication between the podiatrist and the patient. The overlying skin of affected bone often feels warm because of increased vascularity of the diseased bone. The increased vascularity can eventually cause high output cardiac failure.

Bone metabolism is complex and involves organs such as the liver and kidney. Damage to these organs (e.g. oedema and impaired tissue viability) has implications for podiatric management. Signs and symptoms of hypercalcaemia may be seen during periods of immobilisation; these include drowsiness, muscle weakness and hyporeflexia viability.

Thus an understanding of metabolic disorders is necessary for podiatrists so that they may identify the symptoms of these diseases and formulate care plans in established cases.

## REFERENCES

Chantelau E, Leisch A 1994 Footwear, uses and abuses. In: Boulton AJM, Connor H, Cavanagh PR (eds) The foot in diabetes. Wiley, Chichester, pp 99–108.

Diabetes Control and Complications Trial Research Group 1993 Effect of intensive treatment of diabetes on the development and progression of long term complications in insulin dependent diabetes mellitus. New England Journal of Medicine 329:977–986.

DeFronzo RA, Ratner RE, Han J, et al 2005 Effects of exenatide (exendin-4) on glycemic control and weight over 30 weeks in metformin-treated patients with type 2 diabetes. Diabetes Care 28(5):1092–1100.

Edmonds ME 2004 Autonomic neuropathy. In: De Fronzo RA, Ferrannini E, Keen H,

Zimmer P (eds) International textbook of diabetes, 3rd edn. Wiley, Chichester.

Edmonds ME, Foster AVM 2005 Managing the diabetic foot, 2nd edn, Blackwell Science, Oxford.

Faglia E, Dalla Paola L, Clerici G, et al 2005 Peripheral angioplasty as the first-choice revascularization procedure in diabetic patients with critical limb ischemia: prospective study of 993 consecutive patients hospitalized and followed between 1999 and 2003. European Journal of Vascular and Endovascular Surgery 29(6):620–627.

Lazaris AM, Tsiamis AC, Fishwick G, et al 2004 Clinical outcome of primary infrainguinal subintimal angioplasty in diabetic patients with critical lower limb ischemia. Journal of Endovascuar Therapeutics 11(4):447–453.

Mueller MJ, Diamond JE, Sinacore DR 1989 Total contact casting in treatment of diabetic plantar ulcers. Diabetes Care 12: 384–388.

Sanders LJ, Frykberg RG 2008 The Charcot foot: In Bowker JH, Pfeffer MA (eds) Levin & O'Neal's The diabetic foot, 7th edn. Mosby, St Louis, MI, pp 257–284.

UK Prospective Diabetes Study (UKPDS) Group 1998 Intensive blood-glucose control with sulphonylureas or insulin compared with conventional treatment and risk of complications in patients with type 2 diabetes (UKPDS 33). Lancet 352:837–853.

Winkler AS, Ejskjaer N, Edmonds M, Watkins PJ 2000 Dissociated sensory loss in diabetic autonomic neuropathy. Diabetic Medicine 17:457–462.

## FURTHER READING

Bowker JH, Pfeifer MA (eds) 2008 Levin & O'Neal's The diabetic foot, 7th edn. Mosby Year Book, St. Louis, MI.

Edmonds M, Foster AVM, Sanders L 2007 A practical manual of diabetic foot care, 2nd edn. Blackwell, Oxford.

The International Working Group on the Diabetic Foot 2007 International Consensus

on the Diabetic Foot. Available at: http://www.iwgdf.org.

Turner HE, Wass JAH 2009 Oxford handbook of endocrinology and diabetes, 2nd edn. Oxford University Press, Oxford.

Standards of medical care in diabetes. Diabetes Care 2009;32(Suppl 1):S13–S61.

Boulton AJM, Cavanagh PR, Rayman G (eds) 2006 The foot in diabetes, 4th edn. Wiley, Chichester.

Watkins PJ, Amiel SA, Howell SL, Turner E 2003 Diabetes and its management, 6th edn. Blackwell, Oxford.

# Chapter 10

# Management of high-risk patients

*Gordon Burrow*

## KEYWORDS

Alginates
Cleansing/desloughing agents
Complications
Conventional dressings
Diabetes mellitus
Foams
General management
Growth factors
High-risk patients
History taking
Hydrocolloid
Low-adherence dressings
Other approaches to management
Prevention

All patients are at varying levels of risk of acquiring complications following podiatric treatment, the potential being minimised by the podiatrist adopting stringent aseptic/antiseptic techniques before, during and after treatment. Various pathological conditions reduce an individual's healing potential or produce an increased susceptibility to infection and/or necrosis and ulceration. The patient group frequently cited as being at high risk is those with diabetes, but there are other systemic and local pathologies that place patients in the high-risk category (Box 10.1).

Diabetes mellitus affects approximately 750 000 individuals in the UK (1–2% of the population). It is estimated that 6% of people over 65 years of age suffer from diabetes. Four per cent of hospital beds are occupied by people affected by the complications of diabetes, and 20% of those will be hospitalised because of foot pathologies. Fifty per cent of lower-limb amputations are performed due to the complications of diabetes mellitus, and after 3 years only 50% of diabetics who have undergone amputation will still be alive. It is important to note that 15% of the diabetic population has a foot ulcer, and that 84% of leg amputations are preceded by an ulcer. The podiatrist is part of the multidisciplinary diabetic team caring for the patient. Diabetes is a multisystem disease, and without close liaison between all those involved in the patient's care treatment will be submaximal. The diabetic care team ideally comprises a podiatrist, diabetologist, specialist nurse, vascular and orthopaedic surgeons, radiologist, orthotist, microbiologist, general practitioner (GP) and the patient and his or her carers. 'Shared care' of diabetic patients, between the hospital and the general GP should still allow multidisciplinary cooperation between professionals. The complications associated with diabetes that can affect the feet are summarised in Box 10.2.

The Saint Vincent Declaration (1990), aimed to reduce all diabetic lower-limb amputations (resulting from gangrene) by 50% over 5 years. Since the publication of this document it has been shown that

---

**Box 10.1 High-risk categories**

1 Vascular disease:
Arterial (macrovascular and microvascular disorders), venous and lymphatic disease
2 Neurological disease:
Peripheral and central nervous system disease leading to motor, sensory and autonomic signs and symptoms
3 Diseases that compromise the immune system:
Primary: e.g. AIDS, disorders of complement cascade, neutrophils or macrophages
Secondary to drug therapy, e.g. corticosteroids or antimetabolites
4 Arthritides:
e.g. Rheumatoid arthritis, leading to deformity, and possibly reduced sensation, vasculitis and anaemia
5 Metabolic and endocrine disease:
e.g. Disorders of the thyroid or adrenal glands; diabetes mellitus
6 Oedema:
Oedema is associated with many pathologies (venous incompetence, congestive cardiac failure, renal disease). Oedema increases diffusion distance between vessels and tissues. The excess fluid compresses microvessels
7 Haematological disorders:
Anaemia (reduces oxygen carriage), leucocyte dysfunction (compromises immunity)
8 Nutritional deficits:
Either because of malabsorption or reduced intake of essential nutrients, e.g. proteins, vitamins and minerals
9 Psychosocial problems:
Depression, and other states in which the person is unable to care for themselves

---

**Box 10.2 Complications associated with diabetes mellitus that can affect the feet and lower limbs**

1 Vascular:
Accelerated formation of atherosclerosis, preferentially affecting distal arteries
Abnormal vascular endothelium and associated changes in the microvasculature
2 Altered components of blood:
Abnormal erythrocytes that become less deformable and cannot adopt normal flow characteristics in small vessels. Oxygen dissociation is less efficient
Abnormal white blood cells that are less effective in phagocytosing and destroying microorganisms
Abnormal platelet function
3 Neurological:
Abnormal conduction in peripheral nerves, affecting motor, sensory and autonomic modalities. There is resultant deformity and reduced perception of damaging stimuli. Autonomic dysfunction leads to anhidrosis and to abnormalities in blood flow
4 Increased susceptibility to infection:
As a result of ischaemia, neurological changes and abnormal white blood cells (see above)
5 Impaired vision:
Diabetic retinopathy and cataract formation will limit the patient's ability to examine their feet
6 Renal disease:
Oedema may result from renal complications. There is an increased risk of vessel calcification and digital gangrene, particularly in renal transplant patients
7 Effects of abnormal glycosylation of protein:
Collagen and keratin are rendered abnormal by inappropriate glycosylation, and thus interfere with normal wound healing and tissue viability

---

diabetic complications, in type 1 diabetics, can be reduced substantially by strict control of blood glucose concentrations (Diabetes Control and Complications Trial Research Group 1993).

In late 1998 the results from the United Kingdom Prospective Diabetes Study (UKPDS) were published. The UKPDS was the world's biggest and most comprehensive study of type 2 diabetes. It took 20 years to complete and studied 5000 patients in 23 centres in the UK. The results from this study showed that glycaemic control and the control of hypertension have a marked effect on morbidity and mortality in people with type 2 diabetes. Its major conclusions, using existing treatment to establish intensive glycaemic control, were that:

- stroke can be reduced by one-third
- kidney damage can be reduced by one-third
- major diabetic eye disease can be reduced by one-quarter.

The study also demonstrated that:

- 50% of patients with type 2 diabetes show signs of complications by the time of diagnosis
- after 9 years from diagnosis 30% of patients with type 2 diabetes have serious complications
- after 10 years type 2 diabetics have a two-fold greater mortality than the general population.

As stated earlier, the UKPDS demonstrated that a combination of hypertension and diabetes represents a substantially increased risk of morbidity and mortality. It is thought that the prevalence of hypertension in people with diabetes is much greater than in the non-diabetic population; the prevalence may be as high as 40%.

The link between diabetes and hypertension is not fully understood, and may differ between type 1 and type 2 diabetes. Therefore, identifying those at risk will become increasingly important, and the National Service Frameworks for type 1 and type 2 diabetes mellitus will have major impacts on foot care and podiatric provision. Establishing screening programmes to target those people at high risk of developing foot pathologies will be of vital importance and, with diminishing resources, podiatrists and their colleagues from other medical disciplines will be under increasing pressure to preserve tissue viability in diabetics.

## AIMS IN MANAGING HIGH-RISK PATIENTS

The main aims when managing high-risk patients, be they diabetic or not, are:

- to prevent complications (e.g. infection or injury)
- to manage effectively established wounds, infection or necrosis.

## PREVENTION OF COMPLICATIONS

### History taking and assessment

Obtaining a detailed history is paramount, accompanied by a vascular, neurological and biomechanical assessment. History taking includes the recording of medical and surgical details. Any drug therapy (including non-prescription medication) taken by the patient is noted and checked using the current edition of the *British National Formulary*. It is important to make enquiries regarding drug therapy as the underlying condition for which the drug is being administered may impair wound healing (e.g. vitamin B injections for pernicious anaemia). Alternatively, the drug itself may impair wounds healing potential or compromise the patient's immune system (e.g. corticosteroids).

Investigation of vascular and neurological systems does not need to be complicated (see Chs 1 and 5). Non-invasive methods of vascular assessment, such as calculation of ankle–brachial systolic pressure indices, are relatively simple to perform. Doppler ultrasonography provides the practitioner with an opportunity to identify abnormalities in the flow patterns of blood within the vessels. The use of pressure plates/systems can be helpful in locating areas of high pressure loading, particularly in the neuropathic foot.

Simple measurement of blood sugar levels, using a correctly calibrated glucometer, is indicated when there is a family history of diabetes, or when the patient presents with signs and symptoms of diabetes (e.g. recurrent episodes of infection).

Patient education regarding the relationship of their primary systemic pathology to foot health is vital: many excellent educational packs are available, but they must be accompanied by explanations appropriate to the individual patient. Whenever possible, carers should attend, and be involved with, education sessions.

## General points regarding treatment

The practitioner must pay close attention to aseptic/antiseptic techniques. The use of autoclaves for instrument sterilisation is a minimum requirement. Meticulous preoperative preparation of the patient's skin is necessary to effect a rapid reduction in the number of pathogenic transient flora, and to remove gross contamination. The most important preoperative cleansing routine is a thorough application of an alcohol-based preparation; any antiseptic added to the alcohol provides limited improvement to the activity of the solution.

Padding must be accurately shaped, avoiding creases and irregularities. Strapping should be non-constrictive. If caustic medicaments are used they must be applied with great care and their actions monitored closely. Detailed advice regarding suitable footwear and hosiery is essential, and is considered in other chapters. Minor surgical procedures are performed as a last resort, and only after consultation with the patient's GP.

## MANAGEMENT OF ESTABLISHED WOUNDS, INFECTION OR NECROSIS

An ulcer is an example of a wound that, for various reasons, will not heal. Most research pertinent to wound healing is not restricted to ulcers; the general term 'wound' is used in preference to 'ulcer' in the following discussion.

The following wound management strategies are considered:

- examination of the wound
- the use of antiseptics and topical medicaments
- the use of dressings.

## Examination of the wound

A detailed history and examination of the wound occurs at the initial consultation (Box 10.3). At each subsequent visit the wound and the patient's general condition are assessed, any changes being recorded

---

**Box 10.3 History of the wound**

1  The DURATION of the wound
2  Any changes in the SIZE or APPEARANCE of the wound?
3  Any change in the NUMBER of lesions/wounds?
4  Any PREVIOUS INCIDENTS of similar lesions?
5  Any PAIN or ALTERED SENSATION associated with the lesion?
6  The presence of other SIGNS and/or SYMPTOMS that may be related to the wound (e.g. ischaemic changes)
7  Does the patient know the CAUSE of the wound?

---

**Box 10.4 Points to observe when examining a wound**

1  The precise ANATOMICAL SITE of the wound
2  The SIZE of the wound. This should be measured accurately using a commercial measuring device
3  The GENERAL APPEARANCE of the wound and the surrounding tissue (e.g. presence of callus or maceration). Special note should be made of signs of local or spreading infection (cellulitis, lymphangitis, lymphadenitis)
4  The SIDES of the wound. When the walls are undermining the viable tissue the true extent of the wound must be assessed by careful use of a sterile probe
5  The BASE of the wound for the presence of slough, granulation tissue or deeper structures such as bone or tendon. Radiographs are necessary if deeper structures are thought to be involved. The DEPTH of the wound should be assessed. Chronic lesions are associated with fibrous bands tying the base to underlying structures; by gentle manipulation of the wound, the degree of fibrosis may be estimated
6  Any DISCHARGE should be noted and a specimen sent for microscopy and culture. The colour, consistency and odour of discharge should be recorded. The quantity may be approximated by observing dressings and finding out how often they require renewing

---

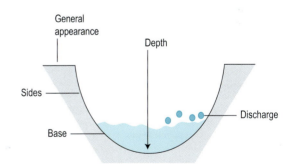

**Figure 10.1** Points to observe when examining a wound.

---

meticulously. The points that will be observed by the podiatrist are summarised in Box 10.4 and Figure 10.1. Photographs provide a detailed permanent record, although this recording method is not always practicable during routine clinical practice. However, pieces of sterile transparent film, often as part of wound-dressing systems, are available. The pieces of film have a grid system to allow accurate measurement and record of the wound, without the risk of contamination and cross-infection. At each visit a subjective, as well as objective, assessment of the wound and the whole patient are made.

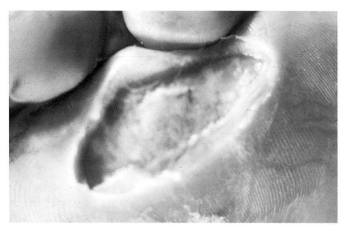

**Figure 10.2** A plantar wound proximal to the toe webbing. This wound has walls that undermine surrounding tissue, making its true size difficult to ascertain. Slough covers its base. The surrounding tissues are macerated.

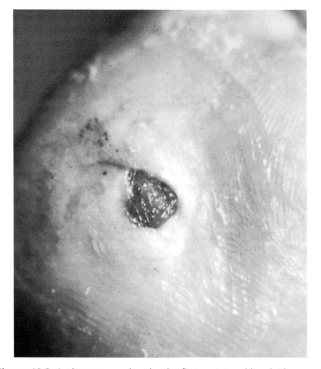

**Figure 10.3** A plantar wound under the first metatarsal head. The wound is shallow and its walls are not undermining surrounding tissue; its base is covered with granulation tissue.

Figures 10.2 and 10.3 illustrate plantar wounds proximal to the toe webbing and under the first metatarsal head, respectively.

## Infection

Diagnosing infection is vital, particularly in the high-risk foot. Without prompt and adequate intervention, tissue, limbs and ultimately the patient his or herself may be severely compromised by severe infection. Swabs are frequently taken from wounds, sent for microbiological examination to diagnose and identify infection and the causative microorganisms, and help in management. Many definitions of 'infection' exist (historically $10^5$ bacteria per gram of tissue has been identi-

fied as the point at which wound healing is inhibited), and the podiatrist needs to understand the principles of what constitutes infection as opposed to wound contamination and wound colonisation:

- wound contamination is where there are microorganisms present in the wound, but they are not replicating
- wound colonisation is where there is the presence of replicating microorganisms, but there are no signs or symptoms of infection
- wound infection is where there is invasion and replication of microorganisms leading to cell injury (e.g. by toxin production or by intracellular replication).

It should be understood that there is a continuum, and the balance between wound colonisation and wound infection is delicate, particularly in the high-risk foot and when ulceration has become chronic.

Although wound swabbing is often considered the 'gold standard' in diagnosing infection, recent opinion advises caution, and swab results may identify only surface colonisation of the wound (Cutting & Harding 1994). It is advocated that, unless attention is paid to 'associated host reaction' (Ayton 1985), treatment may be inappropriate. The signs and symptoms of inflammation, the presence of pus, a change in pain, a change in the appearance of granulation tissue and odour are some of the clinical criteria of 'associated host reaction' used to help diagnose infection.

However, it is important that microbiological specimens, when indicated, are collected in the correct manner, and that all paperwork is completed accurately. As suggested above, all wound surfaces are populated by microorganisms, but not all of these contaminated wounds are clinically infected. Microorganisms obtained from swabs taken from the deepest part of the wound are more likely to be of clinical significance than are those obtained by superficial swabbing. When free pus is unavailable for collection, swabs moistened with sterile saline are generally considered preferable to specimens collected with a dry swab, and the swab should be rotated 360° to ensure that all parts of the collecting head have made contact with the wound. Inappropriate transportation (either by using the incorrect transport medium, keeping the specimen at the wrong temperature, or delaying transport) of the specimen to the laboratory can cause damage. Clinical information provided to the laboratory needs to be full and accurate, including facts such as the patient is diabetic. This latter point is important, as the microenvironment of ulcers associated with diabetes often supports a mixed range of infecting agents, many of which act synergistically, and knowing the patient's medical status will help the laboratory in providing the most accurate report. Advice from the local microbiologist will be invaluable in all these matters.

The recent increase in multiple-antibiotic-resistant strains of microorganisms, such as methicillin-resistant *Staphylococcus aureus* (MRSA), dictate that systemic antibiotics must not be prescribed indiscriminately (Duckworth et al 1988). However, for wounds infected by multiple bacterial strains (particularly diabetic neuropathic ulcers) antibiotic coverage will include drugs active against Gram-positive staphylococci and streptococci, Gram-negative species and anaerobes (e.g. *Bacteroides fragilis*). Where infection has become chronic, or when deeper structures are involved, investigations are required to exclude soft-tissue infection or osteomyelitis. It should be noted that plain film radiographs will not show changes until approximately 2 weeks after bone infection has become established. Bone scans such as $^{111}$In-labelled white-cell scan are much more specific and will show changes early on. However, this method has poor resolution between bone and soft tissues. Other investigations, such as $^{99m}$Tc diphosphonate bone scans, can be used; however, this method has low specificity, as it demonstrates increased osteoblastic activity and increased blood flow to bone. Both these events occur in other pathologies, such as during the active stage of Charcot neuroarthropathy. Magnetic resonance imaging (MRI) is a very sensitive technique for imaging, and distinguishing between bone and soft tissues, but it is not very specific for osteomyelitis. It should also be noted that many imaging techniques are expensive to perform and not always easy to access.

## Management of wounds

There has been much debate about the use of surgical masks, sterile gloves, hats and plastic aprons while treating wounds. Historically, face masks were worn to prevent contamination of wounds by droplets disseminated from the practitioner's nasopharynx. Surveys demonstrate that the incidence of hospital-acquired infection is not affected by the use of face masks (Orr 1981). It is concluded that masks contribute little to protecting wounds, and may increase transmission of *Staphylococcus aureus* by encouraging shedding of colonised skin squames through the rubbing action of the mask on the face (Report of the Infection Control Nurses Association 1984). The most effective method of preventing contamination is to reduce conversation while attending to the wound and to carry out well-organised treatment.

Sterile surgical gloves may be worn, particularly when working on deep wounds, but clean latex gloves are acceptable, providing that they are replaced frequently, and worn only at appropriate times. However, there are problems with latex sensitivity. Most workers in this field advise avoiding the use of powdered latex gloves in order to reduce the number of airborne latex particles. Authorities also recommend wearing gloves for as short a period of time as possible, and advise that hands should be washed after gloves are removed (Ayliffe et al 1999).

Since the insistence of Semmelweis over 150 years ago, it has been well recognised that the practitioner's hands are one of the major vehicles of cross-infection (Rotter 1997). Three levels of hand-washing are recognised: social hand-washing (using soap and water), hygienic hand-washing (with antiseptic hand-wash preparation), and finally surgical hand-washing (a 3-minute hand-wash using an antiseptic). At all levels washing must be performed so that all surfaces of the hands are treated (Taylor 1978).

Many studies confirm that when doctors decontaminate their hands between patient examinations, the rate of hospital infection is also reduced (Larson 1995). An editorial in the *British Medical Journal* (BMJ Editorial 1999) described continuing problems with members of the medical and allied health professions in complying with straightforward hand-washing protocols. In one study doctors were asked to estimate the number of hand-washes they performed prior to patient examination. The practitioners were observed, and although the doctors' own perception of their hand-washing rate was 73% the actual observed rate of hand-washing was only 9% (Tibballs 1996). By adopting a standardised hand-wash technique, using soap and water, the number of pathogenic transient organisms is reduced. Hand rinses containing 70% ethanol are very effective in removing transient organisms (Rotter 1984). Paper hats can prevent skin squames from the scalp contaminating wounds.

Single-use plastic aprons may be worn to prevent contamination of permeable cotton clinic coats. Studies demonstrate a 50% reduction in the number of organisms recovered from clean plastic aprons when compared to the number isolated from a clean cotton garment; the moisture content of cotton supports the growth of bacterial colonies (Report of the Infection Control Nurses Association 1984).

The use of prepacked, sterile instruments, medicaments and dressings is part of normal practice, and aseptic techniques should be employed correctly and with care. Interestingly, papers question the

lack of reliable evidence to support many of the expensive and possibly overcomplicated aseptic practices used by the nursing profession, which podiatry has adapted for its own specialised use (Bree-Williams & Waterman 1996). It has also been shown that such techniques can become ritualised, and potentially dangerous, unless employed logically and with some thought (Merchant 1988).

Disposal of soiled dressings and instruments, unless performed with care, is a major potential source of cross-infection, and local infection-control guidelines must be followed.

The use of instruments on any wound, and the amount of tissue debrided, will depend on the aetiology and clinical state of the lesion at the time of treatment. Ischaemic ulcerations (whether or not they are associated with diabetes) must be treated conservatively; conversely, diabetic neuropathic ulcers (without associated ischaemia) require maximum debridement to encourage healing. It is important when treating neuropathic ulcers (assuming there is an adequate arterial blood supply) with undermining walls to ensure full exploration of the site and to identify the full extent of the wound. In long-standing neuropathic wounds debridement is purported to help stimulate healing to an acute process, thus aiding repair. However, although debridement is widely advocated in neuropathic ulcerations there still needs to be more research to prove and understand its precise role in the wound-healing process.

## Desloughing and wound cleansing agents

### Desloughing agents

Slough (a collection of necrotic material, leucocytes and microorganisms) can become a medium for further bacterial growth; in many cases it is important to try to remove it. In ischaemic wounds, slough tends to be firmly attached to the base of the wound, whereas slough in neuropathic wounds may be less adherent and easier to remove. It is important to recognise the intimate physical relationship that exists between slough and granulation tissue; the problems of disturbing the latter while removing the former must be considered before deciding upon a treatment method.

Desloughing/cleansing agents include the hypochlorite group of chemicals, and enzymes that allow autolytic breakdown of slough by-products generated from the patient's own leucocytes. The hypochlorites interact with protein and it is this reaction that imparts their antibacterial role. It should be noted that the *British National Formulary* no longer recommends the use of chlorinated solutions such as Dakin's solution (Chlorinated Soda Solution, Surgical BPC) for wound cleansing due to their irritant effects.

Preparations containing enzymes are used for desloughing wounds (Forsling 1988). Enzymes, such as streptokinase and streptodornase, degrade fibrin and remove DNA from cell nuclei. Most enzyme preparations are presented as dry powders, which are refrigerated until application, when they are reconstituted with sterile isotonic saline (e.g. Varidase, Lederle). The solution can be held in contact with the wound using gauze and a film dressing, or it can be injected under tough necrotic slough using a syringe. Enzymatic preparations seem to be used less frequently in the UK than elsewhere; however, some workers have found successful results using these products in a small randomised, controlled, double-blinded study (Martin et al 1996).

Cadexamer iodine (Iodosorb, Smith and Nephew UK), contains 0.9% w/w of iodine and exerts a hydrophilic action, acting as an absorbent. The product also helps to remove debris and bacteria from the wound surface by capillary action. The beads swell under the influence of exudate and release the iodine.

Intrasite gel can be used to help remove slough and absorb excess exudate.

Sterile larvae of *Lucilia sericata* (the common greenbottle) are used to deslough wounds (Rayman et al 1998). The way in which the larvae work is not fully understood; however, it is thought they may produce changes in the wound pH, produce natural antimicrobial substances (Pavillard & Wright 1997), and remove necrotic material as part of their normal feeding mechanisms. They reduce pain and odour caused by the wound, and some workers suggest that they may produce growth factors (Prete 1997). Another important attribute is the ability of larval therapy to treat wounds colonised or infected by MRSA (Wise et al 1998).

The larvae are only 2–3 mm long when placed on the wound. They are held in situ by masking the area with a hydrocolloid sheet. The larvae are placed in a carefully shaped hole within the hydrocolloid sheet and then covered with a secondary dressing and left in situ for several days.

## Wound-cleansing agents and antiseptics

The skin around the wound must be cleaned prior to treatment to reduce the number of transient microorganisms present. Solutions of antiseptics, such as chlorhexidine gluconate in alcohol base, are satisfactory. Chlorhexidine gluconate has activity against a wide range of both Gram-positive and Gram-negative bacteria; however, chlorhexidine is not active against fungi, spores or viruses. Iodophors are complexes of iodine and solubilisers (e.g. povidone iodine) and are found in many products, including preoperative skin preparation. Povidone iodine has a wide range of activity against microorganisms, including a sporicidal action.

Wound-cleansing agents are used prior to the application of a dressing. Most authorities advocate that antiseptic wound cleansers are not necessary in a wound management programme and that sterile isotonic saline (0.89%) is the preferred solution for wound cleaning. Wound-cleansing agents are available in sterile, single-use sachets, the use of which is strongly advocated. Solutions are applied to the wound site using sterile gauze. Cotton wool should not be used as fibres are shed onto the wound surface where they act as foreign bodies. Solutions may be applied to difficult sites via a sterile syringe barrel, without the needle attached.

Experiments have demonstrated that wound-cleansing agents, with the exception of isotonic saline, can produce transient closure of capillaries (Brennan et al 1986). Chlorhexidine's effect was minimal. However, in clinical practice, the reduction of capillary blood flow is of very short duration, although the use of sterile isotonic saline is suggested for cleaning the majority of wounds. Interestingly, some recent studies suggest that tap water may be an acceptable alternative to sterile normal saline for cleansing of open wounds (Riyat & Quinton 1997).

## Antiseptics

Over recent years the use of antiseptics in the management of ulceration has been controversial. Most antiseptics have a deleterious effect on the wound microenvironment; they can interfere with wound healing, produce resistance in some microorganisms and produce skin sensitivities if used for long periods of time. However, the debate has been re-opened, and with a newer understanding of the way in which microorganisms behave in a chronic wound environment it is feasible that certain antiseptics may have a role in the management of chronic wounds (Gilchrist 1997).

The use of topical antibiotics is contraindicated; antibiotics should be delivered systemically, but only after the causative microorganism has been identified and its sensitivity to a specific antibiotic ascertained.

## Dressings

There is a continued abundance of new wound dressings, and as technology moves forward more are to be anticipated. It should be stressed that, in many chronic wounds, the failure of a wound-care product to work is the result of underlying pathologies – emphasising the need to assess the patient's general health before deciding on a management strategy. No dressing will heal a wound while the local microenvironment is unsuitable (e.g. oedema and local infection). It is unrealistic to expect all chronic wounds to heal; Turner encapsulates this concept by emphasising the need to consider, before predicting the likely prognosis for wound healing:

> *'factors which will produce a microenvironment associated with the wound that will allow healing to proceed at a maximum rate commensurate with the age and physiological condition of the patient'*

(Turner 1979)

The literature accompanying a wound-care product must be consulted to ensure the suitability of the dressing for individual patients and their wounds. Unfortunately, the price and availability may restrict the use of some products.

The properties of the 'ideal wound dressing' are considered before describing the various groups of products.

'Ideal wound dressings' are:

1. able to remove exudate
2. able to maintain humidity at the wound–dressing interface
3. permeable to gases
4. impermeable to microorganisms
5. able to maintain a suitable temperature at the wound surface
6. able to maintain low adherence at the wound–dressing interface
7. free from contaminants
8. able to maintain a suitable pH
9. other factors, including ease of application, patient acceptability and comfort, and cost.

### 1. The ability to remove exudate

The removal of excess exudate from the surface of the wound is important for three main reasons:

- exudate can act as a hospitable medium for the growth of pathogens
- exudate can macerate the wound – enzymes present in exudate can produce autolysis of surrounding tissues
- exudate can soak dressings and 'strike through' occurs, allowing entry of pathogens, from the outside of the dressing onto the wound surface, by capillary action.

Exudate also possesses desirable actions. Various substances found in exudate (e.g. growth factors) are necessary for successful wound healing.

### 2. The ability to maintain humidity at the wound–dressing interface

Until Winter's seminal work in the 1960s, wounds were kept dry. The rationale for this regimen was to discourage bacterial invasion. In 1962, Winter showed that epithelial movement across a wound was compromised by thick scab formation. Epithelial cells seek a moist surface for movement, and in dry wounds the suitable environment is deep under the scab; in the latter case re-epithelialisation is a slow, energy-consuming process (Winter 1962). It should be noted that dressings that allow 'strike through' can dehydrate wound surfaces.

### 3. Permeability of the dressing to gases

The importance of atmospheric oxygen varies with different stages of wound healing. Early dressings, such as Op-Site (Smith & Nephew), were gas permeable. Under this type of dressing the number of neutrophils in the exudate increased, and the regeneration of epithelial cells increased ten-fold – both these events being beneficial to wound healing.

The effects of hypoxia (reduced oxygen levels) can aid the healing process. Neoangiogenesis (the production of new capillaries, a major component of granulation tissue) is increased in hypoxic environments. Reduced oxygen concentration stimulates macrophages to produce molecules able to stimulate new vessel growth (Silver 1994). Hypoxia is reported to decrease pain, possibly by interfering with the production of prostaglandins and other chemicals.

### 4. The ability to be impermeable to microorganisms

The dressing should be impermeable to the entry of pathogenic microorganisms onto the wound surface; this situation is most likely to occur during 'strike through'.

### 5. The ability to maintain a suitable temperature at the wound surface

After routine cleansing it takes 40 minutes for the surface of a wound to regain its original temperature, and 3 hours before normal cell mitotic function returns (Myers 1982). It is therefore advisable to leave wounds exposed for the minimum time possible during re-dressings (also reducing the risk of cross-infection). It is also wise to avoid using cold solutions for irrigation and cleaning of lesions.

Oxygen dissociation from haemoglobin is impaired when the temperature is reduced by 10°C. Thus, dressings that allow 'strike through' not only allow contamination, and encourage dehydration of wounds, but can cause temperature loss by convection.

### 6. The ability to maintain low adherence at the wound–dressing interface

Dressings that adhere to wound surfaces damage delicate granulation tissue and epithelium when removed. These dressings can become incorporated into granulation tissue and produce foreign body reactions. In addition, patients may experience distress and pain during the change of dressings if the material has become adherent.

Some low-adherence dressings can be responsible for autolytic damage to tissues around the wound site. This is because exudate is unable to travel through the pore structure of the plastic film interface of the dressing.

### 7. The ability to be free from contaminants

The dressing must be constructed from material that can be sterilised and kept in that condition until it is used. Dressings should not contain substances able to cause toxic reactions, or adversely interact with the wound surface. Particulates or fibres shed from a dressing can become incorporated into granulation tissue and produce foreign body reactions.

### 8. The ability to maintain a suitable pH

Oxygen dissociates from haemoglobin most efficiently in an acidic environment (Bohr effect). A low pH (acidic) is important in stimulating neoangiogenesis.

### 9. Other factors, including patient acceptability, ease of application and comfort, and cost

Some early dressings (particularly the occlusive hydrocolloids) were unacceptable to patients because of malodour and exudate formed by the interaction of the dressing components and the wound.

Some dressings are difficult to apply to the contours of the foot as they are designed for use on larger, flatter body surfaces. The judicious use of strapping and conforming bandages helps to overcome these problems.

The cost and availability of some dressings may prohibit their use; however, the cost-effectiveness of a product should always be fully researched.

## Types of dressing for use in podiatric practice

The introduction, and accessibility, of new dressings is changing at such a prodigious rate that a detailed description of individual dressings is inappropriate. This section describes the features of groups of products currently available. It is stressed that, before using any wound-care product, practitioners should make themselves fully aware of the product's indications and contraindications, either by consulting the manufacturer or the current edition of the *British National Formulary*.

## Conventional dressings

Example: Gauze swabs B.P.

The majority of podiatrists use gauze swabs, mainly because of their availability and low cost. The disadvantages associated with gauze dressings include: 'strike through', the shedding of fibres, adherence and incorporation into the wound surface. Gauze is woven from cotton, but newer developments have led to the production of fabrics made from non-woven viscose. Swabs made from viscose are more absorptive and less liable to shed fibres. Filmated swabs have layers of cotton wool between either traditional woven, or newer non-woven, gauze; this improves absorption, but can lead to shedding of fibres onto the wound surface.

The use of paraffin gauze (the older name for which is tulle gras) reduces some of the adverse effects of using gauze; however, granulation tissue can grow through its structure and incorporate the paraffin gauze into the wound.

## Primary wound-dressing films

### Semipermeable adhesive film dressings

Examples: Bioclusive (Johnson & Johnson), Tegaderm (3M), Opsite (Smith & Nephew UK, Cutifilm) (Beiersdorf).

The first low-adherence dressing was Opsite; it was originally developed as an adhesive incise drape for general surgery. These types of film dressing are permeable to gas and water vapour but are impermeable to water. They have no fibres that can be shed into wounds; they are transparent and therefore allow monitoring of the wound site. However, semipermeable adhesive films are non-absorbent.

Such dressings may be used to reduce shear stress over vulnerable areas, such as heels.

### Perforated film absorbent dressings

Examples: Melolin (Smith & Nephew), Release (Johnson & Johnson).

Other low-adherence dressings incorporate an absorptive backing, covered with a perforated plastic film. Although they can absorb wound discharge, they are not suitable for heavily exuding wounds.

However, a secondary absorbent dressing can be used over the top of perforated film absorbent dressings.

## Low-adherent wound contact layers

### Unmedicated

Examples: N-A Dressing (Johnson & Johnson), Tricotex (Smith & Nephew).

These dressings are made from knitted viscose; they are non-absorbent, providing a non-adherent primary wound dressing.

### Medicated

Examples: Bactigras (Smith & Nephew), Serotulle (Seton).

Some low-adherent wound contact dressings incorporate an antiseptic, such as chlorhexidine acetate, in a paraffin or polyethylene glycol base. Research indicates that chlorhexidine is not easily released from its paraffin base. However, it is suggested that dressings with polyethylene glycol more effectively liberate antiseptics; for example, Inadine (Johnson & Johnson) which contains povidone iodine.

## Semipermeable hydrogels

Example: Intrasite Gel (Smith & Nephew).

At present Intrasite Gel is the only hydrogel available on the Drug Tariff. It is composed of a low percentage of carboxymethylcellulose, 80% water and 20% propylene glycol. Structurally, these are hydrophilic polymers that contain a high percentage of water.

There are two basic presentations of semipermeable hydrogels: the first type is in a sheet form (not dissimilar to a thin slice of table jelly); the second is known as amorphous hydrogel and resembles wallpaper paste in texture. Both forms are absorptive; the first type retains its gross structure but swells, the second type absorbs exudate until its substance becomes dispersed in water.

The sheet form of hydrogel consists of approximately 96% water (the percentage varies with individual products), and is transparent, flexible and easily moulded, with mechanical properties that protect delicate granulation tissue. It is gas-permeable but impermeable to water. This form of hydrogel will dehydrate and must be either replaced or rehydrated with sterile isotonic saline to prevent fragmentation of the product. The percentage of water in the original dressing dictates its absorptive power.

The amorphous hydrogels can remove slough by rehydrating dry, necrotic tissue. This type of hydrogel is effective in absorbing exudate and used as a carrier for medicaments such as metronidazole. Hydrogels are kept in situ by applying gauze, or another secondary dressing, over them.

## Hydrocolloids

Examples: Granuflex (ConvaTec), Comfeel (Coloplast), Tegasorb (3M).

These dressings are composed of substances that form a gel when in contact with a wound surface. The constituents vary from manufacturer to manufacturer, but they contain polysaccharides and protein. Thus constituents adhere to, and interact with, the wound surface; these are held on a water-repellent, flexible foam backing, which should not require a secondary dressing. In the early versions of hydrocolloid dressings, interaction between the dressing and the wound surface produced a yellow, semi-liquid and malodorous substance. Contemporary products are more sophisticated. The semi-liquid produced at the dressing–wound interface is protective and absorptive, providing a moist and insulated environment; finally, it forms an impermeable layer. The latter results in an acidic and hypoxic environment conducive to neoangiogenesis. The occlusive environment contraindicates the use of hydrocolloids when a wound is clinically infected – particularly when anaerobe species are isolated. The use of hydrocolloids may also be contraindicated for treating diabetic ulcers.

Hydrocolloids are available in other presentations (e.g. pastes); these are used in wounds supporting a heavy slough. Most manufacturers produce 'wound-management systems'; these involve using desloughing agents, and specific types of dressing at different stages of wound healing.

## Alginate dressings

Examples: Kaltostat (BritCair ConvaTec), Sorbsan (Maersk).

These products are manufactured from calcium and sodium salts of alginic acid, which is derived from seaweed. They represent a very old treatment: sailors used seaweed for dressing wounds and effecting haemostasis centuries ago.

When in contact with blood or exudate, alginate fibres convert, via calcium/sodium ion exchange, into a hydrophilic gel. The gel is absorbent, providing a protective, moist interface to the wound. The relative amounts of mannuronic acid and guluronic acid present in alginate formulations determine the characteristics of the gel that is finally formed once the dressing is in contact with the wound. Dressings with higher concentrations of mannuronic acid form softer gels (Sorbsan); those with higher concentrations of guluronic acid form firmer end products. Generally, alginates are relatively easy to remove, provided the area is irrigated with sterile isotonic saline; however, some situations will require the use of forceps to complete the removal of the dressing. Theoretically, the fibres associated with the dressing present no hazard, as they are biodegradable. There have been some reports of patients experiencing a mild burning sensation when alginates are applied; this could be due to the intensely hydrophilic properties of the product causing a rapid dehydration. The effect can be minimised by moistening the dressing with sterile isotonic saline before application.

## Polyurethane foams

Examples: Lyofoam (Seton), Allevyn (Smith & Nephew).

Marine sponges were probably the earliest forms of foams used as wound dressings: in 1884 Joseph Gamgee introduced an artificial absorbent sponge.

Foams are indicated for treating wounds with moderate amounts of exudate. The manufacturing process produces a dressing with a smooth, low-adherent hydrophilic inner layer and an outer layer of untreated hydrophobic foam. The construction of the outer layer helps reduce 'strike through', although a secondary dressing may be required. Foam dressings are permeable to gases and allow adequate hydration of the wound surface and provide effective thermal insulation.

## Silver agents

Silver-impregnated dressings are a recent introduction. Silver is known to be antibacterial. However, there is some debate as to the possibility of toxicity associated with silver. Further investigations will hopefully clarify the situation for podiatric use.

## Other dressings – the way forward?

Hyaluronic acid, a glycosaminoglycan, promotes cell proliferation (including fibroblasts), and Hyafill has been used with success by some podiatrists.

Platelet-derived growth factors and cytokines (e.g. transforming growth factors α and β₂) have been used to treat diabetic ulcers (Holloway et al 1993). Recent work shows that the chronic wound environment contributes to an increase in the amount of proteases: the relative overproduction of these substances is thought to break down normal growth factors. Hence the development of products that aim to protect available growth factors from protease degradation – one example being Promogran (Smith & Nephew).

Bioengineered dressings such as Dermagraft (Smith & Nephew) have aroused much interest. This product is a human, fibroblast-derived dermal replacement, and early results appear promising. Other approaches involve seeding the patient's own epithelial cells onto a suitable culture medium and using the resultant culture on their wounds (Shakespeare 1991).

Almost any substance imaginable has been used as a wound dressing at some point in history. Some of the older remedies are currently being reassessed using modern scientific methods. Honey, for example, is acidic (approximate pH 3.7), and it may encourage wound neoangiogenesis and may also be bactericidal.

## OTHER ASPECTS OF MANAGEMENT

In people with diabetes, education and advice about preventing secondary complications of the disease is imperative and part of the podiatric management. Despite general consensus among podiatrists and other healthcare professionals that health education plays a vital role in management plans, there is minimal statistically sound evidence to show the most satisfactory method of delivering health education to people with diabetes. This disappointing lack of evidence must not of course stop education programmes, but must motivate podiatrists to find the optimum ways of disseminating information in the most effective manner to people with diabetes and other pathologies that impair tissue viability. It is a matter of urgency that the delivery and content of foot health education is reviewed in the light of evidence-based practice.

The use of padding and orthoses to protect wounds may be indicated; each patient will require a specific prescription, and therefore only general comments can be made.

Soft, cushioning, padding materials are indicated rather than firm, redistributive materials; the use of the latter can compromise capillary blood flow to the edges of the wound. Accurate positioning of pads is vital, and is not always an easy task, particularly when large dressings are applied. As little adhesive as is practicably possible should be placed on the skin; conforming bandages, for example, Kling (Johnson & Johnson) or plastic film sprays can be used to protect vulnerable areas of skin from adhesives.

Replaceable silicone pads (Silipos) of various shapes and sizes are useful in cases where the patient can reach his or her feet, and where there is no danger of the pad constricting a digit, or part of the foot.

When specific areas of high pressure loading are identified, casted insoles constructed from composites of low-, medium- and high-density thermoplastics may be required. These customised insoles are valuable in preventing initial damage occurring. During the last decade many new orthotic materials have been specifically developed for the diabetic foot, and they show promise in the overall management plan.

Footwear and hosiery must be carefully selected and, if necessary, modifications such as stretching or balloon patching executed. Slippers, often a popular choice with patients, are not recommended unless well fitting, as they produce shearing stresses that cause movement of dressings, predispose to falls and reduce activity of the calf muscle pump. Boots made from low-density thermoplastics may be suitable for an immobile patient. Bespoke or semi-bespoke footwear is the answer for many chronic foot problems, or they can be worn as a preventive measure. As a temporary measure, commercially available postoperative boots or sandals can be modified by the addition of felts and sponges. The orthotist is an important link in the provision of special footwear when caring for patients in a hospital setting.

Total contact casting may be indicated when treating neuropathic ulcers. The technique has several variations that allow removal of the cast for inspection of the wound site. The technique must be taught correctly by someone with experience in the technique, and the podiatrist must be confident in the correct application of the cast before attempting to use total contact casts on patients. The introduction of Aircast pneumatic walkers has proved beneficial for some patients; these transfer pressure over the whole of the plantar surface of the foot and support the leg, and they also have a rocker sole. When these methods are used the patient must be provided with an address or telephone number that they may access 24 hours a day, 7 days a week, in case advice is needed.

The patient with an ulcer, open lesion or infection is advised to rest and elevate the affected limb, but the danger of immobility producing a deep vein thrombosis cannot be overlooked. Other problems of immobility are the development of pressure sores and, if the limb is insufficiently elevated, oedema may ensue.

Patients must be discouraged from smoking. Smoking adversely affects wound healing in several ways: it causes vasoconstriction, reduces macrophage and epithelial cell function and reduces immunoglobulin G (IgG) levels (Siana et al 1992).

However, the patient's quality of life, and their compliance, may be adversely affected unless a compromise between ideal and realistic advice is given.

Consideration has been given to the role of multidisciplinary care of the patient, which is crucial during treatment of wounds. The same approach is important once improvement of the wound occurs, so the patient is monitored by professionals, such as district nurses and the GP, who can liaise with each other and the podiatrist in providing patient care.

## CONCLUSIONS

The high-risk patient and their wounds provide a challenge to the podiatrist; the adage 'prevention is preferable to cure' holds true for this group of patients. The challenge is minimised by adopting a multidisciplinary approach to patient care, using expertise gained by other healthcare professionals and by colleagues. It is important that other professions understand the role of podiatry in the care of the high-risk patient, and it is incumbent on the podiatrist to ensure that this information is forthcoming.

Patient education is important, but only if the patient and their carers understand the rationale behind the information that is provided – the responsibility for this lies with the podiatrist.

When wounds develop they must be treated on an individual basis, and only after a full medical history and physical examination of the patient, and their lesion, have been carried out. When selecting wound-care products the practitioner is aided by an understanding of the normal wound healing process and by frequent consultation of the medical and nursing press for new developments.

# REFERENCES

Ayliffe GAJ, Babb JR, Taylor LJ 1999 Nursing aspects of prevention of infection. Hospital-acquired infection – principles and prevention, 3rd edn. Butterworth & Heinemann, Oxford, p. 104.

Ayton M 1985 Wounds that won't heal. Nursing Times 81(46 Suppl):16–19.

BMJ Editorial 1999 Hand-washing. A modest measure with big effects. BMJ 318:686.

Bree-Williams FJ, Waterman H 1996 An examination of nurses' practices when performing aseptic technique for wound care. Journal of Advanced Nursing 23(1):48–54.

Brennan S, Foster ME, Leaper DJ 1986 Antiseptic toxicity in wounds healing by secondary intention. Journal of Hospital Medicine 8:263–267.

Cutting KF, Harding KG 1994 Criteria for identifying wound infection. Journal of Wound Care 3(4):198–201.

Diabetes Control and Complications Trial Research Group 1993 The effect of intensive treatment of diabetes on the development of long-term complications in insulin dependent diabetes mellitus. New England Journal of Medicine 329:977–986.

Duckworth GJ, Lothian JLE, Williams J 1988 Methicillin resistant Staphylococcus aureus: report of an outbreak in a London teaching hospital. Journal of Hospital Infection II:1–5.

Forsling E 1988 Comparison of saline and sreptokinase–streptodornase in the treatment of leg ulcers. European Journal of Clinical Pharmacology 33:637–638.

Gilchrist B 1997 Should iodine be reconsidered in wound management? Journal of Wound Care 6(3):148–150.

Holloway GA, Steed DL, De Marco M, et al 1993 A randomised, controlled, multicentre, dose response trial of activated platelet supernatent, topical CT-102 in chronic, nonhealing diabetic wounds. Wounds. A Compendium of Clinical Research and Practice 5(4):198–206.

Larson EL 1995 APIC Guidelines for hand-washing and hand antisepsis in healthcare settings. American Journal of Infection Control 23:251–269.

Martin SJ, Corrado OJ, Kay EA 1996 Enzymatic debridement for necrotic wounds. Journal of Wound Care 5(7):10–311.

Merchant J 1988 Aseptic technique reconsidered. Care – Science and Practice 6(3).

Myers JA 1982 Modern plastic surgical dressings. Health and Social Services Journal 18 March:336–337.

Orr N 1981 Is a mask necessary in the operating theatre? Annals of the Royal College of Surgeons 63:390.

Pavillard ER, Wright EA 1997 An antibiotic from maggots. Nature 180:916–917.

Prete P 1997 Growth effects of Phaenicia sericata larval extracts on fibroblasts: mechanism for wound healing by maggot therapy. Life Science 60:505–510.

Rayman A, Stansfield G, Woolard T, et al 1998 Use of larvae in the treatment of the diabetic necrotic foot. Diabetic Foot 1:7–13.

Report of the Infection Control Nurses Association Working Party on Ward Protective Clothing 1984. Infection Control Nurses Association.

Riyat MS, Quinton DN 1997 Tap water as a wound cleaning agent in accident and emergency. Journal of Accident and Emergency Medicine 14(3):165–166.

Rotter M 1984 Hygienic hand disinfection. Infection Control 5:18.

Rotter ML 1997 150 years of hand disinfection – Semmelweis' heritage. Hygienic Medicine 22:332–339.

Saint Vincent Declaration 1990 Diabetes Care and Research in Europe. Workshop Report. Diabetic Medicine 7:370.

Shakespeare P 1991 Cultured human skin epithelium for wound repair. Journal of Tissue Viability 1:19–20.

Siana JE, Frankid S, Gottrup F 1992 The effect of smoking on tissue function. Journal of Wound Care 1(2):37–41.

Silver IA 1994 The physiology of wound healing. Journal of Wound Care 3(2):106–109.

Taylor LJ 1978 An evaluation of hand-washing techniques. Nursing Times 74(54):108.

Tibballs J 1996 Teaching hospital medical staff to hand-wash. Medical Journal of Australia 164:395–398.

Turner TD 1979 Products and their development in wound management. Symposium on wound healing, Espoo, Finland, 1–3 November 1979.

Winter GD 1962 Formation of the scab and the rate of epithelialisation of superficial wounds in the skin of the young domestic pig. Nature 193:293–294.

Wise R, Hart T, Cars O, et al 1998 Antimicrobial resistance. BMJ 317:609–610.

# FURTHER READING

Ayliffe GAJ, Lowbury EJL, Geddes AM, Williams JD 1992 Control of hospital infection, 3rd edn. Chapman and Hall, London.

Levin ME, O'Neal LW, Bowker JH 1993 The diabetic foot, 5th edn. Mosby, St. Louis, MI.

Pickup JC, Williams G 1994 Chronic complications of diabetes, 1st edn. Blackwell Scientific, Oxford.

Underwood JCE 1992 General and systemic pathology, 1st edn. Churchill-Livingstone, Edinburgh.

Watkins PJ, Drury PL, Taylor KW 1990 Diabetes and its management, 4th edn. Blackwell Scientific, Oxford.

# Chapter 11

# Podiatric management of the elderly

*Bev Durrant, Janet McInnes, Farina Hashmi and Alistair McInnes*

## INTRODUCTION

Life expectancy has increased dramatically over the last century. This is a result of a combination of decreased infant mortality, significant advances in surgical and medical treatments, and, most importantly, improved social circumstances. These improvements have resulted in an increasingly ageing population, with similar findings repeated across all developed countries. The Office Of Population Statistics predicts a rise in the total population of all four countries of the UK from 59 million in 2002 to 71 million in the year 2031. It is expected that there will be fewer deaths than births and that immigration will outstrip emigration. The ageing population is predicted to continue, with the proportion of those over 65 years old rising from 16% of the population in 2006 to 22% in 2031. The likely consequence of the peak in UK population during these years is that as this group grows older there will be fewer people of working age to support them both financially and practically.

The age group showing the greatest increase in size is the over 80s, who in 2008 represented 4.5% of the total population, with this trend set to continue into the future. The reason for this profile is the reduction in mortality rates for the older age group, which may result from advances in the treatment of cardiovascular disorders and some cancers. In addition, the entire population enjoys generally improved living standards (UK National Statistics 2008).

The costs of the trend towards an increased number of the very elderly are borne by both the individual and by society. Increasingly, podiatrists are joining the debate to consider how these costs can be reduced and how individuals may be supported to grow older successfully. This effort starts with promoting good health in young and middle-aged groups, while at the same time providing a socio-medical framework to assist the elderly to live an optimally fulfilled life. In order to understand and contribute to the debate, a working definition of successful ageing is required.

Rowe and Kahn (1998) have proposed that ageing may be considered in two ways: as 'usual ageing' and as 'successful ageing'. Usual ageing is the normal decline in physical, social and cognitive functioning over time and is affected by extrinsic factors. Successful ageing occurs where both physical function and psychological well-being are only marginally affected and where extrinsic factors play little or no part. Theories of successful ageing are broadly biomedical, psychosocial and lay theories, with some overlap between all three. Successful ageing may be considered as the individual's ability to overcome physical deterioration and mental disability and to optimise a high-quality life expectancy, where extrinsic factors are not negative but play, at best, a neutral or even a positive role. To age successfully one should avoid disease, avoid disease risk factors, remain physically active, maintain satisfactory levels of cognitive functioning and, most importantly, participate in a fulfilling social life (Rowe & Kahn 1998).

However, this may be an unrealistic ambition for many. Although half of elderly people consider that they themselves have aged successfully, one in five are not defined as such by the traditional medical models of health and disease .The socio-psychological view of successful ageing considers important factors such as life satisfaction and participation in life, contentment with one's life both past and present, being able to continue with an active social life and to maintain good personal relationships with friends and family. The personal characteristics required for successful ageing include self-efficacy, a generally positive outlook, effective coping skills and, importantly, the ability to adapt and change when faced with difficult challenges and adverse life events (Baltes & Baltes 1990).

Most elderly people have experienced bereavement and loss. For some, the financial burden encountered following the death of a spouse may require relocation to more affordable accommodation, which brings additional difficulties. Personal resources and characterisation of the individual will largely determine the extent to which transitions in life can be deemed to show successful coping mechanisms.

There have been few studies that have investigated the views the elderly themselves hold on ageing, but in those that have been conducted the elderly define successful ageing as good mental, physical, psychological and social health. They include such features as having financial security, good physical appearance, a sense of humour and spirituality. Important to the elderly is a sense of purpose and of being able to learn new skills and make a contribution (Baltes & Baltes 1990).

In a national survey of 854 people aged over 50 years and living at home in the U.K, 75% of respondents considered themselves as ageing successfully, describing their ageing as either 'very well' or 'well'. The most common factors identified for successful ageing were good physical health and functioning, but most mentioned other factors. For example:

'Successful ageing is to go out a lot and enjoy life, take it day by day and enjoy what you can ... have good health – that is more important than anything else. Keep active – while your legs are moving, get out on them, you need to contribute to society, get involved'

'I don't think about getting old. I just don't feel old and act accordingly'.

(ONS Omnibus Survey, Bowling & Dieppe 2005)

Podiatrists are in an ideal position to contribute to the successful ageing of their patients, and it is the purpose of this chapter to identify and highlight these opportunities. The role of the podiatrist requires the practitioner to take a patient-focused and holistic approach, and therefore encompasses more than the purely technical.

> **Box 11.1 Letter of referral for Mr E (Case study 1.1)**
>
> Dear Podiatrist.
> **Re: Mr E, DOB: 07.04.1922**
> Mr E has thickened nails of both big toe nails. He is unable to cut them and is finding it difficult to manage them by filing. Some time ago they were treated surgically and have been problematic since. I believe that you would be the best person to manage this problem.
>
> The patient has had a left hip and dual knee replacement in recent years and is unable to get down to his feet and is finding it increasingly difficult to mobilise. Mr E has had a number of falls and is seeing the falls-prevention team.
>
> Mr E lives alone in a two-storey dwelling. He has carers visiting twice daily and District Nurses visiting twice weekly for redressing of his chronic venous leg and foot ulcers.
>
> He has had a myocardial infarction (MI); has recently been diagnosed with peripheral vascular disease (PVD), is hypertensive and has hyperlipidaemia. Some years ago Mr E was diagnosed with cancer of the thyroid gland and as a result had a thyroidectomy, for which he is medicated with levothyroxine. I have attached a list of medication that Mr E is currently being prescribed.
> Yours sincerely,
> Dr J Smith
> Thyroxine,
> Co-codamol,
> Furosemide,
> Simvastatin,
> Ramipril

In order that the chapter may focus on the podiatric care of the elderly, the following narrative introduces the reader to two patients whose case studies are outlined briefly. Consideration of the cases will raise questions and issues of interest to the podiatrist, and these are discussed in the appropriate sections. The chapter concludes with advice regarding further reading.

## CASE STUDY 11.1 MR E, DATE OF BIRTH 7 APRIL 1922

The letter of referral shown in Box 11.1 was received from Mr E's GP. An appointment is arranged for assessment. The letter includes a comprehensive history including medical, surgical, social and pharmacological details. This is not always typical and this example allows some preliminary thoughts on the case. When the medical history provided by the referent is incomplete, it is often possible to deduce from the medications listed the nature of the medical problems. Fortunately, in this case we were provided with a very complete referral, and can be confident that assumptions will be reasonable. Mr E is likely to be suffering arthritic pain and possibly stiffness, for which he takes co-codamol; his cardiovascular system is supported by furosemide and ramipril; and thyroid function by levothyroxine. In common with many patients, Mr E takes a statin in order to regularise his blood cholesterol. From an initial consideration it would seem that the short-term podiatric treatment is straightforward and involves nail care.

## NAIL CONDITIONS AND CARE

One of the most common nail conditions that presents in older people is onychauxis, defined as a thickened nail plate. Precipitating factors associated with onychauxis are: onychomycosis, peripheral vascular disease (PVD) and a history of trauma to the nail plate. The trauma may be intrinsic in origin, such as subungual exostosis, or extrinsic, such as inappropriate footwear.

Another type of thickened nail is onychogryphosis. This is a thickened deformed nail plate, in which the deformity progresses to form a curvature of the nail so that it appears to resemble a ram's horn, hence the alternative term for the pathology. As the structural alteration in the shape of the nail originates from the cells within the nail matrix, the causes of onychogryphosis can be similar to those of onychauxis. However, the aetiology of onychogryphosis is most often, but not always, attributed to a single traumatic event. In light of this, gryphotic nails often present in single nails as opposed to several, compared to onychauxis, particularly if the underlying causes are due to systemic disease (e.g. PVD) or infection (e.g. onychomycosis). When all the nails present with this condition, there is often an association with long-term neglect and impaction of the nails within the footwear. This presentation is sometimes seen in the elderly, who are unable to look after their own foot health or who are unwilling to seek assistance from family members.

On examination of Mr E's feet, a diagnosis of onychogryphosis of both first toenails was made by the podiatrist. The clinical signs and history of this particular case match those of the description of onychogryphosis above. It is possible that the single traumatic event was

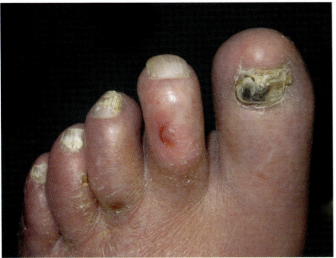

**Figure 11.1** Onychomycosis/onychauxis and superficial digital ulceration.

the nail surgery that Mr E underwent a few years ago. An unfortunate iatrogenic outcome of a total nail avulsion procedure is occasionally deformity of the nail plate resulting from damage to the nail bed and matrix during surgery or the postoperative period.

All the other nails on both feet were thickened and yellow in colour. The differential diagnosis for this could be one or more of a number of conditions: yellow nails syndrome, onychomycosis and onychogryphosis (Figure 11.1). It is not uncommon for two nail pathologies to coexist in older people. Using this case as a specific example, Mr E has chronic venous insufficiency (see below), which is a known aetiology for the thickening and discoloration of toe nails. The primary reason for the referral of Mr E for podiatry care is his inability to reach his feet to cut his nails. This being the case, it could also be speculated reasonably that he may encounter difficulties with foot hygiene. Therefore, in a limb that already has a compromised circulation and consequent alterations in the nail structure the susceptibility for the nail tissue to contract a fungal infection is increased.

Maceration of the skin occurs when the normal regulation of skin water content is disturbed. This may be intrinsic, because of excessive sweating, or extrinsic, when evaporation of moisture cannot take place, for example where the toes are crowded together because of deformity or footwear and/or oedema as in Mr E's case of interdigital maceration (Box 11.2). In addition, older patients sometimes find it difficult to carry out usual foot hygiene and fail to dry properly.

Should the maceration go untreated the skin viability may be compromised, and when subjected to sheer stresses may split to form painful fissures and/or ulceration (Figure 11.2). Once a break in the skin is established there is increased risk of colonisation by bacteria or fungi, and unchecked this may go on to frank infection either as erythrasma, a yeast infection or tinea pedis (see Ch. 24).

A vascular assessment of the lower limbs of Mr E revealed mixed chronic venous and arterial insufficiency (Figure 11.3). This and the condition of the nails, if left untreated for a prolonged amount of time, could potentially affect the soft tissues in the area local to the nail plate.

> **Box 11.2  Condition of the skin on the feet: Mr E (Case study 11.1)**
>
> Closer examination of the skin of the interdigital spaces of all of the toes on both feet reveals damp, soggy, and white-coloured skin (Figure 11.2). Mr E does not report any symptoms associated with these clinical signs.

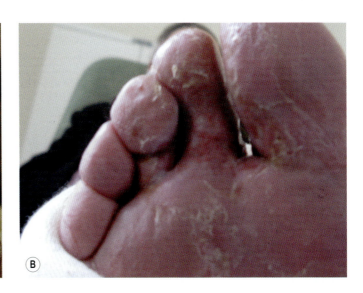

(A)  (B)

**Figure 11.2** (A and B) Interdigital maceration and subsequent ulceration.

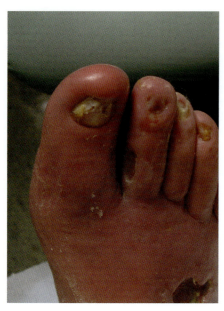

**Figure 11.3** Subungual and periungual ulceration as a result of poor peripheral circulation.

**Table 11.1** Nutritional requirements for ulcer healing

| Nutritional prerequisites for optimal wound healing | Positive effects on ulcer healing |
| --- | --- |
| Carbohydrates | Energy for fibroblast and leucocyte function |
| Protein | Phagocytosis Angiogenesis Collagen synthesis Wound remodelling |
| Vitamin A, C, B12 Complex | Collagen synthesis Macrophage migration Epithelialisation |
| Vitamin K | Clotting cascade |
| Zinc Manganese Copper Magnesium | Cell division Epithelialisation Collagen strengthening |

The soft tissue subungual to the nail may be subjected to increased levels of trauma as a result of the thickened nail plate. With time, this could lead to the formation of a subungual heloma. An evaluation of the footwear along with an examination of the structure and function of the foot may reveal deformities (in the forefoot in particular, such as hyperextension of the hallux in hallux limitus/rigidus and overlapping of the toes in hallux abducto valgus) that would compound the existing pressures already being applied to the soft tissues due to the nail. These are also aetiological factors for the accumulation and impaction of desquamated keratotic tissue and heloma formation in the nail sulci (onychophosis).

In a patient with no PVD and good integrity of the skin, the development of heloma as described above is a common finding. However, in the case of the older lower limb with PVD as a manifestation of the aging process or the secondary complications of systemic disease, the skin's response to the excessive mechanical pressure outlined above is quite different. In this case the GP referral letter already mentions the fact that there are issues regarding impaired venous drainage, chronic venous leg ulcers and poor peripheral arterial supply. The key clinical feature to note is the marked bilateral oedema. The colour and texture of the skin around the feet and ankles display a ruddy cyanotic hue and anhidrotic and trophic changes. These fragile physical features increase the risk of the development of ulceration.

The soft tissues surrounding the nail plate, or indeed below the nail plate, may become inflamed in response to trauma (i.e. *paronychia* and *onychia*). The trauma could be one single event that can render the tissues susceptible to bacterial colonisation. In the older foot this is of significance as systems intrinsic to the host add to the risk of opportunistic infections, consequently introducing a risk of cellulitis and tissue breakdown and, if untreated, ulceration and bacteraemia. A further consequence of repeated minor trauma or undue pressure to a thickened toenail from footwear may be a non-infected subungual breakdown of tissue and a consequent subungual ulceration. To prevent such a condition from occurring, the podiatrist must ensure that the thickened nail is skilfully reduced.

## RISK FACTORS ASSOCIATED WITH THE DEVELOPMENT OF ULCERATION IN THE FEET AND LEGS

The prevalence of venous leg ulcers is reported to range between 0.15% and 0.8% (Callum et al 1986, Cromwell et al 1985). Approximately 20% of patients experience recurrence of the ulcer (Cullum et al 1985). The financial cost of this condition totals £400 million per annum (Bosanquet et al 1993). The cost to the quality of life, however, such as pain, immobility and social isolation leading to depression (see Case study 11.2), is arguably a greater burden.

Considering the nature of the systemic effects in terms of ageing and pathology, Mr E has had a myocardial infarction, is hypertensive, and has hyperlipidaemia and hypothyroidism. The first three conditions form part of the group of multifactorial aetiologies of arterial disease. Part of the vascular assessment revealed the ankle–brachial index to be < 0.6. The pedal pulses were not palpable due to the marked oedema. Doppler assessment followed by a resting period of 20 minutes to assess the degree of ischaemia is recommended (Cullum & Roe 1995).

Venous hypertension leads to capillary distortion and increased capillary permeability. This leads to the classic signs of haemosiderin deposits that can then irritate the skin, causing venous eczema. The increased vessel permeability allows red blood cells to leak into the adjacent skin tissues and often results, over time, in the skin developing a fibrous, woody texture. This atrophied skin acts a barrier to the removal of waste products from the system. Lipid leakage into the skin (lipodermatosclerosis) adds to the fibrotic nature of the skin.

### Health professionals involved in multidisciplinary care

#### Dietician

Protein in the diet is essential for the facilitation of the biochemical process involved in tissue construction (Table 11.1). Advice regarding a balanced diet is indicated (see also Case study 11.2).

*Note*: Podiatrists are well placed to support the 'healthy eating' messages as part of the 'MOT' engaged in promoting health.

## District nurse

The referral letter has already stated the involvement of the district nurse regarding the regular assessment and dressing of the ulcers.

Toe-to-knee, class 2, compression stockings (Moffatt & O'Hare 1995) are often recommended for venous incompetence. When provided they should be renewed and replaced every 3 months to ensure compression consistency. A Doppler assessment would be helpful to ensure that a reduction in hydrostatic pressures is being achieved. However, the PVD experienced by this patient should indicate a cautious approach to this course of action.

## Vascular specialist

It is essential that all members of the team are aware of the results of the regular monitoring of the progression of the PVD. The vascular status of the limb will have an impact on the development of several of the pathologies mentioned already in this section. A difficulty that remains is the lack of a common case record available to all members of the health team working with Mr E. All the medical issues were addressed by the multidisciplinary team in Mr E's case. However, the gold-standard treatment for venous insufficiency and peripheral oedema, which is the application of compression bandaging and/or the use of compression hosiery, was contraindicated for Mr E because of the peripheral ischaemia.

Podiatric treatment is in this case relatively straightforward, comprising careful and skilful reduction of the thickened toenails, advice regarding the most suitable footwear and care of the skin. Of great importance is the need for careful baseline measures to be determined, against which ongoing assessment can be made to note any changes that warrant referral to medical colleagues. In this case, Mr E is seeing the district nurse for the treatment of the venous ulceration, which extends from the dorsal aspect of his foot to the proximal aspect of his leg ulceration, thus requiring toe to knee bandages.

Despite the apparently straightforward podiatric intervention there are a number of other areas highlighted in the referral that are of concern. As a member of the healthcare team, holistic management provides the best opportunities for optimal outcome benefits for the patient. The podiatrist has a responsibility to monitor all aspects of the patient's care and to refer appropriately depending on the need. The management of the patient may include monitoring certain aspects of the patient's care that the podiatrist had not been directly involved in. Nevertheless, good communication with all members of the multidisciplinary team is essential.

The next section deals with some of these areas of holistic care.

## MUSCULOSKELETAL CHANGES

Podiatrists are often involved with the multidisciplinary care of a patient and may liaise with a number of healthcare professionals, and Mr E's case is no exception. Perhaps before analysing what the management may be for Mr E (Box 11.3), it would be beneficial to review the changes that may occur as soft tissues age.

There are a number of physiological changes that occur as a normal consequence of the ageing process. Some of these changes may have a detrimental effect, contributing to the decline in daily activity levels experienced by many older people. These include changes to the integumentary system (see the section on nail conditions, above, and Chs 2 and 3), peripheral vascular system (see the section on vascular assessment, above) and musculoskeletal system (see below and Ch. 8).

---

**Box 11.3 An holistic approach to patient care Mr E (Case study 11.1)**

When Mr E first attended the clinic it was quite obvious that he was experiencing mobility problems. He was initially reluctant to engage with suggestions from members of the clinical team about this. Once his resistance was realised, the clinicians did not pursue this.

Over time, Mr E disclosed more about himself and we were able to engage in conversation regarding his home self-care arrangements. Eventually, Mr E began to see the positive outcomes to some of the interventions provided by podiatry, and he was more willing to accept further suggestions of modifications that could be made to improve his lifestyle.

See the comments on the psychosocial aspects of management in other sections in this chapter.

---

## Muscle tissue

Age-related change in muscle fibre mass is known as sarcopenia, or senile sarcopenia in older adults. This simply relates to the loss of muscle mass that occurs in older people. This loss is related to both the number of muscle fibres and the muscle fibre type. Muscle fibre type is determined by the contractile property of the fibre. Type I fibres, also known as slow twitch fibres, contract more slowly and for longer periods than type II fibres. Type II fibres, also known as fast twitch fibres, contract more quickly but for shorter periods of time.

Slow-twitch, type I muscle fibres are more efficient at using oxygen to generate more fuel (known as ATP) for continuous, extended muscle contractions over a long time. They fire more slowly than fast-twitch fibres and can work for a long time before they fatigue.

Because fast-twitch fibres use the body's metabolism to create fuel, they are much better at generating short bursts of strength or speed than are the slow-twitch muscles. However, they fatigue more quickly.

Muscle mass reduction is thought to decrease by approximately 40% between the ages of 20 and 60 years (Porter et al. 1995), and the maximum contractile strength in both the proximal and the distal muscles. is thought to decrease by 20–40% for both men and women in advancing age (Doherty 2003).

Research suggests that fibre type may have a part to play in both strength and mass reduction in older people. Histological data can help provide a basis for explaining old-age muscle atrophy. A number of studies have confirmed that type II fibre size diminishes as ageing occurs, and some report this to begin as early as 25 years of age. Type II fibre size is thought to reduce from by 20–50%. Type I fibre size appears to be affected much less by the ageing process. (Doherty 2003, Larsson et al 1978, Lexell et al 1988, Roos et al 1997). Furthermore, muscle fibre numbers are also thought to change significantly over time. Lexell and Taylor (1991) conducted a study on whole-muscle cross-sections from the vastus lateralis obtained after postmortem examination, and found that there were 50% fewer type I and type II fibres by the ninth decade of life compared to muscles of a younger population.

In cases where comorbidities and reduced activity levels coexist, the rate at which sarcopenia occurs is thought to increase significantly. (Roubenoff 2000). An advanced rate of sarcopenia will affect muscle strength and thus inevitably a range of activities of daily living (e.g. to climb stairs safely). A resultant reduction in the ambulatory status of the patient may ensue, increasing the frailty of the older person.

## Tendon and ligament

Tendons are composed of mostly collagen, some elastin and a matrix of proteoglycans and mucopolysaccharides in a gel substance. The main function of tendons is to transmit muscle force to the skeletal system. Tendons must be able to withstand significant force, while also adapting to surface structures. This is achieved through the tissue types involved. Collagen gives the tensile strength to the tendon structure, while elastin gives flexibility. This combined function maintains the integrity of the tendon function.

Collagen type I is the main type of collagen present in tendons and ligaments. The building block of collagen type I is the tropocollagen module. Tropocollagen is synthesised by the tenoblast, a type of fibroblast, specially differentiated for collagen formation. The tropocollagen molecule is formed of three helical chains of polypeptides. Four of the tropocollagen molecules form a tendon fibril. As ageing occurs there is an innate process that occurs at a cellular level in the functioning tendon unit.

It is thought that there is a general decline in older age in the number of tenocytes present in older age, and therefore the reparative process may take longer. In addition, there is a general decrease in the organelle content of cells, and it is thought that there is in particular a decrease in the number of protein-synthesising organelles such as endoplasmic reticulum. There is thought to be a general reduction in the capillaries per unit surface area, which during senescence leads to a relative loss of blood flow to the area. This produces tissue hypoxia, lack of nutrition and a decrease in metabolic activity.

These are thought to be some of the main reasons why older people may start to present with soft-tissue symptoms such as tendinosis, particularly where tendons are primarily adapted for weight-bearing activity, such as in the lower extremity. Research has demonstrated that some tendons, such as the posterior tibial tendon, are more susceptible to damage in the older age group.

## Management of change

A number of studies confirm that with inactivity muscle atrophies and its mass reduces, which may ultimately put the patient at risk as a result of muscle-strength decline (Evans 2002, Porter et al 1995, Roubenoff 1989). There is clear evidence that exercise and muscle-strengthening programmes prescribed to older people can have a significantly positive effect on muscle strength (Doherty 2003, Evans 1995, 2002, Roubenoff 2000).

The available information on muscle strength specifically related to the foot is scarce. However, there have been two studies that have both reported similar findings. Endo et al (2002) measured how much force was applied to the toes while leaning forward as far as possible. They found that there are significant differences in toe muscle strength (calculated using a force plate) between age groups, with the younger group showing a 27% muscle strength advantage. Unfortunately, this study was not able to specifically report on muscle strength generated by lesser toe function. This is a significant limitation, as the anatomical functioning of the first toe is distinctly different to the anatomical structures required for lesser toe function. However, the second study, by Menz et al (2006b) used a different protocol and was able to isolate the lesser toes from the first toes, although their findings were similar.

Menz et al (2006b) used a modified paper-grip test and a pressure-sensing system in two groups of subjects: an older group and a younger group. They found that there was a 32% reduction in the muscle strength of the hallux and a 29% reduction for the lesser toes in the older people studied, compared to the younger group. The added benefit of the methodology developed by Menz et al (2006b) is three-fold. It presents a way to assess toe strength in older people

that could easily be used in a clinical setting; it is able to distinguish between the toes and the hallux strength; and it assesses the patient in a seated position, and therefore does not suffer from the balance variable, which is often diminished in the older age group and was not accounted for in the study by Endo et al (2002).

Toe function has an important role to play during the propulsive phase of gait to help resist ground reaction forces and to stabilise the foot against the ground (Bojsen-Møller & Lamourex 1979 Hughes et al 1990, 1979, Mann & Hagy 1979). Until relatively recently, there has been a paucity of available information to confirm the link between toe function and balance. Balance is a significant risk factor for falls (NICE 2004). Recent evidence suggests careful attention should be given to foot assessment when screening patients for balance deficits. Menz et al (2006a) conducted one of the few studies to explore whether foot characteristics are significant determinants of balance and functional ability in older people. The results demonstrated that lesser toe functional strength and ankle flexibility were significantly and consistently associated with performance on functional balance tests. Ankle joint flexibility had previously shown good reliability (Menz et al 2003). Where subjects failed the functional balance tests they also failed the toe strength and ankle flexibility tests. The results indicate that foot and ankle characteristics are significantly related to balance and functional ability in older people.

Nutritional intake of proteins and vitamins, particularly vitamin C, is also thought to be important, and a lack can have significant detrimental effects on muscle, tendon and general soft-tissue synthesis (see box 11.12, and the section on malnutrition in Case study 11.2). Research has shown that additional protein intake by way of supplements may have a positive benefit on muscle mass. In the study by Meredith et al (1992), subjects undertook a 12-week exercise programme, and in addition half the participants were given a calorie-enhancing protein drink that added approximately 550 calories/day. Computerised tomography measurements of midthigh substance revealed that the group that received the calorie supplement had significantly increased muscle mass, indicating that muscle hypertrophy may be increased by the use of dietary supplements.

In addition to maintaining adequate nutrition in order to maintain protein and collagen synthesis, other external factors can also promote increases in both muscle bulk and strength. Fiatarone et al (1994) reported that older people demonstrated a significant increase in muscle bulk and strength following a progressive muscle-resistance exercise training programme. There were added benefits to doing this that were not anticipated at the beginning of the study. These included a spontaneous increase in activity levels, and some of the participants who walked with the aid of a walker were able to be mobile with the use of a walking stick only after the study. Importantly, gait velocity increased, as did general daily activities, stair-climbing power and balance. So even though muscle strength did not increase overall, activity did. This suggests that exercise and correct nutrition in older people may help prevent the adverse effects of senescent sarcopenia, even if a direct impact on strength is not achieved immediately. Although the cause of sarcopenia is multifactorial, strength training represents a consistently and easily implemented way in which to augment, restore and slow down loss of muscle mass and strength in older people (Evans 2002).

From this information a picture is emerging regarding Mr E and his vulnerability. It is clear to see that there are a number of factors that are putting Mr E at risk of a further decline in his mobility. The fact that his PVD prevents him from exerting himself, and that he has significant osteoarthritic changes, means that he is unable to exercise as much as may be considered optimal, and as such is likely to be losing muscle strength and mass. In addition, he lives alone, and this in combination with his decline in mobility may lead to social isolation (see Case study 11.2). Social isolation may have implications for his self-efficacy, which may affect other areas of his well-being such as nutritional status and mental health, as well his overall confidence. All these factors have implications for patients who are at risk of falling, and in the case of Mr E have no doubt been compounded and exacerbated by his history of falls.

## FALLS IN OLDER PEOPLE

Falls in older people are a major public health concern, and the associated financial burden to the tax payer and the NHS is considerable. Research indicates that approximately 647 721 people aged 60 years and over are admitted every year to A&E departments in England for fall-related injuries, and there are 204 424 admissions to hospital for fall-related injuries in the same age group in the UK (NICE 2004). The cost per 10 000 of the population for this amounts to approximately £300 000 for the age group 60–64 years, and increases to an astonishing £1.5 million for those aged 75 years and over. The total cost to the government for falls in the UK is almost £1 billion pounds, 59% of this cost being incurred by the NHS and the remaining 41% being incurred by social services (Scuffham 2003).

Throughout this section the key features and falls risk factors that the podiatrist needs to be aware of when assessing, diagnosing and managing older people will be explored.

### Risk factors associated with falls

Although a large number of older people do fall, this is not an inevitable consequence of ageing. It is the identification of risk and the subsequent management of risk factors that can help in falls prevention.

One of the problems associated with monitoring the number of older people falling is the under-reporting of non-injurious falls. However, a non-injurious fall is often a precursor to a more serious injurious fall, and can often lead to psychological sequelae, such as a fear of further falls, and thus to restricted mobility and social isolation, which in turn lead to further risk of falling (O'Loughlin et al 1993). The National Service Framework for Older People (DoH 2001) clearly identifies key areas of risk for falls. These may be intrinsic (e.g. systemic disease) and/or extrinsic (e.g. surrounding environment). For the purposes of referring to these guidelines, an older person is defined as anyone over the age of 65 years. Risk factors identified in the NICE guidelines include poor balance, visual impairment, Parkinsonism, stroke, gait abnormalities, use of assistive devices, depression, cognitive impairment, environmental factors, mobility impairment/reduced activity, polypharmacy, muscle weakness, low body mass, arthritis, impaired activities of daily living and high alcohol consumption (NICE 2004).

From the information we have for Mr E (Box 11.4), it is clear that he demonstrates multiple risk factors for falls, and would therefore require a multidisciplinary assessment by the falls-prevention team. Mr E's struggle to rise from the chair may be a sign of muscle weakness and/or subsequent loss of mobility, both of which are key risk factors. There is convincing evidence that muscle strength programmes are effective at reducing falls. Overall, the evidence suggests that strengthening exercises not only have a positive benefit to the patient in reducing the number of falls, but also by following an exercise programme, and thus maintaining muscle strength, there is the additional indirect benefit that the individual is able to avoid the unwanted consequences that muscle weakness may bring, such as loss of general mobility, loss of balance and loss of confidence.

A useful indicator of whether a patient may be at risk of falls through motor-strength deficits affecting mobility is the 'get up and

> **Box 11.4 Mobility issues and risk factors for falls: Mr E (Case study 11.1)**
>
> Mr E presented at the clinic using a Zimmer frame to help him mobilise. When he was called from the waiting area it was noted that he struggled to rise from the chair. Eventually, he was able to shuffle forward on the chair and, by moving his centre of force forward, to lift his body weight from the chair and use his Zimmer frame to provide balance, before attempting to walk. He was observed walking with a shuffling, apropulsive gait; he was unable to achieve full knee extension due to his bilateral knee replacements. He had a noticeable limb-length discrepancy, which was later confirmed to be the result of his hip replacement and the osteoarthritis in his other hip. He was wearing his house slippers, which had been slit longitudinally on the dorsal aspect to the elastic, which had become too tight across his foot due to his significant oedema. However, this modification to the slippers resulted in him struggling to keep them in place and fastened whilst walking.

go' test. This simple test does not require any specific training and has been shown to be a useful indicator of functional ability (Podsiadlo & Richardson 1991). The test involves asking the patient to rise from a seated position, walk a specified distance, turn, return to the chair and sit down. A modified version has also been shown to have good sensitivity in predicting falls in community-dwelling older people (Giné-Garriga et al 2009).

The second risk factor that Mr E presents with is his footwear (Figure 11.4). He is wearing his house slippers for all his weight-bearing activity. Mr E has modified the slippers in such a way that they are no longer effective at providing any support, and they are, in fact, more of a hazard than a benefit. Inadequate footwear and poorly fitting slippers are a major concern in any group of patients. However, for an older person the risk of wearing such footwear is undoubtedly increased. Although the link with falls and footwear is not well documented, there is a general consensus that inadequate footwear does have a negative impact on the mobility of older people.

Menant et al (2008) have reviewed the literature in this area and have confirmed that footwear is influential in balance control, and therefore also influences the risk of slips, trips and falls. Shoe style is also thought to be a significant factor. In a prospective study, Gabell et al (1985) concluded footwear to be a major contributory factor in falls. This research revealed that elevated heel height, heavy boots or boots with a cut-away heel were associated with the most significant risks for slips, trips and falls. Similarly, Tencer et al (2004) found that certain measurable properties had a significant impact on falls in older people. They found that in the 61% of falls that occurred outdoors, heel heights of 2.5 cm or more increased the risk of falls as compared with trainer-style shoes.

The fact that Mr E was wearing slippers for all his activities is significant. The evidence suggests that for patients who are at risk of falls their chances of falling are increased by wearing slippers. An investigation into the footwear worn at the time of a falls-related hip fracture revealed that slippers were the most prevalent shoe style. Furthermore, subjects who tripped were more likely to be wearing shoes or slippers with no fastenings, and the most common type of footwear without fastenings was slippers, followed by court shoes (Sherrington & Menz 2003). Another study found that risk of falling was associated with wearing socks or walking around the house barefoot. The authors concluded that older people should be advised to wear shoes indoors (Menz et al 2006).

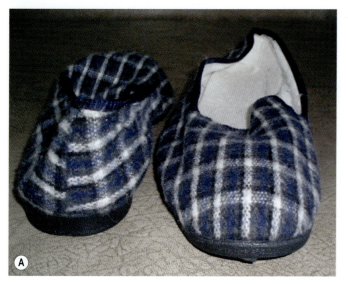
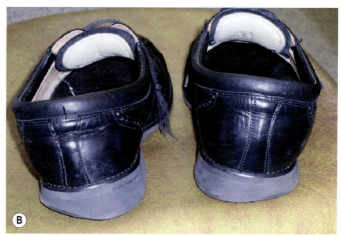

Figure 11.4 Inappropriate footwear often worn by vulnerable older people, causing a falls hazard. (Reproduced courtesy of Jayne Evans, Lead Podiatrist Rehabilitation, Stockburn Memorial Home, Kettering, with permission.)

## What is the ideal footwear style for an older person?

There are a number of footwear companies in the UK, and undoubtedly worldwide, that can provide suitable shoes, at a fraction of the cost of a bespoke shoe, which can usually meet the needs of this patient group (e.g. extra-width and extra-depth shoes).

The evidence for optimal footwear style and design characteristics advice is limited for this group of patients. The evidence suggests that the tread of the sole of the shoe may be a key feature to consider in order to enhance safety. Another is the heel height, which has two likely effects. Firstly, the heel height may influence stability, and certainly this has been evidenced in the literature. Secondly, a lower heel height offers greater ground contact (Menant et al 2008, Menz et al 2001, 2006).

Munro and Steele (1999) suggest that a shoe should comprise a non-uniform sole pattern that offers good friction when worn on walking surfaces typical of the older person's environment. In balance tests carried out in older men it was concluded that optimal stability could be obtained with thin, hard-soled shoes and that trainer-style shoes should be avoided, particularly for those individuals at a high risk for falls. A soft midsole was found to decrease stability, as was a thick midsole. (Robbins et al 1993) However, in a more recent study on a larger population that monitored the falls history of patients over a 2-year period, it was found that athletic shoes to be associated with the lowest risk of falls. This perhaps is linked to the fact that falls are multifaceted events and should be assessed on a variable scale. Conversely, the same study found that going barefoot or in stocking feet increased the risk of falling even after controlling for other factors. Relative to the athletic shoe, other styles of footwear demonstrated a 1.3-fold increase in the risk of falling. Part of the reason for these findings was thought to be connected with the slip resistance of the sole of the shoe.

Menz et al (2001) confirmed that the coefficient of friction (a measure of the friction of materials under controlled conditions) was greatest in men's Oxford-type shoes, and this coefficient was significantly lower for women's fashion shoes. However, none of the shoes tested showed good slip resistance under wet conditions. The authors suggest that a safety standard should be adopted due to the suboptimal performance of the test shoes in wet conditions. Further research suggests that older people do not base their footwear selection on the

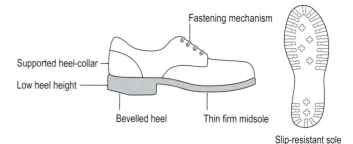

Figure 11.5 Recommended characteristics of shoe style for older people (Menant et al 2008).

premise of safety but rather base their choices entirely on comfort. However, a shoe that is deemed most comfortable has been associated with a shoe that gives a high balance failure rate (Robbins et al 1993). From this it would seem that footwear choice is anything but straightforward, and perhaps help needs to be made available to assist older people to make appropriate footwear choices. This advice needs to take into account the holistic picture of individual circumstances and may include environmental factors and psychosocial factors (see Case study 11.2) as well as medical and surgical history, personal circumstances, in addition to the myriad of other potential risk factors that have be described elsewhere in this section.

The advice given to Mr E regarding his footwear consisted of purchasing new footwear with a soft, giving material for the upper. This was mainly to accommodate the dorsal ulceration and oedematous feet. In addition, the shoe needs to have a secure fastening, and in this case advice was given to purchase a shoe with a Velcro fastening, for two reasons. Firstly, Mr E's oedematous feet fluctuated in size depending on the time of day, and obviously his dorsal foot ulceration was a concern. Secondly, although Mr E had assistance from carers twice daily, he often needed to manage shoeing and unshoeing himself. This was another reason why he had chosen to modify his slippers. Figure 11.5 depicts some of the positive shoe characteristics suggested by Menant et al (2008) that may help prevent falls in older people resulting from inadequate footwear.

Mr E has not complained of balance problems. However, given that he has recently become less mobile, walks with the aid of a Zimmer

> **Box 11.5 Polypharmacy: Mr E (Case study 11.1)**
>
> Taking a pharmacological history revealed that Mr E was taking multiple medications for several different conditions (see Case study 11.1). He took his medications via a dosing system, set up with the local pharmacy. The carers that visited him daily to help with washing and dressing and meal preparation, also assisted him with taking his medication.

> **Box 11.6 Social isolation affecting day to day well being Mr E (Case study 11.1)**
>
> Mr E has found that, while he has felt much better since his medication has been reviewed and modified, he feels that he has lost confidence and spends much of his day in the house. He does have a motorised scooter that he uses for his shopping and trips into town, but he uses this less and less as he feels unstable when manoeuvring himself into the seat. He also experiences occasional dizziness on standing, and is worried that if he was out alone he would fall or faint.
>
> As a consequence, Mr E feels that he is becoming more socially isolated. He no longer sees his regular shopping friends on his weekly trip to the supermarket. He used to have coffee with them afterwards. He now feels that he would be a burden on them and they may not be interested in his conversation, as the majority of it revolves around his ailments! His osteoarthritis prevents him from doing much gardening any more and his daughter has now enlisted the help of a gardener. While this provides some interaction for Mr E, he also says it makes him feel sad, as it forces him to recognise that he is getting older (see Case study 11.2).

frame and is currently taking a combination of medications, the implications for balance deficits are increased.

## POLYPHARMACY

Polypharmacy is defined as taking multiple medications, specifically as taking four or more medications a day or taking four or more medications simultaneously (Box 11.5). NICE (2004) reports that patients taking more than three or four medications are at risk of recurrent falls. However, the probability of an individual receiving a risk-increasing drug has been postulated as being a precipitating factor in the increased incidence of falls in older people, rather than the polypharmacy itself (Ziere et al 2006).

A population-based study examined the use of multiple drug use and falls in the elderly. Data were collected from 6928 individuals aged ≥55 years. Whilst the study did find that the interaction between drugs and the probability that one of the multiple drugs was a fall-increasing drug was significant, it also found that the risk of falling increased significantly with an increasing number of drugs, and after adjustments in the analysis for comorbidities, polypharmacy remained a significant risk factor for falls. However, certain drugs are thought to be risk-increasing drugs, and should be considered as part of a falls risk assessment. Such drugs include sulfonamides and potassium-sparing diuretics, hypnotics, calcium preparations, central-acting obesity products and bioflavonoids. In fact, a total of 28 drugs are thought to be associated with a higher incidence of falling in this group of patients (Ziere et al 2006).

Comorbidities, and in particular long-term conditions, have been cited as a problem for this group of vulnerable adults.

### Long-term disease and older people

In the case of Mr E there are a number of pathologies affecting his day-to-day well-being (Box 11.6). At least three of these have been associated with falls. Hypertension, cardiovascular problems and osteoarthritis have all been associated with increased risk of falls (Lawlor et al 2003).

Lawlor et al (2003) found significant increased risk factors for falls with the number of chronic diseases present. In total 4050 women over 60 years old from 23 GP practices in the UK were studied. The findings suggest that, while there may be pharmacological reasons why people are falling, the fact that this group of people also tend to present with comorbidities may be more significant than the drugs that are used in their treatment.

The study found that, for fully adjusted population statistics, the attributable risk of falls when one chronic disease was present was 32%. There was a significant linear trend of increasing odds of falling with increasing number of chronic diseases. The analysis examined the chronic disease status and the history of falls. There were significant differences found in the women who had a history of at least one fall in the preceding year. Circulatory disease, chronic obstructive pulmonary disease, depression and arthritis were each associated with higher odds of falling, even with adjustment for drug use and other potential confounding factors. The population attributable risk of having had at least one fall in the previous 12 months, estimated from the fully adjusted models, was 6.2% (2.0–10.0%) for coronary heart disease, 6.2% (1.6–10.5%) for circulatory disease, 8.0% (3.3–12.4%) for chronic obstructive pulmonary disease, 9.4% (5.4–13.3%) for depression and 17.4% (10.4–23.9%) for arthritis. The fully adjusted odds ratio of having had a fall in the previous 12 months associated with having at least one of the chronic diseases was 32%.

The study concludes that polypharmacy on its own may not fully explain the higher risk of falling. Chronic disease brings its own set of risk factors, and the two topics are closely related, as the number of medications taken may well increase with the number of chronic diseases, but in some cases it may be the effects of the chronic disease profile itself that is the main risk factor.

A number of Department of Health publications(DoH 2004, 2008a,b) have acknowledged the impact that chronic conditions have on the older population. It is estimated that 15.4 million, or 1 in 3, of the population in England suffer from a long-term condition. Three out of every five people over 60 years old in England suffer from a long-term condition, and due to the ageing population the number of people with a long-term condition is set to rise by 23% (DoH 2008a). This information suggests that Mr E may not be unusual in having three long-term conditions to contend with.

## QUALITY OF LIFE

Osteoarthritis is likely to impact Mr E's activities of daily living (ADLs). Mr A has generalised large-joint osteoarthritis, and this affects his hips, knees and some of the smaller joints in his periphery, including his first metatarsophalangeal joint. His circulatory problems are significant.

Osteoarthritis is a commonly presenting condition for this age group, and knee and hip osteoarthritis are thought to have a significant impact on day-to-day mobility. Large cross-sectional studies have confirmed that large-joint osteoarthritis, present either as a single

---

**Box 11.7 Activities of daily living: Mr E (Case study 11.1)**

Mr E reported no problems with higher functional tasks such as using the telephone, meal preparation or writing his shopping list for the carers, or with basic self-care such as eating and toileting. However, Mr E spends much of his day alone and finds it difficult mobilising, and this has significance especially for his self-efficacy, confidence and long-term ability to maintain independent living.

Mr E confirmed at assessment that the main areas that he found difficulty with were walking any distance, bending to put on and do up his shoes and buttoning up his shirts. Occasionally, due to the shoulder pain caused by his arthritis, he found it difficult to get things down from the top cupboards in the kitchen. His carers have rearranged his food storage to account for this.

Due to his peripheral vascular disease and his venous leg ulceration, and more recently his mixed arterial and vascular tissue breakdown affecting both feet, both interdigitally and on the dorsum, he is finding it increasingly painful to mobilise. The pain adds to his disability, further restricting his daily activities.

---

morbidity or paired with a second condition (comorbidity), increases disability (Boyd et al 2005, Fried et al 1999, Vogeli et al 2007). The effects can range from difficulty getting dressed to mobilising and reaching kitchen cupboards (Box 11.7).

Fried et al (1999) conducted a large cross-sectional study looking into the association of comorbidities and disabilities in older women. Research has already confirmed that osteoarthritis has a significant effect on mobility, and when this is combined with other comorbidities there is a greater risk of mobility and transfer difficulty, ultimately affecting ADLs (Ettinger et al 1994a). Fried et al (1999) used pairing of the original 14 chronic diseases studied. A self-reported, interviewer-administered questionnaire assessed the level of disability, and the findings were grouped into different areas of disability. Statistical analysis revealed that there was a much higher incidence of disability when more than one chronic disease was present. The results show a high incidence of chronic disease, with an average of three diseases per subject. Eighty-one per cent reported two or more chronic conditions. This figure is echoed in more recent research, where an estimated 62% of Americans over the age of 65 years have multiple chronic conditions (Vogeli et al 2007).

Fried et al (1999) reported that 50% of their study group reported difficulty with mobility, 35% with upper-extremity tasks, 22% with self-care tasks and 22% with higher functioning household tasks. The study also showed that when diseases were paired there was a recurrence with specific pairings that was consistently affecting mobility. These included osteoarthritis and high blood pressure, joint arthritis and visual problems, heart disease and cancer, stroke and high blood pressure, and (ranked eighth) arthritis and hearing impairment.

Mr E is a perfect example of someone who lives independently with a number of chronic conditions, and demonstrates difficulty in a number of areas of daily life affecting his ability to perform and maintain his ADLs. Mr E experiences at least four of the conditions studied, and three of the paired conditions that were reported to significantly affect ADLs, with an increasing likelihood of disability. This highlights the need to raise awareness of all healthcare practitioners to be sensitive to the fact that older people can have a range of related conditions, and it is the combination of these that can have a significant impact on their ability to maintain an independent life of a quality that they deserve.

Mr E is able to continue living independently, with the support of domiciliary carers.

## DUTY OF CARE

Case study 11.2 describes a vulnerable woman (Mrs B) in very different circumstances from Mr E. The consideration of psychosocial, cognitive and other factors is not always associated with the role of a podiatrist. However, the case of Mrs B illustrates how important an holistic approach is to patient care.

---

**CASE STUDY 11.2 MRS B, DATE OF BIRTH 11 OCTOBER 1921**

Consideration of the drug history (Box 11.8) offers indications of Mrs B's general health, which bears out a history of type 2 diabetes and hypertension. In addition, Mrs B takes an antidepressant, calcium carbonate and a vitamin B supplement. Part of the role of the healthcare team looking after the elderly is to ensure the general well-being of all patients, and this duty includes taking the opportunity to enquire about the achievement of the expectations of the drug regimen. Often a discussion about the medication can reveal misunderstandings that can be easily resolved (see the sections on falls and polypharmacy).

The primary podiatric assessment suggests that management in the short term must include nail and skin care. (See Chs 2–5 for a more detailed account of skin and nail disorders and lower-limb vascular disorders.)

---

As part of the multidisciplinary health and social care workforce you are required to act in the best interests of your patient and their carers, and it is the duty of podiatrists to work within the Codes of Conduct for Podiatrists as set out by the Professional Regulator, which in the UK is the Health Professions Council. Most podiatrists are also members of a professional body, and as members are expected to abide by that organisation's code of conduct or ethics. As already noted in the introduction to this chapter, the roles and responsibilities of the podiatrist extend beyond the feet to include concern for a patient's health and well-being in general.

When considering the circumstances of Mrs B there are already a number of clues to suggest that this may be a family approaching a crisis, which becomes clearer following your next visit (Box 11.9).

There are many factors that, either singly or in combination, may result in a fall. The consequences of a fall may be grave, and include loss of consciousness, fracture of any bone, haematoma and skin abrasion. A number of validated programmes are available that seek to prevent falls in older people and, where appropriate, to help them to overcome a fear of falling. The greater challenge is where the individual does not recall a previous fall and does not recognise themselves as being at risk of falling, as is the case with Mrs B.

The greatest challenge for the podiatrist is to guide the patient to deciding to seek help from outside the family. Some older patients may be reluctant to seek help, fearing interference from official agencies or being ignorant of the eligibility criteria for and the nature and extent of services available. Frequently, they declare themselves to be coping adequately. One of the most important responsibilities of the healthcare professional is to provide information to patients and clients in order to improve health, prevent illness and, importantly, enable them to maintain their independence.

Great sensitivity and well-developed communication skills are required when discussing these issues with both patients and their carers, as this sort of information provision may be seen to imply a

Mrs B's daughter, Mrs R, requested an appointment for her mother. Up until recently she has been able to look after her mother's foot health but is now finding it increasingly difficult to cope. She makes a request for a home visit after office hours ,when she is able to be present.

On your first visit you are welcomed by Mrs R, who introduces you to her mother as the podiatrist. It soon becomes clear to you that Mrs B is unsure of the purpose of your visit. Following some discussion, where Mrs B seeks to assure you that she is capable of looking after herself, she is finally persuaded to allow you to examine her feet. During the foot examination, the conversation turns to Mrs B's general health and the circumstances of her life, with much of the detail provided by her daughter. An informal referral for podiatry was made previously following advice from the falls team.

Mrs B's story is a very familiar one for a woman of her generation. She is married to her 91-year-old husband, who is unable to leave his chair without difficulty. She has three surviving children, having lost a daughter in an accident some 10 years before, but only her daughter Mrs R lives locally. It becomes clear that this will be a somewhat protracted visit.

Foot and lower-limb examination reveals bilateral *hallux valgus grade 3* (Figure 11.6), hammer *second toes with clawing of all other lesser toes*. There is evidence of *nail dystrophies* including signs of *onychomycosis* and the presence of *onychauxis*. In addition, there is general anhidrosis and diffuse *callus* over the first, second and third metatarsal heads, and *hard corns* over the proximal interphalangeal joints of both fifth toes. Both ankles and legs are *oedematous*, with extensive discoloration and thickening of the skin. There are also excoriations on the anterior aspect of both legs, and both knees are bruised, and Mrs R tells you that Mrs B fell in her bedroom the week previously, which is why she has a black eye. All pulses are palpable, there is *telangiectasia* and *haemosiderosis* and large tortuous *varicose veins*.

Mrs B has type 2 diabetes and is being treated for hypertension. The only occasion when Mrs B leaves the house is when her daughter is able to arrange time off work to accompany her to the surgery, where her family GP and the Community Service offer her annual screening for her diabetes and a review of her medication. Occasionally, she takes a short walk when her grand daughter visits, but these outings are infrequent at best. Mrs R is able to provide a drug list, and asserts that her father ensures that Mrs B takes her medication.

**Drug list**
Aspirin 75 mg once daily
Metformin 850 mg, 3 times daily
Glicozide 80 mg, once daily
Ferrous sulfate 200 mg, once daily
Atenolol 59 mg, once daily
Felodipine 10 mg, once daily
Indapamide MR 1.5 mg, once daily (a.m.)
Adcal D3 chewable, once daily
Paroxetine hydrochloride 20 mg, once daily
Ibandronic acid 150 mg, once monthly

You return, as arranged, 8 weeks later. Mrs B opens the door to you, is clearly not expecting any callers and does not recognise you. She is using a wheeled walker to assist her in getting about the house. Once again she has bruising on her temple and a black eye, and has obviously fallen again recently, although she denies this.

Mrs B is still in her night clothes and has a pair of cloth slippers on her feet; there is a strong smell of urine on her dressing gown. She complains of being very tired and the house strikes you as cool. Mr B would appear to be still in bed at 2 o'clock in the afternoon.

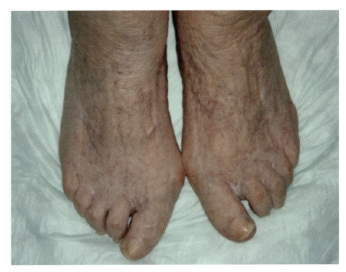

**Figure 11.6** Mrs B HAV grade 3.

## Hypothermia risk

At the second visit by the podiatrist it becomes a concern that Mrs B may be at risk of developing hypothermia (Box 11.9).

Hypothermia occurs when the core (rectal) body temperature falls below 35°C. Should the core temperature fall further, to below 32°C, death is frequently likely to follow. Accidental hypothermia is an unintentional drop in temperature and is suffered by the elderly. Whilst environmental temperature is an obvious cause of hypothermia, significantly low temperatures are not required to precipitate hypothermia in the older individual. It is possible for people suffering from hypothermia to be discovered in bed covered with blankets in a heated room (Woolner & Collins 1992). Most body heat is generated through the normal metabolism of the organs and muscles. Metabolism decreases in the older person; the metabolic rate of those aged over 70 years is estimated to be about half that of a young child (Guyton 1991).

The older individual is particularly susceptible to hypothermia, as there is both a decrease in heat generation and at the same time an increase in heat loss. Generation of heat from muscle activity decreases primarily as a consequence of a 30% reduction in muscle bulk and by a reduction in activity levels by as much as a 50% in people aged 70 years. Other risk factors include inadequate clothing, poor nutrition, depressant drugs, alcohol, or systemic conditions such as hypothyroidism and diabetes. A study by Neil et al (1986) concluded

criticism of a patient's living arrangements and self-care ability. In addition to the statutory agencies, such as the health and social services departments, a number of charities for the elderly and other organisations have helpful leaflets that signpost practical and financial assistance (e.g. Age Concern, Help the Aged, Citizen's Advice Bureau).

that hypothermia was more common in elderly women with diabetes than in the general population, and that 'Diabetes is an important factor to consider when assessing the risk of hypothermia in elderly women, particularly if they are exposed to low environmental temperatures in the home' (Neil et al 1986). Mrs B is consequently at greater risk of hypothermia because of her diabetes, the cool room temperature and her reduced mobility. If suspicion is raised that a patient may be hypothermic, same-day referral to the Social Services is indicated. It is important that re-heating is started immediately by increasing the ambient temperature, with warm drinks and dry clothing and blankets. Although it is Mrs B who is your patient and you have a duty of care for her, it would be wise to reassure yourself that Mr B is not also suffering; alert the family doctor and contact their daughter to explain your actions. If you remain concerned that these first-aid measures are not effective you should consider an emergency admission to hospital by ambulance. A further possible cause of Mrs B's confusion could be dehydration.

## Dehydration

Dehydration is a common finding in the elderly population, both in the community and at the time of hospital admission. The symptoms are insidious and non-specific, and include lassitude, fatigue, muscle cramps and dizziness (due to postural hypotension). Thirst decreases with age and, accompanied by the normal ageing of the kidneys that results in a reduced ability to concentrate urine, the possibility of dehydration is exacerbated. At the same time, urine flow is generally maintained, resulting in further dehydration. Causes of dehydration include multiple medications, especially potent diuretics, antipsychotics, sedatives and non-steroidal anti-inflammatory drugs (NSAIDs). Further risk factors for dehydration include incontinence, lack of mobility, dementia, and consumption of alcohol and caffeine-containing drinks. The possible consequences of dehydration for the elderly are serious; in one American study, 18% of patients whose primary diagnosis on hospital admission was dehydration died within 1 month and a further 30.6% died within 1 year (Warren et al 1994). Even those dehydrated patients who do not die may suffer debilitating medical consequences such as urinary tract infection, bowel obstruction, delirium and cardiovascular symptoms.

Although many of the signs are non-specific there are further key risk factors that should alert the healthcare professional to the possibility of a diagnosis of dehydration. These factors include being female, being over 85 years old, having four or more chronic medical conditions, taking four or more medications, being confined to bed, using laxatives inappropriately and suffering chronic infection (Bennett 2000).

Such patients should be considered at risk of dehydration, and advice should include encouragement to take plenty of water, fruit drinks or non-salty soups. However, you may be suspicious that a patient's failure to recognise you or to recall that an appointment had been arranged may indicate more than confusion resulting from dehydration and hypothermia, but could suggest dementia and depression.

## Dementia and depression

Mental health problems are suffered by 25% of the elderly population, and include depression and anxiety. Dementia affects some 10% of those aged over 65 years, rising to 20% in those over 80 years old. The findings from a systematic review predict that the numbers of affected people will double every 20 years, to 81.1 million worldwide by 2040. In 2009 there are estimated to be 700 000 elderly sufferers of dementia (Ferri et al 2006).

The dementias are a group of diseases defined by clinical cognitive deficits, including memory impairment, an inability to recall previous information or to learn new information, language disturbance (aphasia), impaired ability to carry out motor tasks despite satisfactory motor function (apraxia), failure to recognise and/or identify objects (agnosia), this often in the presence of intact sensory function, and disturbances in executive functioning such as planning and organising.

Any one of these deficits will have a major effect on social and occupational functioning, and will represent a decline from previous functioning. There are many causes of dementia, including metabolic disorders and neurological conditions. However, 70% of cases are due to Alzheimer's disease, which has been described as 'one of the most disabling and burdensome health conditions worldwide' (Ferri et al 2006).

Alzheimer's disease is not only devastating for the individual patient, but also to the family and carers. In addition, there is a considerable cost burden on society for residential care or for support to enable the patient to remain in their own home. Nevertheless, there are encouraging developments in research into the genetic basis of late-onset Alzheimer's disease (Rogaeva et al 2007). In the UK in 2009 the Department of Health launched the Living Well with Dementia Strategy (DoH 2009). The strategy aims to provide 17 key objectives to improve health and social services for both patients and their carers. Linked with dementia is depression. Of the general elderly population 1–4 % has major depression, with twice as many women as men affected ; prevalence and incidence rates double after the age of 70–85 years (Palson et al 2001). The prevalence of minor depression in the elderly is 4–13%. An elderly person is as likely to have depressive symptoms as someone in middle age (8–16%), but a very old person is especially prone to this condition, which may be explained by increasing disability, cognitive impairment, widowhood and a fall in socio-economic status (Blazer 2000). Individuals in residential homes suffer greater rates of all types of depression than the corresponding group who remain living in the community. For a diagnosis of depression to be made, five of the diagnostic characteristics for geriatric depression must be present (Box 11.10).

Symptoms of depression are often present in patients with dementia from all causes. Indeed, depressive syndromes in the elderly are associated with both medical disorders and the side-effects of drug use. Patients who develop sad mood or show diminished interest may have other co-morbidities that are associated with depression, or have pharmacological complications following medication review/ change/ or cessation of medication (Box 11.11):

---

**Box 11.10 Key signs of three types of depressive disorder**

**Dysthymic disorder**

A chronic condition characterised by a sad mood that occurs for most of the day, more days than not, for at least 2 years. The condition is diagnosed if accompanied by two symptoms of major depressive disorder

**Major depressive disorder**

Depressed mood, diminished interest, loss of pleasure in almost all activities, weight loss or gain, insomnia, agitation, fatigue, feelings of worthlessness, inappropriate guilt, recurrent thoughts of death or suicide

**Minor depressive disorder**

At least two of the above symptoms must be present for at least 2 weeks and lead to distress and impaired function that cannot be attributed to a medical condition or bereavement.

**Box 11.11 Some common conditions and drugs associated with depression**

Viral Infection

Endocrine disorders of the thyroid parathyroid adrenal glands

Malignancy, leukaemia, pancreatic cancer

Cerebrovascular disease – e.g. stroke, vascular dementia

Myocardial infarction

Metabolic disorder – malnutrition, vitamin $B_{12}$ deficiency

**Symptoms of depression may emerge within 1 month of commencing or withdrawing from the following medication:**

Antiparkinsonism drugs

Beta blockers

Tamoxifen

Benzodiazepines

Propanolol

Reserpine

Steroids

**Box 11.12 Risk factors for osteoporosis**

- Advanced age
- Low body mass index
- Glucocorticoids
- Rheumatoid arthritis
- Previous low-trauma fracture
- Smoking
- Excessive alcohol consumption
- Parental fracture

The management aims for depression are to reduce distressing symptoms, prevent relapse and improve cognitive function. Importantly, patients should be helped to develop skills to cope with their disability or psychosocial difficulties. A careful assessment and treatment by medical staff of any comorbidity and a review of drug regimens is an important first step in treatment. Coupled with this, both pharmacotherapy and psychotherapy should be considered. Antidepressant drugs such as serotonin selective reuptake inhibitors (SSRIs) have been shown to be effective in this group of patients. Late-life depression is poorly recognised and undertreated, even in the face of evidence to suggest that management outcomes are as successful in the elderly as in younger cohorts. Strategies that include treatments in primary care settings improve outcomes for elderly patients (Alexopoulos 2005).

The symptoms of depression described above include a gradual loss of interest which, when coupled with profound fatigue, may lead to deterioration in motivation to maintain personal hygiene, which often reveals to family and carers that the elderly person may be incontinent.

## Osteoporosis and fracture

Osteoporosis is a major public health issue and the incidence is expected to rise given the ageing of the worldwide population (Cauley et al 2000). The World Health Organization (WHO) has estimated the prevalence of osteoporosis in western women, at any site, as 14.8% in women aged 50–59 years, rising to 70% in women aged 80 years or more (World Health Organization 1994).

Osteoporosis is characterised by low bone mass and deterioration of bone tissue. This is seen on the radiograph as decreased bone density, with thinning of the cortex. There is accentuation of the primary trabeculae and thinning of the secondary trabeculae (McCarthy 2008). This leads to increased bone fragility and increased risk of fracture (Consensus Development Conference 1993). Foot and ankle fractures are among the most common non-spinal fractures occurring in the elderly (Delmas et al 2007). One study found that fracture of the fifth metatarsal was the most common foot fracture, with a prevalence of 56.9%. The incidence of foot fractures was 3.1 per 1000 woman-years (Hasselman et al 2003).

Currently, the diagnosis of osteoporosis is based on the use of dual x-ray absorptiometry (DXA), measured at the hip or spine and defined as a bone mineral density that is 2.5 standard deviations (SD) or more below the average value for a young healthy woman (Hans 2006). Other diagnostic modalities include single-photon or dual-photon absorptiometry (SPA or DPA), which measures bone density in the forearm, and ultrasonography, which may be used to indicate the bone density in the calcaneum (McCarthy 2008).

A new set of WHO diagnostic criteria for osteoporosis, based on a recent analysis of osteoporotic risk factors, will soon be available (Wendling 2006). The use of the new WHO risk factors may enable the diagnosis of osteoporosis to be considered on the basis of these risk factors in the absence of DXA. A list of risk factors for osteoporosis is given in Box 11.12.

An important prospective study of 6174 Swiss women aged 70–85 years has found that the use of diagnostic quantitative ultrasound stiffness index together with four clinical risk factors can identify women at higher risk of osteoporotic fracture. The stiffness index is calculated as a combination of two parameters of bone status at the heel: ultrasound attenuation (in decibels per megahertz) and the speed of sound (in metres per second). The smaller the index, the higher the fracture risks. The four clinical risk factors were older age, history of fracture, recent fall and a failed chair/get up and go test (see earlier in this chapter). The study follow-up period was 2.8 years. The results demonstrated that of the 4710 women who had a higher risk score, 6.1% had an osteoporotic fracture, compared with 1.8% of the 1464women who had a lower risk score (Guessous et al 2008).

This has important relevance for podiatry practice. With an ageing population, many patients seeking podiatry treatment will be of advanced age and may have additional risk factors for osteoporosis. With the use of the WHO diagnostic criteria, podiatrists may be able to identify those patients who may be at high risk of developing osteoporosis and refer them promptly for diagnosis and treatment. This is even more pertinent when there is a suspicion of fracture.

Mrs B takes Adcal to treat her previously diagnosed osteoporosis and reduce the risk of fracture. However, she still has risk factors for falls, and it is apparent from her bruised face that she still suffers from falls.

## Incontinence

Urinary incontinence, or enuresis, is common in the elderly and is distressing and disabling. Patients often complain of being 'caught short' or that they 'can't make it to the loo in time'. The common causes are urinary tract infections, often associated with impaired bladder emptying associated with prostate cancer in men and neuropathic bladder in women. Other causes of incontinence in the older person whose mobility is impaired include potent dieuretics, constipation and infection. Signs and symptoms of infection include a pungent smell, general vague feelings of illness, nocturia and bacteria.

In a sample of 559 subjects aged 65 years and over the prevalence of urinary incontinence was found to be 11.6%. In those 80 years and over the prevalence rose to 21.7%. Those with dementia were more likely to be incontinent than those with normal mental function. In the majority of those aged over 80 years who were incontinent the incontinence was associated with either confusion or a combination of factors. Because incontinent elderly people are commonly frail, with a number of conditions contributing to the disorder, the extent of the disorder needs to be carefully assessed for each patient (Campbell et al 1985).

A quality-of-life study of women with incontinence not surprisingly confirmed that women suffering from all types of urinary incontinence were more socially isolated than those from a comparison group, and that incontinence in women has a detrimental effect on their daily lives and they avoid social contacts (Grimby et al 1993).

## Malnutrition

From age 20 years to age 80 years there is a gradual reduction in the amount of food that people eat (Wakimoto & Block 2001). To eat less food as a response to decreased activity is appropriate. Nevertheless, for the elderly, such a reduction in food intake may place the older person at risk of a pathological weight loss if it is accompanied by the chronic disease known as 'anorexia of ageing' (Wilson & Morley 2003). A major European epidemiological study revealed differing levels of malnutrition in the elderly depending on their living circumstances: prevalence rates for older people living in the community were estimated at 8–13%, for those in nursing homes 19–36% and for those in hospital 30–90% (Raynaud-Simon 2009).

Potter et al (1988) considered mortality rates and body mass index (BMI) across different age ranges and concluded that there is a tripling of mortality in those with a BMI of <18 in the age group 70–79 years as compared with those with the same BMI but aged 20–40 years. Malnutrition in the older population has also been associated with increased hospital stay, discharge destination, infections, gait disorders, falls, fracture pressure sores and poor wound healing (Raynaud-Simon 2009). Objective measures to reach a diagnosis of malnutrition include anthropometry, plasma levels of albumen, weight loss reports and BMI monitoring (Box 11.13).

Any one or combination of the conditions discussed in this section would lead the podiatrist to make a referral to the multidisciplinary health and social-care team.

---

> **Box 11.13 Additional factors that may lead a clinician to suspect the patient may be malnourished (Hanlon et al 2007)**
>
> - Poor oral health, with red seborrhoeic nasolabial folds
> - Lax, pale, dry skin with loss of turgor and pigmented patches
> - Thinning or loss of hair
> - Diminished sensory function
> - Thirst
> - Nocturia
> - Diminished tendon jerks
> - Subnormal body temperature

## CONCLUSION

This chapter has endeavoured to identify some of the issues that must be considered when working with elderly patients. Podiatrists must act as part of the multidisciplinary team and be able to identify warning signs and risk factors that may herald the development of treatable medical problems. Too often in the past health professionals have attributed ill health and disease in the elderly simply to the ageing process, which could be inferred as ageist, and patients have heard the expression from health professionals 'at your age what can you expect'. Older patients deserve careful, holistic assessment across all dimensions of their life, conducted in a sensitive and respectful way and considering their wishes and expectations. The Age Discrimination Act came into force in the UK 2006 primarily to protect older people from enforced retirement, but today is increasingly being used to justify claims for a better deal in health and social care for older people. It was not the intention in this chapter to discuss the foot problems that may affect all the population but perhaps have a higher prevalence in older people, as these are comprehensively dealt with elsewhere. For detailed information of the topics introduced in this chapter, the sources listed in the Further Reading section may be of interest.

## ACKNOWLEDGEMENT

The authors would like to thank Morag McInnes for her assistance in the preparation of this chapter.

---

## REFERENCES

Alexopoulos GS 2005 Depression in the elderly. The Lancet 365:1961.

A Review: Consensus Development Conference: Diagnosis, Prophylaxis and Treatment of osteoporosis. Hong Kong April 1–2 Am J Med Nov 30:95.

Baltes PB, Baltes MM 1990 Successful ageing: perspectives from the behavioural sciences. Cambridge University Press, New York.

Bennett JA 2000 Dehydration: hazards and benefits. Geriatric Nursing 21(2):84–87.

Blazer DG 2000 Psychiatry and the oldest old. American Journal of Psychiatry 157:1915–1924.

Bojsen-Møller F, Lamourex L 1979 Significance of free-dorsiflexion of the toes in walking. Acta Orthopaedica Scandinavica 50(4):471–479.

Bosanquet N, Franks P, Moffatt CJ, et al 1993 Community leg ulcer clinics: cost-effectiveness. Health Trends 25(4):146–148.

Bowling A, Dieppe P 2005 What is successful ageing and who should define it? BMJ 331:1548–1551.

Boyd CM, Darer J, Boult C, et al 2005 Clinical practice guidelines and quality of care for older patients with multiple comorbid

diseases: implications for pay for performance. JAMA 294:716–724.

Campbell AJ, Reinken J, McCosh L 1985 Incontinence in the elderly: prevalence and prognosis. Age and Ageing 14:65–70.

Callam MJ, Ruckley CV, Harper DR, Dale JJ 1985 Chronic ulceration of the leg: extent of the problem and provision of care. British Medical Journal 290:1855–1856.

Callam MJ, Harper DR, Dale JJ, Ruckley CV 1987 Chronic ulcer of the leg: clinical history. British Medical Journal May 294:30.

Cauley JA, Thompson DE, Ensrud KC, Scott JC, Black D 2000 Risk of mortality following clinical fractures. Osteoporosis International 11:556–561.

Cornwall JV, Dore CJ, Lewis JD 1986 Leg ulcers: Epidemiology and aetiology. Br J Surg 73:693–696.

Delmas PD, Marin F, Marcus R, et al 2007 Beyond hip: importance of other nonspinal fractures. American Journal of Medicine 120:381.

DoH 2001 National Service Framework for Older People. National Institute for Clinical Health and Excellence (NICE), London.

DoH 2004 Chronic disease management: a compendium of information. Department of Health, London.

DoH 2008a Ten things you need to know about long term conditions. Department of Health, London. Available at: http://www.dh.gov.uk/en/Healthcare/Longtermconditions/DH_084294.

DoH 2008b Raising the profile of long term conditions care: a compendium of information. Department of Health, London.

DoH 2009 Living Well with Dementia Strategy. Department of Health, London. Available at: http://www.dh.gov.uk/dementia.

Doherty TJ 2003 Invited Review: Aging and sarcopenia. Journal of Applied Physiology 95(4):1717–1727.

Endo M, Ashton-Miller JA, Alexander NB 2002 Effects of age and gender on toe flexor muscle strength. Journal of Gerontology A Biological Sciences and Medical Sciences 57(6):M392–M397.

Ettinger WH, Davis MA, Neuhaus JM, Mallon KP 1994a Long-term physical functioning in persons with knee osteoarthritis from NHANES I: effects of comorbid medical conditions. Journal of Clinical Epidemiology 47(7):809–815.

Evans WJ 2002 Effects of exercise on senescent muscle. Clinical Orthopaedics and Related Research 403:S211–S220.

Fiatarone MA, O'Neill EF, Ryan ND, et al 1994 Exercise training and nutritional supplementation for physical frailty in very elderly people. New England Journal of Medicine 330(25):1769–1775.

Ferri CP, Prince M, Brayne C, et al 2006 Global prevalence of dementia: a Delphi consensus study. The Lancet 366(9503):2112–2117.

Fried LP, Bandeen-Roche K, Kasper JD, et al 1999 Association of comorbidity with disability in older women: The Women's Health and Aging Study. Journal of Clinical Epidemiology 52(1):27–37.

Gabell A, Simons MA, Nayak US 1985 Falls in the healthy elderly: predisposing causes. Ergonomics 28(7):965–975.

Giné-Garriga M, Guerra M, Marí-Dell'Olmo M, et al 2009 Sensitivity of a modified version of the 'timed get up and go' test to predict fall risk in the elderly: a pilot study. Archives of Gerontology and Geriatrics 49(1):60–66.

Grimby A, Milsom I, Molander U, et al 1993 The influence of urinary incontinence on quality of life in women. Age and Ageing 22(2):82–89.

Guessous I, Cornuz J, Ruffieux C, Burckhardt P, Krieg MA 2008 Osteoporotic fracture risk in elderly women: estimation with quantitative heel US and clinical risk factors. Radiology Jul 248(1):179–184.

Guyton AC 1991 Guyton's textbook of medical physiology, 8th edn. Saunders, Philadelphia, PA.

Hanlon P, Byres M, Walker BR, Summerton C 2007 In: Boon NA, Colledge NR, Walker BR, Hunter JAA (eds) Davidson's Principles and Practice of Medicine, 20th edn. Churchill Livingstone, Edinburgh, p. 117.

Hans D, Dargent-Molina P, Schott AM, et al 1996 Ultrasonographic heel measurements to predict hip fracture in elderly women: The EPIDOS prospective study. The Lancet London Aug 24, 348(9026):511–544.

Hasselman CT, Vogt MT, Stone KL, et al 2003 Foot and ankle fractures in elderly white women. Incidence and risk factors. Journal of Bone and Joint Surgery – American Volume 85:820.

Hughes J, Clark P, Klenerman L 1990 The importance of the toes in walking. Journal of Bone and Joint Surgery – British Volume 72B(2):245–251.

Hughes J, Clark P, Linge K, Klenerman L 1993 Nov-Dec A comparison of two studies of the pressure distribution under the feet of normal subjects using different equipment. Foot Ankle 14(9):514–519.

Larsson L 1978 Morphological and functional characteristics of the ageing skeletal muscle in man. A cross-sectional study. Acta Physiologica Scandinavica 457(Suppl):1–36.

Lawlor DA, Patel R, Ebrahim S 2003 Association between falls in elderly women and chronic diseases and drug use: cross sectional study. BMJ 327(7417):712–717.

Lexell J, Taylor CC 1991 Variability in muscle fibre areas in whole human quadriceps muscle: effects of increasing age. Journal of Anatomy 174:239–249.

Lexell J, Taylor CC, Sjöström M 1988 What is the cause of the ageing atrophy? Total number, size and proportion of different fiber types studied in whole vastus lateralis muscle from 15- to 83-year-old men. Journal of the Neurological Sciences 84(2–3):275–294.

Mann RA, Hagy JL 1979 The function of the toes in walking, jogging and running. Clinical Orthopaedics and Related Research 142:24–29.

McCarthy C 2008 Diagnostic imaging. In: Merriman's Assessment of the Lower Limb, Ch. 12. Churchill Livingstone, Edinburgh.

Menant JC, Steele JR, Menz HB, et al 2008 Optimizing footwear for older people at risk of falls. Journal of Rehabilitation Research and Development 45(8):1167–1181.

Menz HB, Lord ST, McIntosh AS 2001 Slip resistance of casual footwear: implications for falls in older adults. Gerontology 47(3):145–149.

Menz HB, Tiedemann A, Mun-San Kwan M, et al 2003 Reliability of clinical tests of foot and ankle characteristics in older people. Journal of the American Podiatric Medicine Association 93(5):380–387.

Menz HB, Morris ME, Lord SR 2006 Footwear characteristics and risk of indoor and outdoor falls in older people. Gerontology 52(3):174–180.

Menz HB, Morris ME, Lord S 2006a Footwear characteristics and risk of indoor and outdoor falls in older people. Gerontology 52:174–180.

Menz HB, Zammit GV, Munteanu S, et al 2006b Plantar flexion strength of the toes: age and gender differences and evaluation of a clinical screening test. Foot & Ankle International 27(12):1103–1108.

Meredith CN, Frontera WR, O'Reilly KP, Evans WJ 1992 Body composition in elderly men: effect of dietary modification during strength training. J Am Geriatr Soc Feb 40(2):155–162.

Moffatt CJ and O'Hare L 1995 Venous leg ulceration: treatment by high compression bandaging. Ostomy/ Care/Wound Management 41(4): 6–8, 20, 22–5.

Munro BJ, Steele JR 1999 Household-shoe wearing and purchasing habits. A survey of people aged 65 years and older. Journal of the American Podiatric Medicine Association 89(10):506–514.

Neil HA, Dawson JA, Baker JE 1986 Risk of hypothermia in elderly patients with diabetes. BMJ (Clinical Research Edition) 293:416–418.

NICE 2004 Clinical practice guideline for the assessment and prevention of falls in older people. Royal College of Nursing, London.

O'Loughlin JL, Robitaille Y, Boivin J-F, Suissa S 1993 Incidence of and risk factors for falls and injurious falls among the community-dwelling elderly. American Journal of Epidemiology 137(3):342–354.

Palson S, Ostling S, Skoog I 2001 The incidence of first onset depression in a population followed from age 70 to 85. Psychology and Medicine 31:613–629.

Podsiadlo D, Richardson S 1991 The timed get up and go test: a basic test of functional mobility for frail elderly persons. Journal of American Geriatric Society 39(2):142–148.

Porter MM, Vandervoort AA, Lexell J 1995 Aging of human muscle: structure, function and adaptability. Scandinavian Journal of Medicine & Science in Sports 5(3):129–142.

Potter JF, Schafer DF, Bohi RL 1988 Hospital mortality as a function of body mass index: an age-dependent variable. Journal of Gerontology 43:M59–M63.

Raynaud-Simon A 2009 Malnutrition in the elderly: epidemiology and consequences. European e-journal of Clinical Nutrition and Metabolism 4:e86–e89.

Robbins S, Gouw GJ, McClaran J et al 1993 Shoe sole thickness and hardness influence balance in older men. Journal of the

American Geriatrics Society 41(9):1011–1012.

Roe BH, Griffiths JM, Kenrick M, Cullum NA, Hutton JL 1994 Nursing treatment of patients with chronic leg ulcers in the community. Journal of Clinical Nursing 3:159–168.

Rogaeva E, Meng Y, Lee JH 2007 The neuronal sortilin-related receptor SORL1 is genetically associated with Alzheimer disease. Nature Genetics 39:168–177.

Roos M, Rice C, Vandervoort AA 1997 Age-related changes in motor unit function. Muscle & Nerve 20(6):679–690.

Roubenoff R 2000 Sarcopenia: a major modifiable cause of frailty in the elderly. Journal of Nutrition, Health and Aging 4(3):140–142.

Rowe JW, Kahn RI 1998 Successful ageing. Pantheon books: New York.

Scuffham P 2003 Incidence and costs of unintentional falls in older people in the United Kingdom. Journal of Epidemiology and Community Health 57(9):740–744.

Sherrington C, Menz HB 2003 An evaluation of footwear worn at the time of fall-related hip fracture. Age and Ageing 32(3):310–314.

Tencer AF, Koepsell TD, Wolf ME, et al 2004 Biomechanical properties of shoes and risk of falls in older adults. Journal of the American Geriatrics Society 52(11):1840–1846.

UK National Statistics 2008. Available at: http://www.statistics.gov.uk

Vogeli C, Shields AE, Todd AL, et al 2007 Multiple chronic conditions: prevalence, health consequences, and implications for quality, care management, and costs. Journal of General Internal Medicine 22(Suppl 3):391–395.

Wakimoto P, Block G 2001 Dietary intake, dietary patterns, and changes with age: an epidemiological perspective. Journal of Gerontology A – Biological Science and Medical Science 56:65–80.

Warren JL, Bacon WE, Harris T, et al 1994 The burden and outcomes associated with dehydration among US elderly. American Journal of Public Health 84:1265–1268.

Wendling P 2006 WHO considers change in osteoporosis criteria. Clinical Endocrinology News 1:13.

Wilson MMG, Morley JE 2003 Invited review: aging and energy balance. Journal of Applied Physiology 95:1728–1736.

Woolner L, Collins KJ 1992 Disorders of the autonomic system. In: Textbook of geriatric medicine and gerontology, 4th edn. Churchill Livingstone, Edinburgh, pp 399–403.

World Health Organization 1994 Assessment of fracture risk and its application to screening for postmenopausal osteoporosis. WHO Technical Report Series 843. WHO, Geneva.

Ziere G, Dieleman J, Hofman A, et al 2006 Polypharmacy and falls in the middle age and elderly population. British Journal of Clinical Pharmacology 61(2):218–223.

## FURTHER READING

Cullum N, Nelson EA, et al. 2001 Compression for venous leg ulcers. Cochrane Database of Systematic Reviews, Issue 2.

Ettinger WJ, Afable RF 1994b Physical disability from knee osteoarthritis: the role of exercise as an intervention. Medicine & Science in Sports & Exercise 26(12):1435–1440.

Frontera WR, Suh D, Krivickas LS 2000a Skeletal muscle fiber quality in older men and women. American Journal of Physiology – Cell Physiology 279(3):C611–C618.

Frontera WR., Hughes VA, Lutz KJ, Evans WJ 2000b Aging of skeletal muscle: a 12-year longitudinal study. Journal of Applied Physiology 88(4):1321–1326.

Fulton MM, Allen ER 2005 Polypharmacy in elderly: a literature review. Journal of the American Academy of Nurse Practitioners 17:123–132.

Guccione AA, Felson DT, Anderson JJ, et al 1994 The effects of specific medical conditions on the functional limitations of elders in the Framingham Study. American Journal of Public Health 84(3):351–358.

Guesseous I, Cornuz J, Ruffieux C, et al 2008 Osteoporotic fracture risk in elderly women: estimation with quantitative heel US and clinical risk factors. Radiology 248:179–184.

Martin RR, Charles LR, Vandervoort AA 1997 Age-related changes in motor unit function. Muscle & Nerve 20(6):679–690.

McPoil TG Jr 1988 Footwear. Physical Therapy 68(12):1857–1865.

McShane R, Areosa Sastre A, Minakaran N Memantine for dementia. Cochrane Database of Systematic Reviews 2006 Issue 2. Art. No.: CD003154. DOI: 10.1002/14651858.CD003154.pub5.

Roe BH, Griffiths JM, Kenrick M 1994 Nursing treatment of patients with chronic leg ulcers in the community. Journal of Clinical Nursing 3(3):159–168.

# Chapter | 12 |

# Paediatric podiatry and genetics

*Krishna Goel and Gordon F Watt*

## KEYWORDS

Acquired deformity

Anatomical anomalies

Biomechanical anomalies/abnormalities

Chromosome abnormalities

Congenital and genetic malformations

Dermatological conditions

Diabetes

Examination and assessment

Family tree

Foot types

Footwear

Growth and development

Infections

Ingrowing toe nails

Knock-knee and bow leg

Medical/surgical conditions

Orthoses

Passive and active exercises

Patterns of inheritance

Podiatric management

Postural anomalies/abnormalities

Principles of human genetics

Role of the paediatric podiatrist

Screening

Tarsal coalition (peroneal spastic flat foot)

Paediatric podiatry differs from general podiatric practice in that the growing foot provides unique problems and challenges that are not encountered in the adult foot. The simple reason for this is that, not only is the foot subject to local problems due to growth, but it is also required to adapt and compensate for developmental change as the general posture develops through a series of changes affecting the whole skeleton – in particular, from the podiatric point of view, changes that affect the spinal posture, position of the pelvis and the long bones of the lower limb. As the foot supports this structure, any changes that take place produce a 'knock-on' effect on the foot, altering its posture, either temporarily or permanently, which can leave it compromised and lead to other pathologies as it attempts to compensate for these changes. Equally, an inherited or acquired problem within the foot can compromise its posture, resulting in changes to the bony skeleton above it. In some instances it may be that both scenarios contrive to compound the situation. The foot can also be affected by the many diseases of childhood, either directly or indirectly, and it is of paramount importance that abnormalities or suspected manifestations of systemic disease are recognised at an early stage and appropriate action taken in order to avoid, reduce or eliminate complications into adulthood. It is, therefore, obvious that, as in the adult foot, the growing foot cannot be considered in isolation from the rest of the body, but unlike the adult foot, where the posture tends to be static, the paediatric foot is in a state of flux as it adapts to change.

Many misconceptions exist related to paediatric foot problems. Unfortunately, foot problems, unless gross or particularly troublesome, traditionally were given low priority, with the result that manageable cases were left untreated and secondary features related to structural pathologies developed. These included chronic intractable plantar keratoses in their many guises, or arthritic states affecting the foot, lower limb and lumbar spine. These problems obviously require treatment, and it is interesting to note that the majority of the elderly population attends a podiatrist, with many requiring hip, knee and foot surgery.

Early recognition and management of actual and potential foot problems in the young would go a long way to reduce these numbers. In an attempt to tackle this problem, successful podopaediatric screening programmes have been established in the past. However, the numbers of elderly currently requiring foot care in the UK have stretched resources to the stage where these services have become a luxury rather than a priority – the result being that actual or potential pathologies easily identified and potentially successfully managed by the podiatrist, but as yet asymptomatic to the patient, are remaining undetected until they become a chronic feature in later life, when palliation rather than cure may be the outcome.

Traditionally, paediatric foot pathologies have been regarded as consisting mainly of verrucae, tinea pedis, ingrowing toenails, corn and callus, and hyperhidrosis/bromidrosis. These conditions do exist commonly and are found often as secondary features associated with structural or functional abnormalities. The misconception that they are the most common paediatric foot problem may be based on the fact that they can be painful, unsightly or antisocial, resulting in treatment being sought. However, the majority of foot problems in the young are inclined to be more subtle and tend to be related to the following broad categories:

- footwear
- foot types
- infections
- injuries
- anatomical anomalies
- biomechanical anomalies/abnormalities
- acquired deformities
- congenital and genetic abnormalities
- postural anomalies/abnormalities
- surgical/medical conditions
- dermatological conditions.

These broad headings will either be referred to specifically under their individual headings or be alluded to within the text. However, before considering these, it is important to have an understanding of the normal chronological growth and development of the lower limb, particularly in the early years of life when change can be dramatic and rapid.

# NORMAL GROWTH AND DEVELOPMENT

In the embryo, the limb buds first appear at about 4 weeks of intrauterine life, becoming segmented into proximal, intermediate and distal parts by the week 6 and digitated by week 7 of gestational age. The thigh, the leg and the foot are recognisable entities by week 9. The feet should reach a nearly neutral position by the end of postovulatory week 11. The positional changes of the feet appear to depend invariably on the skeletal and neuromuscular development.

Ossification starts initially in the larger bones of the leg and foot, extending gradually to the smaller bones (Table 12.1). By the completion of the embryonic stage, all the major neural, vascular and muscular parts of the limb are present and in appearance closely resemble those of an adult.

The majority of children are born with normal feet, both structurally and functionally. It seems that the shape, size and form of feet are genetically determined but are liable to being affected by other factors. However, in some children faulty intrauterine morphogenesis may be responsible for deformity and disability. Also, drugs may have dangerous effects on the developing fetus. The most disastrous drug has been thalidomide, which has caused severe limb abnormalities (Fig. 12.1). The thalidomide tragedy has brought about a thorough reappraisal of all drugs prescribed during pregnancy because of their potential teratogenic effects. Later in life, infection, injury and other systemic diseases may be responsible for foot problems. The conditions present at birth are designated 'congenital disorders'.

Children are not 'mini-adults' and the child's foot is not a small-scale replica of the adult foot. It is comparatively shorter and wider, tapering towards the heel because the hindfoot is less fully developed than the forefoot (Fig. 12.2). As the infant's foot is very malleable, it

**Table 12.1** Ossification timetable

| Bone | Primary centres | Secondary centres | Fusion remarks |
|---|---|---|---|
| Tibia – diaphysis | 7th week | | |
| Tibia – upper epiphysis | At birth | 20th year | |
| Tibia – lower epiphysis | 2nd year | 18th year | Sometimes a separate centre for the medial malleolus appears at the same time |
| Fibula – diaphysis | 8th week | | |
| Fibula – upper epiphysis | 4th year | 25th year | |
| Fibula – lower epiphysis | 2nd year | 20th year | |
| Calcaneum – body | 6th month | | |
| Calcaneum – epiphysis | 6th–10th month | 13th–15th year | |
| Talus | 7th month | | |
| Cuboid | At birth | | |
| Lateral cuneiform | 1st year | | |
| Medial cuneiform | 3rd year | | |
| Intermediate cuneiform | 4th year | | |
| Navicular | 4th year | | |
| First metatarsal shaft | 8th–9th week | | |
| First metatarsal base | 3rd year | 17th–20th year | Sometimes a separate centre for the head appears at the same time |
| Other metatarsal shafts | 8th–9th week | | Sometimes a separate centre for the base of the fifth metatarsal appears at the same time |
| Proximal phalanx shafts | 12th–14th week | | |
| Proximal phalanx bases | 3rd–6th year | 17th–18th year | |
| Intermediate phalanx shafts | 4th–9th month | | That for the fifth toe does not appear until shortly after birth |
| *Intermediate phalanx bases* | | | |
| Distal phalanx of hallux | 3rd–6th year | 17th–18th year | |
| Distal phalanx shafts | 8th week | | |
| Distal phalanx bases | 6th year | 17th–18th year | |

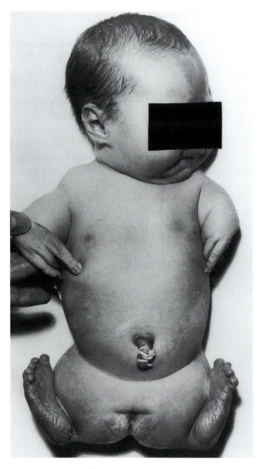

**Figure 12.1** An example of the limb abnormalities caused by thalidomide.

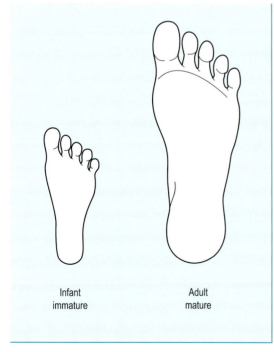

Infant
immature

Adult
mature

**Figure 12.2** The differing proportions between the mature and immature foot.

may allow some congenital deformities to be corrected easily, although it also means that the foot may be deformed by abnormal stresses of weight bearing. The usual age group of children presenting with foot problems ranges from neonate to pre-school, but it is not unusual for problems to present at a much later stage or to be detected by screening programmes during primary school.

In general, the foot tends to appear short, broad, stubby-toed and fat at birth. It may also appear flat due to fatty padding in the medial longitudinal arch area, but during the first year this is gradually absorbed as growth proceeds. To allow normal growth and development it is important to allow the baby freedom of movement to allow for normal muscle development, and therefore tight bedclothes and constrictive foot coverings should be avoided. During the early crawling and walking stages it is also important to allow barefooted walking to encourage normal function. It is best that children do not wear shoes until they are walking competently out of doors. A child will normally sit unaided by 6–8 months and be crawling by 9 months. Some children never crawl, being 'controllers' and provided for by older siblings. Some 'bear-walk' on all fours and others 'bottom shuffle', but the majority of children crawl in the recognised manner. By 12 months they will walk with assistance, by 15 months independently and be running by 18–24 months. It should be remembered, however, that all children are different and that these figures are governed by relatively wide parameters. The child should be allowed to progress at their own rate and not be artificially stimulated, for example by the use of babywalkers. However, it is prudent to seek a specialist opinion should there be any concern over a child's development, particularly if the mother who spends more time with and knows her child better than anyone else is concerned, so that she can be reassured or appropriate investigations undertaken.

## Knock-knee, bow leg and rickets

During this early period the child walks on a broad base and may appear flatfooted with bow legs, and may show lordosis, with bulging of the abdomen with the legs partly flexed at the knees. The feet may be variously abducted or adducted and apparently 'flat'. During gait, the child will lean forward with the arms abducted and partly flexed at the elbows, reminiscent of a tightrope walker.

From 2–6 years of age, developmental knock-knee is evident, with the vast majority of cases resolving spontaneously between the ages of 5 and 6 years as growth progresses, and few cases are seen in 8-year-olds. The abdomen becomes less prominent and the foot type and medial longitudinal arch become more evident.

During this period the general posture is constantly changing as the child experiments with their body image and equilibrium. Most of the developmental changes that take place in the lower limb result in compensation within the foot in the form of subtalar joint pronation. It is very important to establish the cause of this, and in most cases reassurance and footwear advice is all that is required. However, it must always be remembered that the cause may be more serious (particularly if it is unilateral), and a full and thorough examination is always undertaken (see Ch. 1) and appropriate action taken. Decisions regarding orthotic management depend on age, severity and assessment of the posture in general.

### Rickets

By definition, the cause of rickets is an insufficient intake of vitamin D to promote normal bone growth and to prevent the occurrence of specific abnormal changes in bone. In the UK, a dietary intake of 10 µg/day vitamin D (400 i.u.) is accepted. Toddler rickets presents with bow legs in a child who is already able to walk, with or without other signs as found in infantile rickets (Fig. 12.3). In severe rickets

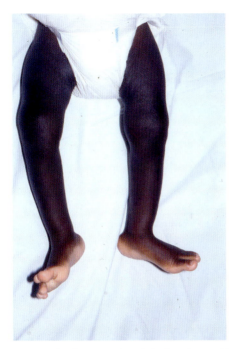

**Figure 12.3** Nutritional rickets. Bowing of the legs in an African child.

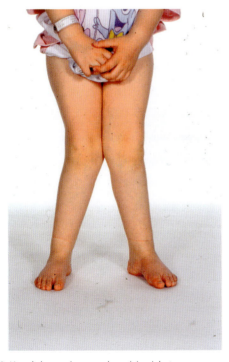

**Figure 12.4** Knock-knees (genu valgum) in rickets.

there may be spinal curvature, coxa vara and bending or fracture of the long bones. The treatment of nutritional rickets requires therapeutic doses of vitamin D. The bony lesions occurring in infants and toddlers may be gross (Fig 12.4), but usually complete healing, followed by virtual loss of significant deformity, occurs as the limb doubles in length as growth continues. Residual compensatory foot problems may persist and require ongoing management.

## Flat foot

Many young children when first standing appear to have flat feet, as the adipose tissue under the medial longitudinal arch is pressed to the ground, the hollow obliterated, and the foot looks flat. This is not pathological and the parents should be reassured.

Older children very frequently have flattening of the medial longitudinal arch on standing but the arch reasserts itself on standing on tiptoe – this is the mobile flat foot and no specific treatment is needed beyond encouraging the child to practise toe walking and walking on inverted feet. As the limb matures, a normal arch will appear. In severe cases a casted foot orthosis may be required.

## Peak rates of growth

Growth continues steadily at varying rates into late adolescence, with peak rates at puberty. The main period of accelerated growth in girls occurs between 8 and 13 years of age, with the peak rate at approximately 12 years of age. The main period of accelerated growth in boys occurs between the ages of 10.5 and 16 years with the peak rate at approximately 14 years of age. Many foot pathologies seen in children, particularly in this age group, are associated in some way with growth, and it is important to be aware of any growth spurts that may be taking place. This age group also tends to be more active physically, putting additional stress on growing tissues. Children under active management by a podiatrist should have their feet and height measured and charted at each visit.

In general, the rate of growth of the feet is constant from birth, increasing by approximately two sizes per year for the first 4 years and then by one size annually thereafter until the mid-teens. Foot growth, however, is very variable between individuals, with some children growing by several sizes in a very short period and others having long periods with no growth, hence the importance of regular measuring when purchasing footwear. It is a noticeable trend that feet are becoming larger, particularly among boys. It is not unusual to find 11-year-old boys with size 11 feet.

## FOOTWEAR

The role of footwear in relation to foot deformity is contentious. Some authorities consider that foot deformity, unless inherited, is solely related to the outcomes of compensations related to biomechanical disorders within the foot or general skeleton, while others hold the view that foot deformity can be caused only by an outside influence such as inadequate footwear. It is likely that, given ideal circumstances, factors from both are responsible but, given the multifactorial influences upon the foot, both intrinsically and extrinsically, and the variations in posture, gait and anatomy between individuals, it is possible that a definitive opinion will never be forthcoming. However, it is reasonable to assume that in the early years of life the foot is so flexible and malleable that it can be influenced by outside forces and hence deformity may result. A good example of this is the (now illegal) practice of Chinese foot binding, in which feet were bound in a prescribed position from birth, resulting in a gross, permanent and disabling deformity. In the older foot, where ossification, posture and neuromuscular control are more established, this may be less likely to occur or more difficult to achieve, but it is interesting to consider that in order to correct certain mobile deformities the principles of Davis' law (Box 12.1) are utilised, in all age groups, by serially encouraging the deformity into a corrected position with appropriate orthotic devices. It could be argued that inadequate footwear does this in reverse or inhibits or negates the action of foot orthoses.

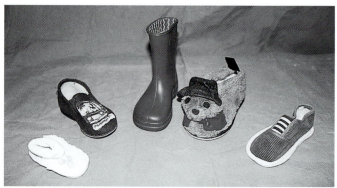

**Figure 12.6** An example of a pram shoe (far left) and other footwear that should only be worn as a short-term measure.

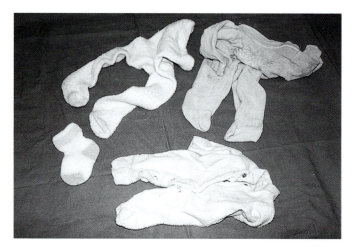

**Figure 12.5** Babygros, sleep suits, stretch tights and socks.

Children's footwear is available in many forms and should always be examined and its suitability considered with every patient. These forms and their associated hazards include:

- Babygros and sleep suits. All babies wear babygros and sleep suits (Fig. 12.5) but consideration is often given to colour, design and general size rather than the suitability regarding foot size. As many of these items are made of cotton, frequent washing may reduce their size. In addition, terry towelling and disposable nappies occupy space, thus further relatively reducing their size. These result in the mobility of the foot being further restricted and the digits held in a flexed position, with the added risk of damage to the periungual tissues.
- Stretch tights and socks (Fig. 12.5). Most attention tends to be paid to the shoes that a child wears, with the hosiery often being neglected. It is possible with very young children that inadequate hosiery may have a more damaging influence than inadequate footwear. This is particularly the case when children learn to dress themselves, where they will 'make' small hosiery fit by stretching it beyond its limits. Equally, hosiery that is too large will accommodate the 'growing room' in shoes, making them relatively too small. Sizing on tights and socks may not correspond with the sizing system used for the shoes.
- Knitted booties. These tend to be knitted with an open weave, which can result in entrapment of a digit and resultant gangrene due to ischaemia. They are commonly found to be too small or too large.
- Pram shoes (Fig. 12.6) are often purchased for special occasions, for example baptisms. This is a harmless practice. Permanent use should be discouraged, as the sizing of many pram shoes is spurious, making accurate fitting by the parents almost impossible and the style of many paying little heed to

the form of a baby's foot. The synthetic materials employed in many are also unsuitable, encouraging excessive sweating and often being worn with hosiery containing a large percentage of synthetic fibres. As stated previously, children do not require shoes on their feet until they are walking competently out of doors.

Exceptions include children born with deformity, such as talipes equinovarus, or neurological conditions, such as hemiplegia, where the foot must be artificially maintained in a corrected or ideal posture. In these circumstances, the footwear would be prescribed professionally on medical or podiatric advice.

## Inadequate footwear

In general, footwear may be inadequate in many differing ways, including being too short, too narrow, having a pointed or a shallow toe box, poor or no retaining medium, inadequate heel stiffener, heel height too high, narrow base to the heel, synthetic uppers and/or lining, or any combination of the above, and not being compatible with the foot it is covering (Fig. 12.7).

Children should always have their feet measured for shoes at a reputable retail outlet by a trained competent shoe fitter. Ideally, both feet should be measured at approximately 2-month intervals and the shoes replaced as required, and not when worn out.

### Plimsolls

Ideally, for everyday wear one pair of shoes should be purchased and worn to destruction. This is not always possible for children at primary school in many areas of the UK. In order to keep the schools quiet and clean, some education authorities require plimsolls to be worn in school all day. At the end of the school day the plimsolls are placed in shoe bags on a peg overnight, with the result that they do not dry out fully and are worn again the following school day. In the meantime, the shoes that have been purchased carefully are hardly worn, while the plimsolls at school are not replaced as the foot grows. The growing foot is, therefore, in a constantly damp environment within a shoe, which cannot be fitted accurately and is often too small. Plimsolls are excellent for the purpose for which they are intended (i.e. gymnastics), but do not provide a suitable environment for a growing foot, and this current practice should be discontinued. Furthermore, plimsolls (Fig. 12.8) do not allow for the changing flare of a young foot, and this may have a damaging influence if they are

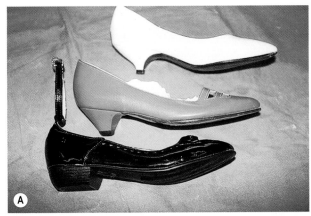

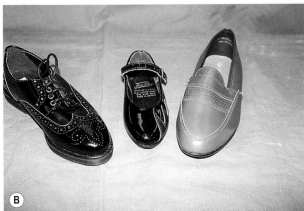

**Figure 12.7** (A, B) Examples of inadequate children's footwear.

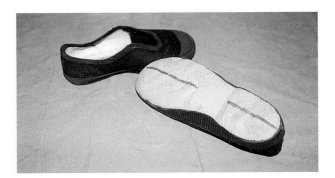

**Figure 12.8** Plimsolls. Note the straight flare, indicated by the straight line through the centre of the heel and sole. In the young child this line should ideally emerge in the lateral distal region of the sole, allowing space in the medial part of the forefoot for the relatively adducted position of the first ray.

worn continually. They are also unsuitable as a vehicle for casted orthoses.

## Babywalkers

These are included here as they relate to the child who is on his or her feet. As alluded to previously, children walk at different ages, and it is best to 'let nature take its course' and allow the child to walk naturally when ready instead of prematurely stressing tissues and loading joints.

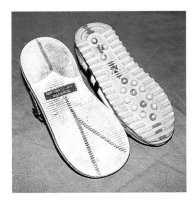

**Figure 12.9** The 'ideal' flare for a young child's shoe (left) compared with that of an unsuitable shoe (both shoes are for left feet).

## Fashion, peer-group pressure and economics

It is important to recognise when managing the case of the teenager that fashion, peer-group pressure and economics play a large part in their social and emotional development, and it is necessary to make compromises regarding footwear or they may be lost as cooperative patients altogether. It is important that the podiatrist working with this age group is acquainted with footwear fashions and costs, to allow them to communicate with the patients at their own level and understand and advise them accordingly.

## Trainers

Much has been said regarding the suitability or otherwise of trainers for all ages of children. In some schools, trainers are the only footwear in evidence, particularly as peer-group pressure dictates specific manufacturers. In general terms, trainers are not a problem, so long as, like any other shoes, the criteria for an adequate shoe are followed. The one criticism of trainers, particularly in the age group of puberty where the feet may be very sweaty, is the high percentage of synthetic materials used, leading to a hyperhidrotic state and predisposing to verrucae, tinea pedis and onychocryptosis.

## FOOT TYPE

Foot types are many and varied, hence the necessity for children to have their footwear fitted by an experienced, competent fitter with a wide range of styles, sizes and fittings. The infant foot, when viewed from below, tends to be triangular in shape (this is particularly obvious in premature children, who may also be late walkers). As the child progresses into adolescence the foot tends to become rectangular, hence the difference in shape between adult and children's footwear, the child's shoe being inflared and the adult's tending to be relatively straight-flared by comparison (Fig. 12.9). The first ray also tends to be in a relatively adducted position at this age, and it is possible that a straight-flared or small shoe may cause or result in soft-tissue pathologies or digital deformity. Typical foot types include:

- *short broad* – the foot is relatively short in relation to its length
- *square forefoot* – all the digits are virtually the same length (commonly found in Down's syndrome).

These are typically robust foot types common in boys. They can present shoe-fitting problems in girls.

The following foot types can be classified as 'at-risk' feet and appear to be more commonly found in females:

- *hypermobile* – this type of foot may be classified as belonging to an individual with hypermobility syndrome, but can loosely be classed as someone who has a greater than 'average' range of joint motion in the feet
- *long slender* – the foot is relatively narrow in relation to its length
- *triangular* – the heel is narrower than normal in relation to the forefoot
- *long inner border* – this speaks for itself and leaves the hallux and associated structures open to trauma.

All the above foot types can appear singly or in any combination, and can present considerable problems for the shoe fitter.

## Low-arched and high-arched feet

Normal feet come in all shapes and sizes and it is important that feet which appear relatively highly arched or low arched due to their inherited architecture are not misdiagnosed as pathological features. There is also the possibility that certain foot types may be the inherited features of different races and cultures.

# INFECTIONS

In general, unless the child has an underlying medical condition, which may make them more prone to infection or diminish their ability to combat it, this does not present as a particular problem. Infections are most commonly bacterial, fungal or viral (see Ch. 3).

With the exception of tinea pedis and verrucae, by far the most common 'paediatric foot' infections dealt with by the podiatrist relate to nail pathologies, either as true onychocryptosis or paronychia. These conditions can occur in any child at any age but are most common among teenagers and children who are immunocompromised (undergoing chemotherapy) or those with lymphoedema (Turner's syndrome), where there is an added risk of cellulitis. Aseptic technique is, therefore, a priority.

Infections from foreign bodies and broken blisters can also be a problem.

## Onychocryptosis (ingrowing toenail)

The most common nail condition found in children is onychocryptosis, but this tends to be mainly associated with teenagers, particularly boys. However, it can occur at any age and is a particular management problem in very young children and babies who may suck their toes. It is important to remember that in this age group failure of conservative podiatric management could result in surgery either with partial or total nail avulsion, requiring the administration of a general anaesthetic. In this age group, such a procedure is normally carried out without ablation of the germinal matrix and this may result in the possibility of the development of involution or onychogryphosis in later life. It is therefore of great importance that all efforts are made to resolve the problem conservatively. In very young children it is unusual to find a 'spur' of nail in the nail sulcus. Apart from the distress caused to the child, unnecessary investigation of the nail sulci using instruments should be considered very carefully and used sparingly so as not to worsen the condition.

Usually the nail plate is found to be triangular in shape, widest distally (as if the nail is too large for the toe), with the periungual tissues hypertrophied, inflamed and fibrosed. There is often no hypergranulation tissue, but there may be evidence of fibrous repair in the area of the lateral nail sulci and a history of long-term antibiotic use.

The condition usually responds to prescription of appropriate footwear and hosiery. With crawlers, it tends to resolve when the child starts walking.

Regular swabbing with 0.5% chlorhexidine in spirit helps to reduce the incidence of infection and helps to 'tone' periungual tissues, making them less prone to damage from trauma. The parents are reassured and the child is monitored regularly with advice to seek treatment should the condition deteriorate. Most cases resolve with a little patience.

Some children are born without nails, which grow in at a later date, and management similar to the above may be necessary as the nails 'erupt' and grow forward until the corners of the free edge are beyond the pulp of the toe.

Many older children are 'at risk' from onychocryptosis due to intrinsic foot abnormalities. In particular, there may be involution of the toenail, hyperextension of the hallux, abduction of the hallux (often with valgus rotation) and subtalar joint pronation (Fig. 12.10). These may occur in any combination, and inadequate footwear and hyperhidrosis may compound the problem.

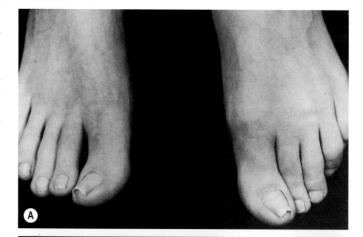

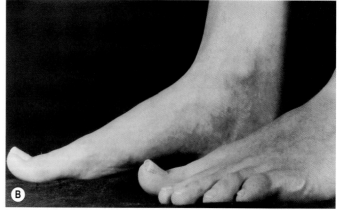

**Figure 12.10** (A, B) An example of 'at-risk' first toenails in an older child due to involution of the nail plate accompanied by hyperextension and abduction of the terminal phalanx.

## ANATOMICAL ANOMALIES

These include anomalies of the sesamoid bones, supernumerary bones and tarsal synostoses.

### Sesamoid bones

These may be classified as additional, bipartite or multipartite.

### Supernumerary bones

These include os trigonum, os tibial externum and os vesalii.

Abnormalities of sesamoid bones and supernumerary bones rarely directly cause problems in the paediatric foot but may result in soft-tissue lesions. Radiography confirms their presence.

### Tarsal coalition (peroneal spastic flat foot)

In tarsal coalitions there is an anomaly of ossification in which adjacent tarsal bones are fused together. Fusion may be bony or cartilaginous. The most common coalition occurs between the calcaneus and the navicular, with union across the midtarsal joint. In a talocalcaneal coalition, fusion occurs between the sustentaculum tali and the talus.

Children with tarsal coalitions may never be aware that they have them. Occasionally, they have distressing painful symptoms and surgery is necessary for adequate relief. Between these two extremes are most children who have little trouble until they enter a growth spurt, when they develop the classic symptoms of the 'spastic flat foot'. This is a painful contraction of the peroneal muscles and occurs as a protective mechanism, resulting in a fixed, everted, abducted foot, which resembles a flat foot and from which it must be distinguished. Diagnosis is not always easy. Examination reveals tender, taut and prominent peroneal tendons, and attempts to invert the foot will be painfully resisted. Specialist radiographs and/or a computerised tomography scan may be necessary to demonstrate the fusion (Fig. 12.11).

Initial therapy consists of resting the foot in a below-knee plaster of Paris cast if necessary, and reserving surgery for those with recurrent or intractable pain.

Long-term follow-up management with casted foot orthoses may be necessary.

## BIOMECHANICAL ANOMALIES/ABNORMALITIES

### Acquired deformity

Virtually any pathology is possible. By far the most common, whether due to footwear or as secondary features of compensation for biomechanical anomalies/abnormalities, are digital deformities, including hammer toe, mallet toe, retracted toe, claw toe and hallux abducto valgus (see Ch. 4). The lesser toes may also be variously burrowed in varus positions with lateral and medial deviations at the interphalangeal joints. There may also be early periarticular thickening and limitation of motion.

Deformity at the subtalar joint due to excessive subtalar joint pronation may result in serious forefoot disruption and deformity, and should always be considered as the cause and either corrected or controlled rather than simply treating the secondary digital deformities.

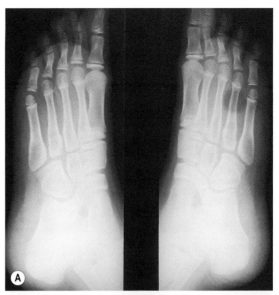

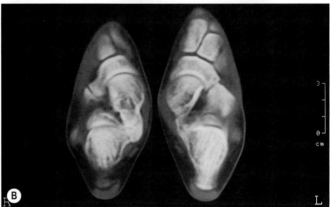

**Figure 12.11** (A, B) Tarsal coalition. Computerised tomography scan of a talocalcaneal bar (B).

### Mucopolysaccharidosis

The mucopolysaccharidoses are lysosomal storage diseases. Mucopolysaccharides (glycosaminoglycans) are complex macromolecular compounds composed of a protein core to which are attached polysaccharide side-chains. In mucopolysaccharidosis IV (Morquio syndrome) the child presents usually at 18–24 months because of gait problems from genu valgum and coxa valga. Contractures of the knees and hips produce a jockey-like stance. The feet are broad and flat (Fig. 12.12). Genu valgum severely impairs gait. Following the birth of an affected child, the parents face a 25% risk that a future child will also have the disease. Prenatal diagnosis and carrier detection with enzyme assays is available.

### Juvenile hallux abducto valgus

As in many other foot problems, footwear has been universally blamed for this condition in teenagers. In almost all cases, a strong family history can be elicited, with a number of predisposing factors being inherited and, given the appropriate set of circumstances, deformity develops. Footwear may aggravate an established tendency to abducto valgus deformity, and may cause bunion formation by friction over the medial eminence of the metatarsal head. The abducto

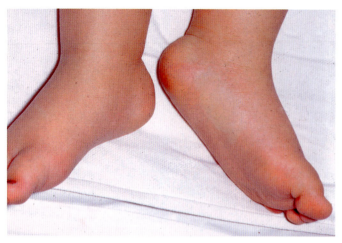

**Figure 12.12** Feet of a child with mucopolysaccharidosis IV (Morquio syndrome).

valgus is often accompanied by adduction of the first metatarsal. Up to 20° of abductus can be normal, but a useful guide to whether surgery is indicated is the position of the sesamoids on a radiograph – no subluxation, no operation. Surgery should not be carried out before the foot is skeletally mature, at about age 14 years. Until then, an orthodigital splint (see Management, p. 295) can control the position of the hallux.

## INJURIES

### Juvenile hallux rigidus

While not common, this condition causes much discomfort to its sufferers, who are usually teenaged males. It is now thought that the aetiology is recurrent minor trauma or a single incident, which produces a chondral injury. The resulting pain and muscle spasm results in loss of extension at the metatarsophalangeal joint. The patient walks on the outer border of the foot to avoid the painful area. Rest in a cast is the recommended first-line treatment, with a proximal phalangeal osteotomy being reserved for those in whom symptoms persist. Appropriate physical therapy and padding and strapping (see Ch. 16) and footwear advice is usually sufficient to effect a cure.

## CONGENITAL ABNORMALITIES

These may arise from two sources: genetic factors, and environmental factors affecting the developing fetus. It is likely that some of these congenital malformations result from a mixture of genetic and environmental factors. Approximately 1 in 50 babies is born with a severe malformation. Malformations are more common in babies born prematurely and possibly in those born to mothers with diabetes. Genetic counselling is vital in the handling of parents whose child has been born with a congenital malformation.

Total correction of some abnormalities may not be possible, and thus residual deformity and handicap remain as a chronic feature in adult life, requiring careful supervision, orthopaedic appliances, and podiatric treatment and monitoring.

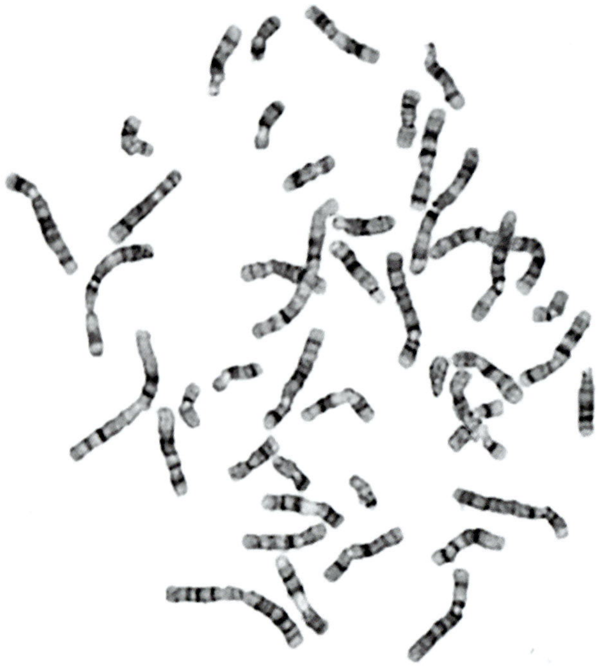

**Figure 12.13** A spread of chromosomes from the nucleus of a single cell.

## BASIC PRINCIPLES OF HUMAN GENETICS

Genetic information is coded in DNA, which is packaged into chromosomes. Each chromosome contains a single DNA molecule consisting of two strands woven together as a double helix. The DNA code on one helix is a mirror image of the other. During cell division, the DNA molecule replicates itself by separating the two helixes and assembling two new double helixes by using the two mirror-image strands as templates. After replication, the DNA is repackaged and the chromosomes are then visible with a light microscope. The chromosomes in one nucleus are shown in Figure 12.13. The chromosomes can then be arranged into a karyotype of matching pairs starting with the largest (numbered 1) down to the smallest (numbered 22). This leaves the sex chromosomes, which are two Xs in a female and an X and a Y in a male. The karyotype of a male is shown in Figure 12.14; it consists of 23 pairs of chromosomes, making 46 in all. When an individual reproduces, only one of each pair will be transmitted to the egg or sperm. Thus the eggs and sperm have only 23 chromosomes and the full complement of 46 is restored at fertilisation.

## GENETIC AND CONGENITAL DISORDERS

Many foot disorders have a genetic or part genetic basis, but it is important to recognise that not all congenital (present at birth) disorders are genetic. Some are caused by the adverse intrauterine effects of drugs or infection. Another example is amputation defects that are caused by intrauterine constrictions.

Genetic disorders may be classified according to whether the underlying abnormality is at the chromosome or the DNA level. Some DNA

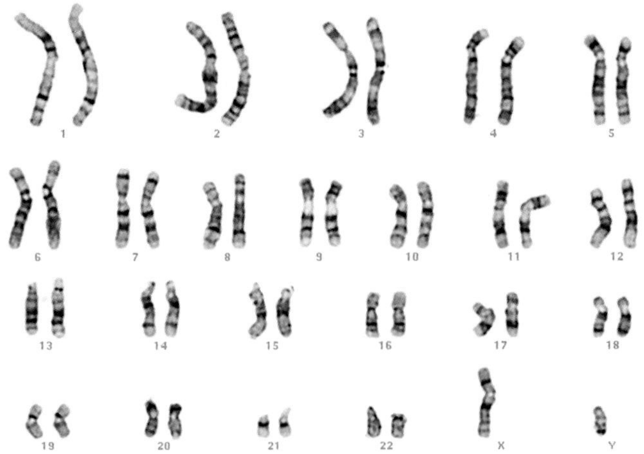

**Figure 12.14** The chromosomes of a nuclear spread arranged into pairs to form a karyotype.

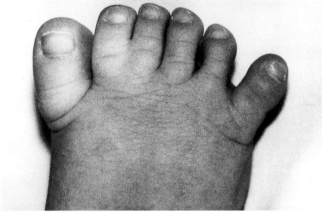

**Figure 12.15** Polydactyly. Note also the partial syndactyly affecting the second and third toes. There is also hypertrophy of the additional 'sixth' toe.

abnormalities in single genes may cause disease, while others work in concert with other genes and environmental effects.

## Chromosome abnormalities

Abnormalities of the chromosomes include deletions, duplications and rearrangements of the genetic material. For example, Down's syndrome is usually caused by having three copies of chromosome 21 instead of two.

## Single-gene disorders

Single-gene disorders are caused by sequence changes (mutations) in the DNA of one gene. Depending on whether a gene is situated on one or other of the sex chromosomes it is called X- or Y-linked. If it is on one of the other chromosomes it is described as autosomal. Depending on whether the mutation needs to be present on the copy (allele) of a gene on both chromosomes or only on one chromosome to cause the disorder, it is described as recessive or dominant, respectively. Thus, each single gene disorder has a pattern of inheritance such as autosomal dominant or X-linked recessive. Each inheritance pattern is associated with predictable recurrence risks for relatives. These patterns of inheritance are illustrated using animated diagrams (University of Glasgow 2009).

## Multifactorial disorders

A complex interaction of multiple genes, each of minor effect, can work together with environmental factors to cause multifactorial disorders such as talipes equinovarus. At present the genetic and environmental components of this disorder are unknown, but twin and family studies reveal the influence of genetics.

## SYNDROMES

Genetic disorders may affect any organ system and a condition might have multiple component features. Recognition that these component features are interlinked (i.e. are a syndrome) is crucial for clinical management. Problems can arise when individual specialists concentrate on single components and no one sees the whole picture. The process is not helped by the variability of many syndromes. The classic textbook descriptions are rare and most patients do not have 'a full house' of clinical features. Syndromes may be caused by single gene, chromosomal, multifactorial, environmental and unknown factors. A major problem requiring the expertise of the medical geneticist is where apparently similar syndromes have different genetic or non-genetic aetiologies with very different recurrence risks for the family.

## The lower limbs

Examination of the musculoskeletal system should commence with observation of the infant or child. The position of the limbs and the gait may give a clue to a problem that is later confirmed on more detailed clinical examination. Having inspected the lower limbs of an infant for signs of dissimilarity in the skin creases, girth, gross abnormalities such as bowing of the legs and length of the limbs, a systemic examination is indicated. Discrepancy in leg length is usually due to muscle wasting or poor development. It may also be due to a neurological problem, but on occasion it is the larger limb which is abnormal due to hypertrophy, lymphoedema or a malformation.

### Polydactyly

This term denotes the presence of supernumerary digits attached either to the hand or the foot. On the foot the extra digits may develop from one metatarsal or there may be complete extra metatarsal segments (Fig. 12.15). Depending on the severity of the abnormality, selective 'amputation' at an early age is indicated to ensure optimum foot function, thus facilitating shoe fitting in childhood and adult life. As in any operation on the foot, it is vital to ensure that any resulting scar is away from pressure areas.

### Syndactyly (webbed toes – zygodactyly)

This term is applied to a total or partial fusion of adjacent digits. It is very common, usually bilateral and often familial. Multiple syndactyly occurs in hands and feet associated with other anomalies, as in Apert's syndrome (an autosomal-dominant disorder – acrocephalo-syndactyly). No treatment is required for webbing (zygodactyly) of the toes (Fig. 12.16).

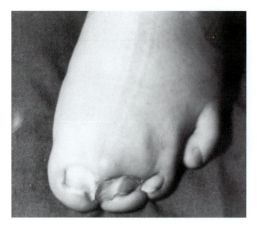

Figure 12.16 Syndactyly associated with Apert's syndrome. Note the potential for toenail problems.

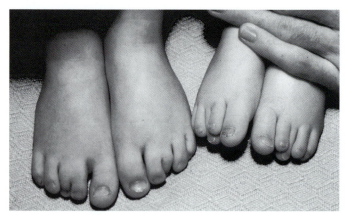

Figure 12.18 The feet of the affected children in Figure 12.17.

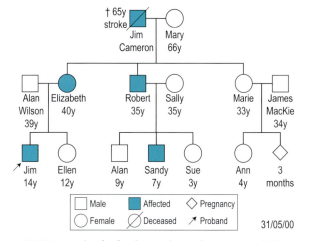

Figure 12.17 Example of a family tree drawn during a consultation.

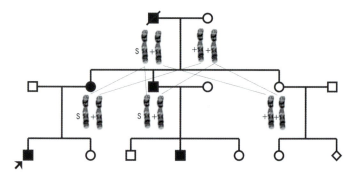

Figure 12.19 Jim Wilson's family tree, with chromosome pairs that contain the syndactyly gene. The healthy copy of the gene is marked '+' and the affected copy marked 'S'.

## ASSESSMENT OF A FAMILY WITH A GENETIC DISORDER

### Drawing the family tree

Normally a family will see a genetic specialist after being referred by a general practitioner, another specialist or by a member of one of the professions allied to medicine, such as a podiatrist. The referring healthcare professional may have the genetic basis of a condition brought to his or her attention by the patient, or may find a clinical sign suggestive of a genetic disorder on examination. Once alerted to the possibility of a genetic disorder, even the non-geneticist should draw a family tree. This is done freehand, using a standard set of symbols, which are shown at the bottom of Figure 12.17.

The family tree, or pedigree, is a very compact way of storing a large amount of family information. Each generation occupies the same horizontal level, and within a generation the birth order is presented from left to right. It is usually easiest to start with the youngest generation at the bottom of the page and then work back to the older generations. This may reveal that other persons in the family are, or might be, affected.

In the family shown in Figure 12.17, Jim Wilson was born with syndactyly of toes 2 and 3. Jim Cameron, Elizabeth and Robert are similarly affected, and his cousin Sandy has a milder abnormality consisting of overriding of toes 2 and 3 (Fig. 12.18). In addition, the affected family members all have complete or partial webbing between the third and fourth fingers but no one has any other congenital abnormality.

### Interpreting the family tree

In Jim's family there are affected members in three generations. We can interpret the pattern that links them together in order to try to work out how the gene is inherited and thus an affected person's risk of passing it on (Fig. 12.19). In this family both males and a females are affected, and so the gene causing syndactyly cannot be on the Y chromosome. There are two instances of a male passing the condition on to a male. Because a male does not transmit an X chromosome to his sons, we can also say that the syndactyly gene is not on the X chromosome. It therefore must be on one of the autosomes. This is called autosomal inheritance.

Looking at the family, it would be extremely unlikely that the partners of affected people (Mary, Alan and Sally) were, by chance, all healthy carriers of the syndactyly gene, and so affected children must have received only a singly copy of the abnormal gene from the affected parent. Because they have developed syndactyly even though they have inherited a healthy gene from the other parent, the syndactyly copy of the gene is said to be dominant to the healthy copy of

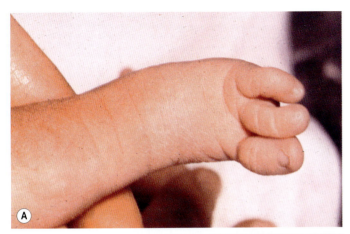

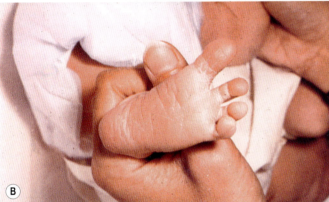

Figure 12.20 Oligodactyly with (A) three toes and (B) four toes.

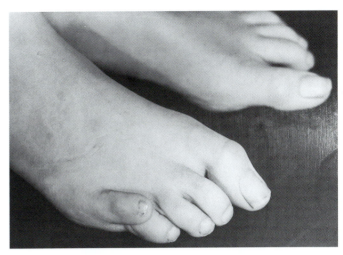

Figure 12.21 Congenital overlapping fifth toe. Note the 'knock-on' effect upon the other digits, particularly the fourth toe.

the gene. The inheritance of syndactyly in this family can thus be said to be autosomal dominant.

## OLIGODACTYLY

This term denotes the developmental absence of one or more digits (fingers or toes) with the total absence of all parts of the digit (i.e. metatarsal parts and all phalanges) (Fig. 12.20).

## CONGENITAL OVERLAPPING FIFTH TOE (DIGITI MINIMI QUINTI VARUS)

In this condition, from birth the smallest toe lies on the dorsum of the base of the fourth toe in a medially deviated position, although the degree of severity is variable (Fig. 12.21). The condition may be bilateral or unilateral. This is the only common toe abnormality in childhood that requires surgical correction on most occasions in order to avoid trouble with shoe fitting. From about 3 years of age a simple surgical correction allows the toe to return to its normal position. Silicone combined props (see Ch. 17) with a sling to the fifth toe may be beneficial if used from a very early stage on moderate to mild deformity, but surgery is usually required. It is important to manage this condition positively, as disruption of the other lesser digits can occur, with associated skin lesions, in later life.

## CURLY TOES

It is normal for the fourth and fifth toes to be a little flexed and curled medially, but if the third toe, instead of being straight, shares this flexed and medial deformity the second toe is usually deformed such that it lies on a higher plane than the others and curls laterally, overlying the third toe. This curious pattern of deformity is very common, being either bilateral or unilateral and variable in degree, but it is seldom a cause of trouble, although tight shoes and socks should be avoided. If the degree of deformity is great the patient will often present complaining of nail pain. However, most cases present for treatment because the parents are concerned due to the unusual appearance of the toes. Digital silicone devices (see Ch. 17) and exercises produce very good results but treatment may be protracted (see Management, p. 296).

Occasionally, a single toe, usually the fourth, is more flexed and adducted than usual, and if it causes pressure on others in the group with the side of the nail discomfort is felt (Fig. 12.22). The toe can be straightened without affecting the growth potential by transferring the insertion of the long flexor tendons to the extensor tendons on the dorsum of the toe. Orthodigital correction with silicone devices and exercises may also be of benefit (see Management, p. 296).

## CONGENITAL FLEXED TOE

This is uncommon and may affect a single toe or two adjacent toes. On walking, the affected toe takes the weight on the distal end instead of the plantar surface. Surgical or podiatric treatment is the same as for curly toe. If the condition is ignored, chronic nail problems due to onychauxis or onychogryphosis may arise.

## METATARSUS ADDUCTUS

In this less common deformity the forefoot is deviated towards the midline in relation to the hindfoot, as in clubfoot but without equinus or inversion. This is best treated as early as possible with serial, well-padded, moulded plasters until the forefoot remains straight. In a

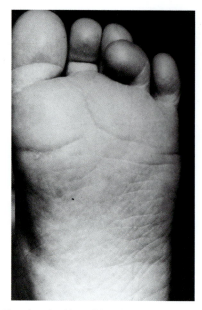

**Figure 12.22** Flexed and adducted fourth toe.

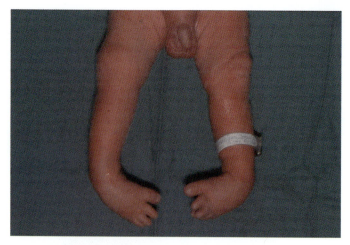

**Figure 12.23** Talipes equinovarus.

small proportion surgical exploration is needed to release the tight medial tether.

## HALLUX VARUS

While this is an extremely uncommon condition in the UK, this is not the case elsewhere, for example in India. Commonly seen with metatarsus adductus, frequently it corrects with growth. Occasionally surgery is necessary for the satisfactory fitting of footwear.

## CONGENITAL TALIPES EQUINOVARUS: CLUBFOOT

This common deformity occurs in 2–4 of 1000 births; that is, it is about twice as common as congenital dislocation of the hip. The male is twice as often affected as the female, and in half the affected children both feet are deformed. The diagnosis is obvious on inspection, with the deformity being in three parts: the heel is drawn up, the foot inverted and the hindfoot adducted (i.e. in an equinovarus position) (Fig. 12.23). In a small minority the deformity is postural and can be corrected easily by manipulation to neutral and beyond (Fig. 12.24). Repeated manipulation is sufficient treatment. The majority have rigidly deformed feet. In most this is the only problem, but clubfoot deformities are also found in conditions such as arthrogryposis, trisomy 18 and spina bifida cystica.

Initially, the treatment is carried out as an inpatient with daily manipulation of each element of the deformity. The correction obtained each day is maintained with the careful application of a Denis Browne splint to the foot (or feet). As the deformity is overcome progressively, the splint may be bent to hold a greater degree of correction and then connected to the other foot (normal or affected) by a connecting bar to hold the correction more effectively. Over a period of 7–14 days the foot will reach the overcorrected position and the baby can be sent home in the splints. It is necessary to continue to maintain an overcorrection by re-manipulation and re-application of

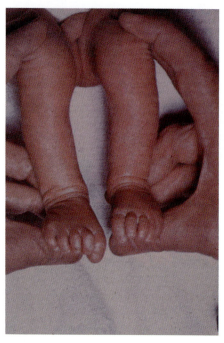

**Figure 12.24** An example of correction of talipes equinovarus by manipulation.

the splints as an outpatient every 2 weeks until the child starts to stand late in the first year. Alternative regimens to hold the correction obtained by manipulation involve the use of Elastoplast strapping or plaster of Paris.

For walking, the splints are discarded and boots with an outer raise to the sole are supplied, with night boots and a corrective bar for night wear. The parents are instructed to manipulate the foot into the over-corrected position. Over the next few years these treatments can be abandoned gradually with a view to the child going to school at 5 years of age with normal footwear and a foot that is slightly smaller and stiffer than usual. If the foot is found to be inadequately corrected during the first year or to be relapsing during later years, a soft-tissue release operation on the medial and posterior aspects of the foot and ankle is needed. About half of the corrected feet will need this procedure, and in a few with severe deformity bony correction will be necessary. In some cases foot orthoses with life-long podiatric management may be required.

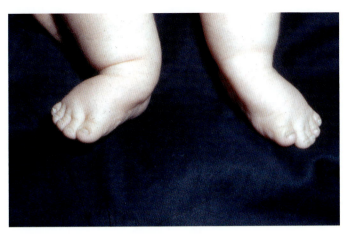

**Figure 12.25** Typical appearance of rocker bottom feet in a case of trisomy 18.

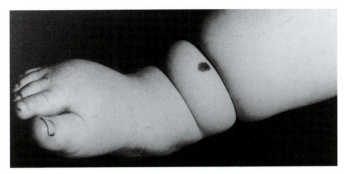

**Figure 12.26** Congenital constriction band syndrome affecting the ankle region.

## TALIPES CALCANEOVALGUS

As the name implies this is exactly the opposite deformity to clubfoot. It is usually the result of in utero posture, in that the foot has been caught in an upturned position with the sole against the uterine wall. The prognosis is excellent, as natural improvement occurs with active movement on release from the uterus. All that is needed is for the mother to manipulate the foot into equinovarus frequently and the deformity resolves permanently within a few weeks. It is important, however, to recognise that this condition is associated in a few with congenital dislocation of the hip and deformity of the tibia.

## VERTICAL TALUS (ROCKER BOTTOM FOOT)

This is a rare deformity known by several alternative names such as 'rocker-bottom foot' and is primarily caused by a dislocation of the talonavicular joint (Fig. 12.25). It occurs in 10–50% of the trisomy 18 syndrome. Correction is surgical and is planned to reduce the dislocation of the talonavicular joint. In the older child, it is more likely that bony correction or fusion will be needed. Foot orthoses may be required to maintain foot posture.

## ONYCHOGRYPHOSIS

Often thought of as an acquired complaint of the elderly, this condition can be congenital – affecting any toe or toes, but usually the first or fifth. It is easily managed conservatively, with the parent/patient being taught how to care for the nails. If the shape of the nail causes trouble and cannot be made tolerable by cutting or filing, radical removal of the nail with phenolisation is indicated (see Ch. 21).

## ARTHROGRYPOSIS MULTIPLEX CONGENITA

This name is used for a congenital condition affecting the joints, which may be localised or generalised. The joints may be either extended or flexed but more often the former, with a severe degree of talipes being present. The muscles are atrophic and fibrous, and the skin is tight so that the limbs resemble hosepipes. Arthroplasty has always failed to provide useful movement and the only treatment is to stabilise the affected joints in a good position.

## CONGENITAL CONSTRICTION BAND SYNDROME

This may result in the congenital absence of toes. The condition occurs in utero, possibly due to floating strands in the amnion wrapping around the affected part. This can result in amputation of the part if it occurs in early fetal life. Congenital constriction band syndrome presents as ring-like concentric bands, which may be deep or shallow. Deep bands affect lymphatic and venous drainage, resulting in oedema that causes the distal portion to enlarge (Fig. 12.26).

## POSTURAL ANOMALIES/ABNORMALITIES

These are considered in the section on examination and assessment (see p. 291), but can be found associated with their individual headings elsewhere.

## SURGICAL/MEDICAL CONDITIONS

### Leg-length discrepancy

It is important to realise that up to 1 cm difference in true length is considered a normal variation. Also, apparent discrepancy exists where limbs are actually the same length, but because of the alignment of one or the other are functionally different. The effects of leg-length discrepancy are either to cause a compensatory pelvic tilt and secondary spinal scoliosis, or to make the child walk on the toes in order to effectively lengthen the leg. The latter response will, in time, result in adaptive shortening of the Achilles tendon.

The importance of these clinical situations is that they impose abnormal stresses on the foot, particularly on the talus. These stresses in turn may lead to changes in the function and structure of the foot with growth, and it is these that are important for the podiatrist.

Leg-length discrepancy may develop due to a variety of causes. In all but rare events, such as arteriovenous malformation (in which the leg overgrows) or occasionally following acute osteitis, the short leg is the pathological one. Shortening may be due to malunion of a fracture, but this is not a progressive shortening as occurs when epi-

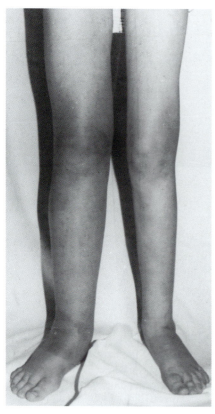

Figure 12.27 Hemihypertrophy of the right leg and foot associated with lymphangioma.

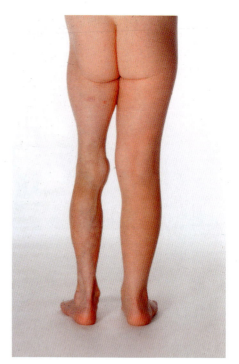

Figure 12.28 Linear scleroderma affecting the leg.

physeal growth plates are damaged by trauma or infection. A flaccid (as opposed to spastic) paralysis deprives a limb of the growth stimulus of muscle contraction, and poliomyelitis has in the past given rise to severe leg-length discrepancy. A length discrepancy of less than 3 cm can be dealt with simply by an appropriate shoe or heel raise, but greater deficiencies may be dealt with by:

- shortening of the longer leg
- retarding growth in the longer leg by destroying or stapling the epiphyseal plates above and below the knee
- lengthening the short leg, usually in the tibial segment, although this requires attention to avoid complications.

Hemihypertrophy ranges from enlargement of a single digit to enlargement of one half of the body. Some cases of limb hypertrophy are associated with a widespread haemangioma or lymphangioma (Fig. 12.27).

## Linear scleroderma

Linear scleroderma occurs as a linear band of hypopigmentation and sclerosis. The legs are most commonly involved and usually in a unilateral distribution (Fig. 12.28). Growth failure may develop in patients with linear scleroderma, affecting a limb because of atrophy of muscle and skin, which in turn affects bone development. Some children may have combined forms, with linear scleroderma on an extremity and morphea on the trunk.

## Localised scleroderma (morphea)

Localised scleroderma is much more common than systemic progressive sclerosis. Morphea usually begins as a circumscribed patch of skin

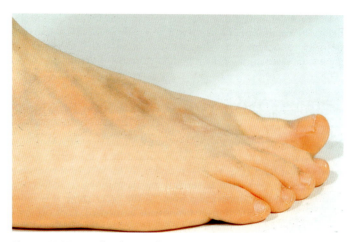

Figure 12.29 Morphea lesion of the right foot.

induration, typically on the trunk, feet or other parts of the body. At onset, the skin is oedematous and warm and has a characteristic violaceous border with an ivory centre. As the skin becomes tight and hard over a joint, range of motion may be limited (Fig. 12.29).

## Pes cavus

There is a wide variation in the height of the arch of the foot, but when this is seen to be marked and unilateral it must be regarded as pathological. The affected leg is often a little thinner and short, and with the raised arch the foot is often smaller. This condition develops in the early years and it is probable that all cases have a neurological cause, mostly due to minor anomalies of the cord in the lumbosacral region. As occasion may justify, investigation by myelography, magnetic resonance imaging or direct surgical exploration will demonstrate a lesion such as an intraspinal lipoma or angioma. In Friedreich's ataxia the characteristic is that of pes cavus associated with hammer toes and also scoliosis. Attempts to deal with the fundamental neurological defect are generally unrewarding and are associated with hazard to continence. Accordingly, attention should be directed to the foot deformity, tackling whichever feature is most troublesome.

## Sever's disease (calcaneal apophysitis)

In many ways this disease is similar to Osgood–Schlatter's disease of the tibial tubercle. The condition troubles children in the age group 10–14 years, with pain at the point of the heel, usually worse during or after athletics. The calcaneal apophysis is tender as the heel strikes the ground, and even on tiptoes is painful due to the pull of the insertion of the Achilles tendon. In half of the children the condition may be bilateral. The diagnosis depends on the history and finding tenderness about the point of the heel. Radiographs are normal. The treatment is simply to restrict activity to a level at which the symptoms are tolerable. Cycling and swimming are useful alternatives to football or netball. An absorbent rubber heel pad to the shoe may cushion heel strike, and in 1–2 years the symptoms will disappear. The affected foot should always be investigated for forefoot/hindfoot malalignment, as this may cause added stress at the insertion of the Achilles tendon and prolong the condition. Appropriate foot orthoses should be prescribed.

In very active children who are actively growing it is not uncommon to encounter Sever's disease, Osgood–Schlatter's disease and pain at the insertion of the plantar fascia to the medial plantar tubercle of the calcaneum occurring concomitantly in the same patient. This should be treated with rest and appropriate foot orthoses.

---

### CASE STUDY 12.1 CALCANEAL PAIN

Andrew is 11 years of age and is in first year at secondary school. He is a very active, robust boy, playing rugby, football and tennis. He also has to walk one mile to attend school. When he started secondary school he became aware of how much more active he was during the school day, travelling between class and going up and down stairs. Also, physical education was much more taxing than at primary school. Six weeks after starting secondary school he noted that his right heel, and to a lesser extent his left heel, became progressively more painful as the day progressed. If he stopped his activities for a few days it improved, but would recur when he resorted to his normal level of activity.

He also complained of occasional pain in the arch of his foot after rugby and football.

On examination his feet were functionally and structurally normal for his age but he did have a degree of excessive subtalar joint pronation associated with a forefoot varus deformity. His feet have grown three sizes in the past year and his mother states that he is increasing in height.

Radiographs of his heel were negative but on examination he complained of pain on palpation along the apophyseal margin of the calcaneum and at the plantar, lateral and posterior point of heel strike, indicating a calcaneal apophysitis. Pain was also elicited at the origin of the plantar fascia at the medial plantar tubercle of the calcaneum, indicating an enthesiopathy.

Both symptoms were associated with growth and increased activity. Andrew was advised to rest, given footwear advice, provided with an appropriate functional foot orthosis and heel lift/cushion. He suffers periods of exacerbation and remission associated with his velocity of growth and level of activity, but with treatment and his awareness of his own 'limit' of activity he is now predominantly pain-free.

---

## Kohler's disease of the navicular

An osteochondritis, similar to Perthe's disease of the hip, Kohler's disease affects the navicular bone, causing vague pain about the midfoot, and locally the part may be tender. Radiographic findings show changes of increased density and collapse of the navicular. With minimal treatment, with temporary supportive padding and strapping or casted supportive foot orthoses, the symptoms will disappear and the radiographic appearances will become normal in 1–2 years.

## Freiberg's disease

In the capital epiphysis of the second (occasionally the third) metatarsal, osteochondritic change similar to Perthe's disease may occur, with the head of the bone becoming enlarged and tender. Radiographs show an irregular increase in density and flattening of the front of the head. This may end up with a large square-shaped metatarsal head, which later in life may need excision, but in childhood no specific treatment is needed as symptoms disappear with rest. However, it is often prudent to 'protect' the area with appropriate padding and strapping as circumstances dictate. This should involve the use of a 1–5 plantar metatarsal pap with a 'U', a 2–4 plantar metatarsal pad, props or dorsoplantar splints. Where there is a forefoot/rearfoot malalignment this should be managed with appropriate foot orthoses – the main objective of all orthoses being to reduce the stresses at the affected metatarsophalangeal joint and maintain it, as far as is possible, in an ideal position functionally.

## Stress fracture of a metatarsal (march or fatigue fracture)

As occurs in the upper tibia, an increase in physical activity may stress a metatarsal (usually the second) and produce an undisplaced self-healing fracture. Local pain, tenderness and swelling will be found, with radiographic changes similar to those seen in the tibia. Moderate rest with supportive padding and strapping for a few weeks will result in cure. Some patients may require a walking plaster.

## Diabetes

Currently, the incidence of diabetes among children in the general population in Scotland is 25 per 100 000 and in England 13 per 100 000 (see also Ch. 9).

Children with diabetes do not require any specialist podiatric care different from that given to other children, as long as their diabetes stays well controlled and they are free from acquired foot infections such as onychocryptosis. However, it is well established that due to the influence of motor, autonomic and sensory neuropathy as they progress through adulthood, those with diabetes are at risk of deformity, infection, ulceration and gangrene. It is therefore important that all diabetic children should be screened by a podiatrist at yearly intervals in order to detect and manage any digital deformities or biomechanical disorders that may be present and thus reduce the risk of potential pressure lesions that may occur in adult life. This also affords the opportunity to provide appropriate health education. All potential future high-risk groups, including those suffering from childhood cancers, neuromuscular disorders and other endocrine and genetic disorders, including Turner's syndrome, should be similarly managed.

## Poliomyelitis

As a result of the introduction of the live oral polio vaccine used for immunisation, only isolated cases of polio are now seen. The disorder is caused by the polio virus, which spreads from the alimentary tract to the central nervous system, particularly the anterior horn cells of the spinal cord. The problems that arise are due to loss of function and the acquisition of deformity, due to the unbalanced pull of muscles no longer opposed by paralysed muscles. The effects of the disease in the lower limb are seen in the muscles, with weakness of inversion, eversion, plantar flexion of the ankle and also foot drop. Each patient's problems are individual. Recovery from the disease is often incomplete. Polio is associated with contracture of muscles causing an equinovarus deformity, pes cavus or permanent foot drop. These conditions may require surgical correction, but will demand considerable attention from the podiatrist owing to abnormal load bearing of the foot and the need for special orthoses and footwear.

## Spina bifida cystica

This is a congenital disorder in which there has been a failure of the posterior spinal elements. The level in the spine at which the lesion occurs relates in some measure to the effects on the patient, but does not equate with their function. Problems arise in the foot in those with sacral lesions, where an imbalance primarily affects the muscles of the foot (Fig. 12.30).

In the legs, the sensory loss may be extensive, depending on the degree of nerve root or spinal cord damage. The motor dysfunction is largely due to root damage giving flaccid paralysis, but areas of spasticity may be present due to higher cord damage with intact lower cord segments and lower motor neuron function, together with a potential to develop severe deformity. Some problems are reasonably predictable: for example, a common level of lesion about L4 will leave the roots of the femoral and obturator nerves largely intact while the sciatic nerve will be paralysed. As a result, the hip, subject to the pull of flexors and adductors but with no extensor or abductor muscle function, will dislocate. At a lower level, active quadriceps, unopposed

by paralysed hamstrings, will produce recurvatum of the knee. The foot may be deformed in any direction, and the loss of the normal weight distribution on the sole of the foot will readily lead to trophic ulceration in the anaesthetic foot.

By a variety of procedures, leg deformity may be controlled and function improved by calliper bracing. Any success in getting the child to stand or walk in some way with various aids depends upon the child's intelligence, the degree of neurological damage and the possible presence of spinal deformity – none of which is under our control. One factor that may be controlled is obesity, which makes standing and walking more difficult. A wheelchair existence is the likely result in many children, and indeed later many may choose this as an easier way of life. The sensory loss gives way to the problems of trophic ulceration. Any ill-fitting appliance or footwear may initiate this, and the ulcer can be very deep as well as slow and difficult to heal. Trophic ulceration is a much more common problem in the second decade of life than the first. Children with spina bifida should be monitored regularly by a podiatrist and treated, referred or advised as circumstances dictate.

## Cerebral palsy

The term cerebral palsy is used to denote a disorder of movement and posture resulting from a permanent, non-progressive defect or lesion of the immature brain. The incidence of cerebral palsy is in the region of 2.5 per 1000 in childhood. The spastic group shows the features of lesions of the pyramidal tracts, such as muscle spasm resulting in spastic postures of the limb. The most common is spastic tetraplegia, in which all four limbs are involved. This group is subdivided into types I and II. In the common type I spastic tetraplegia the legs are more severely involved than the arms. In the much less common type II spastic tetraplegia the spasticity is extremely severe in all four limbs, so that the contractures develop early and disuse muscle atrophy may be masked (Fig. 12.31). As with all of this group of conditions, there is a great need for a team approach to management via all modalities of therapy so that maximum benefit may be gained from each. Inevitably this means that, for the podiatrist, foot care may become a primary treatment.

## Muscular dystrophies

The muscular dystrophies are a group of genetically determined disorders with a common denominator of a progressive degenerative

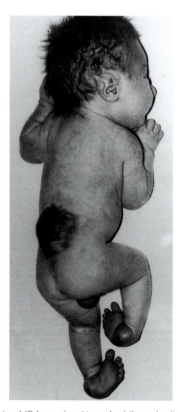

**Figure 12.30** Spina bifida cystica. Note the bilateral talipes equinovarus.

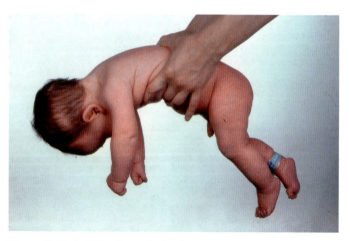

**Figure 12.31** A child with cerebral palsy.

process in the skeletal muscles. These have been subdivided into separate entities mainly on the basis of the distribution and severity of the muscle weakness and their mode of inheritance. Many of these children later develop foot problems and may require help from a podiatrist.

## CASE STUDY 12.2 **RECURRENT INFECTIONS ON THE FOOT**

Adam is now 18 years of age. He first presented as a patient at 8 years old, being referred by his general practitioner who was concerned about chronic recurrent breakdown lesions on the plantar aspect of each heel and recurrent toenail infections. Adam has the less common type II spastic tetraplegia, necessitating permanent wheelchair use and transfer by a helper or his mother. His arterial supply was very poor, as was his venous drainage, due to the dependent position of the feet and the lack of development of a competent arterial supply caused by non-use of the lower limbs. This resulted in chilblains during the winter months, with the feet having a permanent purple appearance and chronic low-grade first toenail infections due to the abnormal and involuntary movement of the toes within the shoes. There was a long history of continued antibiotic use in order to overcome and prevent infection in the feet, which was having a knock-on effect on his general health, with several episodes of chest infections requiring hospitalisation. Positionally, both feet were extremely cavus and inverted, similar to a moderate case of talipes equinovarus, and it was noted that his postural position in his wheelchair was poor due to a kyphoscoliosis. This resulted in chronic overloading of his heels, producing ischaemia and hence breakdown. Mum had great difficulty obtaining appropriate footwear in the high street and Adam had never been assessed by a podiatrist.

Initially, the ulcerated heels were treated with appropriate dressings, addressing the problem as one would with a high-risk diabetic patient, bearing in mind that he was only 8 years old. A new, made-to-measure wheelchair was provided, with appropriate spinal, pelvic and thigh support in order that there were no overload areas on the feet in the footrest. Prescription footwear was provided to accommodate the movement of the toes within the shoes and a casted evazote orthosis was provided for the heels. Digital 2–4 silicone props in Otoform-K™ were also provided to control the movement of the second toe over the hallux and nail plate. The nails responded well to conservative podiatry and regular nail care. Home physiotherapy and massage was arranged in order to improve his venous drainage.

Adam has now been under podiatric care for 10 years. During this time his foot posture has deteriorated secondary to his neuromuscular state, but he has had no further foot infections and a chest infection is now a very rare occurrence. He attends on a regular basis, has his footwear and foot orthoses replaced and wheelchair monitored and adjusted as necessary. He is regarded as a priority patient and is seen immediately if he assesses he has a problem.

There are three important messages in this case. The first is that young children with neuromuscular conditions can be at very high risk of foot problems. Secondly, children do not need to be ambulant to require podiatry, and thirdly, podiatry has a very important role in the holistic management of these patients.

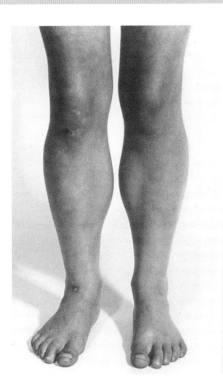

**Figure 12.32** Duchenne muscular dystrophy. Note hypertrophy of the calves.

from birth, the disease usually becomes clinically apparent between the ages of 1 and 4 years. The affected child is slow to walk, falls frequently and has difficulty in getting up or in climbing stairs. Rubbery hypertrophy usually occurs in the calves (Fig. 12.32), quadriceps and deltoids. By the age of 10–12 years most patients need to use a wheelchair for life.

## Hypermobility syndrome

Generalised joint laxity is a feature of the hereditary connective tissue disorders such as Marfan's syndrome, the Ehlers–Danlos syndrome and osteogenesis imperfecta. A patient is considered hypermobile if he or she can perform two of the following three manoeuvres:

- passive opposition of both thumbs to the volar aspect of the forearms
- passive hyperextension of the fingers so they lie parallel to the extensor aspect of both forearms
- active hyperextension of both elbows beyond 180°.

Hypermobility is relatively common in the general population. The term 'hypermobility syndrome' has been coined to define a clinical situation in which there is generalised joint laxity associated with musculoskeletal complaints. In young children this syndrome is observed equally in both sexes, but towards puberty it predominates in girls. The knees are the most frequent sites of complaint but occasionally the ankles may also be affected. The discomfort usually comes after exercise, and the whole clinical picture is consistent with an episode of traumatic synovitis. There is a strong familial tendency to this syndrome and the diagnosis is, therefore, essentially clinical combined with an awareness of family history. The management is largely reassurance as to the absence of serious disease, and activity, which precipitates symptoms, should be avoided if possible. Casted foot orthoses may be of benefit during acute episodes and in maintaining

## Duchenne muscular dystrophy

Compared with other causes of physical handicap, such as cerebral palsy and spina bifida, Duchenne muscular dystrophy is rare. The condition is due to a sex-linked recessive gene with a high mutation rate. Although biochemical and histological abnormality are present

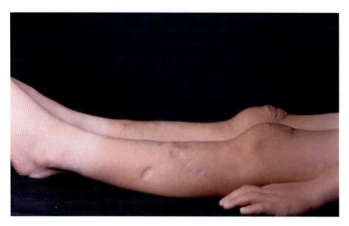

**Figure 12.33** Ehlers–Danlos syndrome. Note genu recurvatum and 'tissue paper' scarring.

foot posture. Most young subjects will grow out of their complaints altogether.

## Ehlers–Danlos syndrome

The disorder is familial and autosomal dominant. The child tends to be slim and underheight, and may have kyphoscoliosis. The hyperextensible joints allow abnormal postures. Genu recurvatum (Fig. 12.33) and pes planus are common. The infant may demonstrate delayed motor milestones, will tend to fall and may sustain recurrent fractures. No specific treatment is available but all foot deformity should be managed as a matter of urgency. Wounds will be slow to heal and will exhibit 'tissue paper' scarring.

## Limb pain of childhood with no organic disease

So-called 'limb pains' or 'growing pains' are more common in childhood than all the other rheumatic diseases put together.

Growth in children involves two phases – 'shooting up' and 'filling out'. A limb may show bone growth followed (not accompanied) by muscle growth. It may be that in such a shooting-up phase extra strain is put on the muscle, which tires easily and gives pain towards the end of the day or during the night when relaxation is incomplete. A history of rheumatic disorders is more common in the families of children with limb pains than in the families of controls, and therefore parents often become worried and feel that their child suffers from rheumatic disease. In two-thirds of affected children limb pains occur during the daytime or evening. In the remainder the pains are predominantly nocturnal and can wake the child and may be severe enough to cause crying. The age group mainly affected is 9–12 years – girls more than boys. The children cite pain between joints – suggesting that the pain is muscular. Most children like to have the area gently rubbed by a parent, which effectively excludes acute rheumatism. With reassurances based on discussion, it should be possible to convince parents that their child does not suffer from a rheumatic disorder. Occasionally, children have psychosomatic musculoskeletal pain and should have a full psychological evaluation. Children with limb pain should respond well to treatment directed towards decreasing the pain and restoring function. Foot orthoses have been found to be of use in some cases, particularly where there is an obvious biomechanical abnormality, but care must be taken not to provide a 'crutch' that is not necessary.

### CASE STUDY 12.3 LIMB PAIN OF CHILDHOOD WITH NO ORGANIC DISEASE AND HYPERMOBILITY SYNDROME

Emma is 7 years old, and since the age of 3 years she has frequently wakened her parents at night, crying and requesting them to rub her legs. This could variably be her knees, outer lower leg, anterior thigh, plantar aspect of the foot and, occasionally, her buttocks. Her mother also gave her Calpol™. Her general practitioner later prescribed ibuprofen, which was taken in the evening before going to bed. Mum could find no pattern in Emma's behaviour or activities that appeared to precipitate an attack, although she knew that she would most likely be attending to Emma during the night after her dance class or a very long day in town. Her general practitioner initially arranged physiotherapy, which made no difference. Emma was then referred to a paediatric orthopaedic surgeon, who found no abnormality. Finally, suspecting a rheumatic disorder, Emma was referred to a paediatric rheumatologist, whose findings were also negative apart from a diagnosis of hypermobility syndrome.

At this point, when Emma was 5 years old, she was referred to a podiatrist because of her foot pain and the suspicion that the limb pain may be associated with abnormal foot posture resulting in an anomaly of gait and general posture, and hence causing muscle pain in an attempt to achieve 'normal' posture.

On examination her feet were markedly hypermobile, with a large degree of forefoot varus and associated excessive subtalar joint pronation. The gait was noticeably apropulsive, with the feet abducted and everted. Advice was given regarding footwear, but this was largely unnecessary as her mother had always suspected that her posture and gait were an issue and had gone to great lengths to obtain the correct footwear. Following subtalar neutral casting and orthotic prescription to control the hypermobility and improve the postural attitude of the foot to the leg and ground, Emma was provided with an appropriate functional foot orthosis and given advice regarding its initial usage. At follow-up 2 weeks later, Emma was pain-free and has remained so to date, with occasional and rare episodes that can be traced to overactivity or unusual activity. She does not get pain after her dance class now and is dancing in competitions.

## Juvenile idiopathic arthritis (juvenile chronic arthritis)

Juvenile idiopathic arthritis (see Ch. 8) comprises a heterogeneous group. It may present as oligoarthritis (Fig. 12.34), systemic arthritis, polyarthritis (rheumatoid factor (RF) negative, antinuclear antibody (ANA) positive), polyarthritis (RF-negative, ANA-negative), polyarthritis (RF-negative, ANA-negative), polyarthritis (RF-positive) or juvenile psoriatic arthritis. Involvement of the joints and soft tissues is a common complication of rheumatoid disease; the extent to which they are affected is varied. In the lower limbs the common joints affected are the hip, knee, ankle and the subtalar joint. There is a wide variety of arthritic foot problems, and leg-length differences are not uncommon. The management of these foot problems depends not only on medical treatment of the arthritis but also on local application of specific measures to the damaged foot. Fortunately, there have been great advances in the prescription of orthoses, involving the development of new materials with appropriate properties, and their use in individual patients for each specific abnormality.

## Psoriatic arthritis

Juvenile psoriatic arthritis has been defined as a form of chronic arthritis with onset before the age of 16 years and occurring in associa-

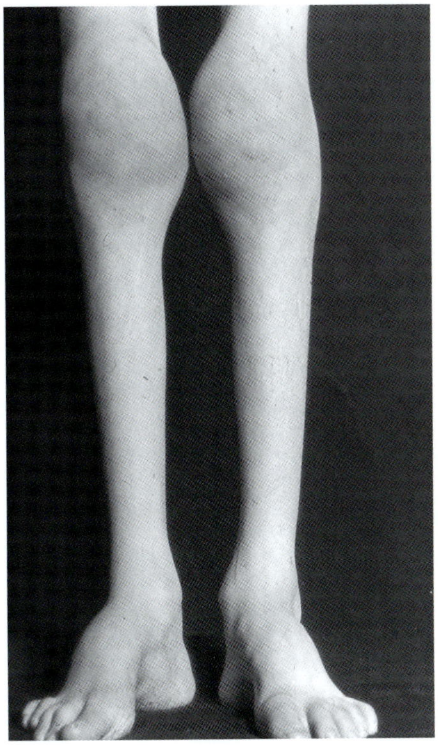

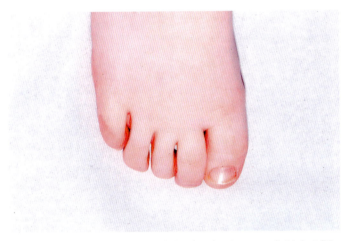

**Figure 12.34** Juvenile idiopathic arthritis (oligoarticular). Note the swollen knees and ankles.

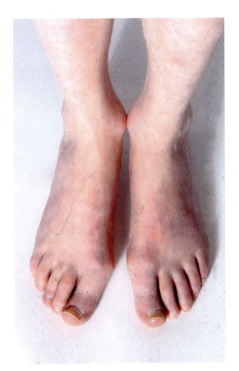

**Figure 12.36** Feet of a boy with Raynaud's phenomenon.

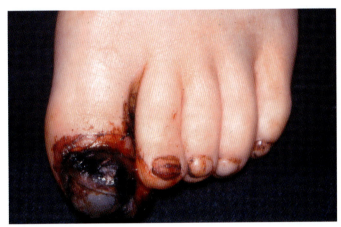

**Figure 12.37** A child with haemophilia showing haemorrhage in the left big toe.

**Figure 12.35** Juvenile psoriatic arthritis showing 'sausage digit' dactylitis.

tion with a characteristic psoriatic rash. The onset of the arthritis is often sudden, with the joint being acutely swollen and painful. Toe or finger joints are frequently involved, often with flexor synovitis, giving a characteristic sausage-digit appearance (dactylitis) (Fig. 12.35). A family history of psoriasis also suggests the diagnosis. These very painful digits respond well to silicone digital devices in the acute phase and also as maintenance therapy.

## Raynaud's phenomenon

Raynaud's phenomenon is prominent in scleroderma. The digits become cold, numb and painful. Local hypoxia leads to cyanosis, resulting in a bluish colour. Raynaud's phenomenon is best treated by keeping the whole body, especially the hands and feet, warm, and by preventing and protecting the body from cold exposure. Feet, especially toes, should be carefully monitored, particularly through the autumn and winter months, with prevention and early management of problems being a high priority (Fig. 12.36).

## Haemophilia

Joint swelling and pain often heralds haemarthrosis, which is the single most incapacitating event in the life of a severe haemophiliac. The correct policy is to encourage the patient to attend hospital at the earliest sign of joint swelling in order that replacement therapy can be given. Where there is joint deformity in the foot, either as a result of bleeding or from some intrinsic primary cause, it is important that appropriate orthotic management is instigated at an early stage in order to limit damage and encourage normal function (Fig. 12.37).

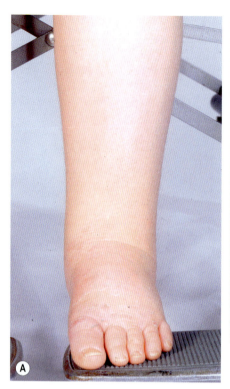
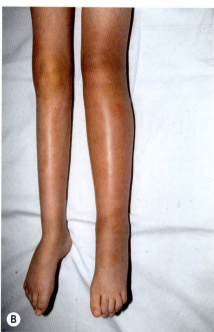

**Figure 12.38** (A, B) Lymphoedema associated with Turner's syndrome.

## Turner's syndrome

Foot problems such as lymphoedema of the lower limb secondary to poor lymphatic drainage and nail dysplasia are well recognised as valuable diagnostic features in Turner's syndrome. Affected girls are at increased risk of ingrowing toenails compared to the general population, and this is due to a number of factors in combination. Typically, the girls have short, broad feet with hyperextension of the great toe, involuted toenails and oedematous periungual tissues, accompanied by subtalar joint pronation resulting in damage to the nail plate and surrounding soft tissues. Due to the poor lymphatic drainage, girls with Turner's syndrome are at increased risk of cellulitis, and thus all cases must be treated diligently and as a matter of urgency (Fig. 12.38).

### CASE STUDY 12.4 THE EFFECTS OF TURNER'S SYNDROME ON THE FOOT

Jane was diagnosed with Turner's syndrome following karyotype testing when suspicions were raised shortly after her birth due to persistent ankle oedema. She also appeared to have no toenails at birth. As a result of her short stature and short and very broad variably swollen feet, appropriate footwear was almost impossible to obtain, with the available shoes being far too long to accommodate the breadth and swelling, resulting in frequent trips and falls. Also, because of involution of the toenails, hyperextension of the first toes, developmental subtalar joint pronation and inappropriate footwear, accompanied by chronic ankle oedema, Jane began to develop ingrowing toenails shortly after she began to walk. This was dealt with initially by appropriate footwear and nail-cutting advice. Girls with Turner's syndrome have a high pain threshold, and may have behaviour difficulties resulting in toenail picking, which compounded the problem in this case. As she became older, the Turner's syndrome features in the foot became more pronounced and the ingrowing toenails more marked and persistent, resulting in one prolonged hospital stay necessitating the administration of intravenous antibiotics to combat a severe cellulitis. Due to chronic lymphoedema, Jane was also managed by bed rest and elevation, which made no difference to the swelling as the lymphatic system could not drain fluid as intended. The most appropriate management would have been normal exercise in order to allow the venous system to drain the excess fluid. Following resolution of the infection and a partial nail avulsion with phenolisation, there have been no further serious episodes, due to diligent and immediate podiatric input if a problem is suspected. Jane's mother has been given advice regarding nail care, contact telephone numbers, oral antibiotics (to be given at the first suspicion of infection) and topical 10% betadine aqueous solution (for children over 2 years old) or 0.5% chlorhexidine in spirit applied on a once-daily basis as prophylaxis.

## Down's syndrome (trisomy 21)

The most significant of the autosomal trisomies is trisomy 21, or Down's syndrome. The features of Down's syndrome are usually evident at birth. Classically, the most striking physical abnormalities are to be seen in the face and skull. During the first years of life, hypotonia and laxity of joints are often evident, but these become less apparent as the child grows older. The first and second fingers and/or toes may be widely spaced (Fig. 12.39). Children with Down's syndrome may have a number of pedal anomalies, including hypermobility with an adducted first ray and severe pes plano valgus compounded by genu valgum, and in some cases they may be overweight. There may also be circulatory compromise, which should be monitored carefully. Down's children are also prone to psoriatic arthropathy and are unlikely to complain of pain; therefore, diligent examination is important.

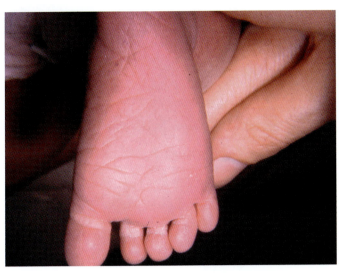

**Figure 12.39** The foot in Down's syndrome. Note the widely spaced first and second toes ('sandal sign').

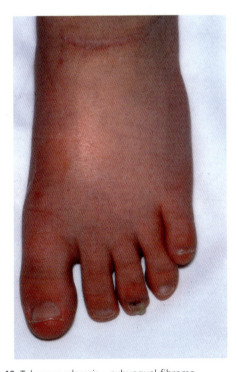

**Figure 12.40** Tuberous sclerosis – subungual fibroma.

## Tuberous sclerosis

This is inherited as an autosomal-dominant condition, and 75% of cases have a positive family history. The characteristic features of tuberous sclerosis are mental retardation from birth, and epilepsy starting usually before 2 years of age. The classical clinical triad consists of edenoma sebaceum, and epilepsy and metal retardation. The skin patches found are shagreen patches over the sacrum, ichthyosis, café au lait spots, subungual fibromas (Fig. 12.40), telangiectasia and vitiligo.

## DERMATOLOGICAL CONDITIONS

The most common dermatological conditions seen in childhood are atopic eczema and dermatitis. Psoriasis may also appear at any age but is more common in the late teens. Juvenile plantar dermatosis is also common in childhood, is associated with atopic eczema, and usually presents around 3–4 years of age and disappears in the teens. Verrucae are also very common, as are blisters; however, fungal infections are relatively uncommon until the teens. Inherited and acquired keratodermas may manifest in childhood, and these and other dermatological conditions are detailed in Chapter 3.

## EXAMINATION AND ASSESSMENT

Children should not be treated as mini-adults and their feet should not be treated as miniature versions of adult feet. Children's feet are constantly being subjected to developmental change due to both intrinsic factors within the foot due to growth, and extrinsic factors within the lower limb and skeleton in general, associated with growth and torsional change within the long bones and postural change within the body, generally. A child's psychological make-up, expectations, perceptions and behaviour are also different from those of an adult, and these factors have to be taken into consideration during the examination. Children may also present with one or more adults whose anxieties and needs also have to be considered. A relaxed, happy and cooperative child is quickly and easily examined.

The needs of a child within a specialist paediatric unit are relatively easily catered for, as such units are geared to being user-friendly, with appropriate decor, toys, games etc., and staff who are well versed in dealing with children. This scenario is less likely within a 'hard' clinical site, and an appropriate area for children should be set aside. The podiatrist should provide a relaxed, stress-free atmosphere and be wary of causing anxiety or distress by words or actions.

Examination and assessment in general has been dealt with in Chapter 1, but due to the specific nature of the problems encountered in examining the paediatric patient it is recommended that the following examination methodology be employed:

- relaxed, stress-free atmosphere
- observe gait and posture with footwear
- subjective questioning of child and/or parent
- measure feet and measure footwear
- examine footwear
- visual examination of foot for skin, nail, soft-tissue and bony lesions
- physical examination of lesions as required
- physical examination of the range, quality and direction of motion in all joints of the foot
- determine foot type
- biomechanical assessment for forefoot/rearfoot malalignment
- observe and assess barefooted gait and general posture
- compare barefooted gait and general posture with foot posture and general findings, comparing right with left
- make a firm diagnosis
- produce a management plan
- provide written literature concerning the complaint and treatments.

This methodology is designed to highlight any lower-limb pathology or developmental change/anomaly that may be present, which can then be investigated and managed further by the podiatrist or referred to the appropriate specialist. It utilises the ASK, LOOK, TOUCH convention, which guides the practitioner through a set diagnostic strategy in order to avoid misdiagnosis or missed diagnoses by making hasty, ill-informed assumptions.

These principles can also be applied in podopaediatric screening programmes, where it is important that nothing is overlooked as there may not be a further opportunity to examine the child.

## Observe gait and posture with footwear

This is easily observed when the practitioner accompanies the patient from the waiting room. It may be the only opportunity to observe the child when they are not aware that they are being watched. If the child is brought to you this opportunity is lost, and you may not obtain a true picture of the gait and posture. Children have a habit of demonstrating a 'Ministry of Silly Walks' type of gait when they are requested to walk, or will walk only when holding a parent's hand – which, with a small child, causes the hand to be held high in the air, with associated changes to their posture and pattern of gait. This may falsely produce or mask features. Very young children tend to be inconsistent regarding posture and gait, as they do not have an established body image and are constantly experimenting. Furthermore, developmental change produces constant, yet subtle, changes in the skeleton for which the child must make allowances to maintain equilibrium.

## Subjective questioning of child and/or parent

This should be done in such a manner that the important facts are obtained without setting a false trail by putting words in the mouth of the child, who may be happy to agree in order to please. Also, remember that the child is not an inanimate object who is detached from the proceedings. It is always important to communicate with children and include them in any discussion. This may be difficult with some overbearing parents or an overly nervous or precocious child.

## Measure feet, measure footwear

The feet and footwear should be measured on compatible gauges in order to determine their relationship. Ideally, the shoes should be approximately two sizes larger than the foot when new (English shoe-sizing system). The use of a foot-measuring board (Fig. 12.41) also affords the opportunity to assess asymmetry of length, width and girth, as well as any other noticeably different features between the two feet, against a linear background. The footboard also provides hard evidence, which can be recorded and charted. Many non-specific foot complaints occur during periods of active growth.

## Examine footwear

This should take into account the degree and pattern of wear and should include the heel, sole and combined heel and sole wear. It should also include any deformation of the uppers and heel stiffener. Typically, a 'normal' adult will wear down the heel of the shoe posterolaterally and this will also be found in older children. However, children undergoing developmental change up to approximately 7–9 years of age may show posterior wear that would be considered abnormal in an adult but is a feature the child will grow out of as change takes place. Each case has to be taken on its own merit, with all factors being taken into consideration. Moderate to severe medial heel wear with possibly forefoot wear and bulging or broken counters generally require some form of intervention and possibly further investigation. This is certainly the case if the problem is unilateral, or associated with pain or a general postural abnormality. Many children will exhibit this pattern of wear but when asked to walk barefooted will appear

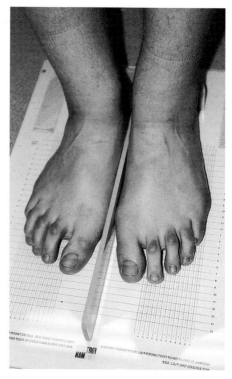

**Figure 12.41** Measuring feet with a foot board during a routine screening session. Note the pressure marks on the dorsal aspect of the interphalangeal joints.

normal. This is often due to the style of shoe with a raised heel and poor counter such that the heel falls off of the shoe medially. A lower heel and firm counter usually produce a 'cure'.

Deformation of the uppers is usually due to deformity of the hallux or lesser toes. There is a habit among some shoe fitters to 'fit large', allowing excessive growing room but making the shoes too spacious on the dorsum of the foot, causing deep creasing. Refitting solves the problem.

The style and suitability of the footwear should also be considered with respect to the child's age and the shape of the foot. If the child is wearing prescription footwear and orthoses this should also be recorded and assessed for suitability.

It is not unusual for children within one family to share footwear, and as a result it is not uncommon to find a child with normal feet wearing footwear suggesting gross deformity, or vice versa.

Also, abnormal wear where the foot is found to be 'normal' may be induced due to habit traits and other activities (e.g. football, cycling, tennis), which can confuse a diagnosis. Children suffering from neuromuscular disease almost always show abnormal wear, and this is widely variable according to the muscle groups affected and the effect upon the general posture and gait. As with all children with abnormal wear on the shoes, these wear marks should always be recorded and charted, as they can be an early indicator of deterioration and thus allow for early intervention.

## Visual examination of foot for skin, nail, soft-tissue and bony lesions

It may be that the presence of these lesions is due to inadequate footwear, intrinsic or extrinsic structural abnormality, or both. It is not unusual to find multiple pressure marks that the child has no concern about (see Fig. 12.41). Bursae and bursitis are also common at the posterior aspect of the heel, the dorsum of the interphalangeal joints of the toes, and the medial and lateral aspects of the first and fifth metatarsophalangeal joints, respectively.

Callus and ulceration are relatively rare unless there is severe deformity, sensory impairment or the footwear is persistently unsuitable, as is often found on return to school after holidays with girls wearing new fashion shoes but not prepared to admit that they are troublesome. These are the individuals who are also most likely to present with fibrous and periarticular thickening associated with footwear. Acute nail conditions are most commonly found in teenagers, particularly boys. However, it is not unusual to find babies with ingrowing toenails. Where there is sensory impairment and/or abnormality of function, either intrinsic, extrinsic or both, there is the possibility of any form of lesion and ulceration.

## Physical examination of lesions as required

*Physical examination of range, quality and direction of motion in all joints of the foot*

This is a skilled assessment requiring considerable experience. All joints, including the ankle, subtalar, midtarsal, metatarsophalangeal and interphalangeal joints, should be examined for range, quality and direction of motion, comparing right with left. In children there should be a considerable range of motion free from crepitus, pain or restriction. It should be remembered, however, that some individuals do not have large ranges of joint motion, and this is perfectly normal in the absence of any systemic disease or injury. In children with juvenile idiopathic arthritis or neuromuscular conditions particular attention should be paid to the range of motion at the subtalar and ankle joints. In children with systemic disease or following trauma, great care should be taken during this part of the examination, as the affected joints may be exquisitely painful to even the slightest movement. The range of motion or deformity (e.g. hallux abducto valgus) in problem joints should be recorded using a goniometer, for charting and comparison at a later date once treatment has been instigated. Young children may not be cooperative and it may be possible only to obtain an impression of any abnormality that may be present. The various foot types discussed earlier in this chapter should be determined.

## Biomechanical assessment, including examination for forefoot/rearfoot malalignment

Biomechanical assessment can be very difficult in the young child for a variety of reasons. This has been discussed previously, but as accurate an assessment as possible should be carried out, including examination for forefoot to rearfoot malalignment. The procedure for assessment is detailed in Chapter 1.

## Observe and assess barefooted gait and general posture

This part of the examination relies heavily on experience and a 'quick eye'. As a general convention, it is usually better to ignore the feet initially as it is best to obtain an impression of the skeleton in general before considering the effect on the foot, or vice versa. Remember that the feet and legs are interdependent – neither should be considered in isolation. A long, well-lit corridor is ideal for this purpose. If the patient is particularly uncooperative, a play area or physiotherapy gymnasium is ideal, where the child can be left to play while the podiatrist sits in a corner and observes. The following factors should be considered when observing gait and posture in children:

- *Head* – size, shape, symmetry, facial expression
- *Shoulders* – level, position
- *Spine* – kyphosis, lordosis, scoliosis, kyphoscoliosis
- *Pelvis* – anteroposterior tilting, posteroanterior tilting, lateral tilting, rotation, asymmetry
- *Hips* – level
- *Femur* – bowing, internal torsion, external torsion
- *Knee* – position of patella (inward, forward, outward facing), genu valgum, genu varum, genu recurvatum
- *Tibia* – internal torsion, external torsion, bowing
- *Foot* – in-toeing, out-toeing, calcaneal deviation, (excessive) subtalar joint pronation, forefoot deformity.

## Comparison

Compare the barefooted gait and general posture with the foot posture and general findings, comparing right with left.

## Diagnosis

Make a firm diagnosis and record measurements for comparison at a later date. Discuss your findings, treatment options and the potential outcomes with the parents or carers, and obtain informed consent to progress with the child's management.

## Produce a management plan

Decide whether to treat (there and then, or at a later date), monitor or refer.

Box 12.2 gives an example of a simple management plan for a 9-year-old girl presenting with onychocryptosis affecting the medial

---

**Box 12.2 Example of a management plan**

**Plan**

**Immediate**
- Footwear advice, with reference to size, heel height and retaining medium
- Conservative management of onychocryptosis. Consider partial nail avulsion if there is no improvement in 2 weeks
- Casted functional foot orthosis with medial forefoot post to control excessive subtalar joint pronation associated with forefoot varus. Review every 3–4 months

**Follow-on once immediate plan established**
- Passive stretching exercises for digits integrated with intrinsic muscle exercises for digits and passive circumduction exercises for hallux for 3 months. Follow with:
  - night splints for hallux abducto valgus?
  - digital 2–4 silicone prop with 1/2 interdigital wedge. Review initially at 6 weeks then 3 months
  - extend review to 3–6 monthly intervals for at least 3 years; sooner if required by patient
  - monitor hallux abducto valgus for several years. Consider future surgical opinion if degree of deformity increases significantly

**Comments**
- Parents advised regarding possible outcomes of onychocryptosis and foot condition generally
- Health promotion material related to footwear, exercises and foot orthoses provided

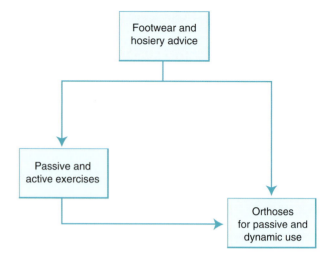

Figure 12.42 Paediatric podiatry management methodology.

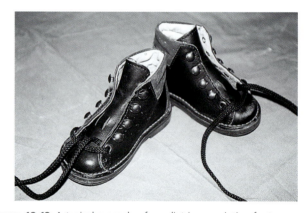

Figure 12.43 A typical example of paediatric prescription footwear.

border of the right first toenail associated with forefoot varus that has resulted in excessive subtalar joint pronation, 15° hallux abducto valgus and claw toes. The footwear was also two sizes too small, with a 5 cm heel and no retaining medium.

## Written information

Provide written literature, which the patient may take home and study at their leisure, concerning the complaint and associated management (Box 12.3).

## MANAGEMENT

Many children with foot pathologies are treated in a relatively ad hoc fashion, with little apparent logic to the management. In order to overcome this, a logical approach is required. Having made a diagnosis, obtained informed consent and formulated a management plan, all children should be managed similarly, utilising a standard convention. This simply involves footwear, exercises and orthoses (Fig. 12.42).

## Footwear advice and prescription

There is little point in attempting to manage a structural foot condition until suitable footwear and hosiery have been obtained or provided. This is equally true for most foot conditions. Where there is a financial burden upon the family, many charities provide footwear for children with proven chronic foot disorders.

Often, children with a disability are 'over-shod' with clumpy, unsuitable and socially unacceptable prescription footwear, which is often unnecessary, and 'off-the-peg' shoes should always be considered where possible. Currently, the available range of trainers is so vast and diverse that, unless the deformity is gross or particularly difficult to manage, it should be possible to find a suitable trainer. This not only improves the podiatric management, providing a suitable vehicle for an orthosis, but it also enhances the child's psychological well-being.

Footwear is such an important issue in the podiatric management of the paediatric patient that, until it is resolved, treatment normally cannot continue. The podiatrist will have to decide whether or not to continue with orthotic management with, say, a teenager, where the effect of the device is being negated by unsuitable footwear due to non-compliance. It may be that the best approach is to leave a long time until the return visit in the hope that their attitude may change in the meantime. Where there is an obvious financial burden on the family, it is probably best to make the most of the situation in the hope that it will improve.

Most hospital orthotic departments supply footwear (Fig. 12.43) but this is sometimes limited and directed more towards the use of rigid ankle/foot orthoses or leg/ankle/foot orthoses. Footwear for more dynamic podiatric use may have to be found elsewhere. As alluded to previously, there are many excellent trainers on the market in both shoe and boot form which provide excellent support for the hindfoot and can almost be regarded as a treatment in themselves with regard to controlling the subtalar joint.

## Passive and active exercises

Once appropriate footwear has been obtained or while attempting to resolve the footwear issue, both passive and active exercises may be prescribed, depending upon need. Passive exercises will help to stretch tightened tissues and mobilise joints and, if necessary, can be complemented by active exercises. Typical examples where this can be employed are digital deformities, shortening of the Achilles tendon, and where there is active disease within the foot, such as the effect of juvenile idiopathic arthritis upon the subtalar joint resulting in rigid or semimobile eversion. Generally this management incorporated with active exercises to re-educate and balance muscle groups is best undertaken by a physiotherapist who can advise the parents on home treatment. This should be incorporated as part of the multidisciplinary approach to care, allowing the podiatrist to concentrate on orthotic management.

Hydrotherapy and physical therapies may also be employed at this stage, but it must always be remembered that the foot is still growing and therefore still possesses epiphyseal plates, which may become damaged, particularly in the very young child. The use of ultrasound therapy is usually contraindicated.

One of the most common reasons for referral is digital abnormalities. Figure 12.44 shows intrinsic muscle digital exercises, which are very effective and relatively easy to perform. Most children under 8 years old find this exercise very difficult, if not impossible. However, it is easy to teach as the child can learn the exercise with their hand initially and then transpose it to their feet. Children showing early stages of hallux abducto valgus can mobilise the joint utilising a passive circumduction exercise to the first metatarsophalangeal joint while maintaining traction on the joint. Active adduction exercises for

the hallux can also be employed in an attempt to maintain or correct the position of the hallux (Fig. 12.45).

## Orthoses for passive and dynamic use

### Night splints

Orthoses for passive use help to maintain correction of deformity obtained dynamically during walking. This may simply be an additional silicone digital device to maintain correction in bed or a night splint to maintain ankle joint extension at 90° where there is tightening of the Achilles tendon.

Night splints for the management of hallux abducto valgus (Fig. 12.46) have been used for many years, often as the only means of correction, with no exercise therapy or orthotic management of the foot. The aetiology of hallux abducto valgus remains contentious. It seems unlikely that a device worn during rest for one-third of the day, with the first toe being subjected to abnormal biomechanical stress and/or the deforming influence of footwear for two-thirds of the day will have a significant effect unless used as part of an integrated management programme as detailed above. Accounts vary as to the efficacy of integrated orthotic management for hallux abducto valgus, as the degree of deformity and accompanying features vary. However, it is suggested that early intervention and a positive approach will provide a better long-term result, and should an osteotomy be required at a later date, after bony maturity, the first metatarsophalangeal joint will have been protected from excessive damage, providing a better long-term outcome.

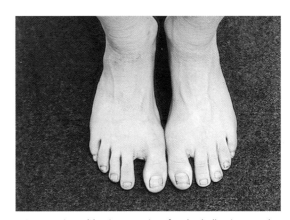

**Figure 12.45** Active adduction exercises for the hallux in a moderate case of juvenile hallux abducto valgus.

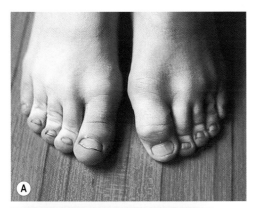

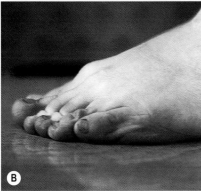

**Figure 12.44** Dorsal (A) and lateral (B) views of digital intrinsic muscle exercises. The action of the lumbrical muscles to flex the metatarsophalangeal joints and extend the interphalangeal joints can be clearly seen.

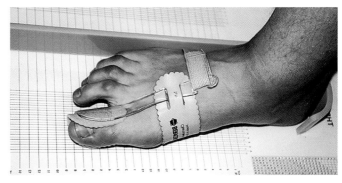

**Figure 12.46** Example of a night splint passively correcting hallux abducto valgus. (Note that night splints should not be used weight bearing.)

## Silicone

The dynamic use of orthotics is provided by silicone in its endless applications for digital management and should normally be reviewed at 6-weekly intervals when actively correcting deformity. When treating very young children, great care should be taken in patient selection and parental advice, as choking may occur if the child puts the device in his or her mouth after removing shoes and hosiery. Silicone devices can also be used for correction and maintenance of position in scalds and burns, where contracture will cause an increase in deformity, or in progressive neuromuscular disorders.

When managing hallux abducto valgus the use of an interdigital wedge in the first interspace should be avoided, as the device tends to act as an extra digit, pushing the other lesser digits laterally, and has little or no effect on the hallux. This condition is best managed with a two to four combined prop to splint the hallux against the lesser toes and thus promote correction.

## Casted foot orthoses

The use of casted foot orthoses forms the mainstay of podiatric orthotic management in children. The type of device, and when to use it, must be the decision of the practitioner according to the findings for each individual child. In general terms, rigid casted orthoses are contraindicated (although semi-rigid devices may be indicated) in children undergoing developmental change, which is at its greatest up until approximately 8 years of age. The majority of cases of subtalar joint pronation relate to compensation for normal physiological change, which should be left well alone unless it is excessive, causing particular secondary problems within the foot, or complicated by other biomechanical disorders. Where the practitioner is unsure, or the parents particularly concerned, the child can be monitored at regular intervals, measurements taken and the parents reassured, with orthotics possibly being used at a later date when the picture is clearer.

Children affected by systemic disease and neuromuscular conditions must be treated positively, each one on their own merit, to control or correct the problem. It is best to cast each child individually and not use 'off-the-shelf' orthoses.

Parents should be given verbal and written advice regarding the use of orthoses, and followed up, initially at short intervals, with the time between follow-ups being gradually extended.

As stated previously, the foot cannot be regarded in isolation, and before embarking on orthotic management the podiatrist must be satisfied regarding the primary seat of the pathology. If there is any concern regarding a more proximal cause of the condition or of systemic disease the child should be referred accordingly. Where bow leg, knock-knee or spinal lordosis is detected outwith the normal developmental stages, or the problem is unilateral, appropriate referral should be made.

## THE ROLE OF THE PAEDIATRIC PODIATRIST

In many ways this differs from the role of the podiatrist in other sectors of podiatry, as there is the opportunity to prevent and correct deformity and maintain normal function, underpinned by footwear prescription and advice and health promotion as part of a multidisciplinary team. Traditional skills in the management of skin, soft-tissue lesions, nail conditions and infections are still necessary but play only a small part. It is not always necessary to indulge in physical treatment, and often 'masterly inactivity' in the form of monitoring, charting and advising over time is the main requirement. When dealing with structural problems the practitioner must always be satisfied that he or she is dealing with a pathological state requiring intervention, and not a 'normal' variant of developmental change.

## REFERENCES

University of Glasgow 2009 OMIM Online Mendelian Inheritance in Man. Department of Medical Genetics, University of Glasgow. Available at: http://www.gla.ac.uk/medicalgenetics/neales.htm.

## FURTHER READING

Goad RN 1997 Pediatric podiatry. WB Saunders, Philadelphia, PA.

Harris EJ 2000 Advances in the treatment of pediatric flatfoot. WB Saunders.

Labovitz JM 2006 Pediatric foot and ankle disorders. Saunders, Philadelphia, PA.

Mini-symposium 2002 The paediatric foot. Churchill Livingstone.

Podopediatrics. Written Symposium. Papers, British Library.

Tax HR 1985 Podopediatrics, 2nd edn. Williams & Wilkins (out of print).

Thomson P, Russel GV 2001 Introduction to podopaediatrics. Churchill Livingstone, Edinburgh.

# Chapter 13

# Sports medicine and injuries

*Donald L Lorimer*

## KEYWORDS

Achilles tendon injuries

Ankle injuries

Association football

Ballet and dance injuries

Baseball

Basketball injuries

Bowling injuries

Children and adolescent sports

Chronic leg pain

Cross-country skiing

Forefoot injuries

Golf injuries

Gymnastics

History taking

Heel pain

Impingement syndrome of the ankle

Marathon running

Muscle cramps

North American football

Overuse injuries

Phases of running

Posterior tendon dysfunction

Psychological factors

Retrocalcaneal exostosis

Rugby football

Skiing injuries

Snowboarding

Step/bench aerobics

Stress fractures

Tennis injuries

Tibial fasciitis (shin splints)

## INTRODUCTION

Sports-related injuries have become a very common entity seen by the podiatrist. With the advent of exercise programmes, as well as amateur and professional sports, it is imperative that the practitioner has the knowledge to diagnose and treat many of the overuse and traumatic injuries seen in the foot and ankle. The continual and ever-expanding study of sports medicine now incorporates a total 'sports medicine team' consisting of the primary care physician, sports medicine subspecialist, physical medicine and rehabilitation specialist, orthopaedist, podiatrist, chiropractor, athletic trainer, physical therapist and massage therapist. The podiatrist is an integral part of this comprehensive, multidisciplinary team using his or her expertise of lower extremity biomechanics to offer conservative management and remedies to the injured athlete.

Many sports involve repetitive action of lower extremity joints and muscle groups, and thus overuse injuries are a common result. The recognition of the foot, ankle and lower extremity injuries, and their

successful treatment, rely upon a proper history of the athlete (see Ch. 1) and a knowledge of the particular sport as well as the anatomical structures and biomechanics involved (see Ch. 15). In addition, a thorough physical examination, prudent clinical judgement and anatomically sound treatment, as well as an early and assertive physical and functional rehabilitation programme, are necessary.

## ATHLETIC PROFILE AND HISTORY TAKING

When treating the athletic patient, the sports medicine practitioner should have a clear-cut understanding of the particular sport of that patient. In addition, it is imperative that the practitioner should also be cognisant of the unusual emotional, physiological, biomechanical and nutritional demands of the athletic patient. The podiatrist should have a working knowledge of the biomechanics and kinetics of that specific sport and the pattern of injury that can occur, as well as the rehabilitation exercises that the athlete should employ to return safely back to sporting activity. In addition, the practitioner should be aware of age-related injuries and their prevention and also general medical factors related to gender. For example, *female triad* is a term used to describe female athletes who have become too serious about exercise and sport (e.g. track stars, ballet dancers). Frequently they do not eat well and lose too much weight to maintain their perceived 'image' and consequently develop anorexia nervosa. As a result of eating poorly, they lose fat from their bodies and develop amenorrhoea, bone density loss, and osteoporosis.

The main focus of the podiatric sports medicine specialist should be to treat the athlete conservatively, avoid surgery whenever possible, and have the athlete return to sports competition healed, and in better condition than before the injury. Special attention should be directed towards improving the athlete's strength, flexibility, proprioception, balance, alignment, power and biomechanical function. There should be good communication between the sports medicine specialist and the athlete, creating an awareness of the mechanism of injury and how that injury can be prevented in the future.

The following questions may be helpful in gaining a specific understanding of the athletic patient:

1. What type of athlete is to be treated? An amateur, high school, collegiate or professional athlete? A recreational athlete? A serious addicted athlete, marathon runner or triathlete? A fitness walker, senior citizen fitness enthusiast, high-impact aerobics exerciser, jogger or 'weekend warrior'?
2. What are the inherent risks of the sport? Will the patient be subject to higher risk for recurrent injury, and what measures can be employed to lower the risk of re-injury?
3. How important is it for the patient to return to a competitive level of the sport?
4. How likely is it that the treatment plan will be successful or fail due to the biomechanics of the sport?
5. Is the injury acute or due to overuse? If it is an overuse injury, how can the underlying cause be corrected biomechanically?
6. Will the treatment plan safely allow the athlete to return to his or her sport, without greater or further risk of injury?
7. When faced with a severe injury, how will the athletic patient deal psychologically with 'exercise withdrawal'? Are there safe cross-training activities that can be recommended to the patient to maintain 'training effect', and yet reduce the chances of recurrent injury?
8. Is the patient compliant and following the training rule of not increasing by more than 10% per week to 2-week periods?

9. Is the patient addicted to their sports and 'overexercising'? Are they subjecting themselves to higher risk of injury? At what stage do they reach too much aerobic activity?

10. Is it safe for a child or adolescent athlete to compete at this level all year round? When do these younger athletes need to rest to allow for recuperation, particularly after injury?

11. What types of overuse injuries are specific to the sport, and how are they recognised?

12. How can sport and aerobic physical activity benefit or be detrimental to the patient?

13. When is it the appropriate time to have an athlete stop that particular sport or change to another sporting endeavour?

Box 13.1 suggests questions that should be asked when taking a history from an athletic patient.

## Past treatment history

There are a variety of sports injuries that may be categorised as acute, chronic but improving (overuse) or chronic and not improving. An understanding of tissue response to trauma is helpful when creating an appropriate treatment plan and anticipating the eventual outcome (Frederson 1996). The aetiology behind the injury may be due to a number of factors: age, physiological preparedness, psychological dependency and, of course, biomechanical considerations.

An acute injury or traumatic injury occurs when an episode stresses tissue beyond its normal physiological limits. These injuries can affect a variety of tissues and anatomical sites, but they all share a common aetiology: repetitive trauma that overwhelms the tissue's ability to repair itself (Herring & Nelson 1987). For example, a tendon ruptures when its tensile strength is exceeded. A ligament ruptures when the normal range of motion of a joint is exceeded. A sprain occurs when there is disruption of the ligamentous structures surrounding the joint. An inflammatory process that usually lasts 24 hours – and is characterised by vasodilatation, local necrosis of tissue, and the release of inflammatory cellular elements such as prostaglandin, serotonin and histamine (Subotnick & Sisney 1999) – follows acute injury. Factors in inflammation can be classified into three categories: vasoactive substances, chemotactic factors, and agents leading to cell and tissue damage (Rodman & Schumacher 1983). After acute injury, the initial inflammatory phase is best treated with the mnemonic RICE (Rest, Ice, Compression, Elevation).

Knowledge of how the patient treated the initial injury, and how that treatment may have affected the condition, is imperative. With early treatment, the practitioner and athlete can reduce the undesirable effects of the acute inflammatory phase. Applications of ice

---

### Box 13.1 Taking the history of the sporting patient (after Boyd & Bogdan 1997)

#### Training history

- How many years have you been running?
- How many miles per day do you average?
- How many miles per week do you run?
- What's your longest run during the week or weekend?
- What pace (in minutes per mile/kilometre) do you average in your workouts?
- Do you do interval training? Track work?
- What type of terrain do you usually run on (dirt, grass, asphalt, concrete, cinder, beach sand, hills, flat, crowned, or track)?
- Do you run on any canted surfaces (on one side of the road, on beaches) or always around a track (in the same direction or opposite directions) clockwise or counterclockwise?
- What time of day do you normally run (a.m., p.m., or midday)?

#### Racing history

- How often do you race?
- Do you compete in 5000 or 10 000 metres or marathons? Do you compete in triathlons?

#### Running shoe history

- In what brand and model(s) of running shoes do you train and/or race?
- How long have you had your present pair(s) of running shoes?
- Approximately how many miles of wear do you have on your present shoe(s)?
- Do you 'build up' your running shoes to keep the outer soles from wearing out too quickly?
- Where does the most outer sole wear occur on your running shoes (inside/outside/back)?
- How do your shoes fit (too long, short, narrow, wide)?
- Do you wear a straight last, curved last or semicurved lasted shoe?
- Do you wear socks when you run? Of what type of material are these made (cotton, acrylic, coolmax)? How many pairs of socks do you wear?

- Are you still wearing the same model shoe more than one time?
- Do any of your pairs of shoes make the problem better or worse?
- Do you wear any orthotics, over-the-counter insoles, special arch supports in your shoes?

#### Pre/post run activities

- Do you stretch before and/or after your run and for how long?
- What type of stretching do you do (describe it precisely)?
- Do you warm-up/warm-down for your runs and for how long?
- Do you do any muscle strengthening exercises (weight training)? Describe them?
- Do you participate in any other sports or any other physical activities (cross-training)?
- Do you use a massage therapist?

#### Injury-related history

- Did you modify your training/racing schedule prior to your injury? Have you increased your mileage significantly in a short period of time?
- Did you run a particularly hard race or have a hard workout immediately prior to your injury?
- Did you switch to another pair of running shoes prior to your injury? How long have you worn them?
- Did you modify your shoes prior to your injury?
- Did you adapt to your new orthotics slowly? Over how long a period?
- Was there any direct trauma associated with your injury?
- Did you have another injury or any discomfort in your feet or legs prior to your injury that you tried to train through?
- Have you attempted to compensate your running gait due to any pain or discomfort?
- Have you cut back on your mileage or pace since your injury? Any results?

decreases pain and inflammation; this allows for early return to range of motion. After the initial vasoconstriction from the use of the ice, a secondary vasodilatation occurs. When combined with early range of motion, and decreased pain, a clearing of the inflammatory cellular elements occurs, thus leading to a decrease in local necrosis. Non-steroidal anti-inflammatory drugs (NSAIDs) are also helpful in decreasing the prostaglandin release, and allow for pain-free range of motion, providing for an early recovery (Aronoff 1982, Obel 1982, Weissman 1982).

## CHRONIC OR OVERUSE INJURIES

Overuse injuries are common in serious athletes and the everyday aerobic exerciser. When analysing the biomechanical factors of aerobic sports, it is easy to see why damage to tissues from cyclic overloading occurs. It has been shown that 30–50% of all sports injuries are due to overuse (Orava 1980b, Renstrom & Johnson 1985). In overuse injuries the cumulative effects of repetitive force lead to microtrauma, which triggers the inflammatory process. Inflammation, although a necessary component in the healing process, can become a self-limiting entity, which can lead to chronic inflammation and eventual destruction of surrounding tissues. Therefore, it is essential to minimise the chronic inflammation so as to prevent repetitive overuse injury or new acute injuries.

When the patient ignores the signs and symptoms of overuse injury (stiffness, soreness, increased temperature of the affected area), and continues to participate in his or her sport despite the injury and advice against further activity, a more serious injury can develop. The concept at this point is to treat the patient aggressively with rest, ice, compression, elevation and cessation of the sport that caused the injury. This is followed by a combination of training and physical therapy to decrease the inflammation, and increase range of motion, while preventing further injury.

The tissue most commonly affected by overuse injuries is the musculotendinous unit. According to Barfred (1971) a tendon is most likely to be injured when:

- tension is applied to it quickly
- tension is applied to it obliquely
- the tendon is under tension before loading
- the attached muscle is maximally innervated
- the muscle group is stretched by exterior stimuli
- the tendon is weak in comparison with the muscle.

During athletic sport participation, when maximum effort is attained, these conditions usually exist. In the case of tendons, the tendon sheath or paratendon may also be involved. As a result of chronic inflammation of the tendon, tenosynovitis, or tendinitis, can occur – leading to a local degeneration and even recurrent injury to the previously damaged tendon and resulting in a partial or even complete tendon rupture.

Bursae are located at sites of friction between tendon and bone, or skin and bone. When a bursa is subject to repetitive trauma due to overuse, it may become inflamed, thus causing effusion and thickening of the bursal wall. The latter is seen clearly in the retrocalcaneal bursitis that commonly develops from shoe irritation.

Bone, which has tremendous strength, is dependent on the forces placed upon it. Wolff's law states that bone is laid down where needed and resorbed where not needed. Loads can be applied to bone in five different directions: tension, compression, bending, shear and torsion.

For the athlete, a stress fracture may be the result of the bone's resorptive process exceeding its reparative process. When osteoclastic breakdown is greater than osteoblastic development weakness will occur, resulting in a stress fracture. In the athlete, the stress fracture is the epitome of an overuse injury and, as such, signals the need for an investigation into training habits, equipment and athletic techniques (De Lee et al 1983).

Bone may fracture as a result of a single, large force, or a number of repetitive, smaller forces. In endurance sports, such as running, which requires repetitive impact movement, the constant force on bone creates a remodelling process, which eventually results in increased bone strength in the direction in which that force is applied. The ability of the bone to withstand repetitive loading depends on the amount of the load, the number of repetitions, and the frequency of the loading. When the fatigue process outstrips the bone reparative process, a stress fracture will usually occur.

## Physical factors

One theory, stated by Nordin and Frankel (1980), is that during continuous strenuous activity muscles fatigue. As the muscles tire they become less able to absorb energy and reduce the stress that is transmitted to the bone. This altered stress distribution allows abnormally high forces to be transmitted to bone, and a stress fracture may develop. A second theory, outlined by Stanitski et al (1978), is that the force of the muscles themselves acting on their attachments to the bone creates the repetitive stress that eventually leads to the failure of the bone. In 1855, Briethaupt, a Prussian military physician, first described swelling combined with foot pain in young military recruits unaccustomed to the rigours of basic training. These injuries were later described as 'march fractures' following their radiographic analysis (Markey 1987).

A stress fracture of the metatarsals is not evident for 2–3 weeks following the injury. The typical clinical picture will be that of swelling seen on the dorsum, redness, and discomfort overlying the involved metatarsal. There will usually be extreme pain elicited on direct digital pressure. Upon creating motion to the metatarsal, pain will be enhanced even further. As a general rule, when in doubt the clinician should suspect a stress fracture even without radiographic evidence until proven otherwise (see also Ch. 22).

Cartilage is composed of collagen, a proteoglycan gel, cells, and 60–80% water. In adults, cartilage contains no blood vessels, lymphatics or nerves. Because of its high metabolic activity, particularly in the production of proteoglycans, the ability of cartilage to repair itself is quite limited. After injury, rather than reproducing hyaline cartilage, the tissue that is synthesised is primarily fibrocartilage. Joint cartilage is normally lubricated and protected from injury by two different mechanisms (Rodman & Schumacher 1983). The hydrostatic mechanism prevails during high loads and at high speed. The second mechanism, the boundary surface phenomenon, occurs during low loads and at low speeds. Cancellous bone helps in the protection of the cartilage by its ability to deform in response to stress. However, when these mechanisms fail damage to the cartilage can occur.

Nerve tissue in the foot is also subject to overuse injury. Large-diameter myelinated peripheral fibres are at risk of compression. In the sporting patient, repetitive loading and motion direct trauma, decreased flexibility, and pathobiomechanics have all been involved in nerve entrapment. Particularly common in the runner, is tarsal tunnel syndrome, which may involve one, two or all three branches of the posterior tibial nerve.

Associated with equinus, or prolonged forefoot strike, intermetatarsal stress may result in perineurofibrosis, producing pain, tingling, numbness and burning from an interdigital neuroma.

With chronic overuse injuries, the question to be asked is: why has the condition not resolved, even when the patient has rested for a prolonged period of time? Factors leading to overuse injuries can be

## Box 13.2 **Factors in overuse injuries**

| Extrinsic factors | Intrinsic factors |
|---|---|
| Training errors | Alignment abnormalities |
| Time (duration) | Femoral neck anteversion |
| Distance | Genu valgum |
| Repetitions (intervals) | Tibial varum |
| Intensity | Pronation |
| Hills | Tibial torsion |
| Surfaces: | Limb length discrepancy |
|   hard (asphalt, concrete) | Muscle weakness |
|   soft (grass, dirt) | Muscle imbalance |
|   track (cinder, composition) | Flexibility |
|   canted track | Previous injury (pull strain, sprain) |
|   crowned road | |
|   shoes and equipment | |

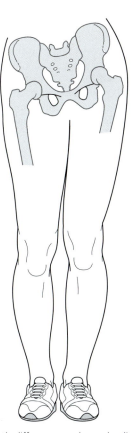

**Figure 13.1** Limb-length difference syndrome leading to groin strain.

divided into intrinsic and extrinsic categories (Renstrom & Johnson 1985) (Box 13.2).

Combined with excessive repetition and impact, these intrinsic factors can lead to breakdown and injury. Malalignment, due to excessive pronation, tibial varum, genu valgum, underlying degenerative joint disease, and other structural abnormalities can lead to abnormal loads on joints, articular surfaces and soft tissue structures. Other intrinsic factors involved in the sports participant are muscle weakness and poor flexibility. As a result, atrophy of muscle groups can occur quite quickly and can be subject to re-injury unless those muscle groups are re-strengthened. When muscle tears or sprains take place scar tissue adhesions will be seen in the form of swelling and stiffness, and quite often instability and weakness. Other biomechanical factors, such as limb-length discrepancies, equinus and lack of flexibility associated with tight muscle groups, can also contribute to chronic recurrent injuries (Fig. 13.1).

## Psychological factors

It has been considered that sports and exercise are endeavours for children, adolescents and young adults. However, with the exercise phenomenon explosion starting in the 1970s and 1980s, people from childhood to the age of senior citizens have discovered the physical and psychological benefits of exercise. And with the 'addicted' generation, attention now also focuses on psychological issues, such as exercise dependency, overtraining, motivation, injury acceptance, social factors, and burnout.

Studies have shown the positive effects from exercise on the mental status of athletes and those who exercise. Hughes (1984) reported that in more than 1000 studies exercise had a positive effect on the participants. A study by Steptoe et al (1989) indicated that moderate aerobic workouts alleviated psychological tension in both normal psychologically healthy people and in those who suffer from moderate anxiety – whereas non-aerobic exercise, such as weight or flexibility training, produced no such effect in either group.

On this evidence, the public should be highly motivated to participate in sports, and be exercisers; however, a study in 1986 showed that in the USA less than 20% of adults aged 18–65 years exercised at sufficient levels. By 1992, the level had increased to only 25% (Le Unes & Nation 1989). Practitioners can provide to the public a means to prevent injury, allowing the participant to continue to exercise injury-free and pain-free. The adult athlete must accept the fact that they will not be able to perform at a similar level as when they were young, and that exercise will continue to offer benefits, and help to increase longevity.

Fear of injury is one of the greatest concerns of most athletes. An estimated 17 million sports-related injuries occur yearly among American athletes (Heel 1993). It is imperative that the sports medicine practitioner or personal trainer helps people to understand that the physical and psychological benefits of activity far outweigh any risks to the body (Dulberg & Gueally 1999).

When injuries do occur the athlete must be able to deal with the physical injury, but also to cope on the psychological level. Once the participant is faced with a long-term injury there may be an initial emotional downturn which, if not recognised early, may eventually turn into a case of sport depression and withdrawal. After injury, the athlete goes through five stages, similar to the grieving process for a friend or relative (Heel 1993). Initially, the athlete experiences denial and disbelief over what has happened. Anger then sets in, followed by downplaying the severity of the injury, leading into the next stage, namely depression. Finally, the athlete comes to accept the true extent of the injury and at last the hope for a committed effort at rehabilitation will begin. Post-injury, fear and anxiety may be the major problem, even though physiologically the athlete is fine. The problem is a condition known as 'phobic response to injury', which can decrease performance and increase the risk of re-injury (Dulberg & Gueally 1999). Sports practitioners can offer support for athletic patients and help them to promote their return to active participation and prevent injuries.

## Patient constraints

Once the sports participant has been injured the practitioner must create a treatment plan that is realistic, so that the patient will be compliant, and complete the treatment in the prescribed time period.

Rest is essential, to allow the healing process to begin and continue through the proper course. Occasionally, a non-impact cross-training regimen (swimming, water jogging, water aerobics, elliptical walker) may be prescribed to allow the participant to continue cardiovascular workout yet avoiding re-injury or further injury.

Nutrition is another important component for both the healthy participant and the injured exerciser. In addition to a balanced diet, nutritional supplements are important to support optimal function. Hydration is just as important to maintain tissue well-being. Water constitutes the majority of body tissue and is responsible for 60% of the average adult's body weight. It is recommended that a typical adult should drink 8–12 glasses of water each day. A simple way to determine how much water should be ingested each day is to calculate two-thirds of body weight in pounds and drink that number of fluid ounces of water per day. As body weight increases, so does the fluid replacement requirement. Exercise generates oxidative stress via free radical toxins that can inflame and irritate tissues, and may increase

potential for injury. After injury, damaged tissues under repair will have greater nutritional requirements and will need additional vitamin and antioxidant intake. Antioxidant supplement would include the regular use of vitamins C and E, β-carotene, zinc and selenium to the recommended daily dose.

To summarise, following diagnosis, a treatment plan (Box 13.3) is initiated, with a follow-up programme (consisting of weight training, cross-training, and rehabilitation). Attainable goals should be laid out for both the participant and the practitioner, with a reasonable timetable for return to activity. Finally, a prognosis is formulated. After the patient's return, there are four possibilities for the patient's condition:

1. no improvement or worse
2. somewhat improved
3. greatly improved
4. completely better.

If the patient is completely better, a gradual return to activity is essential.

---

### Box 13.3 Treatment list (Boyd & Bogdan 1997)

#### Activity modification
- Hard walk programme
- Walk/run programme
- Daily activity only (walking only)
- Reduction of stair/hill walking
- Reduce running partially
- Discontinue speed work
- Discontinue hill work
- Prolonged rest
- Bicycle/swim alternative
- Wheelchair or bedrest
- Crutches or cane

#### Ice/heat therapy
- Contrast baths
- Ice pack after activity
- Ice massage
- Hot water soaks/heat packs
- Deep heat lotion massage

#### Shoes
- Change to shoes that limit pronation
- Change to shoes with more shock absorption
- Modify shoes with built-in changes
- Special shoes
- Stay with same shoes
- Biven shoe, wooden sole shoe

#### Taping, supportive strapping, wraps
- Rest strapping for the midtarsal joint
- Rest strapping for the ankle
- Combination of both
- Figure-of-eight strapping
- Special area taping (digits, etc.)
- Removable ankle wrap
- Removable knee wrap
- Knee immobiliser

- Tubular grip bandage
- Tubular grip bandage with horseshoe padding
- Orthoplast or air cast splints
- Lateral ankle splints

#### Foot inserts/orthoses
- Spenco padding
- Sorbothane padding for the heel
- Foot accommodation (e.g. Korex)
- Felt arch padding or 'D' pads
- Metatarsal support
- Metatarsal bar
- Runner's varus heel wedge
- Heel cup
- Forefoot/rearfoot wedge
- Spenco or arch support
- Cuboid padding
- Heel lifts
- Morton's extension
- Latex shields
- Bunion splints/digital splints
- Biomechanical examination and casting for orthoses
- Dispense orthoses
- Modification of orthoses, if necessary

#### Stretching exercises
- Static stretching programme for home use
- Contracting and relaxing programme for home use
- Contracting and relaxing therapy programme
- Spray and stretch techniques
- 45-minute programme of heat/ice stretch
- Cryostretch programme; stretching after application of cold

#### Stretching and range of movement
- Isometric strengthening
- Theraband or elastic rubber tubing techniques
- Isotonic strengthening

- Isokinetic strengthening
- Upper body isotonic programme
- Range of motion exercises
- Muscle stimulator for home use

**Physical therapy treatment**

- Ultrasound therapy
- Electrogalvanic stimulation
- Electro-acupuncture probe therapy
- Dynamometer muscle test
- Deep friction massage
- Electro-accuscope therapy
- Transcutaneous nerve stimulation

**Medication**

- Aspirin
- Strong anti-inflammatory medication
- Oral steroid therapy for 6 days
- Vitamins
- Oral calcium supplements
- Iron supplements
- Vitamin B$_{12}$ injection
- Short-acting cortisone injection
- Long-acting cortisone injection
- Hyaluronidase injection
- Local anaesthesia diagnostic injection
- Local anaesthesia therapeutic injection
- Diet evaluation

**Special tests**

- Radiographs
- Bone scan
- Computerised tomography scan (CAT/CT scan)
- Xerogram – reverse radiograph for soft tissues
- Arthrogram
- Nuclear magnetic resonance imaging (MRI)

**Surgery**

- Surgical discussion
- Surgical intervention

**Casts**

- Standard below-knee cast
- Removable below-knee casts
- Above-knee cast
- Unaboot cast – calamine lotion compressive bandage

**Miscellaneous**

- Foot manipulation techniques
- Referral to an orthopaedic surgeon
- Referral to a neurologist
- Referral to a physician
- Referral to a chiropractic
- Referral to a dietician
- Referral to a rheumatologist
- Referral to a vascular specialist
- Evaluation

## RUNNING

### The four phases of running

Subotnick (1999f) describes four phases of development that the majority of runners pass through:

- *Phase I* runners are early casual runners who often were never serious runners in the past. Typically, they run 3 miles, 4 or 5 days a week, with a weekly mileage of 12–15 miles. The pace is usually at 8–9$\frac{1}{2}$ minutes/mile. The participant enjoys the sport and finds that it maintains weight control. They find they have more energy at the end of the day, a better mental attitude, and find that running gives them the benefits of aerobic fitness and makes them feel better in general.

- *Phase II* runners are the serious runners, but they tend to be obsessive or compulsive about their running activity. They tend to run 5–7 miles a day, 5 days a week, averaging approximately 30 miles a week. These runners enjoy aerobic exercise and, as a side benefit, develop positive psychological and stress-reduction effects. They enjoy limited competition, and will run 5000- or 10 000-metre road races. Occasionally, they might attempt to run a marathon, for the challenge. These runners are not addicted to running and usually take 2 days off per week. When faced with injuries these runners are very cooperative and are compliant when mileage cut-back is necessary.

- *Phase III* runners are individuals with obsessive–compulsive behaviour. They are frequently psychologically and physiologically dependent on running, as well as on the 'runner's high' they develop from increased endorphin and encephalins that are produced during the runs. These runners are truly addicted to the sport and often use it as a psychological 'crutch'. Many are young, gifted athletes, or 'class' runners, while many are obsessed with physical appearance, and/or weight control. They feel that they are invincible and that injuries are not a reality. They are faced with biomechanical, as well as functional imbalance problems. It is not uncommon to see them with a tight/weak musculature, and with overuse injuries, such as tendinitis, tenosynovitis, myositis, periostitis and/or stress fractures. These patients require a great deal of time and patience, particularly with outlining treatment plans. It is in this group in particular that the sports practitioner should avoid surgical intervention at all costs.

- *Phase IV* runners are usually the ones who have passed through the Phase III stage already and have 'grown out' of that stage in their running careers. They no longer run the sub-8-minute miles but rather are content to run at the 8–8$\frac{1}{2}$-minute mile pace. They no longer have that great desire for serious competition but rather have matured into a more sensible competitive mode that helps to avoid injuries. These patients are very cooperative, and quite compliant post-injury, particularly during rehabilitation.

### The walking–running cycle

Depending upon the sport in which the participant engages, they utilise either the entire walking and running cycle or parts of these cycles (see also Ch. 15). In the case of basketball, dribbling and driving to the basket may involve a quick sprinting run followed by a vertical leap. In alpine skiing, a down-weighting of the feet and legs, which is then followed by up-weighting, translates into a flatfoot on the skis (pronation) followed by a rolling outwards of the foot on the skis (supination). The repetitive action of the lower extremities that occurs during walking or running constitutes the gait cycle. Because the majority of sports require some form of running, it is essential that the practitioner interprets the gait cycle and how it affects the foot and lower extremity.

Walking gait differs from running gait in several ways. Walking is exhibited by a heel contact, midstance (flat foot) and propulsive phase (toe-off), with a base of gait approximately 5 cm between the malleoli (see Ch. 15). With slow walking speed there is a short period of swing phase; however, as walking speed increases there is an increase in swing phase. The duration of double support decreases as walking speed increases, and eventually is eliminated with the transition to running (Bates & Stergiou 1999b). As walking speed increases the contact phase shortens, and as the transition to running occurs the double support phase is eliminated completely, and is replaced by an airborne phase where neither foot is on the ground. It is estimated that the support phase varies from about 60% for slow runners, and 40% for fast runners. The non-support periods range from 40% and 60%, respectively. A single step concludes when the opposite limb makes contact with the ground about midway through the forward swing subphase at about 70–80% of the limb cycle.

To understand locomotion and the gait patterns of walking and running it may be observed that in walking gait the foot and lower limb is always in contact with the ground, whereas in running there is a period of time when the body is 'airborne' with both feet off the ground. In locomotion, there is a mechanical interaction between locomotor structures and an external force – that of gravity. The final product is forward physical movement, and postural stability. Thus, in running, at the heel contact phase the supporting foot must move beneath the centre of mass of the body for stability. In running, the body's centre of gravity must travel in a more vertical direction than it does in walking. During the running heel contact, the base of gait is reduced, creating a varus attitude, thus, compelling the subtalar joint to increase pronation to allow the foot to plantar flex (Fig. 13.2). Locomotion comprises a number of important components; namely, stride length, stride frequency, and their resultant speed. It has been estimated that up to two to three times the body weight passes through the loaded limb during the contact phase of walking. In running, that figure can rise to as high as three to six times the body weight.

Energy transfer takes place when there is a change in frequency of the foot impact, as well as the stride length. It has been shown that at lower or higher speeds greater energy per strike is necessary compared to an intermediate speed. In Rolston's (1993) article on the energetics of human walking, he showed that plotting the energy expenditure versus speed in walking would result in a parabola. The parabolic function demonstrates that there is an optimal minimum at which walking is more efficient than the participant's preferred speed. There is a period immediately after the transition from walking to running, in which energy expenditure will fall to an optimal minimum where frequency and stride length work in harmony to the body's best advantage (Hreljac 1993).

In running, deceleration occurs every time the foot makes contact with the ground. Immediately after contact the forward velocity of the body decreases during a 'breaking phase' of action. In running, this critical phase causes the centre of gravity to be elevated, creating additional potential energy, thus a greater vertical velocity at contact, with even higher kinetic energy. Thus, a braking action of the limb occurs in addition to the impact occurrence of the body in regard to ground reactive forces. Therefore, running is a combination of actions of the lower extremity that involves maintaining forward motion while simultaneously accentuating the centre of gravity against internal and external resistance. In addition, the lower extremities must also

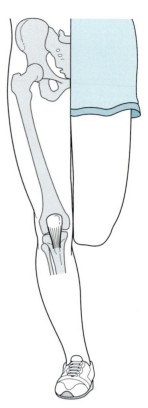

**Figure 13.2** Limb varus while running.

support the body's weight and absorb the impact forces that transcend up the leg during the contact phase. As the speed of the runner increases, energy production and usage increases due to increased forward propulsion and, in addition, muscle contraction that must decelerate the body while simultaneously diffusing impact forces.

Shock occurs after immediate impact of the heel striking the ground as the stance phase of gait begins. As mentioned before, at heel strike ground reaction forces are transmitted into the heel as shock. This shock is usually absorbed and dissipated by the normal motion of the foot and lower limb. It is when that motion is restricted within certain joints of the lower extremity that abnormal degrees of shock are transmitted through the foot and leg and directly into the trunk. One of the key functions of the subtalar joint is to absorb shock at heel contact. The subtalar joint pronates quickly to absorb some of this shock directly. Again at heel strike, additional shock is absorbed by knee flexion. However, the knee cannot flex rapidly unless the tibia can internally rotate faster and farther than the femur. Subtalar joint pronation allows the tibia to rotate faster and farther than the femur, thus unlocking the knee so that it can flex and assist in shock absorption (Steindler 1955). Thus, the subtalar joint is the main means of shock absorption for the foot and lower limb at heel strike. In the runner, who demonstrates increased stride and greater acceleration, additional ground reactive forces will be transmitted through the heel as it hits the ground. The subtalar joint will demonstrate increased pronation, thus increasing the ability of the foot and limb to absorb this increased amount of shock. Therefore, adequate shock absorption cannot occur at heel strike unless subtalar joint pronation can take place (Root et al 1977).

In addition, muscle function is also influenced by the action of the subtalar joint. When subtalar joint motion is limited, a ripple effect of abnormal muscle function can occur. This will impede knee flexion, creating increased impact shock into the lower leg and knee. The action of the posterior tibial muscle at heel contact is to decelerate subtalar joint pronation. However, when the foot and subtalar joint are completely pronated, the posterior tibial muscle will contract with its effect more proximally, rather than distally. Therefore, the knee will remain extended, limiting both its ability to flex and to act in shock absorption. In running, the knee flexes through 35–40° at contact, compared with only 15° when walking.

Subtalar joint pronation lasts longer in the running gait cycle, and readjustment of the foot into supination occurs much later – approximately 70% of the support phase. When the foot demonstrates abnormal pronation of the subtalar joint, pathological shock will develop. The runner or walker experiences increased impact shock up the limb, through the pelvis, and into the spine. This can be prevented when the participant shortens his or her stride, and utilises a flattened foot to eliminate the heel strike, and the remainder of the contact phase. For the foot to become a rigid structure for propulsion it has to function in an adaptive manner longer in the gait cycle, and resupination must occur much sooner.

During propulsion, the centre of gravity must be transferred toward the opposite foot. During transference, force is diminished while motion is maximised. At the end of propulsion, weight is transferred completely to the opposite foot. In walking, the centre of gravity moves over the support limb, whereas in running the limbs move beneath the centre of gravity, thus cancelling out any transference.

In addition to visual observation of walking and running gait, computerised force data sensor systems can be used to measure the distribution of pressure at specific areas on the plantar aspect of the foot. Henning and Milani (1995) used a discrete pressure sensor system in conjunction with a force platform to examine the effects of shoes on ground reactive forces. With computerised pressure technology, the clinician can evaluate the participant's gait in any type of environment. In addition, specific areas of pressure can be determined, including the specific point of heel strike, adaptation and propulsion. This information can be helpful in determining whether the participant is in need of an orthotic device and, when worn, obtain data on the device relative to the foot and/or shoe.

Often, walking and running disorders can be identified using a simple video system. An inexpensive, high-quality digital video camera, in conjunction with a computer and appropriate software can be used to record the participant's gait pattern. The subject can be evaluated in slow motion or freeze-frame to analyse any potential faults in the gait pattern such as leg-length discrepancy, shoulder drop, internal or external femoral rotation, high degrees of tibial varum, or excessive pronation or supination. With slow motion, and having the capability to freeze frame the subject, the clinician can determine specifically when the heel strikes the ground, or whether there is an excessive propulsive phase (equinus) and/or a functional hallux limitus. The recording can also be used to measure stride length, the position of the foot at heel contact, base of gait, and position of the foot during toe-off. This can be performed either on a treadmill, or simply by walking or running down a corridor. This system can be extremely helpful in the education of the patient, in pointing out specific areas of concern, and when walking or running styles can be altered or corrected. In addition, it is a great tool for determining whether an orthotic device might be necessary, while simultaneously educating the patient as to its need and use.

## Marathon running

The marathon is a gruelling 26.2-mile endurance race. As one of the original Olympic events, it continues to rank as one of the most challenging of all track events. The popularity of the marathon has transcended from the elite athlete to the 'weekend warrior'. Men and

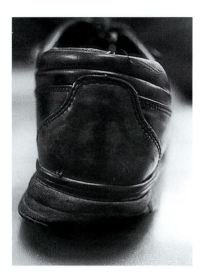

**Figure 13.3** Worn and distorted sports shoe.

women of all ages have focused in on the marathon as the ultimate challenge to compete in and to complete.

During the training period, or before, during or after the marathon, many runners suffer from some type of overuse injury. Some of these runners never even make it to the starting line due to overtraining, running on hard concrete surfaces, worn-out shoes (Fig. 13.3), poor biomechanics, lack of flexibility or recurrent injury.

Many of the overuse injuries that have been mentioned previously will now be examined individually.

---

### CASE STUDY 13.1

#### INSERTIONAL CALCIFIC TENDINOSIS FRACTURE

A 57-year-old male runner first presented with shooting, burning, pulling pains on the posterior aspect of his right heel of 2 months duration. The patient was training for the Houston Marathon in January but was unable to participate in the race because of the pain and took time off, resuming running in March, starting with 3 miles/day. He again experienced soreness in the same region and took 6 weeks off from running. However, when he resumed running the pain started again. His first steps in the morning were painful.

The patient has been running for approximately 5 years and has completed two marathons in 5.5–6 hours.

The patient also indicated that he had suffered from other chronic injuries along the right lower extremity ranging from piriformis syndrome to plantar fasciitis, a groin pull and ankle pain. All of these have been resolved.

The patient had prescription orthotics fabricated 2 years ago to help correct a right out-toeing. He goes to the gym 6 days a week to cross-train, runs two times a week and also does weight lifting.

*Impression.* Achilles tendinitis on the right foot. There is also a limb-length discrepancy, with the right leg being longer than the left, and a collapsing pes plano valgus foot type.

The patient was re-casted for new orthotic devices to treat the chronic left heel pain and prescribed a night splint, NSAIDs and ice massage.

#### BIOMECHANICAL EVALUATION

Vascular and neurological examination – all seemed normal.

Hip range of motion 90° external, 45° internal, equal and symmetrical, bilateral.

Forefoot: L 4° varus; R 5° varus
Rearfoot: L 3° varus; R 3° varus

There was significant limb-length discrepancy, the right leg being 2 cm longer than the left leg. His gait was abducted with significant medial column prolapse in both stance and gait but he denied pain on the posterior central portion of the calcaneus and in the plantar fascia. There was no pain in the midbody of the Achilles tendon.

### ONE YEAR LATER

The insertional Achilles tendinitis flared again. The patient has run three previous marathons, and recently ran the Great Wall of China Marathon. He experienced no pain during the run but now complains of pain during his first steps in the morning and when he steps out of a car. The pain diminishes after one minute of walking. There is pain along the medial–posterior right heel.

Bilateral lateral-projection radiographs revealed a right fracture insertional calcific Achilles tendinosis 'spur', with fragmentation. There was an infracalcaneal exostosis, and a possible previous fracture.

On the left foot there was a retrocalcaneal insertional calcinosis 'spur' but no fracture.

### CONSERVATIVE TREATMENT

- Evaluate and refurbish the orthotic device.
- Therapeutic steroid; local anaesthetic; vitamin $B_{12}$ injection to the medial calcaneal extratendinous.
- Physical therapy: nerve stimulation; ultrasound; deep-tissue, cross-friction massage.
- Cox-2 NSAID; ice massage.
- Recommended to do no impact activity or running for 2 weeks.

## CASE STUDY 13.2

### RUPTURED ACHILLES TENDON

A 69–year-old woman complained of retrocalcaneal insertional calcific Achilles tendinosis. The patient had run/walked numerous marathons, and was participating in the Alaskan Marathon when she began to experience excruciating pain. One month ago, after the race, she stepped off a kerb and began to experience swelling along the posterior tibial and flexor hallucis longus tendons of the right foot, and a strain of the gastrocnemius–soleus. She has been receiving physical therapy and describes pain and tenderness along the posterior tibial and flexor hallucis longus tendons, and the gastrocnemius–soleus muscle group. She also described pain at the posteromedial aspect of the insertion of the Achilles tendon in her right foot.

### MEDICAL HISTORY

The patient had hypertension, arthritis, seasonal allergies, hypercholesterolaemia and gout.

*Past lower extremity history.* Posterior tibial tendinitis, tarsal tunnel syndrome, plantar fasciitis, metatarsalgia and sciatica, on the left foot. She was taking a number of systemic medications: Allopurinol, Avapro, Lopid, Clarityn, Zyrtec, Aleve.

*Social history.* A retired nurse who enjoys walking and jogging for fitness. Denies smoking.

*Family history.* Non-contributory.

### PHYSICAL EXAMINATION

There was pain at the insertion of Achilles tendon and a palpable exostosis on the retrocalcaneal region of the right foot. There was some weakness and pain upon dorsiflexion of the right foot. There was oedema along the posteromedial aspect of the calcaneus and along the medial aspect of the right ankle. The gastrocnemius–soleus muscle group was tight and there was pain along the course of the posterior tibial and flexor hallucis longus tendons. The patient was unable to perform a single heel-raise test.

### LOWER EXTREMITY PHYSICAL EXAMINATION

The patient is 5 feet (152 cm) tall and weighs 124 pounds (56 kg).

*Vascular examination.* The dorsalis pedis and posterior tibial pulses were recorded as +2/4 bilaterally; the capillary filling time was 3 seconds, the toes were warm and the colour was normal; there were no varicosities.

*Neurological examination.* There was mild tingling along the posterior tibial nerve on the left foot; sensation was good, equal and symmetrical; Achilles and patellar deep tendon reflexes were normal; the plantar response was normal.

### LOWER EXTREMITY BIOMECHANICAL EXAMINATION

There was bilateral tibial varum, some collapse of the midtarsal joint and the longitudinal arch with medial column prolapse and talonavicular prolapse.

The foot type was pes planus, the first ray was hypermobile, and ankle joint dorsiflexion was normal. The stance position showed mild abduction with calcaneal eversion.

| | |
|---|---|
| Subtalar inversion: | R 18°; L 30° |
| Subtalar eversion: | R 8°; L 7° |
| Subtalar neutral: | R 3°; L 3° |
| Forefoot: | R 2°; L 2° |

### X-RAY EXAMINATION

Insertional calcific Achilles tendinosis with bone cystic changes, posterosuperior aspect, and right calcaneus.

Loose body bone fragments, with spur formation at the insertional level of the Achilles tendon.

### MRI FOOT AND ANKLE

Presence of focal swelling, with partial disruption of the distal portion of the Achilles tendon near the attachment of the tendon to the posterior aspect of the calcaneus.

No joint effusion. The fibular (peroneal)s, extensor and flexor tendons were normal, with no evidence of inflammatory changes or disruption.

### SURGICAL INTERVENTION

Resection of insertional calcific Achilles tendinosis
Resection of posterosuperior 'step' of the calcaneus
Repair of partial rupture insertion of Achilles tendon
Reattachment with absorbable anchor screw with absorbable suture
Jones compression dressing
Non-weight-bearing posterior splint cast was applied, and with crutches the patient was able to be ambulant postoperatively.

## CHILD AND ADOLESCENT SPORTS

It is estimated that 30 million children and adolescents in the USA participate in organised sports. With this change of focus of children in sport, the number of overuse injuries has increased. Children participate in a particular sport not just for one season but often for many seasons – and in some cases all year round. It is not uncommon to see youngsters and adolescents engaged in a variety of sports (e.g. soccer, football, rugby in the autumn; basketball, swimming, indoor track, hockey, volleyball, gymnastics in the winter; baseball, lacrosse, soccer, cross-country-track in the spring; and swimming, soccer, baseball and running in the summer). Some children who excel in a particular sport may participate in that activity all year round, as seen in gymnastics, ballet dancing, basketball, soccer and baseball. One of the main questions that parents have to ask is: is my child ready to participate in organised sports? There are two aspects to a child's readiness: motivational readiness and maturity or cognitive readiness (Dulberg 1999). Many times the child may be physically ready to master the skills of the sport but may not be intellectually prepared to participate. Determining the right age for the child to participate in a particular sport can often be difficult. Physical-contact sports suitable for one young person who is more physically mature may not be right for another. Similarly, choosing to go on point for one young ballet dancer may be deleterious for another young ballet dancer.

With the increased participation of younger athletes in organised athletic and competitive sporting programmes, there has been a change in the pattern of injuries observed (Maffulli et al 1992, Sterling et al 1991) as well as an increasing number of injuries (Kannus et al 1988, Micheli 1983, 1987, Micheli & Ireland 1987, Micheli & Smith 1982). These include microtrauma overuse injuries as well as acute macrotrauma injuries.

Overuse injuries are not only common in adult athletes. With the volume of training and repetition now being undertaken by many young athletes, normal repetitive processes are eventually overwhelmed, leading to tissue inflammation (Herring & Nelson 1987). In addition to tissue areas that are subject to overuse injuries (i.e. tendons, bones, tendon–bone junctions), other areas in the young athlete also vulnerable to overuse injury include growing tissues. Growth cartilage, found in the youngster at the epiphyseal plate, the articular cartilage of the joint surface, as well as the apophyses at the insertion of the muscle tendon unit, are at risk of overuse injuries. The traction apophysitises involve growing tissue and are particularly evident during the rapid growth during adolescence (Micheli & Fehlandt 1992). Injuries at the traction apophyses may be the result of an acute macrotrauma, creating an avulsion of a portion of the apophysis. The repetitive microtrauma to the youngster will present with pain, swelling, as well as 'apophysitis' where bony or cartilaginous overgrowth occurs. Osgood–Schlatter's disease of the tibial tubercle apophysis is probably one of the most commonly recognised of these injuries in youngsters. Sever's disease or calcaneal apophysitis is another common complaint seen in the child and adolescent. It is usually seen between the ages of 10 and 12 years in boys and girls, occurring more frequently in boys.

A significant amount of growth takes place between the ages of 11 and 15 years, and this is quite often rapid and in spurts. Bone is undeveloped and is not completely ossified until 18–21 years of age. The immature bone can be stressed when muscles are relatively overdeveloped through excessive activity (Ch. 12). A frequent site of injuries in children is where muscles and ligaments attach to bone. Because bone grows faster than the soft-tissue structures mature, frequently there will be restriction in motion as well as muscle imbalances for periods of time while soft tissues adapt to the additional bone development. During puberty, the growth plates are especially soft and weak, and are subject to injury at the end of the growing period as they become more rigid. As the youngster matures, the body changes shape, muscles become bigger, bones become longer and weight increases. Adaptation to these changes, as well as a change in coordination, also takes place as the young athlete matures.

The patient complains of pain located in the posterior medial aspect of the heel which is exacerbated by sports activities where running and high impact are involved (e.g. soccer, basketball, baseball, football and tennis). Hard surfaces can also contribute to the impact shock, and contribute to the complaint. Aetiological factors that are often seen include repetitive microtrauma, a sudden adolescent growth spurt, a tight gastrocnemius–soleus muscle group, a tight Achilles tendon and weak dorsiflexors. Biomechanical factors are also contributory; for example, genu valgum, excessive pronation of the subtalar joint and forefoot varus. It is difficult to make a clear-cut diagnosis of Sever's disease because radiographs show only increased density and a maturing apophysis that may reveal lines that could mimic fractures (see also Ch. 4). Treatment usually begins with rest from the affected sport for a period of time until pain has subsided significantly. In addition, treatment should include exercises for the plantar flexors to improve dorsiflexion of the ankle as well as strengthening exercises for the dorsiflexors of the ankle.

A stretching programme involving the gastrocnemius complex, Achilles tendon and hamstrings is also advised. For children whose feet pronate excessively, and who have tight Achilles tendons, prescription orthotic devices and heel lifts are also helpful, particularly in the pes plano valgus individual. In severe situations where conservative treatment has been exhausted, lower-leg cast immobilisation may be necessary to rest the inflamed apophysis. Another injury to the apophysis that has been described in youngsters is at the base of the fifth metatarsal (Lehman et al 1986).

Another site for traction apophysitis is the tarsal accessory navicular. It is suggested that the formation of the accessory navicular may be the result of an apophyseal separation, similar in nature to Osgood–Schlatter's disease, at the insertion site of the tibialis posterior tendon–muscle unit. Children who suffer from painful accessory navicular bones experience inflammatory traction apophysitis at the insertion site of the posterior tibial tendon into the accessory navicular and the navicular. These children usually demonstrate severe pronation, secondary to a pes planus or flat foot. In cases where there is a hypertrophied navicular, mechanical irritation over the bony prominence may be the cause. With pain associated with traction apophysitis, biomechanical correction, and support of the longitudinal arch and tendon with the use of prescription orthotic devices has proven to be very successful. In addition to anti-inflammatory medications, strength and flexibility exercises directed towards the tibialis posterior muscle–tendon unit, as well as heel walking, are also helpful. For the youngster who suffers from mechanical irritation of the navicular bone, as in skiers, skaters, snow-boarders and horseback riders, a tight-fitting, unrelenting boot is often responsible. The use of accommodative felt oval cavity pads (Ch. 16), or those made from ethyl vinyl acetate (EVA) or polyurethane (Ch. 17), as well as boot modification (Ch. 18), can be very helpful.

For youngsters who suffer from consistent painful accessory navicular bones, aggressive conservative treatment with cast immobilisation is very helpful in relieving pain. Once the cast has been removed, stretching and strengthening exercises are resumed and orthotic devices employed. For those children who have not responded well to conservative management, surgical intervention is recommended. This takes the form of resection of the hypertrophied navicular, with excision of the accessory navicular when present, combined with a transposition of the tibialis posterior tendon in a more mechanically efficient location inferior to the navicular, as described by Kidner (1929). It is not uncommon for a child to be out of sports training and/or competition for up to 6–9 months postoperatively.

When traction apophysitises are recognised early, and the clinician institutes rest, therapeutic exercises and biomechanical correction, these overuse apophyseal injuries can be managed conservatively, allowing the youngster to return to his or her full sports programme. However, in cases where these complaints are neglected, or treated minimally, symptoms, deformity and disability can continue into adulthood.

Some youngsters, as with their adult counterparts, are at high risk of injury. These young athletes, due to morphological difficulties, may break down even with minor trauma. Some of these participants may truly be 'accident-prone' (Lysens et al 1989, Standish 1995, Stanitski 1989). The well-trained young athlete, compared to the novice, is generally more resilient to an equivalent trauma. Standish (1995) states, that any tissue (whether bone, ligament or tendon) will disrupt only when it faces a force greater than its inherent strength.

In the child athlete eight main causative factors for injury have been identified (Betz & Klimt 1992, Boyd & Bogdan 1997):

1. load –the amount of impact to the lower extremity, including training and 'playing' time
2. decreased strength
3. decreased flexibility
4. decreased endurance
5. technique – running stride, arm swing, heel contact, etc.
6. biomechanical abnormalities – pes planus, pes cavus, calcaneal valgus, tarsal coalitions, genu valgum, tibial varum, equinus, tight gastrocnemius–soleus group, posture
7. increased psychological stress
8. equipment – shoes, cleats.

Underlying biomechanical imbalances and weaknesses can play an important role in the onset of overuse injuries in the child or adolescent athlete. As described, excessive pronation due to rearfoot, knee or leg structural abnormality can lead to undue amounts of stress upon tissues and disturb normal alignment, thus reducing shock-absorbing mechanisms. Conservative intervention with antipronatory devices can often solve a simple biomechanically induced overuse injury. These biomechanically corrective appliances can often restore normal alignment and function to the feet and lower extremities. The common overuse injuries occurring in the young athlete include traction apophysitis (Sever's disease), sinus tarsi syndrome, chondromalacia patellae and patellofemoral joint syndrome (where articular cartilage of the joint is damaged), osteochondritis dissicans, stress fractures, avulsion injuries, spondylosis and spondylothesis.

# FOOTBALL – SOCCER

Football is known internationally, but in the USA it is referred to as soccer. Due to the popularity of the sport, the number of football injuries is high. Whereas running involves a unidirectional movement, football, like other sports, requires multidirectional movements in addition to running. In football, manoeuvring and manipulating the ball with the foot, as well as tackling to gain the ball, requires a number of motions of the foot (subtalar joint, midtarsal joint, Lisfranc joint) as well as the ankle. Flexibility is a key component due to the sprinting and changes in direction involved in this sport. Strengthening and conditioning are integral components in soccer. Thus weight training may improve the strength and endurance of the participant, but at the cost of flexibility. It is imperative that the coach or trainer supervises properly to avoid a loss of flexibility in muscle groups.

There are a number of common football injuries incurred from the youth league age to the professional. These injuries include traction apophysitis, which is commonly seen in the active, growing child. Injuries at the traction apophyses may be a result of macrotrauma, in which avulsion of a portion of the apophysis takes place, or an effect of repetitive microtrauma (soccer cleats, hard soccer fields, increased training and running).

Commonly seen in football are injuries to the nail and nail plate, as well as ingrown toenails, blisters and tinea pedis (athlete's foot) infections. Severely involuted nails can be due to a tight toe box in a soccer cleat. In many cases a patient who pronates excessively and who has hallux abductus will develop a close approximation to the adjacent second digit, and with forefoot shoe pressure can also develop an involuted tibial or fibular border of the hallux nail. On occasion these involuted nail borders, complicated by paronychia, may require partial avulsion with or without matricectomy (see Ch. 23).

Plantar fasciitis is a common chronic overuse injury resulting from microtrauma and microinflammation of the plantar fascia. It is located at the calcaneal origin and is usually involved with the medial band of the plantar fascia. In football, due to the stop and run motion, chronic repetitive stress can occur, and this can lead to chronic irritation and inflammation of the plantar fascia. After sudden, violent or 'explosive' movement partial rupture of the plantar fascia can also occur. After repetitive microtrauma, eventual heel spur development may occur. Plantar fasciitis is commonly brought on in football by prolonged training sessions and playing numerous games. Another contributing factor is that the typical football cleat does not have adequate arch support and does not have good shock-absorbing properties for the heel. Football fields may also contribute to the problem, because hard, unrelenting ground surfaces can add increased impact shock to the heel, particularly in the young football player.

Other common injuries seen in soccer play involve stress fractures of the lesser metatarsals (Davis & Alexander 1990, Stanitski et al 1978). There is no age that is immune from this overuse injury. Jones fractures and avulsion fractures at the base of the fifth metatarsal, due to traction of the fibularis (peroneus) brevis tendon, are also seen. Strains of the hamstrings and quadriceps are quite common as a result of continual contraction during play. In youngsters during their growth years, enthesitis at the attachment of these muscles to bone can also occur, particularly in shin splint areas of the tibialis anterior or posterior muscle groups, such as the soleus. Painful inflammation along the lower third of the medial tibia is often seen as a result of Sharpey's fibres being torn away. Chronic shin splints, if left untreated, could eventually lead to medial stress fractures of the tibia as well. A direct blow to the lower leg from an opponent can lead to increased pressure of either the anterior, lateral or posterior medial compartment, and eventual compartment syndrome. Running on uneven surfaces, being kicked by an opponent, or tripping over another player, can easily lead to ankle injury. Most frequently seen is the inversion mechanism sprain as a result of supination of the rearfoot, and plantar flexion of the forefoot. Occasionally, when attempting to block a kick, and sliding the foot and leg towards the ball and ground, a medial, eversion mechanism ankle sprain can occur. Os trigonum fractures of the talus can occur as a result of the player striking the ground, in a hyper-plantar-flexing motion, with the posterior, lateral process wedged between the posterior tibial malleolus and calcaneus. Flexion of the flexor hallucis longus tendon will elicit painful symptoms at the region of the os trigonum. Achilles tendinitis, another common overuse soccer injury, is seen as a result of tight posterior muscle groups and a short/tight Achilles tendon, with a lack of flexibility and inadequate stretching. In youngsters, traction of the Achilles tendon can occur, and in adults insertional calcific tendinosis may also occur. Excessive pronation, and flat football shoes without sufficient cushioning, can also cause and aggravate the condition (Clark et al 1983, Scioli 1994, Talloway et al 1992). Patellofemoral joint syndrome is quite frequently seen in footballers, as is internal derangement of the knee ligaments. Chondromalacia may develop due to the distance run, running on hard ground surfaces, increased Q-angles and excessive pronation, all of which can lead to this overuse syndrome. Women football players with genu valgum and increased Q-angles are highly subject to this injury. Hip injuries are frequently seen, with bursitis, contusions and hip dysfunction being the typical complaints. Groin pain may actually emanate from the hip, lower abdomen and lumbosacral region, or from the groin itself (Renstrom & Peterson 1980, Taylor et al 1991).

Prevention of football injuries can be accomplished with proper supervision and capable coaching in a properly designed training programme (Erstrand & Gillquist 1983a,b). With the preponderance of youth football leagues, careful attention should be given to growing children, as well as to the intensity and duration of the training sessions. Proper football cleat selection, a pre-season training programme as well as a flexibility and stretching programme can dramatically reduce the occurrence of football injuries. Some other helpful means of preventing injuries include proper equipment (shin guards), correct training habits, proper footwear with biomechanical balanced insoles/orthotics, and pre-activity ankle-taping for those with a chronically unstable ankle. It is also important to have a certified trainer and/or sports medicine healthcare professional, and optimal field conditions (dry, level, no divots or cracks).

## GYMNASTICS

Gymnastics is another sport that has seen an increase in interest in the past decade, particularly due to exposure in the amateur and Olympic ranks. About 500 BC, the Spartans gave meaning to the word gymnastics, which translates as 'to perform exercises while naked'.

Facets of gymnastic safety include: pre-assessment of the gymnast; proper warm-up and stretching; physical, psychological and emotional preparedness of both the gymnast and the coach; and proper gymnasium design. The coaches, parents, gymnast and team physicians are all involved in the overall safety of the gymnastic participant.

There are many causes of gymnastic accidents (Wettstone 1982): horse play, failure to spot a slippery area, shoes, aggressive coaching, fatigue, lack of strength and flexibility, lack of kinaesthetic awareness, overexertion, bones, lack of fundamentals and defective equipment.

Plyometrics are dynamic exercises designed to develop power for running, jumping and throwing. These drills include hops, bounds, depth jumps, and jumping with weights and medicine balls (Dyatch Rov 1969, Miller 1980). Plyometrics are based on the principle of the stretch reflex mechanism – that a muscle contracts faster and with more force from a prestretched position than from a relaxed state. Gymnastics has specific strength and power demands, and plyometric exercises are specifically designed to meet these needs (coupled development).

Injuries to the lower extremities in gymnastics can occur on a variety of equipment, and during various movements. It has been shown that nearly all beam injuries to the non-team-level gymnasts (preparation level) occur on the high balance beam (Weider & Ganim 1982). Dismounting from the balance beam, pommel horse or rings can easily result in acute injuries such as a stress fracture, periostitis of the calcaneus, plantar fascia strains or inversion mechanism sprains to the ankle. Proper care and maintenance of these pieces of equipment can help avoid unnecessary injury. The fact that gymnasts train and perform barefooted (except when wearing ankle or foot braces) adds to the high risk of injury that these athletes face.

## BASKETBALL

Basketball is physically demanding, and there is the risk of high-intensity trauma to the lower extremities. Although technically a non-contact sport, basketball could be compared to hockey or football. Quite frequently, physical contact between players, as well as between players and the court, can result in spontaneous acute traumatic injury. Overuse injuries can be the result of poor lower extremity biomechanics, shoes, practice deficiencies and other factors.

Due to the tremendous stresses on the musculoskeletal system of the lower extremity, a basketball player's feet, ankles and knees must absorb high levels of impact shock. These muscles, tendons and ligaments are subject to constant loading forces, and the hamstring and gastrocnemius–soleus muscle groups must activate and 'spring into action' with every vertical leap.

Even the lower back is at risk from hyperextension during shooting and rebounding. Effective recognition and management of acute and overuse injuries will help to increase the effectiveness of later treatment and promote early return to play.

The vast majority of musculoskeletal injuries sustained by basketball players are to the lower extremity (Henry et al 1982, Messina et al 1999, National Basketball Athletic Trainers' Association 1989–90, Ray et al 1991). As in adult players, a 1999 study of Texas high-school basketball players found that ankles were the most common sites of injury in both boys and girls. After the ankles, the next most frequent areas to be injured are the knee and groin. Injuries to the hip and lower back also occur with high frequency.

The fundamental treatment plan for basketball injuries should include the following: proper diagnosis, with early intervention, followed by aggressive treatment that will guard the basketball player from further injury, permit return to activity as quickly as possible and prevent recurrent injury. A basic treatment plan can be divided into three steps:

1. immediate treatment
2. continuing treatment
3. correction of any biomechanical problems (Taylor et al 1999).

At the side of the court, sprains and strains are treated according to the recognised mnemonic RICE (Rest, Ice, Compression, Elevation) (see Ch. 16). Immediate application of ice will help to reduce swelling and the ensuing inflammation. Compression may be by means of a simple elastic bandage, taping, an Air Splint, an ankle brace, or a posterior splint to immobilise the injured site. Elevating the extremity will also help to minimise the swelling and reduce discomfort. By reducing the onset and extent of the swelling, recovery time can be reduced, and this also helps promote early rehabilitation.

One of the more common injuries that basketball players suffer from is toenail injury. Due to rapid acceleration and deceleration, and with twisting and changing of direction, the foot will slide forward in the basketball shoe and cause a jamming of the nail against both the upper of the shoe and the toe box. It is not uncommon for players to be stepped on during a game, and suffer from a typical subungual haematoma fracture of the distal phalanx. Injuries to the nails include ingrown toenails and subungual exostosis secondary to trauma (see Ch. 2).

Blisters are another typical problem in basketball players, usually at the beginning of the season due to friction and shearing forces on the toes and plantar aspect of the foot. Initial treatment should include draining of the blister, while leaving the blister roof in place.

Products such as Second Skin can be used for players who have sensitive skin and a predilection for abrasion and blister formation. Duct tape, which fanatical marathon runners use to prevent blisters, is another remedy that can be employed. To reduce shearing and rubbing, insoles such as Spenco, Superfeet and Sorbothane can be very beneficial. If a biomechanical problem is present wherein abnormal pronation and abduction (pivoting) of the hallux takes place, a soft prescription orthotic covered with the anti-friction insoles can provide even greater defence against blister formation. Marathon runners often apply Vaseline to the skin to reduce friction, and this has also been shown to be helpful.

Other common basketball injuries include: stress fractures of the metatarsals, sesamoids, calcaneus and tibia/fibula; fractures of the os trigonum; avulsion fractures of the navicular and of the base of the fifth metatarsal; cuboid subluxation; heel bursitis; plantar fasciitis–heel spur syndrome; anterior ankle impingement; painful accessory navicular; and ankle sprains. Other acute injuries include Achilles tendon ruptures, knee injuries, contusions to the quadriceps, and muscle pulls and tears, particularly of the gastrocnemius–soleus, fibular (peroneal) and posterior tibial tendons. Frequent overuse injuries seen in basketball include contusions and bursitis of the sesamoid bones, sesamoiditis, hallux rigidus, bunions, interdigital neuromas, Achilles tendinitis, insertional Achilles tendinitis and calcinosis formation, posterior tibial tendinitis, fibularis (peroneus) longus, brevis tendinitis and flexor hallucis longus tendinitis.

With the high incidence of injuries to basketball players, trainers and team physicians have a responsibility to prevent these injuries. Measures include proper training to take into account the fact that a National Basketball Association or college season runs for 6–9 months and that players practise continually – both during the season and in the off-season – for about 11–12 months. The amount of mental and physical stress, in addition to the physical pounding that the players experience during the game itself, can lead to injury. Other means of reducing the incidence of injuries include diet and nutrition, strengthening programmes, travel schedules (jet lag), proper equipment, and a well-designed stretching and flexibility programme.

## BOWLING

It may not generally be expected that bowling would be a sport with frequent injuries. However, the movement of the bowler toward the foul line may lead to injury due to lurching or a heavy awkward gait (Wysocki 1999). When a foot does not track straight ahead with approximately 10° of abduction, balanced flexion at the metatarsophalangeal joint (MTPJ) cannot occur. As a result, the ankle changes the direction needed by this movement. Stress occurs to the foot and ankle, and eventually compensation begins, leading to overuse injuries such as medial band plantar fasciitis, posterior tibial tendinitis, ankle strain, medial knee pain, and hip and lower back strain.

## TENNIS

Tennis is multidirectional, involving both forward and reverse as well as side-to-side motion. As in other court sports, many of the acute injuries in tennis involve a sudden, violent movement from a stationary position, and they usually occur when the player comes to a sudden stop to hit the ball. This can be seen in the movements of rushing to the net, covering the sidelines or retreating to cover the baseline. These multidirectional movements can lead to both acute and overuse injuries. Many of the injuries incurred in tennis involve overuse inflammatory processes; however, traumatic fractures and dislocations, as well as tears and ruptures of ligamentous and tendon structures, are often seen (Ross 1999c). Grand slam exposure, worldwide ranking, junior play, and high school and intercollegiate play have all contributed to the increase in popularity of tennis since the 1960s. Tennis is a sport that demonstrates technique, athletic ability, stamina and agility, and to this end there have been great advances in flexibility, strength training and conditioning (Hageman & Lehman 1988).

Tennis injuries of the lower leg and foot can be divided into two basic categories: acute and chronic. Most of the lower-leg injuries that occur in competitive tennis are chronic in nature and develop from repetitive stress (Leach 1988, Levisohn & Simon 1984, O'Connor et al 1992). The overuse syndrome injury that is seen in tennis, as in other sports, has a common aetiology: a repetitive trauma that eventually interferes with a tissue's ability to repair itself (Herring & Nelson 1987). Microtrauma occurs with overuse, triggering events that ultimately can lead to tissue degeneration (Galloway et al 1992, Greenfield 1990, O'Connor et al 1992). These muscles and tendons are subject to repeated stretching and traction. As a result, a degenerative process develops, wherein the rate of tissue breakdown is faster than the rate of tissue repair. This continual stretching during play can cause fatigue, as is often seen in overuse syndrome. Because of the poor blood supply directed to tendons, repeated subintimal injury and delayed healing are very common. According to Clancy (1982), the Achilles is the tendon most commonly injured in sports.

Overuse injuries suffered by tennis players include tendon injuries, chronic Achilles tendinitis, Haglund's deformity, with chronic bursitis, posterior tibial and fibular (peroneal) tendinitis, posterior and anterior shin splints, compartment syndromes, interdigital neuromas, chronic plantar fasciitis, hallux limitus/rigidus of the first metatarsal phalangeal joint, acute and chronic sesamoiditis, as well as subungual exostosis, with nail deformities. These overuse injuries occur as the musculoskeletal system becomes more and more fatigued due to increased and repeated loads of stress, followed by failure.

In tennis, overuse injuries that may not force the player out of competitive play but will affect performance can be categorised as the 'lesser injuries'. These entities develop as a result of excessive pressures on bony prominent areas, or as a result of the foot or toe(s) jamming against the shoe or toe box – 'tennis toe' or a subungual haematoma. This is one of the reasons why it is so important for the tennis shoe to have adequate room and toe space. Keeping the nails short and trimming them properly will help to delay the onset of 'tennis toe'. Repeated pressure on the sole of the foot or against the digits can lead to blisters, corns and calluses, and these often develop in a competitive game of tennis or when breaking in a new pair of tennis shoes.

Acute injuries to the lower leg, ankle and foot in tennis are also quite common. Racquet sports place an undue amount of stress on the lower leg and the supporting soft-tissue structures. The reason for this increased stress, and potential for acute injury, is the amount of time players spend on the balls of their feet, the extreme ranges of motion that foot and ankle must move through, and the violent nature of these movements (Levisohn & Simon 1984). Two of the more common acute injuries incurred in tennis are spontaneous rupture of the Achilles tendon and of the gastrocnemius muscle. As in basketball, tennis involves a ballistic start from a standing position, which can impose a large force on the Achilles tendon. Barfred (1971) stated that the tendon is subject to injury when (1) tension is applied quickly, (2) the tendon is under tension before loading, and (3) the tendon is weak compared to the muscle. Recurrent injury to the Achilles or any other tendon can cause partial or complete rupture. A tear of the medial head of the gastrocnemius ('tennis leg'), usually occurs in a younger population than those suffering from acute Achilles tendon ruptures. This is the most common injury occurring in male tennis players (Arner & Lindholm 1958, Leach 1988) and is often misdiagnosed as a rupture of the plantaris muscle (Anouche et al 1987, Froimson 1969). This injury often occurs while the player's foot is in plantar flexion with simultaneous supination. This creates tension on the medial head of the gastrocnemius, while relaxing the plantaris and lateral head of the gastrocnemius.

Other acute traumatic injuries include spontaneous rupture of the posterior tibial and fibularis (peroneus) tendons, dislocation or subluxation of the fibularis (peroneus) tendons, and acute compartment syndrome. The most common fractures in tennis are stress fractures of the metatarsals and calcaneal fractures, which occur particularly when landing hard on the court from an overhead jump shot, service or net play. Another stress fracture site due to forced dorsiflexion, during the same shots, is the tibial plateau or distal shaft of the tibia. Occasionally, fractures to the styloid process or os trigonum of the posterior aspect of the talus occur due to a sudden violent movement of the rearfoot when in plantar flexion and inversion, with the posterior process impinged on the tibia.

Ankle sprains are often seen in tennis, particularly in the net game, or when running hard laterally, and attempting to stop quickly to set up to return the shot. The lateral ankle injury is the most frequent, usually affecting the anterior talofibular ligament, followed by the calcaneal fibular ligament, and lastly the posterior talofibular ligament. Another acute trauma to the ankle involves an eversion–plantar flexion and abduction mechanism sprain, affecting the deltoid ligament. If severe enough, this can lead to fracture of the medial malleolus, as in a lateral injury, resulting in avulsions of the fibular apex. Styloid process fractures (Jones) of the base of the fifth metatarsal are also seen in tennis players who have experienced an inversion, lateral ankle sprain. A proximal fifth metatarsal fracture can be categorised into two specific types: (1) a fracture of the tuberosity, and (2) a fracture of the metatarsal shaft within 1.5 cm of the tuberosity (Ross 1999b).

Tennis court surfaces are another factor to consider. The various surfaces can be divided into clay, composition, hard court, wood, carpet and grass. The harder the court surface the greater the stress incurred by the tennis player's feet and lower extremities, while the softer surfaces dampen shock and impart less stress to the knees, ankles and feet. For the older player who suffers from degenerative joint disease, with concomitant foot pathology, a softer surface should be chosen to avoid excessive amounts of stress and shock to the feet and legs. After a player has been injured, it is recommended that softer surfaces be used to allow for rehabilitation, and then to resume play later on harder surfaces.

## GOLF

Foot and lower extremity function is one of the keys to a proper golf swing. To transfer weight and produce an efficient swing proper biomechanical balance of the foot is essential. Most professional golf injuries involve the lower back, followed by injuries to the left wrist and shoulder. Whereas, in male amateur golfers the lower back was the most commonly injured area, followed by the elbow, hand or wrist, shoulder and knee, among female amateur golfers the elbow was the most commonly injured site, followed by the back, shoulder, hand or wrist, and knee (McCarroll & Gioe 1982).

Approximately 10–12% of golf injuries occur in the lower extremity (McCarrol et al 1990). Acute foot injuries in golf are not common. One study showed that in 584 golf-related injuries, 2.1% were foot-related (Cavanaugh & Williams 1983). However, walking the course, pre-existing foot injuries are complicated by repetitive weight transference during swing, and improperly fitting shoes can contribute to foot complaints during golf play.

As recognised by Cavanaugh and Williams (1983), foot function, ground reaction forces and centre-of-pressure position are critical for a proper golf swing. It was shown that the right and left foot function in an entirely different manner, and with no symmetry. During the swing, the right foot begins a rocking movement, and by the end of the swing the golfer begins to apply pressure to the medial border of the hallux, concluding at the distal aspect of the hallux.

The left foot functions asymmetrically by beginning with a pronatory effect on the medial edge and then supinating to the lateral edge of the foot and ankle.

There are numerous foot conditions that the golfer may suffer from, particularly from the shoes they wear; for example, hallux abducto valgus can be a source of irritation in shoes. Hallux limitus/rigidus with dorsal osteophytic lipping of the first metatarsal head can create degenerative joint disease and synovitis. This can cause limitation of motion and stiffness, and prohibit normal pivoting and toe-off during the golf swing. Irritation from the counter of the golf shoe against the posterior aspect of the heel can cause exacerbation of a Haglund's deformity, or retrocalcaneal bursitis. Occasionally, Achilles tendinitis can be a problem, particularly in a middle-aged or older golfer.

Aetiological factors such as excessive pronation, tight Achilles tendon and posterior muscle groups, equinus, combined with uneven terrain and uphill lies, can create additional stretch and torque of the tendon and contribute to the tendinitis. Plantar fasciitis, one of the more common overuse injuries seen in sports, particularly in golfers who walk the course, is due to chronic traction and irritation of the origin of the plantar fascia on the medial plantar condyle of the calcaneus. If left untreated, an enthesopathy will eventually develop, due to hyperpronation, with resulting heel spur formation. Old golf shoes and poor foot biomechanics can lead to this overuse injury. Ankle sprains are not uncommon.

Golfers who walk on undulating fairways, attempt to swing from an uneven or uphill lie, or have excessive supination of the ankle in the follow-through of the swing may suffer from an acute ankle sprain. Morton's neuroma, usually in the third inter-space, is quite common, particularly if walking a great deal or wearing tight-fitting golf shoes with little toe box room. Other conditions that golfers suffer from are blisters, corns tinea pedis, dryness of the skin, heel fissuring and onychomycotic nails.

Golf shoes are important because they act as a base of support for the golf swing by reducing foot slippage and offering lateral stability (Furman 1999). They are found in three basic styles: (1) welted shoes, the classic-appearing shoe, with a leather upper and stitched leather sole; (2) athletic-style shoes, similar to the characteristic athletic shoe; and (3) comfort classic shoes, which are similar to the classic welted shoe, but lighter and with more cushioning.

## AMERICAN FOOTBALL

American football is a contact sport, and more acute injuries occur in this sport than any other (Meewwisse & Fowler 1988, Pritchett 1980). The study by Pritchett revealed that one-third of the injures involved the lower extremities and accounted for one-half of the cost (Welch 1996). It was also noted that nearly half of the injuries reported involved sprains and strains of the ankle, knee and back, as well as contusions of the lower extremity (Kune et al 1980, McCarthy 1989). Other aetiological variables that play a part in American football injuries include the surface of the field (grass versus artificial turf), the size of opponents, speed, style of play and conditioning of the athlete (Skovrm et al 1990). The question of whether artificial surfaces cause more injuries than natural grass, particularly to the knees, ankles, foot and hallux, is continually being explored; however, there is some evidence to support this assertion (McCarthy 1989, Skovrm et al 1990).

One of the more common problems incurred involves the medial and intermediate dorsal cutaneous nerves. As a result of direct trauma, and being 'cleated' (stepped on) by another player, a neuropraxia of these nerves can occur. Another factor in this condition is chronic irritation on the dorsum of the foot due to taping and from the laces of the shoe being too tight. Such neuropraxia is seen quite frequently in American football players who have a cavus foot type with a metatarsal–cuneiform exostosis (instep). Radiating pain extending from

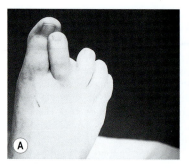 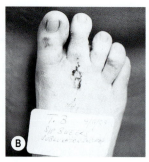

**Figure 13.4** (A) Spontaneous subluxation of the second metatarsophalangeal joint (MTPJ); (B) postoperative repair of spontaneous subluxation of the second metatarsophalangeal joint.

the medial dorsal cutaneous nerve will extend to the medial branch of the saphenous nerve, and to the hallux (McNerney 1990, 1999). Another nerve injury that occurs commonly in American football is interdigital neuroma with entrapment and degenerative fibrosis. This occurs as a result of being on the ball of the foot for a prolonged period of time and a strong propulsive push-off. Tight-fitting shoes are another reason for compression of the nerve, and can create other symptoms. Occasionally, tarsal tunnel syndrome may develop from excessive pronation, traction of the posterior tibial nerve, and direct and indirect trauma to the deltoid ligament region or the nerve itself.

Other traumatic and overuse injuries include turf toe, a traumatic injury to the first MTPJ and the metatarsal–cuneiform joint, which occurs more frequently on artificial surfaces (Clanton et al 1986, Dollar 1978). The term 'turf toe' refers to a hyperextension or a hyper-flexion of the joint, creating a capsular or ligamentous sprain of the MTPJ. Other injuries that can be categorised as turf toe are dislocation and subluxation of the joint, rupture of the intersesamoidal ligament, sesamoiditis, fracture of the sesamoids and capsulitis of the joint (Fig. 13.4). Rodeo et al (1990) evaluated a number of professional American football players and found that 57 of those surveyed had reported symptoms of turf toe. It should be noted that this figure was similar to that for players from other teams who played on a natural grass surface; however, 84% of the players in the series reported that their initial injury occurred on artificial turf. Some of the aetiologies that predispose an American football player to this type of injury include the number of years in professional American football (Rodeo et al 1990), pes planus, decreased pre-injury MTPJ range of motion (Clanton et al 1986), decreased pre-injury ankle range of motion, and shoes too flexible at the shank. Although turf toe is a common injury in football it can occur in any sport that is played on artificial turf (Underwood 1985).

Other injuries commonly seen in American football include Lisfranc's joint injuries, which are also common on artificial turf surfaces, causing pain and swelling of the metatarsal–cuneiform joint. In some cases of violent hyperextension, Lisfranc dislocations and fractures may occur. Ankle sprains, common in all sports, are reported to be the second most common injury in American football, with knee injuries being the most common (Meewwisse & Fowler 1988, Pritchett 1980). Lateral ankle sprains make up the majority of these injuries, involving the anterior talofibular and calcaneal fibular ligaments. Injuries to the tibiofibular syndesmosis are associated with a high morbidity, limiting the player's early return to normal activity (Hopkison et al 1990). Deltoid sprains occur very infrequently, but can be just as serious and disabling. Overuse injuries seen often in American football include intracalcaneal pain, which in younger athletes (described in the younger athlete section) is quite often due to calcaneal apophysis (Sever's disease). Heel spur syndrome and plantar

fasciitis are other frequent overuse injuries in American football. Chronic Achilles tendinitis, insertional tendinosis, shin splints, myositis, bursitis of the foot, ankle and lower leg, and exertional compartment syndromes are typical in this game.

Recommendations for the reduction of overuse injuries in American football are pre-season flexibility and strength exercise programmes, physical therapy, proper selection of stable and motion-control cleats, flexible arch supports, prescription orthotics to control poor biomechanics, anti-inflammatory medication and, when safe, injection therapy.

Skin disorders are prevalent. Thick socks and perspiration can lead to tinea pedis and, with trauma to the nails due to the cleated shoe and constant forefoot push-off, this can cause subsequent onychomycosis. Other skin lesions such as blisters, corns, calluses, intractable plantar keratomas and verrucae may also develop. Conservative management of these disorders in the American football athlete is desirable, except when trauma or conservative measures have failed, when surgical intervention may be necessary.

## RUGBY

A contact sport, historically the forerunner of American football, rugby is played without any protective gear. Injuries to the head, upper extremities and lower extremities are prevalent. The sport requires upper body strength and lower body power.

This sport also requires great athleticism, where speed is needed during sprint running. In addition to running skills, the player must pass and catch the ball, requiring balance and coordination. The training for such an explosive sport is designed to improve stamina and speed.

The training methods in rugby have not necessarily paid sufficient attention to pre-season conditioning, strengthening and flexibility. As a result, tight muscle groups and poor flexibility lead to many acute and overuse injuries such as gastrocnemius–soleus muscle pulls and tears, ruptures of the Achilles tendon, and chronic Achilles tendinitis, plantar fascia strains and chronic plantar fasciitis. Due to biomechanical imbalances, posterior tibial and fibular (peroneal) tendinitis, shin splints and turf toe injuries are seen. Direct trauma to the lower extremity can result in knee injuries, ankle sprains, fractures and compartment syndromes. Tackling on grass, compared to artificial turf, reduces the chances of injuries (as discussed in the section on American football); however, playing rugby often leads to injury. Field conditions (dry versus wet) as well as footwear can have an impact on the incidence of injury in this highly physical, combative, traditional sport.

## STEP/BENCH AEROBICS

Step and bench aerobics as an 'exercise dance' was developed from the high-impact aerobic dance form, which led to an abundance of lower extremity injuries, as a safer form of low-impact dance. By reducing impact shock on the lower extremities the number of injuries seen by the sports medicine practitioner has been dramatically reduced. However, step and bench aerobics can still cause overuse injuries.

Approximately 18 years ago aerobic dance matured into a new form utilising a 'bench' platform and creating a new way to exercise with less impact, while simultaneously allowing for the same, if not better, cardiovascular workout. The exercise routine is centred on a 'step' that is just 43 inches long by 16 inches wide by a minimum of 4 inches high (109 cm × 40 cm × 10 cm). It was thought in the early stages that the higher the step the harder and more vigorous a workout. However, with the elevations of one-, two- and three-block increments the risk of overuse injury is increased.

The development of aerobic shoes has had a great deal of impact on the sport. Over the years, technological advances in design have led to a much more stable, as well as a high-performance, aerobic shoe. Further design changes have led to a new breed of 'cross-trainers'. This popular shoe can be used for aerobic dance and for short-distance running, and it is a favourite among aerobic instructors. With increased running incorporated in the routines, and with dance movements, including lateral movements as well as back peddling, the cross-trainer shoe has proved to be an asset.

Injury prevention, as in all sports, begins with good observation and correction. Most aerobic instructors agree that technique is very important in the avoidance of injuries, and that repetition is dangerous. It has been shown that if an aerobic dance routine is performed at a cadence that is too fast (over 128 beats/minute) participants cannot secure their entire foot on the bench, resulting in strain or pulling of the Achilles tendon, posterior tibial tendon or fibularis (peroneus) tendons. This can also lead to strain of the long plantar fascia or the intrinsic musculature of the plantar aspect of the foot (Ross 1999a). In addition, an over-quick step off the bench can lead to sesamoiditis, stress fractures of the lesser metatarsals as well as the tibia and fibula, tarsal tunnel syndrome and the formation of interdigital neuroma. It has been shown that extending too far back off the bench can lead to a hyperextension of the ankle, with concomitant traction of the Achilles tendon. If left undetected, this overuse injury could eventually develop into a chronic Achilles tenosynovitis and/or insertional calcinosis. It is imperative that instructors observe carefully the participant's knee alignment in relationship to the lower leg, as well as their foot placement on the bench. It has also been shown that striking the floor from the bench with repeated impact can result in overuse patellofemoral joint syndrome or shin splints. It is important that the instructor survey the class before the initial workout to help determine whether any of the participants has a pre-existing overuse injury or a high potential for developing a new injury.

Prevention of injuries should be of paramount importance to the sports medicine specialist, particularly for aerobic enthusiasts who train at high intensity levels and ignore the potential for injury. Quite often aerobic dance participants may have psychological or physiological disorders (e.g. anorexia nervosa, amenorrhoea and osteoporosis). Any one of these conditions can have serious consequences when participating seriously in this sport. The sports medicine specialist should be on alert when interviewing the patient during the history taking, because any one of these diagnoses can render clues regarding the underlying injury. Extreme weight loss and/or stress fractures (particularly in the young female) should alert the sports medicine practitioner to look beyond the easily definable diagnosis and consider referral.

In a preliminary study by Ross (1999a) of 329 participants, 153 claimed that they had suffered some discomfort or pain due to step/bench aerobics, whereas 163 claimed that they were symptom-free. The most common sites for the incidence of injury were the knee, calf, Achilles tendon, foot and shin.

There were a number of recommendations made by the instructors to help prevent some of the typical injuries:

- keep the knees slightly bent, never locking the knee
- bring the foot all the way up to the bench, so that the heel is not hanging off
- keep the knee over the ankle (creating less strain on the knee)
- push off with the heel (not with the knee) with either squats or lunges
- keep the head up and the chest tall (to prevent lower back strain)
- avoid stepping too far back from the bench
- avoid stepping overenthusiastically off the bench
- maintain the same pace and avoid stepping too quickly
- do not be afraid to lower the bench to a level more suitable to your abilities to avoid injury.

## BALLET AND DANCE

Classical ballet had its origins in the Italian Court in the 15th and 16th centuries. The practice of dancing 'en pointe', or on the tips of the toes, was popularised in the early 1830s, and is one of the aetiological factors in the development of foot deformities. Yet it is a ballet form that is practised by young girls and women all over the world. In addition to classical ballet, other forms of dance are also popular. Each form of dance has its own intrinsic character and injury incidence.

Ballet is an elegant and very athletic art form, and ballet dancers can be regarded as elite aesthetic athletes. The athletic artiste must master solitary body positions and specific repetitive movements that are incorporated into a choreographed programme. Dance has a unique set of biomechanical considerations specific to this art form, and with a whole group of distinct injuries connected to the biomechanical demands of the activity.

The sports medicine specialist must be attuned to the high demands and mechanics of the sport as well as the potential for injury and recurrent injury. Quirk (1994) described four main causes of injury in ballet:

1. *Physique.* Due to the unique requirements of ballet, the dancer needs a certain type of body to avoid injury. The female dancer tends to be very slim, with a long back, long legs and exceptional joint mobility, particularly in the spine, hips and feet. The male ballet dancer is inclined to be of light build, muscular, but not as flexible as his female counterpart.

2. *Technique.* Incorrect technique repeated over a period of time, combined with frequent classes and performances, can lead to overuse injuries. Proper technique in ballet has been gradually refined over the years, and movements that often led to injury have been eliminated. A good sports medicine practitioner who is cognisant of ballet movement can easily predict or recognise the technical fault based on the injury.

3. *Overuse.* Ballet is a demanding athletic art, and as a result dancers are expected to work for many hours on any given day, creating the potential for overuse injuries. Combined with a biomechanical fault in physique, or error in technique, an injury can ensue.

4. *Mishaps.* With choreographed, rehearsed routines, the chances of acute injury are remote, as opposed to contact sports. The most frequent acute traumatic injury is the sprained ankle, usually from landing off a jump, or from an intricate ballet movement.

What makes ballet so unusual is the 'turnout' of the feet, or extreme external rotation of the hips. The dancer trains daily by exercising the anterior musculature of the hip to achieve the classic position, referred to as 'well turned out'. The ideal position is that in which the hips and feet are laterally rotated 180° from each other, and where the heel is facing the opposite heel, and the toes are facing in opposite directions. Kravitz and Murgia (1999) suggest that dancers attempt to create the illusion of the desired foot position by tilting the pelvis forward, by laterally rotating the tibia at the knee, or by applying an abductory force to the pedal segment. The pelvic tilt can produce excessive compressive forces on the posterior aspect of the vertebral bodies and discs of the lumbar spine, and can result in lumbar strain injuries.

The rotation of the knee produces excessive strain of the capsule and medial collateral ligament, and can produce medial knee pain. The abductory force created on the foot will then lead to subtalar joint and midtarsal joint pronation, as well as prolapsing of the longitudinal arch. For the pronated dancer, with a collapsed longitudinal arch, difficulty in maintaining position can create pain and a 'rolled in at the ankle' appearance.

The externally rotated position is seen in the five basic positions in ballet. Essential basic movements in ballet comprise the plié, relevé and pointe. The plié exercise consists of deep knee flexion while maintaining the 'toe-out'. Again, the hips are rotated laterally at 180° to each other. Plié is a flexed-knee position. In demi-plié the dancer lowers herself, upper body erect with the knees bent, and with the heels in full contact with the floor. Demi-plié is an important movement used in preparation for a propulsive action phase, as well as in the landing stage when impact forces are being reduced, or at the end of movements such as jumps, turns or leaps. In grand plié, the dancer lowers herself even further, again with the upper body erect, with greater bending of the knees, and as the heels come off the floor weight is transferred to the ball of the foot. In relevé the dancer assumes an erect upper body stance, with the knees extended, and the weight shifted to the balls of the feet. The next position is referred to in French as 'sur les pointes' or 'en pointe'. In going en pointe the dancer assumes a stance position on the toes. Pointe shoes are identical between the right and left. The pointe shoe is constructed of a leather sole with an upper made of canvas, cotton and silk, with a stiffened toe cap made of fabric, glue and stiffened paper (Whiteside 1986). A stiffened shank made of board material is found plantarly to help secure the longitudinal arch. Ribbons are used to hold the shoe on the foot, wrapped around the ankle, and tied at the back. Their half-life can be very short and, once broken, they have to be discarded immediately. In some cases soft, flexible orthotics can be used for additional support and to attempt to achieve neutral control.

When the dancer is en pointe, weight is shifted onto the distal and medial aspects of the first and second rays as the foot is supported by the toe box, the shank, the musculature of the dancer and the intrinsic bony architecture of the foot and ankle (Denton 1997). The demi-pointe attitude is a position in which the dancer stands on the metatarsal heads while the ankle is fully plantar flexed and the MTPJs are maximally dorsiflexed. A forced arch attitude is the same as demi-pointe, with the addition of the knee being flexed.

Overuse injuries in ballet are a common entity. The injuries are specific particularly to dancers, and are not seen in other athletic sports. Specific movements combined with repetitive biomechanical demands on the lower extremities frequently lead to these overuse injuries.

## Tendinitis

Due to the repetitive nature of ballet, tendinitis conditions are common overuse injuries. Flexor hallucis longus tendinitis is a very common injury (Hamilton 1982b). This type of injury frequently occurs as a result of the strain created on the hallux tendon antagonistic to hallux hyperextension while en pointe. The foot is plantar flexed or pointed, with the hallux in maximum plantar flexion. When jumping, leaping or push-off is required, the great toe flexor is required for the completion of this propulsive phase. The flexor hallucis longus is then maximally stretched, followed by contracture along with the

other plantar flexors. Repetitive movement, and jumps with the foot en pointe can lead to fatigue, tendinitis, peritendinitis, tenosynovitis and, if severe and long-lasting, the flexor hallucis longus can spontaneously rupture. Pain and crepitus can be elicited around the medial malleolus. The second most commonly affected tendon is the Achilles tendon, with pain elicited at the distal portion of the tendon and at its insertion. Crepitus upon movement as well as thickening of the tendon and distortion of the surrounding tissues may develop. There are various aetiologies for the onset of Achilles tendinitis. One such mechanism is the repetitive jumping involved in ballet, where a concentric tension is created at push-off, followed by an eccentric force on the posterior muscles and Achilles during the completion of the movement. Not getting the heel down to the floor (as in running equinus injuries) can also lead to this overuse injury. Another interesting entity is that of the dancer who ties her ankle ribbons too tightly around the back of the ankle, and the knot presses directly on the Achilles tendon, thus irritating during these leaping manoeuvres. Extensor tendinitis occurs as a result of overuse of the extensor digitorum longus, and in some cases the tibialis anterior tendons. This is usually seen with increased external rotation and turnout of the foot. Due to excessive pronation, and plantar flexion to achieve additional external rotation and turnout, fibular (peroneal) tendinitis may develop.

Plantar fasciitis is another entity due to a weak arch, barefooted practices, repetitive jumping and landing, as well as attempting to further toe-out with additional pronation. The dancer will often attempt to compensate for this chronic injury, and may develop other areas of injury, such as posterior tibial tendinitis, fibular (peroneal) tendinitis, shin splints, iliotibial band syndrome, as well as hip and lower back pain.

## Posterior and anterior impingement syndrome of the ankle

Posterior impingement of the ankle or talar compression syndrome (Quirk 1982) is much more common in dancers than in athletes. It is seen with maximal plantar flexion of the ankle joint, and occurs with the en pointe position. Pain may be elicited at the posterior aspect of the ankle when the toe is pointed, and is caused by compression of the posterior tubercle of the talus on the posterior distal tibia when the ankle is maximally plantar flexed.

This process can fracture and irritate against the flexor hallucis longus tendon. Flexing or extending the hallux will precipitate a painful response. This usually requires cast immobilisation and, on occasion, may necessitate surgical excision of the bone fragment. Another aetiology is the os trigonum (being separate from the main body of the talus in about 10% of ankles), which may become entrapped and compress the surrounding soft-tissue structures (Quirk 1982, 1994). Anterior tibiotalar impingement syndrome is another complaint experienced when the ankle joint is dorsiflexed. The aetiology of this syndrome may be an exostosis of either the anterior distal tibia or the dorsal neck of the talus. In either scenario, a bony block occurs when an attempt is made to maximally dorsiflex the ankle.

## Shin splints

These are usually seen with pain in the anterior lower third of the tibia, involving the posterior tibial and anterior tibial tendons. Fibularis (peroneus) tendons may also become involved, particularly the fibularis (peroneus) longus, which plantar flexes the first ray and ankle joint. As in any sport with the commencement of conditioning, tendons and muscles that have been inactive initially become 'overused' and inflammation develops. For ballet dancers who are pronators, or who have a pes planus foot type and force the 'turn-out', shin splints can be a recurring problem.

## Ankle sprains and toe sprains

The ankle sprain is the most common traumatic injury seen in ballet. When a dancer performs a leap or jump and lands incorrectly, or on a previously injured ankle, a typical lateral inversion mechanism sprain may occur. When the ballet performer has to place the ankle in a plantar-flexed position during performance or participation, ankle sprains become a common entity (Hamilton 1982a). Lateral ankle injuries usually affect the anterior talofibular ligament, sometimes with or without injury to the calcaneal–fibular ligament. The posterior talofibular ligament is rarely involved, except in severe ankle sprain cases. With dancers who over-pointe, stretching of the ankle collateral ligaments and capsular tissues may occur. This can often lead to symptoms of a sinus tarsi syndrome, rather than a typical ankle sprain. Toe sprains, as in footballers with turf-toe, can also be a frequent occurrence, particularly with dancers en pointe, and who rehearse and perform barefooted (modern dance). A sprain of the collateral ligaments and/or the sesamoid apparatus may occur.

## Stress fractures

This is another common entity for the ballet dancer, again as a result of overuse. With the dancer en pointe, the first and second rays are where weight impact is focused. In the demi-pointe dancer, the entire weight of the body rests on the second metatarsal. As a result, most dancers have a marked hypertrophy of the second metatarsal bones (Quirk 1994). The most frequent site for fractures of the second metatarsal is at the neck, but fractures at the base are also not uncommon. Other areas where stress fractures may occur in the ballerina are the other metatarsals, the lower third of the fibula, and occasionally the talus, calcaneus and navicular.

Fractures of the sesamoids are another injury to suspect, particularly with the dancer who performs a great deal on demi-pointe.

## Hallux limitus

With narrowing of the joint space, metatarsus primus elevatus, osteophytic changes of the first metatarsal head and base of the proximal phalanx, hallux limitus can be a disabling condition for a ballet dancer. Due to increased stress on the first metatarsal phalangeal joint en pointe and in the demi-pointe stance, 'jamming' of the joint occurs, with subsequent stiffness and capsulitis. Surgical intervention may be necessary in cases where there is decreased range of motion and where hypertrophic bone and 'spurs' cause further destruction of articular cartilage. Simple cheilectomy may be all that is needed; however, even plantar-flexor osteotomies may not provide enough dorsiflexion of the joint to provide total relief and normal range of motion.

## Bunion deformities

Although bunion deformities are common among ballet dancers, a normal foot type does not necessarily mean that the dancer will have a predisposition towards developing a bunion. However, the pronated, pes planus, flexible fore-footed dancer will have a greater tendency towards developing a hallux abducto valgus deformity. Ballet, and dancing en pointe, contribute to further deterioration of the joint and a more extensive deformity. Surgery should be an absolute last option for the ballet dancer; however, when symptoms are consistent, and performing dance has become impossible, surgical correction with a distal metatarsal head osteotomy, that is an Austin procedure (Chevron – see also Ch. 23), is a desirable.

## Neuromas

Due to being en pointe and performing in a toe shoe with a rigid toe box, compression of the intermetatarsal nerves can develop, creating irritation and fibrosis of the nerve. Once again, surgery should be reserved for the dancer who suffers from consistent pain and an inability to perform after conservative measures have failed.

## Nail problems

With the dancer's en pointe stance, and the focus of the weight directed to the distal aspect of the hallux, pressure on the nail can be tremendous, and subungual haematoma is a common entity. In addition, formation of a subungual exostosis may cause further irritation of the hallux nail and develop into a thickened, sometimes onychomycotic, nail. The nail may even begin to involute, causing an ingrown nail with paronychia formation. On occasion, when pain is persistent, the ingrown nail, or the thickened nail or spur may have to be removed (see Ch. 21).

## BASEBALL

Although injuries to the throwing arm are quite common in baseball (Magnusson et al 1994, Timmerman & Andrews 1994), lower extremity injuries can be just as unrelenting. Baseball is a throwing, catching, batting and running sport. Injuries to the lower extremity can be categorised by specific injury, and by the position that is played. Typical injuries include muscle pulls and strains, ankle injuries, contusions and fractures by being struck by the ball, either by the pitcher or by being 'fouled-off' by the bat. Runners sliding into the bases or the home plate are predisposed to injury because of a sprinting action creating hamstring pulls, ankle sprains, knee injuries, turf-toe or being 'cleated' by the opposition player.

Many overuse injuries can also develop during the conditioning 'spring-training' season. Due to the running involved, and taking into account the biomechanical lower extremity factors of the player (i.e. genu valgum, tibial varum, pes planus, cavus foot, etc.) common overuse injuries such as chronic Achilles tendinitis, plantar fasciitis, heel spur formation, posterior/anterior shin splints, iliotibial band syndrome, anterior/posterior tibial tendinitis, retrocalcaneal exostosis with bursitis, patellofemoral joint syndrome and hip dysfunction are found.

As in football, basketball, soccer and hockey, strength and conditioning coaches are a key element to the training of these amateur and professional athletes. Running is a key element in the preparation for, and the maintenance of, conditioning during the baseball season. As in most sports, the three training factors involved with preparation and injury prevention are flexibility (range of motion of joints), function and strength. Speed work and interval training are an integral part of the training and conditioning process for the baseball athlete. This is what affords the player the ability to accelerate from home plate to first base, after hitting the ball, or when attempting to steal a base. Running style, gait, stride, limb-length discrepancies and foot type are all part of the evaluation of the baseball player that should be performed by the trainer and/or team podiatrist or sports medicine specialist. When needed, biomechanical correction with soft insoles, or prescription orthotics within the baseball spikes, may be a great asset in the correction of lower leg and foot imbalances.

Special consideration for injury prevention begins with the individual player, and the position played. Pitchers, when delivering the pitch, have a particular set of biomechanical considerations. Technique, leg extension, rotation, weight balanced on one foot, stride and foot plant during delivery are all important factors that can cause faulty mechanics or injury at any time. Slow- and fast-pitch softball pitching have different sets of mechanics, yet they can also be subject to repeated overuse injury. Particular injuries include blister formation on the medial hallux and forefoot, as well as subungual haematoma from the hallux striking the end of the shoe at the end of the delivery of the pitch. For pitchers with excessive pronation on the stance leg, medial knee pain may develop.

Catchers are high-risk players for foot, ankle and lower leg injuries. The catcher, constantly in a crouched position, places his or her entire body weight on the forefoot, creating a great deal of forefoot pressure which can translate into neuroma formation. For a pes planus foot type, or in the case of a pronated catcher, subtalar joint pronation can result in posterior tibial tendinitis, deltoid ligament strain and, combined with the rocking and stretching of the longitudinal arch, plantar fasciitis will often develop. Stretching of the posterior muscle groups, Achilles and plantar fascia is essential for catchers. Catchers are constantly being hit by foul balls off the bat and onto the toes, first MTPJ and beneath the instep protector on the dorsum of the foot.

Batters must have good foot mechanics and position to transfer weight efficiently from one foot to the other when attempting to hit the ball. Batting is a sequence of coordinated muscle activity, beginning with the hip, followed by the trunk and terminating with the arms (Shaffer et al 1993). For a right-handed batter, the right foot (back) is stable in relation to the ground, with the foot supinated and the leg externally rotated. Until the swing is attempted, the left foot is virtually unweighted. As the swing begins, weight transference from the right foot to the left begins. Once the bat is in motion, and has begun to swing forward, the forefoot and hips begin to pivot, further transferring weight from the right foot and leg to the left foot and leg. At the conclusion of the swing, and at the time of contact with the ball, both feet should be pointed forward to the pitcher. Batters, as well as their counterparts behind the plate, are frequently being struck on the foot directly, or by the ball ricocheting off the ground. Often, the ball will strike the instep, medial arch, shin or the great toe, possibly resulting in a painful contusion or haematoma.

Infielders are subject to injuries from sliding runners, spiking them as they slide into base or step across the base. Runners are at risk of hamstring strains as they sprint to the next base, as well as inversion ankle sprains as their foot connects with the base as they slide.

Baseball shoes vary according to level of play and the surfaces being played on. High-school players use rubber cleats, while college and professional baseball players wear metal ones. Rubber cleats are also worn on artificial turf. The configuration of the cleats is three on the forefoot and three on the heel. Baseball shoes should have a strong counter for stability, a rigid shank for longitudinal arch support, a deep toe box to prevent toe irritation, and a flexible sole to allow for quick running speed.

## SKIING

Alpine or downhill skiing is a complex skill that requires controlled pronation, setting the foot, ankle and lower extremity on the inside ski edge. Pronation sets the inside edge of the downhill (control) ski, and allows for the skier to lean inward against the ski, which holds a skidless arc throughout the turn. While balanced on a beam of flexible composite 6.3 cm wide, the skier drives the shin forward against the stiff boot cuff and swings the hips to the opposite direction. The ski rolls onto its sharp steel edge and bites the snow, creating an arc across the hill (Ross & Subotnick 1999). Skiing is like ballet on snow, and the skier encounters many centrifugal and g-forces, as turns are created, while simultaneously attempting to keep the centre of gravity

in line over the centre of the ski. Any variation in normal lower extremity biomechanical balance can alter the skier's ability to develop a controlled turn, thus predisposing the skier to injury if the abnormality is great enough. The three factors that are important in a skier's conditioning and performance are flexibility, strength and proper range of motion. Variable factors such as structural biomechanical deformity, functional deformity or dynamic imbalance of muscle groups can also influence the performance of the skier and help to predict potential injury. When skiers have pre-existing injuries, creating weakness in muscle groups, decreased flexibility and limited range of motion of the involved lower leg joints, the skier's ability to ski efficiently and safely will be significantly diminished. As a result of these compromised factors, an increased muscular effort is required, resulting in skier fatigue. Fatigue has been shown to be one of the main factors in the incidence of downhill skiing injuries (Ross & Subotnick 1999). Skiers will compensate for biomechanical abnormalities by obtaining the use of pronatory forces from other joints (i.e. hips and knees) in order to ski properly. Ross (1985), utilising the electrodynogram (EDG), showed that forces are transmitted from both the forefoot and the rearfoot, which is essential in up-and-down weighting, as well as in the completion of proper turns. Abnormalities such as excessive foot pronation, shortened heel contact and excessive propulsive phase on the toes, extreme forward lean of the boot, including asymmetry between the two feet, were all observed, affecting the skier's effectiveness and performance. Skiers can overcome some of these lower extremity abnormalities, including poor skiing style, poor edge control and foot imbalances, by using various orthotic controls in their ski boots. It has also been shown that custom insoles for mild foot and lower leg imbalances, as well as prescription orthoses for the more severe rearfoot and forefoot abnormalities, could be valuable in helping to provide proper foot bed balance and to improve ski performance and efficiency (Ross & Cohn 1984). It has become widely accepted to use easy-to-customise liners and removable full-length soft support systems within them; custom insoles or prescription orthoses may be substituted for the pre-existing insole.

It is imperative that the foot specialist or sports medicine specialist has a basic understanding of both boot design and skiing performance, in addition to a working relationship with the boot shop and ski boot fitter. The sports medicine specialist can help in the selection of the correct boot by determining foot type and targeting existing areas of biomechanical weakness or physiological defects. The specialist can diagnose bony deformities, stress areas of the foot, biomechanical imbalances, areas of friction and irritation, poor circulation, nerve entrapments and metabolic disorders. With these factors taken into consideration, the boot fitter can help to decide whether the skier will require a boot designed for a wide foot, a flat or high-arched foot, a volume boot, a pure forward entry boot, a hybrid boot (with both overlap and rear entry design), a narrow heel pocket or a thin, thick or adaptable liner.

Tibia varum is a biomechanical abnormality that has a great effect on a skier's ability to ski normally. Tibia varum is a result of an uncompensated varus deformity of the tibia, which transmits instantaneously to the ski–snow interface and causes the skier to ride excessively on the outside edge of the ski. When a skier has more than 8–10° of tibia varum deformity, he or she will have a great deal of difficulty initiating a parallel turn without 'catching' the outside edge of the ski. Skiing on the outside edge is often associated with tips being crossed, which eventually leads to sudden falls (Ross & Subotnick 1999). Today, most high-performance boots provide a boot cuff adjustment to accommodate varying degrees of tibia varum and create a flat ski surface. One of the easiest and most reliable methods of treating tibia varum is to use a full-length, canted, in-boot foot orthosis. This method has the advantage of providing for total foot contact within the boot, thus correcting for biomechanical imbalances within the foot and lower leg. It also has the effect of reducing the friction of the foot against the boot while at the same time affording a comfortable, dependable, balanced foot bed that helps to provide effectual edge control. Other lower-leg and foot abnormalities that can contribute to a skier's difficulty in edge control and performance are tibia valgum, subtalar varus, forefoot varum, forefoot valgum, transverse plane asymmetry and leg-length discrepancies.

Skiers frequently complain that their feet hurt and that they are cold, tight and irritating. Over the years, ski boots have advanced in technological design and performance, and have become quite biomechanically sophisticated. Some of the adjustable features include internal versus external canting systems, adjustable 'spoilers' or shaft-angle adjustments, boot flex, forward lean, internal/external heaters and custom heat-mouldable liners made of EVA. Most ski boots have removable foot beds that may be replaced with custom-made orthoses. Some ski shop devices can be made readily by using an apparatus that places the foot in a semi-weight-bearing neutral position, with knee stabiliser apparatus built into the platform to accurately align the knee over the foot for complete lower leg correction. The traditional orthotic, made from an in-boot cast while the skier assumes a neutral ski stance position, will function much better than the custom insole because it can provide additional correction and stability in the rearfoot, subtalar joint, midtarsal joint and forefoot. It has been shown that control of excessive pronation/supination and locking of the midtarsal joint (stability) will result in better edging and higher performance. The five areas of concern in a boot are:

- zone one, the foot bed
- zone two, the tongue
- zone three, the hindfoot
- zone four, the shaft
- zone five, the forefoot.

The sports podiatrist or specialist should be cognisant of the numerous problems that skiers face, whether they be biomechanical imbalances leading to poor ski technique or performance problems related to foot or boot-fit discomfort. It is imperative to understand the lower extremity biomechanics related to skiing, boot design, boot fitting, and the interrelationship between a ski orthosis and the boot in which it sits.

## Cross-country skiing

Cross-country skiing compared to alpine skiing has a totally different technique and application. In downhill skiing the heel and lower leg are locked in a rigid boot, affording more control to the skier's rearfoot complex. The body's centre of mass is located directly over the rearfoot complex (subtalar joint); with properly aligned joint compressional forces, rearfoot neutrality is maintained. By comparison, cross-country skiing involves a heel that is repeatedly lifted within the shoe from the ski surface and lowered again, allowing for more skier imbalance. Cross-country skiing employs a technique referred to as a 'swing kick and glide'. Using the poles to create upper body stability and propulsion, the heel is kicked upward to maintain forward motion with a forefoot propulsion on the ski. Diagonal stride is created by alternating the opposite arm and leg forward; a ski gait is created similar to walking and jogging (Parks 1989).

Cross-country boots are an intermediary between backcountry and racing boots in both design and support. Compared to the alpine ski boot, the cross-country touring boot has much more freedom of movement, at the expense of much less support. Because sagittal plane motion is the predominant direction of foot and leg action, it is not essential for the touring skier to require stability in the shoe for

exaggerated turns because moderate curves are usually the only ones encountered.

Similar biomechanical considerations for the cross-country skier as for the alpine skier are essential. The patella should be properly aligned over the skis in a bent-knee skiing position. A lighter, flexible orthosis than the bulkier alpine device is preferred. Keeping the devices as thin as possible will provide more room for the foot and toes to function.

## SNOWBOARDING

This relatively new sport is popular with participants of all ages. This winter version of skateboard surfing has its risks, as does alpine skiing. Of the injuries incurred in snowboarding 40% involve the upper extremity while 43% involve the lower extremity. The most common site of injury is the wrist (trauma and fracture), followed by the knee (sprains) and then the ankle (fractures) (Ganong et al 1992). The snowboarder lacks the freedom of individual leg movement, and thus the chance for recovery is much less than in downhill skiing. Unlike alpine skiing, which uses the integration of foot, knee and hip motion, the short pivoting turns involved in snowboarding concentrate the energy on the hips and knees.

Snowboarding boots are quite different from their alpine skiing counterparts. Earlier designs incorporated a soft type of boot, whereas the full hard shell and half-shell are the more recent designs. The soft boot allows for more motion of the foot, so that more injuries are incurred than with the harder designs. The most common injury seen with the soft boot is at the ankle, whereas the rigid full-shell boots protect the ankle but allow for more forces to be transmitted to the knees. This has resulted in a higher frequency of knee injuries.

## FOREFOOT INJURIES

Athletic injuries can be classified by the area in which they occur: the forefoot, midfoot or rearfoot. Forefoot injuries to the athlete can be attributed to the high levels of stress that the ball of the foot has to withstand. These injuries can range from nagging to disabling, depending on the site and the repeated impact to the area. We can further divide the forefoot into medial, lateral and central sections to specify the exact location of the injury. The following is a list of potential differential diagnoses based on mechanical considerations:

- skin irritation secondary to mechanical abrasion
- metatarsalgia
- capsulitis
- bursitis
- sesamoiditis
- tendinitis
- neuritis (neuroma)
- stress fracture
- nail and toe conditions.

The plantar aspect of the foot is subject to friction and shearing forces that create plantar keratomas under the metatarsal heads. Thickened subcutaneous tissue beneath the metatarsal heads offers a protective layer to dampen the shock that is transmitted to the forefoot bones.

Plantar keratomas vary from simple calluses to deep, intractable plantar keratomas, which can be both painful and incapacitating to the athlete.

## Metatarsalgia

Athletes who have equinus deformity or protracted propulsive phases may develop changes in the forefoot – the metatarsal heads change position, becoming plantar flexed and prominent on the plantar aspect of the foot. Metatarsalgia occurs when these protuberant metatarsal heads become painful, and may be either acute or chronic. One of the primary reasons for this painful debilitating injury is that there is loss of the transverse arch, with increased metatarsal stress. As the metatarsal bones begin to sublux in a plantar-grade direction, plantar interdigital nerves are subject to irritation from prominent metatarsal heads. When the metatarsalgia, along with the plantar callus, is due to a pes planus as well as a hypermobile first ray, a more rigid orthotic device would be more advantageous than a softer, accommodative, shock-absorbing device. Metatarsalgia can also result from a rupture of the plantar (volar) plates of the MTPJs, or may possibly be due to a synovial cyst plantar to the MTPJ. This type of injury is seen quite often in martial arts and hard-landing sports such as basketball, tennis and volleyball. Lastly, stress fractures may produce symptoms of metatarsalgia, particularly in the metatarsal shaft regions and the sesamoids.

## Capsulitis

The capsule of the first MTPJ, as well as the lesser MTPJs, may develop inflammation as a result of repeated trauma. This may occur in any of the sports outlined earlier. Typical examples are turf toe involving the first MTPJ in football, capsulitis of the first MTPJ due to pointe stance in ballet, vertical landing on the first MTPJ in basketball, hyperextension inflammation in track sprinting and step aerobics, and direct trauma to the first MTPJ in striking a ball in soccer.

## Bursa formation and bursitis

As a consequence of constant pounding of the second, third or fourth MTPJ, chronic irritation of the periarticular structures can lead to the development of a submetatarsal bursa. This can occur naturally (anatomically) or adventitiously (in response to superficial external irritation) in the subcutaneous tissues. These anatomical bursae are nature's response to a functional need to reduce both friction and shearing. The adventitious bursa will develop in response to soft-tissue structures that are constantly being subjected to great shearing forces. Pain and swelling will usually develop as a result of an inflamed bursa due to mechanical trauma. Chronic irritation may cause the bursa to distend due to the accumulation of synovial fluid within the bursa sac. The sac may be either fixed (attached to fascia or to the capsule) or freely moveable.

In any case, the larger the bursa the greater the chance of irritation and painful symptoms. The abnormal shearing forces may be secondary to hypermobility of the forefoot, of the first and fifth rays, or from the foot sliding forward in the athletic shoes due to improper fit. These conditions can lead to increased friction, inflammation of the plantar tissues, formation of plantar keratomas and, if severe and consistent enough, bursa formation anterior and plantar to the metatarsal heads. Conservative treatment, such as protective padding and/or accommodation incorporated into the forefoot extension of a sport prescription orthotic device, will help to reduce the chronic friction and shearing forces affecting the chronic adventitious bursa.

## Sesamoiditis and fracture

The sesamoid bones of the plantar surface of the first MTPJ are now recognised for their importance in relation to symptoms of pain, gait biomechanics (functional and structural hallux limitus), the particular sport in which the athlete participates, and the footwear that is worn.

The sesamoid bones are isolated bones that lie within the flexor tendons; they have a dorsal concavity and a plantar convexity. The larger and longer tibial sesamoid lies more distally than the smaller, more rounded fibular sesamoid. Both sesamoids lie plantar and within each respective tendinous expansion of the medial and lateral heads of the flexor hallucis brevis muscle (Bojsen-Moller & Flagstad 1976). It has been shown that 10–33% of feet have either a bipartite or multipartite sesamoid (Jahss 1981). The sesamoids have articular cartilage that lies within the tendon and is subject to injury. The sesamoid provides protection and shock absorption for both the joint and tendon. In addition, like any pulley, they increase the musculotendinous mechanical advantage for the first MTPJ, particularly during the propulsive phase of gait. In court sports, as well as in running and other high-impact sports, the high ground reactive forces act on the first MTPJ. Together with constant 'push-off' and pronatory 'pivoting' of the hallux, the sesamoids act by assisting gait, and provide additional flexor strength. It has been shown that forces three times the body weight pass through the sesamoids during weight shift in a normal gait cycle (Drez 1982). Forces are greater beneath the tibial sesamoid, which explains why the tibial sesamoid is involved in more injuries than the fibular sesamoid.

In cases of hallux abducto valgus a lateral shift of the tibial sesamoid will occur, creating a situation in which the medial sesamoid is susceptible to increased forces beneath the first metatarsal head. With the sesamoid vulnerable to these excessive forces, subchondral erosion and/or fracture can occur. In cases of hallux limitus, with a semi-rigid or rigid plantar-flexed first ray, it is not unusual to see sesamoiditis or injury to the sesamoid apparatus.

When injury to the sesamoid does occur, there will be limited movement and pain upon dorsiflexion of the first MTPJ. Routine radiographs with comparison views of the contralateral foot can often determine whether there is an actual fracture or whether it is a bipartite or tripartite sesamoid. An axial 'sesamoidal' view radiograph can aid in determining whether there is deviation of the sesamoids. It can also help to identify whether the tibial sesamoid is more plantargrade, and whether upon weight bearing the standing forces are greater than normal. Additional investigative studies, such as bone scans and computerised tomography (CT) scans, can help determine whether or not a fracture is present.

There are five categories of injury to the sesamoid apparatus. The injuries can be either of the acute nature, such as avulsion fractures, or of the chronic type, involving repetitive stress to the sesamoids or the medial and lateral support structures.

- *Sesamoiditis* – tendinitis of the flexor hallucis longus at the MTPJ, sesamoid bursitis (McBryde & Anderson 1988), synovitis of the MTPJ, chondromalacia, and painful bi- or tripartite sesamoids. This condition is usually due to repetitive stress and compression on the sesamoid and the first MTPJ, rather than to acute injury. It is seen in the cavus foot, plantar-flexed semi- or rigid first ray, functional or structural hallux limitus and forefoot valgus.
- *Stress fractures of the sesamoid* – occur in running sports, court sports and dancing due to high impact and compression. They are characterised by pain, which may limit play or performance. A standard radiograph 3 weeks after injury usually will show the stress fracture to the sesamoid bone. When there is suspicion of a stress fracture, however, it is sometimes not readily seen on a plain film radiograph; a bone scan or CT scan may be necessary. Conservative and early management of this injury is essential. Proper treatment includes 6 weeks of below-knee casting, followed by 6 weeks of protection (surgical shoe, Cam walker or

running shoe). The use of prescription orthoses, particularly for a runner, is necessary to disperse pressure from the area of the sesamoid (dancer's pad), often with a Morton's extension. The orthosis will aid in the prevention of further injury to the remaining sesamoid and prevent further damage to the undersurface of the metatarsal head. When this injury is not diagnosed correctly, or not treated aggressively enough, the fracture may not heal, or may eventually progress to a delayed union at 4 months, non-union fracture at 6 months, or osteochondrosis with possible avascular necrosis. After all conservative measures have been exhausted, and after a prescribed period of time, surgical intervention is indicated, with excision of the non-united fractured sesamoid. Again, orthotic therapy is imperative to provide for normal length of the flexor hallucis longus and brevis tendons.

- *Acute sesamoid fracture* – occurs in dancers and other sports rarely, but can be recognised on plain radiographs because of the sharply defined edges of the fragments (Quirk 1994, Sammarco 1984). These fractures are most frequently seen in the tibial sesamoid and have a transverse compression appearance. In this category, the avulsion fracture is the most common, but it is not unusual to see fractures that are widely displaced. Surgical excision is indicated for fractures that are displaced and do not respond to conservative care.

- *Osteochondritis dissicans* (osteochondrosis, avascular necrosis) – can occur initially or after repetitive stress injury and initial stress fracture. Once fractured, the blood supply to the sesamoid bone is interrupted and this can often lead to avascular necrosis.

- *Chondromalacia of the sesamoid* – occurs as a result of continual synovitis. With chronic synovitis of the plantar first MTPJ, fibrosis will develop surrounding the sesamoid apparatus to the metatarsal head and the plantar capsule. This will lead to a 'freezing' of the sesamoids. The sesamoids will not slide back and forth with the motion of the flexor tendon, and as a result a decreased range of motion will develop, creating a functional hallux limitus and, eventually, a hallux rigidus. Aggressive treatment (i.e. icing, immobilisation, physical therapy, NSAIDs, and a prescription orthosis with a Morton's extension) can prove successful for the athlete, while helping to avoid surgical intervention. This early and proactive treatment plan can allow the athlete to return to action with limited symptoms, restoration of normal gait, and few or no sequelae.

---

## CASE STUDY 13.3

### SESAMOID FRACTURE

A 39-year-old woman presented with a chief complaint of severe pain of 4 months' duration under the ball of her left foot, and directly beneath the first metatarsophalangeal joint. Some years ago a cyst overlying the extensor hallucis longus tendon was excised, with scar tissue formation and possible recurrence. The patient described the previous injury as having broken the base of the fifth metatarsal of her left foot stepping off a pavement. Over 4 months ago she suffered an injury to the tibial sesamoid. Radiographs revealed a stress fracture to the tibial sesamoid.

The patient is a runner who, until the injury, ran on a treadmill for 3 miles two or three times a week, and used a recumbent bicycle and elliptical trainer two times a week. Since the injury the patient has attempted to exercise by walking and running on a treadmill for 3 miles twice a week. However, she continues to experience pain and discomfort. She has begun to exercise with the stair-stepper and walks to work in comfortable dress-heel shoes. She experiences pain when wearing her shoes.

A Cam-walker removable cast boot was applied for 2 months, and prescription orthotics and NSAIDs were prescribed. The patient continued to have pain and discomfort in the region of the plantar first metatarsal head.

A repeat radiograph (anteroposterior/medial oblique) revealed a stress fracture distal to the tibial sesamoid of the left foot with mild distal migration and lateral deviation.

*Past medical history*. Non-contributory to condition (mitral valve prolapse and hay fever).

*Biomechanical*. Past history of ankle sprains.

### PHYSICAL EXAMINATION

Cavus foot type, semiflexible, plantar flexed to normal first ray. Hallux dorsiflexion normal to semirigid. Supinated subtalar joint. Ankle joint dorsiflexion – normal, tibial varum; subtalar joint range of motion – normal.

*Gait analysis*. Right foot abducted. Supinated heel strike, right foot pronates significantly more than the left foot at midstance to toe-off. Circumvention of right foot, left stays rectus, with functional hallux limitus, and plantar-flexing first ray.

### ORTHOTICS AND TREATMENT

The patient's sport orthotics required modification. They were uncomfortable and created too much pressure under the first metatarsal head. In addition, her dress-shoe orthotics required reducing in size to fit properly into her shoes. A dancer's pad was created with accommodation for the tibial sesamoid and first metatarsal head.

It was recommended that the patient cease all impact physical activities to allow bone healing of the fractured sesamoid. A bone stimulator was prescribed for the fractured tibial sesamoid.

### ONE-YEAR FOLLOW-UP

The dress-shoe orthotics required refurbishing as the rearfoot posts had worn down. A metatarsal pad was put on the sport orthotics, creating too much pressure under the tibial sesamoid. There was a contusion fracture of the distal phalanx (fifth digit, left foot).

A radiograph showed a healing fracture of the tibial sesamoid of the left foot. There was no displacement or further migration. There was reduced but continued intermittent pain. A therapeutic steroid injection with vitamin $B_{12}$ was administered to the capsular joint tissues below the tibial sesamoid. Physical therapy was given. A Cox-2 NSAID was prescribed for 7 days. Bone stimulation was continued.

---

## Metatarsal stress fractures

Stress fractures are common injuries among athletes (Devas 1958, Drez et al 1980, Jones et al 1978, Markey 1987, Ting & Yocum 1988). A stress fracture occurs as a result of repetitive cyclic loading with lower forces than those necessary to produce acute fracture (Gilad et al 1985). The term 'fatigue fracture' has also been used to demonstrate the result of mild forces or stress with eventual alteration or disruption of a material, such as bone (Morris & Blickenstaff 1967). Therefore, a stress fracture is not the result of a single occurrence but rather an ongoing process. The end result may be a fracture, but in actuality it is the product of continued applied forces on the bone creating a defect (weakness) by reabsorbing bone in advance of the laying down of new bone (Ross 1999b). Johnson (1964) describes it as a disease process that never involves any strange or new reactions, but only altered relationships in normal reactions. For the athlete, constant change in levels of stress, training methods and environmental factors can create an alteration in the relationship between growth and repair. For the runner, forces of three to six times the body weight occur at heel strike, with an estimated 800-foot strikes impacted on each foot per mile. It is estimated that stress fractures comprise 6% of all injuries to runners (Mann 1986).

There are various stresses that are transferred to bone which ultimately develop into a stress fracture. Devas (1975) has described several types, including:

- compression impaction
- distraction with pulling of the periosteum (shin splint)
- muscle concentration aetiology – when a decreased cellular response, or inadequate remodelling of stressed bone occurs, stress fractures will develop.

Stress fractures occur most often in the central region of the forefoot; however, they may occur in any location depending on the forces. In high-impact sports, stress fractures usually result from repetitive pounding and impact through both the soft tissues surrounding the bone (muscle, tendons and periosteum) and the bone itself. There are many aetiologies for the development of stress fractures. Biomechanical abnormalities, such as excessive pronation (Fig. 13.5), hypersupination, lower extremity malalignment (tibia varum, genu valgum, external or internal femoral rotation) and limb-length discrepancy, can all lead to alteration in normal gait, which can then lead to stress fractures. A second tier of aetiology is the training methods of the athlete. The runner who runs in worn-out shoes, on crowned roads or hard running surfaces, or who inadequately prepares for long-distance events or overtrains, is at high risk of developing a stress fracture. In addition to the metatarsals (third, second, fourth), other areas of the foot and lower leg that are subject to increased stress and fracture are the distal tibia, distal and proximal fibula, navicular, calcaneus, cuboid and sesamoids (Fig. 13.6).

An athlete will present with erythema and oedema overlying the involved metatarsal.

After such an injury, extreme pain upon palpation of the area will usually determine the site of the fatigue fracture. Pain will be elicited upon motion, as well as with the use of a tuning fork overlying the involved bone. Keep in mind that bone callus formation will usually

not be evident on a radiograph for at least 2–3 weeks after injury. After radiographic evaluation, the standard special procedure for early detection is the technetium-99m diphosphonate three-phase or single-phase bone scan. This investigative study can help to detect a fracture within days of the injury. When the athlete presents clinically, it is important to determine from the history the exact mechanism of occurrence of the injury. This can often help to differentiate a stress fracture from another type of injury. When combining the history and the clinical findings, even without radiographic or nuclear study evidence, if there is suspicion of a stress fracture, assume that it is a fracture until proved otherwise.

The treatment of a stress fracture depends on the time at which the diagnosis was made. The clinician should take into account the severity of the stress fracture. In cases of a fresh injury, an Unna boot (soft compression cast) with overlying elastic tape and a postoperative shoe is usually indicated for at least 3 weeks. Ice, elevation and anti-inflammatory medication are also very helpful in reducing symptoms. Follow-up physical therapy treatments of heat (warm gentle whirlpool) and fluidotherapy (dry whirlpool) are helpful in increasing blood flow to the area, which can help to accelerate bone healing. When the fracture is pronounced, cast immobilisation and non-weight-bearing for 4–6 weeks may be necessary. In cases where delayed union (after 6 weeks) is evident, the use of a bone stimulator may be advantageous. When displacement of the fracture is seen, particularly in midshaft fractures, or if angulation takes place, then closed or open reduction with internal fixation is indicated.

Rest, immobilisation and refraining from participation in impact sports for at least 4–8 weeks post-injury is necessary. Metaphyseal stress fractures take the least time to heal, while intra-articular, cortical fractures take the longest. When the athlete is pain-free, he or she is ready to begin rehabilitation, but not necessarily ready to return to sports activity. The athlete must have a full range of motion in the

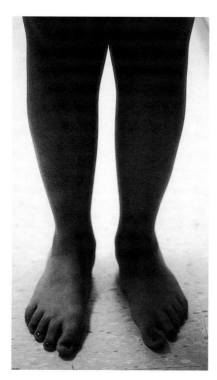

**Figure 13.5** Severe pronation at the subtalar joint.

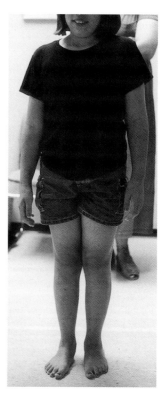

**Figure 13.6** Genu valgum and severe pronation.

joints in the involved injured extremity, and must have redeveloped the flexibility of the muscles of that limb, and developed strength, endurance, proprioception, agility and cardiovascular reserve before returning to full competition. A good training programme will help to lower the incidence of recurrent injury. Cycling between vigorous activity and periods of rest are essential. The use of proper shoes, impact surfaces and orthotics can be important preventive measures in avoiding the recurrence of stress fractures in the athlete.

## Osteochondritis dissicans – Freiberg's infraction

Freiberg's disease (see also Ch. 4) is a sequel to injury of the lesser MTPJs. It is a dorsal trabecular stress injury of the lesser metatarsal heads (Kinnard & Lirette 1989). An osteochondrosis develops as a result of trauma or vascular embarrassment that changes enchondral ossification and ultimately results in an incongruity of the articular cartilage. Freiberg's infraction is such a case where, due to repetitive stress on a long second metatarsal bone, overuse injury to the articular surface occurs.

Examples of sports where there is a high probability of developing such an injury include running sports and impact jumping. The condition can lead to chronic pain and limited function when participating in sport activity.

Smillie (1955) developed a staging classification correlating the physical and radiographic findings, and described various stages of the injury:

*Stage I* represents the earliest form of the disease in which a fissure develops in the epiphysis, considered to be a form of ischaemia (Wiley & Thurston 1981).

*Stage II* represents progression of the subchondral fracture with bone resorption. A collapse of the dorsal central portion of the metatarsal head occurs, with an early alteration of the articular surface. During the healing process, a mild flattening of the head develops, secondary to infraction of the subchondral trabeculae. This also creates (as seen on the radiograph) a small degree of widening of the joint space.

*Stage III* represents a further deformation and collapse of the central portion of the metatarsal head. The medial and lateral projections develop the picture of the uninvolved peripheral portions of the head. The healing process creates a slightly incongruent joint that may or may not be symptomatic. Progressive flattening of the metatarsal head will occur, with osteolysis and further collapse.

*Stage IV* represents further deterioration of the central portion and the peripheral portions of the metatarsal head fracture, thus becoming loose bone bodies. The joint has now become incongruent, with loose bone bodies creating a permanent deformity.

*Stage V*, the end stage of the disease, represents an advanced level of degenerative arthrosis as a result of continued flattening and articular destruction of the metatarsal head. The proximal phalanx has now become more involved, with its base becoming irregular, with osteophyte formation. This is in addition to further narrowing of the joint space, and hypertrophy of the metatarsal head.

There are various theories as to the aetiology of Freiberg's disease. Freiberg (1914) originally concluded that the condition was due to trauma, whereas Kohler (1961) disputed that theory. Smillie (1955) also reported that trauma was the underlying cause, and postulated that the condition was due to a weak foot, with a short, hypermobile first ray. Others have reported a vascular deficiency that can cause necrosis of the metatarsal head (Wiley & Thurston 1981), while other investigators have argued that the epiphysis was underdeveloped for

unknown reasons, although mechanical stress to the abnormal epiphysis eventually caused the final injury (Duthii & Haughton 1981) (see also Ch. 4).

The athlete requires a full range of motion at the MTPJ and, due to this type of deformity, foot function is greatly impaired. The condition resembles that of a second metatarsal stress fracture and compels the clinician to radiograph the foot to differentiate between the two. Conservative management includes rest, cast immobilisation and, in some cases, non-weight bearing with crutches for walking. This is followed by a slow phased return to sports activity, with the use of biodynamic orthoses, with a metatarsal pad or a metatarsal bar (over metatarsals 2–4) to diminish pressure on the second metatarsal head. In some cases, the capsulitis can be treated with injections of corticosteroid with local anaesthetic. Alternatively, homeopathic intra-articular injections of Traumeel or Ruta Graveolens may be used safely, without further weakening the periarticular structures (Subotnick & Sisney 1999).

When conservative measures have failed, surgical intervention is usually required, with many and various procedures advocated. Some include abrasion arthroplasty, with removal of the osteophytes and loose bone bodies and remodelling of the metatarsal head. Others include dorsiflexory metatarsal osteotomies at the metatarsal head, metatarsal head resection and MTPJ replacement with a lesser total joint hinged implant. Orthotic therapy in all cases is also strongly advised.

---

### CASE STUDY 13.4

#### FREIBERG'S INFRACTION

A 14-year-old female cross-country runner presented with pain of 2 weeks duration in her right foot, and 4 months duration in her second toe. She experiences pain when running, with pain in the arch and extending to the ball of the foot. She states that she experiences pain during her track workouts, but had no pain during her workout yesterday. The foot hurts at night, but there is no swelling. She has been applying ice, and did not run for one weekend 2 weeks ago.

The patient has been running since her fifth grade at school. In seventh grade she ran track and cross-country. As a freshman in high school she runs 3200 metres, 2 miles, 1 mile and cross-country. She has run a number of 5-km races. After running 800 metres on her last track workout she began to experience pain. She admitted to experiencing pain after a cross-country. The pain did not persist from the previous day's workout, but pain appears during a track workout.

#### TREATMENT

Two weeks after the initial visit a walking and running gait analysis was performed. The capsulitis in the second metatarsal area was improved. Temporary insoles were supplied, followed by biomechanical evaluation and casting for prescription orthotics. A Cox-2 NSAID was prescribed to be taken every day with meals. Rest from all running activities was advised, with no impact sports to be carried out.

Five weeks later the pain had improved. Repeat radiographs showed no further changes (Fig. A). With walking exercise and short-distance running the patient continues to experience pain. The patient was advised to undertake no further running and no impact exercise, and to return in 4 weeks.

After 9 weeks radiographs showed more flattening of the metatarsal head, and more impaction and narrowing of the second metatarsophalangeal joint space (Fig. B). The patient has continued to walk and occasionally sprint. All running and impact activities were stopped, as was the taking of the Cox-2 NSAID. The patient was now

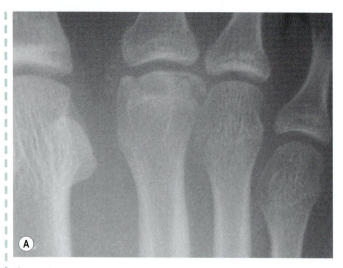

Figure A

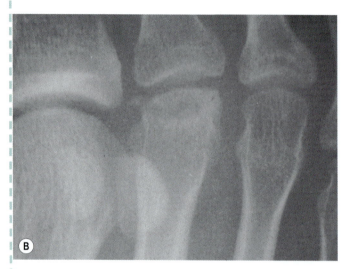

Figure B

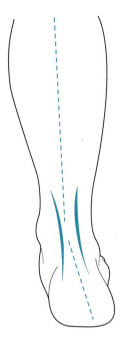

**Figure 13.7** Hyperpronation in the runner.

wearing orthotics and running shoes. The patient was asked to return in 5 weeks.

Fourteen weeks after the trauma the patient was wearing the orthotics continuously. Radiographs showed no further changes. The second metatarsophalangeal joint was no longer inflamed and the swelling was reduced, with much less discomfort. The patient has been compliant and had ceased running and impact activity. A bone scan was ordered to determine the level of osteoblastic/osteoclastic activity, and a bone stimulator was prescribed.

## Morton's neuroma

One of the most common nerve disorders is the interdigital (Morton's) neuroma (see also Ch. 4), which affects the third intermetatarsal and interdigital space, but which can also affect the second intermetatarsal and interdigital space. It is less commonly seen in the first interspace and is occasionally seen in the fourth interspace. Morton's neuroma was described by T. G. Morton in 1876. Distinctive pathological changes such as oedema of the endoneureum, perineural fibrosis, fibrinoid degeneration, demyelination and endoneural fibrosis are often seen.

The athlete will complain of pain, as well as a burning and tingling sensation that radiates distally into the adjacent digits. They will experience symptoms more often after wearing a tight athletic shoe that compresses the metatarsal heads together against the nerve. In running, and particularly in skiing, it is not unusual for the athlete to describe a numbness of the toes and forefoot, with a cramping and occasional shooting pain as well. Occasionally, the athlete will say that they feel a fullness or swelling in the forefoot. They will often be forced to remove their shoe to massage the foot to relieve the numbness and burning pain. The pain often begins as an intermittent soreness and is related to increased athletic activity. If left untreated, the neuroma pain symptoms will become more persistent as well as more severe. It is not uncommon for the pain to be associated with certain shoes.

This condition is manifest during sports activity, particularly during the propulsive phase of gait, when toe-off begins. This is seen in running sports, ballet, aerobic dance, stair steppers and skiing. It is often seen postoperatively following bunion correction, when the patient compensates to the lateral aspect of the forefoot due to a hallux that is functionally limited. It is also seen with athletes who demonstrate a high degree of pronation combined with a forefoot varus (Fig. 13.7). It may also be seen in athletes who have suffered hyperextension injury of the second or third MTPJ, particularly when rupture of the collateral ligaments has occurred. For runners and dancers who suffer recurrent metatarsalgia and capsulitis of the second MTPJ, oedema surrounding the joint will lead to compression of the nerve and a greater incidence of metatarsal head irritation. An abnormal metatarsal parabola can cause impingement (Hoadley 1893), as well as nerve ischaemia (Nissen 1948), trauma and stretching of the nerve.

On physical examination pain will be elicited upon direct pressure to the indicated interspace. Squeezing of the metatarsal heads with the use of medial and lateral compression, together with direct push-up pressure of the nerve in the interspace, will produce a palpable click, known as a positive Mulder's sign, and will often induce symptoms. This is usually pathognomonic for a neuroma within the interspace. Pain may be elicited both distally to the toes and proximally to the tarsal tunnel region. Therefore, the clinician should trace the nerve from the web space to the tarsal tunnel to rule out an impingement or compression of the nerve outside the web space. It is imperative to rule out other possible diagnoses such as stress fractures, neuropathy and lesions within the spaces as well as bone and joint lesions.

Conservative treatment is always recommended, with a variety of injection therapies described. The author uses a combination of long- and slow-acting corticosteroids (dexamethasone acetate and phosphate), a total of 1 ml in combination with 1 ml of 1% lidocaine (lignocaine) plain, 1 ml 0.5% bupivacaine plain, 0.2 ml Wydase and 0.5 ml of vitamin $B_{12}$ with a 27-gauge needle. After the injection, the use of nerve stimulation, ultrasound, and later iontophoresis, in combination with NSAIDs, the application of ice, change of footwear, massage and prescription orthotic use with a metatarsal pad and/or a 'peanut' to spread apart the metatarsal heads has proven very successful. Subotnick (1999b) has reported a 70% success rate using both cortisone and homeopathic injection mixtures. The use of orthotic devices has proven successful in controlling abnormal pronation and excessive transverse plane motion of the forefoot, particularly in the midstance to toe-off phases of gait.

After all conservative measures have been exhausted, surgical excision of the neuroma may be necessary. Excision of the nerve proved successful in 76% of the cases reported by Gaynor et al (1989) and 80% of the cases reported by Miller (1987), with a 7% recurrence rate according to Subotnick (1999b). The author has also found that, by using a $CO_2$ laser, bleeding and fibrosis are reduced, and there is a reduction in postoperative pain and recurrence. However, athletes should be forewarned that a stump neuroma can develop, and this can present an entirely new set of problems. Some surgeons advocate release of the intermetatarsal ligament when the nerve appears compressed, as seen via the endoscopic procedure. In all cases, however, it is strongly suggested to the athletic surgical patient that an orthotic device with a metatarsal pad be worn to prevent recurrence and to prevent the development of a neuroma in an adjacent interspace.

There are many other nerve entrapment disorders of the foot involving nerves – such as the tarsal tunnel – proximally involving the tibial nerve and distally involving divisions of the tibial nerve, medial, calcaneal lateral and the first branch of the lateral plantar nerve. Other nerves involved include the medial plantar nerve, lateral plantar nerve, the higher tibial nerve in the leg or popliteal fossa, deep fibular (peroneal) nerve, superficial fibular (peroneal) nerve, saphenous nerve, sural nerve and the medial common hallucal nerve. All these entities can cause symptoms similar to the interdigital nerve and can result from a variety of sports activities. Proper identification of the involved nerve and early conservative management can often help to prevent unwarranted surgical intervention.

## CASE STUDY 13.5

### SURAL NERVE ENTRAPMENT

A 53-year-old, white man presented with pain and numbness in his left leg and foot. He was preparing for the Amsterdam Marathon, and 2 months ago ran 23 miles in Huntsville Texas. At mile 15 his calf muscle went into cramp up to 4 inches (10 cm) above the heel. He completed the 23 miles and next day there was no pain. On the following Wednesday he ran 6.5 miles. There was no problem for the first 3 miles but he experienced pain during the last 3.5 miles.

The following Sunday he attempted a 10-mile run. Over the first 3 miles there was no pain, but the next 3 miles he ran slowly and walked the last 4 miles in pain. That afternoon numbness developed in his left foot. The patient began applying ice and taking ibuprofen. Ten days later he began massage therapy.

Forty-two days later the patient was continuing with massage therapy twice a week, as well as applying ice and taking 6 tablets/day of ibuprofen 200 mg. The left foot continued to be numb and tingled when touched on the rear 4 inches of the leg above the heel. He attempted slow running and experienced no pain. At day 35 pain began in the left ankle, independently of running. Forty days later the patient ceased all running. The numbness decreased, but the pain increased.

*Past medical and surgical history*. Non-contributory
*Medications*. Ibuprofen
*Allergies*. No known allergies
*Social history*. Geologist, married, denies smoking
*Family history*. Non-contributory

### PHYSICAL EXAMINATION

*Vascular*. DP/PT pulses palpable bilaterally. Capillary filling time within normal limits. Skin temperature and colour within normal limits.

*Neurological*. Deep tendon reflexes within normal limits. Fine touch sensation within normal limits. Plantar response normal, clonus-negative. Numbness along the lateral aspect the left foot, along the course of innervation of the sural nerve. No tingling recreated with percussion of the sural nerve. Mild pain experienced posterior to the lateral malleolus.

*Dermatological*. Skin texture and swelling within normal limits.

*Musculoskeletal*. Muscle strength 5/5 bilaterally. Pain on palpation of the base of the fifth metatarsal of the left foot.

### ASSESSMENT AND TREATMENT PLAN

#### Initial diagnosis

Sural nerve neuritis/neuralgia
Neuropraxia (stretch) sural nerve
Fibular (peroneal) tendinitis
Possible mild tear lateral gastrocnemius and fibres of the Achilles tendon
Possible lateral exercise-induced compartment syndrome

#### Plan

Prescribed Vioxx, d/c ibuprofen
Cease all impact activities, no running
Cross-training, swimming, low-resistance cycle
Physical therapy

### FOLLOW-UP TREATMENT – 1 MONTH

Continued numbness left lower leg and lateral foot
Very little benefit from Vioxx
Numbness and tingling in the heel, extending lateral aspect foot
Numbness lateral to Achilles tendon, left heel, fifth metatarsal
A/P entrapment neuropathy sural nerve, with neuropraxia
Injection 0.5 ml Decadron, 1 ml xylocaine 1% plain
Continue Vioxx, physical therapy

### FIVE-WEEK FOLLOW-UP VISIT

Fibular (peroneal) pain with paraesthesia
Pain posterior lateral malleolus and proximally along lower third of Achilles tendon
Numbness and tingling in lateral calf spreading into the foot

### WHAT TO DO NEXT

Scheduled for consultation with sports medicine physical medicine specialist
Scheduled for consultation with neurologist

### CONSULTATION FINDINGS

*Sports Medicine Physical Medicine Assessment*. Nerve entrapment, left lateral cutaneous nerve-branch sural nerve.

**323**

Ruled out compartment syndrome – condition too focal, pain worse with rest. Hyperaesthesia rather than numbness. No evidence of muscular involvement. Area of injury localises to the superficial posterior compartment rather than the deep posterior compartment. Positive Tinel sign

## PHYSICAL MEDICAL CONSULTATION

*A/P.* Possible muscle tear, some type of stretch injury, resulted in compression of this branch of the sural nerve.

*Recommended.* Limited surgical exploration and decompression of sural nerve. After decompression patient might have full recovery over course of months.

## NEUROLOGY CONSULTATION

*Neurological examination.* Thickened left sural nerve at the ankle.

Positive Tinel sign with palpation below the lateral malleolus. Reduced superficial pain sensation over left ankle and foot. No lower extremity motor or reflex deficits present.

Clinically, left sural neuropathy suspected.

## ELECTROMYOGRAPHIC EXAMINATION

### Motor nerve conduction studies

L Fibular (peroneal) distal latency 6.3 m/s; conduction velocity 42–43 m/s

L Tibial distal latency 5.6 m/s; conduction velocity 41 m/s

### Sensory nerve conduction studies

L Sural distal latency NR; amplitude NR
L Superficial fibular (peroneal) distal latency 4.0 m/s; amplitude 7 volts
R Sural distal latency 4.3 m/s; amplitude 12 volts

### SURGERY (5 MONTHS 3 WEEKS)

*Procedure.* Decompression with neurolysis of adhesions sural nerve left lower leg.

Lysis of adhesions, scar tissue formation gastrocnemius/Achilles tendon 14 cm proximal to tip fibular malleolus.

Skin incision 6 cm length. Lysis, decompression 4–6 cm proximally and distally. 4 mg Decadon. Jones compression dressing.

*Findings.* No tear peritenon, no tear tendon.

Cam-Walker with crutches.

## POSTOPERATIVE COURSE OF EVENTS

*2 weeks.* Less discomfort distal to nerve and posterior to lateral malleolus. Continued numbness and sensitivity from lateral branch of sural nerve to base fifth metatarsal. Cast boot removed – physical therapy twice a week begun.

*4 weeks.* Continued improvement, physical therapy, biomechanical evaluation for orthotics.

*6 weeks.* Physical therapy completed (continued in office on follow-up visits). At times states he is 50% improved. Walking 1 mile. Swimming. Mild pain lateral heel. Numbness still present in lateral midfoot.

*8 weeks.* Mild superficial numbness of dorsum/lateral foot. Ambulating/exercising.

*4 months.* Continued improvement. Less paraesthesia, decreased hyperaesthesia posterior inferior aspect lateral malleolus. No pain along course to base fifth metatarsal. Increased sensation in dorsal lateral aspect. Running 12½ miles/week; 8 min/mile.

*6 months.* Feeling much better. Ran 9 miles/week for 6 weeks. To run 12 miles this week. Mild numbness of lateral third, fourth, fifth digits. Mild numbness of dorsum and lateral aspect of foot. No complaints re. posterior heel. No complaints of pain in fibular (peroneal) groove. No complaints along incision line.

# Hallux limitus and rigidus

In hallux limitus and rigidus (see also Ch. 4), a condition seen frequently in the athletic patient, a limited range of motion of the first MTPJ occurs, creating pain during propulsion. It was first described in 1887 by Davies-Colley as a progressive, degenerative, arthritic condition of the first MTPJ and termed 'hallux flexus'. In 1888, Cotterill proposed the term 'hallux rigidus' to describe this same condition. There are two forms of hallux limitus/rigidus, with various levels of pain. They include a structural hallux limitus and a functional hallux limitus (Root et al 1977). In structural hallux limitus/rigidus a degenerative process of the first MTPJ occurs, which impairs joint motion, leading to ankylosis.

Primary motion of the first MTPJ is in the sagittal plane, where the minimum dorsiflexion range of motion for normal propulsion is about 65–75°. In running sports this figure may actually be greater, because in running there is a prolonged propulsive phase and an elongated stride. To achieve this dorsiflexion, the first metatarsal must plantar flex. With a limitation of plantar flexion of the first ray, the hallux may be able to dorsiflex only 25–30°.

During the propulsive phase the hallux must be stable against the ground, and then act as a rigid lever arm to push off the ground. While the hallux remains stable against the ground, the first metatarsal plantar flexes as the heel lifts off the ground. As the metatarsal head glides over the sesamoid apparatus, the sesamoids begin to migrate distally to the metatarsal head. When the first metatarsal is restricted, and unable to glide along the dorsal aspect of the sesamoid apparatus, the development of a hallux limitus or rigidus will be accelerated. Some examples of these sesamoid conditions include chondromalacia or degeneration of the sesamoids, degenerative breakdown of the articular surfaces of the metatarsal head, and ankylosis of the sesamoid apparatus to the plantar articular condyles of the metatarsal head.

As noted earlier, the first ray must be able to plantar flex for the hallux to ride dorsally over the metatarsal head and dorsiflex. When the metatarsal head is limited in its ability to plantar flex during propulsion, the shift of the first metatarsal in the transverse axis of motion will be inhibited, thus preventing the hallux from dorsiflexing and creating a jamming of the MTPJ dorsally.

There are a number of aetiological, mechanical factors that lead to dorsiflexion of the first metatarsal. Root et al (1977) described several mechanical factors that cause a dysfunctional first ray. Some of these include excessive subtalar joint pronation, a long first metatarsal, hypermobility of the first ray, a dorsiflexed position of the first ray (structural metatarsus primus elevatus) and functional metatarsus primus elevatus.

Dananberg (1986) described how abnormal biomechanical function of the first MTPJ can restrict the body's peak power for forward motion (as may be seen in walking as well as running) over the stance foot. This will lead to compensation occurring at various sites, minimising forward thrust and finally resulting in a decrease in forward momentum. For the athlete, normal range of motion with unrestricted dorsiflexion of the first MTPJ is essential. For sports involving quick acceleration (track, football, soccer), vertical leaping (basketball, volleyball), jumping (aerobics, dance, gymnastics) and quick changes of direction (tennis, court sports, football, soccer) the athlete relies on normal function of the first MTPJ. Certain sports require maximum dorsiflexion of the first MTPJ, such as in step aerobics, to step rapidly on and off the bench from a certain height, and the ballet dancer who must assume the demi-pointe position before going en pointe. The athlete who is limited in that dorsiflexory range of motion will develop dorsal lipping of both the first metatarsal head and the base of the proximal phalanx. In addition, the athlete may begin to compensate for the hallux limitus or rigidus deformity with hyperextension of the hallux interphalangeal joint, external rotation of the lower extremity, or increasing forefoot varus, all of which may lead to increased stress and loads to the foot and lower legs, leading to acute or chronic overuse injuries.

The athlete may present with either non-painful functional or painful structural hallux limitus. In the case of the functional hallux limitus, the patient will demonstrate a normal range of motion of the first MTPJ in weight bearing; however, during gait or running, when the first MTPJ is loaded, a limited range of motion is observed. Kravitz et al (1994) referred to the functional hallux limitus as a 'pre-hallux limitus, which is entirely functional, related to the biomechanical abnormality of hyperpronation syndrome causing unlocking, and metatarsus primus elevatus, where the participant either relates minimal pain or no pain at all. In the case of the structural hallux limitus there is limitation of motion of the first MTPJ, in both the unloaded and loaded state, due to the fact that the first ray is fixed in a dorsiflexed position, or due to a structural metatarsus primus elevatus.

The athlete may present to the clinician with pain and stiffness of the first MTPJ. Many will complain that they are having difficulty pushing off during running and jumping gait. They will often relate that the shoe is beginning to rub a joint that now has become swollen or becoming physically larger. Various sports and the physical demands of these activities may cause increased symptoms, particularly when the first MTPJ is 'pushed' to its limits. As the degenerative disease process begins, further dorsal jamming of the first MTPJ will occur and a 'dorsal bunion bump' will appear. This is followed by a narrowing of the joint space and development of subchondral erosion of the articular surfaces. As a result, greater impingement during push off, fracturing of the dorsal exostosis or lipping may occur, creating loose bone body fragments either floating in the joint or becoming attached via synchondrosis. The athlete will often relate that they feel a painful popping or grinding sensation in the joint during their athletic activities. During the final stages, when ankylosis and joint destruction takes place (Fig. 13.8), as well as fusion of the sesamoid

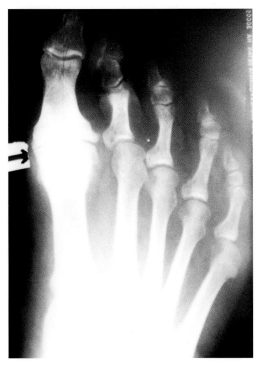

**Figure 13.8** Hallux rigidus of the first metatarsophalangeal joint showing the level of degeneration.

apparatus, consistent pain and swelling will be described. Due to the prominence of bone and/or bursa formation overlying the first MTPJ, an increase in the width and depth of the foot will occur. This will significantly reduce the space available in the shoe, creating additional pressure on the joint. This, in turn, will often lead to compensation, with increased weight bearing to the lesser metatarsals and a reduced loading of the first metatarsal, resulting in metatarsalgia capsulitis and callus formation plantar to the second metatarsal head. Another typical compensatory effect will be the formation of a hallux elevatus or hyperextension of the distal phalanx, which will cause rubbing and irritation of the hallux nail against the toe box of the athletic shoe. This constant pressure on the distal phalanx and nail may cause proliferation of the bone, resulting in a subungual exostosis and a dystrophic nail. Frequently, runners and other athletes will present with subungual haematoma as a result of this distal hallux jamming against the shoe. Evaluation of the shoe and observing wear patterns in both the toe box and the outer-sole of the forefoot will help identify these pathologies.

Radiographic evaluation of the involved foot and joint in the anteroposterior view will reveal typical narrowing of the first MTPJ space, and broadening and flattening of the articular surfaces of both the metatarsal head and the base of the proximal phalanx. In the severe stages osteochondral defects, osteophytic changes of the metatarsal head, subchondral cystic formation and loose bone bodies will be seen. On weight-bearing lateral views, dorsal lipping of the first metatarsal head and base of the proximal phalanx is characteristic. The first metatarsal may appear dorsiflexed when compared to the contralateral side. To further illustrate the deformity, and to demonstrate the restriction of joint function, it is recommended that the clinician perform a stress lateral radiograph (see also Ch. 22). In this image, the patient is asked to raise the heel and stand on the ball of the foot maximally with the hallux stabilised on the surface, similar to a demipointe position. The radiograph will now reveal the degree of dorsal impingement and plantar joint distraction of the joint. Comparing the two views may help to determine just how restricted the joint has become during the midstance to propulsive phase of gait. This may also help to determine whether the athlete is suffering from a functional or a structural hallux limitus.

For athletes with hallux limitus or rigidus deformity, conservative care is always indicated initially. Because the condition is a degenerative as well as a progressive process, conservative management is designed to reduce the biomechanical metatarsus primus elevatus, as well as the dorsiflexory jamming of the first MTPJ. Conservative treatment will offer relief of symptoms, particularly in the early stages, in which minimal degenerative changes of the articular surfaces and joint are seen. However, this treatment plan only diminishes the damage to the joint. It does not alter the progressive nature of the deformity, nor does it restore normal range of motion to the joint.

To begin with, altering shoe selection is advised. A stiffer-soled shoe will help to reduce painful dorsiflexion of the first MTPJ. A rocker-bottom shoe or a metatarsal bar (rocker) proximal to the metatarsal heads will also help to reduce dorsiflexion of the first MTPJ. Again, a shoe with greater toe box room will help to avoid chronic rubbing of the hallux and reduce the pressure on the enlarged first MTPJ. Laces, seams and the tongue of the athletic shoe should also be checked prior to wear to avoid direct pressure and irritation.

In addition to shoe modifications, conservative treatment may consist of NSAIDs, intra-articular steroid or homeopathic injections, physical therapy modalities, with active/passive range of motion exercises and functional orthotic control. The orthosis will help to address the aetiology of the hallux limitus/rigidus development, such as hypermobility of the first ray, metatarsus primus elevatus and increased pronation of the foot. A Morton's extension placed distally plantar to the hallux has been used quite successfully by equalising the height of the hallux and the first metatarsal. This extension can be incorporated in the orthotic device, occasionally with a dancer's pad accommodation for the first metatarsal head, resembling 'kinetic wedge' described by Dananberg (1986).

As in all cases where conservative measures have been exhausted and the athlete continues to have pain, surgical intervention is indicated. There are five types of surgical procedure that can be performed, each classified according to the particular region of the MTPJ where the surgery takes place:

1. remodelling arthroplasty or cheilectomy
2. wedge or transpositional osteotomies of the first metatarsal or proximal phalanx
3. resection arthroplasty
4. joint replacement (implant) arthroplasty
5. arthrodesis or fusion of the first MTPJ.

There is no 'perfect procedure' for cases of hallux limitus and rigidus. However, when treating the athlete or active patient, joint preservation and attempting to achieve maximum motion of the first MTPJ should be the surgeon's goal. Cheilectomy is an excellent procedure when the biomechanics of the first ray are correct; however, decompression and plantar-flexor osteotomies are desired to reduce dorsiflexion stress and jamming of the joint.

For patients who are less demanding in terms of athletic activity, joint fusion can be a consideration.

When degenerative joint disease changes are great, and the older non-competitive participant wants to improve the range of motion and maintain hallux length without placing high stresses on the joint, implant replacement surgery is a viable option. In cases where the total joint prosthesis fails, arthrodesis may be the only remaining viable option.

## Bunion deformity in the athlete

For the athlete, a symptomatic bunion deformity can limit function, reduce performance and be extremely frustrating. Associated with metatarsus primus varus are excessive pronation, hypermobility of the first ray, equinus, hyperelasticity, metatarsus adductus and a strong family history, which are more common in the female population. Even the mention of bunion surgery drives fear into the heart of any athlete. Therefore, the clinician is prudent to consider all conservative measures first before entering any discussion about surgical correction.

The clinician must take into account a number of factors first before considering the surgical option (Baxter 1994b, Pagliano 1997, Subotnick 1999g):

- First, the clinician must determine the extent of the bunion deformity.
- Second, biomechanical evaluation of the lower extremity and foot with gait analysis must be performed to determine the aetiology of the bunion formation.
- Third, in the athletic history, as well as the consultation with the athlete, a determination must be made as to the activity level, plus the short-term and long-term goals of the patient. Note: expectation levels of the athlete are high, and the surgeon must consider these factors, and whether those goals are attainable.
- Fourth, can the athlete return to his or her sport within a prescribed period of time? If not, surgery should be postponed until a suitable time frame can be established.
- Fifth, how compliant will the athlete be to postoperative care? Most athletes are motivated and will usually follow instructions and be aggressive in their physical therapy. However, many athletes want to expedite their follow-up care and rush back

into a physically demanding exercise routine, placing the surgical results at risk.
- Sixth, the psychological status of the athlete must be assessed. Does the athlete have any underlying medical or psychological disorders (e.g. diabetes mellitus, osteoporosis, anorexia/bulimia nervosa, amenorrhoea, depression, anxiety, or compulsive behaviour pattern)? This is important in predetermining whether the athlete is a good candidate for surgical intervention.

In the mildly compensated bunion deformity, with a low intermetatarsal angle (less than 11°) and a low hallux abductus angle (less than 20°), only intermittent symptoms may be present, particularly in sports activity. Neuritis of the saphenous and superficial medial dorsal cutaneous nerve, as well as capsulitis and bursitis, may also be present. With a functional fibular sesamoid in an acceptable position (at least 50% covered by the metatarsal head) and the first MTPJ articulation congruent, the positional compensated bunion deformity should be treated conservatively. The goal for this athlete should be to prevent further progression of the bunion deformity, by proper athletic shoe selection (wide forefoot with adequate toe box room). In addition, the athlete should use a prescription orthosis to limit excessive subtalar joint pronation and hypermobility of the first ray, and also undertake a good stretching programme when equinus of the gastrocnemius or Achilles tendon is identified. As long as the athlete is performing at a normal level and symptoms are controllable, surgery should be avoided, with the clinician reviewing the bunion deformity radiologically (Fig. 13.9) at least once a year.

When the athlete presents with an uncompensated symptomatic bunion deformity, a rapid deterioration of the deformity will often be seen. As a result of excessive pronation and excessive medial column prolapse and instability, retrograde forces upon the hallux and first MTPJ cause further deviation of both the first ray and hallux. Pain will ensue, particularly during the propulsive phase of gait, which is the most important phase for the athlete. With a hypermobile first ray,

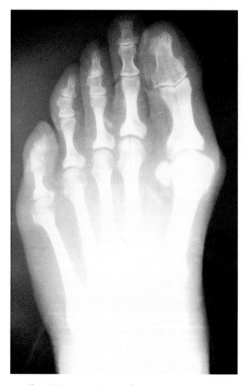

**Figure 13.9** Hallux abducto valgus deformity showing the extent of dislocation of the sesamoids from the articular surface.

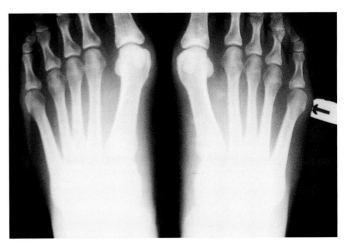

**Figure 13.11** Radiograph showing tailor bunions of the fifth metatarsal.

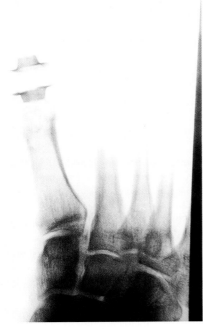

**Figure 13.10** Postoperative view of a repair to a hallux abducto valgus with total joint replacement.

instability of the joint region will occur. In the uncompensated bunion, the first metatarsal head will further increase adduction, dorsiflexion and inversion, as the sesamoid apparatus becomes subluxated laterally and the joint becomes incongruous. The joint becomes unstable and dysfunctional, and as a result other compensatory events occur, such as the development of neuromas, stress fractures, plantarflexed second metatarsals with plantar lesions, varus rotated fifth digits, with hyperkeratotic lesions, tailor's bunions of the fifth metatarsals, as well as compensatory ankle and lower leg pain.

When the symptomatic hallux abducto valgus deformity becomes consistently painful, both in athletic as well as in everyday shoes, and after orthotic use, altering of shoes and all conservative measures have failed, surgical correction should be considered (Fig. 13.10). The surgical procedures to be considered are of two types: the soft-tissue procedures; and the bone procedures, consisting of osteotomies and fusions. For the athlete, the simpler procedures are always recommended over the fusions, Lapidus procedures, Keller arthroplasties and implant procedures. Whenever possible, unilateral correction of the bunion deformity of the athlete is advised, particularly in cases of bilateral osteotomies.

The V-transpositional (Austin – see also Ch. 23) osteotomy (Austin & Leiventhen 1981) has shown to be for the athlete one of the simplest, most consistent procedures with the least complications. There have been a number of modifications to the Chevron (Austin) transpositional osteotomy, with various types of cuts of the first metatarsal head. Fixation of the osteotomy can be accomplished with a variety of techniques, including K-wire, screw, Steinman pin, Biofix (absorbable) and Orthosorb (absorbable) pins. For the athlete, the use of a biodegradable pin, when indicated, is preferable to screws that may need to be removed at a later time. The short Scarf Z-plasty is another excellent procedure for higher intermetatarsal angles. In cases where the proximal or distal articular set angle is high, or where hallux interphalangeus is present, proximal or distal

osteotomies of the hallux (Akin) may be performed to correct the deformity.

For the athletic bunion patient, 6–8 weeks of postoperative progressive care is required before return to activity, with most distal osteotomies. With proper fixation, early return to activity may be permitted with surgical shoes, and assistance with crutches. After 3–4 weeks, stationary bicycling, as well as swimming and water jogging rehabilitation is strongly encouraged. Physical therapy, with active/passive range of motion of the first MTPJ and or hallux interphalangeal joint, is essential for restoration of function. This will help the athlete to return to the athletic sport without previous symptoms, but now with normal function.

## Tailor's bunion

In cases where the athlete has a cavus foot type and high degree of forefoot varus with splaying of the forefoot, it is not uncommon to see a tailor's bunion develop. Both clinical and radiographic evaluation of the deformity to determine the extent of the bowing and rotation of the fifth metatarsal head are required (Fig. 13.11). The lateral bowing or concavity of the fifth metatarsal is a radiographic positional observation secondary to eversion and abduction of the fifth ray (Schepsis et al 1991). For the athlete who has a prominent lateral fifth metatarsal head, irritation due to unyielding athletic shoes (e.g. roller blade boots, ski boots, cycling shoes) can produce an adventitious bursa, entrapment of the lateral dorsal cutaneous nerve or enlargement of the styloid process. If the transverse plane separation between the fourth and fifth metatarsals is minor, and there is a low lateral metatarsal deviation angle, the clinician may choose a simple resection of the lateral prominence of the metatarsal head, with remodelling both laterally and dorsally if necessary. If a plantar lesion is present secondary to hypertrophy of the plantar condyles, the surgeon may decide to resect concomitantly the hypertrophied plantar condyles during the remodelling procedure. For the athlete, this simple procedure can afford an early return to activity because no osteotomy is involved.

However, in cases where there is a great deal of bowing with a high transverse plane separation of the fourth and fifth metatarsal heads, a distal osteotomy should be considered.

Evaluation of the separation should be planned preoperatively to determine whether adequate reduction of the fifth metatarsal deformity can be achieved with a distal osteotomy (Fallet 1990).

There are a number of procedures the surgeon can choose for correction of this deformity, including: oblique sliding osteotomy at the neck (Sponsel 1976), the transverse V (Throchmorton & Bradlee 1978), the medial closing wedge and the Hohmann displacement osteotomy (Hohmann 1951). Various fixation techniques are available, including 0.045- and 0.062-gauge K-wire fixation and 2.0-mm screw fixation. One preferred by the author employs, in conjunction with the transverse V osteotomy, the Orthosorb (half) absorbable pin from dorsal distally (just proximal to the articular surface) to plantar proximally, crossing the osteotomy site. If a second pin (half) is needed it can be utilised from dorsal proximally to plantar distally (opposite direction). When the symptomatic tailor's bunion deformity is a result of significant splaying of the fifth metatarsal, a proximal basal wedge osteotomy may be chosen as the corrective procedure. Postoperative care and rehabilitation is similar in nature to the bunionectomy with osteotomy procedures.

## REARFOOT INJURIES

### Infracalcaneal heel pain

Infracalcaneal heel pain is one of the most common overuse injuries seen by the sports medicine practitioner on a daily basis. It comprises over 12% of the overuse injuries in the foot, and is seen in runners as well as middle-aged walkers who, after a fairly sedentary lifestyle, embark upon a fitness walking programme without commensurate preparation. As in most overuse injuries, underlying causes include improper shoe selection or worn-out shoes, poor biomechanics associated with excessive pronation, increased level of activity and intensity, and atrophy of the plantar fat pad as the athlete begins to age. It is estimated that the fat pad absorbs 20–30% of the heel force at heel strike (Paul et al 1978).

A runner or other athlete will describe pain at the beginning of a run or activity that quickly dissipates as the activity continues. The pain is often described as deep and aching, occasionally described as a burning sensation, or shooting pain down the foot, or up to the ankle. After the so-called 'cooling down' period when the participant has been off his or her feet, pain on the plantar aspect of the heel is once again encountered. The next day, upon rising, the first steps can result in excruciating, hobbling pain until the intrinsic soft-tissue structures of the plantar aspect of the feet have adapted to the floor and stretched out adequately. (Dog owners will have observed their pets arise in the morning and see how instinctively they stretch before they begin to walk.) This type of pain is referred to as *post-static dyskinesia* and is pathognomonic in the diagnosis of heel spur syndrome (Agostinelli & Ross 1977).

*Plantar fasciitis* is inflammation of the plantar fascia as well as the surrounding perfascial structures. The most commonly described painful region is the plantar medial calcaneal eminence, the origin of the plantar fascia. The plantar fascia is a multilayered fibrous aponeurosis, consisting of three bands, the medial, central and lateral, which fan out from the medial plantar calcaneal eminence into each of the plantar toe areas.

The dominant central band originates on the plantar surface of the posteromedial calcaneal tuberosity. The medial component of the fascia covers the abductor hallucis, while the lateral band covers the origin of the abductor digiti quinti, and extends to the plantar plate of the fourth and fifth digits. Passive dorsiflexion of the toes causes tightening of the fascia and allows the medial band to bowstring and become easily visible. Occasionally, a subcalcaneal bursa may form, and may be another cause of the heel pain in the athlete. The bursal sac develops often as a result of acute or chronic trauma,

often related to the athlete's heel landing hard on the floor or ground (volleyball, basketball), or repetitive striking of the ground (running, aerobics, martial arts). In addition, the nerve supply is as important in this syndrome.

The aetiological and biomechanical factors involved in heel spur syndrome are of great value in making a diagnosis (Agostinelli & Ross 1977):

- pes planus
- excessive subtalar joint pronation
- inadequate dorsiflexion (equinus)
- forefoot varus
- flexible forefoot valgus
- functional or structural hallux limitus
- weakness of the plantar intrinsic musculature
- chronic traction of the origin of the plantar fascia
- hypertrophic connective tissue response
- fibrocartilage proliferation
- osseous spur formation
- adventitious bursal development.

The plantar fascia tightens by passive extension of the digits, which then raises the arch. As the plantar fascia is maximally elongated by digital plantar flexion, the longitudinal arch will be greatly depressed. As the plantar fascia is shortened at the time of MTPJ dorsiflexion, the longitudinal arch is then elevated. Hicks (1954) compared the function of the plantar fascia during the propulsive phase of gait to that of a windlass. There are many abnormal foot conditions that can lead to plantar fasciitis, such as pes planus foot, with a decrease in the calcaneal inclination angle, and with excessive subtalar joint pronation, cavus foot, external femoral rotation, inadequate dorsiflexion (equinus), a forefoot varus, or flexible forefoot valgus, and weakness of the plantar intrinsic musculature, which can alter normal biomechanics and lead to heel spur syndrome (Malay & Duggan 1987, Schepsis et al 1991, Ubler et al 1991).

When attempting to define the aetiology of plantar fasciitis the clinician should consider the three major categories: mechanical, degenerative and systemic (Bordelon 1983, Leach et al 1983). Athletes who develop plantar fasciitis as a result of chronic inflammation will develop pain that will extend distally along the entire course of the fascia, with concomitant thickening, and even nodular formation of the fascia. Their heel pain, or *calcaneodynia*, falls into the mechanical overuse category. The older active patient who develops atrophy of the plantar fat pad will also develop increased pronation with age as the medial longitudinal arch begins to prolapse and weaken. The younger athlete with the same foot type may not suffer symptoms due to the compensatory ability of the foot to maintain intrinsic support. However, as age takes its toll, the foot may weaken and become unable to compensate for the additional loads placed upon it. This is a degenerative process that results in an increased level of stress to the plantar fascia and perifascial structures. The result will be pain due to the inability to accommodate for these increased loads.

Repetitive traction of the plantar fascia and surrounding soft-tissue structures, particularly the ligamentous tissues, has been implicated in the development of a symptomatic heel. This repetitive stress will lead to development of chronic irritation of the plantar fascia or, in some cases, an acute traumatic incident can lead to a partial rupture of the fascia. Generally it is not the spur that is the underlying cause of the heel pain but rather the inflammation process of the fascia due to the extreme tension and traction. The 'sharpy fibres' that attach ligaments to bone are stretched in heel spur syndrome, hence the term *enthesopathy* for the micropathology of the associated heel spur syndrome (Agostinelli & Ross 1977). However, the actual spur can be a source of pain, particularly in the older patient who has begun to suffer from atrophy of the plantar fat pad, or even in younger athletes where repeated steroid injections have been employed. In cases of large infracalcaneal heel spurs, any rotation of the calcaneus (i.e. everted rearfoot) can cause increased irritation to the calcaneal tuberosity and make the spur more prominent and subject to trauma. Both conditions can be conservatively treated with Spenco or Sorbethane heel pads or cups, as well as protective shock-absorbing and heel-countered athletic shoes. The use of orthotic devices can also furnish rearfoot balance and cushioning to protect the calcaneus and spur against unwarranted trauma.

A number of other differential diagnoses that need to be ruled out when considering the diagnosis of heel spur syndrome are listed in Box 13.4.

On physical examination some patients may exhibit mild oedema surrounding the plantar fascia attachment at the medial calcaneal tubercle. Deep palpation of the medial band of the plantar fascia, as well as the medial calcaneal tubercle, will elicit a sharp pain, which is typical of heel spur syndrome. When cupping the posterior-inferior portions of the calcaneus with compression, a non-painful test is usually indicative of a possible stress fracture of the calcaneus, rather than heel spur syndrome. A tight plantar fascia will again elicit pain at the attachment at the calcaneus upon passive dorsiflexion of the digits. Midarch plantar fasciitis can be recognised as a separate entity from heel spur syndrome that displays more proximal symptoms. Quite often in long-distance running and in track and field events requiring violent bursts of effort, particularly sprinting, long jump and high jump, as well as basketball and other jumping and landing sports, partial ruptures of the plantar fascia can occur due to overuse and weakening of the collagen tissue. The athlete will present with pain, oedema and ecchymosis. Chronic partial ruptures will develop thickened scar tissue formation surrounding the injury. As a result of the chronic strain, tension and partial tears of the plantar fascia, the resulting scar tissue may organise and become solidified and develop into a singular or multiple plantar fibromas.

After physical examination, a dynamic gait analysis is often very helpful in determining any compensatory action of the symptomatic foot, such as an early heel-off or diminished propulsive phase. The clinician may observe an antalgic gait due to tenderness in the heel region upon heel contact, and may observe excessive pronation in the midstance phase that could be contributing to the traction on the plantar fascia.

Conservative treatment is geared towards both short-term relief of the inflammatory process of the plantar fascia and long-term relief involving correction of biomechanical imbalances. By only treating the initial complaint, and not directing attention to the underlying causes, the patient is doomed to repeated bouts of the overuse injury. The key to treatment of chronic plantar fasciitis is the recognition of aetiology and prevention of recurrent injury. Some of the various factors that should be investigated also involve choice of shoes as well as the discarding of old shoes. Shoes with proper shock absorption, and motion control and stability, can be very helpful in preventing this particular injury. In addition, the surfaces on which the participants play should be evaluated, as hard surfaces contribute to the incidence of injury. Conservative care has been shown to be effective after all measures have been employed. Baxter (1994a) studied 200 patients for over 2 years and found that 95% of them recovered and did not require surgery. Most authors have recommended that 6–12 months of conservative treatment be employed before considering surgical intervention (Box 13.5).

The initial conservative management consists of physical therapies at least three times a week to reduce the inflammation. These therapies are nerve stimulation, ultrasound, iontophoresis (cortisone patches), ice massage and cross-friction massage, and initial treatment with oral NSAIDs, and occasionally a therapeutic steroid injection directed

---

### Box 13.4 Differential diagnosis for heel spur syndrome

**Traumatic**
- Calcaneal fractures
- Post-traumatic arthritis
- Rupture of the origin of the plantar fascia
- Puncture of the plantar fat pad

**Infectious**
- Osteomylelitis of the calcaneus
- Tuberculosis

**Neurological**
- Medial calcaneal nerve entrapment
- Tarsal tunnel syndrome
- Lateral branch of the plantar nerve to abductor digiti quinti entrapment
- Neuropathy secondary to diabetes
- Alcoholic neuropathy

**Metabolic**
- Osteoporosis
- Osteomalacia
- Degenerative osteoarthritis
- Atrophy of the plantar fat pad
- Degenerative arthritis

**Overuse syndromes**
- Plantar fasciitis
- Calcaneal apophysitis (Sever's disease)
- Periostitis
- Calcaneal stress fracture
- Infracalcaneal bursitis
- Achilles tendinitis/peritendinitis
- Retrocalcaneal bursitis
- Tenosynovitis of the flexor hallucis muscle/tendon

**Inflammatory**
- Rheumatoid arthritis
- Juvenile rheumatoid arthritis (juvenile idiopathic arthritis)
- Reiter's syndrome
- Ankylosing spondylitis
- Psoriatic arthropathy
- Gout

**Tumours**
- Simple and aneurysmal bone cysts
- Osteoid osteoma
- Osteoblastoma
- Chondrosarcoma

---

towards the site of the inflammation or the infracalcaneal bursa. The injection consists of 0.5 ml (2 mg) dexamethadexasone acetate, 0.5 ml (2 mg) dexamethasone phosphate, 0.2 ml Wydase, 1.5 ml lidocaine (lignocaine) 1% plain, 1.5 ml bupivacaine 0.5% plain and 0.25 ml cyanocobalamin (vitamin $B_{12}$). This has proven to be most useful with sports injury patients. On occasion, when the use of corticosteroids is not advisable or the limit of three injections has been reached, homeopathic anti-inflammatory medications such as Zeel

## Initial visit

- X-rays
- Ice massage for 20 minutes, 3 times daily
- Contrast footbaths if swelling present, twice daily (see Ch. 16)
- In cases of extreme pain – cortisone injection followed by nerve stimulation/ultrasound treatment
- Achilles tendon, calf muscle, hamstring stretching programme
- Plantar fascia rest strapping and taping
- Temporary insole
- Antipronation shoes if patient runs
- Heel accommodation if plantar pain
- Entrapment of the medial plantar nerve
- NSAIDs for 4–8 days

## Second visit

- Continued physical therapy – nerve stimulation/ultrasound
- Iontophoresis (cortisone) patch
- NSAIDs, if needed, for 4–8 days
- Cease all impact activity
- Biomechanical evaluation/impression casting for orthotics
- Gait analysis
- Plantar fascia rest strapping and taping

## Third visit

- Dispense orthosis
- Continue physical therapy
- Iontophoresis (cortisone patch)
- Evaluate shoe selection
- Possible night splint

If there is no significant improvement, or in cases where recurrence of symptoms has occurred due to activity:

## Fourth visit

- Cortisone injection
- Continue physical therapy
- Check orthotic control
- Possible bone scan
- Cam walker removable cast
- Night splint

If painful symptoms continue:

## Fifth visit

- Third and final cortisone injection
- Below-knee fibreglass cast immobilisation

If symptoms continue with no significant improvement after 6 months to 1 year of conservative care:

## Sixth visit

Surgical consultation

---

(rhus toxicodendron) or Trameel (2.0 ml vials) may be employed. These medications can also be substituted into the 'cocktail' rather than using the cortisone, or for patients opposed to using cortisone (Bordelon 1993). One must be knowledgeable about the metabolism of these drugs and their potential side-effects before prescribing them. It should be emphasised that injection therapy for reduction of acute plantar fascial inflammation is only a temporary treatment and it must be combined with biomechanical orthotic control.

Rest from the activity is most important. Use of orthoses for the control of excessive pronation is essential; however, as the participant's progressive pronation or compression of the orthotic appliance occurs, modifications and adjustments to the device may be necessary. The author advises re-casting the sports patient every 3 years, as the foot will change biomechanically and structurally. In many cases, orthotic control may not be sufficient to eliminate excessive pronation and any other underlying biomechanical factors. Therefore it is prudent that the athlete ceases all impact activity and cross-trains until they are asymptomatic. In cases where there is excessive pronation combined with a shortened gastrocnemius–soleus muscle complex, or tight heel cord, stretching and flexibility exercises are beneficial. Heel cord stretching with the knee both extended and flexed will help to isolate both the gastrocnemius–soleus and the Achilles and allow for reduced equinus in heel strike, and diminish plantar fascial strain. When conservative measures fail to produce a resolution to the complaints, a night splint (a posterior below-knee splint holds the foot at 90° to the leg, and extends the foot and plantar fascia) is used to help prevent contracture of the intrinsic plantar structures. This has been shown to be effective in reducing pain and stiffness when patients take their first steps out of bed in the morning. It is recommended that the night splint be worn at 5° of dorsiflexion for a minimum of 3 months while gradually weaning the patient off the splint in 2-week increments. On occasion, when night splints and aggressive physical therapy have been employed, and symptoms continue to be present, the author frequently applies a below-knee fibreglass cast or employs a below-knee Cam walker removable cast to rest the foot and extremity completely. It should be reiterated that at least 6 months to 1 year of conservative management should be attempted before surgery is even contemplated.

When surgery is indicated there are two approaches that may be employed, depending on the presence of a symptomatic infracalcaneal spur. The heel spur is not the offending problem, but rather the chronic inflammation and enthesopathy of the surrounding fascia. Therefore, plantar fasciotomy, with or without excision of the infracalcaneal spur, is the surgical procedure of choice for chronic unresolved heel pain. This author recommends only a release of the medial third (medial band) of the proximal plantar fascia, leaving the lateral two-thirds of the plantar fascia intact for cases involving pure plantar fasciitis. Endoscopic plantar fasciotomy has proved to be a viable alternative to open surgical plantar fasciotomy. It is generally agreed that there should be minimal invasion of the tissues in an athlete, and that releasing the entire plantar fascia will only destabilise the intrinsic structures and lead to compensatory complaints such as sinus tarsitis, calcaneocuboid joint syndrome, midtarsal joint pain, anterior tendinitis, ankle discomfort and metatarsalgia. In cases where scar tissue thickening of the fascia occurs it may be necessary to excise a section of the proximal plantar fascia.

When there is nerve compression, entrapment, neuritis or a 'minicompartment syndrome', it is important to perform a decompression of the nerve simultaneously at the time of plantar fascia release. This is performed by dividing the abductor hallucis muscle and the fascia and freeing the medial calcaneal nerve (Baxter & Pfeffer 1992, Murphey & Baxter 1985). It is also suggested that if symptoms of a tarsal tunnel entrapment are present further lengthening of the incision is performed proximally, and the tarsal tunnel should be released (Stein et al 1989). If a heel spur is found to be projected into the flexor digitorum brevis muscle or the quadratus muscle, superior to the plantar fascia, then if large enough it should be removed. It is agreed, however, that the spur is indeed not the culprit, and that the spur does not have to be removed on all occasions. This should be explained to the patient fully preoperatively.

Although not a regularly occurring problem in the athlete, entrapment of the medial plantar nerve has been described as a 'jogger's foot' (Murphey & Baxter 1985, Stein et al 1989). The aetiology of this condition involves the fascial covering which, if thickened, may break down or entrap the nerve. The abductor hallucis muscle may also compress the nerve. Tendinitis of the flexor hallucis longus and/or the flexor digitorum longus can also mimic neuritis of the medial plantar nerve.

The typical clinical presentation of the athlete with medial plantar nerve entrapment or neuritis will be similar to the medial calcaneal nerve entity, with burning, radiating sharp pain from the arch to the hallux or second toe, and shooting pain or numbness. Excessive pronation in sports, athletic shoes, ski boots or skating boots that have a high arch or a hard insole and/or rigid orthosis can also irritate the nerve.

## Ankle equinus

Ankle equinus is defined as a limitation of ankle joint dorsiflexion to less than 10° of dorsiflexion of the neutral foot required for normal gait. Without the minimum 10° of dorsiflexion at the ankle, function of the foot will be altered, and compensation at the midtarsal joint will develop (Subotnick 1999e).

Equinus may be present due to either soft-tissue limitation or bony block at the ankle. It may also be a result of congenitally short gastrocnemius muscle, obliquity of the ankle joint or congenital osseous limitation. Previous ankle injury (sprains, fractures or direct trauma) can cause dorsal lipping at either the neck of the talus or the anterior–inferior portion of the tibia, which can prohibit freedom of movement within the ankle mortise. Rubbing, grinding and impingement may occur, causing degenerative changes in the articular surfaces of both the talus and tibia. Performance in sports that require free movement of the ankle mortise can be adversely affected.

Other clinical entities that can result in equinus are traumatic injuries to the posterior muscle groups and myositis, which may cause fibrosis, scar tissue formation and eventual shortening of the muscle belly itself. In cases of long-distance runners, when muscle groups are greatly fatigued and lactic acid levels increase, cramps or tears of the gastrocnemius or soleus muscles can occur, creating scar tissue as well as weakened or contracted muscle groups. There are also cases where children's long bones literally outgrow muscle groups, creating short and underdeveloped muscles. Women wearing high-heeled shoes create an equinus, which can have severe ramifications when exercise is performed. The author recommends female patients to 'kick off' the high heels during the middle of the day and perform some simple stretching exercises. It is essential that they do the same before initiating their exercise routine, particularly if they exercise in the evening after a full day of wearing high-heeled shoes. Equinus can be seen in cases of generalised ligamentous laxity, which can result in gastrocnemius tightness and shortening.

To differentiate between a bony and soft-tissue limitation, the patient is examined in the prone position with the knee flexed. Once the knee is extended, the foot will then begin to plantar flex into an equinus position, creating a soft-tissue contracture of the superficial gastrocnemius. This contracture usually occurs during the last 20° when the knee is going from flexion to full extension. In some cases there may also be a contracture of the soleus muscle. If the limited ankle joint dorsiflexion occurs both when the knee is flexed and extended, then the problem is not a soft-tissue equinus but rather a bony block. This is referred to as *anterior impingement exostosis*. This can be seen on a lateral-projection radiograph with the foot stressed to maximum dorsiflexion.

Some of the clinical features that are seen in equinus involve a variety of gait adaptations. There is some transverse plane abduction of the feet with external femoral rotation at the hip, extended knee flexion throughout the gait cycle, early heel-off, which will aggravate the medial head of the gastrocnemius as well as the Achilles tendon. Other areas of compensation include a shortened stride, abductory twist of the foot and heel, excessive pronation, an elongated propulsive phase and forefoot subluxation, creating medial column prolapse. The ankle, now limited in its ability to dorsiflex, compensates by attempting to use the midtarsal joint. For the midtarsal joint to function efficiently the subtalar joint must be pronated to unlock the midtarsal joint. In addition, contracture of the gastrocnemius–soleus complex will pronate the foot further, which then compensates at the midtarsal joint. As a result, the athlete may have calf leg cramps, digital contractures and rearfoot pain. In addition, subluxation of the knee may also occur, leading to chronic knee pain.

Posterior muscle group equinus in the athlete is also secondary to a combination of tight gravity muscles and weak antigravity muscles. This imbalance between the two groups can lead to further contracture, and additional compensatory action. An aggressive stretching programme and flexibility training, often with a sports physical therapist, trainer and massage therapist, can help to alleviate this dynamic imbalance and afford better heel strike and an overall more efficient gait performance. When observing the wear pattern on the shoes, there will be minimal heel and lateral wear, while excessive wear will be seen at the forefoot and under the ball of the shoe.

In cases of anterior ankle impingement, or ankle bony block, the athlete will complain of pain at the anterior aspect of the ankle or in the Achilles tendon. This can also be seen with hyperostosis of the neck of talus, as the athlete attempts to maximally dorsiflex. The location of the bony block may also have a bearing on the heel strike of the athlete (Subotnick 1999e). An anterior lateral exostosis creates a supinated foot plant, while an anterior medial exostosis will create a pronated foot plant. As the foot and ankle reach a maximum point of dorsiflexion, tension and enthesitis of the Achilles tendon will occur, which will lead to distinct pain either in the tendon or at its insertion.

The conservative treatment for osseous deformity of the ankle is with the use of heel lifts. When conservative measures have been exhausted for a bony ankle equinus, surgical resection, either arthroscopically or via arthrotomy, may be required. Postoperatively the athlete is encouraged to passively remobilise the ankle.

Heel lifts, used concomitantly with a stretching routine, are very helpful for a soft-tissue equinus deformity. The stretching is imperative to prevent recurrence of the posterior muscle group contracture, including the tightening of the heel cord. Those athletes with hypertonicity will benefit from heat treatment.

## Achilles tendon injuries

Achilles tendinitis, or paratendinitis, is a chronic condition seen in running and jumping sports. It is one of the most common injuries in athletes and has been estimated to afflict 6.5–20% of all runners (Clement et al 1984, James et al 1978, Krissoff & Ferris 1979, Subotnick & Roth 1988). Due to its structure as well as the functional demands, the Achilles tendon is susceptible to both acute and chronic injury. Repetitive loading that exceeds the ability of the Achilles tendon to repair may cause tendinitis, whereas the acute rapid loading of the tendon may cause traumatic rupture. Paratendinitis of the Achilles tendon accounts for 20% of all non-specific tenosynovitis or paratendinitis seen in the foot and ankle. Some of the aetiological factors of acute or chronic Achilles tendinitis are irritation of the heel against the counter of the shoe, excessive pronation, limb-length discrepancy and a tight gastrocnemius–soleus complex as a result of inadequate stretching. Also involved are conditions such as Haglund's deformity and a short Achilles tendon. The repetitive loading seen in long-distance marathon running and the traction of the tendon–muscle unit due to jumping, hill running, or running on uneven or hard surfaces may also contribute. Similarly, an increase in running mileage, intensity of interval speed running and the start of a running or athletic programme after a prolonged period of inactivity can all be factors.

Other factors include running or athletic shoes that show excessive outer-sole wear, inner soles that are crushed down and heel counters that are distorted and create an unstable heel strike or midstance phase of gait. Biomechanical considerations that can contribute to Achilles tendinitis and paratendinitis include lower extremity malalignments, such as tibial varum, compensated gastrocnemius–soleus equinus or ankle block equinus, and a cavus foot with excessive supinated heel strike. These factors will lead to unusual lateral shoe wear, which then causes hyperpronation at midstance, creating higher levels of torque on the Achilles tendon.

Other compensatory biomechanical factors, such as rearfoot varus, forefoot varus, forefoot valgus with a plantar-flexed first ray, and varus condition of metatarsals two to five, also contribute to pathologies of the Achilles tendon.

Overuse injuries of the Achilles tendon result from the inflammatory process in the tendon tissue as well as the paratendon. Inflammation is the direct result of repetitive microtraumatic forces. The inflammatory process is a necessary component of the healing process. In many cases, acute inflammation is productive, whereas chronic inflammation can be destructive and disabling. The key is early treatment of this overuse disorder to prevent the injury from becoming irreversible.

After initial vasoconstriction and haemostasis, local vasodilatation takes place, leading to the release of capillary fluid. Prostaglandin production due to inflammation causes vasodilatation, which then produces oedema. Histological changes within the tendon constitute the underlying reason for the pain and pathological conditions in the tendon (Astom & Rausing 1995). In cases of chronic Achilles tendinitis, nodules comprised of mucoid degeneration will appear, together with longitudinal fissures within the tendon itself.

The areas most commonly involved in Achilles tendinitis are:

- The myotendinous junction.
- The area of the Achilles tendon approximately 8–10 cm proximal to the distal insertional region of the calcaneus and ankle joint. Lagergren and Lindholm (1958) noted that the area 2–6 cm above the calcaneal insertion had the poorest blood supply, which substantiates the fact that most non-insertional Achilles tendon injuries occur in this region. For participants over the age of 35 years, overuse tendinopathy in this region increases dramatically. This is due to the blood flow by approximately 40% at this age. Carr and Norris (1989) showed that there was a significant reduction in the number, as well as the mean percentage of area occupied by, blood vessels in this region.
- The insertional region of the Achilles tendon into the posterior aspect of the calcaneus, with or without calcinosis. Clain and Baxter (1992) categorised the entities into insertional and non-insertional tendinitis. Insertional tendinitis will usually involve the adjacent bursa, and includes anatomical changes within the tendon, such as thickening, microscopic tearing, calcinosis within the tendon body, and fraying as a result of a Haglund's deformity or other enthesopathies.

The triceps surae combine to form the Achilles tendon. The Achilles is the largest and strongest tendon in the body. It is estimated that the tendon receives up to 7000 N of force (Clain & Baxter 1992). While running, the Achilles tendon is subjected to constant extreme forces with tensile loads of up to eight times the body weight. The medial head of the gastrocnemius is the main component during running, whereas the soleus, which lies deep to the gastrocnemius, is subject to early disuse atrophy secondary to undertraining and/or immobilisation. The Achilles tendon places the insertion of the soleus medial to that of the gastrocnemius on the calcaneus. In addition, there is a medial insertion of the Achilles tendon on the calcaneus. Because the tendons of the gastrocnemius and soleus do not have a parallel configuration, the theory is that the shear stress between the two tendons creates an area of potential weakness, and eventual rupture due to attrition (Christensen 1953).

The triceps surae are the main decelerators of the leg, a major supinator of the subtalar joint, a plantar flexor of the ankle and a stabiliser of the rearfoot. In sports such as gymnastics and ballet, the muscle complex assists in maintaining a variety of movements and positions.

The Achilles tendon does not have a synovial sheath, rather it is surrounded only by a peritenon. The peritenon as well as the tendon is subject to acute trauma, chronic overuse or disease entity. Peritendinitis of the Achilles tendon may occur as a result of athletic shoe counter irritation, a sudden increase in running or workout intensity, or prolonged running or walking. Microvascular studies of this body indicate that there is an area of relative avascularity just proximal to its insertion into the calcaneus. As a result, this region is highly vulnerable to Achilles tendinitis, peritendinitis and eventual rupture.

Chronic traction, irritation, and inflammation of the Achilles tendon will present as tenosynovitis, or a partial or complete rupture. Microscopically, an abnormal Achilles tendon of an athlete suffering from chronic tendinopathy differs from a normal tendon. First there is a loss in collagen continuity, and an increase in ground substance, vascularity and cellularity (fibroblasts and myofibroblasts). In those who suffer from chronic overuse pathologies of the tendons, inflammatory cells are absent (Khan et al 2000).

Although Achilles tendinitis is rare, acute primary tendinosis will be recognised as pain over the posterior aspect of the Achilles tendon. *Paratenonitis* is a more accurate term for this condition, which presents as an inflammation of the paratenon, whether lined by synovium or not. Chronic tenosynovitis will cause fibrosis of the paratenon, creating pain upon motion. This condition has been referred to as *adhesive tendinopathy*. It is associated with intratendinous degeneration (Jarvinen et al 1997) and produces the crepitus or, as Subotnick (1999d) refers to it, the 'glue' that forms between the tendon and paratenon. The clinician will feel swelling and inflammation in the paratenon. The tendon should be checked completely to rule out any small tears or 'dells' in the tendon. Any thickness or egg-shaped appearance of the tendon may be a clue as to pathology within the tendon itself, or partial rupture. When palpating the paratenon, localised oedema is more indicative of a tenosynovitis. Investigative studies such as magnetic resonance imaging (MRI), ultrasound or even xerograms may assist in making the correct diagnosis.

Paddue et al (1976) classified Achilles tendon pathology into three distinct entities based on the clinical and histological findings seen at the time of surgery:

- peritendinitis
- peritendinitis with tendinosis
- pure tendinosis.

Peritendinitis is a pathology of the highly vascular paratenon. The condition has also been described by Kvist and Kvist (1980) as fibrin adhesions organised between the paratenon and the tendon itself. When peritendinitis and tendinosis is seen in combination, there will be a significant change in the tendon morphology itself. The Achilles tendon will become thicker, softer and yellowed. Paddue et al (1976) and Kvist and Kvist (1980) described cleavage planes as well as vascular budding from the paratenon invading the tendon. The third classification, referred to as pure tendinosis, is seen in cases of acute ruptures of the Achilles tendon. Paddue et al (1976) described mucinoid degeneration and lipomatous infiltration of the collagen fibres, with patients who had no prodromal symptoms prior to rupture. In those subjects who did suffer Achilles tendon pain prior to rupture, a specific zone of histiocytic infiltrate and capillary infiltration was seen.

Obtaining a thorough history from the patient will often help to determine the underlying cause of the injury and the level of activity (i.e. miles run, length of time involved in workouts, intensity and competitiveness). Subjective findings, such as the type of pain, its character and when it occurs (before, during or after activity), are also important. Previous treatment, particularly localised corticosteroid injections, should be noted.

The clinical examination should involve the evaluation of both Achilles tendons, as well as a comparison of both lower extremities. The clinician should examine for signs of swelling, erythema, thickness of the tendon or paratenon, nodules and any bony abnormalities. On occasion, ossification within the tendon body itself may occur. The ankle joint range of motion should be evaluated to rule out equinus. This examination should take place with the forefoot supinated and with the knee both flexed and extended. The difference between the symptomatic leg versus the contralateral asymptomatic leg should be noted. During the examination, the practitioner should look, feel and listen for any palpable or audible crepitus surrounding the tendon, while actively or passively putting the foot and ankle through the range of motion. The combination of an accurate history and thorough physical examination can help to determine whether the injury is an insertional or non-insertional tendinitis, or a combination of the two.

In the acute stage of Achilles paratendinitis, the complaint will be unilateral. Clancy et al (1992) defined tendinitis of less than 2 weeks duration as acute, 3–6 weeks duration as subacute, and more than 6 weeks duration as chronic. The symptoms are usually local; the affected tendon becomes two to three times its normal size, with soft-tissue swelling, crepitus and restricted pain upon movement. Any presence of nodular formation above the insertion may be indicative of microscopic tears or small ruptures of some of the tendon fibres. The pain will be most discrete above the tendon insertion, precipitated by overuse activity and relieved quickly by rest.

Treatment for the acute stage of Achilles tendinitis and paratendinitis consists of a decrease in activity or an attempt to eliminate the overuse.

When running or activity continues, reducing mileage, eliminating all hill and interval training, avoiding uneven running surfaces, and ceasing all jumping or bouncing repetitive sports is required. Ice or contrast whirlpools after activity, as well a consistent pre- and post-exercise stretching programme, should be adhered to.

Measures to reduce the inflammation include anti-inflammatory medications, icing (3–4 times daily of no more than 20 minutes duration), analgesics and heel lifts (except in cases of unilateral Achilles tendinosis and/or paratendinitis secondary to limb-length discrepancy, where only the short limb is raised). Physical therapy modalities consist of iontophoresis nerve stimulation of the muscle–tendon unit and ultrasound, together with biomechanical correction and prescription orthoses to reduce excessive pronation and pull upon the Achilles tendon. Shoe selection is also important, with a flexible athletic shoe and moulded Achilles pad to prevent irritation of the tendon. Homeopathic injectable medications in combination with local anaesthetic can be administered followed by deep soft-tissue cross-friction massage. This will assist in breaking up scar tissue and adhesions painlessly and improve circulation to the region. After a period of time, a mild stretching programme can be initiated, with strengthening of the anterior and posterior muscle groups.

All running and other physical impact athletic activity must cease for at least 4–6 weeks. A non-impact cross-training programme consisting of bicycling, elliptical trainer, swimming and deep water jogging can be substituted during the recuperative phase. Failure on the part of the athlete to adhere to the recommended rehabilitation programme can result in chronic adhesive inflammation, and ultimately focal degeneration of the tendon, which can lead to chronic tendinitis and partial or complete rupture of the tendon. In cases where the conservative measures have continued to be ineffective, the tendon and extremity can be rested by using a cast to immobilise the area or a removable Cam walker.

In the subacute stage, diffuse swelling along the tendon is indicative of thickening of the paratenon. Crepitus can be palpated upon movement of the tendon. The participant will relate symptoms of pain, particularly upon rapid acceleration. Fibrosis of the paratenon secondary to tenosynovitis will create pain upon motion. Treatment is similar to the acute phase, with aggressive physical therapy and cross-friction massage. On occasion, when this phase occurs, local anaesthetic injections with or without homeopathic medication can be administered to achieve lysis of the adhesions along the course of the paratenon. Adjunctive treatment with cast immobilisation should also be considered for this particular overuse injury (Box 13.6).

For the patient with the chronic stage of tenosynovitis, after self-treatment of the condition for a period of time, they will have been referred to the sports podiatrist or specialist for definitive diagnosis by their physical therapist or primary care physician. This condition responds well to physical therapy and becomes asymptomatic. However, a return to activity causes the symptoms to recur.

Examination in chronic tendinitis will usually reveal residual focal thickening and nodularity of the tendon. The participant will relate pain after activity but not during the sport. They will have pain at rest and stiffness upon rising and taking those first steps in the morning. After a period of time of walking the stiffness and pain seem to subside. Quite often the patient may never develop an acute stage, but the condition may rapidly become chronic. Crepitus at the myotendinous junction may be palpated, and in some rare cases a stenosing tenosynovitis of the synovial sheath may develop, indicating a much more advanced stage of inflammation. Kvist et al (1987a) found high levels of fibronectin and fibrinogen in the connective tissue and vascular walls of the paratenon in chronic paratenonitis, which is indicative of an immature form of scar tissue. This inflammatory infiltrate, if left untreated, will undergo fibrotic changes from early fibrin organisation, resulting in chronic Achilles paratenonitis. Clinically, chronic oedema and hyperplasia of sections of the paratenon will be seen, with fibrous adhesions, chronic pain and disability (Kvist & Kvist 1980, Kvist et al 1987b).

Conservative management of chronic tenosynovitis in an athlete is the best plan. Treatment should consist of aggressive physical therapy with deep cross-friction massage. Physical therapy consists of galvanic nerve stimulation, ultrasound, contrast temperature whirlpool and, as an adjunctive measure, iontophoresis (see also Ch. 16). Application of cold can also be helpful. This treatment plan should be carried out for a minimum of 3–4 weeks. Other measures that can be beneficial include NSAIDs, trigger point injections, or intralesional injections of lignocaine and bupivacaine with or without added homeopathic medication to produce lysis of the adhesions.

Other measures to be taken include shoe evaluation for the wear pattern on the outer soles and to see whether the shoes are stable or distorted, gait analysis, and an active programme of stretching (flexibility) and strengthening. Biomechanical correction should be considered, either through the use of temporary insoles or permanent control orthoses. A final measure is the use of a removable or below-knee non-weight-bearing cast to immobilise the area.

## Box 13.6 Achilles tendinitis: treatment

### Initial visit

- Thorough history with check of underlying factors
- Check flexibility of hamstrings, gastrocnemius, soleus, Achilles tendon stretches
- Evaluate shoes: check heel outer-sole wear, lateral or medial forefoot, heel to ball ratio; check heel counter, and for distortion of the shoe
- Check for swelling, tenderness; physical therapy-electro galvanic stimulation (PT-EGS), ultrasound, iontophoresis and ice
- Home ice massage
- NSAIDs for 2 weeks
- Check training habits – modify programme, eliminate hill running and speed work
- Gait analysis, biomechanical correction, heel lifts, temporary orthoses
- Lateral weight-bearing radiograph – rule out insertional calcific tendinosis, intratendon calcification and bony ankle block

### Second visit

- Re-evaluate swelling, tenderness; PT-EGS, ultrasound three times a week for 3–4 weeks
- Re-check flexibility – evaluate stretching programme – ice after activity, hot whirlpool
- Continue stretching programme – ice massage, cross-friction massage
- Biomechanical evaluation and orthotic casting
- Cross-training recommendation – no impact or propulsion, bicycling, elliptical trainer, swimming, aqua-jogging
- Check new athletic shoes
- NSAIDs – second week

### Third visit

- Dispense orthoses: check for proper biomechanical control
- Continue PT-EGS, ultrasound, iontophoresis and ice massage
- Consider tendinosis, tendosynovitis, partial rupture, retrocalcaneal bursitis, gout, plantaris rupture, posterior ankle capsulitis, os trigonum, fracture status process – posterior talus
- Gait analysis with orthotic devices and new shoes
- Continue cross-friction massage therapy

### Subsequent visits

- If pain continues – consider cast immobilisation
- If all conservative measures fail – consider surgical intervention

Alternative diagnostic methods to predict muscle function as well as chronic traction and strain of the Achilles tendon include a Cybex dynamometer, which provides an isokinetic method of evaluating muscle strength over a range of angular velocities. Electromyography provides electrophysiological evaluation of dynamic muscle function and reveals the maximum fibre use during activity with increased resistance being applied. Computerised gait analysis, with force plates, and video will also help to provide valuable data on the biomechanics as well as muscle kinetics during the various phases of gait. Lastly, MRI will help to determine the points of focal degeneration of the tendon and provide information about the volume of the gastrocnemius–soleus complex.

In cases where all conservative measures for treating chronic paratenonitis and tenosynovitis fail, surgical tendolysis is a viable alternative. The surgery is performed to expose the paratendon and to excise all chronic inflammatory tissue surrounding the Achilles tendon.

All fibrous adhesions should be released, with dissection of the surrounding subcutaneous tissue. The surgeon should take care to maintain the blood supply of the surrounding subcutaneous tissues. Preservation of normal paratendon tissue should be made, with abnormal tissue being resected. Examination for any nodules within the tendon body should be made, and if any tendinosis is seen within the tendon, both should be surgically excised.

If there are any calcific deposits, or an insertional calcific tendinosis is present, the calcific deposits are excised and the tendon remodelled. This may require an incision into the tendon down to the bone, with partial avulsion of the insertion of the Achilles tendon to identify and remove the calcific tendinosis.

Postoperative care consists of a posterior splint cast, non-weight-bearing for the first week, followed by a removable cast boot or immobilised fibreglass casting for 4–6 weeks. The cast and foot is held at a mild equinus for the first week, and then at a 90° angle neutrally for the second week, with slight dorsiflexion beginning in the fourth week. The postoperative course will depend highly on the extent of the surgery and tendon dissection.

## Partial rupture of the Achilles tendon

A partial rupture injury will present with extreme pain and swelling over the injured section of tendon. There will be more pain with this injury than with chronic resistive paratenonitis or tenosynovitis. In many cases the partial tear will be difficult to differentiate from the chronic paratenonitis. Bleeding, ecchymosis and pinpoint tenderness overlying the location of the partial tear will indicate the severity of the injury. Immediate care for this injury includes rest, ice, elevation of the limb, anti-inflammatory medication (after 48–72 hours from the time of injury) and the application of a posterior splint cast to allow for maximum swelling. This is followed by the application of a below-knee non-weight-bearing cast to immobilise for 4 weeks, if the condition is severe. The advantage of the posterior splint is that the cast can be removed to allow for the application of physical therapy modalities. In both cases the cast should be applied, avoiding equinus, and set at a 90°, neutral position. This will help to avoid contracture of the posterior musculature and allow for a quicker restoration of function and flexibility. A vigorous physical therapy programme designed to improve flexibility, strength and balance, while reducing scar tissue and adhesions, should be instituted 4–6 weeks following injury. It is recommended that the athlete refrain from all impact, propulsive activities for at least 6 weeks, with non-impact cross-training sports being recommended. As the athlete slowly returns to activity, ice should be used after participation to avoid chronic tendinitis and scar tissue formation, together with cross-friction massage. Occasionally, anaesthetic injections with or without combination homeopathic medication can be used to break down any adhesions overlying the partial rupture site.

## Acute complete rupture of the Achilles tendon

Acute Achilles tendon rupture usually occurs in poorly conditioned middle-aged men who quite often are the 'weekend warriors', not engaged in athletic activities on a consistent basis. On occasion, it may affect those participants who have taken oral or injectable corticosteroids. The most frequent site of the tendon rupture will be 2–6 cm from the calcaneus (Fig. 13.12). The injury will occur normally during a rapid eccentric loading (push-off), with the knee extended, as the foot and ankle are landing in dorsiflexion with a contracted soleus muscle. At 8% strain, the tendon fails and breaks the collagen cross-

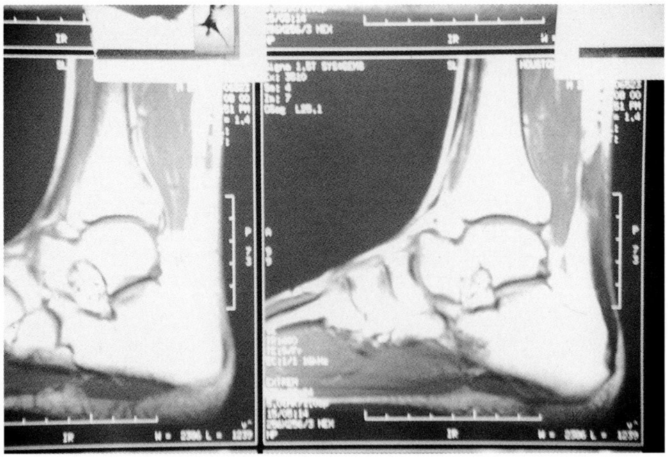

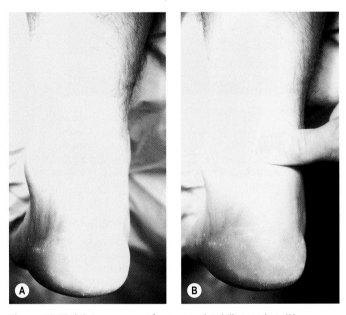

Figure 13.12 Typical site of a ruptured Achilles tendon.

**Figure 13.13** (A) Appearance of a ruptured Achilles tendon; (B) palpation of the site of rupture of an Achilles tendon.

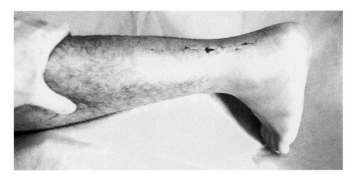

**Figure 13.14** The Thompson test for a ruptured Achilles tendon.

links (Soma & Mandlebaum 1994). The tendon is at great risk if tension is applied too rapidly, if the tendon is under tension before further loading, or if the tendon is weak compared to the muscle. Participants will often say they felt a pop in the back of the leg, and that it felt as if someone hit them in their calf or tendon. On occasion, a direct traumatic blow to the Achilles tendon can create the rupture. In the acute rupture, pain will be present but will not be the major presenting complaint, which will instead be the onset of swelling, ecchymosis, a palpable gap in the Achilles tendon, and a diminished or complete inability to plantar flex the foot (Fig. 13.13). The patient will be unable to continue play at the time of injury and will no longer be able to continue athletic activity. The Thompson test is used to determine whether there has been a complete rupture of the tendon. The test is performed by squeezing the gastrocnemius–soleus firmly in the prone position, where the normal reaction should be plantar flexion. When there is a complete rupture of the Achilles tendon, plantar flexion will not occur (Fig. 13.14). The patient may substitute the intact posterior tibial or fibular (peroneal) muscles or the flexor digitorum longus to plantar flex the ankle. However, they will be unable to perform the single heel raise test, indicating a marked reduction in strength due to the tendon injury.

A number of clinicians advocate closed treatment, with cast immobilisation in plantar flexion to reapproximate the frayed tendon ends to allow for healing (Lea & Smith 1968, 1972). They cite good functional results without the morbidity of surgical intervention, in addition to a more rapid return to activity, avoidance of the necessity for admission to hospital and lower healthcare costs (Ingles et al 1976, Mahan & Carter 1992). However, the closed cast treatment carries with it a higher rate of re-rupture, 10–29% being reported. This ultimately will reduce the ability to perform on the athletic court or field, and is not advised for the active athletic patient (Bradley & Tibone 1990, Carden et al 1989). Of even greater interest, Ingles et al (1976) found that, upon isokinetic testing, the non-surgical subjects in their study achieved only 62–67% of strength and endurance, compared to 88–100% in the surgically corrected group.

This conservative form of treatment is reserved for the patient who is not attempting to return to high levels of athletic activity or demanding functional performance. With these factors in mind, and the fact that the athletic patient who does not have surgery is at high risk for re-rupture, surgical primary repair is recommended. With improved surgical technique and postoperative rehabilitation, surgical repair now has reduced morbidity, and allows patients to return to their pre-injury level of participation (Soma & Mandlebaum 1994). For the athlete, many clinicians recommend primary surgical repair for complete ruptures.

The surgical procedure is combined with an aggressive postoperative active range of motion programme to recreate a level of functional performance that was present before injury. The complication rate from this surgery has been as high as 20% for minor incidents, and 12% for major incidents, with recent rates being as low as 2% (Willis et al 1986). The reported complications include infection, adhesions, sural neuroma, delayed wound healing with or without necrosis, re-rupture and continued pain. In the study by Soma and Mandlebaum (1994), 100% of patients returned to athletic participation 12 months after surgical repair and had no functional deficit on isokinetic testing. It has also been reported that, after surgical repair, approximately 75% of high-performance athletes and 90% or more of recreational athletes can be restored to competitive level activity (Singer & Jones 1986).

A number of surgical procedures for repair of the Achilles tendon have been described. Reapproximation of the torn tendon ends is the great challenge. The majority of these ruptures when operated on are discovered to be located just distal to the musculotendinous junction, and demonstrate a frayed appearance. Surgical repair may include the following:

- open primary repair with direct suturing (Nistor 1981)
- fascial turn down flaps (Ingles et al 1976)

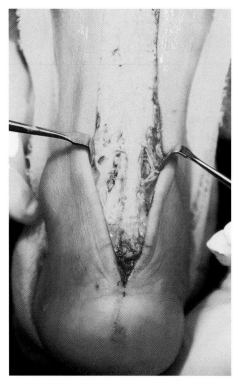

**Figure 13.15** Longitudinal incision over the site of a ruptured Achilles tendon.

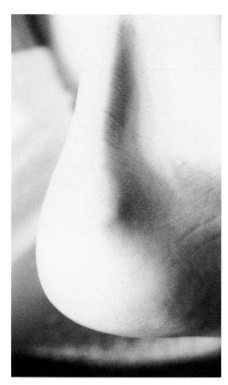

**Figure 13.16** Haglund's deformity.

- plantaris weave (Mahan & Carter 1992, Schuberth et al 1984)
- percutaneous repair (Subotnick & Vogler 1999a)
- peroneus brevis transfer (Turco & Spinella 1987)
- tensor fascia lata wrapping (Fig. 13.15).

Turco and Spinella (1987) identified five factors that challenge successful repair of the Achilles tendon:

1. suturing of the shredded tendon
2. re-establishment of physiological tension
3. weakness associated with a lengthened tendon
4. revitalising an ischaemic injured tendon
5. difficulty obtaining secure fixation when the insertion is avulsed from the calcaneal tuberosity.

When attempting to secure the distal portion of the tendon or graft to the calcaneus this author has found the Mitek GII™ bone/tissue anchor with Mersaline, or the newer Mitek Panaloc™ bone/tissue anchor with Panacryl (Johnson & Johnson), to be useful. Both tissue anchors help to increase the pullout strength of the suture from the calcaneus to the tendon, and can help prevent re-rupture.

Postoperatively, the patient is placed in an above-the-knee non-weight-bearing, posterior splint cast, at a mild equinus, to allow for immediate postoperative swelling. Following the first week, the cast is removed and the joint taken through gentle passive and active range of motion exercises. After 2 weeks, when the sutures are removed, the patient is placed in a below-knee, posterior splint cast, which can be removed daily to allow for range of motion exercises. From weeks 3 to 5 a gentle return to progressive weight bearing is begun.

The patient can then be placed in a Cam walker removable cast, maintaining mild plantar flexion to neutral position. Physical therapy rehabilitation actively begins at the sixth week postoperatively, combining early range of motion with progressive resistance exercises. This has been shown to help attain a successful repair with maximum strength of the Achilles tendon unit, while minimising atrophy of the muscle and tendon, the key being early return to physical activity with minimal sequelae.

## Insertional Achilles tendinitis and calcific tendinosis

Many athletes involved in running, jumping sports, skiing and skating relate pain at the insertion of the Achilles tendon and its insertion into the calcaneus. This is normally associated with hypertrophy of the posterior portion of the calcaneus, a prominent posterosuperior angle of the calcaneus, retrocalcaneal bursitis, Haglund's deformity, an insertional traction exostosis, with ossification or spurring at the site of the Achilles tendon, as well as calcification within the tendon body (Fig. 13.16). In cases where a retrocalcaneal exostosis or hypertrophied posterior aspect of the calcaneus is present, shortening of the Achilles tendon will occur, placing strain on the tendon, as well as chronic irritation, due to increased shoe pressure. Using a lateral-projection radiograph (see Ch. 22), a hyperostosis directed superiorly into the tendon may be seen (Fig. 13.17). Fracturing or fragmentation of the spur may occur as a result of chronic traction forces of the Achilles tendon. A violent impact of the foot on the ground while participating in a sporting event, or a forced eccentric contraction of the gastrocnemius–soleus and Achilles due to excessive dorsiflexion, may also contribute to the formation of fractures along this spur. Microavulsions at the level of the insertion due to excessive traction forces of the Achilles tendon may result in the same pathology (Fig. 13.18). Although the exact aetiology of the calcific tendinitis and tendinosis is not known, the condition is thought to be related to age, overuse, trauma and enthesopathies, and it has a high occurrence rate (Subotnick & Vogler 1999a).

Anatomically the posterosuperior prominence or the bursal projection of the calcaneus functions to lengthen the lever arm of the Achilles tendon, increasing the mechanical advantage of the gastrocnemius–soleus when the ankle is dorsiflexed. At the same time, the

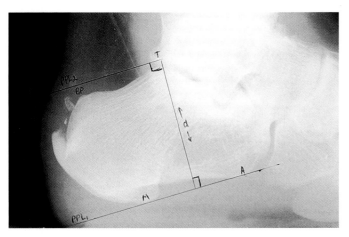

**Figure 13.17** Insertional calcific Achilles tendinosis in Haglund's deformity.

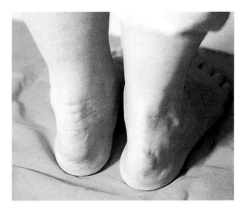

**Figure 13.19** Insertional calcific Achilles tendinosis in Haglund's deformity showing the typical appearance.

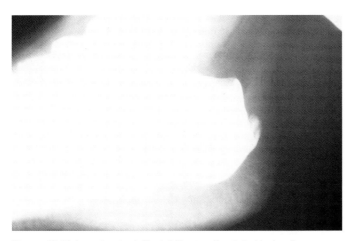

**Figure 13.18** Insertional calcific Achilles tendinosis in Haglund's deformity.

retrocalcaneal bursa protects the Achilles from the posterosuperior aspect of the calcaneus when the ankle is once again dorsiflexed.

It is estimated that the Achilles tendon is subject to forces as great as 900 kg during periods of intense physical activity. The same pathological changes as seen in the calcaneal origin of the plantar fascia are also seen within the tendon and at its insertion.

Microscopic changes include fibrinoid and myxomatous degeneration, fibrosis, and eventual metaplastic calcification with resultant thickening and nodularity of the tendon (Saxena 1996). Also of interest is the fact that after the third and fourth decades of life, blood flow to the tendon shows a significant decrease. The reduced blood flow primarily affects the region of the Achilles tendon 2–6 cm superior to its insertion, which relates to the most frequently ruptured site (DiStefano & Nuron 1972, Lagergren & Lindholm 1958). Rarely, distal tears of the Achilles tendon through areas of calcification, just proximal to the insertion, have been associated with a posterosuperior calcaneal prominence, referred to as a *calcaneal step*, which irritates the tendon upon ankle dorsiflexion (Fig. 13.19).

Upon physical examination, a retrocalcaneal exostosis at the insertion of the tendon, with or without calcification within the Achilles tendon, is noted. The patient will describe a dull aching soreness or pain, sometimes with radiating pain along the sural nerve tract. Tenderness will be localised to the area of the insertion with the peri-

osteum surrounding the calcaneus. The practitioner should compare the two heel regions, with thickening of the Achilles tendon clearly seen at the insertion. Again, the participant will describe pain upon activity that can be reproduced upon active/passive ankle joint range of motion, as well as upon direct palpation. Schepsis et al (1994) noted that there will be a decrease in the range of ankle joint passive dorsiflexion on the afflicted side. On palpation, the practitioner may note discrete crepitus upon ankle joint range of motion as a result of chronic inflammatory infiltrate and fibrin deposition throughout the tendon.

Conservative management of the insertional tendinitis and calcific tendinosis is similar to a painful Haglund's deformity. Physical therapy modalities consisting of ice massage, oral anti-inflammatory medications, nerve stimulation, ultrasound, iontophoresis, viscoelastic heel lifts and removable or hard below-knee cast immobilisation are highly recommended. Of even greater importance is a stretching and strengthening programme, with emphasis on the gastrocnemius–soleus complex,. If an inflamed retrocalcaneal or insertional bursa is present, a single injection of corticosteroid or homeopathic medication may be given, followed by cessation of all physical activity for 2 weeks. Athletic shoe modification with accommodative padding surrounding the posterior heel counter may be employed to lessen the friction and irritation to the posterior prominence of the calcaneus. An orthosis with a mild heel raise can neutralise the irritation to the heel and prevent it becoming chronic. If all conservative measures fail to relieve the pain and irritation to the insertional area of the tendon, surgical intervention may be the only option.

The surgical approach for repair of the posterior calcaneal exostosis and or insertional Achilles calcific tendinosis is dependent on the site, either medially, laterally, or both. Various authors have advocated that, with the patient in the prone position, a single longitudinal midlinear, two incision, medial and lateral linear approach, or a curvilinear and mildly oblique incision may be used. When the retrocalcaneal spurs are present at the insertion, then a midline tendon-splitting approach is advised, which allows for adequate exposure to the calcaneus, to resect the spur (Saxena 1996, Schepsis et al 1994) (Fig. 13.20).

In cases where the spur is central and the calcification is within the tendon and its insertion, the midline, tendon-splitting incision is best option. This approach minimises underscoring, and allows equal medial and lateral halves of the tendon to remain intact to the calcaneus distally. The medial and lateral bodies of tendon are then reflected, allowing for adequate inspection of the site and resection of any intratendinous calcification. For deeply inflamed retrocalcaneal bursae, paratendinosis and superior calcaneal steps, a 'deepening split tenotomy' may be required. After resection of the exostosis and intra-

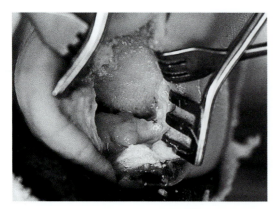

**Figure 13.20** Insertional calcific Achilles tendinosis in Haglund's deformity showing retrocalcaneal exostosis.

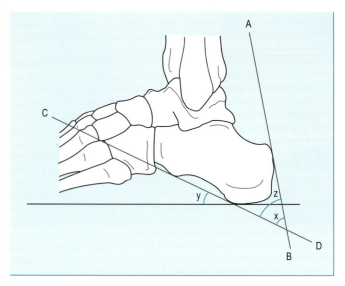

**Figure 13.21** Relationship angles of Haglund's deformity: x = superior calcaneal tuberosity angle (Fowler & Philip 1945); y = calcaneal inclination angle; z = total angle.

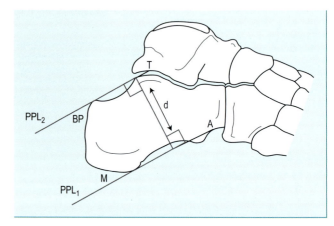

**Figure 13.22** Parallel pitch lines (PPL) to determine the prominence of the bursal projection (BP, or posterosuperior prominence). PPL$_1$ is the baseline, tangential line to the anterior tubercle (A), and the medial tubercle (M) of posterior tuberosity; the perpendicular d is drawn between PPL$_1$ and the posterior lip of talar articular facet (T). The bursal projection (BP) touching or below PPL$_2$ is normal, not prominent.

tendinous calcification, the two halves of the Achilles tendon are reattached using a Mitek-GII™ bone/tissue anchor with Mersaline non-absorbable suture, or the newer Mitek Panaloc™ bone/tissue anchor with absorbable Panacryl suture. To reinforce the repair of the tendon, additional absorbable 2-0 Vicryl is used to reinforce the anchoring of the tendon to the bone.

There are many opinions as to how long the patient should be non-weight bearing postoperatively, and to what degree the ankle should be rested with immobilisation. This author finds the first week to be most important, and in this time the patient is placed in a non-weight-bearing, posterior, splint cast with the ankle at 90° or slight equinus, moving with the assistance of crutches. This is followed in the second week with a semi-weight-bearing fibreglass cast, with the ankle held at neutral position, again moving with crutch assistance. At the end of the second week the sutures are removed and the patient may have the fibreglass cast repeated or be advanced to a removable Cam walker cast boot. Physical therapy modalities similar to those used in repair of the Achilles are encouraged, with active/passive range of motion of the ankle beginning in the third to fourth week postoperatively.

With the advanced use of tissue anchors for securing the Achilles tendon, athletic patients can progress at a much faster rate than before to their preoperative status.

## Retrocalcaneal exostosis (Haglund's deformity)

This refers to a hypertrophy or prominent posterosuperior–lateral border of the calcaneus, secondary to chronic mechanical irritation of the shoe heel counter. As the gastrocnemius–soleus complex acts to decelerate the body as it moves forward over the foot during the propulsive phase of gait, the heel is in contact with the counter of the shoe. This friction and irritation will then lead to the formation of an exostosis. Other secondary biomechanical causes of a retrocalcaneal exostosis include a compensated rearfoot varus, cavo varus, and frequently a forefoot varus, creating a supinated heel strike, which can also lead to irritation of the posterosuperior shelf of the calcaneus. Other factors that contribute to the formation of an exostosis include the inclination angle of the calcaneus, which determines the volume of the posterosuperior aspect of the calcaneus involved in shoe contact. The pitch or degree of adduction of the calcaneus may contribute to the formation of the exostosis more laterally. Due to chronic irritation, as well as the formation of a bursa, a superficial Achilles tendon bursitis or retrocalcaneal bursitis can occur. In some cases, a hyperkeratotic lesion or, when severe, an intractable plantar keratoma lesion can develop over the retrocalcaneal bursa and exostosis.

Using a lateral weight-bearing radiograph the practitioner can evaluate and determine the retrocalcaneal bursal projection, either by posterior calcaneal angle (Fig. 13.21) or by parallel pitch lines (Fig. 13.22). Keck and Kelly (1965) observed that an increase in the parallel pitch lines, and not in abnormal posterior calcaneal angle, determined the degree of posterior heel bursitis. Ruch (1974) pointed out the mechanical function of the posterior calcaneal projection that occurs with ankle joint dorsiflexion, and drew particular attention to the direct relationship this has with an increased calcaneal inclination on the posterosuperior prominence. Fowler and Philip (1945) described another radiographic assessment to determine the posterior bursal projection. It consists of evaluating a superior calcaneal angle, the x angle (Fig.13.21), which is subtended by lines drawn from the bursal projection to the posterior tuberosity (AB), and from the medial calcaneal tuberosity to the anterior calcaneal tuberosity (CD). They regarded an angle of greater than 75° to be pathological; however, the angle does not take into consideration the relationship between the calcaneus and the sole of the foot. Pavlov et al (1981) also described another set of criteria for evaluating the shape and pitch of the calcaneus. They used both the Fowler and Philip posterior calcaneal angle and the parallel pitch lines (PPL) to determine the prominence of the bursal projection and the pitch angle (calcaneal inclination angle). They describe a *Haglund syndrome* on a radiograph as:

- positive parallel pitch lines (Fig 13.22)
- a cortically intact bursal projection
- loss of the retrocalcaneal recess, indicating a retrocalcaneal bursitis
- thickening of the Achilles tendon
- loss of the distinct interface between the Achilles tendon and the pre-Achilles fat pad, indicative of Achilles tendinitis.

The bursal sac contains a small amount of fluid. The normal retrocalcaneal bursa will accept 1–1.5 ml of fluid, and can be seen using bursography (Frey et al 1982). The chronic irritation, as previously described, will lead to an inflammation of the bursa, resulting in a thickening of the bursal wall, with effusion. The subcutaneous bursa is shaped like a horseshoe and is located between the skin and Achilles tendon. The purpose of the bursa is to protect the Achilles tendon and the underlying calcaneus from external pressures. Traction of the insertional region of the Achilles will also contribute to the calcification of the tendon, and with a vertically extended spur may be seen within the substance of the Achilles tendon, as it inserts into the calcaneus, leading to further inflammation of the bursa. This condition can lead to avulsions of the Achilles tendon and/or spur due to fractures and traction overloads. It is believed that the aetiology of retrocalcaneal exostosis or calcific tendinosis is age-related and due to overuse trauma, enthesopathy; it has a high occurrence rate (Fox et al 1975) (Fig. 13.23).

The development of a retrocalcaneal exostosis may be the result of a separate centre of ossification at the posterior angle of the calcaneum (Hoerr et al 1962). This independent ossification centre may be a small portion or fragment of the calcaneal apophysis and may grow separately from the calcaneal apophysis. Another possible aetiology involves traction apophysitis in adolescents. Repetitive traction of the Achilles tendon at its insertion to the calcaneal apophysis, combined

with a compensated rearfoot varus, and heel counter irritation due to sports activity, can contribute to the hypertrophy of the retrocalcaneal and posterosuperior regions of the calcaneus. Chronic irritation can cause further hypertrophy and exostosis formation in later years.

Conservative treatment for symptomatic retrocalcaneal exostosis, similar to the treatment for Achilles paratenonitis, will provide temporary relief. Treatment consists of padding the shoe counter, softening or eliminating the counter via open-back shoes, and inserting a one-quarter to three-eighths inch (6–9.5 mm) heel lift (intended to raise the heel prominence above the counter to reduce shoe counter pressure). The heel height of the shoe has an important influence upon symptoms (Henegham & Pavlov 1984). Raising the heel in the shoe helps to decrease the calcaneal inclination angle, which then alters the position of the bursal projection away from the heel counter. Other forms of conservative care include NSAIDs, particularly during the acute inflammatory phase, ice massage, where the symptoms manifest, and stretching exercises, with special attention to the hamstrings, gastrocnemius–soleus complex and Achilles tendon. Orthoses are particularly helpful in controlling the imbalance in the rearfoot and preventing irritation between the heel and counter. Runners are advised against speed work, to reduce mileage and to avoid hill training. Although local steroid injections are contraindicated, in cases where a retrocalcaneal bursa is present an injection of short-term corticosteroid combined with local anaesthetic can be utilised. The injection should be performed very cautiously, perhaps once, exercising caution to avoid injecting into the tendon (Subotnick & Vogler 1999b). As it is known that local steroid injections can lead to rupture of the Achilles tendon, the injection should be well placed within the bursa and never within the Achilles tendon or its insertion. Following the injection, physical therapy including nerve stimulation, ultrasound, superficial massage and, in lieu of an injection, iontophoresis can be performed two or three times a week for 3–4 weeks. The athlete, and in particular the runner, should be advised to avoid all running, jumping, skiing or any impact activity for at least 2–3 weeks following the injection. They are also advised to participate in cross-training activities that will not cause tension on the Achilles or irritation of the bursal area or retrocalcaneal exostosis. In some severe cases, cast immobilisation or a removable Cam walker cast is recommended. The advantage of the removable cast is that it may be removed daily for access to physical therapy. These conservative measures will prove successful in the majority of cases; however, when all conservative treatment has been exhausted and symptoms continue to plague the athlete's performance, surgical repair is recommended. The procedure may be performed either under general anaesthesia or under local anaesthetic with intravenous sedation. The procedure is similar to that performed for insertional tendinosis and calcific tendinitis. Postoperative care again parallels the previously described procedure.

## ANKLE INJURIES

Acute sprains to the ankle are one of the most common injuries seen by the practitioner. The lateral ankle complex is the most frequently injured anatomical structure in athletes, comprising 38–45% of all injuries (Garrich 1982). The incidence of inversion injuries has been estimated at 1 per 10 000 persons per day (Brooks et al 1981, McCullock et al 1985).

Ankle sprains contribute to one-sixth of the sports injury loss time (Garrich 1982, Garrich & Requa 1973). Ankle sprains consist of 85% of all ankle injuries, with 85% of them being inversion sprains of the lateral collateral ligaments (Baldwin & Tezlaff 1982). Eversion mechanism sprains involving the deltoid ligament or medial collateral

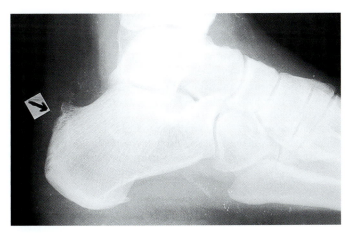

**Figure 13.23** Superior process exostosis calcinosis.

ligament constitute 5–6% of all ankle sprains, while syndesmosis injuries account for the remaining 10% (Baldwin & Tezlaff 1982). Frequently occurring ankle sprains can result from specific sport activity. The sports with the highest proportion of sprains at the ankle are volleyball with 82% and basketball 79%; football, racquetball and dance had more than 70%. Tennis, soccer and aerobic dance had more than 65% of the sprains reported. Sports with a lower frequency of ankle sprains were skiing, ballet and figure skating, each with less than 35%, and the sport with the fewest sprains among their ankle injuries was cycling, with 20% (Garrich & Requa 1988). There is no difference between men and women in the incidence of ankle sprains when comparing injuries sustained from engaging in similar activities (Garrich & Requa 1988). Recurring ankle sprains have always been a concern for the athlete. It has been shown that previous ankle sprains will create a higher potential for future injury (Glick et al 1976).

Many athletes will either ignore or self-treat the injury first, and seek attention only if the ankle continues to be swollen and painful and limits competitive participation. Many ankle injuries when seen are either undiagnosed, inadequately treated or, due to a lack of compliance, go on either to re-injury or chronic instability. Residual symptoms or recurrent sprains occurred in 42% of patients in one study (Bosien et al 1955). Ankle sprains in the athlete require proper and early diagnosis, as well as an extensive rehabilitation programme to return the athlete to his or her normal competitive status. Without such a treatment plan these injured ankles will be left weak and unstable and seriously subject to recurrent injury.

## Anatomy

Three major ligament groups provide the support for the ankle group: the superficial and deep portions of the deltoid ligament, the tibiofibular ligaments, and the lateral ligament complex. The lateral ankle ligament complex of the ankle consists of three individual ligaments: the anterior talofibular ligament (ATFL), the calcaneofibular ligament (CFL) and the posterior talofibular ligament (PTFL). The other support ligaments of the lateral ankle region are the lateral talocalcaneal ligament (LTCL), the ankle syndesmosis, with its ligaments, and the subtalar joint and its ligaments. The collateral ligaments of the ankle are arranged anatomically to afford joint dorsiflexion and plantar flexion, while concomitantly not restricting subtalar joint inversion or eversion. In addition to supporting and stabilising the ankle, allowing for sagittal plane dorsiflexion and plantar flexion, they aid in proprioception.

The ATFL is the most anterior ligament of the ankle. It consists of an upper and lower band and is intracapsular and intra-articular. It lies in a transverse plane crossing from the anteroinferior surface of the fibula to the body and neck of the talus just anterior to the lateral malleolar articular facet. The medial articular surface of the talus or medial facet articulates with the opposite medial facet of the medial malleolus. The lateral articular surface of the talus or triangular lateral talar facet articulates with the analogous lateral facet of the fibular malleolus. The dorsal surface of the talus is also known as the 'trochlear surface', and the inferior surface of the tibia, which articulates with the trochlear surface of the talus, is referred to as the 'tibial platform'. That space lying between the lateral articular surface of the talus and the medial articular surface of the fibular malleolus is referred to as the 'lateral gutter', and the opposite space between the medial malleolus and medial surface of the talus is called the 'medial gutter'.

The ATFL is a flat quadrangular ligament that is closely developed within the joint capsule, and is the most frequently injured of the three. The ATFL runs parallel to the long axis of the talus when the ankle is in neutral or dorsiflexion, but more perpendicular to the long

axis of the talus in equinus (Leonard 1949). This anatomical design leads to a very tight ligament throughout plantar flexion. The ATFL has been shown via biomechanical testing of the ankle ligaments to have the lowest yield force and ultimate load of the lateral collateral ligament complex (Siegler et al 1988). The ligaments are usually injured, with the anterior talofibular being first, followed by the CFL, and lastly the PTFL. The extent of the injury will depend on the level of plantar flexion and inversion forces, as well as the position of the ankle when the foot strikes the ground. In 20% of the population the ATFL is absent, leading to potential instability, and acute and recurrent sprains of the lateral ankle.

The CFL is a taut ligament that originates on the distal inferior surface of the fibula. It descends to an insertion on the tubercle of the lateral portion of the calcaneus. It inserts in a posteroinferior direction under the fibularis (peroneus) tendons. It lies in the sagittal plane approximately 90° inferior to the ATFL. The CFL is an extracapsular, round, cord-like structure that is finely attached to the joint capsule and to the medial surface of the fibular (peroneal) sheath. The ligament is separated from the joint capsule by a thin fatty layer. It possesses the highest elastic strength of the three collateral ligaments, having a higher yield force and ultimate load than the ATFL (Siegler et al 1988). The CFL crosses over the superior portion of the ankle as well as the subtalar joint, and lies perpendicular to the long axis of the talus when the ankle is in neutral or in dorsiflexion. The ATFL and CFL create an angle of 105° when the subtalar joint is in neutral position. The CFL has the greatest resistance to inversion, and in cases of inversion mechanism injury both the ligament and the attached fibularis (peroneus) tendon sheath will be involved.

The PTFL, the strongest of the three lateral collateral ankle ligaments, is the least commonly injured ligament. It is an intracapsular structure, is trapezoidal in shape, and originates proximally from the posterior aspect of the fibular malleolar fossa and attaches distally to the posterior surface of the talus, the lateral tubercle of the posterior process of the talus and to the os trigonum, when present. The PTL has the highest yield force and ultimate load of the three ligaments (Siegler et al 1988).

The lateral talocalcaneal ligament is a smaller ligament that crosses over the lateral aspect of the subtalar joint, and may also be torn in cases of inversion mechanism injuries of the ankle. Another important structure subject to injury is the syndesmosis, which consists of the anterior and posteroinferior tibiofibular ligaments, the interosseous ligament and the interosseous membrane. In external rotation injuries the syndesmosis is frequently injured. The syndesmosis is one of the initial structures to be damaged in either a supination eversion injury or a pronation eversion injury.

The ankle is most stable in dorsiflexion, allowing the talus to be securely locked in the ankle mortise while providing for additional stability against inversion stresses. When the ankle plantar flexes there is more anterior talar translation (drawer) and talar inversion (tilt) (Johnson & Markold 1983). Although the ATFL is the main talar stabiliser, when the ankle is in a plantar-flexed position the talus will be held less securely and will be more unstable in the ankle joint mortise. In this position the ATFL will be under greater tension and subject to higher risk of injury.

In addition to the ATFL being subject to higher loads with inversion and plantar flexion, the CFL may also be subject to injury during high loads in increased inversion. Occasionally, discrete tears in the CFL occur if the foot is forcefully dorsiflexed and inverted. The PTF rarely suffers from injury except in severe cases of total dislocation of the ankle joint. Brostrom (1964, 1966) showed that 20% of inversion ankle injuries involve both the ATFL and CFL.

Ankle ligament injuries may be classified into one of three grades according to pathology, function and instability:

- *Grade I.* A grade I ankle sprain is indicative of an injury in which the ATFL is stretched and some microscopic ligament fibres are torn, but no macroscopic ligament tears are present and the ankle joint is stable. Patients present with mild swelling, mild or no haemorrhage or ecchymosis along the lateral margin of the ankle, pin-point tenderness overlying the injured ligament, mildly restricted range of motion and possible inability to fully weight bear.

- *Grade II.* The grade II ankle sprain is a more moderate injury to the lateral collateral ligaments and consists of a definite complete tear of the ATFL, with a partial tear of the CFL and a mild to moderate ankle instability. Clinical examination reveals moderate swelling and tenderness along the anterolateral aspect of the ankle, restricted range of motion, haemorrhage, ecchymosis and mild instability.

- *Grade III.* The grade III sprain is a severe injury signified by complete rupture of both the ATFL, with capsular tear, and the CFL. Clinical findings reveal marked swelling, haemorrhage with severe ecchymosis along the lateral margin of the ankle and heel, and discrete tenderness overlying the ATFL, CFL and the anterolateral capsule. There will also be moderate to severe laxity of the ankle, with typical anterior drawer or talar inversion tilt demonstrated on testing, indicative of the instability of the joint.

Special tests can be performed to determine ankle instability (Fig. 13.24). The anterior drawer and talar tilt (inversion stress) tests are manual stress tests designed to evaluate the integrity of the ATF and CFL. The anterior drawer test is performed with the patient's knee flexed at least to 45° to relax the gastrocnemius. When patients extend the knee, this tends to alter the resistance to movement of the talus on the tibia. The patient's heel is grasped posteriorly and the tibia is stabilised anteriorly with the other hand. As the calcaneus is pulled forward, a posterior force is placed on the tibia. This will allow the practitioner to translate the foot forward at the tibiotalar joint. A positive anterior drawer will reveal a so-called 'suction sign' overlying the anterolateral aspect of the ankle (between the lateral margin of the fibula and the talar trochlea), with greater than 4 mm of anterior displacement when compared to the contralateral uninjured ankle. This reveals incompetence of the ATFL (Anderson et al 1952, Schon & Ouzounian 1991). The talar tilt test is performed by grasping the lateral aspect of the calcaneus with one hand, while the medial aspect of the tibia is stabilised with the other hand.

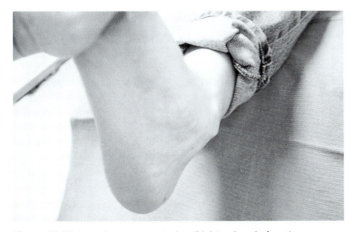

**Figure 13.24** Inversion stress posterior tibial tendon dysfunction.

## CASE STUDY 13.6

### LATERAL ANKLE INSTABILITY

A 28-year-old woman presented with a complaint of repeated right lateral ankle sprains and pain of several months duration. One month later she began describing pain along the medial aspect of her right arch and heel. The patient has had previous trauma to the right ankle, with a subsequent avulsion loose bone body of the medial malleolus.

The patient has been taking self-prescribed NSAIDs and applying ice to the ankle and arch/heel.

Temporary insoles were recommended with an NSAID and stretching exercises.

The patient wears Birkenstock sandals.

### PAST MEDICAL HISTORY

The patient had a history of asthma and ocular toxoplasmosis. Her past surgical history included anterior cruciate ligament repair in the right knee, septorhinoplasty, T&A.

*Injuries.* Fracture left arm at 4 years old, repeated ankle sprains over the years.

*Medicines.* Orthotricycline, over-the-counter NSAIDs, vitamins.

*Allergies.* None known.

*Social history.* Married, works as a cardiac rehabilitation exercise physiologist, does not smoke, no special diet.

*Family history.* Mother had hallux abducto valgus, diabetes, heart problems.

### TREATMENT PLAN

Two months after her initial visit the patient had a cast taken for Birkenstock inserts. The patient stated that her plantar fasciitis had improved but she continued to experience pain along the lateral aspect of her right ankle.

Four months later she still had recurrent pain to the plantar fascia and the abductor hallucis muscle, secondary to excessive pronation, and weakness of the longitudinal arch. She continued to have pain along the lateral column of the right foot in the area of the adductor digiti quinti.

A therapeutic steroid injection was given in the right heel.

Five months later she continued to have infracalcaneal heel pain in the right foot.

The injection was not very helpful, but a second injection was given with the addition of physiotherapy. A Cox-2 NSAID was prescribed, with ice treatment and stretching. The patient was told to cease all impact activity. She was about to leave on a vacation during which she would be walking often.

Six months after the initial visit the patient reported that the therapeutic steroid injection had been beneficial, but the pain had recurred and there seemed to be no improvement; however, compared to the first visit there was definite improvement.

On her vacation she walked excessively and now has significant pain and discomfort.

Physical therapy was given. The prescribed Cox-2 NSAID had not been effective, and the patient has begun to take over-the-counter NSAIDs. The patient was doing stretching exercises and applying ice, as well as receiving physiotherapy and cross-friction massage therapy.

An MRI scan was ordered to evaluate the ankle and heel; in addition, a night splint and neuromuscular stimulator were ordered. As a result of the review of the MRI a Cam-walker boot was ordered.

Seven months after the initial visit the patient continued to use the Cam-walker boot and continued to have infracalcaneal heel pain and ankle pain.

She continued to have physiotherapy treatment which seemed to produce a small improvement. Pain levels according to the therapist were 5/10, with a long gait, and right ankle plantar flexion was 4/5.

An attempt was made to increase strength, particularly with regard to right inversion and plantar flexion, and to improve prolonged standing and gait.

Seven and a half months after the initial visit the patient continued to have pain, which was increasing in severity and consistency. The patient had difficulty walking, with distinct pain in the right heel. A therapeutic steroid injection was attempted again (last of three).

Eight months after the initial visit the patient continued to have chronic plantar fasciitis, with no relief after exhaustive conservative care and physiotherapy. The patient had been cooperative, undertaking stretching, using ice, wearing orthotics, taking NSAIDs, and undergoing a series of three injections, with no improvement noted. Surgical intervention was recommended.

Nine months after the initial visit surgical correction was performed.

*Procedures.* Endoscopic plantar fasciotomy with decompression of the medial calcaneal nerve branch of the right heel. Arthroscopic evaluation of the right ankle. Partial synovectomy. Repair of the anterior talofibular ligament of the right ankle with Panaloc absorbable tissue anchor and Panacryl suture.

A below-knee fibreglass posterior splint cast was applied to the right leg.

### POSTOPERATIVE COURSE

One week after the operation the post-splint cast was removed. The area was re-dressed and the patient was fitted with a below-knee fibreglass non-weight-bearing cast.

Two weeks after the operation there the patient reported no pain and the cast and the sutures were removed. There was minimal oedema and no erythema. The limb was placed in a below-knee Cam-walker boot and a CPM machine was ordered. Physiotherapy was to commence in one week.

Two months after the operation the incision had healed well, and the scar overlying the anterior talofibular ligament repair was reduced. The incision overlying the right heel had completely healed, but had left some scar tissue thickness. As a consequence of this there was some compensating gait to the forefoot and the lateral side of the foot. It was recommended that the patient wear a running shoe with an ankle brace. The range of motion of the ankle has improved and lateral ankle stability has been restored. There was mild discomfort in the right heel and arch following the operation. There was no pain in the right ankle. The patient was able to resume work on light duties.

Three months after the operation the patient's gait was compensating, with a shortened heel strike, an extended forefoot contact phase, and to the lateral column. There was compensatory pain to the forefoot, along the fifth metatarsal head, and fifth metatarsal–cuboid joint.

A biomechanical evaluation was performed for a prescription sport orthotic device.

Heel pain has resolved and the scar is minimal.

The ankle is symptom free and is now stable.

With the ankle at 0° of dorsiflexion, the examiner inverts the calcaneus to its maximum. Under normal conditions, talus inversion is limited; however, when there is excessive excursion of the talus, the ATFL is suspected of rupture. Additional lateral dimpling is indicative of CFL injury or rupture. These tests should be performed with comparison with the contralateral side to rule out ligamentous laxity of an uninjured patient. In cases of acute injury local anaesthesia may be needed to perform the test adequately while preventing involuntary guarding by the patient.

Radiographic evaluation should be performed in addition to the anterior drawer and inversion talar tilt ankle joint stress views, and should include anteroposterior, lateral and mortise views of the ankle

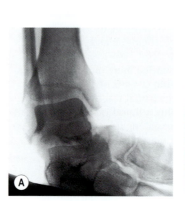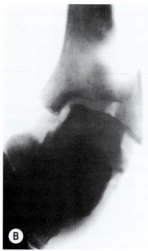

**Figure 13.25** (A) Talar tilt ankle instability; (B) talar tilt ankle instability with inversion stress applied.

joint (Fig. 13.25). A stress inversion of 5–10° or greater of the injured versus uninjured side is considered to be pathological. An inversion stress of 18° or greater between the two sides is indicative of a double ligamentous injury (Pearlman et al 1992).

Karlsson et al (1989) found that anterior translation of the talus of 10 mm and talar tilt of 9° or more reliably indicate mechanical instability. The anterior drawer and inversion stress tests afford only a value in degrees and not a clinical picture. Ankles that have ligamentous laxity, or have higher than normal numerical values may indeed be normal and not show clinical signs of instability. Therefore, the clinician should not hold these study values to be a substitute for further investigation, nor should they be an empirical determinant for surgical intervention. An injury that produces syndesmosis can be evaluated using an external rotation stress radiograph. Widening of the tibiofibular clear space on the anteroposterior and mortise views of more than 6 mm indicates diastasis (Harper & Keller 1980).

Additionally, the extensor retinaculum and periosteal structures may also be involved in lateral ankle sprains. Upon radiographic evaluation the practitioner may notice an avulsion or osteochondral fracture associated with an inversion sprain. An avulsion fracture of the posterior aspect of the distal tibia can also be a sign of an injury causing syndesmosis.

There are a number of other tests that can be performed to determine ligamentous injury and ankle instability. These include:

- Ankle arthrography, which radiographically reveals leakage of contrast dye from the lateral ankle joint and capsule. To obtain an accurate finding, this test should be performed within 48 hours of the injury to be truly effective. In addition, the exact location of the injury can also be determined. With rupture of the deltoid ligament, leakage of the dye will be inferior to the tip of the medial malleolus, radiating superiorly along the medial aspect of the ankle.
- Peroneal tenography, which can be used to determine injury to the CFL. As mentioned earlier, the CFL is closely attached to the fibres of the peroneus tendon sheath, so that rupture of the CFL will show contrast dye extravasated from the tendon sheath into the lateroposterior recess of the ankle joint.
- MRI examination, which has become the benchmark for non-invasive investigation of collateral ligament injury and instability. MRI can help to pinpoint specific soft-tissue injury

such as to the ligaments, capsuler or tendon, without exposing the patient to unnecessary radiation. MRI will determine the nature of both the medial or lateral ankle ligament injury by reflection of T1- and T2-weighted imaging. These studies will show oedema, haemorrhage, alteration of normal ligament contour (wavy) and interruption of ligament structure. A three-plane study can help to reveal rupture of the lateral collateral ligaments, deltoid ligament, peroneus or posterior tibial tendon. The clinician and radiologist can collaborate by using the history of the injury and MRI findings to determine the extent of the injury.

- CT scans can be used to determine osseous injuries to the ankle that may not be seen on a radiograph. One of the advantages of CT scans is their precise recreation of minute injuries, such as osteochondritis dissicans, small avulsion fractures and loose joint bodies (*joint mice*).
- Arthroscopic evaluation of the injured ankle may be used as another investigative as well as therapeutic tool. With arthroscopic visualisation, excision of small bone fragments, hypertrophied synovium, chronic synovitis and osteochondral defects, as well as repair of soft-tissue and bony impingement syndromes can be performed, rendering the patient free of ankle pain (Jarvin & Fercel 1994).

Initial conservative treatment for an acute lateral ankle injury, as well as chronic ankle instability, has proven to be most reliable. The focus of attention for the patient is on functional rehabilitation (range of motion, muscle strengthening and proprioceptive training). Specific areas of strengthening should include the fibular (peroneal) muscles, with stretching and flexibility of the Achilles and anterior tendon groups. Initial treatment should include rest, ice, compression and elevation (RICE), and NSAIDs. Initial conservative treatment may also include short-term cast or Cam walker immobilisation to allow the capsular and ligamentous structure to heal. On occasion, continued passive motion machine (CPM) treatment may help to restore the range of motion in the sagittal plane. High-top athletic shoes, taping before sporting events, air splints, ankle braces and orthoses may all aid in the prevention of recurrent ankle injury. Sports that involve side-to-side movement may predispose to recurrent injury, and thus may force the participant to cross-train during the rehabilitation programme (Box 13.7).

In some cases the athlete may experience residual pain and swelling for 6 weeks after the initial sprain due to injury of the ligaments and inflammation of the ankle joint. Pain on palpation may be elicited overlying the ATFL, sinus tarsi and CFL. Inversion of the subtalar joint may also elicit pain. In severe ankle sprains, ankle ligaments may not heal properly, there may be malalignment of the ankle joint, capsular tissues may heal with fibrosis and scarring, with associated hypertrophied synovitis. Chronic lateral ankle instability with recurrent sprain in the athlete is estimated to develop in approximately 20% of the injuries, regardless of the treatment (Moller-Larsen et al 1988, Rijke et al 1988). The athlete who suffers from chronic lateral ankle instability is subject to chronic pain, swelling, inflammation, recurrent injury and reduced functional stability of the ankle. Subotnick (1999c) states that this, in turn, creates a psychological fear of re-injury, impairing maximum performance as well as causing loss of training time. If, after investigative studies have been performed and exhaustive conservative care has been rendered, recurrent injury prevails and performance is hindered, surgical repair of the athlete's unstable ankle may be required.

Surgical repair for chronic lateral ankle instability can be classified as either reparative or reconstructive. Reparative procedures involve re-establishing damaged ligamentous structures, whereas reconstructive procedures involve re-routing harvested tendons or grafts

---

### Box 13.7 Ankle sprains: treatment

#### Initial visit

- History, mechanism of injury, determine severity of injury: radiographs if fracture is suspected – fifth metatarsal base, beak of calcaneus, os trigonum, fibular neck, fibular and tibial malleolus
- Galvanic nerve stimulation if acute injury or swelling
- Contrast foot baths, ultrasound if chronic swelling
- Compression stocking or Unna boot for acute injury with surgical shoe
- Ankle brace, air splint, or Cam walker removable cast for more severe ankle injuries
- Weight bearing as tolerated, with crutches if able to be performed

#### Second visit

- Continue contrast footbaths, Unna boot with compression wrap
- Increase range of motion – therabands, towel
- Continue physical therapy – nerve stimulation, ultrasound and iontophoresis – if swelling is present
- Begin stretching exercises, Achilles, gastrocnemius–soleus, hamstrings, anterior groups
- Gait analysis – check for compensation (correct when seen)
- Check lateral shoe wear or lateral distortion of heel counter
- When swelling is reduced, test for ankle instability (inversion stress, anterior drawer) and ankle strength

#### Third visit

- Begin ankle strengthening (progressive programme) – fibularis (peroneus) and posterior tibial muscles
- Increase ankle joint range of motion
- Continue contrast footbaths
- Continue physical therapy – nerve stimulation, ultrasound
- Start toe raises, comparing affected and unaffected sides
- Ankle strapping if needed

#### Fourth visit

- Progressive ankle strengthening – fibularis (peroneus) muscles
- Continue contrast footbaths, stretching range of motion
- Teach strapping technique to patient
- Encourage wearing of high-top athletic shoes, ankle brace, ankle strapping
- Fabricate orthoses for biomechanical imbalances – rearfoot and forefoot varus
- Begin proprioceptive exercises – roller-beam, side-to-side running, cutting drills

#### Subsequent visits

- Test ankle strength
- If chronic recurrent sprain, repeat ankle stress tests and order MRI evaluation
- If ankle instability continues to be present consider stabilisation procedure

---

to substitute for failed ligaments (Schon & Ouzounian 1991). Reconstructive procedures can be divided according to the number of ligaments being strengthened. Single-ligament reconstruction will involve the ATFL, whereas double-ligament reconstruction (which is performed to correct anterolateral rotary instability) reconstructs the ATFL and CFL; a triple-ligament reconstruction rebuilds all three lateral collateral ligaments. Many surgical procedures have been described for repair of lateral ankle instability. The Brostrom (1965) procedure is one of the most popular, involving periosteal augmentation flaps to repair stretched out or torn ATF and CF ligaments. This repair is performed without fibularis (peroneus) tendon or other tissue harvesting, thus minimising surrounding ankle tissue damage while reconstructing the ligaments in their true physiological orientation.

Arthroscopic surgical repair of ruptured lateral collateral ankle ligaments with the use of soft-tissue anchors has been a significant advance in the treatment of chronic instability in the athlete. Although technically more difficult to perform than the open stabilisation procedures, this procedure has negated the need for tendon harvesting, minimises the disturbance of adjacent soft-tissue structures and enhances recovery by reducing recovery time. For the athlete, all these are very important factors.

This author is quite aggressive with the postoperative treatment of these delayed primary ligament repairs. Initially, a Jones compression dressing with a posterior splint is utilised to hold the foot and ankle in 0° ankle joint dorsiflexion to provide stability and control immediate postoperative oedema. Seven days postoperatively the patient returns for the first dressing change, and the splint is replaced by either a fibreglass cast or removable cast brace. The advantage of the cast brace is that it allows for gentle CPM to begin at 7–10 days postoperatively. This motion helps to prevent the occurrence of postoperative adhesions, capsulardesis and reduced ankle joint range. The Cam walker is worn for 4–6 weeks postoperatively, followed by a more aggressive physical therapy programme involving muscle strengthening, flexibility and proprioception exercises. After 2–3 months the patient is allowed to slowly return to activities. An ankle brace and orthoses are highly recommended to initially provide for additional lateral support and to help improve early restoration of proprioception.

# LEG INJURIES

## Chronic leg pain in the athlete

Chronic sports-related leg pain is a problem that many athletes experience. In the past, chronic lower leg pain was often regarded as 'shin splints' and recognised as an overuse injury due to excessive training or competitive-level participation. Today, the sports medicine specialist can target the underlying aetiology behind the development of the lower leg pain and determine the precise diagnosis. The goals for the specialist are specific: early and accurate diagnosis, a proper treatment plan, a specific rehabilitation programme, and prevention of recurrent injury.

There are many origins of sports-related lower leg pain. Tissues such as bone, muscle, tendon or insertion, ligament, nerves, arteries, veins and even skin can be the source of lower leg pain. The pain can be classified as traumatic or atraumatic in origin. Atraumatic exercise-induced injuries include medial tibial stress syndrome, stress fractures, gastrocnemius–soleus muscle strains, iliotibial band friction syndrome, tendinitis; compression syndromes (e.g. chronic compartment syndrome, nerve entrapment syndromes (fibularis (peroneus), tibial, popliteal)), arterial occlusion (popliteal artery syndrome) and radiculopathies, and muscle–fascial injuries, including fascial herniations, muscle soreness and muscle cramps. A number of authors have evaluated these conditions and have shown that a significant number of sufferers are athletes, particularly runners (Clanton & Schon 1993, Jones & Jones 1987, Orava & Puranen 1979, Styf 1989).

## Tibial fasciitis – shin splints

Tibial fasciitis is an overuse inflammatory condition localised to the posteromedial crest of the tibia, with occasional involvement of the anterior crest of the tibia. Among runners and other athletes. This has been shown to be the most common cause of lower leg pain among runners and other athletes (Clanton & Schon 1993).

Tibial fasciitis is commonly referred to as posterior and anterior shin splints (Siocum 1967). The syndrome has been recognised as a medial tibial stress syndrome, resulting from overuse of the soleus fascia as it inserts on the posteromedial crest of the tibia, or the periosteal tissue beneath the posterior tibial muscle. Medial tibial stress syndrome may be due to either periostitis of the tibia or insertional fasciitis of the posterior tibial or soleus muscle; however, the clinician must exclude other possible entities, such as muscle strain of those same muscles, tibial stress fracture, deep posterior compartment syndrome and direct blunt injury to the muscle or bone. Detner (1986) developed a classification and management system for medial stress syndrome, dividing the overuse injury into three categories:

- *Type I* represents a stress fracture or stress reaction of bone.
- *Type II* identifies a chronic periosteal reaction due to excessive pulling of the soleus fascia.
- *Type III* is associated with posterior tibial or posterior compartment syndrome. This is often seen with running as well as jumping sports.

Medial tibial stress syndrome (MTSS) is due to overuse or beginning an exercise programme too vigorously. There has been general agreement that certain underlying biomechanical factors contribute to the development of MTSS. Excessive pronation of the foot, as well as exercising on hard surfaces, may enhance eccentric contractions of leg muscles and contribute to the development of MTSS (Michael & Holder 1977, Richie et al 1993, Vitasalo & Kvist 1983). For runners who are excessive pronators, prolonged muscle strain and fatigue will develop. As pronation increases due to elongation of the running gait cycle, there will be a need for increased supination by the posterior tibial tendon. In the shin splint syndrome, abnormal pronation will lead to fatigue of the muscles and reduce shock absorption. With traction enthesopathy along the lower third of the tibia, pain will develop due to the periostitis at the muscle attachment. This will create increased pressure on the fascia by the tendon unit, focused on the fascia–periosteum interface along the tibial crest. Impact shock transmits with every running or jumping step that is taken. These 'shock waves' are transmitted along the tibia, interfering with healing of the 'stress reaction' along the fascia–periosteum attachment. This will lead to further injury of reparative bone cells, and prevent remodelling of damaged bone. Without adequate rest time the process continues, and can worsen to the point where a stress fracture may occur.

The duration of symptoms can be divided into:

- less than 2 weeks (acute)
- 2–6 weeks (subacute)
- more than 6 weeks (chronic).

The location of the symptoms is divided into posteromedial, anterior and combination. The severity of the symptoms uses the functional pain scale grades 1 to 4:

- *Grade 1* represents pain upon palpation of the medial tibial crest, with no pain during activity or running.
- *Grade 2* is indicative of pain or discomfort after activity or running, but not during activity or running.
- *Grade 3* reveals pain both during running and residual discomfort after -activity or running.
- *Grade 4* demonstrates pain and discomfort while engaged in simple walking and the patient will be unable to run without symptoms.

Participants will describe recurrent pain along the posteromedial border of the middle and distal third of the tibia, which will have a gradual onset and is exacerbated by activity and running and relieved by rest. There will be no pain or symptoms in the foot or ankle. Mild swelling may be present. Physical examination reveals pain upon palpation along the posteromedial border and to a lesser degree along the anterior margin of the tibia.

The pain can range in severity from a dull ache to severe pain, particularly with prolonged activity. Neurovascular status is unaffected by MTSS.

Radiographic findings are usually negative for MTSS, except for mild localised thickening of the cortex. On occasion, the clinician may want to order a triphasic bone scan to differentiate between a simple shin splint and a stress fracture. Bone scans normally will reveal localised periostitis. Occasionally, MRI evaluation may help to pinpoint the exact location of the injury.

## Treatment

In the majority of cases of MTSS early conservative treatment will lead to a successful outcome. All sporting activity should be ceased immediately, accompanied by icing, immobilisation and, if necessary, NSAIDs. The patient is advised not to resume activity until they walk without pain.

A four-phase treatment programme is recommended for patients suffering from MTSS:

- *Phase 1*, the acute phase, is directed towards decreasing pain and inflammation. The treatment as described above is designed during the acute phase, and can last days to weeks.
- *Phase 2*, the rehabilitation phase, is focused on decreasing the pain and swelling even further, while attempting to decrease or prevent the formation of scar tissue, strengthen the deep fascia–bone interface, and maintain flexibility of surrounding soft-tissue structures. Deep compartment muscle exercise can help to strengthen the deep fascia–bone interface, while reducing the tension force to the deep facial insertion.
- *Phase 3*, the functional phase, is designed to strengthen the fascia–bone interface and to prevent the tibia from experiencing excessive tension forces. This may be accomplished via the use of orthotics, strapping and taping, as well as the use of neoprene sleeves.
- *Phase 4*, the return-to-activity phase, is aimed at returning the athlete to his or her desired sport and level of participation.

The clinician should consult with the athlete as to the preventative measures that should be taken to protect them from further injury. This prevention programme can be designed by:

- evaluating the patient biomechanically and observing their running gait
- assistance in proper shoe selection
- creating a strengthening programme for weak muscle groups
- establishing flexibility and a stretching programme with the aim of improving range of motion in joints
- following a reasonable training programme that is consistent with the athlete's physical abilities and goals.

Box 13.8 suggests a treatment regimen for shin splints.

## Stress fracture of the tibia and fibula

Stress fractures or fatigue fractures of the tibia and fibula are frequently seen in runners (Colt & Spyropoulos 1979, McBryde 1985, Markey 1987, Shelbourne et al 1988). The tibia is the bone most commonly involved (Belken 1980, Bennell et al 1996, Morris & Blickenstaff 1967). Morris and Blickenstaff (1967) used the term *fatigue fracture*

---

### Box 13.8 Shin splints: treatment

**Initial visit**

- Ice massage to painful shin areas
- Radiograph, if chronic swelling
- Neoprene shin sleeve
- Biomechanical evaluation with gait analysis if not painful
- Athletic shoe evaluation
- Antipronation shoe selection if a runner
- Varus heel wedge or temporary insole support
- Ankle strapping, muscle strengthening exercises for rearfoot invertors
- Rest with cross-training to avoid pain and further injury

**Second visit**

- Two weeks of physical therapy – ultrasound, iontophoresis if needed
- Radiographic evaluation if a stress fracture is suspected
- Flexibility and strengthening home exercises
- Consider functional orthoses if excessive subtalar joint pronation is noted
- Continue to rest and cross-train (non-impact activities)
- NSAIDs
- Ice massage with neoprene shin sleeve

**Third visit**

- Dispense functional foot orthoses
- Continue physical therapy modalities to help reduce pain, inflammation and swelling
- Re-test muscle strength and consider manual resistance exercises, isotonic exercises to increase strength, and eccentric (plyometric) exercises to improve speed work
- Order technetium-99m or triphasic bone scan to rule out stress fracture
- If pain continues, consider walking with crutches with a Cam walker removable cast
- Cross-training (swimming, water running, stationary bicycle)

**Fourth visit**

- If pain continues, consider possible compartment syndrome
- Repeat bone scan and evaluate radioactive uptake pattern
- Check to ensure functional foot orthoses are properly controlling excessive pronation and abnormal motion with current shoes
- Evaluate shoes and consider alternative shoe recommendation
- Consider non-weight-bearing Cam walker or cast immobilisation and walking with crutches

**Fifth visit**

- If pain continues, consider test for compartment syndrome
- If test is positive, consider surgical intervention with fasciotomy
- If bone continues to be negative, continue prolonged rest
- Continue to treat any signs of pain, swelling and tenderness with physical therapy modalities
- Check to see what cross-training activities are being followed and if patient is compliant
- If bone scan is positive, non-weight-bearing cast immobilisation and walking with crutches should be employed

to describe the application of mild forces or stress with eventual alteration or disruption of a material, such as bone. Therefore, a stress fracture is not the result of a single occurrence but rather an ongoing process. A fracture may be the end result, but it is the product of continued applied forces on the bone creating a weakness by resorbing bone in advance of the laying down of new bone. Stress fractures have been described in many sports (Morris & Blickenstaff 1967, Orava 1980a, Radel et al 1992).

There have been a number of explanations for the development of stress fractures. The first hypothesis (Stanitski et al 1978) contends that stress overload causes muscle fatigue, creating a loss in shock absorption and allowing excessive forces to be transmitted to the underlying bone. The second hypothesis (Taunton et al 1981) states that stress fractures occur secondary to repeated muscular forces acting on the bone. Cortical and cancellous bone each have intrinsic properties. When a force, either compressive or tensile, is applied to the bone, stress is generated within the bone. Strain is then produced by a relative change in length. The stress–strain relationship is linear until the yield length is reached. The linear portion represents the elasticity of the bone, whereas beyond the yield strength the bone is irreversibly deformed, until it reaches the breaking point. It is at that point that the bone collapses in compression and separates in tension. A stress or fatigue fracture can occur due to repetitive small loads, or from a single large load. During these load cycles, microfractures develop that are transmitted through the bone until loads increase sufficiently to cause microstress fractures, which produce symptoms or a fracture. Compression, tension and rotation are some of the forces applied to the bones by other bones, ligaments, and muscle origins and insertions. An example of this principle was shown by Devas and Sweetnam (1956) who showed that stress fractures of the fibula are due to the contraction of the calf muscles that pull the fibula toward the tibia. In this case, the tension above the distal fibula is maximised due to a rigidly attached fibular malleolus.

Wolff's law prescribes that bone remodels to the stress placed upon it in fairly predictable patterns. When osteoclastic activity outweighs osteoblastic activity, the bone is in a weakened state. An athlete who continues to exercise is at higher risk of developing a stress fracture until bone remodelling is complete. Complete cessation of all athletic activity is essential to allow the bone to remodel and thus be able to withstand stress that will be applied at a later time. Markey (1987) described two 'phases' of stress fractures. The first phase, characterised by osteoclastic activity, and radiographically noted by its rarefaction or lucency, is referred to as the *fracture phase*. The second phase, described as the *healing phase*, is shown radiographically to have increased sclerosis, cortical thickening and/or callus formation. Another term used to describe the response of bone remodelling to stress prior to stress fracture is a *stress reaction* (Jones et al 1989).

Stress fracture of the tibia may occur either at the medial plateau or the shaft. Approximately half of all stress fractures in athletes occur in the shaft of the tibia (Morris & Blickenstaff 1967). In ballet dancers, the middle third of the tibia is involved (Miller et al 1975) and in runners the area most frequently affected is the middle and distal thirds of the tibial shaft (Devas 1958, Devas & Sweetnam 1956). Stress fractures may also occur at the medial malleolus due to distance running or basketball or American football (Shelbourne et al 1988).

Stress fractures of the fibula generally occur in the lower third of the bone (Barrows 1940, 1948, Devas & Sweetnam 1956). Stress fractures are also seen in the proximal third of the fibula (Blair & Manley 1980), and are thought to occur as a result of the powerful muscle forces of the soleus, posterior tibial, fibular (peroneal) or flexor hallucis longus across the fibula during jumping exercise (Symeonides 1980).

Usually the athlete will describe a significant change or increase in their workout schedule. For the runner, this will be demonstrated by a sudden increase in mileage, inadequate footwear or change of shoes, downhill running, harder running surfaces or greater intensity (speed).

The athlete may have just resumed a training programme after injury, or be unprepared at the commencement of a new training programme. There is a gradual, onset of pain that develops over several weeks. The pain will usually begin after stressful activity and then recede upon rest. In runners, pain will usually be described as occurring towards the end of the run, with the intensity increasing and ultimately reaching a point where the pain becomes so severe that the athlete has to cease running. With rest, the runner will ordinarily experience relief; however, on the resumption of running the pain will reoccur, to the point where it occurs during everyday walking. The key for the clinician is to recognise the onset of a stress fracture and advise the athlete to refrain from all activity, otherwise a return to training or competition could result in a season-ending injury.

Physical examination will reveal an area of well-localised tenderness overlying the tibia or fibula. There will be pain on palpation, percussion pain, increased warmth, oedema or erythema. The patient will be unable to perform the one-legged hopping test without pain, and when treated with ultrasound the pain will be elicited.

Initially after injury, radiographs will be negative; however, after 2–3 weeks of symptoms subtle changes may be evident. These changes will include a periosteal reaction, denoted by a cortical radiolucency indicating bone resorption, followed by an increase in radiodensity, indicating cortical bone formation and thickening. A technetium-99m bone scan is most helpful when plain radiographic films are negative and the clinician suspects a stress fracture. In cases of stress fracture there will be an increased local uptake of contrast medium, which can stay positive for over a year despite the fact that healing has taken place. A triphasic or triple-phase bone scan can offer additional insight into the nature of the injury – whether it is a soft-tissue injury or a fracture, or an acute or chronic injury (Rupani et al 1985).

Treatment includes rest for at least 6–8 weeks, and if severe and chronic, 12 weeks may be necessary to allow for adequate bone healing and to prevent further injury. With rest, symptoms will resolve, and substitute cross-training activities are recommended. In the case of competitive athletes, prolonged cast immobilisation and walking with crutches may be required. On occasion, for a delayed healing fracture or malunion, pulsating electromagnetic fields (bone stimulation) may be employed to accelerate the bone-healing process (Rettig et al 1988). After a sufficient period of rest the participant can then proceed to a period of supervised rehabilitation. Again, it is essential that the clinician emphasise to the athlete the consequences of too early a return to weight-bearing activities. A slow, progressive return to full-impact activity is advised, with periods of rest or cross-training to allow for adequate recovery. The type and location of the fracture will help to determine the length of time before return to competition. For some anterior midtibia fractures an entire year of non-impact activity may be required before a return to full competition standard (Clanton & Solcher 1994). The athlete is not encouraged to return to activity until they have no symptoms of tenderness, and have achieved full range of motion and near-normal strength from their rehabilitation programme. A semirigid pneumatic-type tibial brace that allows the athlete a speedier return to competition than conventional treatment has been used, and continues to be scrutinised (Box 13.9).

The more serious anterior midshaft tibia stress fracture initially described by Burrows (1956) commonly goes on to delayed or non-union (Green et al 1985, Rettig et al 1988) and may go on to complete fracture (Brahms et al 1980). Conservative treatment for this extreme case may prove difficult and may require surgical excision, with bone grafting, as well as percutaneous drilling and/or intramedullary rodding (Barrick & Jackson 1992).

## Box 13.9 Tibial stress fractures: treatment

### Initial visit

- Radiographic evaluation if pain has been present for 2–3 weeks
- Technetium-99m or triphasic bone scan if radiographs are inconclusive, suspicion of fracture, or pain present less than 2 weeks
- Check athletic shoes for wear pattern and shock absorption
- Stop all running and all impact activity; rest for 2–3 months to allow fracture to heal
- Local physical therapy techniques to help reduce swelling and muscle soreness during rest
- Flexibility and range of motion exercises
- Cross-training activities (swimming, water-running, stationary bicycle) to maintain training effect
- Perform gait analysis if patient is able to perform without pain
- Make a return appointment when the patient has been pain-free for at least 2 weeks to re-evaluate the condition and to analyse possible biomechanical aetiology that will cause inadequate shock absorption

### Second visit

- Biomechanical evaluation – check for poor mechanics and for inadequate shock absorption
- Recommend shoes with better shock absorption and antipronation control
- Check bone scan results, if performed
- Consider Spenco, Sorbothane or Superfeet insoles for increased padding in shoes
- Continue non-impact cross-training activity if patient is pain free
- Outline gradual return to activity programme if patient is pain free
- Have runner patients refrain from all uphill and downhill running and interval training, reduce mileage and choose proper athletic shoes
- Continue physical therapy if any swelling or tenderness is present
- If pain returns with activity, or patient is unable to perform one-legged hopping test, arrange for follow-up appointment

### Third visit

- Repeat radiograph to see if tibial or fibular stress fracture is not healing
- Check for *dreaded black line*
- Consider other sources of pain – compartment syndrome, shin splints, muscle strain, fibular (peroneal) nerve entrapment
- Continue physical therapy programme if pain persists
- If fracture is seen, cast immobilisation with non-weight-bearing walking with crutches
- Treat the localised tenderness and swelling, and when asymptomatic begin return to walk/run programme
- If pain persists with return to exercise activity, arrange for follow-up visit

### Fourth visit

- Consider testing for compartment syndrome
- Consider repeat of the technetium-99m or triphasic bone scan and evaluate for fracture or delayed union
- Consider possible radiculopathy with pain referred from lower back
- Consider prolonged period of rest with non-impact activities

The key to success for the athlete is prevention. Recognising the aetiological factors that would lead to this type of injury is essential – for instance, biomechanical considerations (leg-length discrepancy, high tibial varum, tibial torsion, excessive pronation or cavus foot type), muscle imbalances, distorted, worn-out athletic shoes, and inappropriate training programmes should all be evaluated.

## CASE STUDY 13.7

### TIBIAL STRESS FRACTURE

A 29-year-old female runner presented with shin splint pain of 2 years duration. In addition, she had an iliotibial band injury 6 months ago from running. She has been running for about 2 years and started training for marathons. She saw a podiatrist for this problem about 2 years ago and had prescription orthotics made. These helped but did not resolve the condition completely, and she continued to have posterior shin splint pain.

She stated that she could run up to 7 miles without pain, but over that distance the onset of pain begins. Physical therapy has been attempted in the past, along with a strengthening programme for weak anterior group muscles. During her gym workouts she noticed no significant improvement. She ran in a half-marathon, but states that she could hardly walk or run after she completed the race.

### X-RAY ANALYSIS

Anteroposterior and lateral weight-bearing radiographs of both feet revealed pronation of the subtalar joint, bilateral adduction of the talus with accessory navicular bones, bilateral varus rotation of the fifth digits, bilateral mild metatarsus primus elevatus, and bilateral midtarsal joint prolapse.

### BIOMECHANICAL EVALUATION AND GAIT ANALYSIS

Barefooted and running gait analysis revealed right foot abduction, excessive subtalar and midtarsal joint pronation, right foot > left foot, and an abductory twist in the right foot.

### TREATMENT PLAN

Improve existing orthotic devices by refurbishing and increasing rearfoot posting correction.

Technetium-99m bone scan to rule out a stress fracture along the medial posterior aspect of the tibial crest.

Vioxx 25 mg once daily with food was prescribed, together with icing, stretching exercises and rest from running.

Repeated technetium-99m bone scan in 3 months.

## Acute and chronic compartment syndrome

Chronic compartment syndrome (CCS), less common than the acute compartment syndrome (ACS), can sometimes be confusing and make the diagnosis rather difficult. CCS is a condition that results from abnormally high intramuscular pressure during exercise or shortly afterwards. It may also be defined as a condition in which increased pressure within a limited anatomical space compromises the circulation and function of the tissues within that space, resulting in temporary or permanent damage to muscles and nerves (Matson 1975). ACS is generally secondary to trauma, although rarely it may develop due to vigorous exercise. CCS is an exercise-induced condition, with recurring symptoms when exercise is resumed and reduced symptoms when exercise is ceased. In a study by Detner (1986) of the 100 consecutive operative cases of CCS approximately 70% involved runners.

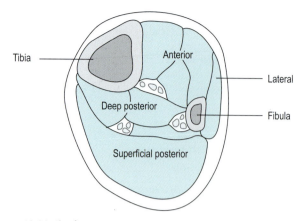

Figure 13.26 The four compartments of the leg.

## Anatomy

The leg is divided into four compartments: the anterior, lateral, deep posterior and superficial posterior (Fig. 13.26). Each compartment is separated from the others by osseous and fascial boundaries, except for the superficial posterior compartment, which has no osseous boundary and is separated only by fascia. The nerves, blood vessels and muscles are encased in compartments surrounded by non-stretch structures. The anterior compartment fascia extends from the anterior fibular (peroneal) septa and encompasses the anterior crest of the tibia. The deep posterior compartment fascia inserts into the postero-medial crest of the tibia and generally intersects the deep transverse fascia, soleus fascia and superficial posterior compartment fascia to form the intermuscular septum.

Everyday activity will result in an increase in capillary filtration to supply much-needed blood to the muscles. The muscles consequently will expand by 20–25% of their normal resting volume. Anteriorly, the crural fascia can expand to permit this increase in tissue volume. Compartment syndrome is caused by an increase in tissue pressure to a critical level, resulting in compromised tissue perfusion (Ashton 1975, Matson 1975). Physiologically, circulation to the microvasculature is impeded, creating a compromised condition of the intra-compartmental musculature. Intracellular and extracellular fluid accumulation within the fascial space occurs. Venous and lymphatic compromise contributes to increased tissue pressure, creating further vascular compromise.

The typical history of the athlete with CCS is one of induced pain during exercise, or immediately upon conclusion of exercise, overlying the involved compartment. Pain will dramatically decline upon rest in the early stages. An aching or cramping pain will be described, even during simple walking. In the runner, however, pain will develop after a certain distance, time or intensity. Other symptoms may include shooting pains and leg weakness, with an inability to dorsiflex the foot (foot-drop), numbness and tingling to the leg, dorsum and plantar aspect of the foot, burning of the compartmental nerve, pain upon stretching of the involved muscles or tendons, a lump formation, or muscle herniation of the leg. Four nerves, each with sensory components, are present within the four lower leg compartments. It is rare to see all four compartments affected simultaneously but it is common to see bilateral involvement. The two compartments most commonly involved are the anterior and deep posterior compartments. Rorabeck (1986) postulated that compartment syndrome of the tibialis posterior could be regarded as a fifth compartment. With signs and symptoms of compressive neuropathy of the superficial and/or deep fibular (peroneal) nerves, the clinician should pay particular attention to those compartments. Muscle herniations through

fascial defects have been found at a higher rate in compartment syndrome patients (approximately 30–60%) and can be a source of chronic pain with or without related nerve entrapment or compartment syndrome (Clanton & Schon 1993).

Radiographic evaluation is helpful to rule out other conditions that may be present, such as stress fractures, periostitis, occult bone tumours or acute trauma. MRI is advantageous because it provides a non-invasive means of assessing intracompartmental pressures simultaneously in all compartments (Amendola et al 1990). Another entity that may mimic a chronic compartment syndrome is intermittent claudication, which refers to a complex of symptoms characterised by pain in the muscles of the lower extremity with exercise; therefore, vascular examination may be required to rule out arterial insufficiency to that limb.

The diagnosis of CCS is first made on clinical evidence; however, measuring the intracompartmental pressure provides reproducible, objective documentation that is needed to confirm the diagnosis of CCS. There are four requisites necessary before the diagnosis of compartment syndrome can be made:

- a limiting anatomical envelope
- an increase in tissue pressure
- compromised circulation
- neuromuscular dysfunction.

There are a number of measuring systems that can be used to record pressures at rest, before and after exercise, and during exercise. They include the needle manometer, wick catheter, Rorabeck's slit catheter and McDermott's solid state transducer intracompartmental (STIC) catheter (for dynamic measurement of intracompartmental pressure) (Detner et al 1985, Mibarak 1981, Pedowitz et al 1990). CCS has also been described as an exertional compartment syndrome. Mibarak (1981) and Pedowitz et al (1990) developed criteria for the diagnosis utilising the wick catheter measurement of compartment pressure as follows. Utilising a wick or slit catheter technique under sterile conditions, the catheter is inserted into the involved compartment using local anaesthesia, and compartment pressures are then monitored at rest and during exercise. The presence of the catheter creates an exercise environment that produces pain, and eventually causes the subject to stop the exercise. Three pressures are recorded: the resting pressure, the pressure during exercise and the pressure after exercise – (1) pre-exercise pressure greater than 15 mmHg, (2) 1 minute post-exercise pressure greater than 30 mmHg, (3) 5 minutes post-exercise pressure greater than 20 mmHg. After 5 minutes the pressure levels should return to their pre-exercise levels. Levels can be monitored and, if the pressure exceeds the resting value by two times during exercise, a diagnosis of recurrent compartment (ACS or CCS) syndrome can be made.

If the ACS or CCS is confirmed, the goals of the athlete must be considered. If the athlete can reduce activities to a tolerable symptom level, surgery is not indicated. Conservative measures at this point are of little benefit, and the treatment indicated is surgical decompression by means of a fasciotomy of the involved compartment. The athletic patient should be thoroughly informed that they are at risk of developing an acute exertional compartment syndrome and that surgery has its inherent risks. Adequate decompression of the involved compartment is essential, without injury to the neurovascular structures or muscles below. Surgical decompressive fasciotomy has a 90% probability of producing significant improvement in or resolution of the symptoms (Martins et al 1984, Rorabeck et al 1988, Styf 1988). After fasciotomy there can be a decrease in strength by up to 20% of the compartment's muscles (Garfin et al 1981, Mozan & Keagy 1969). The trade-off is that muscle weakness is usually offset by the tremendous pain relief and improved performance that the athlete will later achieve.

## Muscle soreness

There are a number of additional lower leg problems that are exercise-induced. They do not fit into the category of overuse injuries or claudication syndromes; however, they have just as important an effect on the athlete. They include muscle soreness or *delayed-onset muscle soreness* (DOMS) (Armstrong 1984). Symptoms of DOMS usually increase in intensity within the first 24 hours after exercise, and peak at 24–72 hours, and subside over the next few days. DOMS can result from an overexertion of skeletal muscles, and although many people may experience DOMS, few ever seek medical attention.

## Muscle cramps

Muscle cramps may occur in both the athlete and non-athlete alike. With muscle cramps, there is pain, a tightening of the muscle group, or both. Cramp is usually due to muscle fatigue, and the accumulation of metabolites during strenuous exercise, such as marathon running, triathlon swimming, cycling or running, or any other sport that involves prolonged muscle use or intensity. In some cases muscle cramps may require further investigation regarding their cause. Limb-length discrepancies, muscle weakness and inadequate preparation are just some of the potential aetiologies of cramp.

## Muscle herniations

Muscle may bulge or herniate through normal fascial openings, through congenital fascial defects or via traumatic openings. Normal openings occur at the lateral or anterior compartment and in the deep posterior compartment. Congenital and traumatic herniations occur in the anterior and lateral compartments, and rarely overlying the medial or posterior leg.

## Posterior tibial tendon dysfunction in the athlete

The posterior tibial tendon (PTT) is one of the main dynamic stabilisers of the hindfoot against valgus (eversion) deformity, and as such it is subject to repetitive overuse injury such as peritendinitis and rupture (Plattner 1989). PTT dysfunction has been described frequently as a form of progressive degeneration that may develop due to biomechanical conditions, such as excessive pronation. Often, PTT dysfunction is due to an intrinsic abnormality of the tendon. In cases of PTT dysfunction in which chronic tenosynovitis is a common predisposing factor, rupture of the tendon may often be seen (Mueller 1984). This is a chronic condition ranging from early swelling and pain, to chronic inflammation, to ultimate rupture. When the condition continues and chronic peritendinitis develops, the inflammatory process can cause the tendon to degenerate, gradually elongate, develop interstitial tears, and eventually rupture (Johnson & Strom 1989, Plattner 1989).

PTT dysfunction may have its origins in overuse, secondary to biomechanical and structural weaknesses, or may result from traumatic injury. With the increased participation in exercise and sport by people of all ages, the incidence of PTT tendinopathy has increased tremendously, particularly in older participants and in sports such as tennis, aerobic dance and walk/jogging.

### Anatomy

The tibialis posterior muscle arises from the interosseous membrane and the adjacent surfaces of the tibia and fibula in the proximal third of the leg. The PTT is formed in the distal third of the leg encased in its own tendon sheath by the gathering of large muscle units

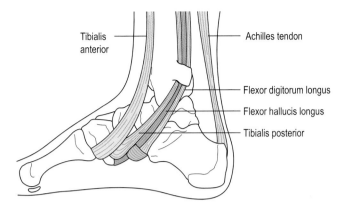

**Figure 13.27** Anatomy of the medial longitudinal arch, illustrating the course of the posterior tibial tendon.

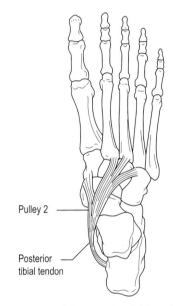

**Figure 13.28** Insertion sites of the posterior tibial tendon.

(Fig. 13.27). The PTT travels posterior to the medial malleolus and anterior to the flexor digitorum longus, posterior tibial artery, vein and nerve, and flexor hallucis longus tendon, beneath the flexor retinaculum.

The tibialis posterior has multiple insertion sites on the plantar–medial aspect of the foot (Fig. 13.28). The most important insertion site is into the navicular tuberosity, with additional extensions into all three cuneiform bones, as well as the bases of the second, third and fourth metatarsals. As a result of this complex anatomical design and insertional attachment, the PTT is regarded as a plantar flexor of the ankle as well as a dynamic inverter (stabiliser) of the foot. During gait, the contraction of the tibialis posterior muscle creates subtalar inversion, locking both the calcaneocuboid and talonavicular joints and creating a rigid lever for forward propulsion of the foot over the metatarsal heads.

When the tibialis posterior does not function properly, inversion of the rearfoot will be greatly diminished. This will enable the overpowering of the gastrocnemius–soleus muscle group and will act on the medial column, more specifically the talonavicular joint. With this loss of PTT function, the fibularis (peroneus) brevis muscle and tendon act independently, which then creates a dynamic abduction and eversion force. As these dynamic forces occur (the action of the gastrocnemius–soleus muscle on the talonavicular joint, and the unopposed pull of the fibular (peroneal) brevis muscle and tendon), a gradual attenuation of the medial static constraints of the longitudinal arch occurs (Mann & Thompson 1985). Disruption of the tendon can result in a loss of integrity of the secondary soft-tissue support structures, namely, the deltoid ligament, talonavicular capsule and spring ligament of the mid- and rearfoot. These secondary static and dynamic restraints then become weaker, developing less mechanical advantage than the posterior tibial tendon, which eventually fails with repeated stress. This deformity of the tendon will create an increase in the valgus deformity of the calcaneus. The progressive deformity results in a medial subluxation (plantar flexion and adduction of the talus), calcaneal valgus and Achilles tendon rotation. Eventually, as this deformity of the PTT progresses, tightening of the Achilles tendon and heel takes place, contributing to the creation of an equinus deformity. Over a period of time of PTT dysfunction, a chronic malalignment of the talonavicular joint, medial column and rearfoot will occur. This flexible deformity continues to become more rigid and fixed with time. The relative strength of the tibialis posterior muscle is a function of its large cross-sectional area, and is greater than two times the strength of its primary antagonist, the fibularis (peroneus) brevis muscle (Sutherland 1966). Because the PTT has a short excursion, elongation of just 1 cm makes the tendon ineffective as the primary dynamic restraint to the longitudinal arch (Sutherland 1966). The deformity usually progresses to a painful flatfoot deformity, with pain described along the longitudinal arch, heel, medial ankle and sinus tarsi (Ross 1997).

## Aetiology

The appearance of a unilateral flatfoot in the adult is a principal manifestation of PTT dysfunction (Funk et al 1986, Johnson 1983, Trevino & Baumhauer 1992). The PTT sheath may become inflamed, producing pain, swelling and tenosynovitis along its course. Tibialis posterior tendinitis can be traced to a number of aetiological factors:

- trauma
- overuse
- inflammatory disorders
- degenerative tendon disease
- infection
- iatrogenic (steroid injections)
- anatomical variations
- shoe distortion (breakdown).

Overuse injuries can be seen in the runner or in other sports that involve excessive pronation and rearfoot imbalance. Inflammation of the tendon and sheath is directly related with strenuous athletic activity, and may occur in all age groups. A clinical picture of tenosynovitis affecting the PTT is seen as an overuse injury. Trauma often involves pronation, external rotation with possible fracture, and complete rupture of the PTT. An os tibiale externum or accessory navicular may also predispose the athlete to posterior tibial tendinitis, in particular following eversion-mechanism ankle injuries.

## CASE STUDY 13.8

### POSTERIOR TIBIAL TENDINITIS

A 44-year-old woman complained of pain along the course of the right posterior tibial tendon, and a pinpoint of tenderness over the right navicular bone. She also complained of pain along the lateral aspect of the fifth metatarsal base of the right foot.

The patient has been a runner for many years, and first presented 7 years ago with chronic tenosynovitis of her right Achilles tendon.

She had a thickened tendon and paratenon with scar tissue formation. The condition was diagnosed on MRI as chronic tendinitis/tendinopathy within the distal Achilles tendon, as well as fluid accumulation/bursitis in the pre-Achilles bursa.

### TREATMENT PLAN

All running and impact activities were ceased and physiotherapy treatment was arranged for chronic posterior tibial tenosynovitis, together with the application of ice and stretching exercises. Cox-2 NSAIDs were prescribed.

The patient's old prescription orthotics were evaluated and found to be worn. The rearfoot and forefoot posts needed to be replaced. The original orthotic was 7 years old and a new biomechanical evaluation for prescription orthotics was performed.

### BIOMECHANICAL EVALUATION

Medium arched foot type on and off weight bearing; first ray hypermobile and plantar flexed to dorsiflexed on weight bearing. Dorsiflexion of the hallux was normal.

Ankle joint dorsiflexion was limited to normal.

*Subtalar joint range of motion.* Inversion: right 20°, left 20°. Eversion: right 3°, left 2°. Subtalar neutral: right 2°, left 2°. Forefoot: right 2° varus, left 2° varus.

*Gait analysis.* Early heel lift-off, with an extended forefoot contact phase. Supinated heel strike, right > left, with lateral column impact. Tibial varum with mild abduction of the right foot. Pronation of the subtalar joint at midstance to toe-off phase of gait, right > left.

### RESOLUTION OF POSTERIOR TIBIAL TENDINITIS

The patient's pain had resolved after physiotherapy, rest from running and the use of new prescription orthotics. She had resumed her running and activity programme, with no recurrence of her previous complaints. She experienced no further pain on the navicular, the lateral base of the fifth metatarsal or the posterior tibial tendon.

## History, physical examination and clinical findings

The history, physical examination and clinical findings of PTT dysfunction in the athlete reveal an overuse condition that, if diagnosed early in its course, can be treated successfully without further sequelae. The athlete with PTT disruption presents with a progressive acquired deformity of the foot and will have a painful flatfoot and difficulty in running or walking normally. The majority of PTT patients describe a gradual onset of the symptoms and the deformity, with disruptions of the PTT most commonly developing in women over 40 years of age (Funk et al 1986, Johnson 1983). Although the cause of PTT dysfunction is not known absolutely, it is believed to be multifactorial, with overuse being the underlying cause, resulting in a progressive degeneration and attenuation, with eventual partial or total rupture occurring when that tensile threshold has been reached. It has been suggested that the zone of hypervascularity between the medial malleolus and the navicular tuberosity is one of the major contributing factors in the development of PTT dysfunction (Frey et al 1990). This is also regarded as the most frequent site of degeneration. An underlying biomechanical weakness can be detected, such as a hypermobile first ray, an unstable medial column and longitudinal arch, and a functional calcaneal valgus. A poor biomechanical design of the tendon, as in a flexible flatfoot, will also predispose the tendon to mechanical abrasion as it courses around the malleolar pulley. In addition, leg-length discrepancy with asymmetrical pronation creating compensation also may be another contributing factor to the development of PTT dysfunction. This condition can be seen clearly when runners who pronate excessively run on one side of the road and back on the other side, or who constantly run in one direction (e.g. clockwise) on a track. This in itself creates a compensated short limb, and with the combined pronatory effect and flexible flatfoot the ingredients for PTT overuse injury are just right. It is rare to see ruptures of the PTT in young patients; however, traumatic PTT have been reported in the young athlete (Conti 1994, Woods & Leach 1991).

A clinical picture of PTT tenosynovitis reveals diffuse swelling, tenderness, warmth and pain at the medial aspect of the ankle and along the course of the tendon, into the medial proximal calf region. Patients will notice a progressive collapse of their longitudinal arch, ambulating on their medial ankle. It is often noted that abnormal shoe wear occurs towards the medial aspect of the outer sole of the heel. The runner, or other athlete, will describe fatigue in the early part of their activity, and a reduction in their ability to withstand prolonged activity. In some cases the athlete may be unable to participate altogether due to the pain and weakness of the foot.

Pain will be elicited over the medial aspect of the ankle by active inversion of the foot against resistance. Genu valgum of the knee may be seen, which can contribute to the painful flatfoot. The symptomatic foot will be abducted and will have a prolapsed or collapsed longitudinal arch. The athlete who presents with overuse injury and degeneration of the PTT will usually complain of pain distal to the medial malleolus. Radiographs are rarely useful in the evaluation of tenosynovitis (Kettlekamp & Alexander 1969). In advanced cases of PTT dysfunction lateral recess impingement involving the calcaneofibular ligament will occur, creating possible fibularis (peroneus) tendon irritation. In addition, a sinus tarsitis can develop with PTT dysfunction simultaneously.

Approximately half the patients with PTT recall a history of localised trauma (Mann 1993). It is essential to determine the exact location of the injury. Traumatic injuries that create partial or complete ruptures of the tendon will have focal pain at the insertion of the navicular bone. A traumatic eversion injury will affect both the spring ligament and the talonavicular capsule. Avulsions of the PTT at the insertion site of the navicular are not uncommon. Frequently, symptoms are related to athletic activity, with gradual weakness, fatigue and loss of strength during the propulsive (push-off) phase of gait. As a result of the instability of the medial column, deltoid ligament or spring ligament (plantar calcaneocuboid) insufficiency may contribute to the development of PTT dysfunction.

When PTT dysfunction has reached the final stages, pes plano valgus deformity will progress, causing a lateral shift in pain due to calcaneofibular impingement. Quite often the medial foot and ankle pain will resolve (Myerson 1996). In cases where the PTT has ruptured, inflammatory symptoms may be absent, while pain may be the major presenting complaint (Banks & McGlamry 1987). This can develop into an acquired flatfoot deformity, with inversion weakness or an inability of the rearfoot to invert at all. Weakness of the PTT can be seen by having the patient attempt to invert the rearfoot against a held plantar-flexed and everted position. This test isolates the PTT and attempts to neutralise the effect of the flexor hallucis longus and anterior tibial tendons from inverting the foot. It is helpful to be able to palpate the PTT posterior to the medial malleolus and feel it contract during inversion. A palpable contraction of the tendon with an acquired flatfoot deformity usually indicates that there is no rupture of the tendon. Rather, tendinitis, a partial tear of the PTT, rupture of the deltoid ligament or rupture of the spring ligament may be present. In some cases, excessive hypermobility of the talonavicular joint may be due to attenuation of the medial capsule and spring ligament complex.

Other tests for confirming injury to the PTT are the *single-heel raise test* and the '*too-many-toes*' sign (Kerr & Henry 1989). A classic triad of deformities on weight bearing presents on physical examination:

- valgus deflection of the heel
- loss in height of the medial longitudinal arch
- abduction of the forefoot ((too-many-toes sign).

This triad reveals a lack of supination of the foot and inversion of the heel when attempting to rise up on the toes. Thus, an inability to lift the heel off the ground is indicative of PTT dysfunction.

Other symptoms may include midlongitudinal arch pain, secondary to increased stress on the PTT, creating a weakened condition and allowing for an overpulling of the fibularis (peroneus) tendons. A significant degree of tension is produced on the surrounding ligamentous tissue, thus creating a soft-tissue shear of the talonavicular, calcaneocuboid and Lisfranc's joints. The end result, subluxation of the lateral midtarsal joint, then occurs, creating forefoot abduction. The tibialis anterior will then become the dominant overpowering force, allowing a forefoot supinatus to develop. This increased tension on the PTT causes a change in the vascularity and a weakening of the tendon as it courses behind the distal–posterior aspect of the medial malleolus. The most hypovascular region of the tendon begins at 40 mm from its insertion to the navicular tuberosity, 1–1.5 cm distal to the medial malleolus, and extending proximally for 14 mm (Frey et al 1990, Johnson 1983, Mann & Thompson 1985).

Radiographic evidence is not a necessity before making the diagnosis of PTT dysfunction (Funk et al 1986, Mann & Thompson 1985, Rey 1953, Teasdale & Johnson 1994); however, it is important in the staging of the deformity (Teasdale & Johnson 1994). Standard anteroposterior and lateral weight-bearing radiographs of both feet, including weight-bearing radiographs of the ankle, should be performed to evaluate the athlete who has developed an acquired flatfoot deformity secondary to PTT dysfunction.

Early in the process the radiographic findings will be normal to minimal changes in the angle. As the deformity progresses, anteroposterior views will reveal a lateral subluxation of the talonavicular joint as the navicular slips laterally upon the talar head (Johnson & Strom 1989). The lateral view shows plantar flexing of the talus, decreased height of the longitudinal arch, collapse of the medial column, and prolapse of the talonavicular, naviculocuneiform and metatarsal cuneiform joints. The axial view may reveal a valgus deformity of the calcaneus. Weight-bearing anteroposterior views of the ankle are also important, particularly in the later stages of the deformity, to determine whether there are any arthritic changes or whether talar tilt is present.

Tenography, CT and MRI have been used to determine the nature of the injury and the level of pathology to the PTT (Alexander et al 1987, Beltran & Moscure 1990, Hogan 1993, Rosenberg et al 1986). Tenography has been useful in the past to evaluate the PTT, but it is an invasive procedure and has not always had positive results (Alexander et al 1987, Funk et al 1986). It can be helpful, however, when there is a rupture of the tendon and the site cannot be located, or if adhesions and fibrosis have developed. However, injection of the contrast dye into the PTT sheath can often be a difficult procedure. CT is directed more towards identifying osseous lesions and has been used to identify severe soft-tissue injuries or abnormalities of tendons.

More recently, advances in the detection of the PTT injury and dysfunction have been achieved through the use of the MRI (Conte et al 1992, Rosenberg et al 1986). Due to its superior soft-tissue contrast resolution, MRI provides a more complete view of the pathological changes than does CT (Conte et al 1992). MRI is the method of choice in the determining of pathological changes of the PTT. An additional advantage of MRI is that there is no risk to the patient from exposure to ionising radiation.

A variety of staging and classification systems have been developed for specific paratendinous structures. Funk et al (1986) developed a classification of four types of pathology involved with PTT dysfunction:

1. avulsion from its insertion along the navicular tuberosity
2. a midsubstance tendon rupture
3. discontinuity of tendon tears without complete rupture
4. an isolated tenosynovitis of the PTT (no tear of the tendon).

Conte et al (1992) also advanced a classification system of tears (types 1 to 3) of the PTT based on MRI. The classification reflects structural features and abnormal signals within the substance of the tendon:

- in type I, the magnetic resonance image reveals one or two fine, longitudinal splits in the tendon, without patterns of degeneration
- in type II, a wider longitudinal split in the tendon is seen, with intramural degeneration
- in type III, there is more diffuse swelling and uniform degeneration of the tendon; some strands of the tendon may remain intact, or the tendon may be replaced with scar tissue formation.

Johnson and Strom (1989) devised a classification system for the staging of PTT dysfunction which has been modified by Myerson (1996). They classified PTT dysfunction abnormalities into three distinct stages, based on the presence or absence of rearfoot or transverse tarsal deformities, and the ability to achieve flexible reduction of the involved articulation.

- *Stage I* reveals a normal length PTT affected by inflammation and associated peritendinitis or tendinosis. There is usually chronic medial ankle pain and swelling. The single heel raise test can be performed as the tendon is intact (Fig. 13.29). Only a mild weakness and minimal deformity are present in this stage.
- *Stage II* is a progressive process in which inflammation and degeneration occur, resulting in an elongated, attenuated PTT. As a result, secondary deformities develop as the midfoot pronates and abducts at the transverse tarsal joint. In addition, there will be a compensatory forefoot varus deformity. The longitudinal arch begins to flatten, whereas the rearfoot articulations remain normal in the non-weight-bearing state.
- *Stage III* is characterised by a condition in which a rigid rearfoot and forefoot deformity develops. The rearfoot will be rigidly everted, and the forefoot abducted.
- *Stage IV* demonstrates a valgus angulation of the talus, with concomitant degeneration of the ankle.

Funk et al (1986) reported that if the inflammatory process of PTT dysfunction is not interrupted by either surgical or non-surgical means, a persistent tenosynovitis (stage I) will progress to stages II and III.

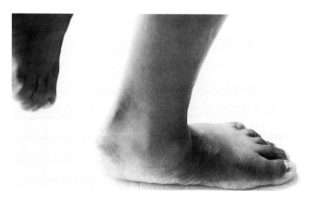

**Figure 13.29** Posterior tibial dysfunction – single heel raise test.

In cases of acute athletic injury to the PTT, conservative non-surgical treatment is valuable in the initial stages, particularly in the presence of various underlying medical conditions that might preclude surgical intervention. Although conservative treatment may be of great benefit in the early stages, there is no guarantee that it will arrest the degenerative process. The initial treatment for PTT injury includes rest, ice, elevation, compression, NSAIDs and various types of immobilisation. In the later stages of acute PTT tenosynovitis a cast is usually indicated for several weeks or even months. The patient may be permitted to walk while wearing the cast or removable boot. However, the more practical approach is to be non-weight bearing. A comprehensive biomechanical evaluation of the lower extremity and a gait analysis should be performed in patients who have developed a flatfoot deformity. A semirigid orthosis with medial control to decrease hyperpronation and eversion of the heel and subtalar joint during the midstance phase of gait or running is prescribed. In the later stages of PTT dysfunction, an articulated ankle–foot orthosis is recommended. Physical therapy has been used as an additional treatment in reducing pain, inflammation, oedema and crepitus in the tendon sheath. On occasion, corticosteroid injections into the sheath have proved helpful in the immediate reduction of symptoms, but these injections may cause focal necrosis and lead to spontaneous rupture of the tendon, and thus their general use is contraindicated (Fadale & Wiggins 1994, Myerson 1996).

Surgical intervention is indicated only in severe cases of chronic tenosynovitis or tendon disruption that have not responded to conservative treatment. In cases of chronic tenosynovitis, characterised by changes in the sheath with degenerative changes in the tendon (as in stage I), debridement is indicated, with incising of the tendon sheath and excising of hypertrophied synovium, and decompression. This will help to decrease painful symptoms and permit improved function. The same condition is seen in attenuation of the Achilles and fibularis (peroneus) tendons. If the tendon is hypertrophied, an elliptical resection with repair can be performed. In cases in which partial tears have occurred, debridement followed by repair is required. In some cases an enlargement of the osseous groove inferior to the medial malleolus may be indicated. The objectives of the procedure are to reduce the girth size of the tendon and to provide an enlargement of the fibrous osseous groove to improve function of the tendon. Proximal Z-lengthening, tendon grafting and the Cobb procedure (taking the distal half of the anterior tibial tendon) are other procedures for direct repair of the PTT.

Postoperatively, the foot is immobilised, first in a pressure dressing followed by application of a posterior splint cast. The foot is placed in a plantar-flexed attitude to reduce stress and traction on the tendon and to allow for early passive range of motion. The patient is immobilised for a period of 3 weeks, followed by mild dorsiflexion and plantar flexion, in addition to inversion–eversion, beginning with passive range of motion and advancing to active range of motion.

In cases of chronic tenosynovitis secondary to PTT malposition, with a hypertrophied and/or accessory navicular, a modified Kidner procedure (rerouting of the tendon, with resection of the hypertrophied navicular bone and/or accessory bone) can be done using a Mitek GII or Panaloc (absorbable anchor) with Panacryl (Surgical Products, Inc., Westwood, MA) tissue anchor. The use of one or two tissue anchors to support the tendon attachment against the denuded bone helps to secure the tendon and improve the mechanical advantage of the tendon. This procedure assists in decreasing both strain and traction on the PTT in an athletic patient who does not need a tendon transfer or arthrodesis procedure, and affords a much earlier return to competitive participation (Ross 1997).

In severe stage II cases, transfer of the flexor digitorum longus (FDL) tendon is utilised. The procedure involves excision of the incompetent tendon or ruptured remains. While positioning the foot in plantar flexion and inversion, a side-to-side anastomosis of the PTT to the FDL tendon is performed and then into the navicular, together with partial translocation of the tibialis anterior into the navicular. The pulley posterior to the malleolus is recreated by repair of the flexor retinaculum (Funk et al 1986, Sutherland 1966). The distal stump of the FDL is tenodesed to the adjacent flexor hallucis longus. Tenodesis of the more proximal segment of the FDL to the myotendinous junction of the PTT is indicated only if the posterior tibial muscle has a normal colour and good elasticity (Goldner et al 1974, Johnson 1983, Mann & Thompson 1985). Immobilisation after this procedure may vary from 8 to 12 weeks.

Although the triple arthrodesis is regarded as the procedure of choice for patients with a severe deformity of the rearfoot with associated posterior tibial tendon dysfunction, long-term studies show that the procedure can lead to degenerative joint disease of the ankle and to the distal unfused joints. This is not a procedure for the athletic or extremely demanding active individual.

Athletic patients who are properly diagnosed as having PTT dysfunction and who are treated early in the onset of the disease with aggressive conservative management have a much more favourable prognosis and are able to return to sports participation much sooner. Even in cases where surgical intervention is inevitable, conservative treatment can serve as a stopgap measure.

## Fibular (peroneal) tendinitis and tenosynovitis

The fibularis (peroneus) tendons and their synovial components can develop various conditions that may result in inflammation, pain, swelling or instability of the lateral ankle and lower extremity (Hatch 1994). Some of these conditions are a result of overuse, faulty athletic shoes, inappropriate training methods or traumatic injuries from a variety of sports that involve side-to-side or torsional activity. The fibularis (peroneus) tendons lie in a common synovial sheath, inferior to the superior fibular (peroneal) retinaculum, and then distally separate into their own sheaths. A thin mesomembrane separates the two tendon sheaths in the region of the fibular (peroneal) sulcus. The floor of the common sheath shares a close anatomical relationship with the talocalcaneal and calcaneofibular ligaments. Tears of the fibular (peroneal) retinaculum can result in anterior dislocation or recurrent subluxation of the fibularis (peroneus) tendons during impact exercise.

The fibularis (peroneus) tendons act by everting and plantar flexing the foot. They are also the primary lateral stabilisers of the ankle joint. Three types of injury to the fibularis (peroneus) tendons can occur in the athlete: overuse tendinitis, chronic subluxation and acute rupture. Biomechanical considerations, such as a plantar-flexed lateral column, can develop into a chronic subluxation of the cuboid, a fibular (peroneal) cuboid syndrome, or the two together. A forced dorsiflexion–eversion mechanism injury to the foot and ankle can result in acute traumatic fibularis (peroneus) tendon subluxation. This condition is seen in medial ankle sprains and is characterised by pain, chronic fibular (peroneal) tendinitis and instability of the ankle.

Fibular (peroneal) tendinitis is related to the pulley action of the lateral malleolus on the fibularis (peroneus) tendon. Mechanical stresses acting on the fibularis (peroneus) tendons as they course through the retrofibular sulcus cause a decrease in vascularity, chronic inflammation and degenerative changes. The athlete who presents with chronic fibular (peroneal) tendinitis will have pain in the retromalleolar area in addition to oedema and tenderness overlying the course of the tendon. When the clinician attempts to evert the foot against resistance pain will be produced overlying the tendon complex and lateral ankle.

Patients with chronic fibular (peroneal) tendonitis will relate a history of postinversion ankle injury, which was not severe enough to require immediate treatment at the time of injury. In addition to pain and tenderness along the course of the tendons, there may also be synovial oedema in the region. The task for the clinician is to determine whether one or both of the tendons are involved in the postinversion fibular (peroneal) tendinitis.

Treatment of painful, tender fibular (peroneal) tendinitis includes decreased activity, NSAIDs, ice massage and physical therapy. In some more severe cases, cast immobilisation may be necessary. Biomechanical factors should be considered, with orthoses being used to correct excessive supinated heel-strike. Rearfoot varus posting with a flange along the lateral margin of the device will assist in limiting stress on the fibularis (peroneus) tendons and limiting their traction.

In cases of a subluxing cuboid or fibular (peroneal) cuboid syndrome, cuboid manipulation may be performed. When pain is elicited along the plantar aspect of the foot from the cuboid to the first metatarsal, fibular (peroneal) cuboid syndrome should be suspected. Accommodative orthoses are recommended, with a 3–6 mm heel lift and a soft pad with a dancer's cut-out under the first metatarsal. This allows relaxation and lengthening of this short tendon, preventing repeated traction and irritation. In a more severe case of fibular (peroneal) cuboid syndrome, in addition to manipulation of the cuboid a below-knee cast is applied, followed by active physical therapy and manipulation.

MRI or sonography of the lateral ankle region can assist in diagnosing chronic fibular (peroneal) tenosynovitis, focal degeneration and attenuation of the fibularis (peroneus) tendons. Standard radiographs may show an enlarged calcaneal tubercle, which may be responsible for chronic irritation, impingement and chronic synovitis. A CT scan can help in defining the retrofibular sulcus and assist in the planning of a surgical procedure to help correct the chronic subluxation of the fibularis (peroneus) tendons.

## Subluxing fibularis (peroneus) tendons

The retrofibular groove is a shallow sulcus within which the fibularis (peroneus) brevis sits. Although the fibularis (peroneus) longus shares a common synovial sheath with the brevis, it does not make contact with the sulcus. The fibular (peroneal) complex is maintained by superior perineal retinaculum. Excessive tension on the fibular (peroneal) tendons while the foot is dorsiflexed and everted creates a slippage of the fibularis (peroneus) brevis tendon laterally and anteriorly, forcing the longus tendon with it into the synovial sheath. In addition to the subluxation of the fibular (peroneal) tendons, a rupture of the superior retinaculum may also develop. Pain and tenderness will occur along the course of the tendons, and recreating the same movement will usually reproduce a subluxation of the fibular (peroneal) tendons laterally and anteriorly across the fibular malleolus. Chronic subluxation will be accompanied by an audible click or pop as the tendon displaces and then relocates into the groove. Athletes who suffer from this disorder will often describe a feeling of ankle instability, that their ankle will 'give way'. There are two types of subluxation in fibular (peroneal) tendons: chronic recurring and traumatic. In the case of traumatic subluxation, the superior retinaculum is ruptured as a result of subluxation of both the brevis and the longus in a forward direction, applying a tearing force on the retinacular sheath. Sports such as skiing, basketball, soccer and ice skating will often be responsible for a forced dorsiflexion, inversion mechanism injury, resulting in a powerful reflex muscular contracture of the fibular (peroneal) tendons. Inadequate treatment at the time of injury can result in a chronic subluxation. Ankle instability usually accompanies subluxation of the fibular (peroneal) tendon, and the ankle mortise should be checked. An acute fibular (peroneal) tendon subluxation will cause rupture of the superior fibular (peroneal) retinaculum together with an avulsion 'fleck fracture' at its insertion along the lateral border of the fibular malleolus. Chronic subluxation seldom requires treatment, although acute traumatic subluxation does require conservative treatment, in the form of a non-weight-bearing below-knee cast held at 90° for at least 4 weeks. Stress examination with inversion talar tilt measurements will help to determine whether a concomitant ankle stabilisation procedure is required.

When conservative management fails after chronic fibular (peroneal) dislocation, surgical repair is required. A variety of surgical procedures have been described in addition to the repair of the superior fibular (peroneal) retinaculum. They include posterior fibular groove reconstruction utilising a periosteal flap (Zoellner & Clancy 1979), rerouting of the fibular (peroneal) tendons under the calcaneal–fibular ligament (Sarmiento & Worf 1975), and a number of bone block reconstruction procedures.

An os peroneum in the athlete in combination with chronic fibular (peroneal) tendinitis can be a painful limiting injury, requiring surgical excision of the ossicle. The os peroneum is located lateral or deep to the fibularis (peroneus) longus, and in some cases is an integral part of the syndosmosis or synchondrosis at the cuboid (Sarratian 1983). Particular care must be taken to avoid severing any of the fibres of the fibularis (peroneus) longus during surgery.

Although rupture of the fibular (peroneal) tendons is rare, a partial tear or rupture is more common in cases of recalcitrant fibular (peroneal) tendinopathy. This occurs as a result of collagen fibre breakdown, focal degeneration and attenuation of the tendon fibres. These ruptures occur between the cuboid and the lateral malleolus, and may extend proximally to the myotendinous junction. Primary surgical repair is recommended to prevent instability of the ankle and overpowering of the invertors, leading to a foot that is unable to evert and plantar flex normally.

## Overuse knee injuries

Overuse knee injuries are commonly seen in the practice of sports medicine. They occur when alignment is altered and when normal synchronous movement of the foot and lower extremity are altered. Examples of the causes of injuries of this type are a change or breakdown of footwear, unrelenting hard running surfaces, training, competitive techniques, equipment and biomechanical factors.

The athlete's knee is frequently injured as a result of both direct trauma and overuse injury. Some of the common causes of knee pain in the sport participant include meniscal tears, patellofemoral joint instability, patellofemoral maltracking, patellar tendinitis, ligamentous injury (ACL, MCL, PCL, LCL), osteochondral injury (cartilaginous), chondromalacia patellae, and degenerative joint disease in the older exerciser. Some less common conditions are apophysitis of the tibial epiphysis (Osgood–Schlatter syndrome), discoid meniscus and knee plica, and some less common sources of knee pain in the athlete include (medially) semimembranosus tendinitis, pes anserinus bursitis, tibial collateral ligament bursitis and saphenous nerve entrapment. Anteriorly, less common sources of knee pain include Hoffa's disease (proliferation of the fat pad following injury to the knee joint) and, laterally, iliotibial band syndrome, popliteus tendinitis and instability proximally of the tibiofibular joint. As the number of participants in sports and exercise increases, the sports medicine specialist is seeing these less common entities more frequently.

## Definition

An overuse knee injury is a chronic, atraumatic injury, portrayed by chronic knee pain secondary to participation in sport. The athlete will deny any history of acute trauma to the knee joint. The physical examination will not reveal any instability of the knee joint due to ligamentous injury, and there will not be any signs of the knee joint locking or marked oedema, which would indicate meniscal damage or loose bone bodies within the joint. On occasion, there might be an accumulation of fluid around the joint, with tenderness in various areas surrounding the knee. Radiographic or arthroscopic evaluation of the knee usually does not reveal any pathological changes.

## Symptoms

Pain may be present in the knee, or may be localised to the medial or lateral collateral ligaments, superior or inferior patellar tendon or the retropatellar region. The location of the pain may vary according to the individual and may be intermittent in nature, fluctuating from day to day. Sporting activity may exacerbate this resting knee pain. The participant with overuse knee pain may describe a feeling of weakness, aching or stiffness, which may at times be sharp and quite severe. Pain will be diminished or even extinguished by rest but will begin again once activity is resumed. Many runners and other athletes will be able to participate in their sport pain free, although pain may be experienced in the later stages of the activity or immediately afterwards. In the history, the patient may remember a particular episode that contributed to the overuse injury. Seen particularly in running, aerobics and alpine skiing, the pain is often associated with a change in terrain or running surface, or with too quick a return to a normal training programme after a prolonged period of inactivity.

## Signs

Physical examination will reveal some form of biomechanical malalignment of the lower extremity and feet. Such malalignments include femoral anteversion, genu valgum or varum, tibial varum, subtalar varus, rearfoot varus or valgus, forefoot varus or valgus, and excessive pronation (Fig. 13.30). Muscle imbalance or muscle weakness can also have a bearing on overuse injury. This may also include atrophy of the quadriceps muscle group, weakened or tight hamstring muscles, or a tight gastrocnemius–soleus complex, despite the fact that

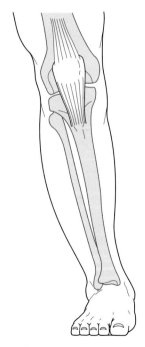

**Figure 13.30** Tibial varum.

there are no signs of ligamentous injury, meniscal insufficiency, internal derangement or swelling of the knee joint. Often this condition does not reveal any true pathology of the knee joint. For this reason, the clinician must obtain the proper athletic training history and observe the gait thoroughly.

## Treatment

When abnormal pronation is the underlying cause, the foot imbalance must be corrected to re-establish a more normal lower leg alignment and neutrality of the knee. In this fashion, during propulsion the knee will be properly aligned and stable in propulsion. To correct this lower leg and structural imbalance, a functional orthosis must be employed. This will help the athlete to compensate for the structural abnormality and achieve a more 'normal' efficient gait.

## Biomechanical causes of knee injuries

Various overuse knee injuries occur when the foot has to compensate for structural deformities in the lower leg or foot. This compensation is in the form of abnormal pronation of the subtalar joint, increasing the speed, or altering the amount of pronation or modifying the point in the gait cycle at which it normally occurs. Changes in subtalar joint pronation may have an adverse effect on the function of the lower limb, and later develop into chronic knee pain. The knee is the most common site for running injuries (James et al 1978, Van Mechlen 1992).

The knee joint is recognised for its design as an integral part of the impact-absorbing mechanism during running (Wosk & Voloshin 1981). Indirect shock absorption by knee flexion is also dependent on subtalar joint pronation (Root et al 1977). The knee is a ginglymoarthroidal-type joint, and for it to change to a flexed position transverse rotation between the tibia and femur must occur. At heel strike the knee is fully extended, and it must flex quickly to absorb the shock generated by heel strike. McMahon et al (1987) concluded that vertical stiffness increased with running speed and that at any given speed this stiffness could be reduced in a controlled fashion by running with greater knee flexion than normal. They also determined that the transmission of mechanical shock due to impact was very sensitive to the degree of knee flexion. At 35–45% of the support phase of the gait cycle, maximum pronation occurs in addition to maximum knee flexion. It is at the maximum point of flexion that the knee joint has its greatest degree of mobility and instability. Internal knee joint structures such as the ligaments and the menisci are at great risk of injury with the knee in this position. As pronation of the subtalar joint and flexion of the knee are initiated by ground reactive forces, shearing forces of the tibia will increase, and these combined with femoral rotation lead to knee injuries, the incidence of which has increased in recent years (Van Mechlen 1992).

During the propulsive phase, knee extension creates a more stable knee joint, as now the knee is subject to increased amounts of stress secondary to an extended lever arm. Due to synchronised knee and hip extension, a more effective use of the hip muscles occurs. This allows for a more effective propulsive phase of gait.

As the leg prepares for propulsion, the pelvis and the femur begin to rotate externally in phase with each other. The tibia will also attempt to rotate externally; however, an excessively pronated foot will prevent this from occurring. Twisting of the knee will develop, with the proximal portion of the knee joint rotating externally, while the distal portion of the joint is prevented from externally rotating and therefore develops an internal rotation. These effects of torque on the knee joint are at their greatest and most damaging after the midstance phase of gait when the foot is maximally pronated.

The efficiency of the biarticular gastrocnemius muscle is highly dependent on the degree of flexion at the knee. During the time the knee is fully flexed or extended, the displacement of the origin of the muscle produces a relative lengthening or shortening of the muscle, which is equal to or exceeds its length of contraction (Bates & Stergiou 1999a). Therefore, during the time the knee is extended, the gastrocnemius is passively stretched and is at its maximum efficiency, creating a power transfer from the quadriceps to the ankle. Conversely, when the knee is flexed, the gastrocnemius is relaxed and loses most of its efficiency. In this scenario, the soleus is the only active muscle, and it is very difficult for this to function without a knee that is extended during the process.

Malalignment and torque will then contribute to strain or injury to the structures of the knee, both intra-articularly and/or extra-articularly, as the demands of the sport increase. Impact injuries to the knee are also seen in knee malalignment conditions, as well as being as a result of the surfaces upon which the athlete performs.

## The patellofemoral joint

This joint is subject to mechanical overuse injuries. The patella acts to decrease the friction of the quadriceps mechanism as it passes over the distal femoral condyles (Ficat & Hungerfred 1977); the patella acts as the sesamoid of the knee (Fig. 13.31). It works in a pulley-like groove on the femur, and serves as a fulcrum for the action of the quadriceps muscles. It guides the quadriceps complex and centralises the various actions of the four muscles of the quadriceps. These forces are then transmitted to the patellar tendon. The purpose of the patella within the extensor apparatus is to protect the tendon from friction and allow the extensor apparatus to withstand high compressive loads. The patella lengthens the extensor arm, providing a mechanical advantage for the quadriceps (Kaufer 1971).

Stability of the patellofemoral joint is due to a number of factors, including patellofemoral congruency, static ligamentous stabilisers and dynamic quadriceps and hamstring muscle stabilisers (Goodfellow et al 1976, Kaufer 1971). The patellotibial and the patellofemoral medial and lateral ligaments maintain proper tracking and keep the patella in the femoral groove (Kaplan 1962). The failure of any one of these stabilising factors will cause a malalignment and allow for unfavourable patellofemoral articulation, which will subsequently lead to increased loading on the articular surfaces.

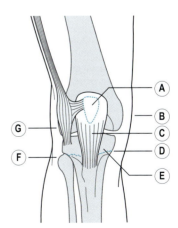

**Figure 13.31** Overuse knee injuries: patellofemoral syndrome.
(A) semimembranosus/semitendonosus tendinitis, (B) patellar tendinitis, (C) tibial plateau stress fracture, (D) Osgood–Schlatter disease, (E) biceps femoris tendinitis, (F) popliteal tendinitis, (G) iliotibial band friction syndrome.

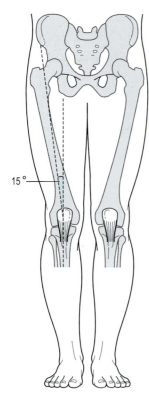

**Figure 13.32** The Q angle.

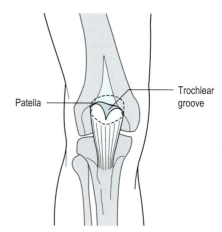

**Figure 13.33** Patella and trochlear groove.

## Patellofemoral problems in runners

Patellofemoral joint pain is one of the most common stress-related injuries experienced by runners. Running biomechanics will guarantee a relatively smooth tracking of the patella in the femoral groove, and therefore it is unusual for the runner to experience an acute traumatic injury to the joint.

'Runner's knee syndrome' is a mild lateral subluxation of the patella, and should not be mistaken for chondromalacia patellae. Runner's knee can often be caused by an increased Q angle, or be due to excessive pronation of the foot (Fig. 13.32). Lateral shearing forces due to a malposition of the vastus medialis will cause subluxation of the patella over a runner's career, and consequently will establish a new position for the patella to sit, thus creating an uneven pressure on the lateral surface of the femoral condyle. The patella will change shape appropriately as stress acts on it, causing it to adapt to this new position. Excessive pronation in running causes internal rotation of the tibia, thus increasing the impact shock to the patellofemoral joint region, leading to runner's knee pain.

Runner's knee syndrome develops because of poor running mechanics, malalignment problems, an increased Q angle, tibial varum, internal tibial torsion, a weakened quadriceps muscle group, hard running surfaces and faulty shoes. Women, due to their increased Q angle secondary to an anatomically wider pelvis, are at greater risk of suffering from this disorder. The use of prescription orthoses can help realign the foot, thus reducing the Q angle and torque, torsion and stress to the knee joint.

## Chondromalacia patellae

Chondromalacia patellae has been associated with abnormalities of patellar tracking as well as changes in the contact forces of the patella. Malalignment with recurrent subluxation of the patella is probably one of the most common causes of chondromalacia (Outerbridge &

Dunlop 1975). In cases where recurrent subluxation of the patella occurs, there will be damage to the patellar articular cartilage. High Q angles create greater tensile stress on the medial and, more specifically, the odd facet of the patella. Tensile fatigue has a direct effect on the medial or odd facet, contributing to the formation of an 'open' chondromalacic lesion. A 'closed' lesion of the patella is a result of a high Q angle combined with normal compressive forces producing high shear stress. A third lesion located over the lateral facet consists of a very firm, sclerotic cartilage. High compressive contact stresses act on the lateral facet in this patellar tracking disorder.

Chondromalacia is caused by a combination of factors that eventually push the patella out of its groove on the femur. These factors include: weakness of the vastus medialis muscle; an increased Q angle, creating an overpowering of the vastus lateralis muscle; and malalignment of the lower limb, creating excessive foot pronation and leading to increased tibial torsion and increased stress on the knee.

Chondromalacia is a degenerative process on the retropatellar surface. This has been classified in stages, from an early onset to an advanced stage of arthritis (Key et al 1999):

- Stage I – a softening or degeneration of the articular cartilage
- Stage II – a cleaving of the articular cartilage
- Stage III – cleaving and fronds of the articular cartilage
- Stage IV – a wearing away of the articular cartilage to subchondral bone.

On physical examination, the runner will complain of generalised, deep knee pain. In some cases, pain may be associated with the tracking areas of the patella, or the undersurfaces of the femoral condyles. The knee may be swollen, with a chronic effusion of synovial fluid. In severe cases, the clinician may elicit a positive patellofemoral grinding test. As previously mentioned, a high Q angle may be seen, as well as a patella that is malaligned. Quadriceps muscle testing will reveal a weak vastus medialis and a high insertion into the patella. The most important radiographic view is the axial or 'skyline' view, also known as the 'sunrise' or 'sunset' views. The infrapatellar view will consistently reveal the inferior surface of the patella in relation to the femoral condyles, without other bone projections obscuring the view. By taking views of both knees simultaneously, the clinician can determine both the morphology and the position of the patella in relation to the trochlear facets (Fig. 13.33). Radiographs may reveal osteophytic 'spurs'.

To make the correct diagnosis of chondromalacia patellae, several differential diagnoses should be eliminated. These include: chronic synovitis, meniscal lesions, fat pad syndrome, pre-patellar bursitis, retropatellar bursitis, infrapatellar tendon tendinitis, medial synovial plica syndrome, pes anserinus bursitis and sprain of the retinaculum.

Conservative treatment is the most prudent plan, consisting of salicylates, NSAIDs, patellar stabilising devices, icing, ultrasound, nerve stimulation, massage, and a change of running programme and running surfaces. Intra-articular steroid injections are not recommended, as collagen and protein synthesis is reduced. Quadriceps exercises and iliotibial band stretching are highly recommended, particularly if the patient is a runner. Realignment of the maltracking patella can be accomplished with the use of orthotic therapy. Steadman (1979) has stated that pronation of the foot increases the patellofemoral angle, creating pressure and symptoms in the patellofemoral joint, and that either soft or rigid orthotics can be helpful in this disorder.

Surgical intervention consists of a lateral release with a concomitant medial imbrication of the vastus medialis to achieve a proximal realignment. Arthroscopic local debridement of the articular lesion is helpful if confined to one facet or if the chondromalacia is grade II or III in severity (McCarroll et al 1983).

## Knee plica

The synovial plica is an embryonic fold or septum traversing the anterior compartment of the knee, and separating the suprapatellar pouch from the main body of the knee. In the embryo, the kneecap is surrounded by a large bursa that differentiates into the prepatellar, suprapatellar and the infrapatellar bursae (Fig. 13.34). These bursae can completely resorb during adulthood and fall into folds superiorly, laterally and medially. Commonly found in runners, these lesions can be asymptomatic, or can cause a great deal of pain and discomfort. Early in the course of patellofemoral pain the clinician should examine for the presence of a synovial plica. In athletic activity, trauma, overuse or long-distance running can cause the plica to become inflamed, thickened and fibrosed. A large plica can fold under the patella and cause lateral displacement. A medially fibrous type plica may also mimic a meniscal tear. This same plica can extend transversely across the joint and can insert into the medial aspect of the infrapatellar fat pad. During running, when the knee flexes and extends, this fibrous plica will run across the medial femoral condyle and create a great deal of pain.

The examiner can feel a shelf while the knee is flexed at about 30–40° and the thumb is rolled over the medial side of the patella. This test, referred to as the 'thumb roll', will elicit a snap or click that will be painful and strongly guarded. Arthroscopic evaluation may determine that the meniscus is normal, while a thickening of the synovial fold indicates that a synovial plica is present. This lesion may be excised arthroscopically, and the procedure has been proven to be very successful in eliminating knee pain in the athlete.

## Iliotibial band friction syndrome

Iliotibial band friction syndrome is a painful, debilitating overuse injury that affects runners, particularly long-distance runners such as marathon runners and ultra-runners, and cyclists. This inflammatory disorder is an overuse injury caused by excessive friction from the iliotibial band (ITB) as it passes over the lateral femoral excrescence and possibly at Gerdy's tubercle (Fig. 13.35). The injury develops as the knee flexes and extends during running, creating a friction 'rub' over the lateral femoral condyle, which is responsible for the inflammatory response. As the iliotibial tract passes distally, it remains in contact with the lateral intermuscular septum of the quadriceps muscles and inserts into a tubercle on the lateral tibial condyle. Some suggest that the ITB acts as an anterolateral stabiliser to the tibia (Kaplan 1958, Terry et al 1986). In extension, the ITB lies anterior to the lateral epicondyle of the femur, and as flexion over 30° occurs, the ITB passes over the condyle. Another underlying factor is that of significant tightness of the ITB, which is prevalent among many athletes and runners. Those runners who suddenly increase their mileage, increase intensity or include hill training in their programme are subject to developing this overuse injury. Runners who have biomechanical abnormalities such as a high degree of tibial varum, who are excessive supinators on heel strike, or who have hyperpronation after midstance are also more prone to this overuse injury. The pain will often be most intense at heel strike, while attempting to decelerate the limb (Nobel 1980). At the onset of the disorder, pain may develop after an extended run. When runners warm up adequately, painful symptoms seem to diminish. However, in more severe or chronic cases, the lateral knee will hurt even while running – the longer the

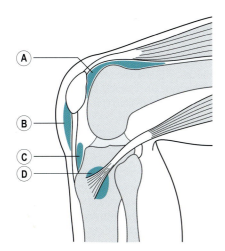

**Figure 13.34** Bursae at the knee: (A) suprapatellar; (B) pre-patellar; (C) infrapatellar; (D) pes anserinus (lateral view).

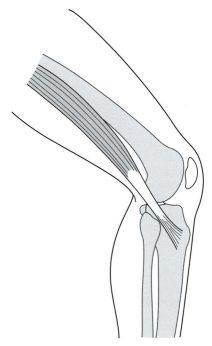

**Figure 13.35** Insertion of the iliotibial band (lateral view).

distance run, the more severe the pain – with residual post-run effects. Other aetiological factors involved in the disorder include genu varum, an abnormally prominent lateral femoral epicondyle, and internal tibial torsion.

The ITB is a thickening of the fascia lata that extends from the iliac crest to insert into the lateral tibial condyle. The band is developed by insertions from the tensor fascia lata and gluteus maximus muscles. The syndrome is due to the inflammation of the ITB and bursa as well as the underlying periosteum of the lateral femoral condyle. Other differential diagnoses include patellofemoral dysfunction, biceps femoris tendinitis, popliteus tendinitis, lateral plica, lateral meniscus injury, degenerative joint disease and stress fracture.

The clinical presentation of ITB friction syndrome is generally tenderness at the point where the ITB slides over the lateral excrescence or at Gerdy's tubercle. Pain may also extend along the course of the ITB, and may radiate proximally or distally. On occasion, soft-tissue swelling may be present, and there may also be palpable crepitus present at the same site. A positive ITB test will confirm the diagnosis. The test is performed by the clinician placing a varus stress upon the knee, and then fully extending and fully flexing it. During extension the ITB slides anteriorly, and during flexion it passes posteriorly. It is this sliding over the femoral excrescence that reproduces the pain. Another way of reproducing the pain is by means of the Nobel test: the lateral femoral epicondyle is palpated by the thumb, where no pain had been elicited previously. On occasion, if needed, MRI or an ultrasound scan can be employed to confirm the diagnosis (Ekman et al 1994).

Treatment for the early stages of the condition includes adequate stretching and warm-up, with heat or topical rub before a run, followed by additional stretching and ice massage afterwards. An ITB stretching programme is highly recommended for athletes with ITB friction syndrome (Box 13.10).

In addition to the ITB stretching, rest or altering activity (e.g. shortening the duration of the training activity, avoiding hills, shortening stride length, changing directions on a circular or banked track, and running back on the same side of a crowned street) is advised, with controlling the inflammation process being the ultimate goal. Cyclists may need to change the height of their seat or their foot position on the bicycle pedal (Holmes et al 1993). When pain persists when running, alternative training programmes should be instituted, such as swimming, aqua-running and weight training. Cycling may exacerbate the ITB pain, and therefore should not be done.

Symptomatic treatment may also include iontophoresis, with a cortisone preparation. Bursal cortisone injections may also be employed in more severe cases. Again, initially ice should be used, followed by heat, whirlpool, ultrasound and NSAIDs. If the patient cannot run or exercise without pain after a course of alternative exercise and treatment, total rest for 4–6 weeks is recommended. For the most part, the great majority of athletes will respond favourably to conservative care (Box 13.11). Correction of biomechanical abnormalities may require only a simple insole or longitudinal arch support. However, in cases where there is an uncompensated inverted rearfoot, a prescription orthosis may be needed to prevent an excessive supinated heel strike, thus reducing the traction and stress on the ITB.

After 12 months of unsuccessful conservative treatment, surgical intervention may be considered. Release of the ITB at its attachment to the patella is one particular procedure that may be employed, as may a bursectomy.

## Popliteus tendinitis

The popliteus muscle originates from the lateral femoral condyle and has a wide insertion on the posterior tibia above the soleal line. It passes superolaterally and anteriorly under the arcuate ligament,

> ### Box 13.10 Iliotibial band stretching programme
>
> Each exercise to be done __ times a day; __ repetitions for each exercise.
>   Hold each stretch for 5–10 seconds.
>
> #### Hip abductor stretch
>
> Stand with the legs straight, feet together. Bend at the waist toward the side opposite of the leg to be stretched. The unaffected knee may be bent.
>
> #### Iliotibial band stretch
>
> Stand with knees straight, cross the leg to be stretched behind the other as far as possible. Stretch to the side of the leg in front.
>
> #### Iliotibial band stretch
>
> Same stance as above. Slightly bend the back knee. Move the trunk toward the unaffected side and the hips toward the affected side. Stretch will be felt along the outside of the bent knee.
>
> #### Iliotibial band stretch/hamstring stretch
>
> Stand with knees straight. Cross the legs so that the affected knee rests against the back of the unaffected leg. Turn the trunk away from the affected side as far as possible, reaching and attempting to touch the heel of the affected leg.
>
> #### Iliotibial band stretch
>
> Lie on the unaffected side with your back a few inches from the table edge. Bend the unaffected hip to maintain balance. Straighten the affected knee and place the leg over the edge of the table so the leg hangs straight. Let gravity pull the leg down, causing the stretch.
>
> #### Iliotibial band stretch
>
> Lie on the affected side with the knee locked and the leg in a straight line with the trunk; bend the upper knee. With your hands placed directly under the shoulders to bear the weight of the trunk, push up, extending your arms as far as possible. The affected leg must be kept straight to get maximum stretch in the hip.

forming a tendon about 1 cm distal to the joint line. The tendon functions by:

- maintaining internal rotation of the tibia on the femur
- aiding the posterior cruciate ligament in preventing forward displacement of the femur on the tibia
- derotating the knee joint at the beginning of flexion (Barnett & Richardson 1953, Basmajian & Lovejoy 1971).

This muscle will help stabilise the femur against forward displacement on the fixed tibia, particularly when running downhill.

For runners who run on a track, or a banked track, pain may be experienced on the lateral aspect of the knee, due to the internal rotation of the tibia on the femur.

Popliteus tendinitis is an overuse injury that is commonly seen in athletic individuals, particularly downhill runners and skiers, and those with excessive pronation.

Physical examination will reveal localised tenderness overlying the tendinous origin and along the lateral femoral condyle.

Treatment includes NSAIDs and restricting all downhill running, application of ice for acute symptoms, followed by whirlpool or moist heat, ultrasound, knee stretching and strengthening exercises. Alleviating stress to the popliteus is imperative. This can be accomplished by changing the side of the road or direction of running on a banked track, and by running uphill, not downhill.

## Box 13.11 Iliotibial band syndrome: treatment

### Initial visit

- Physical examination – perform Nobel's compression test
- Check for excessive iliotibial band tightness – Ober's test
- Rule out meniscal disease and other differential diagnoses
- Check for tibial varum, excessive rotation or varus stress
- Perform walking and running gait analysis
- Check shoe wear pattern and/or distortion
- Check for limb-length discrepancy
- Prescribe iliotibial band stretching programme
- Quadriceps strengthening programme with adductor strengthening programme
- Ice massage to injured area
- Alter athletic activity

If not improving significantly or re-flare with activity:

### Second visit

- Begin physical therapy: ultrasound, iontophoresis, followed by ice massage
- Test for extensive rotation with foot/ankle taping
- Recommend stability/motion control shoes and heel lift for limb-length discrepancy if seen
- Continue stretching programme
- Massage therapy
- Prescribe NSAIDs
- Rest from all running or cycling activities if pain persists

If re-flare with return to activity:

### Third visit

- Consider possible meniscal disorder or collateral ligament injury
- Order MRI or CT scan
- Orthopaedic referral

## Hamstring tendinitis

Injuries to the hamstring are due to a short flexor group. An athlete who does not stretch routinely or adequately is prone to a hamstring strain. Therefore, it is imperative that before engaging in any athletic activity the hamstring muscle group should be properly stretched. This is of particular importance before sprinting, running or during pre-season training. Careful attention during running to overstriding and/or oversprinting can help to prevent a hamstring injury.

Injury to the hamstring can occur at any site along its course. A strain will occur as a result of a sudden overextension of a tight hamstring, and be located either at the hip or the knee. Once a hamstring has been injured it will always be vulnerable to re-injury due to its intrinsic weakness.

On clinical examination, the hamstring will appear to be tight, and in cases where a partial or complete rupture has occurred there will be swelling, ecchymosis and/or haematoma formation. Pain will be elicited at the site of the injury, which is most commonly at the midthigh, or at the ischial tuberosity. A marathon runner who had experienced a cramp early in the race may have gone on to a partial rupture in the later stage of the race. Consequently, the runner will have pain against resistance, and may be unable to bear weight without excruciating pain.

In addition to tight hamstring muscle groups, repeated hamstring 'pulls' should alert the sports practitioner to the possibility of biome-

chanical malalignment. Examples include excessive subtalar pronation, genu valgum, internal rotation of the tibia, short limb and pelvic tilt.

In cases of internal tibial torsion, the origin of the hamstring and the insertion will be stretched and twisted, particularly in the latter stages of the propulsive phase of running. This also can be an underlying cause of injury, but will not be apparent to the untrained eye.

In cases of recurrent strain or pulls, or in chronic hamstring tendinitis, a biomechanical evaluation is essential to rule out poor foot imbalance and lower limb malalignment. In addition, muscle testing is also important to determine whether, for instance, the quadriceps muscle group is stronger than and overpowering the hamstring group. Muscle strengthening and flexibility exercises are essential to prevent recurrent injury. In some cases certain forms of sport may need to be altered or eliminated to prevent further injury. A daily stretching exercise programme to maintain flexibility and a pre-exercise warm-up should be part of the normal routine.

## Groin injury/strain

A groin strain can be an extremely painful and debilitating injury, and it is commonly seen in sports such as soccer, football, tennis, rugby, and in sprinters, long-distance runners and other track and field events. The term *groin strain* incorporates many other conditions that cause pain in the groin region. The groin pain may occur suddenly, or be brought on by a series of traumas secondary to overuse. The structures involved in this area include the adductor muscles, inguinal ligaments, the pubis symphysis and ramus, the gracilis, the iliopsoas and the piriformis. A groin injury may be a result of a sudden violent overstretching of the leg in abduction and external rotation, particularly when there is an opposing force.

A groin injury may develop suddenly or insidiously, and the associated pain may be sharp or dull. In many cases the structure(s) involved may be difficult to identify. The injury presents in the early stages with a mild ache, following activity, which is then relieved by rest, but quickly returns during the subsequent period of activity. As the injury becomes more chronic, the pain will increase in severity, begin earlier in the activity and take longer to subside, until it reaches a point where there is a constant dull ache or pain. At this stage even walking may be painful. To test for the site of the pain, passive and active assisted motion of the patient's hip with the leg extended in all directions, particularly abduction and external rotation, followed by careful palpation of the groin structures to pinpoint the site of injury is required.

For the most part, unless the injury was attributed to a sudden traumatic event, one should suspect a biomechanical origin. The most common aetiology for this biomechanical injury is a limb-length discrepancy, where the short limb pronates for a longer period of time than the longer limb. The hyperpronated foot creates a scenario in which increased internal rotation of the limb occurs, tilting the pelvis forward on that side. This effect on the limb, including the adductor muscle group and the iliopsoas, is to function with a twist, as the pelvis tilts downward. The adductor serves an important purpose in providing stability for the pelvis, particularly in sprinting as well as long-distance running. Functional control of the abnormality is essential to prevent recurrent or further injury.

Rest is the key to allow for healing of the groin strain or injury. Once the athlete stops all activity, pain subsides and the condition will resolve. In addition to rest, physical therapy, anti-inflammatory medication, and a well-designed and properly supervised rehabilitation programme should be part of the athlete's post-injury care to return to a competitive level. Another goal in the treatment of groin injuries is to re-establish biomechanical control to the foot and limb. Limiting excessive pronation of the foot will assist in eliminating the twist in the leg, and in addition help to reduce some of the adverse effects of the limb-length difference. The use of orthotic devices will help to achieve this goal, while simultaneously helping to correct the pelvic tilt. The addition of a 4–7 mm heel lift to correct that imbalance or leg-length discrepancy is advised. To prevent groin injuries, the pelvis and lower extremity must be conditioned to withstand forces generated by the patient's particular sport. Strengthening the groin muscles with exercise performed against resistance, and repetitions to build strength as well as endurance will help prevent recurrent injury. To maintain range of motion, special stretching exercises of the groin incorporating proprioceptive neuromuscular facilitation techniques should be used (Pink 1981).

## LEG-LENGTH DISCREPANCY

Anatomical leg-length discrepancies are a result of the overgrowth or undergrowth of long bones. Functional limb-length discrepancies develop from a malpositioning of the various joints of the lower extremity. When a muscle group of one limb is shorter or overpowers the contralateral side, a functional limb-length discrepancy can develop. Another example is a hyperpronated foot that is more pronated than the contralateral foot, which creates a functional limb-length discrepancy and a lateral pelvic tilt.

A leg-length difference can be either anatomical or physiological. An anatomical leg-length difference describes a true anatomical difference that exists between the two legs. There is no variation in its measurement. The leg-length difference is seen in both the neutral calcaneal stance position and the relaxed calcaneal stance position. On the other hand, a physiological leg-length difference is the result of some other structural area or deviation that has had an effect on the leg length. Examples of a physiological leg-length difference include muscle imbalance and scoliosis, as well as abnormal biomechanics of the foot, which may originate above the pelvis or below the ankle.

Functional leg-length discrepancy may occur in sports where an overdevelopment of one limb produces a difference. Unilateral conditions such as these include iliotibial band syndrome, unilateral patellofemoral joint syndrome or chondromalacia, unilateral shin splints, unilateral posterior tibial tendinitis or Achilles tendinitis. Chronic heel pain in one foot versus an asymptomatic opposite heel is a clear clue that the patient may have a limb-length difference. It is incumbent on the clinician to perform a full biomechanical evaluation to determine where the asymmetry lies.

The biomechanical evaluation should include a measurement of both limbs so that the examiner can quantify the difference between the two. The measurement is taken from the anterior superior iliac spine to the medial malleolus. The femoral component should be measured at the joint line of the femur and the tibia. Knowing the anatomical landmarks and being consistent when measuring the two limbs is important. Measurements of the limb and limb segments, in both neutral and relaxed stances, can eliminate the foot as the source of the limb discrepancy. When examining the foot, evaluate both the forefoot and the rearfoot to determine whether there has been an injury or previous surgical intervention that might have led to some asymmetry.

An excellent way to determine whether there is an asymmetry in body position or gait is to watch the patient stand and walk while wearing a pair of shorts or swim suit. Start at the head and continue the observation down from the shoulders while looking for any tilt. The tilting of a shoulder could be indicative of a short side where the shoulder is tilting.

Look to see if the neck is curved. If a double scoliosis is present, there will be no 'shoulder drop'. Next, look at the hips and pelvis and observe once again any tilt that might be present. Observe the hands to see if they are symmetrical, or if one hand is lower than the other during stance and gait. Draw a line down the spines of the vertebrae and, using a goniometer, measure the degree of deviation. Compare the scapulae and the sacral region, and look for any dimples. Rotation and twisting of the body takes place in the transverse plane; women are more prone to scoliosis than men, and thus these rotations may be more prevalent in women. Arm swing should alert the clinician to an asymmetry of the pelvis, with the opposing arm swinging more with the shorter leg.

It is very common for compensations for leg-length difference to be seen in the feet. The shorter side will supinate and maintain weight bearing on the outside of the foot while attempting to lengthen the limb. It can also function in an equinus position to prevent shortening of the limb. Conversely, the opposite will occur on the long-limb side. This foot will pronate more than normally to shorten the limb, and this will be evidenced by excessive medial shoe wear. It is estimated that 4–6 mm of shortening can occur with pronation at the subtalar joint.

Observe the runner or athlete in his or her running gait, and determine whether the stride is equal in comparison from both limbs. A shoulder drop, bouncing of the body or a short gait on one side versus the other shows an equinus gait and a short limb.

When an athlete relates a unilateral complaint (i.e. heel pain or knee pain), immediately suspect a limb-length discrepancy and check for any underlying aetiology. In the case of the heel pain the underlying cause could be a medial or lateral collateral ligament strain, or a muscle strain of the pes ansersartorius muscle insertion. A tight Achilles tendon or gastrocnemius–soleus complex secondary to one limb pronating more than the other is also indicative of a short limb.

## THE FEMALE ATHLETE TRIAD

For some women participating in sporting activities there is the risk of developing one or more of the three medical disorders that have been described as the *female athlete triad* (American College of Sports Medicine 1992, Nattiv et al 1994, Yeager et al 1993). The female athlete triad refers to the interrelatedness of disordered eating, amenorrhoea and osteoporosis, all of which could lead to significant morbidity and even to a high rate of mortality. The young female athlete who has a burning desire to excel in her sport, and yet feels pressurised to fit a specific athletic image to reach those goals, is at great risk of developing an eating disorder. This in turn can lead to menstrual dysfunction and subsequent early-onset osteoporosis. Each disorder alone is potentially dangerous; however, the three components of the triad together can raise the potential for a serious impact on the athlete's health and cause an increase the risk of mortality.

- Disordered eating refers to the various abnormal eating patterns, including the following behaviour disorders: (i) binge eating, purging, or both; (ii) food restriction; (iii) prolonged fasting; (iv) use of diet pills, diuretics, laxatives; (v) other abnormal eating behaviours.
- Amenorrhoea (secondary) can be defined by the absence of at least three to six consecutive menstrual cycles in women who have already begun menstruating.
- Osteoporosis, as defined for this group of young female athletes, refers to premature bone loss and inadequate bone formation, resulting in low bone mass, microarchitectural deterioration, increased skeletal fragility and an increased risk of fracture (Yeager et al 1993).

Due to the associated health problems, there has been a need to define the scope of the female athlete triad. The benefits of regular exercise are not in question; however, those adult and adolescent female athletes who develop disordered eating patterns, amenorrhoea and/or osteoporosis are at great risk of premature mortality. It is unknown how many young female athletes are affected by the triad of disorders. However, it has been reported that the prevalence of eating disorders in young female athletes is 15–62% (Rosen & Hough 1988, Warren et al 1990).

It is imperative that the sports physician continues to give the message of the importance of regular exercise and its many benefits. However, the health professional who works with female athletes should be aware of the possibility of the triad of disordered eating, amenorrhoea and osteoporosis in all female athletes.

## SPORTS SHOES

With the worldwide popularity of exercise participation and the desire of shoe manufacturers to capture a segment of the market, the explosion in the type and number of sports shoes available can be confusing. Shoe technology and design continue to change, and patients should be advised to visit a speciality athletic shoe shop where the sales staff know the intricacies of the shoes on sale. It is useful to recommend a number of different shoe companies and models to the patient. With that recommendation, the sales staff will know whether the patient needs a motion control, stability or cushioning shoe, and not just sell them a popular shoe. It is useful to establish a relationship with a speciality store.

The evolution of the running shoe over the past 30 years began with a shoe that was durable, the outer sole of which would not wear out too quickly. Next came the cushioning revolution, where most runners were looking for shock absorption and cushioning. In the last few years, the emphasis has been on function and support. Most running shoe magazines describe the important characteristics of shoes: rearfoot counters with reinforcement and stability, combination midsoles with EVA and polyurethane for durability, and stronger midfoot shanks for motion control. Some shoe designs include shock-absorbing mechanisms, stabilisers, antipronation and antisupination mechanisms, gel packs in the forefoot and rearfoot for added cushioning, rollbars for added stability, and varus wedges for additional biomechanical balancing of the forefoot. These features are very nice, but the question remains of how much protection the runner, athlete or patient needs, and how expensive a shoe is desired. If there is a prescribed orthosis for the patient, that in itself will help make a good shoe even better.

### Shoe manufacture

There is now a shoe for just about every sport (see also Ch. 18). Although the shoes may vary greatly in terms of their specifications, their inherent structure is basically the same throughout (Fig. 13.36).

### Lasts

As with most other footwear, sports shoes are made on lasts. The process that follows may be slip lasting, where the upper of the shoe is stitched around the last with the closure being along the length of the sole. Shoes made using this process are flexible and lightweight; they do not give much control of the foot, and are usually chosen for racing.

Another process is board lasting, where the upper is stitched to a board that has the shape of the inner sole. This produces a much

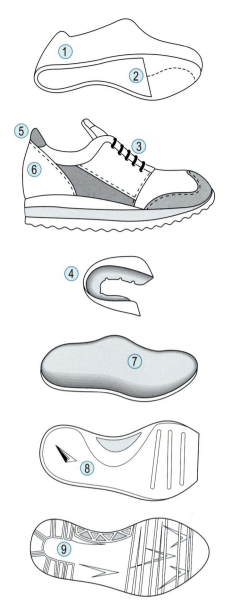

**Figure 13.36** Parts of the sports shoe: (1) last; (2) combination last construction; (3) upper – synthetic material and mesh for ventilation; (4) motion control device; (5) Achilles flex notch; (6) heel counter; (7) inner sole, removable; (8) midsole; (9) outsole.

firmer shoe, which gives the foot much more stability and is a good base for orthotics. However, it may require some time for the shoe to be 'worn in'.

A third form is combination lasting, in which the front part of the shoe is slip lasted and the part of the shoe from just behind the metatarsal heads to the heel is board lasted. This combination gives good stability, but because of the more flexible forepart is not so heavy and difficult to wear at first (Fig. 13.37).

### Shape of the last

There are three basic shapes of last, the first of which is the straight or semi-straight last. This has only the slightest inflare along its medial border and is considered the most supportive; it should be chosen for overpronating low-arched and pronating feet.

The second, and most common, shape is the semicurved last, which has a greater degree of inflare along the medial border. It offers some

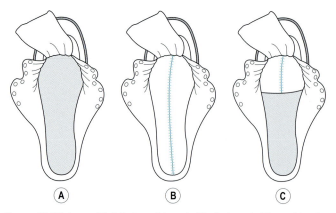

**Figure 13.37** Lasts: (A) fully board lasted; (B) slip lasted; (C) combination lasted.

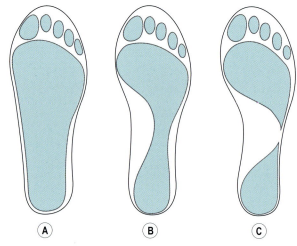

**Figure 13.38** Lasts: (A) semi-straight last; (B) semicurved last; (C) curved last.

medial support but not quite as much as the straight last, and is used for the vast majority of the population.

The third type of last is the curved last, which is used for racing shoes and lightweight trainers, as it has the greatest amount of inflare along the medial border and provides the least amount of support. It is chosen for higher arched feet that tend to be more rigid and for mid- to forefoot strikers. The shoe is flexible and lightweight (Fig. 13.38).

## Other factors

### The heel counter

This part of the shoe probably gives the shoe most of its stability; if the counter is soft and flexible then stability at the heel is lost, however well the rest of the shoe is built. It is usually made from a board type of material or a plastic, and should not compress with manual pressure.

### The tongue

This is designed to protect the foot from the laces, but is tending to be excluded from shoe design at present as a separate entity, and is being incorporated in the upper or the inner sleeve of the shoe. Its function remains the same.

### Insole

This is usually a moulded or contoured thin piece of material, often made from EVA, with a towelling or fleecy top cover, which conforms to the sole of the foot. It provides comfort and gives some stability, preventing the foot from moving within the shoe. It is often removable and can easily be replaced with shock-absorbing materials and orthotics.

### Outsole

This is sometimes referred to as the 'top sole' because, in the method of construction, it is one of the final components to be added when the shoe is on the last and upside down. It provides grip and durability, with differences in tread and pattern that can be chosen according to different needs. Treads with wider spaces are less easily clogged when running off-road. The materials are usually carbon rubber, which is a heavy and durable material for weighty people or rugged activity, or blow rubber, which is lighter and less durable but has more cushioning and is suitable for racing and lightweight people and activities.

### Midsole

This is often considered to be the foundation of a running shoe; it provides cushioning and stability. It can be made from EVA (which provides more cushioning) or polyurethane (which has greater durability), or combinations of the two, and may have various devices added. These can include gel, air sacs, tubes and other such mechanisms, all of which can add to the cost of the shoe. The durability of the midsole depends greatly on the weight of the individual, the mileage covered and any biomechanical problems.

### Upper

This is mostly made from synthetic material and mesh to produce ventilation and a lightweight shoe. Recent materials include Lycra and neoprene, which are comfortable, durable and supportive. Recent advances using these materials have seen the introduction of a sleeve or semi-sleeve, which encloses the foot within the shoe, rather like a glove, and allows the standard shoe to fit many more foot shapes.

Laces have been replaced with many other types of fastening and closure, including Velcro, straps, belts, screws and wheels. One shoe even includes a canister of carbon dioxide, which inflates the innersole to improve the fit of the shoe around the foot.

## Scientific evaluation

Shoe manufacturers invest a lot of time and money in testing shoes and materials for their shock-absorbing properties and ability to reduce trauma. There is an awareness of the causes of trauma, and attempts are made to incorporate materials that will reduce it. Similarly, manufacturers have gained an awareness of the effects of foot function, mechanics and overpronation as a cause of injury, and attempt to incorporate mechanisms to improve foot function and control excessive pronation. Much dependence is placed on current computer technology, and efforts are being made to produce more reliable data concerning the function of the foot in the shoe.

## Features of a good sports shoe

1. Select a shoe with a toe box that has adequate height over the toes and 2 cm of length from the ends of the toes.
2. There is not a standard width or length fitting to cover all makes of shoe; therefore, the selection of the shoe remains a matter of the judgement of the person who is going to wear it. The correct width is necessary to avoid squeezing the forefoot, and the shoe

should not be too loose as this will cause fatigue of the forefoot. It should be possible to 'pinch' 2 cm of the upper material over the ball of the foot to ensure a good fit.

3. Balance and equilibrium in the shoe are necessary to avoid excessive stresses and forces, which could interfere with the normal motion of the foot and limb during running. If the shoe tilts towards the medial border most of the motion will be in that direction, causing overuse syndrome. Always check that the heel counter is perpendicular to the supporting surface of the shoe.

4. Good flexibility of the shoe at the ball of the foot is important to avoid fatigue of the muscles of the lower leg and to avoid tendon strains. If the shoe does not flex at the correct position, arch fatigue or foot strain may result. A shoe should bend easily at the ball of the shoe using the power of one finger alone.

5. The position of the heel counter and its rigidity are important factors for controlling the direction of the forces on the foot during the heel contact phase of the running cycle.

6. Weight and softness of the shoe are closely related, as most lightweight shoes are made from soft midsole materials. Such shoes are adequate for a lightweight person who has good foot structure and who hits the ground hard, but they tend to fatigue and warp after 300–400 km of use. With less midsole protection, the insoles must be made from soft resilient materials, especially at the forefoot.

7. Shoes have a shelf life after which time their component materials, such as the EVA in the midsole, become hard and the glues harden and become brittle. It is not necessarily wise to purchase two pairs of shoes unless they are used concurrently.

## REFERENCES

Agostinelli J, Ross JA 1977 Infracalcaneal heel pain in the athlete. Sports Medicine and Rehabilitation, Clinics in Podiatric Medicine and Surgery 14(3):503–509.

Alexander IJ, Johnson RA, Kerquist TH 1987 Magnetic resonance imaging in the diagnosis of disruption of the posterior tibial tendon. Foot and Ankle 8:144.

Amendola A, Rorabid Ch, Bellett D 1990 The use of magnetic resonance imaging in exertional compartment syndrome. American Journal of Sports Medicine 18:29–34.

American College of Sports Medicine 1992 The female triad: disordered eating, amenorrhea, osteoporosis: call to action. Sports Medicine Bulletin 27:4.

Anderson KJ, LeCocq JF, LeCocq EA 1952 Recurrent anterior subluxation of the ankle. Journal of Bone and Joint Surgery 34A:853, 860.

Anouche Y, Parker R, Seitz W 1987 Posterior compartment syndrome of the calf resulting from misdiagnosis of a rupture of the medial head of the gastrocnemius. Journal of Trauma 27:678.

Armstrong RB 1984 Mechanisms of exercise-induced delayed onset muscle soreness: a brief overview. Medical Science Sports Exercise 16:529.

Arner O, Lindholm A 1958 What is tennis leg? Acta Chirologica Scandinavica 116:73.

Aronoff AM 1982 The use of non-narcotic drugs and other alternatives of analgesic as part of a comprehensive pain management program. Journal of Medicine 13:191.

Ashton H 1975 The effect of increased tissue pressure on blood flow. Clinical Orthopaedics 113:15.

Astom M, Rausing A 1995 Chronic Achilles tendinopathy. Clinical Orthopaedics and Related Research 316:151.

Austin DW, Leiventhen EO 1981 A new osteotomy for hallux valgus. Clinical Orthopaedics 157:25–30.

Baldwin FC, Tezlaff J 1982 Historical perspectives on injuries of the ligaments of the ankle. Clinics in Sport Medicine 1(1):3–12.

Banks AS, McGlamry ED 1987 Tibialis posterior rupture. Journal of the American Podiatric Association 77:170.

Barfred T 1971 Experimental rupture of the Achilles tendon: comparison of various types of experimental rupture in rats. Acta Orthopaedica Scandinavica 42:528–543.

Barnett CH, Richardson AT 1953 The postural function of the popliteus muscle. Annual Physical Medicine 1:177–179.

Barrick EF, Jackson CB 1992 Prophylactic intramedullary of the tibia for stress fracture in a professional athlete. Journal of Orthopedics and Trauma 6:241–244.

Barrows HJ 1940 Spontaneous fractures of the apparently normal fibular in its lowest third. British Journal of Surgery 28:82–84.

Barrows HJ 1948 Fatigue fracture. Journal of Bone and Joint Surgery 303:266–279.

Basmajian JV, Lovejoy JF 1971 Functions of the popliteus muscle in man. Journal of Bone and Joint Surgery 53A:557–562.

Bates B, Stergiou N 1999a Forces acting on the lower extremity mechanism associated with running injuries. In: Subotnick SI (ed.) Sports medicine of the lower extremity, 2nd edn. Churchill Livingstone, Edinburgh, pp 176–177.

Bates B, Stergiou N 1999b Normal patterns of walking and running. In: Subotnick SI (ed.) Sports medicine of the lower extremity, 2nd edn. Churchill Livingstone, Edinburgh, p. 157.

Baxter DE 1994a The heel in sport. Clinics in Sports Medicine, Foot and Ankle Injuries 13(4):683–693.

Baxter DE 1994b Treatment of bunion deformity in the athlete. Orthopedic Clinics of North America, Foot and Ankle Injuries in Sports 25(1):33–39.

Baxter DE, Pfeffer GB 1992 Treatment of chronic heel pain by surgical release of the first branch of the lateral plantar nerve. Clinics in Orthopedics 279:229–236.

Belken SC 1980 Stress fractures in athletes. Orthopedic Clinics of North America 11: 735.

Beltran J, Moscure JC 1990 Magnetic resonance imaging of tendons. New Diagnostic Imaging 30:11–182.

Bennell RL, Malcolm SA, Thomas SA 1996 The incidence and distribution of stress fractures in competitive track and field athletes – a twelve month prospective study. American Journal of Sports Medicine 24:211.

Betz M, Klimt F 1992 Requirements and risk profile of soccer-playing children: orthopaedic aspects. Schweiz A: Sports Medicine 40:169–173.

Blair WF, Manley SR 1980 Stress fractures of the proximal fibula. American Journal of Sport Medicine 8:212–213.

Bojsen-Moller F, Flagstad KE 1976 Plantar aponeurosis and internal architecture of the ball of the foot. Journal of Anatomy 3:599–611.

Bordelon RL 1983 Subcalcaneal pain. Clinical Orthopaedics 177:49.

Bordelon RL 1993 Heel pain. In: Mann RA (ed.) Surgery of the foot and ankle, 6th edn. CV Mosby, St Louis, pp 837–847.

Bosien WR, Staples OS, Russell SW 1955 Residual disability following acute ankle sprains. Journal of Bone and Joint Surgery 37A:1237–1243.

Boyd PM, Bogdan RJ 1997 Sports Injuries. In: Lorimer DL, French G, West S (eds) Neale's common foot disorders; diagnosis and management, 5th edn. Churchill Livingstone, Edinburgh, pp 198–201.

Bradley JP, Tibone JE 1990 Percutaneous and surgical repairs of Achilles tendon rupture, a comparative study. American Journal of Sport Medicine 18:188–195.

Brahms MA, Fumich RM, Ippolito VD 1980 Atypical stress fracture of the tibia in a professional athlete. American Journal of Sport Medicine 8:131–132.

Briethaupt MD 1855 Zurpathogic desmonschlicen Fusses. Medicinisch Zeitungen 24:169.

Brooks SX, Potter BT, Rainey JB 1981 Treatment for partial tears of the lateral collateral ligament of the ankle: a prospective trial. British Medical Journal 282:606–607.

Brostrom L 1964 Sprained ankles: I: amateur lesion in recent sprains. Acta Chirurgica Scandinavica 128:483–495.

Brostrom L 1965 Sprained ankles. Acta Chirurgica Scandinavica 130:560.

Brostrom L 1966 Sprained ankles: V: treatment and prognosis in recent ligament ruptures. Acta Chirurgica Scandinavica 132:537–550.

Burrows HJ 1956 Fatigue fracture of the middle of the tibia in ballet dancers. Journal of Bone and Joint Surgery 388:83–94.

Carden DG, Noble J, Chalmers J 1989 Rupture of the calcaneal tendon – the early and late management. Journal of Bone and Joint Surgery 71B(1):100–101.

Carr AJ, Norris SH 1989 The blood supply of the calcaneal tendon. Journal of Bone and Joint Surgery 71B(1):110–113.

Cavanaugh PR, Williams KR 1983 The mechanics of foot action during the golf swing and its implications for shoe design. Medical Science of Sports Exercise 15:247–255.

Christensen I 1953 Rupture of the Achilles tendon. Acta Chirurgica Scandinavica 106:50–60.

Clain MR, Baxter DE 1992 Achilles tendonitis. Foot and Ankle 13(8):482–487.

Clancy WG 1982 Tendinitis and plantar fasciitis in runners. In: D'Ambrosia R, Drez D (eds) Prevention and treatment of running injuries. Charles B Black, Thorofore, NJ.

Clancy WG, Neidhart D, Brana RL 1992 Achilles tendonitis in runners: a report of five cases. American Journal of Sport Medicine 2(2):46–57.

Clanton TO, Schon LC 1993 Athletic injuries to the soft tissue of the foot and ankle. In: Mann RA, Couglin MJ (eds) Surgery of the foot and ankle, 6th edn. CV Mosby, St Louis, MI, p. 1105.

Clanton TX, Solcher BW 1994 Chronic leg pain in the athlete. Clinics in Sports Medicine 13(4):743–759.

Clanton TO, Butler JE, Eggert A 1986 Injuries to the metatarsophalangeal joints in athletes. Foot and Ankle 7:162.

Clark TE, Frederick EC, Cooper LB 1983 Effects of shoe cushioning upon ground reaction forces in running. International Journal of Sports Medicine 4:247.

Clement DB, Faunton JE, Smart GW 1984 Achilles tendinitis and peritendinitis: etiology and treatment. American Journal of Sport Medicine 12(3):179–184.

Colt FW, Spyropoulos E 1979 Running and stress. British Medical Journal 2:706.

Conte S, Michelson J, Jahss M 1992 Clinical significance of magnetic resonance imaging in preoperative planning for reconstruction of posterior tibial tendon ruptures. Foot and Ankle 13:208.

Conti SF 1994 Posterior tibial tendon problems in athletes. Orthopedic Clinics of North American 25:109.

Cotterill JM 1888 Stiffness in the great toe in adolescents. British Medical Journal 1:1158.

Dananberg HJ 1986 Functional hallux limitus and its relationship to gait efficiency. Journal of the American Podiatric Medical Association 76:11.

Davies-Colley MR 1887 Contraction of the metatarsophalangeal joint of the great toe. British Medical Journal 1:728.

Davis AW, Alexander IJ 1990 Problematic fractures and dislocation in the foot and ankle of athletes, fractures. Clinics in Sports Medicine 9(1):163–181.

De Lee JC, Evans JP, Julian J 1983 Stress fractures of the fifth metatarsal. American Journal of Sport Medicine 11:349–353.

Denton J 1997 Overuse foot and ankle injuries in ballet. Clinics in Podiatric Medicine and Surgery, Sports Medicine and Rehabilitation 14(3):525–532.

Detner DE 1986 Chronic shin splints: classification and management of medial tibial stress syndrome. Sports Medicine 3:436–446.

Detner DE, Sharp R, Sufit RL 1985 Chronic compartment syndrome, diagnosis, management and outcomes. American Journal of Sport Medicine 13:162–170.

Devas MB 1958 Stress fractures of the tibia in athletes or 'shin soreness'. Journal of Bone and Joint Surgery 40B:227–239.

Devas MB 1975 Stress fractures. Churchill Livingstone, Edinburgh.

Devas MB, Sweetnam R 1956 Stress fractures of the fibula, a review of fifty cases in athletes. Journal of Bone and Joint Surgery 38B:818–829.

DiStefano VJ, Nuron JE 1972 Achilles tendon rupture: pathogenesis, diagnosis, and treatment by a modified pullout wire technique. Journal of Trauma 12:671–677.

Dollar JD 1978 The introduction of new pathologies associated with athletic performance on artificial turf. In: Rinaldi RR, Sabice ML (eds) Sports medicine. Futura, Mt Kisco, NY, p. 107.

Drez D 1982 Forefoot problems in runners. Symposium on the foot and leg in running sports. CV Mosby, St Louis, MI, 73–75.

Drez D, Young JL, Johnston RD 1980 Metatarsal stress fractures. American Journal of Sport Medicine 8:123–125.

Dulberg H 1999 Children and sports. In: Subotnick SI (ed.) Sports medicine of the lower extremity, 2nd edn. Churchill Livingstone, Edinburgh, p. 15.

Dulberg HN, Gueally J 1999 Psychological considerations. In: Subotnick SI (ed.) Sports medicine of the lower extremity, 2nd edn. Churchill Livingstone, Edinburgh, p. 213.

Duthii R, Haughton G 1981 Constitutional aspects of the osteochondrosis. Clinical Orthopaedics 158:19–27.

Dyatch Rov VM 1969 High jumping track technique. Journal of Technical Track and Field Athletics 36:1123–1158.

Ekman EF, Pope T, Martin DF, Curl WW 1994 Magnetic resonance imaging of ilio-tibial band syndrome. American Journal of Sport Medicine 22:851–854.

Erstrand J, Gillquist J 1983a Soccer injuries and their mechanisms: a prospective study. Medical Science in Sports 15:267.

Erstrand J, Gillquist J 1983b The avoidability of soccer injuries. International Journal of Sports Medicine 4:124.

Fadale PD, Wiggins ME 1994 Corticosteroid injections: their use and abuse. Journal of the American Academy of Orthopedic Surgery 2:133–140.

Fallet L 1990 Pathology of the fifth ray, including the tailor's bunion deformity. Clinics in Podiatric Medicine and Surgery 7:689.

Ficat P, Hungerfred D 1977 Disorders of the patello-femoral joint. Williams & Wilkins, Baltimore, OH.

Fowler A, Philip JF 1945 Abnormality of the calcaneus as a cause of painful heel. British Journal of Surgery 32:494–498.

Fox JM, Blazineme Jobe FW, Kerlan RK, et al 1975 Degeneration and rupture of the Achilles tendon. Clinical Orthopaedics 107:221–224.

Frederson M 1996 Common injuries in runners: diagnoses, rehabilitation and prevention. Injury clinic. Sports Medicine 21:49.

Freiberg A 1914 Infraction of the second metatarsal bone – a typical injury. Surgery, Gynecology & Obstetrics 19:191–193.

Frey C, Rosenberg Z, Sheriff M 1982 The retrocalcaneal bursa: anatomy and bursography. Foot and Ankle 13:203, 207.

Frey C, Sheriff M, Grunidge N 1990 Vascularity of the posterior tibial tendon. Journal of Bone and Joint Surgery 72:884.

Froimson A 1969 Tennis leg. Journal of the American Medical Association 209:415.

Funk CC, Cass JR, Johnson RA 1986 Acquired adult flat foot secondary to posterior tibial tendon pathology. Journal of Bone and Joint Surgery 68A:95–102.

Furman AF 1999 Golf injuries. In: Subotnick SI (ed.) Sports medicine of the lower extremity, 2nd edn. Edinburgh: Churchill Livingstone, pp 719–724.

Galloway M, Jokl P, Dayton O 1992 Achilles tendon overuse injuries. Clinics in Sports Medicine 11:771.

Ganong RB, Heneveld EH, Bernanek SR, Fry P 1992 Snowboarding injuries: a report on 415 patients. The Physician and Sports Medicine 20:114.

Garfin SR, Tipton CM, Mubarak SJ 1981 The role of fascia in maintenance of muscle tension and pressure. Journal of Applied Physiology 51:317–320.

Garrich JG 1982 Epidemiologic perspective. Clinics in Sports Medicine 1:13–18.

Garrich JG, Requa RK 1973 Role of external support in the prevention of ankle sprains. Medicine and Science in Sports: 200–203.

Garrich JG, Requa RK 1988 The epidemiology of foot and ankle injuries in sports. Clinics in Sports Medicine – Foot and Ankle Injuries 7(1):29–36.

Gaynor R, Hake D, Spinner S 1989 A comparative analysis of conservative versus surgical treatment of Morton's neuroma. Journal of the American Pediatric Medical Association 79:27–30.

Gilad M, Ahronson Z, Stein M 1985 Unusual distribution and onset of stress fractures in soldiers. Clinical Orthopaedics 192: 142–146.

Glick JM, Gordon RB, Nishinoto D 1976 The prevention and treatment of ankle injuries. American Journal of Sport Medicine 4:136–141.

Goldner JL, Keats PR, Bassett FA 1974 Progressive talipes equinus due to trauma or degeneration of the posterior tibial tendon and medial plantar ligaments. Orthopedic Clinics of North America 5:39–51.

Goodfellow J, Hungeford DA, Woods C 1976 Patellofemoral joint mechanics and pathology to chondromalacia patellae. Journal of Bone and Joint Surgery 58B: 291.

Green NE, Rogers RA, Lipscomb AB 1985 Non-unions of stress fractures of the tibia. American Journal of Sport Medicine 13:171–176.

Greenfield B 1990 Evaluation of overuse syndromes. In: Donatelli R (ed.) The biomechanics of the foot and ankle: contemporary perspectives in rehabilitation, 153.

Hageman CE, Lehman RC 1988 Stretching, strengthening and conditioning for the competitive tennis player. Clinics in Sports Medicine 7(2):211–228.

Hamilton WG 1982a Sprained ankles in ballet dancers. Foot and Ankle 3:99.

Hamilton WG 1982b Stenosing tenosynovitis of the flexor hallucis longus tendon and posterior impingement upon the os trigonum in ballet dancers. Foot and Ankle 3:74–80.

Harper MC, Keller TS 1980 A radiographic evaluation of the tibia fibular syndesmosis. Foot and Ankle 1:84–89.

Hatch DJ 1994 Chronic stenosing fibular (peroneal) tenosynovitis. The Lower Extremity 1:197.

Heel J 1993 Psychology of sports injury. Human Kinetics Publishers, Champaign, IL.

Henegham MA, Pavlov H 1984 The Hagland painful heel syndrome. Clinical Orthopaedics 187:228.

Henning EM, Milani TL 1995 In-shoe pressure distribution for running in various types of footwear. Journal of Applied Biomechanics 11:299.

Henry JH, Lureau B, Neigut D 1982 The injury rate in professional basketball. American Journal of Sport Medicine 16–18.

Herring SA, Nelson KL 1987 Introduction to overuse injuries. Clinics in Sports Medicine 6:225–239.

Hicks JA 1954 The mechanics of the foot: the plantar aponeuroses and the arch. Journal of Anatomy 88:25–31.

Hoadley AE 1893 Six cases of metatarsalgia. Chicago Medical Record 4:32–37.

Hoerr NC, Pyle DI, Fracis CC 1962 Radiographic atlas of skeletal development of the foot and ankle: a standard reference. Charles C Thomas, Springfield, IL.

Hogan JF 1993 Posterior tibial dysfunction and MRI. Journal of Foot and Ankle Surgery 32:467–472.

Hohmann A 1951 Fuss und bien. JF Bergmann, Munich, p. 145.

Holmes JC, Pruitt AL, Whalen NJ 1993 Iliotibial band syndrome in cyclists. American Journal of Sport Medicine 21:419–424.

Hopkison WJ, Pierre P, Ryan JB, Wheeler JH 1990 Syndesmosis sprains of the ankle. Foot and Ankle 10:325.

Hreljac A 1993 Preferred and energetically optional gait transition speeds in human locomotion. Medical Science Sports Exercise 25:1158.

Hughes JR 1984 Psychological effects of habitual aerobic exercise: a critical view. Preventative Medicine 13:148.

Ingles AE, Scott NW, Sculco TP 1976 Ruptures of the tendo-Achilles – an objective assessment of surgical and non-surgical treatment. Journal of Bone and Joint Surgery 58A(7):990–993.

Jahss MD 1981 The sesamoids of the hallux. Clinical Orthopaedics 57:88–97.

James SL, Bates BT, Osternig RL 1978 Injuries to runners. American Journal of Sport Medicine 6(2):40.

Jarvin JS, Fercel RD 1994 Arthroscopy of the foot and ankle. Clinics in Sports Medicine 13(4):761, 783.

Jarvinen M, Joza L, Kannus P 1997 Histopathological findings in chronic tendon disorders. Scandinavian Journal of Medical Science and Sports 7(2):86–95.

Johnson EE, Markold KL 1983 The contribution of the anterior talo-fibular ligament to ankle laxity. Journal of Bone and Joint Surgery 65:81.

Johnson LG 1964 Morphologic analysis in pathology. In Frost HM (ed.) Bone biodynamics. Little Brown, Boston, MA.

Johnson RA 1983 Tibialis posterior tendon rupture. Clinical Orthopaedics 177: 140–147.

Johnson RA, Strom DE 1989 Tibialis posterior dysfunction. Clinical Orthopaedics 239:196–206.

Jones BH, Harris JM, Vihn TN 1989 Exercise-induced stress fractures and stress reactions to bone: epidemiology, etiology and classification. Exercise Sports Science Review 17:379.

Jones DC, Jones SL 1987 Overuse injuries of the lower extremity, shin splints, iliotibial band friction syndrome and exertional compartment syndrome. Clinics in Sports Medicine 6:273–290.

Jones SL, Bates BT, Osternig LR 1978 Injuries to runners. American Journal of Sport Medicine 6:40–50.

Kannus P, Nittynaki S, Jarvinen M 1988 Athletic overuse injuries in children. A 30-month follow-up study at an outpatient sports clinic. Clinical Pediatrics 27: 333–337.

Kaplan EB 1958 The iliotibial tract. Journal of Bone and Joint Surgery 40A:817–832.

Kaplan EB 1962 Some aspects of functional anatomy of the human knee joint. Clinical Orthopaedics 23:18.

Karlsson J, Bergsten T, Lansinger O, et al 1989 Surgical treatment of chronic lateral instability of the ankle joint. American Journal of Sport Medicine 17:268–274.

Kaufer H 1971 Mechanical function of the patella. Journal of Bone and Joint Surgery 53A:1551.

Keck SW, Kelly PJ 1965 Bursitis of the posterior part of the heel. Journal of Bone and Joint Surgery 47:267.

Kerr R, Henry D 1989 Posterior tibial tendon rupture. Orthopedics 12:1394.

Kettlekamp DB, Alexnder HH 1969 Spontaneous rupture of the posterior tibial tendon. Journal of Bone and Joint Surgery 51A:759–764.

Key JD, Johnson D, Jarvis G, Ponsonby D 1999 Knee and thigh injuries – chondromalacia patellae. In: Subotnick SI (ed.) Sports medicine of the lower extremity, 2nd edn. Churchill Livingstone, Edinburgh, pp 308–309.

Khan KM, Cook JL, Taunton JE, Bonar F 2000 Overuse tendinosis, not tendinitis. The Physician and Sports Medicine 28(5): 38–47.

Kidner FC 1929 The pre-hallux in its relation to flat foot. Journal of Bone and Joint Surgery 11:831.

Kinnard P, Lirette R 1989 Dorsiflexion osteotomy in Freiberg's disease. Foot and Ankle 9:226–234.

Kohler A 1961 The sesamoid bones of the foot: borderlands of the normal and early pathology in skeletal roentgenology. Grune & Stratton, New York, pp 684–691.

Kravitz SR, Murgia C 1999 The mechanics of dance and dance related injuries. In: Subotnick SI (ed.) Sports medicine of the lower extremity, 2nd edn. Churchill Livingstone, Edinburgh, pp 645–655.

Kravitz SR, LaPorta A, Lawton JH 1994 KL progressive staging classification of hallux limitus and hallux rigidus. Lower Extremity 1(1):55.

Krissoff WB, Ferris WB 1979 Runners injuries. Physician and Sports Medicine 7(12):55–64.

Kune JS, Narechania MS, Sachtjen KM, Clancy WC 1980 Tartan turf on trial. American Journal of Sport Medicine 8:43.

Kvist H, Kvist M 1980 The operative treatment of chronic calcaneal paratendonitis. Journal of Bone and Joint Surgery 62B(3):353–357.

Kvist M, Jorza J, Kvist H 1987a A chronic Achilles paratendonitis in athletes: a histological and histochemical study. Pathology 19:1.

Kvist MH, Lehto MV, Jaroenen M, Vuist HT 1987b Chronic Achilles paratenonitis: an immunohistologic study of fibronectin and fibrinogen. American Journal of Sport Medicine 16:616.

Lagergren C, Lindholm A 1958 Vascular distribution in the Achilles tendon. Acta Chirurgica Scandinavica 116:491–495.

Le Unes AD, Nation J 1989 Sports psychology: an introduction. Nelson-Hall, Chicago, IL.

Lea RB, Smith L 1968 Ruptures of the Achilles tendon. PORR 60:15–118.

Lea RB, Smith L 1972 Non-surgical treatment of Achilles tendon rupture. Journal of Bone and Joint Surgery 54A:1398–1407.

Leach RE 1988 Leg and foot injuries in racquet sports. Clinics in Sports Medicine 7(2):359–370.

Leach RE, Dilorio E, Hurney RA 1983 Pathologic hindfoot conditions in the athlete. Clinical Orthopaedics 177:116.

Lehman RC, Gregg JR, Torg E 1986 Iselin's disease. American Journal of Sport Medicine 14:494–496.

Leonard MH 1949 Injuries of the lateral ligaments of the ankle. Journal of Bone and Joint Surgery 31:373–377.

Levisohn S, Simon H 1984 The knee and lower leg in tennis: conditioning, sports medicine and total fitness for every player. CV Mosby, St Louis, MI, p. 179.

Lysens RJ, Ostynms MS, Vanden-Auweele Y 1989 The accident prone and overuse prone profiles of the young athlete. American Journal of Sport Medicine 17:612–619.

McBryde AM 1985 Stress fractures in runners. Clinics in Sports Medicine 4:737.

McBryde AM Jr, Anderson RB 1988 Sesamoid foot problems in the athlete. Clinics in Sports Medicine 7(1):51–60.

McCarroll JR, Gioe TJ 1982 Professional golfers and the price they pay. The Physician and Sports Medicine 10:54–70.

McCarrol JR, Gidonoghve DH, Grana WA 1983 The surgical treatment of chondromalacia of the patella. Clinical Orthopaedics 175:130.

McCarrol JR, Rettig AC, Shelbourne RD 1990 Injuries in the amateur golfer. The Physician and Sports Medicine 3:18.

McCarthy P 1989 Artificial turf: does it cause more injuries? The Physician and Sports Medicine 17:159.

McCullock PG, Holden P, Rolson DJ 1985 The value of mobilisation and non-steroidal anti-inflammatory analgesia in the management of inversion injuries of the ankle. British Journal of Clinical Practice 29:69–72.

McMahon TA, Valiant G, Trederick ED 1987 Groucho running. Journal of Applied Physiology 87:236.

McNerney JE 1990 Sports medicine considerations of lesser metatarsalgia. Clinics in Podiatric Medicine and Surgery 7:645.

McNerney JE 1999 Football injuries. In: Subotnick SI (ed.) Sports medicine of the lower extremity, 2nd edn. Churchill Livingstone, Edinburgh, pp 739–746.

Maffulli N, Chan D, Aldridge MJ 1992 Overuse injuries in the olecranon in young gymnasts. Journal of Bone and Joint Surgery 74:305–308.

Magnusson SP, Gleim CW, Nicholas JA 1994 Shoulder weakness in professional baseball pitchers. Medical Science Sports Exercise 26:5.

Mahan KT, Carter SR 1992 Multiple ruptures of the tendon Achilles. Journal of Foot Surgery 31(6):549–559.

Malay DS, Duggan GE 1987 In: McGlamry ED (ed.) Heel surgery comprehensive text book for foot surgery. Williams & Wilkins, Baltimore, OH, pp 264–284.

Mann RA 1986 Biomechanics of running. In: Nicholas J (ed.) The lower extremity and spine in sports medicine. CV Mosby, St Louis, MI, pp 396–411.

Mann RA 1993 Flatfoot in adult. In: Mann RA, Coughlin MJ (eds) Surgery of the foot and ankle, 6th edn., Vol. 1. Mosby-Year Book, St Louis, MI.

Mann RA, Thompson FM 1985 Rupture of the posterior tibial tendon causing flat foot: surgical treatment. Journal of Bone and Joint Surgery 67A:556–561.

Markey KL 1987 Stress fracture. Clinics in Sports Medicine 6(2):405–425.

Martins MA, Backaert M, Vermaut G 1984 Chronic leg pain in athletes due to a recurrent compartment syndrome. American Journal of Sport Medicine 12:148–151.

Matson FA 1975 Compartment syndrome – a unified concept. Clinical Orthopaedics 113:8.

Meewwisse WH, Fowler PO 1988 Frequency and predictability of sports injuries in intercollegiate athletes. Canadian Journal of Sports Science 13:35.

Messina DF, Farney WC, De Lee JC 1999 Incidence of injury in Texas high school basketball. American Journal of Sport Medicine 27(3):294–299.

Mibarak SJ 1981 Exertional compartment syndrome. In Mibarak SJ, Hargens AR (eds) Compartment syndromes and Volkmass's contracture. WB Saunders, Philadelphia, PA, pp 209–226.

Michael RH, Holder LE 1977 The soleus syndrome: a cause of medial tibial stress (shin splints). American Journal of Sport Medicine 5:191–193.

Micheli LJ 1983 Overuse injuries in children's sports: the growth factor. Orthopedic Clinics of North America 14:337–360.

Micheli LJ 1987 The traction apophysitises. Clinics in Sports Medicine 6:389–404.

Micheli LJ, Ireland ML 1987 Prevention and management of calcaneal apophysitis in children: an overuse syndrome. Journal of Pediatric Orthopedics 7:34–38.

Micheli LJ, Fehlandt AF Jr 1992 Overuse injuries to tendons and apophyses in children and adolescents. Clinics in Sports Medicine 11:713–726.

Micheli, LJ, Smith AD 1982 Sports injuries in children. Current Problems in Pediatrics 12:1–54.

Miller EH, Schneider HJ, Bronson JL 1975 A new consideration in athletic injuries: the classical ballet dancer. Clinical Orthopedics 111:181–191.

Miller J 1980 Plyometric training for speed. National Strength and Conditioning Association Journal 2:20–22.

Miller SJ 1987 Morton's neuroma. In: Comprehensive textbook of foot surgery, Vol. 1. Williams & Wilkins, Baltimore, OH.

Moller-Larsen F, Wethelund JO, Jurik AG 1988 Comparison of three different treatments for ruptured lateral ankle ligaments. Acta Orthopaedica Scandinavica 59:564.

Morris JM, Blickenstaff LB 1967 Fatigue fractures. Charles C Thomas, Springfield, IL.

Morton TG 1876 A peculiar and painful affection of the fourth metatarsal phalangeal articulation. American Journal of Medical Science 71:37–45.

Mozan LC, Keagy RD 1969 Muscle relationship in functional fascia. Clinical Orthopaedics 67:225–230.

Mueller TM 1984 Ruptures and lacerations of the tibialis posterior tendon. Journal of the American Medical Association 74:109–119.

Murphey PC, Baxter DE 1985 Nerve entrapment of the foot and ankle in runners. Clinics in Sports Medicine 4:753.

Myerson M 1996 Adult acquired flat foot deformity: treatment of dysfunction of the posterior tibial tendon. Journal of Bone and Joint Surgery 78A:780–792.

National Basketball Athletic Trainers' Association, Injury Report, 1989–1990.

Nattiv A, Agostini R, Drinkwater B, Yeager KK, 1994 The female athlete triad. The interrelatedness of disordered eating, amenorrhea and osteoporosis. Clinics in Sports Medicine 13(2):405–418.

Nissen RL 1948 Plantar digital neuritis in Morton's metatarsalgia. Journal of Bone and Joint Surgery 30B:84–94.

Nistor L 1981 Surgical and non-surgical treatment of Achilles tendon rupture – a prospective randomized study. Journal of Bone and Joint Surgery 63A(3):394–399.

Nobel CA 1980 Ilio-tibial band friction syndrome in runners. American Journal of Sport Medicine 8:232–234.

Nordin M, Frankel VH 1980 Basic biomechanics. Lea & Febiger, New York.

O'Connor F, Sobel J, Nirschl R 1992 Five-step treatment of overuse injuries. The Physician and Sports Medicine 20:128.

Obel AO 1982 Practical therapeutics: the newer non-steroidal anti-inflammatory drugs. East African Medical Journal 59:366.

Orava S 1980a Stress fractures. British Journal of Sports Medicine 14:40–44.

Orava S 1980b Extremity injuries due to sports and physical exercise. A clinical and statistical study of non traumatic overuse injuries of the musculoskeletal system of athletes and keep-fit athletes. Thesis, University of Owler, Finland.

Orava S, Puranen J 1979 Athlete leg pain. British Journal of Sports Medicine 13:92.

Outerbridge RE, Dunlop JAY 1975 The problem of chondromalacia patellae. Clinical Orthopaedics 110:177.

Paddue G, Ippolito E, Postacchini F 1976 A classification of Achilles tendon disease. American Journal of Sport Medicine 4(4):145–150.

Pagliano JW 1997 Angular surgical corrections for hallux valgus. Clinics in Podiatric Medicine and Surgery, Sports Medicine and Rehabilitation 14(2).

Parks RM 1989 Podiatric sports medicine care for the cross-country skier. Presentation at American Academy of Podiatric Sports Medicine Meeting, Phoenix, AZ, May 1989.

Paul IL, Munro MB, Abernathy PJ 1978 Musculoskeletal shock absorption: relative contribution of bone and soft tissues at various frequencies. Journal of Biomechanics 11:237–239.

Pavlov H, Heneghan M, Hesh A, et al 1981 The Hagland syndrome: initial and differential diagnosis. Diagnostic Radiology 144:83–88.

Pearlman DD, Bodberg J, Kalish JR 1992 Chronic ankle conditions. In: McGlanry ED, Bands AS, Downey MS (eds) Comprehensive textbook of foot surgery. Williams & Wilkins, Baltimore, OH, pp 1014–1022.

Pedowitz RS, Hargens AR, Mubarak ST 1990 Modified criteria for the objective diagnosis of chronic compartment syndrome of the leg. American Journal of Sport Medicine 18:35–40.

Pink M 1981 Contra-lateral effects of upper extremity proprioceptive neuromuscular facilitations patterns. Physical Therapy 61:1158.

Plattner PF 1989 Tendon problems of the foot and ankle. Postgraduate Medicine 86(3):155–170.

Pritchett JW 1980 High cost of high school football injuries. American Journal of Sport Medicine 8:197.

Quirk R 1982 Talar compression syndrome in dancers. Foot and Ankle 3:65.

Quirk R 1994 Common foot and ankle injuries in dance. The Orthopedic Clinics of North America, Foot and Ankle Injuries in Sports 25(1):123–133.

Radel NJ, Tertz CC, Krommal RA 1992 Stress fractures in ballet dancers. American Journal of Sport Medicine 20:445–449.

Ray JM, McComb W, Sternes RA 1991 Basketball and volleyball. In: Reeder B (ed.) Sports medicine: the school-aged athlete. WB Saunders, Philadelphia, PA.

Renstrom P, Johnson RJ 1985 Overuse injuries in sports: a review. Sports Medicine 2:316–333.

Renstrom P, Peterson L 1980 Groin injuries in athletes. British Journal of Sports Medicine 14:30.

Rettig AC, Shelbourne RD, McCarroll JR 1988 The natural history and treatment of delayed union stress fractures of the anterior cortex of the tibia. American Journal of Sport Medicine 16:250–255.

Rey JA 1953 Partial rupture of the tendon of the posterior tibial muscle. Journal of Bone and Joint Surgery 35A:1006–1008.

Richie DH, DeVrieis HV, Ende CR 1993 Shin muscle activity and floor surfaces in dance exercise: an electromyographic study. Journal of the American Podiatric Medicine Association 83:181.

Rijke AM, Jones B, Vierhut PA 1988 Injury to the lateral ankle ligaments of athletes: a post-traumatic follow-up. American Journal of Sport Medicine 16:256.

Rodeo SA, O'Brien S, Warren RF, Wickiewicz TL 1990 Turf-toe: an analysis of metatarsophalangeal joint sprains of the great toe in professional football players. American Journal of Sport Medicine 18:280.

Rodman GP, Schumacher HR (eds) 1983 Primer on the rheumatic diseases. Arthritis Foundation, Atlanta, GA.

Rolston HJ 1993 Energetics of human walking. In: Herman RM, Griller S, Stein PSG, Stuart DC (eds) Neural control of locomotion. Medical Science Sports Exercise 25:1158.

Root ML, Orien WP, Weed JH 1977 Normal motion of the foot and leg in gait, normal and abnormal function of the foot, Vol. II. Clinical Biomechanics Corp, Los Angeles, CA, p. 152.

Rorabeck CH 1986 Exertional tibialis posterior compartment syndrome in athletes. Clinical Orthopaedics 208:61–64.

Rorabeck CH, Fowler PJ, Nott L 1988 The results of fasciotomy in the management of chronic exertional compartment syndrome. American Journal of Sport Medicine 16:224–227.

Rosen LW, Hough DO 1988 Pathogenic weight control behaviors of female college gymnasts. The Physician and Sports Medicine 16(9):141.

Rosenberg Z, Feldman F, Singson R 1986 Fibular (peroneal) tendon injuries: CT analysis. Radiology 161:743–748.

Ross JA 1985 Computerized gait analysis in skiing: the electrodynogram and its use in the ski industry. Ski.

Ross JA 1997 Posterior tibial tendon dysfunction in the athlete. Clinics in Podiatric Medicine and Surgery, Sports Medicine and Rehabilitation 14(3):479–488.

Ross JA 1999a Step/bench aerobic dance and its potential for injuries of the lower extremity. In: Subotnick SI (ed.) Sports medicine of the lower extremity, 2nd edn. Churchill Livingstone, Edinburgh, pp 657–660.

Ross JA 1999b Tennis injuries. In: Subotnick SI (ed.) Sports medicine of the lower extremity, 2nd edn. Churchill Livingstone, Edinburgh, pp 729–738.

Ross JA 1999c Tennis injuries – stress fractures. In: Subotnick SI (ed.) Sports medicine of the lower extremity, 2nd edn. Churchill Livingstone, Edinburgh, pp 733–734.

Ross JA, Cohn S 1984 If the boot fits you probably have a custom insole. Ski, October.

Ross JA, Subotnick SI, 1999 Alpine skiing In: Subotnick SI (ed.) Sports medicine of the lower extremity, 2nd edn. Churchill Livingstone, Edinburgh, pp 671–686.

Ruch JA 1974 Haglund's disease. Journal of the American Podiatry Association 64:1000–1003.

Rupani HD, Holder LE, Espinola DA 1985 Three-phase radionucleotide bone imaging in sports medicine. Radiology 156:187.

Sammarco HG 1984 Dance injuries. Contemporary Orthopaedics 8(4):15–27.

Sarmiento A, Worf M 1975 Subluxation of the fibular (peroneal) tendons. Journal of Bone and Joint Surgery 57A:115–116.

Sarratian SR 1983 Anatomy of the foot and ankle. Lippincott, Philadelphia, PA.

Saxena A 1996 Surgery for chronic Achilles tendon problems. Journal of Foot and Ankle Surgery 34:294.

Schepsis AA, Leach RF, Gorzyca J 1991 Plantar fasciitis, etiology, treatment, surgical results and review of literature. Clinical Orthopaedics 266:185–196.

Schepsis AA, Wagner C, Leach RE 1994 Surgical management of Achilles tendon overuse injuries: a long-term follow-up study. American Journal of Sport Medicine 22:611.

Schon LC, Ouzounian TJ 1991 The ankle. In: Jahss MH (ed.) Disorders of the foot: medical and surgical management. WB Saunders, Philadelphia, PA, pp 1435–1441.

Schuberth JM, Dockery GL, McBride RE 1984 Recurrent rupture of the tendo-Achilles repair by free tendinous autograph. Journal of the American Podiatry Association 74(4):157–162.

Scioli MW 1994 Achilles tendinitis. Foot and Ankle Injuries in Sports 177–182.

Shaffer B, Jobe FW, Pink M, Perry J 1993 Baseball batting: an electromyographic study. Clinical Orthopaedics 292:285.

Shelbourne RD, Fisher DA, Rettig AC 1988 Stress fractures of the medial malleolus. American Journal of Sport Medicine 16:60–63.

Siegler S, Block J, Schneck CD 1988 The mechanical characteristics of the collateral ligaments of the human ankle joint. Foot and Ankle 8:234–242.

Singer K, Jones D 1986 Soft tissue conditions of the ankle and foot. In: Nicholas J, Hershman E (eds) The lower extremity and spine in sports medicine. CV Mosby, St Louis, MI, pp 498–525.

Siocum DB 1967 The shin splint syndrome – medial aspects and differential diagnosis. American Journal of Surgery 114:875.

Skovrm ML, Levy IM, Agel J 1990 Living with artificial grass: a knowledge update, part 2: epidemiology. American Journal of Sport Medicine 18:510.

Smillie I 1955 Freiberg's infraction (Koehler's second disease). Journal of Bone and Joint Surgery 393:580.

Soma CA, Mandlebaum BR 1994 Achilles tendon disorders. Clinics in Sports Medicine 13(4):811–823.

Sponsel KH 1976 Bunionette correction by metatarsal osteotomy: preliminary report. Orthopedic Clinics of North America 7: 809.

Standish WD 1995 Lower leg, foot and ankle injuries in young athletes. Clinics in Sports Medicine 14(3):654.

Stanitski CL 1989 Common injuries in preadoloscent and adolescent athletes, recommendations for prevention. Sports Medicine 7:32–41.

Stanitski CL, McMaster JH, Scanton PE 1978 On the nature of stress fractures. American Journal of Sport Medicine 6(6):391–396.

Steadman JR 1979 Non-operative measures for patellofemoral problems. American Journal of Sport Medicine 7:374.

Stein M, Shlamkovitch N, Finestone A 1989 Marcher's digitalgia paresthetica among recruits. Foot and Ankle 9:312.

Steindler A 1955 Kinesiology. Charles A Thomas, Springfield, IL.

Steptoe A, Edwards S, Moses J, Mathews A 1989 The effects of exercise training in mood and perceived copying ability in anxious adults from the general population. Journal of Psychosomatic Research 33:537.

Sterling JC, Calvo RD, Holden SC 1991 An unusual stress fracture in a multiple sport athlete. Medical Science Sports Exercise 3:298–301.

Styf J 1988 Diagnosis of exercise-induced pain in the anterior aspect of the lower leg. American Journal of Sport Medicine 16:165–169.

Styf J 1989 Chronic exercise-induced pain in the anterior aspect of the lower leg: an overview of diagnosis. Sports Medicine 7:331–339.

Subotnick SI 1999a Clinical biomechanics, ankle joint. In: Subotnick SI (ed.) Sports medicine of the lower extremity, 2nd edn. Churchill Livingstone, Edinburgh, pp 133–134.

Subotnick SI 1999b Foot injuries – Morton's neuroma. In: Subotnick SI (ed.) Sports medicine of the lower extremity, 2nd edn. Churchill Livingstone, Edinburgh, pp 18–219.

Subotnick SI 1999c Foot injuries – pathology of the lesser metatarsophalangeal joints. In: Subotnick SI (ed.) Sports medicine of the lower extremity, 2nd edn. Churchill Livingstone, Edinburgh, pp 220–221.

Subotnick SI 1999d Foot injuries, tendinopathy of the triceps surae. In: Subotnick SI (ed.) Sports medicine of the lower extremity, 2nd edn. Churchill Livingstone, Edinburgh, p 241.

Subotnick SI 1999e Surgical intervention in the foot and ankle chronic lateral ankle instability with recurrent ankle sprains. In: Subotnick SI (ed.) Sports medicine of the lower extremity, 2nd edn. Churchill Livingstone, Edinburgh, p. 578.

Subotnick SI 1999f The four phases of running. In: Subotnick SI (ed.) Sports medicine of the lower extremity, 2nd edn. Churchill Livingstone, Edinburgh, pp 17–18.

Subotnick SI 1999g Hallux valgus and bunions – surgical intervention in the foot and ankle. In: Subotnick SI (ed.) Sports medicine of the lower extremity, 2nd edn. Churchill Livingstone, Edinburgh, pp 218–219.

Subotnick SI, Roth WE 1988 Achilles tendonopathy. In: Jay R (ed.) Current therapy in podiatric surgery. CV Mosby, St Louis, MI, p. 293.

Subotnick SI, Sisney P 1999 General concepts of injury. In: Subotnick SI (ed.) Sports medicine of the lower extremity, 2nd edn. Churchill Livingstone, Edinburgh, p. 201.

Subotnick SI, Vogler HW 1999a Surgical intervention in the foot and ankle. In: Subotnick SI (ed.) Sports medicine of the lower extremity, 2nd edn. Churchill Livingstone, Edinburgh, p. 242, pp 520–532.

Subotnick SI, Vogler HW 1999b Surgical intervention of the foot and ankle – retrocalcaneal exostosis (Haglund's deformity). In: Subotnick SI (ed.) Sports medicine of the lower extremity, 2nd edn. Churchill Livingstone, Edinburgh, pp 528–531.

Sutherland DH 1966 An electromagnetic study of the plantar flexors of the ankle in normal walking on the level. Journal of Bone and Joint Surgery 48A:66.

Symeonides PP 1980 High stress fractures of the fibula. Journal of Bone and Joint Surgery 62B:192–193.

Talloway MT, Joke P, Dayton OW 1992 Achilles tendon overuse injures. Clinics in Sports Medicine 771–782.

Taunton JE, Clement DB, Webber D 1981 Lower extremity stress fractures in athletes. The Physician and Sports Medicine 9:77.

Taylor DC, Meyers WC, Maylan JA 1991 Abdominal musculature abnormalities as a cause of groin pain in athletes. American Journal of Sport Medicine 19:239.

Taylor PM, Gordon A, Lowe MR 1999 Basketball injury. In: Subotnick SI (ed.) Sports medicine of the lower extremity, 2nd edn. Churchill Livingstone, Edinburgh, pp 691–696.

Teasdale RD, Johnson RA 1994 Surgical treatment of stage I posterior tibial tendon dysfunction. Foot and Ankle International 15:646.

Terry GC, Hughston JC, Norwood LA 1986 The anatomy of the ilio-patella band and ilio-tibial tract. American Journal of Sport Medicine 14:39–45.

Throchmorton JK, Bradlee N 1978 Transverse v sliding osteotomy: a new surgical procedure for correction of tailor's bunion deformity. Journal of Foot Surgery 18:117.

Timmerman LA, Andrews JR 1994 Undersurface tear of the ulnar collateral ligament in baseball players, a newly recognized lesion. American Journal of Sport Medicine 22:33.

Ting A, Yocum L 1988 Stress fractures of the tarsal navicular in long-distance runners. Clinics in Sports Medicine 7(1):89–101.

Trevino SG, Baumhauer JF 1992 Tendon injuries of the foot and ankle. Clinics in Sports Medicine 11:727–739.

Turco VJ, Spinella AJ 1987 Achilles tendon ruptures – fibularis (peroneus) brevis transfer. Foot and Ankle 7(4):253–259.

Ubler WB, Goldberg C, Chamber TJ 1991 Functional biomechanical affects in running athletes with plantar fasciitis. American Journal of Sport Medicine 29:6671.

Underwood J 1985 Turf: just an awful toll. Sports Illustrated 63:48–59.

Van Mechlen W 1992 Running injuries: a review of the epidemiological literature. Sports Medicine 14:320.

Vitasalo JT, Kvist M 1983 Some biomechanical aspects of the foot and ankle in athletes with and with out shin splints. American Journal of Sport Medicine 11:125–130.

Warren BJ, Stanton AL, Blessing DL 1990 Disordered eating patterns in competitive female athletes. International Journal of Eating Disorders 9:565.

Weider A, Ganim R 1982 Cleveland clinic gymnastics injury survey, 1982. Cleveland Clinic, Cleveland, OH.

Weissman G 1982 The biochemistry of inflammation. Journal of the Mississippi State Medical Association 23(3):66.

Welch TF 1996 N.A.T.A. high school football injury study. N.A.T.A. News, April:16.

Wettstone G 1982 What is gymnastic safety? International Gymnast 36.

Whiteside P 1986 Characteristics of various pointe shoes. Journal of the American Podiatry Association 76:570–571.

Wiley J, Thurston P 1981 Freiberg's disease. Journal of Bone and Joint Surgery 63B: 459.

Willis CA, Washburn S, Cauzzo V 1986 Achilles tendon rupture – a review of the literature comparing surgical versus nonsurgical treatment. Clinical Orthopaedics 207:156–163.

Woods L, Leach RE 1991 Posterior tibial tendon rupture in athletic people. American Journal of Sports Medicine 19:495.

Wosk J, Voloshin A 1981 Wave attenuation in skeletons in young healthy persons. Journal of Bone and Joint Surgery 14:261.

Wysocki RJ 1999 Bowling injuries. In: Subotnick SI (ed.) Sports medicine of the lower extremity, 2nd edn. Churchill Livingstone, Edinburgh, pp 711–717.

Yeager RR, Agostini R, Nattiv A, Drinkwater B 1993 The female athlete triad: disordered eating, amenorrhea, osteoporosis (Commentary). Medical Science Sports Exercise 25:775.

Zoellner G, Clancy W 1979 Recurrent dislocation of the fibular (peroneal) tendon. Journal of Bone and Joint Surgery 61A:291–294.

# Chapter | 14 |

# Basic biomechanics of gait

*James Watkins*

## KEYWORDS

Biomechanics
Centre of gravity
Centre of pressure
Force
Forms of motion
Gait
Gait cycle
Gait analysis
Ground reaction force
Load
Mass
Mechanics
Musculoskeletal system
Stability
Strain
Stress
Units of force
Weight

## INTRODUCTION

There are two basic forms of movement, linear and angular. Linear motion, also referred to as translation, occurs when all parts of an object move the same distance in the same direction in the same time. When the movement is in a straight line the motion is called rectilinear translation. When the movement follows a curved path the motion is called curvilinear translation (Fig. 14.1). Angular motion, also referred to as rotation, occurs when an object or part of an object, such as an arm or leg, moves in a circular path about a line in space, referred to as the axis of rotation, such that all parts of the object move through the same angle in the same direction in the same time (Fig. 14.1). Most whole-body human movements involve a combination of linear and angular motion. For example, while walking the head and trunk experience more or less continuous linear motion as the segments of the arms and legs experience angular motion (Fig. 14.2). Movement of a multisegmented system involving linear and angular motion of one or more segments, such as the human body when walking, is usually referred to as general motion (Watkins 2007).

All movements and changes in movement are brought about by the action of forces. A force may be defined as that which alters or tends

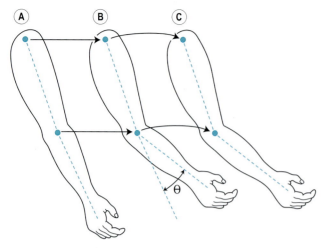

**Figure 14.1** Forms of motion. Between positions A and B the upper arm experiences rectilinear translation and the lower arm and hand experience angular rotation (angle θ) about the elbow joint. Between positions B and C the whole arm experiences curvilinear translation.

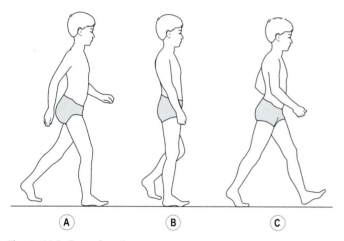

**Figure 14.2** General motion.

to alter an object's state of rest or type (form, speed, direction) of movement. Human movement is brought about by the musculoskeletal system (skeleton, joints, skeletal muscles) under the control of the nervous system. The bones of the skeleton are joined together in a way that allows them to move relative to each other. The skeletal muscles pull on the bones in order to control the movement of the joints and, thereby, the movement of the body as a whole. By coordinated activity between the various muscle groups, forces generated by the muscles are transmitted by the bones and joints to enable the individual to maintain an upright or partially upright posture and bring about voluntary controlled movements (Watkins 1999).

Mechanics is the study of the forces that act on objects and the effects of the forces on the size, shape, structure and movement of the objects. Biomechanics is the study of the forces that act on and within living organisms and the effects of the forces on the size, shape, structure and movement of the organisms. Biomechanics of human movement is the study of the relationship between the external forces (due to body weight and physical contact with the external environment) and internal forces (active forces generated by muscles and passive forces exerted on other structures such as bones and joints) that act on the body, and the effect of these forces on the movement of the body (Watkins 2007).

## CONTACT FORCES AND ATTRACTION FORCES

There are two types of force, contact forces and attraction forces (Watkins 2007). Contact forces result from contact of one object with another. For example, when standing upright the articular surfaces of the hip, knee and ankle joints exert compression (pressing, pushing) forces on each other. Similarly, skeletal muscles exert tension (pulling) forces on bones in order to control joint movements. Attraction forces, such as magnetic force, tend to move objects towards each other (positive attraction) or away from each other (negative attraction).

### Mass and weight

The mass of an object is the amount of matter (physical substance) that comprises the object. In the metric system of measurement the units of mass are the gram (g) and kilogram (kg), and in the Imperial system of measurement the most common unit of mass is the pound (lb) (Watkins 2007). The mass of an object is the product of the volume and density (concentration of matter, or mass per unit volume) of the object. For example, a golf ball and a table tennis ball have a similar volume (occupy the same amount of space) but the density and, consequently, the mass of a golf ball is much greater than that of a table tennis ball. Every object in the universe attracts every other object with a force that is directly proportional to the product of the masses of the two objects and inversely proportional to the square of the distance between them. This relationship is encapsulated in Newton's law of gravitation, which may be expressed algebraically as:

$$F = (Gm_1m_2)/d^2$$

where $F$ is the force of attraction, $G$ is the constant of gravitation, $m_1$ and $m_2$ are the masses of objects 1 and 2, and $d$ is the distance between the two masses. It is difficult to imagine that a force of attraction exists between any two objects, but the magnitude of the force is usually extremely small and of no practical significance. However, there is one object, the Earth, that exerts a significant force of attraction on every other object. The force of attraction that the Earth exerts on an object is referred to as the 'weight' of the object. Weight forces always act vertically downwards. From Newton's law of gravitation, the weight $W$ of an object of mass $m$ is given by:

$$W = m(GM/d^2) = mg$$

where $M$ is the mass of the Earth and $d$ is distance between the centre of the Earth and the object on its surface. The term $GM/d^2$ is usually referred to as gravity ($g$), which is the acceleration due to the Earth's gravitational field. As the Earth is not a perfect sphere $d$ varies slightly at different points on the Earth's surface. Consequently, $g$ also varies slightly, with an average value of 9.81 m/s².

### Units of force

In the metric system the unit of force is the newton (N). A newton is defined as the force acting on a mass of 1 kg which accelerates it at 1 m/s², i.e. 1 N = 1 kg × 1 m/s². As the acceleration due to gravity is 9.81 m/s², it follows that the weight of a mass of 1 kg, referred to as 1 kgf (kilogram force), is given by:

$$1\ kgf = 1\ kg \times 9.81\ m/s^2 = 9.81\ N$$

A mass of 1 kg is equal to 2.2046 lb, i.e. 1 kgf = 2.2046 lbf (pound force). The kgf and lbf are gravitational units of force. Body weight is often recorded in kg or lb, which are units of mass. While this makes no practical difference, the correct units for weight are kgf and lbf (Watkins 2007).

## Scalars and vectors

All quantities within the physical and life sciences are either scalar or vector quantities. Scalar quantities, such as area, volume and temperature, can be completely specified by magnitude, but vector quantities, such as displacement, velocity and force, require a specification in both magnitude and direction. A vector quantity can be represented diagrammatically by a straight line with an arrowhead. The length of the line, with respect to an appropriate scale, corresponds to the magnitude of the quantity, and the orientation of the line and arrow head, with respect to an appropriate reference axis (usually horizontal or vertical), indicates the direction. Figure 14.3a shows the force vectors of the weights of the individual body segments and Figure 14.3b shows the force vector indicating the weight of the whole body.

## CENTRE OF GRAVITY

The human body consists of a number of segments linked by joints. Each segment contributes to the total weight of the body (Fig. 14.3a). Movement of the body segments relative to each other alters the weight distribution of the body. However, in any particular body posture the body behaves (in terms of the effect of body weight on the movement of the body) as if the total weight of the body is concentrated at a single point, called the centre of gravity (Fig. 14.3b). The concept of centre of gravity applies to all objects, animate and inanimate.

The position of an object's centre of gravity depends on the distribution of the weight of the object. For a regular-shaped object with uniform density the centre of gravity is located at the object's geometric centre. However, if the object has an irregular shape or nonuniform density, like the human body, the position of the centre of gravity will reflect the mass distribution and it may be inside or outside the body (Fig. 14.4). Movements that involve continuous change in the orientation of the body segments relative to each other result in continuous change in the position of the centre of gravity.

## MUSCULOSKELETAL SYSTEM FUNCTION

'Posture' refers to the orientation of the body segments relative to each other and is usually applied to static or quasi-static positions such as sitting and standing. When standing upright there are two forces acting on the body, body weight and the ground reaction force (Fig. 14.5a). The ground reaction force is the force exerted by the ground on the body; when standing upright the ground reaction force is equal in magnitude but opposite in direction to the body weight. The combined effect of body weight and the ground reaction force is a compression load that tends to collapse the body in a heap on the ground. This compression load increases with any additional weight carried by the body (Fig. 14.5b). To prevent the body from collapsing while simultaneously bringing about desired movements, the movements of the various joints need to be carefully controlled by coordinated activity between the various muscle groups. For example, when standing upright the joints of the neck, trunk and legs must be stabilised by the muscles that control them, otherwise the body would collapse. Consequently, the weight of the whole body is transmitted to the floor by the feet, but the weight of individual body segments above the feet

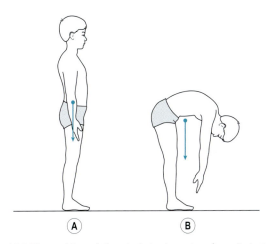

**Figure 14.4** The position of the whole-body centre of gravity in two different body postures.

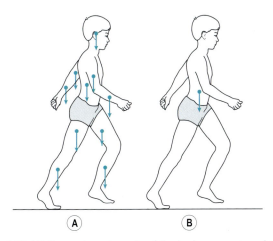

**Figure 14.3** (A) The centres of gravity of the body segments and the lines of action of the weights of the segments. (B) The centre of gravity of the whole body and the line of action of the weight of the body.

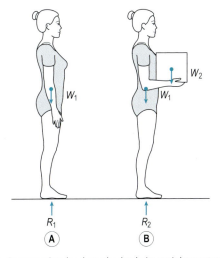

**Figure 14.5** Compression load on the body in upright postures. $R_1$ and $R_2$, ground reaction forces; $W_1$, body weight; $W_2$, weight of box. $R_1 = W_1$. $R_2 = W_1 + W_2$.

(head, arms, trunk and legs) is transmitted indirectly to the floor by the skeletal chain formed by the bones and joints of the neck, trunk and legs.

Transmitting body weight to the ground while maintaining an upright body posture illustrates the essential feature of musculoskeletal function, i.e. the generation (by the muscles) and transmission (by the bones and joints) of forces. In biomechanical analysis of human movement, the forces generated and transmitted by the musculoskeletal system are referred to as internal forces, and forces that act on the body from external sources, such as body weight, ground reaction force, water resistance and air resistance, are referred to as external forces. The musculoskeletal system generates and transmits internal forces to counteract (in static and quasi-static postures) or overcome (during purposeful movements) the external forces acting on the body in order to maintain upright posture, transport the body and manipulate objects, often simultaneously (Watkins 1999).

## STABILITY

In mechanics, an object is said to be stable with respect to a particular base of support when the line of action of its weight intersects the plane of the base of support, and it is said to be unstable when this line does not intersect (Watkins 2007). With regard to human movement, the terms 'stability' and 'balance' are often used synonymously. Maintaining stability of the human body is a fairly complex, albeit largely unconscious, process (Roberts 1995). When standing upright, the line of action of body weight intersects the base of support formed by the area beneath and between the feet (Fig. 14.6A,B). The size of the base of support can be increased by moving the feet further apart. For example, moving one foot to the side increases side-to-side

stability (Fig. 14.6C) and moving one foot in front of the other increases anteroposterior stability (Fig. 14.6D).

In general, the lower the centre of gravity and the larger the area of the base of support, the greater the stability. The recumbent position is the most stable position of the human body, as it is the position in which the area of the base of support is greatest and the height of the centre of gravity is lowest. The recumbent position is also the position that requires least muscular effort (energy expenditure), as all the body segments are directly supported by the support surface (i.e. no muscular effort is necessary to maintain the position of the body segments). In general, the smaller the base of support, the greater the number of joints that need to be controlled and, therefore, the greater the muscular effort. For example, it is usually easier, in terms of muscular effort, to maintain stability when standing on both feet than when standing on one foot. Similarly, it is usually less tiring to sit than to stand, and less tiring to lie down than to sit.

A person recovering from a leg injury may use crutches or a walking stick in order to relieve the load on the injured limb. The use of crutches or a walking stick also increases the area of the base of support and makes it easier for the user to maintain stability (Fig. 14.6E,F).

## CENTRE OF PRESSURE

The ground reaction force is distributed across the whole of the area of contact between the feet and the floor. Figure 14.7A shows the contact area when standing barefoot on both feet; the contact area is much smaller than the area of the base of support. Figure 14.7B shows the contact area when standing on the left foot, and Figure 14.7C shows the contact area when standing on the left foot with the heel raised off the ground. In Figures 14.7B and C, the contact area is very similar to the base of support. Whereas the ground reaction force is distributed across the whole of the contact area, the effect of the ground reaction force on the movement of the body is as if the ground reaction force acts at a single point, which is referred to as the 'centre of pressure' (just as the whole weight of the body appears to act at the whole-body centre of gravity in terms of the effect of body weight on the movement of the body).

If it was possible to stand upright and perfectly still (i.e. with the centre of gravity stationary), the centre of pressure would be stationary and the line of action of body weight would pass through the centre of pressure. However, during normal upright standing, the line of action of body weight and the centre of pressure rarely coincide. During normal upright standing, the centre of gravity sways continuously (along an irregular path in the horizontal plane) about a mean

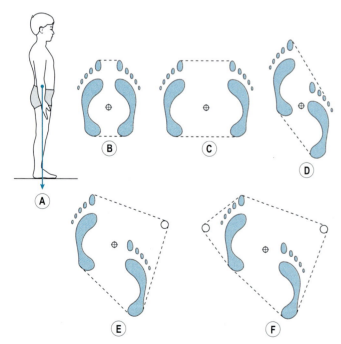

**Figure 14.6** Line of action of body weight in relation to the base of support. (A, B) Standing upright. (C) Standing upright with feet wide apart. (D) Standing upright with the left foot in front of the right foot. (E) Use of a walking stick in the right hand. (F) Use of crutches or two walking sticks.

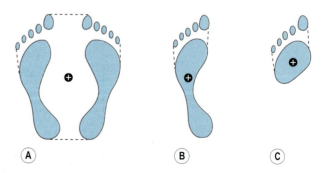

**Figure 14.7** The location of the centre of pressure in relation to the base of support when (A) standing upright on both feet, (B) standing on the left foot, (C) standing on the left foot with the heel off the floor.

position (Winter 1995). The position and speed of movement of the centre of gravity is continuously monitored by visual (eyes), vestibular (ears) and somatosensory (skin and musculoskeletal system) receptors (Peterka 2002). The central nervous system integrates the sensory input and produces appropriate motor output (to change the activation of the muscles that control the joints, especially the hips, knees and ankles) to change the location of the centre of pressure and the magnitude of the ground reaction force which, in turn, counteracts the sway of the centre of gravity and maintains balance (Horak 2006). Winter et al (1998) reported that for a group of ten young adults (mean age 26 years) the mean amplitude of oscillation (sway) of the centre of gravity about the mean position in quiet standing (2 minutes duration) was $0.41 \pm 0.30$ cm in the anteroposterior direction and $0.17 \pm 0.09$ cm in the mediolateral direction. The corresponding mean amplitude of oscillation of the centre of pressure was $0.43 \pm 0.11$ cm in the anteroposterior direction and $0.18 \pm 0.08$ cm in the mediolateral direction. The mean difference between the line of action of body weight and the centre of pressure was $0.07 \pm 0.02$ cm in the anteroposterior direction and $0.05 \pm 0.01$ cm in the mediolateral direction.

## LOAD, STRAIN, AND STRESS

A load is any force or combination of forces applied to an object (Watkins 2007). There are three types of load: tension, compression and shear (Fig. 14.8). Loads tend to deform the objects on which they act. Tension is a pulling (stretching) load that tends to make an object longer and thinner along the line of the force (Fig. 14.8A,B). Compression is a pushing or pressing load that tends to make an object shorter and thicker along the line of the force (Fig. 14.8A,C). A shear load is comprised of two equal (in magnitude), opposite (in direction), parallel forces that tend to displace one part of an object with respect to an adjacent part along a plane parallel to and between the lines of force (Fig. 14.8A,D). The cutting load produced by scissors and garden shears is a shear load, while the cutting load produced by

a knife is a compression load. It is also a shear load that forces one object to slide on another (Fig. 14.8E). The sliding or tendency to slide is resisted by a force called 'friction', which is exerted between and parallel to the two contacting surfaces. The three types of load frequently occur in combination, especially in bending and torsion (Fig. 14.8A,F,G). An object subjected to bending experiences tension on one side and compression on the other. An object subjected to torsion simultaneously experiences tension, compression, and shear.

In mechanical terms, the deformation of an object that occurs in response to a load is referred to as 'strain'. For example, when a muscle contracts it exerts a tension load on the tendons at each end of the muscle, and consequently the tendons experience tension strain (i.e. they are very slightly stretched). Similarly, an object subjected to a compression load experiences compression strain, and an object subjected to a shear load experiences shear strain. Strain denotes deformation of the intermolecular bonds that comprise the structure of an object. When an object experiences strain, the intermolecular bonds exert forces that tend to restore the original (unloaded) size and shape of the object. The forces exerted by the intermolecular bonds of an object under strain are referred to as 'stress'. Stress is the resistance of the intermolecular bonds to the strain caused by the load.

The stress on an object resulting from a particular load is distributed throughout the whole of the material sustaining the load. However, the level of stress in different regions of the material varies depending on the amount of material sustaining the load in those regions; the more material sustaining the load, the lower the stress. Consequently, stress is measured in terms of the average load on the plane of material sustaining the load at the point of interest.

### Tension stress

Figure 14.9A shows a person standing upright with the line of action of body weight slightly in front of the ankle joints. In this posture, stability is maintained by isometric contraction of the ankle plantar flexors, as shown in the simple two-segment model in Figure 14.9B. If the force exerted by the ankle plantar flexors is 350 N (in each leg) and the cross-sectional area of the Achilles tendon at P in Figure 14.9B is 1.8 cm² (square centimetres) then the tension stress on the tendon at P is given by:

$$\text{Tension stress at P} = 350\,\text{N}/1.8\,\text{cm}^2$$
$$= 194.4\,\text{N/cm}^2 \text{ (newtons per square centimetre)}$$

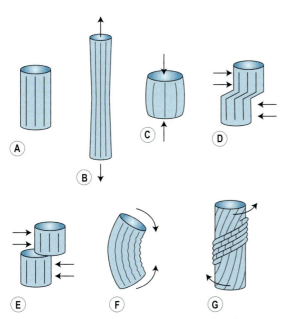

**Figure 14.8** Types of load. (A) Unloaded. (B) Tension load. (C) Compression load. (D) Shear load. (E) Shear load producing friction. (F) Bending. (G) Torsion.

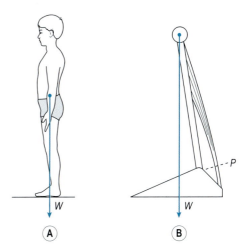

**Figure 14.9** Tension load on the Achilles tendon.

In the metric system the unit of stress is the pascal (Pa), which is defined as the stress produced by a force of one newton uniformly distributed over an area of one square metre (1 Pa = 1 N/m$^2$). Since 1 N/cm$^2$ = 10 000 Pa, the tension stress on the Achilles tendon is equivalent to 1 944 000 Pa or 1.944 MPa (megapascal = 10$^6$ Pa).

## Compression stress

When standing barefoot, as in Figure 14.7A, the ground reaction force exerts a compression load on the contact area of the feet. In an adult the contact area is approximately 260 cm$^2$ (both feet) (Hennig et al 1994). For a person weighing 686 N (70 kgf), the compression stress on the contact area of the feet (on a level floor, contact area perpendicular to the compression load) is given by:

$$\text{Compression stress} = 686 \text{ N}/260 \text{ cm}^2$$
$$= 2.64 \text{ N/cm}^2 = 26\,400 \text{ Pa}$$
$$= 26.4 \text{ kPa (kilopascal} = 10^3 \text{ Pa)}$$

Compression stress is usually referred to as 'pressure'. By raising the heels off the ground the contact area is approximately halved. Since the compression load (body weight) is the same as before, it follows that the pressure on the reduced contact area is approximately doubled.

## Shear stress

Many of the joints, especially those in the lower back and pelvis, are subjected to shear load during normal everyday activities such as standing and walking. For example, in walking there is a phase when one leg supports the body while the other leg swings forward (Fig. 14.10). In this situation the unsupported side of the body tends to move downward relative to the supported side subjecting the pubic symphysis to shear load. The area of the pubic symphysis in the plane of the shear load is approximately 2 cm$^2$. If the shear load at the instant shown in Figure 14.10 is, for example, 20 N, then the shear stress on the joint is given by:

$$\text{Shear stress} = 20 \text{ N}/2 \text{ cm}^2$$
$$= 10 \text{ N/cm}^2 = 100\,000 \text{ Pa} = 100 \text{ kPa}$$

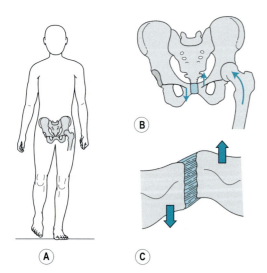

**Figure 14.10** (A) Standing on the left leg. (B) Load distribution on the pelvis. (C) Shear load on the pubic symphysis.

## GAIT CYCLE

In walking and running, a step is defined as the movement of the body from contact of one foot with the ground to contact of the other foot with the ground. A stride is defined as the movement of the body during two successive steps. The gait cycle refers to the movement of the body during a single stride. The gait cycle of the right leg begins with right heel strike (contact of the ground with the right heel), which initiates the stance phase of the right leg (i.e. the period of the gait cycle when the right leg is in contact with the ground). The first part of the stance phase is a period of double support (i.e. when both feet are in contact with the ground) (Fig. 14.11). This period of double support lasts for approximately 10% of the cycle, and after this point the left foot leaves the ground (referred to as toe-off) and the left leg swings forward. During the swing phase of the left leg the right leg supports the body on its own; this period lasts for approximately 40% of the cycle, and is referred to as the 'single-support phase' of the right leg. At the end of the swing phase of the left leg the left foot contacts the ground and another period of double support ensues. At approximately 60% of the cycle the right foot leaves the ground to begin its swing phase, while the left leg experiences a period of single support. The cycle is completed by heel strike of the right foot.

### Trajectory of the centre of gravity

During walking, the movement of the body as a whole is reflected in the movement of the whole-body centre of gravity, which tends to follow a fairly smooth up-and-down side-to-side trajectory. When viewed from the side, as shown in the upper part of Figure 14.11, the centre of gravity moves up and down twice during each gait cycle, with the low points of the trajectory occurring close to the midpoints of the double-support phases and the high points of the trajectory occurring close to the midpoints of the single-support phases. When viewed from overhead, as shown in the lower part of Figure 14.11, the trajectory of the centre of gravity follows the support phases, moving right during the period from the midpoint of single-support of the left leg to the midpoint of single-support of the right leg, and moving left during the period from the midpoint of single-support of the right leg to the midpoint of single-support of the left leg. Orendurff et al (2004) investigated the effect of walking speed on centre of gravity displacement in ten adults (7 men and 3 women, age range 21–45 years, mean age 26.9 ± 5.7 years). The results showed that the vertical excursion (up-and-down range of motion) of the centre of gravity increased with increasing speed from approximately 2.7 cm at 0.7 m/s (slow walk: 1.6 mph) to approximately 4.8 cm at 1.6 m/s (moderate walking speed: 3.6 mph). In contrast, the mediolateral excursion (side-to-side range of motion) of the centre of gravity decreased with increasing speed from approximately 7.0 cm at 0.7 m/s to approximately 3.8 cm at 1.6 m/s.

### Ground reaction force

The trajectory of the centre of gravity reflects the magnitude and direction of the ground reaction force. When standing upright the ground reaction force is equal in magnitude but opposite in direction to body weight (i.e. the resultant force acting on the body is zero) (Fig. 14.12A). To start walking or running (or to move horizontally by any other type of movement such as jumping or hopping) the body must push or pull against something to provide the necessary resultant force to move it in the required direction. In walking and running, forward movement is achieved by pushing obliquely downward and backward against the ground. Provided that the foot does not slip, the

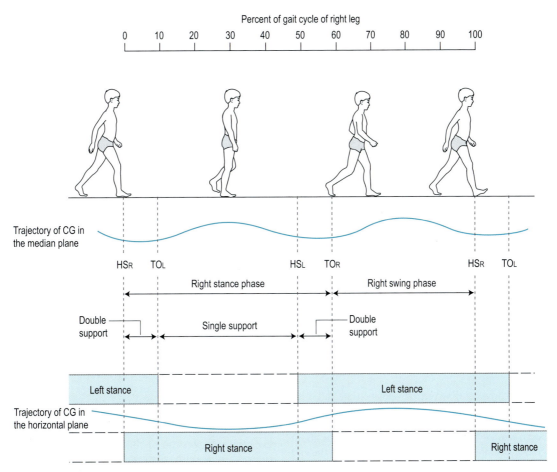

Percent of gait cycle of right leg

Figure 14.11 Gait cycle. CG, centre of gravity; HS, heel-strike; TO, toe-off.

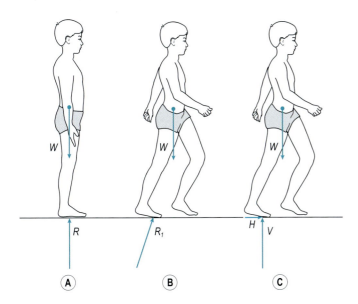

Figure 14.12 Ground reaction force. (A) Standing upright: $W$, body weight; $R$, ground reaction force. (B, C) Push-off in walking: $R_1$, ground reaction force; $H$, horizontal component of $R_1$; $V$, vertical component of $R_1$.

leg thrust results in a ground reaction force directed obliquely upward and forward, which moves the body forward while maintaining an upright posture (Fig. 14.12B). To understand the effect of the ground reaction force it is useful to resolve it into its vertical and horizontal components (Fig. 14.12C). The vertical component counteracts body weight, (i.e. the resultant vertical force acting on the body remains close to zero) and the horizontal component (resultant horizontal force) results in forward movement.

## Components of the ground reaction force

Figure 14.12C shows the vertical and anteroposterior (forward–backward) components of the ground reaction force, but there is also a third component, the mediolateral (side-to-side) component (Fig. 14.13). When walking straight forward, the mediolateral component is normally very small, resulting in little side-to-side movement of the body. Figure 14.14 shows the vertical, anteroposterior and mediolateral components of the ground reaction force (force–time curves) exerted on each leg during the gait cycle. The movement of the centre of gravity during the gait cycle (as in any movement) is determined by the resultant force acting on it. During a period of single-support, the resultant force acting on the centre of gravity is determined by body weight and the ground reaction force exerted on the grounded foot. During a period of double-support, the resultant force acting on the centre of gravity is determined by body weight and the ground reaction forces exerted on both feet.

Figure 14.15 shows the force–time curve of the resultant vertical component of force acting on the centre of gravity during the gait

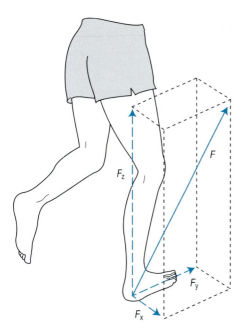

**Figure 14.13** Mediolateral ($F_X$), anteroposterior ($F_Y$) and vertical ($F_Z$) components of the ground reaction force ($F$).

cycle, together with the corresponding vertical velocity–time and vertical displacement–time curves. At heel strike (HS) the centre of gravity is decelerating downwards (downward velocity decreasing: phase D in Fig. 14.15) due to plantar flexion of the ankle, which starts about half-way through the heel-off (HO) to toe-off (TO) period. At the end of phase D, the vertical velocity of the centre of gravity is zero and it is at the lowest point in its trajectory; this corresponds to the midpoint of the double-support period. This is followed by a phase of upward acceleration of the centre of gravity (upward velocity increasing: phase A in Fig. 14.15). Maximum upward velocity of the centre of gravity occurs at the end of phase A, which is followed by a phase of deceleration upward (upward velocity decreasing: phase B in Fig. 14.15). At the end of phase B the vertical velocity of the centre of gravity is zero and it is at the highest point in its trajectory; this corresponds to the midpoint of the single-support period. This is followed by a phase of downward acceleration of the centre of gravity (downward velocity increasing: phase C in Fig. 14.15). Maximum downward velocity of the centre of gravity occurs at the end of phase C, which is followed by a phase of deceleration downward (downward velocity decreasing: phase D in Fig. 14.15). Heel strike of the other foot occurs during phase D, which terminates at the midpoint of double-support; the sequence of phases A, B, C and D then repeats.

The vertical component of the ground reaction force exerted on each leg is characteristically dominated by two smooth peaks, with the rise and fall of each peak taking up about half of the stance phase (Fig. 14.14). The rise and fall of the first peak roughly corresponds to the period from HS to HO, and the rise and fall of the second peak roughly corresponds to the period from HO to TO.

Like the vertical component, the anteroposterior component is normally characteristically dominated by two smooth peaks, the rise and fall of which correspond to the rise and fall of the two peaks of the vertical component. The resultant anteroposterior component of force acting on the centre of gravity during the gait cycle (following an analysis similar to that described above for the resultant vertical component) acts backward from the midpoint of double-support to HO (a braking force), indicating deceleration of the centre of gravity (i.e. the forward speed of the body is decreased). In the HO–TO period the resultant anteroposterior component acts forward, indicating forward acceleration of the centre of gravity (i.e. the forward speed of the body is increased).

The resultant mediolateral component of force acting on the centre of gravity during the gait cycle acts medially during single-support stance and changes direction during double-support (i.e. from medial on the right foot to medial on the left foot during the left HS–right TO period) (Fig. 14.14).

In addition to the characteristic smooth phases of the vertical, anteroposterior and mediolateral components of the ground reaction force, all three components are often characterised by single or multiple transient spikes soon after heel strike, which reflect the impact of the heel with the ground (see $F_Z$ in Fig. 14.14). Shock-absorbing footwear will reduce or eliminate these transient spikes (Czerniecki 1988).

## Path of the centre of pressure

As indicated in Figure 14.14, the magnitude and direction of the ground reaction force change continuously during the gait cycle. Figure 14.16A shows the change in the resultant ($F_{YZ}$) of the anteroposterior ($F_Y$) and vertical ($F_Z$) components. Due to the dominance of $F_Z$, the change in $F_{YZ}$ from HS to TO reflects the double-peaked $F_Z$–time component in Fig. 14.14. $F_Z$ always acts upward, so that the progressive change in direction of $F_{YZ}$ from upward and backward at HS to more or less vertical at HO to upward and forward at TO is largely due to the change in the direction of $F_Y$ from backward (HS to HO) to forward (HO to TO) (Fig. 14.14).

During stance, the foot essentially rolls forward from heel to toe such that the contact area between foot and ground, and consequently the centre of pressure of the ground reaction force on each foot, change continuously, as shown in Fig. 14.16B–F (Hansen et al 2004).

## GAIT ANALYSIS

Walking is a fundamental form of human movement that normally provides the foundation for the development of other movements, including running, hopping, jumping and throwing (Malina & Bouchard 1991, Winter 1990). The importance of walking is reflected in the vast amount of research on the subject over many decades (Sutherland 2001, 2002). Children normally walk for the first time (i.e. take their first few steps without support) when they are 12–14 months old (Malina & Bouchard 1991). At this stage of development the child has the strength to maintain an upright posture and move the body forwards, albeit briefly, but the dynamic balance that is characteristic of mature gait takes much longer to develop (Clark & Phillips 1993). Consequently, a child's initial efforts at walking are characterised by short, stiff-legged, jerky steps, with a relatively wide base of support and arms held outstretched at the sides for balance. As balance improves, the width of the base of support gradually decreases, steps gradually lengthen and the arms gradually become coordinated with the legs in the mature alternate swinging action. Most children establish a mature gait (i.e. mature walking action) by 4 years of age (Adolph et al 2003, Malina & Bouchard 1991).

## Diagnosis of gait disorders

The initial examination of a patient presenting with a gait disorder tends to be concerned with a review of patient records, confirmation of the current general health status of the patient and identifying the symptoms of the patient's current problem. Identification of symp-

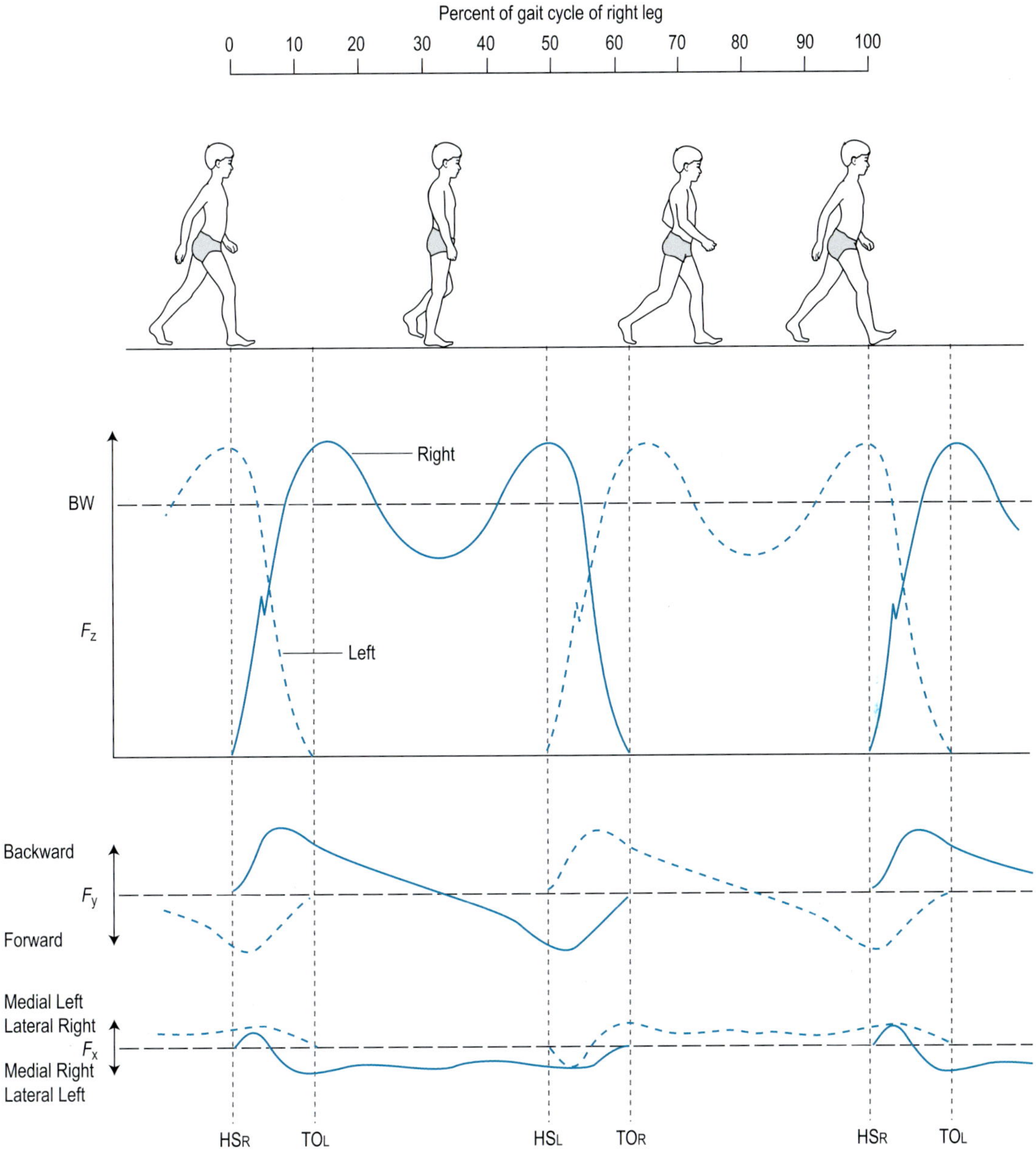

**Figure 14.14** Mediolateral ($F_X$), anteroposterior ($F_Y$) and vertical ($F_Z$) components of the ground reaction force ($F$) during the gait cycle. BW, body weight; HO, heel-off; HS, heel-strike; TO, toe-off.

toms normally involves a verbal description of the symptoms by the patient and a visual/physical examination by the clinician. In many cases, the main symptoms, subsequent diagnosis and proposed treatment are fairly clear. For example, a diabetic patient with peripheral neuropathy may present with an ulcer over the head of the first metatarsophalangeal joint (Caselli et al 2002). The diagnosis would probably be prolonged excessive pressure due to neuropathy resulting from diabetes. The immediate treatment would probably be to relieve the pressure on the ulcerated area in order to promote healing. Further treatment would probably involve modification of the patient's footwear to reduce the pressure on the affected area and thus reduce the risk of further damage following recovery (Praet & Louwerens 2003, Zimny et al 2003). Diagnosis of many other gait problems, especially those without obvious lesions, is not likely to be so straightforward.

Walking is a whole-body activity and the ability to walk normally depends on adequate joint flexibility, adequate strength and appropri-

ate neuromuscular coordination, especially in the trunk and legs. Consequently, deficits in joint flexibility, muscle strength or neuromuscular coordination are likely to affect gait. Deficits may be temporary, such as following an injury, or permanent, such as the result of a neurological disorder. Minor deficits can usually be compensated for, largely unconsciously, by slight changes in gait that have no significant adverse effect on the individual. However, when deficits result in significant adverse effects on gait, then some form of treatment is indicated (Perry 1990). In these cases, diagnosis normally involves some form of gait analysis.

## Qualitative gait analysis

In the first instance, gait analysis normally involves a qualitative analysis, i.e. an analysis based on visual observation from the side, front and rear of the patient walking at their preferred speed (Perry 1990).

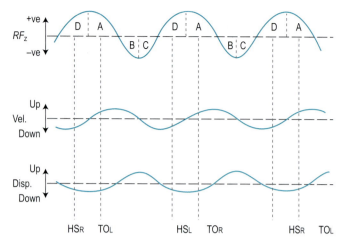

**Figure 14.15** Resultant vertical component of force ($RF_Z$) acting on the whole-body centre of gravity during the gait cycle, and the corresponding velocity and displacement curves.

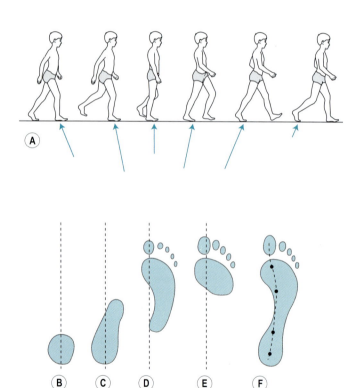

**Figure 14.16** Movement of the centre of pressure along the plantar surface of the right foot during the stance phase of the right leg. (A) Change in the magnitude and direction of $F_{YZ}$ (resultant of $F_Y$ and $F_Z$). (B, C, D, E) Plantar contact area at heel-strike right, middle of double-support, heel-off right, and heel-strike left. (F) Path of the centre of pressure and location of the centre of pressure at the points corresponding to B, C, D and E, respectively.

During the observation, the clinician attempts to identify gait abnormalities on the basis of comparison of the patient's movement with a mental image of what he or she would expect to see in a normal gait. Qualitative analysis is subjective in the sense that no direct objective measures of gait are made. However, the degree of subjectivity depends to a considerable extent on the knowledge and experience of the observer. Figure 14.17 shows a 63-year-old female at different

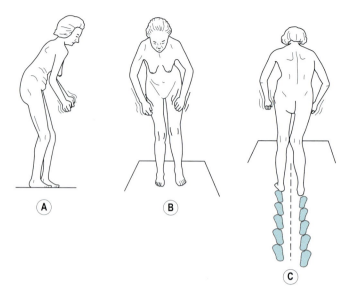

**Figure 14.17** Side (A), front (B) and rear (C) views of a 63-year-old female with Parkinsonism during gait. (Adapted from Ducroquet et al 1968.)

points in the gait cycle. She has a stooped posture with the trunk bent forward. She shuffles her feet with short rapid steps as if she is going to fall forward. Her hands tremor constantly and her trunk and head lurch from side to side with each step. She clearly has an abnormal gait, which would be noticeable to a trained observer. However, the diagnosis might be more difficult. In this case the main cause is Parkinsonism. Figure 14.18 shows the front, overhead and rear views of a 17-year-old female during the gait cycle. She looks down to see where she is going to place her feet. She has a wide base of support, but the step angle is closed. Her trunk is oriented to the left and oscillates from side to side with each step. The gait is clearly abnormal, and in this case the main cause is Friedrich's ataxia.

In many other cases, gait abnormalities are more difficult to detect, especially when changes occur gradually over time. Figure 14.19 shows side and front picture sequences of the right gait cycle of the same child suffering from Duchenne's muscular dystrophy at early (5 years), transitional (7 years 6 months) and late (8 years 2 months) stages in the development of the disease (Sutherland 1984). Note the progressive development of lordosis, a wide base of support, equinus foot strike of the right foot and irregular arm action.

Appropriate treatment clearly depends upon accurate diagnosis, which in turn depends on the quality of information available concerning the patient's condition. In general, the more objective the gait analysis and the more objective the assessment of functional deficits (joint flexibility, muscle strength, coordination), the more accurate the diagnosis is likely to be. Objective gait analysis is usually referred to as quantitative gait analysis.

## Quantitative gait analysis

The movement of the body during the gait cycle, as in every other movement, is the direct result of the internal and external forces acting on the body. The movement of the body as a whole (i.e. the movement of the whole-body centre of gravity) is determined by the resultant external force (i.e. the net effect of all the external forces acting on the body). During gait, the external forces acting on the body are body weight (a constant force acting vertically downwards) and the ground reaction forces. During double support, there will be a ground reaction force acting on the left foot and another ground reaction force

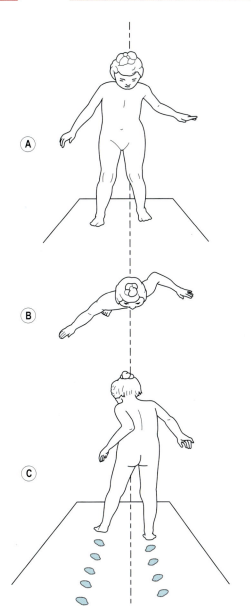

**Figure 14.18** Front (A), overhead (B) and rear (C) views of a 17-year-old female with Friedriech's ataxia during gait. (Adapted from Ducroquet et al 1968.)

time) of the centre of gravity. Kinematics is the branch of mechanics that describes the motion of objects in terms of displacement, velocity and acceleration. Kinetics is the branch of mechanics that describes the forces acting on objects. A kinetic analysis describes the cause of the observed kinematics (Watkins 2007). Figure 14.15 shows the kinetics ($RF_Z$–time curve) and corresponding kinematics (velocity–time and displacement–time curves) of the vertical movement of the centre of gravity during the gait cycle.

During the gait cycle, body weight is constant in magnitude and direction, but the ground reaction forces (in double support) or ground reaction force (in single support) are continuously variable in magnitude and direction. This is due to the continuously variable muscle forces (sequencing and intensity of muscular activity). The magnitude and direction of the ground reaction forces directly reflect the response of the neuromusculoskeletal system to the need to maintain upright posture, balance and forward locomotion. Consequently, normal patterns of muscular activity during gait are directly reflected in normal ground reaction force–time patterns and vice versa. Figure 14.21A shows the line of action of the ground reaction force $R$ acting on the right foot of a 10-year-old boy just after right heel-strike while walking with a normal gait at his preferred speed. At this point in the gait cycle, the line of action of $R$ normally passes (in the YZ plane) in front of the transverse axis through the hip joint, very close to or just behind the transverse axis through the knee joint and behind the transverse axis through the ankle joint. Consequently, $R$ tends to flex the hip joint due to the turning effect of $R$ about the transverse axis through the hip joint. The turning effect of a force about a particular axis is referred to as the 'moment' of the force. The size of the moment is the product of the magnitude of the force and the moment arm of the force (i.e. the perpendicular distance between the line of action of the force and the axis of rotation). In Figure 14.21A, $d$ is the moment arm of $R$ about the transverse axis through the hip joint. The hip flexor turning moment exerted by $R$ (i.e. $R \times d$) is normally resisted by the hip extensors so that the normal action of slight hip extension between heel-strike and foot-flat occurs under control. However, weak hip extensors would tend to result in hip flexion instead of hip extension. In this case, the weak hip extensors may be compensated for by a shortened step involving reduced knee extension and a flat foot contact, which would tend to direct $R$ closer to the transverse axis through the hip joint (i.e. reduce the moment arm of $R$) and, therefore, reduce the size of the hip flexor moment exerted by $R$ to a level that the hip extensor muscles could cope with (Fig. 14.21B). Figure 14.21A,C illustrates a similar compensation at the ankle joint. Just after heel-strike, $R$ normally exerts a plantar flexor moment on the ankle joint, as in Figure 14.21A. This plantar flexor moment is normally resisted by the dorsiflexors of the ankle joint and results in the normal action of controlled plantar flexion from heel-strike to foot-flat. However, weak dorsiflexors would tend to result in rapid uncontrolled plantar flexion. In this case, the weak dorsiflexors may be compensated for by a shortened step involving a flat foot contact, which would tend to direct $R$ neutral to the ankle, thereby preventing the development of a plantar flexor moment (Fig. 14.21C).

Force–time analysis, as described in relation to Figure 14.21, is extremely helpful in identifying abnormal patterns of muscle activity in the diagnosis and treatment of gait abnormalities (Cerny 1984). The method is dependent on being able to accurately locate the centre of pressure, i.e. the point at which the whole of the ground reaction force acting on the foot can be considered to act. However, the ground reaction force does not act at a single point; it is distributed across the whole of that part of the plantar surface of the foot that is in contact with the support surface. Since the plantar contact area and the magnitude of the ground reaction force both vary continuously during the gait cycle, it follows that the average pressure on the plantar contact area also varies. Furthermore, the pressure across

acting on the right foot. During single support, there will be only one ground reaction force (i.e. the force acting on the supporting foot). Figure 14.20A shows the external forces acting on a 10-year-old boy at a point during terminal stance while walking at his preferred speed. There are two external forces, body weight acting at the centre of gravity and the ground reaction force acting at the centre of pressure on the right foot. The resultant external force, which determines the acceleration of the whole-body centre of gravity, is shown in Figure 14.20B,C; it is clearly much smaller in magnitude (reflected in the length of the line representing the force vector) than body weight or the ground reaction force and acts in a forward–upward direction.

In clinical practice, the three components of the ground reaction force(s) can be measured by having the patient walk across a force plate or, preferably, two adjacent force plates so that the ground reaction forces on each foot can be measured separately (see Fig. 14.14). The force–time curves can be numerically integrated to determine the change in velocity (velocity–time) and displacement (displacement–

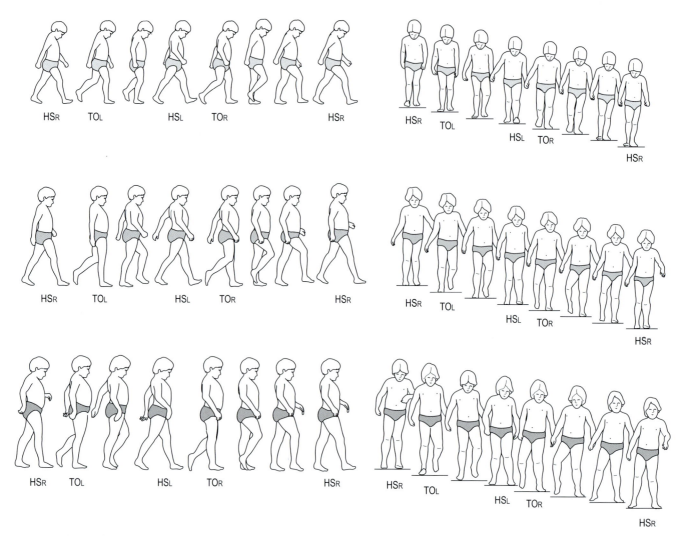

**Figure 14.19** Side and front picture sequences of the right gait cycle of the same child at different stages of Duchenne's muscular dystrophy. (Top) Early stage, 5 years of age. (Middle) Transitional stage, 7 years 6 months. (Bottom) Late stage, 8 years 2 months. (Adapted from Sutherland 1984.)

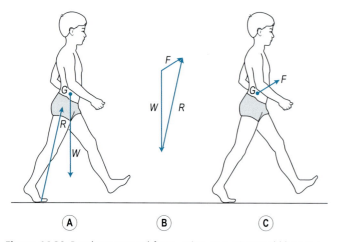

**Figure 14.20** Resultant external force acting on a 10-year-old boy at a point during push-off of the right foot while walking at preferred speed. (A) External forces acting on the boy. (B) Vector chain method of determining the resultant external force. (C) Resultant external force acting on the boy. G, centre of gravity; W, body weight; R, ground reaction force acting on the right foot; F, resultant of W and R.

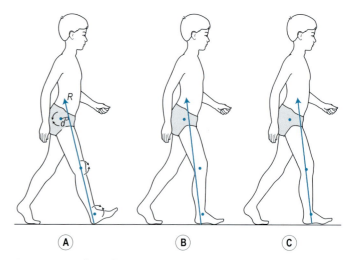

**Figure 14.21** Effect of muscular activity on the line of action of the ground reaction force during gait. (A) Line of action of the ground reaction force (R) in relation to the transverse (mediolateral) axes through the hip, knee and ankle joints; d, moment arm of R about the transverse axis through the hip joint. (B) Possible compensation for weak hip extensors. (C) Possible compensation for weak ankle dorsiflexors.

the plantar contact area also varies quite considerably, as all parts of the plantar contact area do not transmit the same amount of load. The variation in load across the plantar contact area is due to the shape and structure of the foot. The feet of normal children are not as stiff as those of adults due to the relatively greater proportion of cartilage to bone; this tends to distribute the ground reaction force more evenly across the plantar contact area (Hennig & Rosenbaum 1991). In contrast, neurological disorders such as muscular dystrophy and hemiplegia tend to alter the shape and flexibility of the foot arches, which tends to accentuate local differences in plantar pressure, especially in the forefoot (Femery et al 2002, Meyring et al 1997). Consequently, in clinical practice, local pressure measurements (the variation in pressure over the contact area) are more useful than average pressure measurements.

Hennig et al (1994) measured the peak plantar pressure at seven plantar locations in 125 children aged between 6 and 10 years walking slowly while barefoot. Compared to adults (Hennig & Rosenbaum 1991) the children showed considerably lower peak pressures at all plantar locations. The mean body weight to plantar contact area ratios (standing upright on both feet) for the children and adults were 1.66 N/cm² and 2.63 N/cm², respectively, and the lower peak pressures for the children when walking were mainly attributed to their relatively larger feet. Dynamic activities tend to result in greater plantar pressures than static or quasi-static activities. Rozema et al (1996) measured peak pressure on the plantar surface of the foot as a whole and at seven plantar locations (heel, midfoot, heads of the first, second, and fifth metatarsals, hallux, other toes) in 12 healthy adults (mean age 26 years, range 20–33 years) wearing the same type of shoe while performing six activities of daily living (standing, slow and fast walking, slow running, walking up and down stairs, rising from sitting in a chair, walking in a circle). All except the sitting tasks showed significantly higher pressures in all regions of the foot compared to standing, with the exception of pressures in the heel region while walking up and down stairs.

Excessive plantar pressure on any part of the foot will reduce, and may occlude, blood flow to the affected area, resulting in ischaemia. If prolonged, this condition can have serious consequences, such as ulceration or gangrene. Patients with peripheral neuropathy (lack of sensation to pressure and pain), which is often the result of diabetes mellitus, are particularly at risk. In such cases, assessment of local peak pressure is essential for diagnosis and treatment (Mueller et al 2003).

Assessment of local peak pressure is a widely used tool for assessing normal and abnormal foot conditions (Orlin & McPoil 2000). There are basically two types of measurement system: platform systems and insole systems. Platform systems consist of instrumented surfaces (e.g. Emed sensor platform, Musgrave footprint system) or mats (e.g. F-Scan) located in or on a level walkway. The main disadvantage of platform systems is that the patient has to target the instrumented area of the platform, which may be fairly small (e.g. 20 cm × 30 cm). Consequently, many trials may be required in order to record natural movement. Insole systems are based on sensors that are worn inside the shoe in the form of discrete sensors (taped to target sites on the skin) or multiple sensors built into an insole (e.g. Emed Pedar System, RScan, F-Scan). Insole systems are usually linked to a data logger worn on a belt at the patient's waist. The main disadvantage of insole systems is the extent to which the discrete sensors or insoles and linked data logger impair natural movement.

Most platform systems and insole systems are based on a matrix of multiple adjacent sensors (usually 2–5 sensors/cm²). Each sensor measures the force acting on it at the sampling frequency set by the operator (usually 50–100 Hz for walking). The instrumentation computes the pressure on each sensor (force/area of the sensor) and outputs the plantar pressure pattern in two or three dimensions, graphic such as those in Figures 14.22 and 14.23.

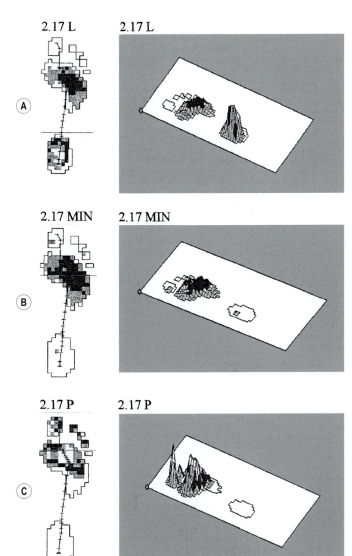

| | Contact time (%) | Load (N) | Area (cm²) | Pressure (kPa) |
|---|---|---|---|---|
| A | 26 | 472 | 45.1 | 104.6 |
| B | 52 | 233 | 35.8 | 64.9 |
| C | 81 | 548 | 36.9 | 148.3 |

Contact time = time of contact of the foot with the floor during stance = 555 ms
Body weight = 395 N
Load = vertical component of the ground reaction force
Area = area of contact between the plantar surface of the foot and the floor
Pressure = average pressure on the contact area

**Figure 14.22** Two- and three-dimensional plantar pressure patterns on the right foot of a healthy 15-year-old female at three points during the right stance phase while walking at preferred speed.

Figure 14.22 shows the two- and three-dimensional plantar pressure patterns on the right foot of a healthy 15-year-old female at three points during the right stance phase while walking barefoot at her preferred speed on a Musgrave platform. Figure 14.22A corresponds to the instant of peak vertical ground reaction force between foot-flat and midstance (26% of contact time). Figure 14.22B

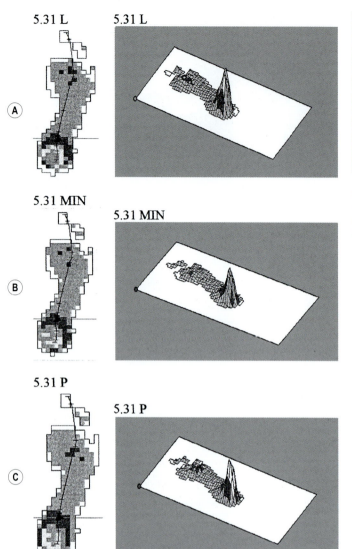

5.31 L     5.31 L

A

5.31 MIN     5.31 MIN

B

5.31 P     5.31 P

C

| | Contact time (%) | Load (N) | Area (cm$^2$) | Pressure (kPa) |
|---|---|---|---|---|
| A | 23 | 584 | 70.4 | 82.9 |
| B | 47 | 514 | 72.3 | 71.0 |
| C | 74 | 563 | 77.9 | 72.2 |

Body weight = 495 N
Contact time = time of contact of the foot with the floor during stance = 778 ms
Load = vertical component of the ground reaction force
Area = area of contact between the plantar surface of the foot and the floor
Pressure = average pressure on the contact area

**Figure 14.23** Two- and three-dimensional plantar pressure patterns on the right foot of a 13-year-old male with juvenile idiopathic arthritis (including right-foot involvement) at three points during the right stance phase while walking at preferred speed.

corresponds to the instant of minimum vertical ground reaction force between foot-flat and heel-off (52% of contact time). Figure 14.22C corresponds to the instant of peak vertical ground reaction force between midstance and toe-off (81% of contact time). The load, contact area and average pressure acting on the foot at each instant are shown in the table accompanying Figure 14.22. Figure 14.22A–C shows the normal progression of the centre of pressure from heel to toe and the accompanying changes in contact area and pressure. Figure 14.23 shows the two- and three-dimensional plantar pressure patterns on the right foot of a 13-year-old male with juvenile idiopathic arthritis, including right-foot involvement, at three points during the right stance phase while walking barefoot at his preferred speed on a Musgrave platform. Figure 14.23A–C corresponds to 23%, 47% and 74% of contact time, respectively, i.e. roughly equivalent to

the same points in time (proportion of contact time) as in Figure 14.22. The load, contact area and average pressure acting on the foot at each instant are shown in the table accompanying Figure 14.23. It is clear that the plantar pressure patterns of the subject with juvenile idiopathic arthritis (Fig. 14.23) are markedly different from those of the normal subject (Fig. 14.22). The most noticeable differences are in the lack of progression of the centre of pressure in the subject with juvenile idiopathic arthritis (most of the weight is taken on the heel throughout the stance phase) and in the increased size of the contact area in the juvenile idiopathic arthritis subject (most of the plantar surface is in contact with the floor throughout the stance phase). The plantar pressure patterns of the juvenile idiopathic arthritis subject presumably reflect neuromusculoskeletal adaptations to minimise pain.

## REFERENCES

Adolph KE, Vereijken B, Shrout PE 2003 What changes in infant walking and why? Child Development 74:475–497.

Caselli A, Pham H, Giurini JM, et al 2002 The forefoot-to-rearfoot plantar pressure ratio is increased in severe diabetic neuropathy and can predict foot ulceration. Diabetic Care 25(6):1066–1071.

Cerny K 1984 Pathomechanics of stance: clinical concepts for analysis. Physical Therapy 63(12):1851–1859.

Clark JE, Phillips SJ 1993 A longitudinal study of intralimb coordination in the first year of independent walking: a dynamical systems analysis. Child Development 64:1143–1157.

Czerniecki JM 1988 Foot and ankle biomechanics in walking and running: a review. American Journal of Physical Medicine and Rehabilitation 67:246–252.

Ducroquet R, Ducroquet J, Ducroquet P 1968 Walking and limping. A study of normal and pathological walking (trans. from French edition (Paris 1965) by Hunter WS, Hunter J). Lippincott, Philadelphia, PA.

Femery V, Moreto P, Renaut H, et al 2002 Measurement of plantar pressure distribution in hemiplegic children: changes to adaptive gait patterns in accordance with deficiency. Clinical Biomechanics 17:406–413.

Hansen AD, Childress DS, Knox EH 2004 Roll-over shapes of human locomotor systems: effects of walking speed. Clinical Biomechanics 19:407–414.

Hennig EM, Rosenbaum D 1991 Pressure distribution patterns under the feet of children in comparison to adults. Foot and Ankle 11(5):306–311.

Hennig EM, Staats A, Rosenbaum D 1994 Plantar pressure distribution patterns of young children in comparison to adults. Foot and Ankle 15(10):35–40.

Horak FB 2006 Postural orientation and equilibrium: what do we need to know about neural control of balance to prevent falls? Age and Ageing 35(Suppl 2):ii7–ii11.

Malina RM, Bouchard C 1991 Growth, maturation, and physical activity. Human Kinetics Corp, Champaign, IL.

Mueller MJ, Hastings M, Comean PK, et al 2003 Forefoot structural predictors of plantar pressures during walking in people with diabetes and peripheral neuropathy. Journal of Biomechanics 36:1009–1017.

Meyring S, Diehl RR, Milani TL, et al 1997 Dynamic plantar pressure distribution measurements in hemiparteic patients. Clinical Biomechanics 12:60–65.

Orendurff MS, Segal AD, Klute GK, et al 2004 The effect of walking speed on center of mass displacement. Journal of Rehabilitation Research & Development 41(6A):829–834.

Orlin MN, McPoil TG 2000 Plantar pressure measurement. Physical Therapy 80(4):399–409.

Peterka RJ 2002 Sensorimotor integration in human postural control. Journal of Neurophysiology 88:1097–1118.

Perry J 1990 Pathologic gait. In: Greene WD (ed.) Instructional course lectures, Vol. 29. America Academy of Orthopaedic Surgeons, Rosemont, IL, pp 325–331.

Praet SFE, Louwerens J-WK 2003 The influence of shoe design on plantar pressures in neuropathic feet. Diabetic Care 26(2):441–445.

Roberts TDM 1995 Understanding balance: the mechanics of posture and locomotion. Chapman and Hall, London.

Rozema BA, Ulbrecht JS, Pammer SE, Cavanagh PR 1996 In-shoe plantar pressures during activities of daily living: implications for therapeutic footwear design. Foot and Ankle International 17(6):352–359.

Sutherland DH 1984 Gait disorders in childhood and adolescence. Williams & Wilkins, Baltimore, OH.

Sutherland DH 2001 The evolution of clinical gait analysis. Part 1: kinesiological EMG. Gait and Posture 14:61–70.

Sutherland DH 2002 The evolution of clinical gait analysis. Part 2: kinematics. Gait and Posture 16:159–179.

Watkins J 1999 Structure and function of the musculoskeletal system. Human Kinetics, Champaign, IL.

Watkins J 2007 An introduction to biomechanics of sport and exercise. Churchill Livingstone, Edinburgh.

Winter DA 1990. Biomechanics and motor control of human movement. Wiley, New York.

Winter DA 1995 Human balance and posture control during standing and walking. Gait & Posture 3(4):193–214.

Winter DA, Patla AE, Prince F, et al 1998 Stiffness control of balance in quiet standing. Journal of Neurophysiology 80:1211–1221.

Zimny S, Schatz H, Pfohl U 2003 The effects of applied felted foam on wound healing times in the therapy of neuropathic diabetic foot ulcers. Diabetic Medicine 20(8):622–625.

# Chapter 15

# Structure and function of the foot

*James Watkins*

## KEYWORDS

Ankle joint

Arch support mechanisms

Midtarsal joint

Modelling

Pronation

Rearfoot complex

Structural adaptation

Subtalar joint

Supination

Windlass

## INTRODUCTION

The main function of the foot is to transmit loads between the lower leg and the ground. In static and, in particular, dynamic situations, such as walking, running, jumping, and landing, the foot is subjected to large loads, which, unless effectively transmitted, would be likely to excessively overload not only the foot but also other parts of the musculoskeletal system (Watkins 1999).

In dynamic situations the foot is required to act as both a shock absorber, to cushion the impact of contact of the foot with the ground, and as a propulsive mechanism to propel the body in the desired direction (Blackwood et al 2005). The foot often performs these functions on a variety of support surfaces. Whereas floor surfaces tend to be firm and level, there are many other situations, such as in cross-country running, where the surface of the ground is neither firm nor level, but continually changes in terms of slope, evenness and hardness. The ability of the foot to function effectively in relation to such diverse environmental constraints is due to its structure, in particular to its arched shape and complex movement capability.

## SKELETON OF THE FOOT

The foot consists of 7 tarsals, 5 metatarsals and 14 phalanges (Fig. 15.1). The tarsals constitute the tarsus, which forms the rear part of the foot. The foot articulates with the lower leg at the ankle joint (talocrural joint), i.e. the joint between the tibia, fibula and talus. The talus, the second largest tarsal, has a convex pulley-shaped articular surface on its superior aspect, called the trochlear surface of the talus, that articulates with the trochlear surface of the tibia. The trochlear surface of the talus is continuous with articular surfaces on its lateral and medial aspects that articulate with the lateral malleolus and medial malleolus, respectively.

The inferior aspect of the talus articulates with the anterior half of the superior aspect of the calcaneus by means of two or, in some cases, three articular facets, which together constitute the subtalar joint (talocalcaneal joint). The anterior aspect (head) of the talus articulates with

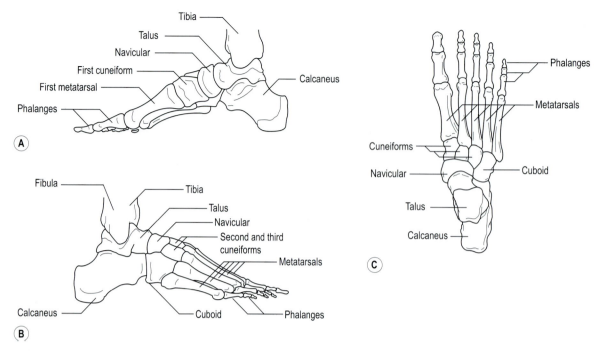

**Figure 15.1** The bones of the right foot. (A) Medial aspect. (B) Lateral aspect. (C) Superior aspect.

the posterior aspect of the navicular, on the medial aspect of the foot, to form the talonavicular joint. The anterior aspect of the calcaneus articulates with the posterior aspect of the cuboid, on the lateral aspect of the foot, to form the calcaneocuboid joint. The calcaneocuboid and talonavicular joints are continuous with each other and constitute the midtarsal joint, also referred to as the transverse tarsal joint (Czerniecki 1988). The anterior aspect of the navicular articulates with the posterior aspects of the three cuneiforms (medial, middle, lateral), which lie side by side and articulate with each other. The posterior two-thirds of the lateral aspect of the lateral cuneiform articulate with the medial surface of the cuboid. The anterior aspects of the medial, middle and lateral cuneiforms articulate with the bases of the first, second and third metatarsals, respectively. The anterior aspect of the cuboid articulates with the bases of the fourth and fifth metatarsals. The joints between the four anterior tarsals and the metatarsals are referred to as the tarsometatarsal joints. The lateral four metatarsals are similar in length, but tend to increase in girth from the second to the fifth. In comparison, the first metatarsal is usually shorter, but has a greater girth than the other four. The metatarsals are collectively referred to as the metatarsus. The heads of the metatarsals articulate with the proximal phalanges of the toes to form the metatarsophalangeal joints. The great toe (also referred to as the big toe or the hallux) is composed of two phalanges and each of the other toes is composed of three phalanges. The phalanges of the toes become progressively shorter from proximal to distal.

In addition to the tarsals, metatarsals and phalanges, a number of small accessory bones and sesamoid bones occur during fetal life ( Anwar et al 2005, Williams et al 1995). There are normally about ten irregular-shaped accessory bones distributed around the tarsus; most of these bones fuse with one of the tarsal bones prior to skeletal maturity. There are normally about 12 sesamoid (seed-shaped) bones. Each sesamoid bone is partially embedded in a tendon or ligament, with the free surface of the bone forming a synovial joint with a bone over which the tendon or ligament slides during normal function. In addition to preventing the tendon or ligament from rubbing on the adjacent bone, sesamoid bones tend to increase the mechanical effi-

ciency (leverage) of the associated musculotendinous unit or ligament. The two most important sesamoid bones of the foot, which contribute significantly to stabilising the foot during propulsion (see the section on the windlass mechanism later in this chapter), are the sesamoids in the plantar aponeurosis (see later section on arches of the foot) beneath the base of the first metatarsophalangeal joint; the medial sesamoid is shown in Figure 15.1A.

## MOVEMENTS OF THE ANKLE AND FOOT

Many of the 26 bones in each foot articulate with two or more other bones such that there are approximately 40 joints in each foot. Consequently, most movements of the foot involve a large number of joints, and the movement of individual joints in each movement is difficult to describe. However, as in most movements of the body, there tends to be high degree of functional interdependence between the joints of the foot, especially between the intertarsal and tarsometatarsal joints, such that movement of one joint tends to bring about fairly predictable movement in adjacent joints (Kitaoka et al 1997a, Nester 1997, Singh et al 1992). A group of joints with a relatively high degree of functional interdependence is called a joint complex (Peat 1986). The term 'rearfoot complex' is frequently used to describe the functional interdependence between the ankle, subtalar and midtarsal joints (Bowden & Bowker 1995, Downing et al 1978, Nester 1997).

### Ankle joint

The ankle joint is a hinge joint that facilitates rotation about an axis of rotation which runs approximately 20° anterosuperiorly in the sagittal plane with respect to the horizontal plane and 20° anteromedially in the horizontal plane with respect to the coronal plane (Fig. 15.2) (Singh et al 1992). Consequently, the movement of the ankle joint is triplanar (i.e. movement occurs simultaneously in the sagittal,

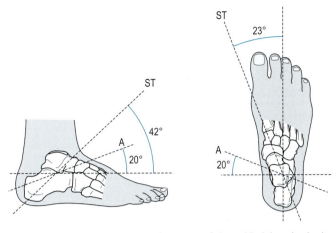

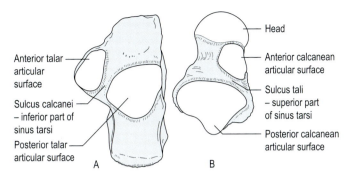

**Figure 15.4** Articular surfaces of the right subtalar joint. (A) Superior aspect of the right calcaneus. (B) Inferior aspect of the right talus.

**Figure 15.2** Orientation of axes of rotation of the ankle (A) and subtalar (ST) joints.

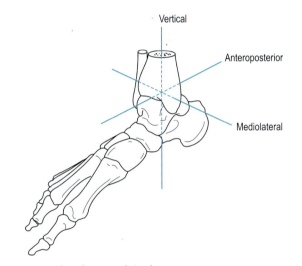

**Figure 15.3** Reference axes of the foot.

coronal and horizontal planes), with movement predominantly in the sagittal plane. Movement in the sagittal, coronal and horizontal planes occurs about the mediolateral, anteroposterior and vertical axes, respectively (Fig. 15.3). Sagittal plane motion of the foot about the ankle joint is usually referred to as plantar flexion and dorsiflexion. In dorsiflexion, sometimes referred to as true flexion of the ankle, the dorsal (superior) surface of the foot is drawn closer to the shin. In plantar flexion, sometimes referred to as extension of the ankle, the plantar (inferior) surface of the foot is pushed further away from the shin (pointing the toes).

## Subtalar joint

The subtalar joint is part synovial and part syndesmosis. The anterior synovial part of the joint is separated from the posterior synovial part of the joint by a funnel-shaped channel called the sinus tarsi. The sinus tarsi runs more or less horizontally in an oblique posteromedial to anterolateral direction (Fig. 15.4) with the funnel opening out laterally. The posterior talar articular surface of the calcaneus is convex and articulates with the reciprocally shaped concave posterior calcanean articular surface of the talus. The anterior talar articular surface of the calcaneus (located on the superior aspect of the sustentaculum tali)

is concave and articulates with the reciprocally shaped convex anterior calcanean articular surface of the talus. Whereas Figure 15.4 shows only one articular surface in the anterior synovial part of the subtalar joint, there are frequently two adjacent articular surfaces. Four distinct variations in the number (one or two), shape and orientation of the anterior synovial articular surfaces have been identified (Valmassy 1996). The syndesmosis part of the subtalar joint consists of a broad interosseous talocalcanean ligament, which runs obliquely downward and laterally from the sulcus tali (superior part of the sinus tarsi) to the sulcus calcanei (inferior part of the sinus tarsi). The interosseous talocalcanean ligament becomes taut in eversion (Williams et al 1995). Distal to the anterior end of the sinus tarsi is another broad ligament called the cervical ligament. The cervical ligament runs obliquely upward and medially from the anterior superior aspect of the calcaneus to the lateral aspect of the neck of the talus. The cervical ligament becomes taut in inversion (Williams et al 1995).

Like the ankle joint, the movement of the subtalar joint is triplanar. Inman (1976) showed that the orientation of the axis of the joint varies considerably between individuals, with a mean orientation of approximately 42° anterosuperiorly in the sagittal plane with respect to the horizontal plane and 23° anteromedially in the horizontal plane with respect to the sagittal plane (Fig. 15.2).

## Pronation and supination

In contrast to the ankle and subtalar joints, there would appear to be little empirical information on the movement of the midtarsal joint, which is composed of a biplanar/biaxial saddle joint (calcaneocuboid) and a triplanar/triaxial ball-and-socket joint (talonavicular) (Blackwood et al 2005). However, it is clear that the rearfoot complex facilitates triplanar movements of the foot, which are referred to as pronation and supination (Fig. 15.5) (Kitaoka et al 1997a, Nester 1997).

Pronation involves simultaneous abduction (vertical axis), dorsiflexion (mediolateral axis) and eversion (anteroposterior axis) (Fig. 15.5A,B). Similarly, supination involves simultaneous adduction, plantar flexion and inversion (Fig. 15.5B,C). The orientation of the rearfoot axis varies considerably, with a mean orientation of approximately 51° anterosuperiorly in the sagittal plane with respect to the horizontal plane and 18° anteromedially in the horizontal plane with respect to the sagittal plane (Downing et al 1978).

Using 13 cadaver specimens (mean age 65 years, range 20–89 years) and a magnetic tracking measurement system, Kitaoka et al (1997a) investigated the contribution of the ankle joint, subtalar joint, talonavicular joint and first metatarsal–navicular joint to pronation, supination, dorsiflexion and plantar flexion. The results are shown in Table 15.1. As expected, the ankle is the major contributor (47.2%) to the

**Table 15.1** Contribution of movement between the navicular and first metatarsal (met–nav) and movement of the ankle, subtalar and talonavicular joints to pronation, supination, dorsiflexion and plantar flexion (adapted from Kitaoka et al 1997a)

| Joint | PRONATION | | SUPINATION | | PRONATION–SUPINATION | | DORSIFLEXION | | PLANTAR FLEXION | | DORSIFLEXION–PLANTAR FLEXION | |
|---|---|---|---|---|---|---|---|---|---|---|---|---|
| | Degrees | % | Degrees | % | Degrees | % | Degrees | % | Degrees | % | Degrees | % |
| met–nav | 13.6 ± 3.9 | 43.3 | 3.3 ± 1.5 | 4.4 | 16.9 | 15.9 | 1.7 ± 1.1 | 6.9 | 11.8 ± 5.5 | 19.1 | 13.5 | 15.6 |
| tal–nav | 7.6 ± 3.3 | 24.3 | 39.3 ± 11.8 | 52.5 | 46.9 | 44.2 | 3.5 ± 1.8 | 14.3 | 12.7 ± 8.4 | 20.6 | 16.2 | 18.8 |
| Subtalar | 2.5 ± 1.7 | 8.0 | 23.3 ± 7.3 | 31.1 | 25.8 | 24.3 | 2.7 ± 1.7 | 11.0 | 6.5 ± 4.2 | 10.5 | 9.2 | 10.7 |
| Ankle | 7.6 ± 4.7 | 24.3 | 8.9 ± 4.6 | 11.9 | 16.5 | 15.5 | 16.6 ± 4.8 | 67.8 | 30.6 ± 7.9 | 49.7 | 47.2 | 54.8 |
| ROM | 31.3 | 100 | 74.8 | 100 | 106.1 | 100 | 24.5 | 100 | 61.6 | 100 | 86.1 | 100 |

ROM: range of motion
Pronation: from neutral to full pronation
Supination: from neutral to full supination
Dorsiflexion: from neutral to full dorsiflexion
Plantar flexion: from neutral to full plantar flexion
Pronation–supination: range from full pronation to full supination
Dorsiflexion–plantar flexion: range from full dorsiflexion to full plantar flexion

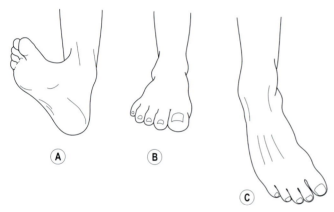

**Figure 15.5** Supination and pronation of the foot. (A) Full pronation. (B) Neutral position. (C) Full supination.

plantar flexion–dorsiflexion range of motion, but there are significant contributions from the other components. The subtalar joint is often regarded as the major contributor to the pronation–supination range of motion, but the results of the study indicate that the contribution of the subtalar joint (24.3%) is less than that of the talonavicular joint (44.2%).

The movements of supination and pronation as described above refer to movements of the rearfoot complex when the foot is not weight bearing. When the foot is weight bearing, these movements are constrained, depending on the magnitude and distribution of the ground reaction force acting on the plantar part of the foot. Under weight-bearing conditions the most noticeable movements of the foot occur about an anteroposterior axis through the foot (similar to inversion and eversion). For this reason, in describing the movement of the foot under weight-bearing conditions the terms supination and inversion are sometimes used synonymously, as are the terms pronation and eversion. However, the actual movements of the foot under weight-bearing conditions are modifications of supination and pronation and, as such, involve simultaneous triplanar movement in all the joints of the rearfoot complex.

## ARCHES OF THE FEET

The tarsals and metatarsals are arranged in the form of two longitudinal arches (medial and lateral) and a single transverse arch. The medial longitudinal arch is formed by the calcaneus, talus, navicular, the three cuneiforms, and the first, second and third metatarsals. The lateral longitudinal arch, which is much flatter than the medial arch, is formed by the calcaneus, cuboid, and the fourth and fifth metatarsals. In combination, the longitudinal arches form a single arched structure between the posterior inferior aspect of the calcaneus and the heads of the metatarsals. The transverse arch runs across the foot from medial to lateral and is formed by the anterior five tarsals and the bases of the metatarsals. The shape of the arch is due to the cuboid, the lateral and middle cuneiforms, and the bases of the middle three metatarsals, which are wedge shaped inferiorly in coronal section.

The arched shape of the foot is maintained by ligaments (passive support) and muscles (active support). Although the ligaments and muscles are not very elastic, they are sufficiently so to enable the arches to flatten slightly following contact of the foot with the ground, such as following heel-strike in walking or running, and then recoil (restore their normal shape) following the impact. Consequently, the arches function like springs in order to help cushion impacts with the ground.

### Passive arch support

The ligaments on the plantar aspect of the foot are very strong and can normally maintain the arches of the foot in upright posture in the absence of assistance from muscles (Hicks 1961, Kitaoka et al 1997b). The main ligaments that support the arches of the foot are:

1. The deep plantar calcaneocuboid ligament, also referred to as the short plantar ligament, runs from the anterior tubercle of the calcaneus to the plantar surface of the cuboid posterior to the groove for the tendon of the peroneus longus (Fig. 15.6). This ligament supports the calcaneocuboid part of the midtarsal joint.

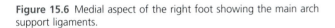

Figure 15.6 Medial aspect of the right foot showing the main arch support ligaments.

Labels: Deltoid ligament, Interosseous ligament, Spring ligament, Long plantar ligament, Short plantar ligament, Plantar aponeurosis, Transverse metatarsophalageal ligament

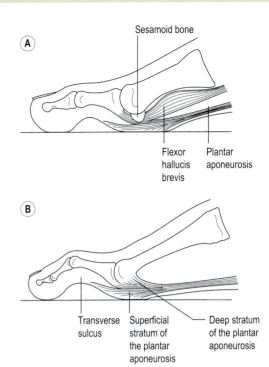

**Figure 15.7** Sagittal sections through the first (A) and second (B) metatarsophalangeal joints.

Labels: Sesamoid bone, Flexor hallucis brevis, Plantar aponeurosis, Transverse sulcus, Superficial stratum of the plantar aponeurosis, Deep stratum of the plantar aponeurosis

2. The superficial plantar calcaneocuboid ligament, also referred to as the long plantar ligament, runs from the plantar surface of the calcaneus between the posterior and anterior tubercles to the plantar surface of the cuboid anterior to the groove for the tendon of the peroneus longus and to the bases of the second to fifth metatarsals (Fig. 15.6). This ligament supports the calcaneocuboid part of the midtarsal joint and the lateral four tarsometatarsal joints.

3. The plantar calcaneonavicular ligament, also referred to as the spring ligament, runs from the anteroinferior aspect of the sustentaculum tali (of the calcaneus) to the plantar surface of the navicular (Fig. 15.6). The plantar calcaneonavicular ligament supports the medial part of the subtalar joint (anterior synovial part) and the talonavicular part of the midtarsal joint.

4. The deltoid ligament (medial collateral ligament of the ankle joint) fans out from the anterior, medial and posterior aspects of the medial malleolus to attach onto a more or less continuous arc formed by the navicular, the spring ligament, the sustentaculum tali and the talus (Fig. 15.6). The deltoid ligament supports the medial aspects of the ankle and subtalar joints.

5. The interosseous talocalcanean ligament is the syndesmosis part of the subtalar joint, described earlier.

6. The plantar aponeurosis is a broad fan-shaped ligament that spans the whole of the tarsus and metatarsus from the posterior tubercles of the calcaneus to the bases of the proximal (first) phalanges (Fig. 15.6). Just anterior to the tarsometatarsal joints, the plantar aponeurosis splits into five separate bands, one to each toe. As each band passes the plantar surface of the corresponding metatarsophalangeal joint, it splits into a superficial stratum (layer) and a deep stratum (Fig. 15.7). The superficial stratum attaches to the skin of the transverse sulcus, which separates the toes from the sole. The deep stratum divides into two slips that attach, one medially and one laterally, onto the proximal plantar surface of the base of the proximal phalanx of the corresponding toe, thus forming an arch for passage of the tendon of the flexor hallucis longus (first toe) or corresponding tendon of the flexor digitorum longus (second to fifth toes) to the distal phalanges (Williams et al 1995). The medial and lateral slips of the plantar aponeurosis to the proximal phalanx of the hallux merge with the tendons of the medial and lateral parts of the flexor hallucis brevis. Each tendon contains a sesamoid bone that forms a synovial joint with the plantar aspect of the head of the first metatarsal. The plantar parts of the capsules of the metatarsophalangeal joints are thickened, and are referred to as plantar plates or plantar pads (Briggs 2005). The plantar plates are connected in series by deep transverse intermetatarsal ligaments and by a superficial continuous transverse metatarsophalangeal. The plantar aponeurosis slips to each toe merge with the corresponding plantar plate and adjoining section of the transverse metatarsophalangeal ligament.

Mechanically, the plantar ligaments support the arches of the feet in two ways, as a beam and as a true arch (or truss) (Hicks 1961). Figure 15.8A shows the type of strain experienced by a loaded beam, i.e. compression strain on the upper surface and tension strain on the lower surface. This is similar to the strain on the tarsals and metatarsals imposed by the type of arch support provided by the long plantar ligament, short plantar ligament, spring ligament, interosseous talocalcanean ligament and deltoid ligament (Fig. 15.6 and Fig. 15.8B). The strain on a true arch is different to that on a beam. In a true arch the ends of the arch must move further apart if it is to become flatter and the strain on the segments of a true arch is basically compression between the segments (Fig. 15.8C). This is similar to the strain on the tarsals and metatarsals imposed by the type of arch support provided by the plantar aponeurosis (Fig. 15.6 and Fig. 15.8D).

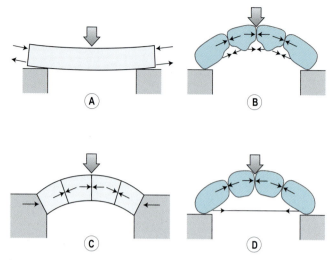

**Figure 15.8** Beam and arch support mechanisms. (A) Strain on a horizontal beam when vertically loaded. (B) Strain on the bones of the foot and beam support mechanism when the foot is vertically loaded. (C) Strain on the components of a true arch when vertically loaded. (D) Strain on the bones of the foot and true arch support mechanism when the foot is vertically loaded.

## Active arch support

The passive ligamentous beam and true arch support mechanisms are normally assisted by the muscles of the lower leg and foot. In relation to arch support, muscles that are located entirely (have their origins and insertions) within the foot are referred to as intrinsic muscles. Muscles that have their origins in the lower leg and insertions in the foot (i.e. cross the ankle joint) are referred to as extrinsic muscles.

The effect that a particular muscle has on the arches (i.e. tendency to raise or flatten) depends on the tendency of the muscle to:

1. Plantar flex or dorsiflex the intertarsal, tarsometatarsal and metatarsophalangeal joints. Plantar flexion of any of these joints will tend to raise the arches and reduce the strain on the plantar ligaments. Dorsiflexion of any of the joints will tend to flatten the arches and increase the strain on the plantar ligaments.
2. Increase or decrease the ankle joint reaction force. In weight bearing, the weight of the body is transmitted to the feet via the ankle joints. Consequently, the effect of a particular weight-bearing activity (standing, walking, running, hopping, jumping, etc.) on the foot arches is determined by the magnitude of the ankle joint reaction forces; the greater the ankle joint reaction forces, the greater the tendency to flatten the arches, and vice versa. As demonstrated by Hicks (1961), the further forward the line of action of body weight in relation to the ankle joint, the greater the magnitude of the ankle joint reaction force and, therefore, the greater the tendency to flatten the arches.

On the basis of these criteria, Hicks (1961) classified all the intrinsic and extrinsic muscles into four groups:

- Direct arch raiser, i.e. a tendency to plantar flex one or more of the intertarsal, tarsometatarsal and metatarsophalangeal joints. This group includes all the plantar intrinsic muscles and the flexor hallucis longus, flexor digitorum longus, peroneus brevis, peroneus longus and tibialis posterior.
- Indirect arch raiser, i.e. a tendency to shift body weight backward (toward the ankle joint), which tends to reduce the magnitude of the ankle joint reaction force and, therefore,

reduce arch flattening. This group includes the extensor hallucis longus, extensor digitorum longus and tibialis anterior.
- Direct arch flattener, i.e. a tendency to dorsiflex one or more of the intertarsal, tarsometatarsal and metatarsophalangeal joints. This group includes the extensor hallucis longus, extensor digitorum longus and tibialis anterior.
- Indirect arch flattener, i.e. a tendency to shift body weight forward (in front of the ankle joint), which tends to increase the magnitude of the ankle joint reaction force and, therefore, increase arch flattening. This group includes the flexor hallucis longus, flexor digitorum longus, peroneus brevis, peroneus longus, tibialis posterior, gastrocnemius and soleus.

## Interaction of the arch support mechanisms

Whereas it is generally accepted that the passive (beam and true arch) and active (muscle) mechanisms both contribute significantly to arch support (Norkin & Levangie 1992), the relative contribution of the mechanisms in different weight-bearing activities has yet to be determined. This lack of information reflects the difficulty of measuring the forces in the ligaments and forces in vivo. Most studies of the arch support mechanisms have been based on cadavers. For example, Kitaoka et al (1997b) investigated the role of the plantar ligaments in the stability of the longitudinal arches of the feet under normal loading (upright standing posture) using 19 cadaver specimens (mean age 71 years, range 20–89 years). It was found that sectioning all the main plantar ligaments (long plantar ligament, short plantar ligament, spring ligament, interosseous talocalcanean ligament, plantar aponeurosis, deltoid ligament) resulted in complete collapse of the longitudinal arch. The arch did not collapse after sectioning any single ligament, but progressive collapse did occur when the ligaments were sectioned consecutively. The effect of sectioning individual ligaments on the degree of arch collapse (reflected in dorsiflexion of the intertarsal and tarsometatarsal joints) varied considerably between specimens, which suggested that the contribution of each ligament to arch stability varies between individuals. This is, perhaps, not surprising considering the variation in the size, shape and alignment of the bones of the feet in normal healthy individuals (Åström & Arvidson 1995).

Whereas cadaver studies provide useful information on the passive arch support mechanisms, they do not provide information about the contribution of active support mechanisms or the relative contribution of the passive and active mechanisms. Research is clearly needed in this area.

## THE WINDLASS MECHANISM OF THE FOOT

As described earlier, the plantar aponeurosis spans the whole of the tarsus and metatarsus by linking the inferior aspect of the calcaneus with the plantar surfaces of the bases of the proximal phalanges of the toes (Fig. 15.6). Consequently, extension of the metatarsophalangeal joints winds the plantar aponeurosis around the heads of the metatarsals, like a cable being wound around a windlass, which simultaneously raises the longitudinal arch (Fig. 15.9). This action is referred to as the windlass mechanism of the foot (Hicks 1954). Flexion of the metatarsophalangeal joints unwinds the plantar aponeurosis and lowers the longitudinal arch; this action is referred to as the reverse windlass (Aquino & Payne 2000).

The reverse windlass action is a feature of the loading phase (from heel-strike to foot-flat) and much of the single-support phase in gait. During this period, the rearfoot complex normally pronates, which unwinds the plantar aponeurosis and lowers the longitudinal arch.

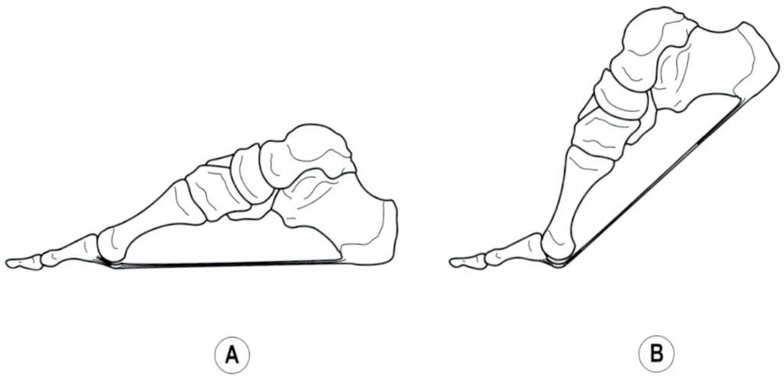

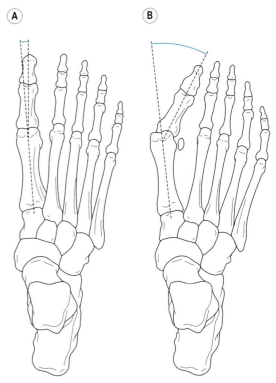

**Figure 15.9** The windlass effect of the plantar aponeurosis resulting from dorsiflexion of the metatarsophalangeal joints.

This movement is associated with extension of the midtarsal joint, which is sometimes referred to as 'unlocking' the midtarsal joint (Blackwood et al 2005, Sobel et al 1999). In the foot-flat position the tension in the plantar aponeurosis exerts a flexor moment on the proximal phalanges (pushes the pads of the toes against the ground), which extends the length of the base of support and, consequently, reduces the pressure on the plantar surfaces of the heads of the metatarsals. In addition, the tension in the plantar aponeurosis, in association with tension in the intrinsic muscles, prevents excessive flattening of the longitudinal and transverse arches and provides a stable base of support.

The windlass action is a feature of the push-off in gait (from heel-off to just before toe-off). During this period, the rearfoot complex normally supinates in association with extension of the metatarsophalangeal joints (Fig. 15.9B). These actions raise the longitudinal arch, which stabilises the foot and provides a firm base of support for the push-off. The windlass movement is associated with flexion of the midtarsal joint, which is sometimes referred to as 'locking' the midtarsal joint (Blackwood et al 2005, Sobel et al 1999).

The windlass action during push-off in gait is most effective (rapid initiation and completion of arch raise) when the leverage of the plantar aponeurosis is maximum. This occurs when (i) the sesamoids are located in their normal position beneath the head of the first metatarsal (Fig. 15.7A) and (ii) the long axes of the first metatarsal and phalanges of the hallux are more or less in line (Fig. 15.10A). Not surprisingly, this would appear to be the normal orientation of the sesamoid bones and first metatarsophalangeal joint, as significant non-alignment of the first metatarsal and proximal phalanx seems to be rare in children (Kilmartin 1991).

With increase in age, many people develop hallux valgus, also referred to as hallux abducto valgus (Thomas & Barrington 2003). Hallux valgus is a complex progressive condition that is characterised by lateral deviation (valgus abduction) of the hallux and medial deviation of the first metatarsophalangeal joint (Fig. 15.10B). Unless treated, hallux valgus results in a progressive increase in the hallux abductus angle (i.e. the angle between the long axes of the first metatarsal and proximal phalanx) (Fig. 15.10B). When the hallux abductus angle is less than 15°, the condition tends to be asymptomatic. However, increases in the hallux abductus angle above 15° tend to be associated with increasing pain and discomfort around the first metatarsophalangeal joint (Easley & Trnka 2007, Menz & Lord 2005).

Relative to the first metatarsophalangeal joint, any increase in the hallux abductus angle will tend to displace laterally the lines of action of the plantar aponeurosis and tendons of the intrinsic and extrinsic muscles that cross over the first metatarsophalangeal joint from the metatarsal to the hallux. Consequently, the sesamoid bones will also be displaced laterally relative to the first metatarsophalangeal joint, resulting in subluxation of the joints between the sesamoid bones and

**Figure 15.10** (A) Superior aspect of the right foot with a hallux abductus angle of approximately 5°. (B) Superior aspect of the right foot with a hallux abductus angle of approximately 35°.

the head of the first metatarsal (Fig. 15.10B). Subluxation of these joints will decrease the leverage of the windlass about the first metatarsophalangeal joint and, consequently, tend to result in increased force in the muscles supporting the arches during push-off in order to compensate for the loss in leverage of the windlass. The increased muscle force will tend to increase the hallux abductus angle and, consequently, increase (i) the pressure on the articular surfaces between the medial sesamoid and the head of the first metatarsal, (ii) the strain on the intertransverse ligament and metatarsophalangeal ligament between the first and second metatarsophalangeal joints, and (iii) the pressure exerted by the shoe on the medial aspect of the first metatarsophalangeal joint (Tanaka et al 1997). This pattern of loading, if prolonged, is likely to result in discomfort, pain, inefficient gait, impaired balance and an increased risk of falling, especially in the elderly (Menz & Lord 2005).

## STRUCTURAL ADAPTATION OF THE MUSCULOSKELETAL SYSTEM

In any body position other than the relaxed recumbent position, the musculoskeletal system is likely to be subjected to considerable loading. In response to the forces exerted on them, the musculoskeletal components experience strain (i.e. they are deformed to a certain extent), and the greater the force, the greater the strain. Under normal circumstances the musculoskeletal components adapt their external form (size and shape) and internal architecture (structure) to the time-averaged forces exerted on them in order to more readily withstand the strain (Carter et al 1991). However, when the degree of strain experienced by a particular component exceeds its strength, it becomes injured. Consequently, there is an intimate relationship between the structure and function of the musculoskeletal system (Watkins 1999).

## Structural adaptation in bone

The last 30 years have produced much of the present knowledge concerning the adaptation of musculoskeletal components to changes in time-averaged load (Frost 1988a,b, 1990). However, the fundamental concepts concerning the adaptation of bone were established over 100 years ago (Gross & Bain 1993). In 1892, Julius Wolff (1836–1902) summarised the contemporary views of bone adaptation to changes in time-averaged load in what came to be known as Wolff's law (Wolff 1988). Wolff's law, which has been shown to be more or less correct, hypothesised that bone adapts its external form and internal architecture to the time-averaged load exerted on it in an ordered and predictable manner to provide optimal strength with minimal bone mass.

The adaptation of bone to time-averaged load is referred to as 'modelling'. In normal growth and development, modelling has been estimated to account for 20–50% of the dimensions of mature bones (Frost 1988b). Some of the load experienced by bone is due to the weight of body segments. However, this source of loading is small relative to the loads exerted by muscles (Schoenau & Frost 2002, Watkins 1999). From birth to maturity, bone has the capacity to model external form and internal architecture. However, the capacity to model external form gradually decreases and virtually ceases at maturity. The capacity to model internal architecture also decreases with age, but is retained to some extent throughout life. In general, bone adapts to changes in time-averaged loads by increasing or decreasing bone mass to maintain an optimum strain environment. In bone, the optimum strain environment is characterised by minimal flexure (or bending) strain and an even distribution of stress (usually compression stress) across articular areas. An even distribution of stress across articular areas is maintained by modelling in accordance with the phenomenon of chondral modelling (Frost 1973).

## The chondral modelling phenomenon

All bones that develop from hyaline cartilage via endochondral ossification experience chondral modelling, i.e. the rate and amount of new bone formed by hyaline cartilage depends on the amount and form of load exerted on it. Chondral modelling applies to articular cartilage, epiphyseal plates, insertions of tendons and ligaments, apophyseal plates, end plates in symphysis joints, and sesamoid bones (Frost 1979).

In a long bone the size and shape of the epiphyses and metaphyses, and consequently the orientation of the epiphyses of a bone to its shaft, are determined by chondral modelling in articular cartilage and epiphyseal plates. When a synovial joint is maximally congruent, the loading on articular cartilage and epiphyseal plates tends to be evenly distributed. Incongruence results in an unequal distribution of load across articular cartilage and epiphyseal plates. If prolonged, such unequal loading results in modelling to restore maximal congruence. However, the actual changes that occur depend on the extent of the changes in the patterns of loading on the articular cartilage and epiphyseal plates. If the changes in loading remain within the normal range, then a negative-feedback mode of modelling is invoked, resulting in restoration of normal congruence with normal or slightly abnormal alignment of the bones. However, if the changes in loading are outside the normal range, then a positive-feedback mode of modelling is invoked, which aggravates the condition, resulting in progressively worsening malalignment.

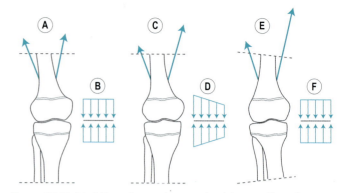

**Figure 15.11** Modelling of metaphyses and epiphyses: effect of negative-feedback mode in relation to an abductor–adductor imbalance at the knee.

## Modelling of metaphyses and epiphyses

A functionally normal joint is a congruent joint that transmits loads across the articulating surfaces in a normal manner. An anatomical malalignment at the knee, or any other joint, will be functionally normal if the malalignment stabilises (does not get progressively worse). In these cases, the anatomical malalignments represent normal modelling in response to abnormal patterns of loading. The skeletal adaptations ensure normal transmission of loads across the joints. Figure 15.11 illustrates the effect of negative feedback in relation to abductor–adductor muscle imbalance at the knee. Figure 15.11A represents a knee with normal balance between the abductor and adductor muscles (i.e. the resultant horizontal force at the knee is zero). This situation is associated with normal alignment between the femur and tibia and an even distribution of load across the articular surfaces and epiphyseal plates (Fig. 15.11B). Figure 15.11C shows the same knee with an abductor–adductor imbalance such that there is a net medially directed horizontal force at the knee tending to increase the degree of genu valgum. Figure 15.11D shows the unequal pattern of loading on the articular surfaces and epiphyseal plates associated with the muscle imbalance. Assuming that the unequal loading is within the normal range, the negative-feedback mode is invoked. The rate of growth of the lateral aspects of the epiphyses and metaphyses is increased and the rate of growth of the medial aspects of the epiphyses and metaphyses is decreased such that normal congruence is restored (with net zero horizontal force at the knee) at the expense of an abnormal alignment between the femur and tibia (i.e. much reduced genu valgum or even slight genu varum relative to most individuals) (Fig. 15.11E,F).

Whether or not a particular joint is anatomically malaligned during childhood, the only time when it may become painful (excluding injuries and pathological conditions not due to loading) is during adulthood, when the bones are no longer capable of modelling in response to abnormal loading. In most adults, abnormal patterns of loading are the result of an increasingly sedentary lifestyle in which body weight gradually increases and muscle strength gradually decreases.

## Modelling of articular surfaces

Minor incongruences between articular surfaces in synovial joints tend to result in large changes in the compression stress experienced by different parts of the articular surfaces (Calhoun et al 1994). This is especially the case in joints with pulley-shaped articular surfaces such as the ankle joint (Fig. 15.12). Under normal circumstances, the subtalar joint contributes to inversion and eversion of the foot (Fig.

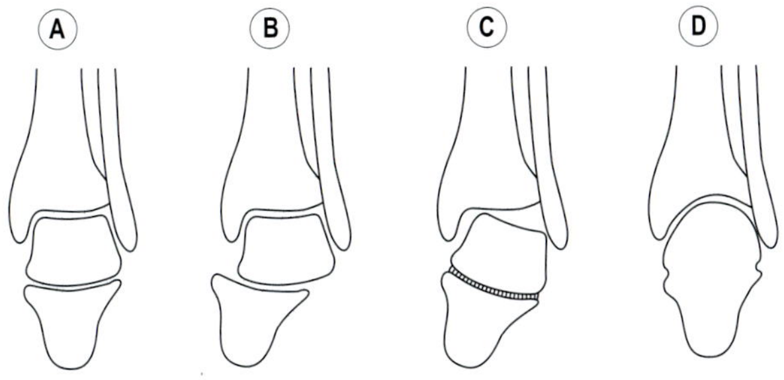

**Figure 15.12** Modelling of articular surfaces.

15.12A,B). However, if movement at the joint is absent or limited, inversion and eversion of the foot twists the talus in the tibiofibular mortise, resulting in excessive compression stress on those parts of the articular surfaces that remain in contact (Fig. 15.12C). The excessive loading on the impinging areas reduces or halts growth in these areas, while growth of the unloaded areas proceeds at the normal rate. Consequently, the shapes of the articular surfaces adapt to the abnormal loading conditions by forming a rounded surface in the coronal plane rather than a pulley-shaped surface, and the ankle joint as a whole resembles a ball and socket joint rather than a hinge joint (Fig. 15.12D) (Frost 1979).

# REFERENCES

Anwar R, Anjum SN, Nicholl JE 2005 Sesamoids of the foot. Current Orthopaedics 19: 40–48.

Aquino A, Payne C 2000 The role of the reverse windlass mechanism in foot pathology. Australasian Journal of Podiatric Medicine 34(1):32–34.

Åström M, Arvidson T 1995 Alignment and joint motion in the normal foot. Journal of Sports Physical Therapy 22 (5):216–222.

Blackwood CB, Yuen TJ, Sangeorzan BJ, Ledoux WR 2005 The midtarsal joint locking mechanism. Foot and Ankle International 26(12):1074–1080.

Briggs PJ 2005 The structure and function of the foot in relation to injury. Current Orthopaedics 19:85–93.

Bowden PD, Bowker P 1995 The alignment of the rearfoot complex axis as a factor in the development of running induced patellofemoral pain. Journal of British Podiatric Medicine 50:114–118.

Calhoun JH, Li F, Ledbetter BR, Viegas SF 1994 A comprehensive study of pressure distribution in the ankle joint with inversion and eversion. Foot and Ankle International 15:125–133.

Carter DR, Wong M, Orr TE 1991 Musculoskeletal ontogeny, phylogeny, and functional adaptation. Journal of Biomechanics 24(Suppl 1):3–16.

Czerniecki JM 1988 Foot and ankle biomechanics in walking and running: a review. American Journal of Physical Medicine and Rehabilitation 67:246–252.

Downing BS, Klein BS, D'Amico JS 1978 The axis of motion of the rearfoot complex. Journal of the American Podiatric Association 68:484–499.

Easley ME, Trnka H-J 2007 Current concepts review: hallux valgus part 1: pathomechanics, clinical assessment, and nonoperative management. Foot and Ankle International 28(5):654–659.

Frost HM 1973 Orthopedic biomechanics, Vol. 5. Charles C Thomas, Springfield, IL.

Frost HM 1979 A chondral modelling theory. Calcified Tissue International 28:181–200.

Frost HM 1988a Structural adaptations to mechanical usage: a proposed three-way rule for bone modelling. Part I. Veterinary and Comparative Orthopaedics and Traumatology 1:7–17.

Frost HM 1988b Structural adaptations to mechanical usage: a proposed three-way rule for bone modelling. Part II. Veterinary and Comparative Orthopaedics and Traumatology 2:80–85.

Frost HM 1990 Skeletal structural adaptations to mechanical usage: four mechanical influences on intact fibrous tissues. The Anatomical Record 226:433–439.

Gross TS, Bain ST 1993 Skeletal adaptation to functional stimuli. In: Grabiner MD (ed.) Current issues in biomechanics. Human Kinetics Corp, Champaign, IL.

Hicks JH 1954 The mechanics of the foot. II. The plantar aponeurosis and the arch. Journal of Anatomy 88(1):25–31.

Hicks JH 1961 The three weight-bearing mechanisms of the foot. In: Evans FG (ed.) Biomechanical studies of the musculoskeletal system. Charles C. Thomas, Springfield, IL.

Inman VT 1976 Joints of the ankle. Williams & Wilkins, Baltimore, OH.

Kilmartin TE, Barrington RL, Wallace AW 1991 Metatarsus primus varus, a statistical study. Journal of Bone and Joint Surgery 73B(6):937–940.

Kitaoka HB, Luo ZP, An K-N 1997a Three-dimensional analysis of normal ankle and foot mobility. American Journal of Sports Medicine 25(2):238–242.

Kitaoka HB, Ahn T-K, Luo ZP, An K-N 1997b Stability of the arch of the foot. Foot and Ankle International 18(10):644–648.

Menz HB, Lord SR 2005 Gait instability in older people with hallux valgus. Foot and Ankle International 26(6):483–489.

Nester CJ 1997 Rearfoot complex: a review of its interdependent components, axis orientation and functional model. The Foot 7:86–96.

Norkin CC, Levangie PK 1992 Joint structure and function: a comprehensive analysis. F.A Davis Company: Philadelphia.

Peat M 1986 Functional anatomy of the shoulder. Physical Therapy 66:1855–1865.

Roberts TDM 1995. Understanding balance: the mechanics of posture and locomotion. Chapman and Hall, London.

Schoenau E, Frost HM 2002 The 'muscle–bone unit' in children and adolescents. Calcified Tissue International 70:405–407.

Singh AK, Starkweather KD, Hollister AM, et al 1992 Kinematics of the ankle: a hinge axis model. Foot and Ankle 13(8):439–446.

Sobel E, Levitz SJ, Caselli MA 1999 Orthoses in the treatment of rearfoot problems. Journal of the American Podiatric Medical Association 89(5):220–233.

Tanaka Y, Takakura Y, Takaoka T, et al 1997 Radiographic analysis of hallux valgus in women on weightbearing and nonweightbearing. Clinical Orthopaedics and Related Research 336:186–194.

Thomas S, Barrington R 2003 Hallux valgus. Current Orthopaedics 17:299–307.

Valmassy RL 1996 Clinical biomechanics of the lower extremity. CV Mosby, St Louis, MI.

Watkins J 1999 Structure and function of the musculoskeletal system. Human Kinetics Corp, Champaign, IL.

Williams PL, Bannister LH, Berry MM, et al (eds) 1995 Gray's anatomy. Longman, Edinburgh.

Wolff J 1988 The law of bone modelling (trans. Maquet P, Furlong R). Springer Verlag, New York. [Originally published as: Wolff J 1892 Das gesetz der transformation der knochen. A. Hirschwald, Berlin.]

# Chapter 16

# Clinical therapeutics

*Maureen O'Donnell, Donald L Lorimer, Christine M Skinner,*
*Anne Whinfield and Asra Ahmad*

## THE THERAPEUTIC MANAGEMENT OF SUPERFICIAL LESIONS

The role of the podiatrist has broadened to include many aspects of healthcare that were previously either the sole prerogative of medical practitioners or were not available to patients at all. However, a recent survey indicated that 'core podiatry' is still the major role of podiatrists (Farndon et al 2002). The major factor that causes patients to seek out the skills of a podiatrist is a superficial lesion that is often a source of much pain, disability and partial loss of, or altered, foot function. Many of these conditions are unique to the feet and deserve particular consideration as clinical entities in their own right. Therefore, it is important that the efficient and effective treatment of these lesions should always be a first priority in the management of the patient, whether or not the underlying deformity or dysfunction is amenable to correction.

The patient's first concern is to obtain relief from pain and anxiety. The podiatrist's ability to treat such conditions successfully may well determine the patient's willingness to cooperate in further therapeutic measures, which may be necessary to deal with the underlying problem.

This chapter discusses a range of therapeutic measures for treating these conditions, but it is presumed that any underlying pathology or other causative factor, such as footwear, will also be assessed, diagnosed and managed. Any systemic diseases that the patient has, as well as the therapeutic measures to treat them, should be noted, and the treatment proposed for the foot modified accordingly, if necessary. Padding and strapping, in most cases an integral part of clinical therapies, may be used as the principal therapeutic method. The principles upon which this is based provide the rationale for orthoses in the continuing management process.

### Operating

Nothing is more important for the quick relief of pain related to skin and nail pathologies than skilful operating, and this aspect of podiatric management should never be underestimated or undervalued as it is a factor that will impress the patient with the practitioner's skill.

Pain during operating should be negligible and almost immediate relief should be provided unless the tissues are inflamed. Essential elements in painless operating are: maximum immobilisation of the area being reduced by correctly applied skin tension; the selection of appropriate scalpels; and the optimum level of reduction of pathological tissue. It is always difficult to define the optimum level of reduction, but the central consideration is to avoid breaking the skin while at the same time avoiding leaving areas of hard skin that will soon act as an irritant. All scalpels and instruments should be sterile (see Ch. 24). When painless reduction of the pathological tissue with scalpels is impossible, as in heloma neurovasculare and verruca pedis, the use of scalpels should be reduced to the minimum in the first instance, with recourse to caustics or keratolytic agents to facilitate the removal of the keratinised layers and to allow further reduction of the lesion on a return visit. Measures to reduce pain while operating may be either a topical application or an injection of a local anaesthetic (see Ch. 20). Topical applications of anaesthetic substances are said to be effective in certain situations, but can take up to 90 minutes to be effective (Elson & Paech 1995).

Protective padding and strapping will assist in relieving any postoperative tenderness.

### Medicaments

With the exception of local anaesthetics and a limited range of prescription-only medicines (POM) taken orally, therapeutic preparations used in podiatry are topical applications. They may have a specific function, as in chemical caustics, antifungal agents and antiseptics, but in general they also have a palliative effect.

Topical therapy can be said to provide relief of symptoms and, more importantly, protection while the skin heals. Many of the agents used lack scientific explanation of their mode of action and are employed because they are known to have been effective in previous treatments. The fact that suitable agents are used empirically should not detract from their credibility but encourage the practitioner to establish links that may add to the understanding of their mode of action. The form in which an agent is used, its method of application, the state of the substrate, the site of the lesion and the patient's state of health are all factors to be considered in the selection of a suitable agent. The paramount concern should be to treat the lesion quickly, using the minimum quantity of medicament to achieve the desired effect.

Long-term use of medicaments should be avoided, as some agents, or the base in which they are delivered, may cause contact dermatitis. Where application over a long time is unavoidable, as in the case of emollients or keratolytics in hyperkeratosis, the practitioner should be aware of this possibility and should minimise the risk by monitoring (and recording changes) and suggesting the use of alternatives.

In the treatment of specific conditions the patient should be advised to follow the treatment regimen and not to supplement, reduce or vary the treatment. The patient should be advised that if the use of a medicament causes any adverse effect then its use should be discontinued and the advice of the practitioner sought.

## Dressings

Dressings give an area of protection from friction, pressure and infection. Dressings are normally sterile and are mainly used on areas where the epidermis has been breached. Sterile dry dressings are available in a variety of sizes and packages, and are packed to facilitate the 'no-touch' technique. These dressings may be used with a medicament. The availability of environmental and interactive dressings for use on open lesions is worthy of consideration because of the many disadvantages ascribed to traditional dressings.

## Padding and strapping

Many foot problems are biomechanical in origin and mechanical therapy has a vital role in their management to correct function. The therapeutic use of padding and strapping covers both short-term treatment with adhesive padding and strapping and long-term management by orthoses with footwear advice, modification to footwear or specialised shoes.

In the short term, adhesive padding, correctly chosen and applied with appropriate strapping, almost invariably gives immediate relief from pain. In many instances, the adhesive padding may be adapted into replaceable, non-adherent, clinical padding until custom-made orthoses have been prescribed and manufactured for the patient.

The long-term use of clinical padding is inefficient in terms of durability and hygiene, and thus it must always be a short-term solution. The combination of clinical padding and then orthoses affords the most effective means of controlling biomechanical disorders. The management process should be carried out with the full understanding and cooperation of the patient. Patient compliance is essential.

Adhesive padding protects by several means: correction, deflection, cushioning, or by removing tensile or shearing stresses from the epidermis and subcutaneous tissues. Corrective padding is normally used when there is sufficient joint function available to realign the joint. It will improve anatomical alignment and reduce or eliminate abnormal stresses. Appropriate strapping is applied with the padding to assist correction. Padding that protects by deflection or cushioning is also adhered by strapping, but in this instance there is little or no alteration to the position of the underlying deformity. The role of strapping is to secure padding closely to the foot in the correct position. Padding or strapping used to remove either shearing or tensile stresses from the epidermis is normally of a thin stretch-type material.

Clinical padding may be applied directly to the foot in adhesive or replaceable form, fitted into the footwear as an insert, or built into a corrective or protective orthosis. The wide range of materials available to the podiatrist provides a choice of thicknesses and densities, from the very firm to the very soft, depending on the therapeutic objective. Firm materials are required for correction of function and deflection of pressure. Softer materials are required to provide shock absorption or cushioning for tissues subjected to abnormal stresses, or where there is atrophy of the subcutaneous tissues due to age, or debilitated by disease, and is subject to trauma and ulceration.

Silicone and thermoplastic materials can also be used as a medium- or long-term measure to follow clinical padding and strapping (see also Ch. 17).

## Review periods

Review of progress in clinical practice and the outcome of the review should be recorded in comprehensive notes in the patient's records, completed at the time of treatment and supplemented, if necessary, by photographs or accurate charting. The management of podiatric conditions is dependent on the practitioner's ability to assess progress and to modify treatment strategies as required, and unless each stage is clearly recorded this cannot be said to have been achieved.

The length of a review period depends on factors such as patient compliance and the practitioner's ability to evaluate the information received. Attention must be paid to the legal issues relating to the accurate recording of treatment strategies and updating all changes that have occurred in the patient, including medical disorders and drug therapy.

A change of treatment strategies may be required if there is a change in medical or social history. If there is no improvement in the condition, the podiatrist must reconsider the original treatment strategy, or re-evaluate the diagnosis, and adapt the management strategy or refer to another professional in the medical field, as appropriate. All changes made must be recorded fully.

## Case records

Properly maintained case records are of inestimable value in refuting allegations of malpractice. Litigation is an increasingly common fact of life for all practitioners, and the main weapon in the defence of such allegations, after the adherence to proper accepted practice procedures, is the well-maintained clinical case record (*Podiatry Now* 1999a).

In all cases emphasis must be placed on an accurate and detailed medical history being taken and recorded in full, and updated at each subsequent visit (see Ch. 1).

Case records should be written up immediately after the treatment has been completed, detailing all that has been carried out in the treatment of that patient and listing all the changes that are necessary to update the case record (*Podiatry Now* 1999b). Time should be allocated for the completion of the record at the end of each episode of episode of care. The format of the record should be adequate for full reporting and abbreviations used only if they are part of an accepted and published norm. Case records should also indicate that informed consent was obtained from the patient or, in the case of a minor, the parent or guardian. The records should be stored in a safe and secure place.

## CONTROL AND TREATMENT OF THE HYPERKERATOSES

### Pathological callus

This should be removed carefully with a suitable scalpel in order that the areas are cleared of thickened stratum corneum. It is considered by some practitioners that callus that produces no discomfort should not be removed. This is referred to as 'physiological' callus. Care should be taken to ensure that the patient does not have loss of sensation due to an underlying medical condition, or the formation of ulceration under the area of callus.

A common cause of sensory loss to the feet is diabetes, and if callus is not removed it may lead to breakdown of tissue as a result of compression of underlying blood vessels, leading to a local ischaemia. Conversely, its removal should be carried out in a manner to ensure that the skin is not breached.

### Postoperative antisepsis

Postoperatively, a broad-spectrum antiseptic should be applied to the skin, the choice of agent depending on the state of the patient's skin. Some antiseptic agents are inactivated in the presence of blood, serum or pus, others will inhibit the development of most bacterial organisms, while others will be bactericidal to one specific type. Depending on the activity required, the choice may be between an antiseptic that acts quickly and has a long duration of action or one whose action builds up slowly to optimum effectiveness.

There is a variety of postoperative topical antiseptic agents from which the practitioner may choose (Dollery 1999). *Chlorhexidine digluconate* exerts its effect on the bacterial cells through interaction with the acidic phospholipids of the cell membranes (Broxton et al 1984). Chlorhexidine is also particularly useful in preoperative skin preparation as well as a postoperative agent. It is effective against a range of Gram-negative and Gram-positive bacteria (Davis et al 1954). For skin disinfection it is generally used at 0.5% in 70% iso-propyl alcohol (Dollery 1999), although more commonly industrial methylated spirit is used instead of isopropyl alcohol. For use as a preoperative hand-cleansing agent it should be used at 4% in water (Lowbury & Lilly 1973).

*Iodine* is useful as a skin preparation and may also be used postoperatively (Wyss & Strandsov 1945). Its use is facilitated in the buffered iodophor form (povidone iodine), which reduces the adverse effects associated with iodine applied to the skin. Povidone iodine is usually used at 10% in an aqueous or alcoholic base. Its action is through the oxidation of the amino acids in proteins (Alexander & Nishimoto 1981). In rare cases there may be local sensitisation as a result of application of iodine compounds. It should be discontinued and avoided in patients with known allergy.

*Tincture of benzoin compound* (10% benzoin in alcohol) was previously used commonly as an antiseptic agent (Martindale 1999) but as its action is not quantifiable its use has been superseded. It can be useful in producing a sticky surface when painted onto the skin to help to secure adhesive padding in the treatment of verrucae with acids, but painting with flexible collodion or spraying with polyurethane dressing spray (Opsite, Smith & Nephew) is better for that purpose. It is sometimes used in the treatment of fissures, particularly around the heel.

The use of *tea tree oil* (the essential oil of *Melaleuca alternifolia*) has become more common. The name Ti-tree oil has also been used for melaleuca oil (Martindale 1999); this is a name also used for oil obtained from the Cordyline plant, indigenous to New Zealand. It has been used in Australia as a topical application and is reported to have a wide spectrum of antimicrobial activity (Carson & Riley 1993). The minimum inhibitory concentration for *Staphylococcus aureus* was found to be 0.08% (Walsh & Longstaff 1987). Other studies have found that concentrations of between 0.05% and 1% are effective against a range of pathogens, including *Staphylococcus aureus* (Altman 1988). (See also the section on treatment of fungal infections later in this chapter.)

### Emollients

The use of emollient substances is the best method of long-term management of dry skin, softening the skin by providing an oily layer on the surface to retain moisture (Holden et al 2002). To gain the maximum effect most agents need to be applied after a footbath, when the skin will have a higher water content, and the application should be repeated frequently (McHenry et al 1995). The patient can usually do this himself, and it is most effective in preventing the dry skin from fissuring. Many proprietary emollients are available for this purpose, and contain substances such as lanolin. Where the hyperkeratosis is widespread and associated with extreme anhidrosis, the use of an emollient with an occlusive dressing overnight, in addition to regular applications by the patient during the day, may give better results. Recent reports of trials of a hydrogel emollient substance (Doublebase™) suggest that this could be acceptable for frequent application (Wynne et al 2002). Frequent application of emollient substances to the feet is difficult to sustain as it usually interferes too much with the patient's daily routine.

Washing with soap products can cause problems by weakening the lipid barrier (Cork 1997). Care has to be taken to ensure that soaps and cleansing products do not contain lauryl sulfate, which is a detergent agent that has been shown to have irritant properties (Tupker et al 1997).

### Astringents

Astringent agents should be used to improve the state of moist skin. This helps to prevent secondary problems such as fissuring and blistering, which may lead to bacterial or fungal infection. Mild astringents in solution such as 3% salicylic acid in industrial methylated spirit or limited applications of 3% formalin aqueous solution may be applied. Alternatively, two or three crystals of potassium permanganate can be dissolved in a footbath and the foot immersed for not more than 5 minutes. A useful measure of the limit of the effectiveness of potassium permanganate is to observe the colour change from pink to a brownish hue. Astringent agents can cause skin irritations.

### Silicone implants

The loss of plantar fibrofatty tissue is a cause of pain in pressure-related foot disorders and also in ulceration of neuropathic feet. Clinical and histological findings indicate that liquid silicone replicates the resiliency of plantar fat and is retained in situ with exceptional stability. It is deposited using a relatively simple injection procedure that offers a safe and effective treatment for foot problems associated with excessive weight bearing. As a soft-tissue substitute, fluid silicone reduces or eliminates pain and prevents diabetic foot ulceration.

About 5% of those who were treated reported increased comfort after only one implant, with the majority improving after the third, fourth or fifth visit when up to 1 ml had been implanted. Patients frequently became able to walk barefoot without pain, and most resumed previous activity levels. Ninety per cent of simple flat fibrous calluses improved greatly, or disappeared within several months. Sixty-five to eighty per cent of keratoses with deeper central cores also improved or were eliminated, but more slowly. Frequently seen were calluses that did not appear much smaller than when first injected; however, patients stated that there was less or no pain.

## Heloma durum (hard corn) of the digits

These occur on the dorsal aspect and apices of the lesser toes, in the nail sulci associated with pressure from the nail plate or at the lateral edge of the nail, particularly of the fifth toe. Because footwear pressure is the initiating factor in the majority of cases, advice in this respect is mandatory. It is essential to eradicate the nucleus with a scalpel at the earliest stage. Enucleation should remove all the keratinised epidermal cells so that the underlying tissue can be restored to a better condition. Enucleation normally can be accomplished at the first visit, provided there is not extreme pain and tenderness. Difficulty in removal due to impacted keratin layers may be facilitated by the application of 5% potassium hydroxide aqueous solution, for its mild keratolytic action, for a few minutes prior to reduction.

Enucleation of the corn may be followed by the application of a mild keratolytic agent. With little underlying fibrofatty tissue, the choice of agents is limited, with those that are more penetrating being contraindicated. If complete reduction of the nucleus has not been achieved with a scalpel, the application of 15–30% salicylic acid ointment in a white soft paraffin may be used. This keratolytic used at the above concentrations will produce a slow and painless structural alteration of keratinised tissue, softening and macerating it. The action of this medicament is slow and cumulative, and for this reason it should be left in situ for a period of 5–7 days and the coagulum completely removed before further treatment is initiated. This treatment may need to be repeated two or three times at weekly intervals to facilitate eradication of the nucleus. Prolonged treatment with salicylic acid may cause dermatitis. Application should be made using a masking plaster to prevent spread of the agent to surrounding tissue. When the application of salicylic acid in ointment form is not practicable, the base may be changed to collodion or spirit, and this can be applied directly to the area by means of an applicator stick without masking the surrounding tissues. This method may also be used in the nail sulcus with low concentrations of the acid. The addition of padding to deflect pressure away from the area in conjunction with footwear advice or modification is necessary. When complete reduction has been achieved, 25% or 50% silver nitrate solution may be applied. This protein precipitant will 'shrink' the walls of the cavity, and repeated applications in conjunction with expert scalpel action will return the tissues to normal, provided that compression stress to the area has been eliminated. Thereafter, patients should be encouraged to restore elasticity to the area by the regular use of emollients.

The presence of peripheral neuropathy, vascular insufficiency, impaired immune response or the effects of long-term steroid therapy on healing will make the application of caustics or any medicament with the ability to cause breakdown of tissue undesirable. However, a mild exfoliant such as 10% salicylic acid in collodion can be used to facilitate enucleation, but the patient should be monitored closely.

Electrosurgery (described later in this chapter) can also produce good results with intractable lesions in carefully selected patients.

## Heloma durum (hard corns) on the plantar metatarsal area

These are usually chronic in nature and may be associated with common structural deformities such as pes cavus (under the first and fifth metatarsal heads), hallux limitus/rigidus (under the second or fifth metatarsal heads and the interphalangeal joint of the hallux), and hallux abducto valgus (under the second and third metatarsal heads). The chronic nature of these lesions results in fibrotic changes to the underlying dermal tissues because of the inflammation of the tissues as a result of trauma caused by overloading due to abnormal gait patterns. Such lesions may prove difficult to eradicate successfully in the long term because the tissues at the weight-bearing area have lost their elasticity. They will respond to attempts to increase pliability, but the main emphasis in management must be on deflective and protective padding and orthotic therapy, with correction of function where possible.

Silver nitrate or salicylic acid may be used as a caustic treatment in a similar method to that discussed above for digital lesions.

### CASE STUDY 16.1 CAUSTIC TREATMENT FOR PLANTAR CORNS

The patient was a 50-year-old man who had a history of foot pain for which he had sought treatment that had taken the form of removal of the plantar callus. This had been carried out on a frequent basis, gradually reducing from monthly to almost every 2 weeks. The patient had moved from another part of the country and was seeking treatment to keep him mobile. Each foot had very large plantar corns over the first metatarsophalangeal joint and smaller versions over the fifth metatarsal, showing the classic plantar lesions of pes cavus. He was able to wear footwear that had sufficient toe depth and there were no toe lesions. His feet were otherwise trouble-free.

After removal of the nucleus of the corns on both feet it was decided to apply a mild caustic in the form of 20% salicylic acid in white soft paraffin to each of the lesions. This was applied through a plaster mask in a manner similar to a treatment for verrucae. The area was protected with a double-wing plantar metatarsal pad made from 5mm semi-compressed felt and secured with an occlusive strapping. The patient was advised to keep the dressing dry and return in 1 week.

On his return and the removal of the dressings, the area was white and macerated. and this tissue was easily removed leaving a very healthy looking and pliable area. It was decided that it would be better to leave the area uncovered and allow the patient to apply a suitable emollient, which had also been applied postoperatively, to the plantar surface of both feet. Non-adhesive protective padding was made from felt and elastic net bandaging in the form of a double-wing plantar metatarsal pad to transfer the patient's weight away from the points of the lesions. The patient was seen after 2 weeks, when he reported that his feet had been reasonably comfortable and trouble-free apart from some pressure on his fifth toes.

When these were examined it was obvious that the plantar padding had been too thick, thus raising the foot too close to the upper of the shoe. There was some build up of tissue on both plantar areas, which was removed. An emollient was applied, and insoles with a double-wing plantar metatarsal pad were supplied, these having been made from shapes taken at the previous visit. The patient was given another appointment 2 weeks later.

On his return the patient reported only a very low level of discomfort and the amount of hard skin that had recurred was small. He was given a return appointment for a month later and arrangements were made for a more permanent form of insole to be supplied. On his return he reported very little pain and, although there was a small build up of hard skin over the areas where the lesions had been, this was not very great. He was supplied with the permanent insoles, which he found very comfortable, and was told that he need not make an appointment until he was of the opinion that he needed treatment. He did not return for 4 months, and then the amount of hyperkeratotic build up was small. The patient was pleased to be freed from very regular appointments and has continued with only a 6-monthly review appointment.

## Interdigital heloma

These lesions are evidence of compression occurring between opposing interphalangeal joints due to abnormal digital alignment or to the base of a proximal phalanx pressing on an adjacent metatarsal head with subsequent pressure on the overlying tissues. These lesions may be exacerbated in some cases by hypermobility of the feet and excessive pronation, with consequent constriction of the toes from footwear. Although a lesion may be limited to the 4/5 interdigital space, it should be borne in mind that the causative factor may well be a biomechanical problem in the rearfoot, such as a rearfoot varus, and complete resolution depends on the elimination of the problem, which is not always possible. Interdigital helomas may also be associated with hyperhidrosis, which determines their consistency as hard (heloma durum) or soft (heloma molle), and which, if present, needs to be controlled. Their enucleation requires skilful operating, especially when they are situated in the fourth web space.

Heloma molle respond well to the application of 20% silver nitrate solution following enucleation. As this has the apparent effect of reducing sweat production, it also toughens up the epidermal tissue of the lesion and makes reduction easier on the return visit. Silicone orthodigital splints or interdigital wedges are the most effective form of padding when the lesion is due to pressure from opposing interphalangeal joints. When the lesion is in the web space, realignment of the metatarsal to the base of the opposing phalanx is required.

## Vascular and neurovascular heloma

Lesions of this type are found over interphalangeal joints and plantar to the metatarsal heads. They are characterised by the protrusion of vascular and neural structures into the overlying hyperkeratosis and the objective of treatment is to destroy these elements by cautery. The presence of nerve filaments and capillaries close to the surface makes these lesions highly sensitive and liable to bleed. Operating on these lesions is extremely painful and this usually prevents complete reduction. Superficial callus should be reduced without causing haemorrhage but, should this occur, treatment with caustics must be delayed until the wound has healed. Any operating may be assisted by the preoperative application for 5 minutes of 5% potassium hydroxide solution to soften the overlying callus. These lesions often have multiple small nuclei that cause further problems in reduction. A local anaesthetic will be indicated if extensive excision or electrosurgery to the lesion is contemplated, but progressive chemical cautery is the less traumatic treatment. Whichever method is chosen, these lesions are by the nature of their pathology extremely difficult to eradicate.

In vascular lesions, applications of 50% silver nitrate solution, following reduction without haemorrhage, are effective over several weekly visits. This substance may cause intense pain when used for neurovascular corns. Salicylic acid is also of use in lower concentrations (20% or 25% in white soft paraffin) when tissue breakdown is unlikely.

Electrocautery may also be used in the treatment of such lesions. Local impairment of circulation may make its use more problematic,

and while early results seem encouraging, longer term evaluation is needed.

## Heloma miliare (seed corns)

These lesions are commonly associated with anhidrosis and may appear on any area of the plantar surface of the foot. They are not associated with pressure, and common sites are the medial longitudinal arch and the heel. They often present difficulties in management due to high recurrence rates regardless of a high level of expertise in enucleation. Some authorities suggest that, if pain is not a feature, treatment should consist of control by the application of emollients or urea-containing compounds, such as 10% urea cream, which affects the keratin linkages and increases the moisture content of the epidermal cells. However, success is more likely if the corn is reduced prior to treatment with a medicament. The area can be softened preoperatively with 5% potassium hydroxide. Patients should be advised on the use of emollients for the long-term management.

## Palmoplantar hyperkeratosis

This condition and its associated punctate form present problems in management.

The condition produces keratotic thickenings, which can cause severe discomfort and interfere with the gait cycle. When it appears in large plaques surrounded by an inflammation, its operative removal is often limited by the discomfort, which may be minimised by the application of 5% potassium hydroxide solution. This agent also helps when reducing the punctate form by scalpel, but it is seldom possible to remove all the hypertrophic material. In many instances, complete removal causes the patient discomfort for several days following treatment.

The management of this condition consists of simple reduction of the hyperkeratotic areas, and daily use by the patient of emollients, either by rubbing in daily or by occlusion overnight. The use of a cushioning insole often gives added relief from pain.

## SHORT-TERM PADDING THERAPY

## Digital padding for the lesser toes

In most instances this should be used either to redistribute the pressure from the lesion or to correct toe function. The application of ointments to digital lesions also necessitates the use of appropriate padding to contain the medicament by redirecting the pressure away from the site of the lesion.

The common deformities of the lesser toes are hammer, mallet, clawed, retracted toes and digiti quinti varus. These deformities may be purely local as a result of footwear restricting the functioning of the toes over a period of years, or secondary as a result of rearfoot or forefoot structural pathology.

Regardless of the cause, conditions such as clawed or retracted toes arise because of excessive extension or flexion. In addition, there may be degrees of axial rotation and medial or lateral deviation. Digital padding should be designed to exert maximum correction, because the toes are only rarely fixed and some degree of correction is almost always possible. The correction achieved in the majority of cases is functional and not structural. Permanent correction can take place only when the foot is held in the correct position by ligamentous and muscular action, without any external help. However, in the young, supple foot opportunities for full correction are increased. These conditions do not usually affect one digit in isolation and, although one

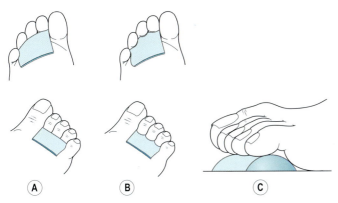

**Figure 16.1** (A) Combined dorsoplantar splint. (B) Adapted combined dorsoplantar splint to obtain deflection from dorsal and apical lesions. (C) Bolster pad for digits 2–4 when correction cannot be achieved. The bolster deflects pressure away from the apices.

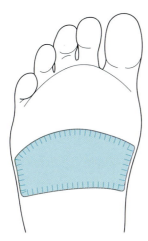

**Figure 16.2** Metatarsal bar.

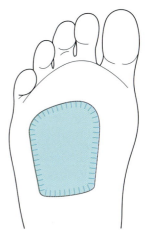

**Figure 16.3** A 2–4 plantar metatarsal pad which may be placed over the metatarsal heads or immediately proximal to them.

digit only may be affected with a hard corn, functional correction is obtained in most cases by regarding the middle three toes as one functional unit and, where necessary, correcting and protecting all three simultaneously through one device.

The major element in claw and retracted toes is an imbalance between the extensor and flexor muscles and it is logical to control these elements by combined dorsoplantar splints (Fig. 16.1A,B). This will exert a reciprocal corrective pressure on the deformities. In a full dorsoplantar splint for the middle three toes, the dorsal pad exactly covers the proximal phalanges and controls any excessive flexion. The plantar pad underlies the intermediate and distal phalanges and controls any excessive flexion. Body weight immobilises the plantar pad against the sole of the shoe, and the dorsal pad is held firmly by pressure from the upper of the shoe. The whole splint is securely in contact with the toes, correcting unwanted deviation in the interphalangeal joints, while the metatarsophalangeal joints are left to function normally. If there is limitation, particularly of dorsiflexion, at the metatarsophalangeal joints, then plantar padding is required in addition to the digital padding to hyperextend the digits. This padding takes the form of a metatarsal bar (Fig. 16.2) or a plantar metatarsal pad behind metatarsals two, three and four (Fig. 16.3) to realign the metatarsophalangeal joints and deflect pressure away from the metatarsal heads if they are receiving excessive pressure. In addition, where there is some contracture of soft tissue, exercises or manual stretching should be initiated to encourage an increase in the range of motion.

The clinical padding used is firm felt (usually semi-compressed and 3–5 mm in thickness) and held in place with adhesive strapping. A standard format is shown in Fig. 16.1A, but the basic shape can be adapted to deflect pressure from lesions on the dorsal aspect or the apices of the digits (Fig. 16.1B). The plantar pad can be extended as a prop under the fifth toe, or under the proximal phalanx of the hallux to correct hyperextension of the distal phalanx. In addition, the splint can be made replaceable, but as this is not secured to the foot, slippage of the pad may reduce the functional correction. The shape and thickness of each pad is determined by the patient's footwear, as is the relative degree of correction or protection required.

Felt padding is a short-term measure for these splints, and it is more effective to manufacture them in silicone materials (see Ch. 17). Silicone can be shaped into retaining grooves interdigitally, which controls any axial rotation and medial or lateral deviation of the digits. The digits must be held in the corrected position until the silicone hardens. Because of the need for precision in the sizing and fitting of orthodigital splints, several important points need to be observed when this technique is used:

- the full thickness of the dorsal pad must not extend any further proximally than the base of the proximal phalanges, nor any further distally than the proximal interphalangeal joints (except if extended to include an oval cavity pad to protect a lesion).
- the proximal edge of the plantar pad should conform to the plantar fatty pad of the foot, particularly where the fatty pad has been pulled distally due to the toe deformities. The full thickness of the pad should fit behind the pulp of the toes.
- the pads must be thick enough to engage the pressure of the sole of the shoe on the plantar prop and the pressure of the shoe upper on the dorsal shield in order to maintain correction of the digits.
- the medial and lateral edges of the pads should not overlap onto the first and fifth toes when all the toes are in a normally constricted position inside the footwear.
- good positional control of the plantar prop is maintained by allowing a concavity in each side of the pad to accommodate the pulp of the first and fifth toes.
- footwear should be of adequate length to accommodate the increased length of the foot with the toes in the corrected position, particularly if combined with a plantar pad to realign the metatarsophalangeal joints. In order to prevent crowding of the toes, the toe box of the shoe must be of the correct dimensions. Other points of good-fitting footwear are mandatory.

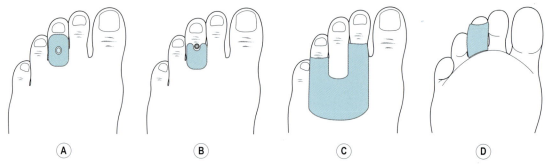

**Figure 16.4** Single-digit padding. (A) Oval cavity pad. (B) Crescent pad. (C) 'U-pad. (D) Single prop. This padding is generally used to protect a lesion by deflection.

In fixed deformities of the lesser toes in the older patient the splints are primarily for protection, by deflecting pressure away from dorsal and apical lesions, and they will have no functional correction, although they may prevent further deformity. These pads are of similar dimensions but are shaped to mould to the position of the digits (Fig. 16.1C) and act as a 'bolster' on the plantar surface of the digits, removing the pressure from the apices. In children this form of padding should be firm and slightly oversized to ensure maximum correction. Digital photographs are an excellent method of referencing correction.

Single-digit padding is sufficient when there is a fixed hammer or mallet deformity affecting only one digit. The fifth toe is particularly susceptible to pressure on the dorsal aspect from footwear when the digit is subluxated or in an adducted and varus position. Single padding will primarily have a protective role for dorsal, apical or interdigital lesions. These can take the form of oval cavity pads, crescent pads, U-shaped pads (which may be in replaceable form) or props to the plantar surface of the toes, which may be shaped in the form of a crescent at the distal portion to protect lesions (Fig. 16.4). The use of silicone devices should be initiated as soon as possible for the reasons stated above. The material is moulded directly to the foot, and this obviates any need for casting. The surgical option should be considered where feasible.

## Plantar metatarsal padding

The range of movement in the metatarsophalangeal joints is crucial in determining the therapeutic objective, and consequently the function, shape and material of the padding required. In the presence of chronic fixation, subluxation or dislocation of these joints, plantar metatarsal padding is designed to palliate the consequential overloading of particular metatarsal heads by redistributing the excessive load or by protecting them with a cushioning material. The cushioning effect is important in the elderly when there is atrophy of the fibrofatty pad underlying the metatarsal heads. In cases of mobile toe deformities in which the metatarsal heads are plantar flexed by the retracted phalanges, metatarsal padding assists in correcting the alignment of the affected metatarsophalangeal joint, particularly if combined with the use of digital dorsoplantar splints.

Footwear must be examined prior to the application of any padding and strapping to assess if it will accommodate the increased bulk of any padding and the increased length of the foot, which results when corrective padding is applied. Initially, plantar metatarsal padding is used in its adhesive or replaceable form, but it is readily convertible for long-term use into the more durable form of metatarsal braces, or as one component of an accommodative insole or functional orthosis.

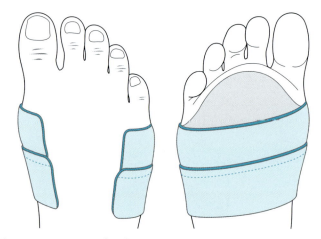

**Figure 16.5** Strapping for plantar metatarsal padding.

The basic plantar metatarsal pad (Fig. 16.3) is shaped to cover the heads and approximately two-thirds of the shafts of the middle three metatarsals in order that, on weight bearing, they are relatively dorsiflexed, provided they are sufficiently mobile. The shape conforms closely to the underlying metatarsals, avoiding impinging on the first and fifth metatarsal heads, and taking into account variation in the metatarsal formula. The full thickness of the pad lies directly under the metatarsal heads and it is bevelled off from there in all directions, being carefully graduated on its proximal and distal edges to ensure that it is securely adhered without any irregularities to cause discomfort under load. In addition to improving the alignment of the middle three metatarsals, it provides slight deflection away from the first and fifth metatarsal heads and it relieves symptoms of metatarsalgia. The improvement in the position of the clawed or retracted toes needs to be maintained with digital dorsoplantar splints.

With plantar padding, metatarsal strapping is used to control excessive splaying of the forefoot. The strapping encircles the metatarsus immediately behind the first and fifth metatarsal heads, non-stretch material normally being preferred. A half-metatarsal ('half-met') strapping may often be sufficient. This leaves the dorsum free, the ends terminating on the dorsum of the first and fifth shafts after traversing the plantar surface. Felt padding should be occluded with strapping by the application of two or three 5 cm wide straps half overlapping each other, the lateral edges covered with 'side straps' and with good anchorage to the skin (Fig. 16.5).

Adaptations of the basic plantar metatarsal pad include single-wing pads (SW/PMP) (Fig. 16.6A), double-wing pads (DW/PMP) (Fig. 16.6B) and U-section cut-outs (U/PMP) (Fig. 16.6C).

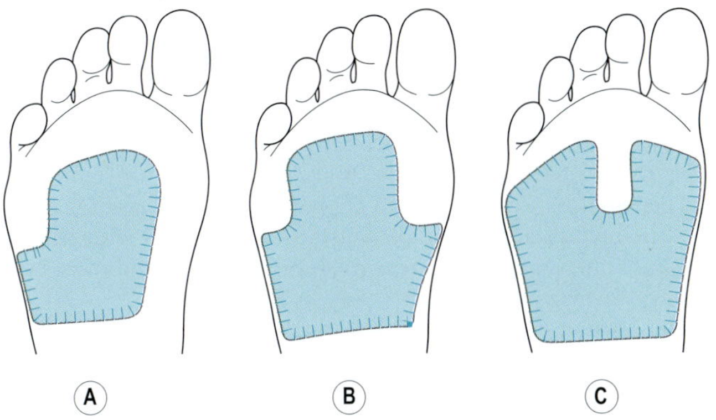

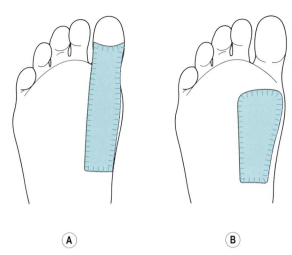

**Figure 16.6** Plantar metatarsal padding. (A) Single-wing plantar metatarsal pad to the fifth metatarsal head. (B) Double-wing plantar metatarsal pad to the first and fifth metatarsal heads. (C) 'U-shaped plantar metatarsal pad.

**Figure 16.7** Shaft pads. (A) Long-shaft pad to the first metatarsal and proximal phalanx. (B) Short-shaft pad to the first metatarsal.

Winged pads are designed to protect either or both of the first and fifth metatarsal heads from overloading. This pad will deflect pressure from the first and fifth metatarsal heads onto the second, third and fourth metatarsal heads and down the shafts. When adhered to the foot, the wing is reverse bevelled, the thickness of the wing fitting immediately around and behind the metatarsal head or heads. For an SW/PMP to the first metatarsal head, the lateral edge of the pad is located over the area between the fourth and fifth metatarsal shafts. The medial edge of a SW/PMP to the fifth metatarsal head is located over the area between the first and second metatarsal shafts. With a medial wing, the overall width of the pad must conform closely to the medial curve of the footwear so that no overlap of full-thickness material on the upper of the shoe is permitted, as this would tighten the vamp. The extra width required for anchorage is well bevelled and moulded around the metatarsal shaft. Full thickness will be under the middle metatarsal heads. This pad can be adapted to increase metatarsophalangeal function by the addition of a metatarsal bar or, if the first and fifth metatarsals are plantar flexed, by the addition of adapted shaft pads to those metatarsals, the distal aspect of the shafts stopping immediately proximal to the metatarsal heads.

The 'U-section pad is similar to a PMP but is extended across all five metatarsals with the 'U-shaped section reverse bevelled and cut out over any one of the middle metatarsal heads. The function is to deflect pressure from a particular metatarsal head to the other metatarsal heads and the shafts. A modified shaft pad may also be added behind the U-section to dorsiflex the metatarsal if motion is available. This pad follows the line of the toe webbing, but enough space is left distally to accommodate the strapping and it extends approximately two-thirds of the way down the shafts.

Metatarsal bars (Fig. 16.2) are functionally corrective pads and are designed to realign the metatarsophalangeal joints, increase toe function and deflect some pressure from the metatarsal heads onto the metatarsal shafts. They are ineffective in high-heeled shoes. When adhered to the foot, the distal margin of the pad is reverse bevelled, with the full thickness of the pad fitting immediately behind the metatarsal heads. The pad is contoured to the metatarsal formula and extends two-thirds along the metatarsal shafts. It is adhered with non-stretch occlusive strapping.

Shaft pads (Fig. 16.7) may be used for any metatarsal, although they are most commonly applied to the first, and can be described as either long- or short-shaft pads. Long-shaft pads (Fig. 16.7A) are used almost exclusively to the first metatarsal and extend to the interphalangeal joint where it is normally crescent shaped and reverse bevelled at that point. The purpose of a long-shaft pad is to increase the weight bearing through the metatarsal head, limit motion at the metatar-

sophalangeal joint and deflect pressure away from the interphalangeal joint. They are used in hallux limitus/rigidus. Short-shaft pads (Fig. 16.7B) stop distal to the metatarsal heads, the convex contour mimicking the metatarsal head with the full thickness of the pad lying directly over the metatarsal head. They are designed to increase the load to a particular metatarsal and realign the metatarsophalangeal joint. Perhaps the most common use is with a first metatarsal that is incompetent. They are used in conjunction with interdigital wedges to treat interdigital corns in the web space.

## THE TREATMENT OF VERRUCA PEDIS

Warts on feet have been recognised as a condition for many years, one of the first descriptions of the condition being given at the beginning of the 1st century AD by Celsus (Spencer 1961). The first recorded use of the term verruca was by Sennertus (Bunney 1982). Any review of their history shows a bewildering variety of 'cures', most of which were based on the theory of transferring them to another object (Bunney 1982). It was not until the latter part of the 19th century that the concept of infective agents was postulated (Payne 1891), and not until the first decade of the 20th century that the causative organism was finally identified (Cuiffo 1907). The idea of a virus was not accepted until the 1950s, when they could be identified as a result of the invention of the electron microscope (Strauss et al 1950). Verrucae are known to regress spontaneously, and it is thought likely that this is due to immunological responses (Chang 1990). However, every practitioner knows that verrucae can remain unresolved for several years and that he or she will be required to treat the lesions. Verrucae may occur as single large lesions or be multiple, usually small or mosaic, giving a distinctive appearance to the skin. A useful rule to follow is that if they are pain-free, treatment should be avoided in the hope of spontaneous regression occurring. Active treatment is indicated when pain is acute, when spread of the virus to other areas is observed, when the risk of cross-infection is high to others, and when non-treatment would entail unacceptable limitations on activities such as swimming, games and athletics. Plastic waterproof socks are available for such activities to guard against cross-infection but are of little value in keeping dressings dry.

If treatment is to be commenced, it is essential to assess the patient's general health status and ensure that an accurate analysis is made of the potential risks. The treatment should be carried out effectively, as the longer the time taken to reach a satisfactory conclusion the greater the risk of producing a verruca that seems to become resistant to treatment and also of causing unnecessary pain to the patient. Most skin warts are caused by human papilloma viruses (HPV). More recent research suggests that plantar warts are associated with HPV-1 and HPV-4 (Doorbar et al 1986, Galloway 1989, Howley 1988). There is less consensus about the causative organisms for mosaic verrucae. Research suggests that HPV-1 is only found in the sole of the foot in heavily keratinised areas (Howley 1988). These warts are highly infectious, are found mainly in teenaged children and are usually associated with minor trauma (Chang 1990). Although one foot only may be affected, both feet should be kept under observation during treatment as a check against cross-infection. However, whatever the causative organism, the format of treatment for warts on the feet falls into clearly defined methodologies.

## The treatment of verrucae

The principal measures are centred on cell-destruction techniques. These include chemical cautery, cryotherapy and electrosurgery. There has been some interest in techniques to produce cell-mediated immunity. In some instances, interactive dressings, astringents and homeopathic remedies are used when possible tissue breakdown is not desirable, as in the case of the 'at-risk' patient. A number of practitioners are using actual cautery or curettage with promising results.

### Chemical cautery

This retains an important place in the treatment of verrucae, and produces rapid results with minimal discomfort to the patient. Fundamentally, the acids are designed to irritate the skin at the level of the dermoepidermal junction, thus separating the verruca from the skin.

The fact should be clearly established with the patient before treatment that chemical therapy can, and usually does, cause pain, and may result in tissue breakdown. It should be emphasised that ,while such symptoms can be upsetting, they are not a sign of the treatment having gone wrong and can be dealt with swiftly and effectively by the practitioner who applied the caustic substance. The stronger acids such as monochloroacetic acid and pyrogallic acid are particularly liable to cause tissue breakdown and pain. Although these acids can be accurately confined to the lesion on initial contact, whether in ointment or solution form, when absorption into the tissues occurs there is less control over spread or depth (Fig. 16.8). Extreme care and good clinical judgement should be employed by the practitioner in the application of these agents.

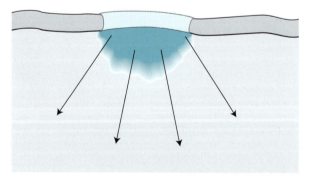

**Figure 16.8** Absorption of acid into the tissues (arrows show directions of spread). Although the application of the medicament is controlled at the surface, spread cannot be controlled through the tissues.

The substances available for use include various preparations of salicylic acid, monochloroacetic acid, trichloroacetic acid and potassium hydroxide, their caustic actions being strictly confined on application to the verruca tissue. The use of substances such as nitric acid and pyrogallic acid has largely been discontinued. The choice of agent depends on a number of factors, as each agent has a different action and penetration potential. When applying any caustic agent it cannot be overemphasised that the patient must be supplied with comprehensive written instructions regarding what to do should there be an adverse reaction.

**Site.** A lesion on a non-weight-bearing area is usually superficial, so liquid caustics are useful (e.g. salicylic acid preparations in collodion, trichloroacetic acid solution or a saturated solution of monochloroacetic acid used sparingly) are useful.

A verruca on a weight-bearing area is deeper as the weight of the patient and the resistance of the ground push the verruca below the surface, and thus both liquid and ointment preparations are suitable. Care must be exercised in the use of caustics where there is little underlying adipose tissue in order to avoid causing a severe tissue breakdown or producing an inflammatory reaction in an underlying joint. In such a situation, less penetrating caustics or strong astringents are indicated.

In certain cases, where the verruca is on a site unsuitable for padding, treatments involving ointments cannot be carried out.

**Number and size.** This influences the form and strength of the medicament to be used. Large verrucae respond well to ointment preparations. However, when numerous growths are present, masking is difficult. A large growth surrounded by smaller satellites may be treated with 60–75% salicylic acid ointment, and the satellites either ignored or treated with toughened silver nitrate alone or in conjunction with trichloroacetic acid. In general, caustic in ointment form or in solution is indicated for one or more large growths, while multiple small verrucae are more easily treated with solutions. Cryotherapy or electrotherapy offer alternative single treatments for any type of verruca.

**Skin texture.** If the skin is moist, solutions of caustics are preferable, as there is no necessity to confine them within padding, which would be contraindicated in the presence of hyperhidrosis. Fair-skinned people seem to be less tolerant of the action of some acids and often react adversely to silver nitrate. Tissues that are thin, dry and atrophied due to age or a systemic disorder do not tolerate acids and are liable to breakdown.

**Circulation.** When the arterial supply is reduced, as in the case of diabetes or atherosclerosis, ulceration of the area must be avoided because healing is delayed and bacterial infection could supervene. For the same reasons, similar care must be taken to avoid ulceration in the case of impaired venous circulation, which results in the tissues being oedematous. In such instances, caustics should be avoided and astringents or mild keratolytic agents employed.

**Neuropathy.** An inability to experience pain is a contraindication to any medicament likely to cause an inflammatory action or tissue breakdown. In such cases astringents or mild keratolytic agents should be employed.

**Availability of patient.** When powerful acids are used, it is essential to ensure that the patient is able to return within 7 days or at a time sooner if considered necessary by the practitioner. Otherwise, use an alternative form of treatment such as cryotherapy or one of the other 'one-off' treatments. A final option would be one of the mild keratolytic agents. The use of home treatments is another possibility, provided the patient will adhere to the treatment regimen.

**Age.** Young children are often nervous, as well as seeming to have low pain thresholds. Their skin tends to be hyperhidrotic and they are normally very active, engaging in swimming or various other sporting activities. Their involvement in the latter areas usually means that 'one-off' solutions have to be used.

**Previous treatments.** The practitioner should establish which medicaments have been used previously in order to reduce the risk of continuing a non-effective treatment or a treatment where there has been an adverse reaction. A history of treatment that has not cleared the condition usually predicts that the verruca will be slow in responding to treatment.

All of the above must be taken into account when deciding on the preferred method of treatment. Ointments or pastes will spread to normal surface tissue unless contained by masking of the adjacent healthy tissue. The surrounding skin should be painted with substances such as tincture of benzoin compound or Opsite™. The area should be masked with thick waterproof adhesive plaster through which a hole has been cut slightly smaller than the surface area of the verruca. (A light application of silver nitrate to the periphery of the lesion using a silver nitrate stick (95% or 75%) prior to the application of the masking tape gives added protection from lateral penetration of the tissues by the caustic.) The ointment is then applied through the hole in the plaster to the verruca and sealed in with waterproof strapping to ensure close contact. Estimating the amount of the agent to be applied is always a matter of judgement, but it is important that the amount is not excessive, encouraging it to spread laterally. Alternatively, if more medicament is required after the initial masking tape is in position a felt pad with an aperture of the same size is placed over the verruca and the ointment placed into the aperture to the required amount, which will help to contain the ointment. If the first method is adopted, then padding with a cavity to deflect pressure away from the area of the verruca and relieve pain should be applied, particularly if the lesion is on a weight-bearing area. The padding should then be covered totally with zinc oxide plaster, left in position for up to 7 days and the patient advised to keep the whole area dry to prevent spread of the acid (Fig. 16.9).

An instruction sheet must be given and explained to patients receiving verruca treatment (see Ch. 27). The information should include issues of hygiene while keeping the dressing and the area dry, the method of treatment used, specific instructions relating to any antidote to the medicament applied, what to do in case of pain from breakdown of tissue, emergency telephone numbers, etc.

At subsequent visits, the necrosed tissue is removed under strict antiseptic conditions. It is unlikely that one application will have resolved the substance of the verruca and subsequent applications of

the caustic should be made and repeated as necessary until complete resolution has been achieved. The state of the skin should be taken into account when continuous treatments are required, as maceration, either with the spread of salicylic preparations or with continual application of plaster to the skin, may require a different approach for a period of time.

As stated earlier, the objective of treatment with acids is to produce an aseptic necrosis and resultant sloughing of the verruca tissue. With carefully controlled dosages and spacing of treatments, this should be a relatively pain-free process.

If tissue breakdown does occur, further applications of an acid should be stopped until healing has occurred. The ulcer should be treated appropriately with a suitable antiseptic agent to prevent infection, or with a sterile dressing, and the patient advised not to remove the dressing. Deflective padding should be applied to remove direct pressure on the area. The patient should be seen at frequent intervals until the pain and inflammation subsides which, as it is aseptic in origin, should be rapid. It is important to monitor the patient well at this stage, as there have been many examples where the patient has considered their painful problem was not being well managed and sought advice from other sources. Such interventions usually result in the lesion being misdiagnosed and inappropriate treatments being applied.

## Disadvantages of treatment with chemical therapy

- It can be time consuming for both the practitioner and the patient, with frequent short review dates of up to 7 days when using acids in ointment form. This is expensive for all concerned and is not seen as cost-effective treatment.
- Padding applied continuously leaves the tissues macerated.
- Hygiene is problematical because the area must be kept dry.
- The rate of penetration of the acid cannot be predicted easily, and there is always the possibility of tissue breakdown, which is painful and may leave scarring.
- No single chemical treatment can guarantee rapid results.
- All forms of treatment will cause a degree of discomfort or pain and inconvenience.
- Hyperhidrosis is a contraindication to the use of ointments because padding containing the acid will not be secure on a moist skin and thus there will be spread of the acid to normal tissue.

## Therapeutic agents for chemical cautery

### Salicylic acid

Applied topically, salicylic acid has a keratolytic action, and it is also bacteriostatic and fungistatic (Davis & Marks 1976). It has a relatively low systemic toxicity, and no special effects on the gastrointestinal tract, liver or kidneys as a result of topical applications have been recorded. There are reports of salicylates crossing the placental barrier in rodents (Dollery 1999).

It has continued to be one of the main agents used in the treatment of verrucae because it is available in many forms (ointments, pastes, solutions and in collodion) and concentrations (from 20% to 75%). In all its preparations salicylic acid remains one of the most effective treatments for verrucae, with success rates of 65–70% (Bunney et al 1976). It is readily available in many proprietary forms from chemists for home use.

The mode of action of salicylic acid is unclear, but it is thought to affect the linkage mechanism between the cells of the stratum corneum (Dollery 1999). In higher concentrations it produces an increasingly potent and rapid keratolytic effect on the stratum corneum, causing maceration and epidermolysis.

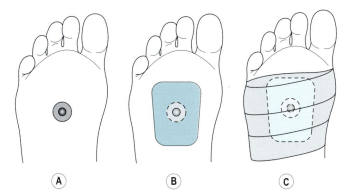

**Figure 16.9** Masking of the tissues to limit the contact area of the acid. Padding and occlusive strapping are used in the application of ointments in the treatment of verrucae.

On non-keratinised tissue it has a rapid destructive action and causes breakdown of tissue. The epidermal tissues often appear intact but, when they are removed, tissue breakdown is observed in the deeper tissues.

In solution or a collodion base, only a limited amount of the salicylic acid comes into contact with the verruca at any one time, and it is easily confined to the area of the verruca and will produce a mild localised action. It is most commonly used on small lesions where there is little subcutaneous tissue, or on sites where padding is difficult (e.g. in the nail sulcus). The preparation is normally applied by the patient on a daily basis and, provided the application is restricted to the area of the verruca, it has a slow, painless action. The podiatrist should remove the resultant coagulum every 14–21 days as part of the monitoring process. This obviates the need for very frequent time-consuming return visits. The patient can bathe daily prior to application and there is no need for padding, although a small plaster to prevent cross-infection may be used to cover the area. The ointment and paste forms contain higher concentrations of salicylic acid and must be confined by masking the area, and the use of padding to direct pressure away from the site of application. They produce a more localised drastic action when used on single verrucae at a site where there is adequate fibrofatty padding. The action of salicylic acid can be enhanced by combining it with monochloroacetic acid. This can produce a violent reaction and should only be used with care and in carefully selected patients. The monochloroacetic acid is usually used in saturated solution form and should be applied first. Continued use of salicylic acid may lead to a local dermatitis.

Life-threatening effects have been reported from the use of topical applications of salicylic acid (Davis et al 1979, Shupp & Shroeter 1986). To produce toxic reactions large areas of skin need to be covered. The concentration of the agent and the use of occlusive dressings are also factors (Dollery 1999).

## Monochloroacetic acid

This is available in solution or crystal form. It acts by hydrolysing proteins, converting the protein to soluble amino acids and peptides. It has a rapid penetrating action and may cause considerable pain. It is not unknown for patients to suffer from lymphangitis following treatment with this acid. It should only be used where there is adequate subcutaneous tissue, its use should be avoided over joints (periostitis or synovitis may result) and it is contraindicated in the very young, the nervous or elderly patients. It should never be used on a diabetic patient, in those with peripheral vascular disease or in cases where healing is impaired due to the high risk of tissue breakdown.

Prior to application the superficial keratinised layers should be removed without breaching the superficial capillaries. The saturated solution should be applied by means of an applicator stick directly and accurately to the verruca (Watts 1968). Care must be taken to confine the application exactly to the verruca tissue and not allow it to run over onto the surrounding skin. If necessary, the surrounding skin can be protected by petroleum jelly as a masking material until the solution has been absorbed into the tissue. Once the saturated solution of monochloroacetic acid has dried into the lesion the petroleum jelly should be removed to allow the application of an adhesive dressing.

It is suggested that crystals of monochloroacetic acid may be combined with salicylic acid ointment, but the practitioner should be aware that mixing of these agents in these forms may be a breach of the 1968 Medicines Act. As a matter of practicality, crystals are difficult to contain and their action may spread to other areas of the foot, producing a very deep penetrating ulcer with destruction of tissue. The action of monochloroacetic acid is neutralised by 5% potassium

hydroxide solution or sodium bicarbonate (1 in 80 solution), and this will work provided it is applied before the acid has been completely absorbed into the tissues (Read 1978). If the patient complains of pain some hours after application of the acid, he or she should use a saline footbath and return to the practitioner for review of the situation as soon as possible. Pain after such a short time is indicative of a violent inflammatory reaction associated with tissue breakdown.

## Trichloroacetic acid

This protein precipitant forms a barrier to its own penetration and is superficial in its action. Its action is slow and controlled if used at its usual concentration of 10%. In contrast to monochloroacetic acid, it can be used as a saturated solution where there is little adipose tissue between the verruca and underlying structures. It is ideal on shallow growths and mosaic verrucae. It should be painted on using an applicator stick, with the surrounding area protected by paraffin jelly, and allowed to dry.

## Potassium hydroxide

This is prepared in pellet form which contains 85% potassium hydroxide. It should be stored in airtight containers as it is hygroscopic. It is an extremely strong alkali that penetrates very deeply and rapidly. It is indicated in the treatment of large, single verrucae when rapid action is required but the patient is unable to return at regular intervals, provided there is adequate adipose tissue underlying the site of the verruca and the patient's state of health is good. The action of the caustic must be stopped before the patient leaves the surgery. It is a method that does not require padding or strapping, except to redistribute pressure after treatment, and therefore it can be used in the presence of hyperhidrosis. As with any penetrating caustic, potassium hydroxide should not be used on the previously mentioned 'at-risk' patients. As it absorbs water to dissolve itself, the following method of application is appropriate:

- all overlying callus should be reduced and the foot immersed in lukewarm water for up to 5 minutes prior to application and the foot thoroughly dried. The tissues will have absorbed additional fluid, which will facilitate the action of the potassium hydroxide (McHenry et al 1995). The skin surrounding the verruca should be protected with petroleum jelly or a similar substance to prevent spread of the potassium hydroxide in solution to healthy tissue.
- the pellet should be held with plastic forceps and applied gently to the verruca for a maximum of 2 minutes. The time necessary may well be less, and is often best judged by the patient's comments regarding pain, the occurrence of which indicates that the potassium hydroxide has reached the dermoepidermal junction. When pain is experienced the process should be stopped immediately. Care should be taken to avoid breaking the pellet in case parts of it lodge anywhere that could cause damage to the patient or the operator.
- the tissues will rapidly develop a white, macerated appearance. Following application of the agent, the foot should again be immersed in tepid water for a few minutes, and on removal the resultant jelly-like tissue can be carefully removed with a scalpel. The area should then be examined with a magnifying glass to establish if total clearance has been achieved. If there is any remaining verruca tissue, a small reapplication of potassium hydroxide should suffice, although this is unlikely and usually unnecessary.
- the area should then be treated with 5% acetic acid to neutralise any remaining potassium hydroxide. This is not an infallible one-off treatment because it is difficult to identify with

the naked eye any remaining verruca. Finally, the area should be covered with a sterile dressing plus the application of a broad-spectrum antiseptic, such as povidone iodine. The patient should be reviewed within 1 month, or sooner if there are any adverse reactions.

## Single-treatment techniques

These treatments have become more common in the management of verrucae, mainly as a result of improved apparatus, particularly in the cases of cryotherapy and electrosurgery. Such methods produce results quicker in all but the most intransigent lesions, and the function of the return appointments is to monitor and evaluate the success of the treatment and, if necessary, to dress any ulceration that has arisen as a result of the treatment. Although classed as single-treatment techniques, there is no absolute guarantee that resolution will be achieved in one session, and caution should be exercised when describing them as such to patients.

Single-treatment techniques are:

- cryotherapy, using liquid nitrogen or nitrous oxide
- electrosurgery, using coagulation, desiccation or fulguration, by 'hot-wire' cautery, or with electrosurgical units
- curettage.

### Cryotherapy

Cryotherapy is a method of treatment that uses profoundly low temperatures to destroy the tissues. Patients should be carefully selected prior to this procedure, and those who have poor healing abilities, low pain thresholds or abnormal sensitivity reactions to cold should be excluded. Cryotherapy can be applied to a verruca of any size and on almost any site, as the depth of destruction can be controlled using clinical judgement. The major disadvantages are the possibly painful nature of the treatment, acute inflammatory reactions in some patients and the initial monetary outlay for the equipment. These are offset by the fact that it is a relatively safe and easily controlled procedure, as the operator can observe the growth of the ice-ball in the tissues and know that the zone of demarcation will be the 'halo' around it. There is a sharp zone of demarcation, with normally a relatively small inflammatory response. When the underlying blister, which usually results, has resolved there should be no scarring. If the blister remains intact until healing has occurred the risk of infection is minimal. The therapy is easy to use on sites where ointments are not indicated. It has a high success rate, does not consume much surgery time and does not entail frequent return visits. Padding is, usually, only necessary to relieve pressure after treatment, if the verruca is on a weight-bearing area.

There are now two main methods available to produce localised freezing of tissue. Nitrous oxide, with a release of temperature of $-88.5\,°C$, is employed in apparatus using the Joule–Thompson principle. The various probe sizes available allow accuracy and safety in the application. It is useful to be aware of a loss of freezing capability at the tip of the probe, which is usually at a higher temperature (less cold) than the release temperature of the gas.

Liquid nitrogen has an operating temperature of $-196\,°C$. The apparatus available for its use is similar to the type of equipment available for nitrous oxide, and recent advances in manufacturing have made this technique more easily used. Due to the even lower release temperature, it is much more efficient than nitrous oxide.

For cryosurgery to be successful the rate of freezing of the tissue must be rapid and all the cells to be destroyed must reach a temperature of less than $-20\,°C$. At this stage there should be intracellular formation of large ice crystals, which are necessary to rupture the cell membranes and cause their death. If the freezing rate is lower (above $-20\,°C$) the ice crystals may form in the intercellular spaces and the cell itself may survive.

Prior to the application of the probe it is useful to remove all overlying callus to facilitate the conduction of cold into the tissues. The following procedure may then be adopted.

A detailed explanation of the treatment should be given to the patient, including appropriate instructions for them to follow after treatment (see Ch. 27). This should include the use of analgesics for any postoperative pain associated with the inflammatory reaction that will occur, and advice on self-treatment to burst the blister if it becomes filled excessively with fluid and causes pain.

The apparatus should be checked for the correct pressure prior to treatment in order to achieve a fast freeze. Manufacturer's instructions should be adhered to in this respect.

A probe size equivalent to that of the verruca should be selected and a conducting medium such as a macrogol jelly (e.g. KY jelly) applied to the probe tip. The probe is applied with light pressure at right angles to the verruca. If the pressure is too great the tissue surrounding the verruca will be blanched and it will be difficult to identify the 'halo' when it appears.

Begin the freeze, and release the slight pressure when the KY jelly turns white. This colour change should not be mistaken for the halo, which is seen as a yellowish white ring to the outside of the frozen KY jelly. This halo identifies the extent of the tissue being frozen, and is referred to as the 'ice ball'. At this point the probe tip will be adhered to the tissues and cannot be removed until the probe tip has defrosted. Normal time of freeze is between 30 seconds and 2 minutes, depending on the size of the lesion and the method chosen. Liquid nitrogen requires less freezing time than nitrous oxide. Timing of the freeze should begin once the halo is seen. The depth of cryonecrosis beyond 2–3 mm is not usually possible because the ice formed within the tissues acts as an insulator to further penetration of cold.

Allow the tissues to thaw at normal room temperature. When normal colour returns a repeat freeze should be carried out. A repeat freeze is more destructive of tissue than a single freeze. A third freeze is not normally required unless the lesion is very large or the freezing rate has been low. Thaw cycles are normally of 1–2 minutes. Freeze times are longer on the plantar aspect of the foot, where the epidermis is thicker. On the dorsum of toes 30 seconds is often adequate. In this area, because of the thinner epidermis, the cold passes more quickly through the tissues and this can be observed by the growth of the ice ball. If this extends beyond the margin of the verruca by more than 2 mm, freezing should be discontinued.

Silver nitrate may be applied over the verruca if desired to harden the superficial tissues and prevent rupture of the blister. Apply a protective dressing to the area, which usually requires padding on weight-bearing surfaces.

The patient should be seen again in 1 week to assess the effectiveness of the treatment. At this stage a blister should have formed around the entire lesion. The lesion may be cut out at this stage and the resultant ulcer treated with an appropriate broad-spectrum antiseptic until healing is complete. Alternatively, the patient may be left for up to 6 weeks, when the blister will have resolved, and the dead verruca tissue can then be removed with a scalpel. The advantage of the latter approach is that there is less danger of infection if the blister remains intact.

There are few dangers associated with cryosurgery other than accidental spillage of liquid nitrogen or accidental contact with freezing probes. The use of nitrous oxide equipment produces large volumes of the gas, which must be vented outside the building. The risk of abortion in early pregnancy has been noted in anaesthetists, due to prolonged exposure to nitrous oxide gas (Crawford & Lewis 1986, Donaldson & Meecham 1995).

## CASE STUDY 16.2 **CRYOTHERAPY IN THE TREATMENT OF VERRUCA PEDIS**

A 16-year-old schoolboy attended the surgery with a single large verruca on the plantar surface of his right heel. He was a keen swimmer and did not wish to suspend his swimming activities for any length of time. He was fit and healthy, and it was decided after discussion with him and his parents, who were present, that the best route of treatment would be to use cryotherapy.

Using liquid nitrogen apparatus the verruca was given three 30-second freezes, allowing the area to thaw fully between each freeze. Towards the end of the third freeze the patient complained of the pain being quite severe, but he managed to bear the discomfort until the freeze was completed. As the verruca was on an area of the heel that was going to be subjected to a lot of pressure, a 5-mm thick Poron heel pad was made for the right shoe. This had a hollow excavated on the undersurface to correspond with the lesion on the plantar surface of the heel, and thus redirect the weight-bearing area away from the site of the freeze. The patient and his parents were then given an advice sheet (see Ch. 27) and were also taken through the salient points that could be expected as a result of the treatment, in particular that there would be the formation of a deep blister at the site of the lesion. The heel was painful when the patient walked on it but he considered that the discomfort was not too great.

The patient returned after 7 days, as arranged, and reported that the pain had gradually subsided to a level where it was only a problem if he landed heavily on the heel but, otherwise, he had been walking normally. The appearance of the verruca was much changed and there was clear evidence of deep blistering. It was decided that, as the blister was intact, it would be better to leave it for another week. This time when the patient returned there was no discomfort and the blister was opened, all the exudate cleaned out and the appearance suggested that the area was clear of verruca. The ulcerated area was covered with a sterile dry dressing and the patient given an appointment for 4 days later. On his return the verruca was clear and the area had closed and had settled down well.

The use of cryotherapy had allowed the patient to swim all the time during the treatment, except for the days when a sterile dressing was applied after the ulcerated area was cleared. As a single treatment skilfully applied the use of liquid nitrogen is recommended, particularly in areas where there is adequate subcutaneous tissue.

## Electrosurgery and radiosurgery using cutting, coagulation, desiccation and fulguration

Electrosurgery is the use of electrical energy in the form of a high-frequency current applied locally with a metal instrument for the removal or destruction of tissue (Stedman 1990).

The term 'radiosurgery' is also sometimes used to describe electrosurgical treatment. This is because some machines operate at a radiowave frequency.

### Background

It may have been in Ancient Egypt that heat was first used to control bleeding. Throughout history, heated metal instruments have been used to destroy tissue and stop haemorrhage. While early instruments were heated on a fire for cauterisation of tissue, the development of tools heated by an electric current enabled greater control. This is known as *electrocautery*. Instruments currently used for electrocautery consist of a handpiece with switch and platinum wire electrode. With the advent of machines to produce an alternating and high-frequency current, it became possible to cut and coagulate tissue using the principles of *diathermy* (Brown 2000, Sebben 1988b). Standard diathermy

is based on the principle of two large thin plates (electrodes) being placed on the body over the treatment area. A high-frequency electric current is passed to the patient, and tissue resistance results in local heating. Standard diathermy causes mild local heating, as the heat is dispersed over the large area of the electrodes. Electrosurgical machines also operate on the principle of diathermy, but one of the large electrodes is replaced by a small electrode. While the same current is applied to both electrodes, it has a higher concentration in the small electrode. Resistance of body tissue to the electrical energy causes an increase in molecular heat. This results in evaporation of the cell fluids, and destruction of the tissue (Cresswell 1992) (Fig 16.10).

For several decades, electrosurgery has been a popular treatment modality amongst dermatologists and other medical specialists (Sebben 1989). Podiatrists have also recognised the advantages of using electrosurgery to perform a number of minor surgical procedures, and electrosurgical units are now a well-established tool in many podiatry clinics. Electrosurgery is frequently used in podiatry for the treatment of cutaneous lesions. Research has shown that electrodesiccation is a successful method of treating chronic corns (Anderson & Burrow 2001, Whinfield & Forster 1998, Wilkinson & Kilmartin 1998). Investigators have demonstrated electrosurgery to be a useful treatment option for removal of resistant verrucae (Lelliott & Robinson 1999, Valinsky et al 1990, Wyre & Stolar 1977). Electrosurgery may be used to destroy the nail matrix after nail surgery procedures. Anecdotal evidence indicates there is less postoperative pain and a faster healing time with electrosurgery compared to some other methods such as phenolisation. One study reported a success rate of over 98% after 73 matrixectomy procedures were carried out using radio wave correction; there were no incidences of regrowth or postoperative discomfort (Hettinger et al 1991, Zuber 2002). Training and practice in the technique, as well as standardisation of treatment parameters, are thought to be important factors in achieving good results (Zuber 2002). Further controlled trials are needed to determine the long-term effectiveness of this procedure.

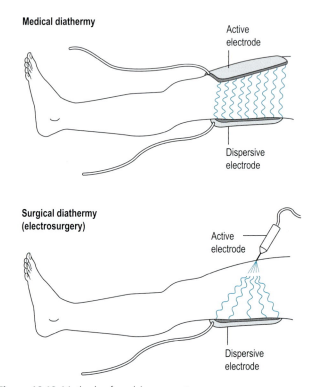

**Figure 16.10** Methods of applying current.

## Electrosurgical physics

An understanding of electrophysical principles is necessary in order for the practitioner to make safe and optimum use of electrosurgery.

The effect of applying electrical current to tissue is modified by changes to the:

- frequency
- current
- waveform
- shape and size of the electrode(s).

**Frequency.** The energy required to perform electrosurgery is provided by a high-frequency alternating current. High-frequency currents set up alternating electrical fields of electromagnetic waves that switch so rapidly that there is no time for the actual flow of electrons. A rapid 'to-and-fro motion of molecules is thus produced (Sebben 1988a). When in contact with body tissue, friction from the tissue's resistance to this motion results in the residual effect of the production of heat. The effect on the tissues will vary according to the frequency level. The use of frequencies below 500 kHz results in muscle contraction or electric shock, known as the faradic effect. As the frequency increases, this effect begins to disappear. Electrosurgery units vary in the frequency level at which they operate; the exact frequency obtainable is specific to each machine. To cut tissue, an optimum frequency level of 3.8 MHz has been recommended (Maness 1978). Electrosurgery units operating within this spectrum convert electrical current into controlled energy in the radiowave frequency (Brown 2000, Ellman International Inc 2007, Niamtu 2001). The term *radiosurgery* is often used for treatment using these wavelengths. Radiofrequency waveforms do not cause a faradic effect (Hettinger 1997). The chart shows a range of electrical frequencies and their respective uses (Fig 16.11).

**Current.** For most procedures, a low current at high voltage is passed to the patient through the electrodes. Altering the voltage or amperage will affect the amount and depth of heating. When current passes through tissue with a high resistance, such as muscle, a greater heating effect will result than when it is applied to tissue with a low resistance, such as bone (Bennett 1988). The heating effect also increases with the amount of time for which the current is applied.

**Waveform.** Electrosurgery units produce an oscillating wave known as a sine wave (Sebben 1989). *Pure* sine waves are described as a continuous, regular oscillation of electromagnetic energy (Sebben 1988b). The focused oscillations of a pure sine wave are used for tissue section or cutting. This waveform gives the least lateral heat and least tissue damage. A *damped* (also known as *rectified*) wave can be described as intermittent pulses of voltage that rapidly return to zero after each burst of activity. The intervals between each pulse can be varied to produce different degrees of damping. Slightly damped, or

blended, waves may be used for cutting with coagulation. Markedly damped waves are required for fulguration (spark gap or hyfrecation), desiccation and coagulation, in which more lateral heat is produced (Fig 16.12).

**Electrode selection.** Electrosurgery units often require two electrodes to complete the circuit. One emits the current (emitting electrode) and one disperses the current (dispersive electrode) (Sebben 1989). To destroy tissue, a small emitting electrode or probe is used to concentrate the heating effect. The smaller the area of the probe applied the greater the tissue damage. The dispersive electrode is placed in contact with the patient. It carries the same amount of current as the emitting electrode, and must therefore be relatively large to prevent unwanted tissue damage. It also offers a return pathway of least resistance should the equipment malfunction or the patient touch a conductive surface during the procedure. Electrosurgery units operating at the higher and radiowave frequencies do not require a dispersal plate. The use of an antenna is usually recommended for optimum effectiveness. This acts as an aerial and concentrates energy at the operating area. Contact of the antenna with the patient is not required as it is not a grounding plate, and there is no opportunity to shock or burn the patient (Niamtu 2001). There is no danger if the antenna plate is not used, but power settings may need to be increased (Hettinger 1997). The heating effect created at high frequencies occurs in the tissues only, so when it is in use the active electrode remains cold (Brown 1995).

## Equipment

Spark-gap generators were the first instruments to use high-frequency alternating currents. They produced a spark that burnt the surface of the tissue to produce the superficial charring known as hyfrecation.

Today a wide range of electrosurgical units is available. Many of them are small, portable units suited to small surgery use. Some machines are suitable for desiccation, fulguration and coagulation, but cannot be used to cut tissue. For those professionals who do not wish to use a cutting current, these lower power units may best serve their needs (Sebben 1988b). Electrosurgical units operating at radiowave frequencies are designed to perform a range of procedures and may be used to successfully cut, desiccate and coagulate tissue (Ellman International Inc 2007).

Active electrodes (probes) are usually supplied with the machine but they can also be purchased separately. Various shapes and sizes

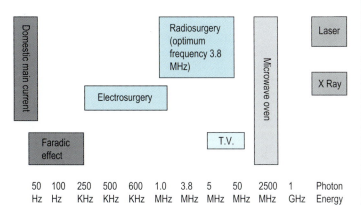

**Figure 16.11** Range and Uses of Electrical Frequencies.

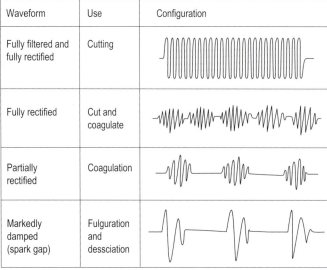

| Waveform | Use | Configuration |
|---|---|---|
| Fully filtered and fully rectified | Cutting | |
| Fully rectified | Cut and coagulate | |
| Partially rectified | Coagulation | |
| Markedly damped (spark gap) | Fulguration and desciation | |

**Figure 16.12** Waveforms.

**411**

are available, facilitating a range of procedures. For example: *needle* electrodes to make incisions, *loop* electrodes for excising tissue, *ball* electrodes for coagulation and desiccation, *rod* electrodes for fulguration and desiccation, and *matrixectomy* electrodes for desiccation of the nail matrix. Matrixectomy electrodes consist of a narrow flat plate, the upper side being insulated to prevent damage to the proximal nail fold (Brown 2000). Probes are available in disposable, sterile packs, or as reusable items that can be sterilised.

When a high-frequency current is passed through the electrode, the electrode remains sterile and thus should not become contaminated during use. (Brown 2000, Ellman International Inc 2007). However, Bennett and Kraffert (1990) have suggested that bacterial transfer could take place from one patient to another via the electrodes. Active electrodes should be either disposable or designed for re-use with standard sterilisation techniques such as autoclaving.

Operation of the unit may be either by a foot pedal or a button on the handpiece. Some handpieces can be treated with gas sterilisation. Alternatively, surgeons may employ single-use disposable coverings or gauze to maintain sterility of procedure (Broughton & Spencer 1987).

It is important to follow the manufacturer's advice with regard to the use of electrosurgical units, due to the number of different machines available and the variation in safety and operational requirements between them.

## Safety

When used correctly, electrosurgery is a safe procedure. The main dangers during use of an electrosurgical unit are from the rare occurrence of unintentional grounding, burns and the risk of explosion. Unintentional grounding can be avoided by good use of the dispersal electrode and the removal of metal objects from the work area. The patient's chair should not contain metal that could be easily touched during treatment. Work trolleys should have glass or plastic surfaces.

Burns may occur if the dispersal plate is poorly applied, the patient has metal implants or there is intense scar tissue between the plate and the leg. The danger is much less in podiatry, where anaesthesia is local and the patient is conscious. If a patient complains of heating anywhere in the body, treatment should be stopped until the source has been found and the problem solved.

Although emergency equipment should be available in case of accident, pressurised cylinders such as oxygen should not be kept in the room where electrosurgery is being carried out.

If the preoperative antiseptic contains alcohol the skin surface should be completely dry before applying the activated probe. Failure to do this will cause the residual alcohol on the skin to ignite, which may alarm the patient.

## Patient selection

With few exceptions, local infiltration or nerve blockade anaesthesia is required before treatment. Care must therefore be taken to ensure that patients are suitable for the administration of local anaesthetics. As a wound is created, desiccation of a corn or verruca is not recommended where healing is severely compromised. Electrosurgery should not be carried out if the patient has a metal implant between the lesion to be treated and the site of the dispersal plate. Where the manufacturer does not advocate the use of a dispersal plate, their advice should be sought before proceeding. Caution is advised when operating in very close proximity to bone tissue, due to its high conductivity (Ellman International Inc 2007). Consideration should be given to the potential risk of interference with pacemakers. Modern pacemakers are considered safe from the effects of electrosurgery, but advice should be sought from the patient's medical consultant before treatment is given.

## Procedures

Before undertaking electrosurgical procedures the technique has to be learned, and it is advisable that an individual using the technique for the first time undertakes training. It is also important to note that individual manufacturer's instructions may vary slightly and adaptations to the procedure should be made accordingly.

**Cutting**. To cut tissue, an undamped or mildly damped current with a very fine emitting electrode is used (Sebben 1989). Cutting current is a valuable tool for surgical procedures due to its speed, efficiency and lack of trauma to the surrounding tissues (Hettinger 1997).

While tissue section can be carried out with some lower power electrosurgery machines, most successful results will be achieved with a unit that provides the optimum cutting frequency of 3.8 MHz. Modern radiosurgery machines using a pure filtered waveform operating at this frequency can generate several different waveforms (Ellman International Inc 2007). To cut tissue, no pressure is required as cells are vaporised in the path of the radiowaves, causing them to split apart. Use of a wire or loop electrode to incise tissue therefore results in less trauma to surrounding tissues than does the use of a cold scalpel (Brown 2000).

In podiatry, loop or wire electrodes are a popular choice for removal of unwanted lesions such as verrucae, skin tags, cysts, benign growths, hypergranulation tissue or pyogenic granuloma. The operator can control the amount of tissue removed and, where bleeding is a problem, can modify the waveform to produce a small amount of lateral heat to coagulate small blood vessels whilst cutting.

Unlike desiccated or fulgurated tissue, lesions that have been removed using this procedure can be sent for histological analysis.

**Fulguration**. The word fulguration derives from the Latin 'fulgur', which means lightning. For electrofulguration, a high voltage damped waveform is used. If the electrode is activated whilst held just above the skin surface, a stream of sparks can be drawn from the electrode to the point of treatment. This produces a superficial charring of the tissues. Tissue damage is shallower than with desiccation, as the superficial carbonisation acts as a barrier insulating the tissue from deeper current penetration. The wound therefore tends to heal very quickly (Laughlin & Dudley 1992). The electrode should be precisely positioned to avoid an electrical 'arc' being diverted to adjacent tissue areas with higher conductivity or to metal instruments. The amount and depth of tissue destruction is dependent on current intensity, length of time of application, the density and the moisture content of tissue, and distance of the electrode from the operating area.

Fulguration is sometimes used for destruction of verrucae and is a useful method for removing shallow skin lesions. If a lesion is destroyed with fulguration, it cannot be examined histologically, unless a preliminary biopsy is taken.

**Desiccation**. The word desiccation is from the Latin 'desiccare', meaning to dry. An intermittent, damped waveform with a relatively high voltage and low current is used (Sebben 1989). Heating within the tissues causes the water in the cells to evaporate, leaving them shrunken, shrivelled and with nuclei condensed and elongated (Bennett 1988). Low power settings confine the damage to the upper layers of skin, and result in separation at the dermoepidermal junction (Hainer 1991a,b, Sebben 1988b, 1989). Desiccated tissue has a 'white cap' appearance. Scarring is usually absent or minimal, although higher power settings may result in some scarring due to damage to deeper tissues (Hainer 1991a,b, Sebben 1988b, 1989). The probe is held in contact with the skin, causing a radial spread of current. Electrodesiccation and fulguration may occur simultaneously to some extent, depending on the application. Use of some machines that employ a high voltage can result in superficial charring due to arcing, particularly around areas of high resistance as the current 'jumps' to tissue with a higher conductive capacity (Broughton & Spencer 1987).

It is advisable to keep the treatment area moistened with sterile saline solution. Most modern units are designed to enable electrodesiccation to take place without the problem of arcing.

Desiccation is an excellent treatment for the destruction of unwanted lesions such as chronic corns and verrucae. As with fulguration, once desiccated the lesion cannot be examined histologically unless a preliminary biopsy is performed.

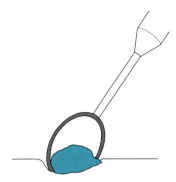

**Figure 16.13** Placement of loop electrode to cut/coagulate lesion (e.g. verruca).

---

## CASE STUDY 16.3 **MANAGEMENT OF CHRONIC HARD CORN**

A 43-year-old male taxi driver was referred to the advanced therapy clinic. He reported a 7-year history of recurrent pain associated with a hard corn in the ball of his left foot. The symptoms were most severe when he was standing, walking or driving his taxi cab. Regular scalpel enucleation of the corn at his local podiatry clinic afforded temporary relief of pain, but had failed to resolve the problem. He had received footcare advice. His footwear was satisfactory and he was wearing the recommended cushioning insole. The patient was keen to find a longer term solution to the problem.

On examination, a lesion consisting of callus overlying a central hard corn was present on the plantar surface of the left foot over the third metatarsophalangeal joint. The area was sensitive to firm pressure. There was no obvious functional or biomechanical abnormality. The patient was in good general health, and his medical history was unremarkable. He was not taking any medication.

The procedure for electrodesiccation was explained to the patient. He was given written information about the treatment and a postoperative advice sheet.

**PROCEDURE**

On the day of surgery, a tibial block was administered, using 2 ml mepivacaine hydrochloride. Whilst awaiting anaesthesia, overlying callus was reduced and any remaining corn tissue enucleated. Desiccation was carried out using a 2 mm ball probe. The section of desiccated tissue (approximately 7 mm × 5 mm × 4 mm) was removed. The wound was dressed and the patient was advised to rest the foot for 48 hours.

**3 DAYS POSTOPERATIVELY**

The patient admitted he had returned to work 2 days after treatment due to staff shortage. Despite the additional trauma to the wound, he had felt only mild postoperative discomfort. The wound was clean.

**4 WEEKS AFTER SURGERY**

A slight eschar had formed over the wound and this was debrided with a scalpel.

**6 WEEKS AFTER SURGERY**

The wound was fully healed. The patient stated that he could walk and drive without discomfort.

**REVIEW AT 6 MONTHS**

A thin layer of callus was present over the area that had been treated. This was asymptomatic. The patient was pain-free and he stated he was 'highly satisfied' with the electrodesiccation treatment.

---

**Coagulation.** The term coagulation derives from the Latin term 'coagulare', meaning to clot. It is achieved electrosurgically using a current relatively lower in voltage and higher in amperage than for desiccation. The intermittent, damped current and a larger emitting electrode produce less intense heat over a larger area (Sebben 1989). The mass temperature created in the tissue cells is sufficiently high to cause coagulation of cell protein.

Ball or flat probes are often used to coagulate small blood vessels and stop bleeding, with the electrode held in light contact with the area to be coagulated. The method is often used for haemostasis of small blood vessels during and after surgical procedures such as cutting or desiccation.

Very precise haemostasis may be obtained by using bipolar forceps. Each forcep blade is connected to the radiosurgical unit so that the current passes between the two blades. This may be useful in microsurgery to coagulate individual vessels.

### Electrosurgical treatment of verrucae

Verrucae can be removed by cutting with a loop electrode, or desiccated using the procedure described for desiccation of chronic corns (see below).

The use of high-frequency radiosurgery units is recommended for optimum cutting results. When excising a verruca using a loop electrode, a rapid, smooth, 'sweeping' movement with the loop can effectively peel off progressive layers of the epidermis. The operator can control the depth and area of treatment, and thus remove selected areas of diseased tissue (Fig 16.13). A ball probe and lower setting may then be used where haemostasis is required.

### Nail bed ablation

Excellent results have been reported using radiosurgery for ablation of the germinal nail matrix. The technique is similar to that used with phenolisation, except that the matrix is destroyed electrically (Brown 2000). The procedure is facilitated by using a specially designed matrixectomy electrode that is insulated on one side to prevent damage to the overlying eponychium. The tourniquet remains in place following partial or total nail avulsion. Using the setting recommended by the unit manufacturer, the probe is held lightly over the nail bed and activated for 2–4 seconds. The probe is moved and the process is repeated until all areas of the germinal epithelium have been treated. Normally bleeding is not a problem, due to the desiccating effect. Patient preparation, safety precautions and postoperative care are carried out as for other electrosurgical and nail surgery procedures (Fig 16.14).

### Suggested procedure for desiccation of heloma durum (hard corn)

A suggested procedure for electrodesiccation of a corn is set out below. Success in this technique depends on accurate treatment of the lesion. It is advisable that the individual using the technique for the first time undertakes training. Poor results may be due to the formation of excessive scar tissue through improper use of the machine, and to incomplete desiccation.

1. The procedure is explained to the patient and a written information sheet regarding postoperative management provided. Jewellery and rings, especially those near the operative site, should be removed. A local anaesthetic is administered.

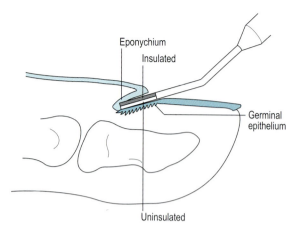

**Figure 16.14** Placement of the dorsally insulated matrixectomy electrode.

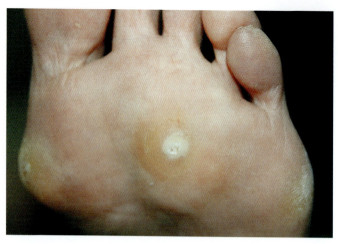

**Figure 16.16** After electrodesiccation is completed. Heloma durum showing the 'white-cap' effect.

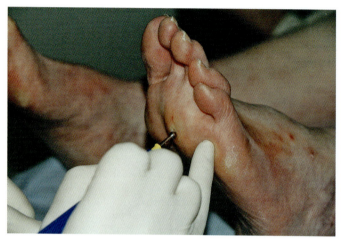

**Figure 16.15** A 4-mm probe held in contact with plantar heloma durum prior to electrodesiccation.

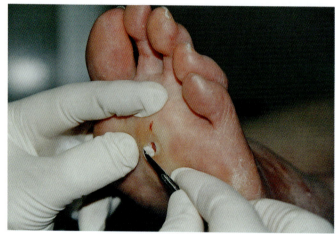

**Figure 16.17** Removal of desiccated tissue.

Local infiltration is generally adequate, but for plantar lesions a tibial blockade may be preferable. Overlying callus or corn is reduced with a scalpel.

2. A suitable probe is selected. For the dense nucleus of a small corn a 2-mm ball probe is appropriate. A larger probe is more suitable for peripheral callus or larger lesions. Probes may be changed during the procedure, but the machine should be switched off when doing so.

3. If a dispersal plate is recommended by the manufacturer, this is positioned carefully according to the instructions provided.

4. Set the electrosurgery unit to the minimum setting advised for this procedure by the manufacturer.

5. Swab the area to be treated with sterile saline; this is repeated throughout the procedure to allow maximum desiccation and to prevent superficial charring.

6. Place the ball electrode at the margin of the lesion and hold at 90°, just touching the skin. If pressure is exerted unnecessarily tissue damage may occur, and if skin contact is not maintained hyfrecation may take place, hindering penetration to deeper tissues (Fig 16.15).

7. Depress the foot or hand switch and release after approximately 2 seconds. A blanching of the tissues should occur. This indicates desiccation. If blanching has not occurred, reset to the next higher setting until blanching is seen. Blanching may take

some seconds to emerge, so do not readjust the setting until you are sure of the result. Once the blanching has been achieved, the process is repeated around the lesion periphery, with each area of blanching interconnecting, until a complete outer ring of white tissue is formed. Continue the process in decreasing circles, overlapping each circle until the whole lesion is desiccated. This will have produced a blanched area or 'white cap' effect (Fig 16.16).

8. Use the blunt edge of a scalpel to work around the periphery of the blanched area to loosen it – desiccation will have caused separation at the dermoepidermal junction. Using a pressing and lifting motion, carefully remove all the desiccated tissue to reveal the underlying dermis (Fig 16.17).

9. Using a lower setting and a ball probe, perform haemostasis as required.

## INFLAMMATORY CONDITIONS

### Perniosis (erythema pernio, chilblains)

Chilblains represent one of the conditions in which intervention to control the inflammatory process is necessary in order to prevent additional tissue damage. Theoretically, chilblains can be divided into four stages, but the initial stage, the *cyanotic* stage, often passes unnoticed. The hyperaemic stage is noticeable on examination and is symptomatic. This is followed by the *congestive* stage, after which the lesion may resolve or pass to the *ulcerative* or broken chilblain stage. In the *hyperaemic* stage the areas affected are variously described as being red, hot, burning, itchy or painful. At this stage the patient tends to scratch the area and cause a break in the skin. The application of cold compresses is essential to control the symptoms of this stage, and to reduce the volume of tissue fluid and blood in the area and diminish the possibility of broken chilblains. Cool evaporating dressings such as gauze dressings saturated with witch hazel are invaluable. At the congestive stage the principle of treatment is to stimulate the local circulation with rubefacients, vasodilator creams or the application of heat. Care must be taken that the peripheral circulation is adequate to cope with the effect of the application of any of the above. Any counterirritants or heat applied locally will cause an increase in cellular metabolism, with a resultant increase in waste products. Cells require an adequate blood supply to deliver oxygen to meet the increased demands of the cells and an adequate drainage system to remove the waste products. The action of a mild rubefacient with gentle massage to the area can be used to stimulate locally when the circulation is impaired, which is the case in many older patients. If appropriate, heat can be applied via the use of an infrared heat lamp, wax baths or a warm footbath. Numerous proprietary rubefacients and vasodilators are available.

In elderly patients the risk of tissue breakdown is increased. The most common site for broken chilblains is any area receiving excessive pressure or friction. The dorsum or apices of the digits are particularly at risk, as is the medial aspect of the first metatarsal joint in association with hallux abducto valgus, and the lateral aspect of a prominent fifth metatarsal head. The objective when this stage is reached is to encourage healing and prevent the entry and spread of infection. In the majority of cases the site is tender and the surrounding tissues cyanotic due to a generally impaired blood supply. Where the area has ulcerated in a younger healthy individual, due usually to trauma, the surrounding tissues exhibit the signs of an acute inflammation. Healing is achieved by removal of pressure from the area, which should include deflective padding and, if necessary, advice on footwear. Infection is prevented by the application of a topical antiseptic or interactive dressing. Patients who have circulatory or sensation impairment should be monitored very closely and, if deemed necessary, referred to their general practitioner for antibiotic therapy.

Patients who are subject to chilblains should be advised about preventive measures. These should not be limited to the foot but should include advice on keeping the legs warm with the use of trousers, and extra thick tights in ladies and the use of 'long johns' in men.

If prolonged exposure to cold is unavoidable, the feet should be warmed slowly. Warm-lined footwear and thick woollen socks (or two pairs of fine socks) should be worn, provided they are not constricting by tightening the shoes and causing further local areas of ischaemia.

Thermal insoles can be manufactured and inserted within the footwear to retain heat. If the footwear or hosiery becomes wet it should be changed as soon as possible, because damp cold appears to precipitate the formation of chilblains more readily than dry cold conditions. The circulation can be stimulated by means of rubbing in a cream or ointment specially formulated for the treatment of chilblains, many of which contain an antipruritic agent. Some studies have shown the use of systemic therapy such as nifedipine to be of advantage in the treatment of chilblains, and this may prove of benefit to the patient with severe chilling and the complications of ulceration. However, it should be used only if prescribed by a general medical practitioner.

## Ulceration

The management of established ulceration is discussed fully in Chapter 10.

## TREATMENT OF DISORDERS OF THE SWEAT GLANDS

## Hyperhidrosis

A hyperhidrotic skin loses its natural elasticity and cannot withstand tensile and shearing stresses, resulting in fissures and blisters. Furthermore, it is an ideal substrate for fungal and bacterial infections to become established and is a source of embarrassment to the patient.

In the management of hyperhidrosis it is important to appraise all footwear worn by the patient and also the demands of their occupation. Instances exist where a patient's sensitivity to sweating and foot odour has led to them enclosing their feet in occlusive footwear when the reverse approach was indicated. Occupational factors are less easily controlled, but a willing approach by the patient can often improve the condition, in particular patient compliance with regard to the use of footwear (the avoidance of moisture-retaining materials) and hosiery (wool or cotton) that will absorb the sweat and prevent it lying on the skin. Various treatment strategies can be adopted for general hyperhidrosis of the feet depending on the severity of the condition. These can range from the application of dusting powders, to swabbing with an astringent lotion, to the administration of footbaths containing an astringent medicament. For general, more severe hyperhidrosis a small number of crystals of potassium permanganate dissolved in a footbath is an effective, cheap and easily obtained treatment. Care should be taken not to make the solution too strong or a brown discoloration of the skin will result, and it may even induce skin irritation (Martindale 1999). If the hyperhidrosis is severe, daily footbaths with tepid water, a few crystals (usually two or three, but no more than four) of potassium permanganate (enough to turn the water pale pink) for 15 minutes at a time over a period of a few weeks should result in a dramatic reduction in sweat symptoms. When maceration has ceased, the footbaths should be reduced to twice weekly. Footbaths containing 3% formalin may also be used, but care must be taken to avoid overuse due to the higher incidence of allergic reactions with this treatment (Martindale 1999). In less severe cases, contrast footbaths in conjunction with lotions and powders are effective.

Spirit-based astringent agents (e.g. 3% salicylic acid) may be applied interdigitally if there is excessive maceration, and the application of dusting powders is advantageous, particularly those that contain an antifungal agent. Cases of salicylate poisoning have been reported following excessive application of salicylic acid compounds, and long-term application of these substances on the skin should be avoided (Martindale 1999). Interdigital fissuring should be treated rigorously with astringent antiseptics. There are many astringent, antiseptic and antifungal agents available commercially, including insoles that are absorbent and deodorising. The patient should be advised to dispense with shoes and socks whenever possible, or to wear sandals, to pay particular attention to foot hygiene, to change hosiery daily and to alternate footwear.

This condition is rarely a short-term problem, and it cannot be permanently cured by any of the above treatments. However, patient compliance with management is easily achieved in this condition because of the discomfort. If the excessive sweating is not isolated to the foot but is more generalised, help should be sought from a medical practitioner. It may be that the condition cannot be treated, but underlying factors such as stress and diet may be controlled.

# Anhidrosis

Many instances of anhidrosis result from poor peripheral blood supply in the elderly or in diabetic patients with autonomic neuropathy. Where this is the cause, little more can be done than to apply emollients regularly, preferably daily after washing. The choice of emollient matters little, as the purpose is to prevent moisture loss from the skin. Hydrous lanolin, E45 cream, white soft paraffin, urea-based preparations or proprietary medicaments incorporating lanolin are suitable. It is useful to remember that long-term use of lanolin can cause skin sensitisation reactions (Martindale 1999).

The main complication of anhidrosis is the formation of fissures due to the reduction of epidermal elasticity and applied tensile stress. These can become a considerable problem, causing much pain and disability, as well as being a site for the entry of infection. Fissuring is most commonly found on the borders of the heel, and is associated with callus formation.

Treatment consists of careful reduction of the callus at the edges of the fissures, and treatment with an antiseptic cream and an occlusive dressing for a few days. If the anhidrosis is severe, and is associated with thickening of the stratum corneum, a thick layer of emollient occluded and left in situ overnight is a suitable treatment. If fissures are open and infected, antiseptic emollient dressings are indicated until the lesion heals, followed by the regular application of emollients.

# TREATMENT OF FUNGAL INFECTIONS

Fungal infection is the most common type of infection seen by the podiatrist and is usually caused by *anthropophilic* (man to man) fungi (see also fungal infections in Ch. 3). The source of the dermatophytes can also be *zoophilic* (animal to man) or *geophilic* (soil to man). The superficial fungal infections are most commonly caused by dermatophytes or ringworm infections and superficial candidosis. The names given to fungal infections are variable, and include ringworm, tinea and dermatophytosis. Most dermatophyte infections that involve skin are confined to the stratum corneum, and rarely extend beyond the stratum granulosum unless there is hair follicle involvement. When hair follicles are involved, the infection is present in the dermis and there is destruction of the hair follicle. In the dermis the fungi are surrounded by phagocytes or giant cells. Nail involvement with the superficial mycoses affects the epidermal tissue under the nail plate and causes modification of the epidermal cells and nail dystrophy. The dermatophytes include *Trichophyton*, *Epidermophyton* and *Microsporum*. *Candida albicans* is a normal inhabitant of the mouth, intestine and vaginal mucosa but established infections may involve skin or nails of the feet. Interdigital infections with *Candida* are more commonly seen in warmer countries or in warmer weather, but onychomycosis due to *Candida* is more commonly seen in colder climates. Most *Candida* infections are endogenous, but under certain circumstances the disease is transmitted from person to person.

The healthy adult has a high level of immunity to fungal infections. This natural resistance is of a non-specific type and depends on genetic factors, age, nutrition and hormone balance. Another determinant is the mechanical barrier of intact skin surface secretions (fungicidal fatty acids in sweat and in sebaceous material). If the skin is degraded in any way, thin and devitalised, hyperhidrotic, fissured, blistered or abraded, then the likelihood of infection becoming established is enhanced. The underlying cause(s) should be addressed and the fungal infection treated. Patients who have diabetes appear to be particularly prone to fungal infection of the feet, particularly interdigitally. Patients on long-term antibiotic therapy are susceptible to fungal infections due to the reduction in the normal skin commensals that compete with the fungi for adherence sites. Immunosuppression through illness, drugs or a congenital condition will also predispose to an increased incidence of infection, either with the dermatophytes or *Candida*.

# Tinea pedis

Tinea pedis is most commonly found in adults, being relatively uncommon in children. The common causative organisms in the UK, in order of frequency, are: *Trichophyton rubrum*, *Trichophyton interdigitale*, *Epidermophyton floccosum*, Microsporum *canis* (cat and dog ringworm), *Trichophyton verrucosum* and *Trichophyton mentagrophytes*. Less frequently the following may be isolated: *Trichophyton tonsurans*, *Trichophyton erinacei* and *Microsporum gypseum*. *Scopulariopsis brevicaulis* can cause onychomycosis in nails that are already affected by a pathological process such as onychauxis or onychogryphosis, and is most commonly found in the first toenail. Other fungi that can be isolated from dystrophic nails are *Aspergillus*, *Fusarium* and *Pyrenochaeta* species. *Candida albicans* can affect skin and nail, particularly at the base of the nail plate under the eponychium, where it is very difficult to eradicate due to its inaccessibility. Interdigitally, *Candida* infections are frequently secondary to dermatophyte infections with associated fissuring. A severe *Candida* infection – *chronic mucocutaneous candidosis* – is a relatively uncommon chronic condition that presents in childhood and affects the mouth, skin and nail. In the foot it is associated with hyperkeratotic areas and dystrophic nails.

The only positive means by which the infecting organism can be identified is by laboratory diagnosis. Superficial mycoses will be identified by direct microscopy and culture. In skin mycosis the skin scrapings should be taken from the active margin of the skin affected, and if vesicles are present the active fungal cells will be contained in the roof of the blister, which should be removed completely for analysis. Prior to removal of scrapings for mycological examination the skin should be swabbed with alcohol to remove any medication that may have been applied. Scrapings from nails should be from the under surface and as far proximally as possible. Fungi in the distal portion of the nail may not be viable if the infection is active proximally, and scrapings taken from that area frequently produce negative results on culture.

Infection of the host by the fungi is due to penetration of keratinised cells. Fungi are able to enter the keratinised cells by producing enzymes that can degrade or split the keratin, and the fungal hyphae are then able to penetrate between the keratinocytes. Consideration of the epidemiological factors involved in dermatophyte infections is relevant when considering the treatment of tinea pedis. The incidence rises in winter with the wearing of occlusive footwear. The main areas where conditions are suitable for transmission of infection are swimming pools, communal changing areas such as sports halls and schools, industrial shower rooms used by employees after work (e.g. miners or servicemen), or any area where there are liable to be infected skin squames on floors. Dermatophytes can survive for months if not years in desquamated skin cells. If the infection is zoophilic and the infected human has a cat or dog, the infected material is likely to be from the home and the spread can occur directly from the pet or from chairs, floors or floor coverings. An atypical mycosis may have been acquired by a patient who has travelled abroad, particularly outside Europe. This should always be taken into account if an unusual clinical picture is seen.

General issues regarding treatment should be to identify the probable source, if possible, and to provide advice on avoidance, foot hygiene and type of footwear. Advice should be given to eliminate barefoot contact with all surfaces that are liable to be contaminated. Personal foot hygiene should be of the highest standard, the feet should be meticulously dried, and the shared use of towels or footwear should be avoided. The type of footwear worn by the patient should be considered and, if occlusive footwear cannot be entirely avoided because of his or her occupation, the wearing of open sandals should be advised whenever possible to allow free circulation of air. Hosiery should be changed daily, and shoes should be regarded as a potential source of reinfection and treated with a fumigating agent (e.g. 10% formalin solution). If formalin is used, care must be taken to aerate the shoes prior to use to avoid irritation caused by the agent. Disinfection of shoes is easily achieved by placing formalin in a shallow container, such as a tin lid, inside the shoe, placing the shoes inside a plastic bag and leaving for 24 hours. Provided the ambient temperature is about 15°C, the inside of the shoe will be exposed to a high concentration of formalin. The shoes should be exposed to the air for some hours after such treatment to minimise the risk of hypersensitivity reactions (Martindale 1999).

## Clinical features of tinea pedis

The clinical picture varies with the severity, site and infecting organism. In its mildest form tinea pedis may be confused with erythrasma and the symptoms negligible. In the more severe form there is associated inflammation, maceration, fissuring, bleeding, blistering and the possibility of a superimposed bacterial infection. Regardless of severity, similar treatment strategies should be adopted to prevent spread of the fungal infection.

The interdigital areas are most commonly affected in the first instance, particularly the third and fourth web space. The appearance can vary from simple scaling of the skin with minimal itching, to macerated raw areas with spread of the infection to the undersurface of the toes or to the dorsum of the foot with blistering and inflammation. There may well be a superimposed bacterial infection with Gram-negative bacteria, commonly of the *Pseudomonas* type. Blistering is usually associated with *Trichophyton interdigitale*.

The sole of the foot in the area of the medial longitudinal arch may be affected. The skin in this area tends to be dry, flaky and inflamed, with associated blistering. Differential diagnosis is with pustular psoriasis and eczema. Tinea pedis may spread to the whole of the sole and encroach on the medial and lateral borders of the foot and the dorsum of the toes. In this instance it is described as a moccasin-type fungal infection due to this typical distribution. The common infecting organism in this type of dry, scaly infection is *Trichophyton rubrum* or *Epidermophyton floccosum*.

Fungal infections associated with hyperkeratosis are commonly found in the heel area, which appears dry, with fissuring and surrounding inflammation. Treatment of this area involves reduction of keratin, either by scalpel and/or with a keratolytic agent, and the application of a fungicidal preparation.

Fungal infections can spread to any area of the skin or to the nails. It is essential that treatment is effective to prevent spread and reinfection. Treatment should be continued for several months after the clinical signs and symptoms have subsided in an effort to prevent recurrence. The use of fungicidal powders as a prophylactic measure should be continued indefinitely in patients who are susceptible to infection.

## Treatment

Fungicidal preparations are dispensed in various forms. They can be applied topically as creams, ointments, lotions, aerosol sprays and powders. Fungicides are effective if the infection is not widespread or involves nails. The time taken to clear the infection is normally about 4 weeks, but the relapse rate is high. This is not surprising if the source of infection has not been identified and eliminated.

A wide variety of antifungal preparations are available without prescription. The choice of base depends on the state of the skin. Ointments are normally avoided on moist surfaces because of their occlusive property. Lotions are less occlusive and are indicated inter-

digitally, on pustular areas and over large areas. Dusting powders must be used in conjunction with either an ointment or a lotion when a fungal infection is present but may be used alone as a prophylactic measure when infection has cleared. Powders may also be used inside footwear and hosiery. All of the above should be applied sparingly to the affected areas two or three times daily, with thorough washing between applications.

In some instances other actions are required in addition to the application of a fungicide. If inflammation is present, a preparation containing hydrocortisone may be required, and this is useful in the treatment of eczematous areas which are secondarily infected with fungi. Preparations of this type should be used for a few days only, until the inflammation has subsided, and then a routine fungicidal preparation applied. They should be used with care in children and in pregnancy. Overdosage in topically applied steroid preparations can occur if used long term over large areas. If a mild bacterial infection is present the antifungal agent should be combined with a bactericidal agent, even though some fungicidal agents are effective on some Gram-positive and Gram-negative bacteria. Alternatively, if the bacterial infection is extensive or severe it should be cleared with antiseptic preparations, or antibiotic therapy if necessary, before commencing treatment with a fungicidal preparation. Keratolytic agents may also be combined with a fungicidal preparation for areas with associated hyperkeratosis.

Some preparations exert a fungistatic/fungicidal action by a variety of mechanisms. Some agents used in the treatment of superficial mycoses may have little or no direct action on the fungi at the concentrations employed and their beneficial actions are not related to their direct action on fungi. For example keratolytics reduce the infection by causing desquamation of the infected keratinised cells.

Antiseptic antifungal preparations tend to have a weak action on both types of infection, and they are often messy to apply and can stain the skin. Resorcinol is both bactericidal and fungicidal and also has mild keratolytic properties, but it should not be applied to large areas of the body, used in high concentrations, or used for long periods as it can be absorbed through the skin (Martindale 1999). It is usually applied as a 1–10% concentration in an ointment, cream or lotion. Anaflex cream, which contains 10% polynoxylan, is reputed to have an antifungal action. It is an ideal medicament to use initially when there is a coexistent bacterial infection, before changing to a medicament with a more definitive antifungal action.

Keratolytic preparations to assist in removing the stratum corneum used to be employed but their use has now been discontinued.

The practitioner and patient have a wide choice of specific antifungal preparations for topical therapy. The following are some of the most commonly used preparations.

### Undecenoic acid

This drug is primarily fungistatic, although fungicidal activity may be observed with long exposure to high concentrations of the agent. It is effective against the common pathogens in superficial mycoses of the feet. Concentrations as high as 10% may be applied to the skin. Preparations are not usually irritating and sensitisation to them is uncommon. It is beneficial in retarding fungal growth in tinea pedis but the infection frequently persists despite extensive treatment with preparations of the acid and zinc salts. At best the clinical cure rate is 50%, which is much lower than the rate achieved with tolnaftate and the imidazoles. Preparations that contain undecenoic acid are Monphytol, Mycota, Phytocil and Tineafax.

### Tolnaftate

This is effective in the treatment of cutaneous mycosis caused by a wide range of the Trichophyton species, *Epidermophyton floccosum* and several of the *Microsporum* species. It is ineffective against *Candida*, but less so in the presence of hyperkeratotic lesions. It occasionally causes skin irritation (Martindale 1999). In tinea pedis the cure rate is about 80%. It is available as Tinaderm and Timoped.

### The imidazoles

These have a broad-spectrum antifungal activity and are effective, topically, against nearly all the fungi of clinical interest in podiatry. They are also effective against some bacteria and protozoa. Acquired resistance to imidazoles rarely occurs, and has been seen only with *Candida albicans*. The imidazoles are active at the cell-wall level of fungi. They inhibit the incorporation of acetate into ergosterol (which is important for the integrity and function of the fungal cell membrane). This causes leakage of cellular contents, and the uptake of essential nutrients is impaired. This explains their selectivity for fungi and the low toxicity to human cells. They are more effective than the undecenoates and tolnaftate in treating superficial skin mycoses. *Candida* fungal infections may also be treated by topical application of the broad-spectrum antifungal preparations 1% clotrimazole (available as Canesten), 1% econazole (available as Ecostatin and Pevaryl) and 2% miconazole (available as Daktarin and Dermonistat).

Any of the above drugs that contain hydrocortisone or nystatin are available only on prescription. Examples of these are Tinaderm M (tolnaftate), Quinoderm cream with 1% hydrocortisone (benzoyl peroxide and potassium hydroxyquinoline sulfate), Daktacort (miconazole) and Econacort (econazole). Others in the azole group that are available as topical therapy, but are prescription-only medicines, include Exelderm (sulconazole) and Nizoral (ketoconazole).

The most popular topical fungicidal agent to date is terbinafine (Lamasil). This is an allylamine antifungal preparation that blocks ergosterol formation in the cell membrane through inhibition of squalene epoxidase. It is effective against the dermatophytes and *Candida*. It is also available as an oral preparation and, in this form, is usually only taken for about 2 weeks to eradicate skin infections. The other drugs most commonly used systemically are fluconazole and itraconazole, and the azoles, which block ergosterol formation in the cell membrane and produce good results with eradication of the fungus from nails after only 3 months of treatment. Of these three, fluconazole is the least effective in the treatment of nails and terbinafine the most cost effective (Arca et al 2002). Griseofulvin, which is incorporated into keratin and blocks the intracellular microtubules, has a low (40%) success rate, even after 12 months of therapy. Because of this and its systemic side-effects, it is now rarely used.

### Tea tree oil

Tea tree oil (oil from the plant *Melaleuca alternifolia*) has become more commonly used in podiatry for the treatment of a number of conditions. It is considered to have an antifungal action, which may make it useful in the topical treatment of fungal infections. There are some issues to be resolved in the determination of the level at which it is antifungal and how this could affect the levels at which it sensitises human skin (Benger et al 2004).

## Tinea unguium (onychomycosis)

### Clinical features of tinea unguium

Fungal infection of the nails occurs in 2–5% of the population (Arca et al 2002). In dermatophyte infections of the nail, the clinical appearance is variable depending on the stage of infection. Initially, only the distal or lateral edges of the nail will be affected, and a white discoloration spreading proximally with some onycholysis will be seen. When the disease is established, the nail will be thickened and crumbly, with a yellowish discoloration. Eventually, the whole nail plate may be involved. Onychomycosis frequently coexists with skin

infection, often results from spread from the skin, and represents 30% of all mycotic infections of the skin (Goodfield et al 1992). A vigilant practitioner will be alert to the early signs of infection, and early treatment rate with topical applications of a fungicide will lead to a higher cure. Differential diagnosis is with psoriatic nails, onychauxis and onychogryphosis. The commonest cause of onychomycosis is *Trichophyton rubrum* and occasionally the cause is *Trichophyton interdigitale*. There are other dermatophytes of the *Trichophyton* and *Microsporum* genera that normally cause scalp infections but which may infect the nails and cause an atypical appearance of pitting, ridging and splitting of the nail plate. *Scopulariopsis brevicaulis* also causes a form of onychomycosis, which usually affects the first toenail. The nail has a brownish appearance, and is not crumbly. It infects nails that have previously been traumatised (on rare occasions it can affect the interdigital spaces). Other fungi that may affect dystrophic nails are *Aspergillus*, *Fusarium* and *Pyrenochaeta*.

Nail infections are very difficult to eradicate with topical applications of fungicidal preparations because the infection initially affects the nail on the undersurface and the nail bed is also infected (see Ch. 2). The nail itself acts as a barrier to the absorption of any cream or lotion, and even when the nail is thinned down as far as possible to facilitate this process treatment is still extremely protracted. Creams or lotions should be applied daily and are more effective if the nail plate is occluded because this enhances penetration of the medicament. However, this leads to further problems with maceration of the surrounding tissues. Patient compliance often fails due to the time taken to eradicate the infection, which may be 12–18 months, if ever. The success rate is extremely low with this method of treatment.

Alternatively, the nail plate may be avulsed with or without phenolisation of the matrix. If the latter method is used the nail bed must be treated with a fungicidal cream to eliminate the infection from this area or from any modified nail tissue adhering to the nail bed. This must be achieved prior to regrowth of the nail. During the regrowth period the podiatrist must remove modified callus from the nail bed to ensure that infection is totally eradicated. This is a more effective, although more radical, form of treatment than topical preparations only, and is suitable if only one or two nails are affected. When the use of local analgesia is contraindicated, medical avulsion may be attempted with the use of 40% urea cream, and thereafter topical antifungal preparations applied as described above. Although this procedure is painless, success in avulsion is not guaranteed. The surrounding tissues must be protected from the urea cream by the application of an occlusive dressing such as Tegaderm or Opsite, which is also applied over the cream to contain it, followed by the application of a tubular gauze dressing. The medicament should be left in situ for 7 days, and frequently a further application is necessary to achieve complete avulsion.

Systemic treatment of onychomycosis is now probably the treatment of choice in adults. Any of the creams or lotions mentioned above for the treatment of tinea pedis may be used in the treatment of onychomycosis.

In addition, there are preparations that are specifically for nail infections, such as borotannic complex. This may be used in conjunction with salicylic acid, methyl salicylate and acetic acid. The method of action of borotannic complex is that, on application to the nail, the solvents within the complex evaporate at body temperature, leaving a clear film of the active agent over the infected area. Perspiration will dissolve the active complex, which then ionises to produce a local area of low pH (approximately 2.0), which is fungicidal. Borotannic complex is available in a clear, straw-coloured paint as Phytex and Onychocil. With both these preparations the manufacturers do not recommend occlusive dressings. Another drug, amorolfine, differs chemically from other antifungals and affects most superficial fungi. It is available as Loceryl, which is a lacquer that is painted over the affected nail plate. Tioconazole is available in solution for use in onychomycosis. It is applied topically to the infected nail. It also contains an undecenoic acid base. The diffusion of tioconazole into human nail tissue is facilitated by long-chain fatty acids and alcohols. Because of the undecenoic acid present in the solution, tioconazole penetrates the nail plate extensively. Unfortunately, success rates are disappointing.

## Candidosis

*Candida* infections can affect both skin and nail (see Chs 2 and 3). The most common sites in the foot to be affected are the interdigital spaces and the nail. In appearance the web spaces are extremely macerated with open fissures, and have a distinctive yeasty odour. The infection may be secondary to a dermatophyte infection, but in contrast to the dermatophyte infections it is unlikely to spread. Paronychia as a result of a *Candida* infection is usually chronic in nature and is caused by *C. albicans* or *C. parapsilosis*. The nail folds and surrounding tissues are grossly inflamed and painful. The affected border of the nail will exhibit onycholysis and there will be a discharge of pus. Staphylococcal and Gram-negative infections may coexist; therefore, bacteriological identification should also be sought. The nail plate itself may become infected in association with paronychia. The nail plate will not become thickened, but onycholysis and destruction of the distal end of the nail plate may result. This condition is more common when Raynaud's disease, chronic chilblains or Cushing's syndrome are present. It is unusual to find associated skin symptoms elsewhere on the foot.

Most of the superficial *Candida* infections respond to topical applications of the azoles, terbinafine or Nystatin. For paronychia the treatment should be in solution form to enable it to run into the nail folds, and treatment should be continued for 3–4 months. Oral therapy with terbinafine, itraconazole or ketoconazole is necessary when the nail plate is involved.

## PHYSICAL THERAPY

Physical therapy can be defined as the treatment of disease or injury by physical means such as light, heat, cold water, electricity, massage and exercise (*Gould Medical Dictionary*, 4th edn).

Physical therapy can be used effectively, in conjunction with padding, tension strapping and an orthotic device, as a management strategy in podiatric practice without the use of pharmacological preparations or invasive treatments. Conditions such as plantar fasciitis associated with an overpronated foot can benefit greatly from a treatment regimen that involves both ultrasound therapy and padding in the short term and orthoses in the longer term (see Ch. 17).

Assessment of the patient prior to the commencement of any treatment regimen is essential (see Ch. 1) and the findings of the assessment will influence the choice and method of treatment.

Factors that require consideration include the condition requiring treatment, as this will determine whether heat or cold should be used and its method of application. The vascular status of the lower limb should also be considered, as certain treatment methods are contraindicated if the patient has an impaired arterial supply. The condition of the skin should be assessed, as thin fine skin will not tolerate extremes of temperature. Underlying medical problems such as diabetes, or the existence of a pacemaker, will also influence the method of treatment chosen. The availability of the patient and the ability of the patient to understand the nature of the treatment will determine the regimen to be undertaken. The age of the patient will also determine the use of certain treatment modalities.

## Heat and cold

Heat and cold have been used as a method for the treatment of trauma since 400 BC. The local physiological effects of heat and cold help many of the adverse local pathological changes that occur as a result of the tissue damage. Subsequently, the cardinal signs and symptoms of inflammation (rubor, calor, dolor and tumour) may be reduced, healing assisted and rehabilitation time improved.

## Heat

Heat may be applied to the skin by:

- *conduction* – heat is transmitted between objects of different temperatures that are in contact with each other. For example, a hot pack applied to an area of skin will induce a rise in the temperature of the cooler skin surface, and vice versa for an ice pack.
- *radiation* – an object when heated emits infrared rays (and possibly also visible and ultraviolet rays), which travel away from their source of production until they encounter a material that absorbs them without heating the intervening medium. For example, dry heat in the form of infrared lamps.

### Physiological effects

There are mainly three different specific physiological actions of heat on the tissues, and many other indirect effects.

- *Expansion* – this is the result of kinetic energy producing greater movement of the molecules within a substance so they then move further apart and expand the material.
- *Acceleration of chemical action* – Van't Hoff's law (Kitchen 2002) states that any chemical reactions involved in metabolic activity are increased by a rise in temperature . The converse is also true, that cooling slows the rate of reaction.
- *Reduced viscosity of fluids* – the molecules in viscous fluids are strongly attracted to one another. Heating increases the kinetic movement of these molecules and reduces their cohesive attraction – this makes the fluid less viscous. Consequently, there will be a local and remote increased blood flow due to temperature rise, stimulation of the neural receptors in the skin or tissues and an increase in metabolic activity. The application of external heat to restricted body areas produces many changes in the tissues by local, general or remote effects.

The parameters that determine the extent of physiological response to heat, include:

- site of area exposed
- intensity of radiation
- relative depths of absorption of specific radiation
- integrity of cardiovascular and nervous systems
- structure of skin and subcutaneous tissues
- age of the patient
- functioning of neural, hormonal and chemical control of blood vessels
- functioning of the patient's thermoregulatory centre
- thermal conductivity, density and specific heat of living skin and tissue
- pathophysiology of the area to be treated
- temperature variation
- rate of rise or fall of temperature
- duration of tissue temperature elevation or reduction.

As a result of the application of heat and the subsequent temperature increase in the tissues there will be specific changes in certain organs. The local effects of heat on the skin will lead to vasodilatation of the blood vessels at temperatures up to 42°C (blood flow increasing by four to five times that of resting level). If the heating is prolonged for more than 30 minutes the blood flow reaches a plateau and then declines.

There will also be an increase in tissue metabolism. The increase in metabolism is greatest in the region where most heat is absorbed, which is in the superficial tissues. As a result of this increased metabolism there is an increased demand for oxygen and nutrients. There will also be an increased output of metabolites and waste products. Conversely, the metabolism decreases with a drop in temperature. When heat is used as a method of treatment it must be remembered that heating of tissues above 45°C causes irreversible damage of tissue proteins and death of tissues.

## Increased blood supply

Heat has a direct effect on the blood vessels, causing vasodilatation, particularly in the superficial tissues where the heating is greatest. This has a particular benefit in the treatment of chronic inflammatory conditions. Heat has a direct effect on the smooth muscles of the arterioles and venules, causing them to dilate. Stimulation of superficial nerve endings can also cause a reflex dilatation of the arterioles, with a resultant increased flow of blood through the area. There will also be increased capillary membrane permeability, escape of plasma proteins into tissue spaces and a change in both hydrostatic and osmotic pressures. As a result of the increased permeability of the vessels there will be cell migration into tissue spaces, thereby increasing the number of phagocytic cells able to counteract tissue damage.

The application of heat stimulates lymphatic drainage, leading to reduction in swelling and removal of waste products. Superficial vasodilatation causes erythema of the skin, which appears as soon as the area becomes warm and begins to fade soon after the exposure to the heat finishes. Erythema resulting from exposure to ultraviolet irradiation takes longer to appear and can persist. Note that, while mild heat can aid removal of unresolved exudate, inflammatory products and oedema, vigorous heating will damage the tissues and produce further inflammatory reaction.

Heat also has physiological effects on other tissues. At normal tissue temperatures collagen primarily exhibits elastic properties and only minimal viscous flow, but when heated to 39–44°C the viscous flow becomes more dominant and tension relaxes markedly. This leads to a residual elongation of these tissues. Joint stiffness is often associated with changes in the viscoelastic properties of joints. Heat can reduce joint stiffness, while cold increases the stiffness of joints. Apart from stimulating the tissues, heat produces definite sedative effects on sensory nerve endings. Cold reduces nerve conduction, and thus relieves pain.

A skin temperature of about 45°C is critical for evoking pain and reflex responses. It is also critical for producing cutaneous burns. Pain is related to skin temperatures only, whereas tissue damage is related to both skin temperature and the duration of the hyperthermic episode, which starts the chemical reactions towards the production of burns.

## Generalised effects of heating

When an area of the body is exposed to more than a minimal amount of heat or cold the effects do not remain localised. Vasodilatation from heat spreads to adjacent areas. The remote effects of heat occur as a result of stimulation of the body's heat-regulating centre in the hypothalamus. There is increased sweat production due to an increase in the activity of the sweat glands throughout the body. When generalised sweating occurs there is increased elimination of waste products. The application of heat will also speed up the clotting time of blood. Heat may be applied to a localised area of damage to help reduce the inflammatory reaction of the tissues. It is indicated in cases of acute and subacute inflammation; inflammation associated with sepsis; acute muscle spasm, and chronic traumatic inflammatory conditions such as foot strain, osteoarthritis of the metatarsophalangeal joints and plantar fasciitis.

To maximise the effectiveness of the treatment in the aforementioned situations, appropriate short-term padding and strapping (see later in this chapter) should be used, followed by the fitting of an orthosis and, where appropriate, footwear advice (see Chs 17 and 18). It is important to remember that, when choosing heat as a method of treatment, attention should be paid to dosage and technique.

## Heat therapy

### Infrared radiation

Infrared radiation forms part of the electromagnetic spectrum. Its wavelength is longer than that of visible light, and thus it cannot be seen. Artificial infrared radiation is generally produced by passing an electric current through a coiled resistant wire, and it can be used clinically as either a luminous or non-luminous source (Charman 1990).

**Effects.** The heat is produced when body tissues absorb infrared rays. The non-luminous generator produces long rays (>12 000 Å) and is absorbed in the tissues of the epidermis. The luminous generator produces shorter rays (7700–12 000 Å), which penetrate to the dermis and subcutaneous tissues. Luminous rays can cause irritation of the tissues; however, the use of a red glass filter can eliminate this irritation. The application of infrared rays leads to a local rise in temperature with a subsequent increase in the blood supply to the area, relief of pain, muscle relaxation and elimination of waste products.

**Safety precautions.** Prior to use, all manufacturer's instructions should be read carefully and the electrical safety of the equipment checked regularly by appropriately qualified staff; the equipment should meet the required standards regarding the safety of medical electrical equipment (IEC 2009). It is essential to assess the suitability of the patient, ensure that they are fully aware of the nature of the treatment, and report any inappropriate heating or discomfort. As the radiation is absorbed by mucous membranes such as the eyes, the patient should be issued with a pair of dark goggles or advised to avoid looking directly at the lamp to protect the eyes.

**Method/application.** The lamp should be preheated. The patient should be sitting in a comfortable position and advised to remain still and not to touch anything. The lamp should be positioned so that its rays strike the part to be treated at a right angle and at a distance of 18–24 inches (45–61 cm) (or according to manufacturer's instructions). Cover the surrounding tissues with white paper towels to protect them. Ensure that the lamp is not positioned directly over the part to be treated, as there is a danger of the generator falling onto the patient and causing burns. The process of heating should be comfortable, and constant monitoring of the patient is essential. Changing the distance of the lamp from the area to be treated, if no control switch is available, can alter the intensity of heat delivered. The duration of treatment should be 15 minutes and it may be repeated on a daily basis.

**Indications for use.** Infrared radiation can be used effectively for chronic musculoskeletal and traumatic conditions such as sprains, strains, plantar fasciitis and arthropathies.

**Contraindications.** Skin that has had liniment, oil or embrocation cream applied to it recently should not be treated with this form of heat as this may enhance the heating effect and cause superficial blistering. Acute inflammation, evidence of bleeding, sepsis, other skin conditions or circulatory impairment are also contraindications.

**Hazards**. Infrared radiation may cause damage to the tissues if used at excessive levels over long periods or if used at very high intensities. There is a danger of burns, blistering and permanent pigmentation (erythema ab igne). When dealing with any piece of electrical equipment there is always the danger of electric shock to either the patient or clinician. All health and safety precautions should be observed.

## Ultrasound

Sound is mechanical vibration to which the human ear responds in the range 20 000–30 000 Hz. Unlike other forms of mechanical energy, sound cannot travel through a vacuum. It can only be transmitted through media such as solids, liquids or gases.

The mechanical vibrations set up a waveform motion which, when passing through a medium, causes alternate compression and distension of its particles. Only the form of the waves moves forward, while the particles through which they pass merely move back and forth around a mean point. The progression of a sound wave through a medium depends on the transfer of energy from one particle to the next.

Ultrasound is defined as inaudible, acoustic, mechanical vibrations of high frequency (usually 1–3 MHz) that produce thermal and non-thermal physiological effects (Gann 1991). Ultrasound is generated by a transducer, a device that transforms one form of energy into another. The most commonly used transducer in ultrasound is crystal quartz, which changes electrical energy into mechanical energy using the piezoelectric effect. The voltage across the ultrasound transducer may be applied continuously over the entire treatment time (continuous mode) or in short bursts (pulsed mode). The energy in an ultrasound wave is characterised by intensity. This is the energy crossing a unit area perpendicular to the wave in unit time. The units used in medical ultrasound are watts per square centimetre ($W/cm^2$).

The energy of the longitudinal wave will produce the mechanical effects of compression and rarefaction in the tissues through which it passes.

**Thermal effects**. When ultrasound travels through tissues a percentage of it is absorbed, leading to the generation of heat within the tissues. As the waves pass through the different tissues or media of the body (skin, muscle, tendon, etc.) they are subject to varying refractions and scatter. As a result, the intensity of an ultrasound beam decreases as it penetrates deeper into the tissues – the 'half-value distance'. The half-value depth for soft, irregular connective tissue is approximately 4 mm at 3 MHz but about 11 mm at 1 MHz. The amount of absorption will depend on the nature of the tissue, the vascularity of the area and the frequency of the ultrasound. Tissues with a high protein content absorb ultrasound more easily than do those with a high fat content.

The higher the frequency the greater the absorption (Young & Dyson 1990). Structures heated preferentially are periosteum, superficial cortical bone, joint menisci, fibrotic muscle, tendon sheaths and major nerve roots. It is important that the clinician has a good knowledge of the structures that lie between the ultrasound equipment head, the injured tissues and the deeper tissues. Because of the application of the ultrasound there will be an increase in tissue temperature, increased vasodilatation, and increased cell metabolism, with a resultant decrease in joint stiffness and pain relief.

**Non-thermal effects/physical properties**. There are situations in which ultrasound produces physical effects on biological tissues but without a significant increase in temperature. Such situations would include bone repair, stimulation of tissue regeneration and soft-tissue repair (Dyson & Pond 1970). The mechanisms involved in the physical or non-thermal effects are the result of cavitation, acoustic streaming or standing waves.

- *Cavitation*. Ultrasound can cause the formation of microsized bubbles or cavities in gas-containing fluids (Ayme & Carstensen 1989). These bubbles can be either useful or dangerous. Cavitation may be unstable and collapse of the bubbles will occur, resulting in an excessive rise in local temperature. This can best be avoided by continually moving the treatment head and by using intensities below 3 $W/cm^2$. Stable cavitation is not dangerous and can have beneficial effects. As a result of cavitation there is localised, unidirectional, small fluid movement around the vibrating bubble. This small fluid movement around cells (microstreaming) is believed to play a role in the therapeutic effect of ultrasound (Dyson & Pond 1970). Modifying the ultrasound beam results in microstreaming whereby the permeability of the cell membrane and the direction of movement of molecules into cells is influenced.

- *Acoustic streaming*. This describes the unidirectional movement of a fluid in an ultrasound field. Acoustic streaming can accelerate tissue repair as a result of increased capillary permeability, stimulation of activity of mast cells and fibroblasts, and the increased production of growth factors by macrophages (Maxwell 1992).

- *Standing waves*. When an ultrasound wave encounters the interface between tissues with different acoustic abilities (e.g. bone and muscle) reflection of a percentage of the wave will occur. The reflected wave can interact with oncoming waves to form a standing wave field in which the peaks of intensity of the waves are stationary and are separated by half a wavelength. This causes gas bubbles to collect and cause damage to endothelial cells and tissue in the immediate area. This can be avoided by moving the head of the transducer continuously throughout the treatment.

**Method of application**. Ultrasound can be applied either directly or indirectly to the area being treated (Robertson & Ward 1996).

*Direct application* is achieved by placing the treatment head in contact with the skin via a coupling gel recommended by the manufacturer of the equipment. The treatment regimen is selected and the machine switched on. It is essential to maintain continuous contact between the whole of the treatment face and the skin to avoid damage to the quartz crystal in the transducer. While maintaining an even pressure, the treatment head is moved in a circular or figure-of-eight motion over the surface.

*Indirect application* is achieved by immersing the area to be treated in a water bath. The water acts as the conductor between the tissue and the transducer. This method is particularly useful for irregular surfaces such as the dorsal aspect of the foot and the first metatarsophalangeal joint. The foot should be placed in a non-metallic basin containing water, preferably distilled water to avoid air bubbles but this is not essential. The dosage is selected and the treatment head is moved continually and parallel to the part in a circular motion about a $\frac{1}{4}$ inch (about 6 mm) from the skin.

Ultrasound therapy can also be used in conjunction with topical non-steroidal anti-inflammatory preparations. This method is considered to improve the management of a variety of musculoskeletal conditions and acute sports injuries. It is thought that ultrasound may enhance the penetration of some drugs across the skin by the process of phonophoresis (Benson & McElnay 1994).

**Suggested treatment dosages in podiatry**. These are as follows:

- Intensity:
  - low (0.25–0.5 W/cm2) for recent and acute conditions
  - medium (0.8–1.0 $W/cm^2$) for chronic conditions.

- Frequency:
  - high frequencies are absorbed more rapidly and therefore are more suitable for superficial tissues
  - low frequencies penetrate deeper.
- Time:
  - start with a short time (e.g. 3 minutes); this can be increased in subsequent applications.
- Pulsed/continuous mode:
  - continuous – thermal effect (chronic conditions)
  - pulsed – non-thermal effects (acute conditions).

**Indications**. Ultrasound can be beneficial in the treatment of soft-tissue injuries, inflammatory conditions such as painful hallux limitus, and rheumatic and arthritic conditions.

**Contraindications**. The use of ultrasound is contraindicated when infection is present in the area, as there is danger of the infection spreading. Ultrasound should never be used if there is a history of deep venous thrombosis, as there may be a risk of embolism. As with other forms of heat therapy, ultrasound is contraindicated in peripheral vascular disease. Other contraindications include the presence of tumours or tuberculosis, or if the patient has recently received radiotherapy, has haemophilia or if there is a suspected fracture. Ultrasound should never be used over the epiphyseal plate in a growing child as it may affect the growth of the limb (Oakley 1987).

---

### CASE STUDY 16.4 **MANAGEMENT OF PLANTAR FASCIITIS**

A 55-year-old woman was referred by her general practitioner (GP) complaining of pain on weight bearing in the region of the right heel which increased on walking. The pain radiated along the medial longitudinal arch in the foot.

The patient was overweight, worked full time in a local supermarket and her normal footwear was a court shoe with a 2-inch heel. Jack's test, whereby the hallux is dorsiflexed putting maximum tension through the plantar fascia and the medial attachment of the facia to the calcaneum, elicited the characteristic diagnostic pain of plantar fasciitis. Examination also revealed limited ankle dorsiflexion (less than 10°) and excessive subtalar joint pronation.

Her GP had prescribed Ibuprofen 400 mg, which had reduced the initial acute symptoms. She had no other medical problems, and the vascular and neurological status was normal on assessment. The patient was advised on appropriate footwear and a course of ultrasound therapy was administered twice weekly. Following the first ultrasound treatment the patient had a bow strapping applied to the foot and a Slimflex insole inserted into the footwear. The patient was shown stretching exercises for the plantar fascia and Achilles tendon. The patient was referred to the dietician for advice on an appropriate diet.

The patient complied with the footwear advice and stretching exercises. Subsequently, a casted orthosis, comprising an ethyl vinyl acetate (EVA) shell with a meniscus in deflective material at the heel, was manufactured, and this limited the subtalar joint pronation; The patient's symptoms subsided after a period of 4 weeks. Her weight gradually decreased, and after 4 months she was pain free.

---

## Cold

Cold has the converse effect of heat. The topical application of cold has an effect on the sympathetic adrenergic nerve fibres, causing constriction of the arterioles and venules and resulting in vasocon-striction. Cold will reduce the metabolic rate of tissues and there will be a lowered demand for oxygen and nutrients. Cold will also reduce the effect of the chemical mediators of inflammation, minimising the inflammatory process. Therefore, there will be a decrease in vascular permeability, an increase in the viscosity of blood, a reduction in the leakage of exudate from the vessels and consequently a reduction in the amount of swelling (Lehmann & DeLateur 1990).

Cold is useful in the initial treatment of acute trauma such as sprains, as it will limit the initial inflammatory response and thus limit tissue swelling and pain. However, the use of cold therapy should be avoided in patients who are elderly, have peripheral vascular disease, Raynaud's disease and sensitivity to cold, peripheral neuropathy or cardiovascular disease.

### Cryotherapy/cold therapy

Cryotherapy is the therapeutic application of cold. Cold can be used in podiatric practice in a variety of different circumstances, ranging from an application of an ice pack for an acute traumatic incident to the destruction of skin lesions such as verrucae (see previously in this chapter). Cold can be a very effective treatment in the acute stages of an inflammatory response.

The physiological effects of cold have been previously described. It can be applied to the area in various forms:

- crushed ice in towels or cloths
- ice cube packs/frozen peas
- frozen gel packs
- cold or cooling sprays
- iced water
- cryogenic equipment.

#### Ice packs

Crushed ice or ice cubes can be placed onto the affected area between layers of a dampened towel for approximately 10–15 minutes. The towel will prevent an ice burn on the tissues. Unopened packets of frozen peas or sweet corn are also useful if quantities of crushed ice are not available. These easily mould round the area, especially the ankle or dorsum of the foot, but must be separated from the skin by a layer of towel or cloth.

Gel packs (3M) are available in different shapes and sizes and are particularly useful when dealing with sports injuries as they have the benefit of being able to be used either hot or cold. The gel does not solidify when frozen, and therefore can be easily moulded to the affected area. The packs can be stored in the freezer compartment of a refrigerator.

#### Cold sprays

Cold sprays are most effective in the initial stages of a traumatic injury. They are applied to the area in short applications of 5–10 seconds over a 2–3 minute period. The skin is cooled quickly by the evaporation of the spray.

Sprays have a very limited use in podiatric practice but can be useful when dealing with sports injuries as they can be readily available at the sports field.

---

## FOOTBATHS

Footbaths can be used effectively in podiatric practice as an alternative treatment regimen as more than one surface can be treated at a time, which is especially useful when treating hands and feet.

## Methods of application

### Cold footbaths

Immersion of the foot for 5–10 minutes in a bath containing cold water with ice added can be a very effective treatment for acute traumatic injury. Care must be taken when using this treatment as the patient can experience extreme pain.

### Contrast footbaths

Contrast footbaths are an alternative regimen whereby the foot is placed alternately in warm water and cold water. The foot should be initially placed in the warm water (45–48°C) for 10 minutes and then plunged into the cold for 1 minute. It is then placed back in the warm water for 2 minutes and then the cold water for 1 minute. This procedure is continued for 20 minutes, finishing with the cold.

### Warm water footbaths

Warm water footbaths are useful for providing diffuse local heat and can also be used as a vehicle for various medicaments. The water should be maintained at a constant temperature of 45°C. It may be necessary on a few occasions to give the patient a footbath for general hygiene purposes. In these cases a suitable detergent such as Hibiscrub (4% w/v chlorhexidine) can be added to the water. Sodium bicarbonate or sodium chloride may be added to the water as antidote in the event of an adverse reaction to strong acids.

### Hypertonic footbaths

A hypertonic footbath may be used when sepsis is present to facilitate the drainage of pus from the wound by osmosis. It also dehydrates the protoplasm of the bacteria.

One hundred grams of either magnesium sulphate or sodium chloride should be dissolved in 5 litres water. The temperature should be kept constant at 46°C for 10–15 minutes.

### Antiseptic astringent footbaths

A footbath containing potassium permanganate crystals or Permitabs is useful in the treatment of hyperhidrosis or bromidrosis. A few crystals of potassium permanganate, sufficient to turn the water pale pink, or one Permitab are dissolved in a basin of water at 38°C. The footbath should be used once or twice a day for 10–15 minutes, depending on the severity of the condition.

**Contraindications.** Footbaths are contraindicated if the patient has impaired arterial supply, neuropathy or thin friable skin. Footbaths should also be avoided if there is a break in the skin, fungal infection or verruca.

## LASERS

The use of lasers for therapeutic reasons such as pain reduction, tissue healing and verrucae pedis is becoming increasingly popular. The uptake of this treatment modality was originally slow, although there has been an increasing amount of research now which focuses on the changes at cellular level that such treatment imparts.

The word LASER is an acronym for:

Light
Amplification by
Stimulated
Emission of
Radiation

**Table 16.1** Lasers: common features

| Component | Function | Example |
|---|---|---|
| Energy source | Excites the lasing medium to the levels required to produce laser radiation | Electric charger (depending on lasing medium) |
| Lasing medium | Absorbs energy and subsequently gives off excess energy as light | Solid crystal, gas, liquid, semiconductor |
| Structure | Central chamber with two mirrors at either end, containing lasing medium. This increases the amplification of the lasing medium and makes the light more coherent | Hand-held probe |

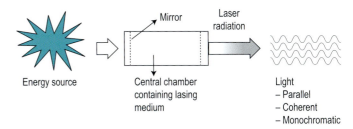

**Figure 16.18** Some of the important features of laser light.

There is a variety of different types of laser available, each of which is used for various conditions. Table 16.1 shows the features that are common to all types of laser.

## Properties of laser light

A combination of properties makes laser light unique, allowing the treatment of specific conditions. The beam from a single probe has a narrow bandwidth (usually 660–950 nm), and the photons are in-phase, with very little divergence. Each photon carries the same amount of energy, resulting in the light being consistent and uniform.

Some of the important features of laser light are listed below and in Figure 16.18.

- Monochromatic: narrow bandwidth; single wavelength
- Coherent: the light waves move in step and are constant over time
- Collimated: the beams of light are parallel (produce a small spot size over a relatively large distance).

Prior to use of any course of laser therapy, the wavelength, pulse frequency and energy must be considered.

The power is the strength or power output of the laser. The power density is the light-output power per unit area of the target, and is measured in watts per centimetre squared (W/cm²). It can be calculated using the following formula:

$$\text{Power density} = \frac{\text{probe power (W)} \times \text{time (s)}}{\text{area of irradiation (spot size; cm)}}$$

The energy density is the total amount of energy conducted into the tissues, measured in joules per centimetre squared ($J/cm^2$).

The pulse frequency is the number of pulses per second. When a laser is pulsed, the laser light power varies between the peak output of the pulse and zero.

The wavelength has a biological effect; it is therefore important to use the correct wavelength for the right indications (Baxter 1994).

## The effect of laser light

Treatment with laser therapy produces biochemical and photobiological effects within the cells and tissues. Together, these stimulatory effects are known as biomodulation (Turner & Hode 2002). Local metabolic changes occur, such as increased inflammatory response, effects on the immune system and increased formation of capillaries, as well as a number of other effects that are of therapeutic value.

The radiation emitted by a laser is athermic. However, the biomodulation effects have been shown to be dose-dependent. The laser dose is calculated as:

$$Dose = \frac{power \times time}{area}$$

## Safety

As with any other electrical equipment, the laser machine must be checked and serviced regularly. Local rules should be drawn up that detail the safe use of the unit.

Only authorised users who have undergone approved training should provide laser treatment. The treatment should be given in a confined area with no uncovered windows or shiny surfaces or mirrors in order to prevent reflection of the light. A warning sign should be mounted outside the area of treatment and should be clearly visible. Both the patient and practitioner must wear goggles designed specifically to filter the wavelengths emitted by the laser machine and to protect against damage to the eyes.

The laser machine must be switched off when unsupervised and not in use, and it must be calibrated regularly.

## Treatment technique

It is important that the practitioner has a good knowledge of anatomy to ensure that the correct area is treated. The painful area should be pinpointed each time and the target area should be in its optimum position to receive treatment.

The patient should be advised of a possible flare up after the treatment (described later). To be able to monitor the treatment effects effectively, it is advisable to use adequate outcome measures.

The laser probe should be held at 90° to the skin. An appropriate technique, such as holding the probe still in one area or moving it over the skin, should be used depending on the area being treated. The probe should be in contact with the skin; the distance between the probe and treatment area should be minimal in order to prevent divergence of the beam and, therefore, ineffective treatment. Light reaching tissues from a distance (not in contact) aims over a larger area and is more superficial. Close-contact light penetrates deeper and over a localised area. This is demonstrated in Figure 16.19.

The light distribution in the tissues depends on the wavelength, with shorter wavelengths producing small rounded distribution and longer ones having an elongated ball effect (Turner & Hode 2002).

To prevent cross-infection the end of the probe should be wiped and any thin clear film can be used as a barrier. For the treatment of ulcerated lesions the clear inside sterile packing of wound dressings is useful for this purpose.

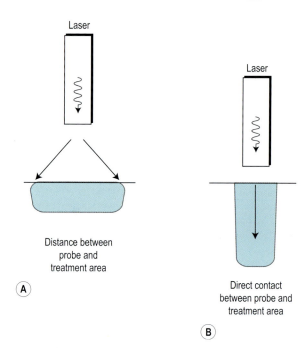

**Figure 16.19** (A) Light reaching tissues from a probe not in contact with the skin aims over a larger area and is more superficial in its effect. (B) With the probe in close contact with the skin the light penetrates deeper and over a more localised area.

## Contraindications

The following is a summary of some of the cautions and contraindications associated with laser therapy:

*Contraindications*:

- direct treatment of the eye (unless by qualified personnel within the area)
- treatment over pregnant uterus
- presence of active neoplasm
- area of haemorrhage
- transplants.

*Cautions*:

- treatment over the epiphyseal lines of the bones of children
- irradiation of gonads
- photosensitive tissue.

## Laser in patient management

Laser therapy can be used for an increasing number of conditions, either alone or in conjunction with other treatment options.

There are a variety of probes available to produce light with different characteristics, the hand held probe and the cluster probe are the most commonly used. The manufacturer's advice should be adopted when pulses and treatment doses are considered.

*Indications*:

- trigger points and acupuncture points
- bone repair
- verrucae pedis
- pain relief (acute and chronic)
- myofascial pain and dysfunction
- rheumatoid arthritis
- osteoarthritis
- neuralgias
- soft-tissue and overuse injuries
- wounds

- bed sores
- burns
- scar tissue.

When using laser as part of any treatment plan, the patient must be informed of the effect it may have on their condition. The patient may experience pain flare-up due to the cellular changes taking place – pain becomes acute when the healing process starts. It is important that the patient be informed of this before treatment commences so that they are aware of what to expect. They should be advised that the pain may increase but should then reduce to less than the original level. Some patients may not experience any increase in pain after the treatment.

The treatment should be adapted to the patient's needs, and its effect should be reviewed at each treatment session and adapted accordingly. It can be included as part of a treatment plan; for example, in wound healing, regular debridement, padding and dressing will also be done.

Studies have shown that non-steroidal anti-inflammatory drugs (NSAIDs) and steroids inhibit the effect of laser therapy, and this should be taken into consideration when the therapeutic effect is reviewed.

Laser promotes wound healing by stimulating the cellular effects that result in wound healing. It can be administered first around the periphery of the wound, and then moved slowly across the open wound. The skin absorbs and scatters the light so that the open-wound area will receive a lower dose than the area surrounding it. The dosage should be adjusted according to the type of wound being treated (Ashford et al 1995).

Wounds treated by laser may initially appear to deteriorate, and there may be an increase in the amount of discharge produced, and the patient must be informed of this prior to treatment. The wound may appear to be larger, which is generally due to the slough clearing and granulation tissue developing. It is essential to ensure that, while treating with laser, wound-care interventions such as regular debridement and dressings continue.

---

## CASE STUDY 16.5 **MANAGEMENT OF HEEL PAIN**

A female patient presented with a 7-month history of heel pain. The pain was at its worst first thing in the morning and eased off on weight bearing. The patient had already been given footwear advice and undergone a full biomechanical assessment of the lower limb and was wearing corrective orthoses. She was stretching her calf muscles daily. The patient's initial visual analogue scale (VAS) score for pain was 8, and this had reduced to 5 after the above treatments.

On examination, the medial side of the heel was painful on palpation, although the patient reported that the whole heel was painful. The patient was given a weekly course of laser treatment. All other treatments were continued. The first two laser treatments comprised using a mixture of the cluster and the point probe. The point probe was used over the area that was painful on palpation, and the cluster over the heel area.

### REPORT AFTER FIRST TREATMENT

Pain had increased for 2 days but then decreased to less than the initial level. Original pain returned a day before the next treatment was due. VAS = 4.

### REPORT AFTER SECOND TREATMENT

The patient reported that the pain was now around the medial side only. Surrounding pain had gone. Pain had again increased for 2 days and then reduced to less than the original level, and had stayed low. VAS = 2.

### REPORT AFTER THIRD TREATMENT

Treatment was provided with the point probe only. The pain did not increase after the treatment and was felt only for a few days. VAS = 1–2.

### REPORT AFTER FOURTH TREATMENT

The patient reported no pain during the week. An occasional twitch was felt around the area. The patient was discharged.

---

# MAGNETOPULSE

Magnetic field therapy has a historical connection with China, as healing properties were claimed for lodestone in some early Chinese medical literature.

Work by Franklin, Lavoisier, Galvani and Volta on electromagnetism, and research into electromagnetism by Michael Faraday, led to a theory relevant to the explanation of cellular behaviour. Their investigations laid the foundations for the piezoelectric effect of bones and connective tissue, as well as the biophysical explanations for nerve and muscle function (*Magnetopulse Systems Manual*).

Towards the end of the 1960s, serious investigation was stepped up into the possible effects of magnetic fields on humans. This was given added impetus with the substantial financial and research facilities of NASA and Soviet space research centres. The loss of calcium from bone can now be partly attributed to the weak magnetic fields, as found in space.

Magnetopulse therapy aims to influence the electrical activity across the group of cells being treated and to stimulate a faster natural healing rate. It has two basic functions: first, to suppress the symptoms of an injury or illness, such as inflammation with associated pain; and, second, to treat the cause of the same condition by increased blood flow to the injured area.

Magnetopulse can be used in podiatric practice in the treatment of sports injuries, osteoarthritis and rheumatoid arthritis.

## Contraindications

Magnetopulse is contraindicated in pregnant women and in those with tuberculosis or a viral illness. It should not be used (i) in juvenile diabetes, (ii) if there is a history of thrombosis, (iii) if the patient is susceptible to haemorrhage, or (iv) if the patient has a pacemaker.

When using magnetopulse the clinician must take certain precautions: remove all watches and ensure that the machine is kept away from all other electronic equipment such as computers.

## Operation of magnetopulse equipment

There are 19 magnetic field intensity settings and 19 modulation frequency settings.

**Start**. Pressing a single momentary-action button, marked 'start', provides the signal to the applicator coils and starts an adjustable countdown timer. When high frequencies are selected, it may not be possible to notice the usual pulsation.

At the end of the selected time the system will automatically stop and an audible tone will sound, indicating the end of the treatment.

**Stop**. Pressing a single momentary-action button, marked 'stop', ends the treatment before completion of the set time.

The treatment regimen is flexible in increments of 1 minute, from 0 to 90 minutes, and the output is 120 VA/50 Hz. Magnetopulse

**Table 16.2** Suggested magnetopulse treatment regimens

| Stage 1 | Stage 2 | Stage 3 |
|---------|---------|---------|
| Use this stage for acute cases. Treat once a day for 3 days and then every second day. When the condition improves, gradually increase the intensity, and then move to stage 2 | Use for subacute conditions | Use for chronic conditions |

**Table 16.4** Ankle sprain: suggested magnetopulse treatment regimen

| Stage | Intensity | Frequency | Time |
|-------|-----------|-----------|------|
| 1 | Low<br>30 | 1st<br>1 | 30 min<br>30 min |
| 2 | Low<br>30 | 2nd<br>5 | 30 min<br>30 min |
| 3 | Low<br>30 | 3rd<br>12 | 30 min<br>30 min |

**Table 16.3** Osteoarthritis: suggested magnetopulse treatment regimen

| Stage | Intensity | Frequency | Time |
|-------|-----------|-----------|------|
| 1 | Low/medium<br>20 | 1st<br>1 | 15 min<br>15 min |
| 2 | Low/medium<br>60 | 2nd<br>5 | 20 min<br>20 min |
| 3 | Low/medium<br>80 | 3rd<br>25 | 20–30 min<br>20–30 min |

machines can be obtained with either two or four treatment pads; the method of application will therefore vary.

## Method: machine with two pads

1. Place the applicator over the area to be treated (this should be well supported).
2. Plug the applicators into the treatment sockets at the back of machine.
3. Select the frequency and intensity.
4. Press the start button.
5. The machine will run for 30 minutes – to stop earlier press the stop button.

## Method: machine with four pads

1. Place the applicators over the area to be treated.
2. Plug the applicators into either or both treatment output sockets on the front of machine.
3. Switch the machine on using the power switch on the front.
4. Select the time and frequency.
5. Select the intensity (5–95%).
6. When the settings are complete, start treatment by pressing the start button.
7. The stop button may be used to stop the treatment at any time.

## Indications

Magnetopulse can be used in the management of the following conditions often encountered in podiatric practice: osteoarthritis, rheumatoid arthritis, ankle sprains, haematoma and bruising, bursitis, tendinitis. Suggested treatment regimens are given in Table 16.2, and examples of use are given in Tables 16.3 and 16.4.

# NON-THERMAL ELECTROTHERAPY

## Faradism – muscle stimulation

Faradism involves the use of a low-frequency current (50–100 Hz). It is a faradic-type interrupted direct current with a pulse rate of 0.1–1 ms. This would produce a tetanic muscle contraction, which would be very uncomfortable, so the current is surged to produce alternate contraction and relaxation of the muscles similar to the normal contraction of muscles that have a normal nerve supply.

It is used to facilitate muscle contraction when the patient finds it difficult to produce effective muscle action. This may be because of inhibition due to pain after injury, postoperatively or arthritis. It may be used to re-educate a muscle action. This could be after prolonged disuse, as in flat foot, or incorrect use, as in abductor hallucis in hallux abducto valgus. It is also used to stretch and loosen adhesions and to improve venous and lymphatic drainage.

Large multifunction machines can produce faradism, but the most useful are small, portable, battery-operated machines with automatic surging.

## Technique

1. To help contract the calf muscle, possibly after trauma or immobilisation, two metal or rubber electrodes are placed, one above each other, over the muscle belly and held in place by straps or bandage. Patients are warned that first they will feel a prickling sensation, and then the muscle will contract and the foot will plantar flex, and they will not be able to do anything to stop it. Patients are asked to contract the muscle with the machine, as they get used to it; the power is then turned gently down so that the patient is contracting on their own.
2. To stimulate the intrinsic muscles, a footbath with ½ inch (13 mm) of water is used. One electrode is placed under the heel and the other under the metatarsal heads. The patient is instructed in the same way. To stimulate the abductor hallucis using the bath, one electrode is placed under the medial side of the heel and a button electrode is used on the motor point of abductor hallucis.

## Electrodes

1. Metal plates – often made from pure tin (for high conductivity) on layers of soaked lint.
2. Rubber electrodes – impregnated with graphite for conduction.

**3.** A disc or button electrode covered with lint for individual muscle stimulation.

Faradism is a passive exercise but can cause muscle fatigue, so 5 minutes' treatment is the average to start with.

## Interferential

Two medium-frequency alternating currents of different frequencies from 400 Hz to 4250 Hz are applied to the body. Where the currents cross they 'interfere' with one other and set up a beat frequency. This is a low-frequency current. The two currents can be varied between 0 and 250 Hz to produce different physiological effects.

### Relief of pain

There may be an effect on the pain gate of short-duration pulses at 80 Hz. Endorphin release can be activated by 2.5 or 130 Hz. The pumping action on the blood vessels speeds up the metabolic rate and the removal of metabolites (0–100 Hz or 0–250 Hz).

### Motor stimulation

There will be contraction of muscle between 0 and 100 Hz. This is deeper in the tissues than is the case with faradism, although 0–50 Hz can be effective for the more superficial layers, but the patient cannot contract with it.

The pumping action is very effective for the absorption of exudate.

### Technique

The site for treatment is assessed. Two pairs of electrodes with colour-coded leads are placed diagonally opposite each other, making sure that the two currents cross at the part to be treated. Damp sponge pads are placed on the skin under the electrodes so there is no chance of an electrical burn. The electrodes and pads are held in place with straps or bandages.

The power is turned up, with the patient telling the therapist as soon as a tingling is felt. It must be comfortable. The treatment time is 10–20 minutes.

### Contraindications

The treatment should not be used in patients with thrombosis or pacemakers, and care should be taken with patients with heart conditions and tumours.

Interferential therapy is a useful therapeutic tool in the treatment of many foot conditions, including sports injuries, trauma, arthritic problems and soft-tissue problems such as plantar fasciitis.

---

### CASE STUDY 16.6 **MANAGEMENT OF SHIN SPLINTS**

A 21-year-old male took up running as part of a fitness regimen. After training for 2 weeks he developed pain in the lower medial aspect of the tibia. The area of pain corresponds to the origin of the posterior tibial muscle and radiates distally following the course of the tendon. On examination, pain and tenderness are elicited on palpation of the posterior medial border of the tibia. Following a biomechanical assessment there is evidence of a 5° forefoot varus, with abnormal compensatory pronation at the subtalar joint. A diagnosis of a posterior tibial shin splint is made.

A treatment plan was initiated comprising a course of ultrasound therapy (0.5 W/cm$^2$, low frequency, pulsed for 3 minutes increasing after two applications to 5 minutes). A subtalar neutral cast was taken and a functional orthosis consisting of a rigid shell with medial posting was prescribed. It was arranged for the patient to attend the clinic three times a week for the following 6 weeks. A temporary Slimflex insole with medial EVA wedging was inserted into the patient's footwear and he was advised to discontinue running until the inflammatory process had subsided. The patient did not report any adverse reaction to the ultrasound therapy on his second visit. The functional orthosis was fitted on the third visit and the symptoms had resolved in 6 weeks.

---

## ACUTE AND CHRONIC INFLAMMATORY CONDITIONS

Inflammatory states arising from trauma and/or bursitis may require two methods of treatment complementing each other.

The first aims to reduce and control inflammation and swelling by the application of cold when the inflammation is in the acute stage. This is achieved by cold compresses or ice packs. When the inflammation is chronic, and congestion of the area is evident, mild heat in the form of ultrasound is recommended. Therapeutic laser or magnetopulse therapy are invaluable to hasten the healing process. A major advantage of magnetopulse is that padding and strapping need not be removed during treatment.

The second method is to support and rest the affected part by the use of padding and strapping. Padding can be applied directly to the foot or inserted into the patient's footwear as a transitional stage pending the manufacture and fitting of orthoses. Although orthotic therapy is essential in the longer term, immediate relief or reduction of pain is primarily achieved by padding and strapping.

### Tension strappings

Figure-of-eight strapping for the foot and ankle is shown in Figure 16.19. This strapping may be used for various conditions:

- to support a sprained or weak ankle, either inversion or eversion sprains
- to support a strained foot
- to limit painful movement in the subtalar and midtarsal joints
- to relieve tensile stress on the plantar fascia and its calcaneal attachment.

Depending on the structures that need to be supported or rested, the strapping can be applied in order to invert the foot and to support the structures on the medial aspect of the foot and ankle. Medial support is required, with or without the addition of valgus padding or D-pads, in cases of sprain of the deltoid ligament, acute or chronic foot strain and plantar fasciitis. Conversely, it may be applied in such a way as to support the structures on the lateral side of the foot and ankle. Lateral support is required, with or without a tarsal platform or 'filler pad', in cases of sprain of the external lateral ligaments of the ankle, and in some cases of pes cavus with associated postural instability. It may also be applied to hold the foot in a neutral position and to reduce tensile stress on the plantar aspect of the foot, and limit the motions in all directions. This is indicated in arthritis of the tarsal region.

The strapping of choice is a 5 cm (2 inches) or 6.25 cm (2½ inches) elastic adhesive bandage. This is preferred to non-stretch strapping, particularly where oedema is present, as it is less con-

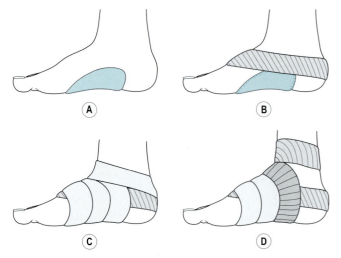

**Figure 16.20** Figure-of-eight strapping for the foot and ankle. (A) Valgus or 'D-pad. (B) Non-stretch strapping applied first to invert the heel. (C) Figure-of-eight elastic strapping. (D) Second application of non-stretch reinforcing strapping.

stricting. If hyperhidrosis is present or the patient is allergic to this material it may be applied over a soft cotton bandage. In order to prevent the plaster sticking to hair on the dorsum of the foot, cotton wool can be dragged across the sticky surface of the strapping to that area only. There will be some stretch of the material during walking but, if necessary, this can be minimised by the addition of two pieces of non-stretch strapping to reinforce and prolong the support given. Of necessity, these strappings are for short-term use only, and should not be reapplied if the skin becomes extremely macerated or signs of allergic dermatitis appear. If reapplication of adhesive plaster is contraindicated but support or limitation of movement is still required, the same strapping may be applied utilising crepe bandage. This will reduce the support that can be achieved and it is also a bulkier form of strapping, which may cause constriction in the footwear, but is a valuable alternative.

## Medial support

- If required, apply a valgus or D-pad (Fig. 16.20A).
- Anchor the first non-stretch strap anteroposteriorly to the lateral side of the foot, pass it around and behind the calcaneum and as low down on the heel as possible. Apply sufficient tension to invert the heel before securing the end of the strap along the medial and dorsal aspect of the first metatarsal, which must be held in plantar flexion. This locks the calcaneum into eversion by supinating the subtalar joint (Fig. 16.20B).
- From immediately behind the base of the toes on the dorsum of the foot (to prevent swelling occurring here), apply the stretch strapping laterally and obliquely round the forefoot to complete one turn of the metatarsus, and then continue round the tarsus with upward tension on the medial border before encircling the ankle and heel as low down as before in order to maintain maximum inversion.
- Continue across the front of the ankle and once more round the tarsus from lateral to medial before again encircling the ankle at a higher level. The second strap should overlap the first by half its width and should also cover the malleoli well so that it may be finally secured to the leg above the ankle (Fig. 16.20C).

- Apply the final reinforcing strap of non-stretch strapping to form a 'figure-of-eight' around the tarsus and the malleoli, the lower loop proving a supporting cradle or 'stirrup' while the upper affords a firm attachment to the leg above the ankle (Fig. 16.20D).

The strapping should just avoid the anterior margin of the plantar fatty pad, leaving it free to change shape on weight bearing, otherwise the edge of the strapping cutting across the fatty pad will cause discomfort.

Depending on the degree of support or correction required, valgus padding may be incorporated into this dressing, with it being applied to the foot before the strapping is in place, or alternatively it may be inserted into the shoe. Firm supporting footwear must be worn at all times with this strapping, the unshod foot never being allowed to bear weight. This strapping will give support for up to 10 days before requiring renewal.

## Lateral support

The technique is similar to the strapping for medial support but the strapping is applied in the reverse direction, the upward tension being exerted on the lateral side of the foot, which is held in eversion. No preliminary reinforcing strap is necessary to evert the foot, but the final reinforcing strap should be applied as previously described, but in the reverse direction. Additional lateral support can be provided if necessary by fitting a tarsal platform into the shoe.

## Neutral support

The object of this strapping is to restrain painful movement in the tarsal joints. The most comfortable position of the foot should first be established by passive manipulation. No preliminary reinforcing strap is necessary. The flexible bandage is applied as for medial support but without the medial tension. The final reinforcing strap is applied with approximately equal tension on the medial and lateral borders of the foot before being secured to the leg above the ankle. Additional mediolateral support can be provided, if required, by fitting a combined tarsal platform and valgus pad into the shoe – the 'tarsal cradle'.

Care must be taken when applying any restricting strapping to the foot when oedema is present or gravitational swelling occurs towards the end of the day. Advice should be given regarding elevation of the limb, but if the swelling is severe enough to cause discomfort or restrict the circulation to the digits the patient should be advised to cut through the strapping on the dorsal aspect up to the level of the base of the metatarsals. This will relieve some of the pressure, while the strapping will continue to give some support to the foot and ankle. If this is insufficient, the strapping must be removed or reapplied in the form of a crepe bandage, which can be removed by the patient and reapplied the following morning.

Orthotic techniques appropriate as follow-up to 'figure-of-eight' foot and ankle strappings may be any of the following: elastic anklets, corrective or palliative orthoses incorporating valgus, tarsal platform or combined tarsal cradle support, buttressed heels and wedged heels. Unlike the strapping, however, all such devices provide only passive support or correction.

## Valgus padding

Valgus padding, so-called because it is used in cases of valgus foot, has two separate but related elements, a plantar cushion and a medial flange. The plantar cushion fills the concavity of the longitudinal arch, with the object of affording support to the joints and the muscular and ligamentous attachments, which become strained in abnormal pronation. It is essentially palliative in function.

The medial flange extends towards, and if necessary over, the prominences of the sustentaculum tali and the tuberosity of the navicular. Its function is to encourage some degree of inversion of the foot and thereby some correction of abnormal pronation. This is achieved by the pressure of the padding against the firm counter of the shoe. Where such correction is possible, it should be initiated primarily by means of medial heel wedging, but the medial flange is often necessary to supplement the correction.

It follows, therefore, that the design of valgus padding must be varied considerably to meet individual needs. When applied directly to the foot it is constructed of a compressed felt material in either 5 mm or 7 mm thickness.

## Applications

- As part of a figure-of-eight strapping for foot strain, a thin felt pad having both elements is usually required (Fig 16.20A).
- As a temporary palliative orthosis or shoe insert, the plantar element alone may be adequate to control symptoms.
- As a permanent feature of an accommodative insole for pes plano valgus, both elements are usually required in combination with medial heel wedging. The shape, texture and density of the materials used must be varied to suit the needs of each patient and will depend on whether the objective is correction or palliation.
- In metatarsalgia and in hallux rigidus, with the addition of metatarsal padding or a shaft pad, respectively.

Valgus padding is contraindicated in the presence of occlusive arterial disease, as it may compress and occlude the plantar arteries and exacerbate or initiate the symptoms of intermittent claudication in the foot. Nor should the plantar element be used alone and continuously as a form of so-called 'arch support'. The degree of compression of the plantar soft tissues entailed in the attempt to provide direct support to the skeletal arch in that way is likely to produce an unacceptable degree of wasting of the plantar soft tissues. Control of the calcaneal eversion by heel wedging and the medial flange incorporated into an orthotic device is the preferred therapy in chronic abnormal pronation.

## Tarsal platform (filler pad)

The tarsal platform or 'filler pad' (Fig. 16.21) is never applied to the foot except as a short-term measure. It is mainly used as a component of orthoses or as an insert in footwear. Its main function is to bring the lateral border of a highly arched foot into firm contact with the waist of the shoe. By raising the floor level to the foot, it enlarges the weight-bearing area and to that extent relieves the loading on the heel and the metatarsal heads. It also tends to evert the foot and is useful where there is peroneal strain.

The basic design is that of a platform of firm material extending the full width of the insole from the anterior margin of the heel seat to just behind the tread (Fig. 16.21A). It fills the empty space between the lateral border of a highly arched foot and the waist of the shoe. There is no contact between it and the plantar aspect of the medial longitudinal arch, the bulk of the padding on the medial side serving only to anchor it more firmly to the waist of the shoe. It is the limitation of contact to the lateral border only that tends to evert the foot, thus stabilising the ankle in cases of abnormal inversion. The medial portion of the padding also provides the base for additional valgus padding where this is needed to form a tarsal cradle.

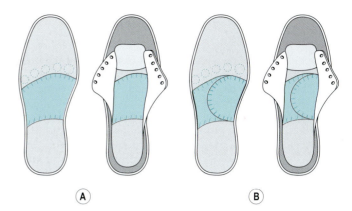

**Figure 16.21** Tarsal platform (filler pad) and extended to tarsal cradle. (A) Tarsal platform on leatherboard insole. (B) Tarsal cradle (combination of platform and valgus or 'D-pad).

When required, the anterior edge of the platform may be thickened to form a metatarsal bar, or may be extended under the three middle metatarsal heads to form a 'double-winged' metatarsal pad to protect the first and fifth metatarsal heads, or extended as shafts under the first and fifth to protect the middle three, or extended as a shaft under the first alone in hallux rigidus.

## Applications

- In *pes cavus*, to redistribute weight from the heel and metatarsal heads.
- In *persistent ankle sprain*, to stabilise the foot by obviating forced inversion.
- In *painful heel*, in conjunction with a heel cushion. The combination is more effective than heel cushioning alone and is indicated in all such cases regardless of the height of the longitudinal arch.
- In *metatarsalgia* and plantar lesions in conjunction with suitably shaped metatarsal padding.
- In *tarsal arthritis* in conjunction with valgus padding to form a tarsal cradle.

## Tarsal cradle

This (Fig. 16.21B) is a combination of a tarsal platform and a valgus support superimposed on it. It provides support for both the medial and the lateral borders of the foot and restrains the movements of inversion and eversion. Its main use is in tarsal arthritis when it may be used to augment the effect of a neutral figure-of-eight strapping. Like the tarsal platform it is not applied to the foot but is used as a component of an insole or as an insert in the footwear.

It also has an important application in restraining hypermobility and elongation of the foot in cases of abnormal pronation associated with calcaneocuboid subluxation. The cuboid underlies the front of the calcaneus by a process that extends from its medial, plantar and posterior aspect. Pressure on this process as the calcaneus everts causes some axial rotation of the cuboid and consequential hypermobility of the fourth and fifth metatarsal. In such cases, support to the lateral segment of the foot is necessary in addition to that provided to the medial segment. The tarsal platform element under the cuboid stabilises the lateral segment much as the valgus element stabilises the medial segment, the entire foot thus being cradled and stabilised much more effectively than by valgus support alone.

## Padding and strapping for hallux abducto valgus

The padding and strapping selected for this condition depends on the cause of the condition, and the mobility and age of the patient. The cause should always be considered, and the structure, shape and application of the padding related to the cause. It is beneficial to use adhesive padding as a temporary measure prior to the manufacture of orthoses, and the size and shape of the footwear must be given full consideration for the short- and long-term management of the condition. Strapping may be used on a younger patient with incipient hallux abducto valgus in order to lessen the deviation of the hallux and thereby relieve strain on the periarticular tissues and protect the medial eminence from shoe pressure. In an established case of hallux abducto valgus where correction is impossible, podiatric management consists of protection of the medial eminence by means of a felt crescent or oval cavity pad. The efficacy of this form of deflective padding depends on the degree of deformity present. If the degree of deformity is great, then footwear modifications in the form of balloon patches are essential to relieve pressure on the area. Often it is not the medial eminence that is the cause of discomfort but the resultant areas of overloading on the plantar aspect of the foot and the pressure on toe deformities. The most common site of corn/callus on the plantar aspect is on the second, third and fourth metatarsal heads or any combination of the same. This is due to an incompetent first metatarsal and toe deformities. The padding/orthosis applied should relate to the cause of the overloading. In this instance a short shaft to the first metatarsal combined with a metatarsal bar should increase the loading through the first metatarsal head and realign the lesser toes, if sufficient movement is available.

In a younger patient, where there is still mobility in the joint and passive movement can return the angulation to near normal, it is imperative that a biomechanical assessment be carried out to ascertain whether an underlying malalignment, such as forefoot varus, may be responsible for abnormal foot function and the development of the hallux abducto valgus. In this instance, although strapping may be used, as suggested above, it is imperative that a functional orthosis is in situ as soon as possible to prevent further deformity from occurring. This management strategy should include the use of an exercise regimen, night splints if appropriate, correction of any lesser toe deformities associated with the condition (see silicone devices) and precise footwear advice pertinent to the individual patient. Silicone devices in the form of an orthodigital splint embracing the middle three toes and an interdigital wedge for the first cleft eliminates any possibility of the lesser digits being abducted by the wedge, as they are firmly fixed against the sole of the shoe by the superimposed weight. For this reason, the interdigital wedge in this form also exerts better control on the hallux to prevent further lateral deviation.

The strapping of choice is adhesive stockinette, or similar, which has one-way stretch only. This is cut into a flask or butterfly shape and the anterior ends are first adhered to the hallux and secured there by a narrow strapping. The non-stretch dimension of this material must lie anteroposteriorly. The main part of the stockinette is then drawn back over the joint with sufficient tension to correct the line of the hallux to the extent required. The 'wings' are then stretched laterally across the dorsal and plantar surfaces of the metatarsal and adhered, covering any padding that has been applied to the joint (Fig 16.22).

## Padding and strapping for hallux limitus/rigidus

The acute form of hallux rigidus is occasionally seen in the younger age group, often associated with a sports injury or repeated minor

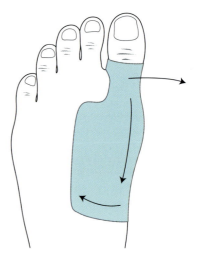

**Figure 16.22** Flask strapping to realign hallux abductus. The strapping is adhered around the hallux, below the interphalangeal joint; the hallux is passively moved from its abducted position, and the strapping is then applied with sufficient tension over the prominence and the medial side of the foot before being stretched laterally.

trauma due to a biomechanical dysfunction, but it is relatively uncommon. It is an extremely painful condition and is associated with inflammation and muscle spasm, traumatic synovitis and subsequent capsular contraction, mainly on the plantar surface. Untreated cases, or where there is repeated minor trauma, may display some marginal dorsal osseous lipping and may progress to chronic hallux limitus/ rigidus. This often depends on the effectiveness of the treatment at the acute stage, as well as on the cause. The clinical features are a rapid onset associated with pain and stiffness in the first metatarsophalangeal joint. The patient has great difficulty in weight bearing on the area and walks with the foot in a supinated position. Although the joint has inflammatory changes these are not always obvious superficially. The great toe is frequently held in a plantar-flexed position due to muscle spasm.

The treatment of acute hallux rigidus consists of an appropriate physical therapy to reduce the inflammation and pain in the joint and rest. If acutely inflamed, the patient may find contrast footbaths more beneficial prior to the application of heat. In severe cases rest will consist of total non-weight bearing and may require a plaster cast, although this is a rare occurrence. On occasion, hydrocortisone injections into the joint may be required. Normally, padding or strapping to reduce movement and relieve pressure on the first metatarsophalangeal joint on weight bearing is sufficient. A single-wing metatarsal pad is often the most readily tolerated padding, as it relieves the load on the painful joint, facilitates the inverted position of the foot that is adopted in such cases, and thus helps to minimise dorsiflexion at the joint. As soon as the pain and muscle spasm have been relieved, discontinue the padding and strapping but continue the heat therapy and restore normal movement in the joint by gentle traction and circumduction exercises. It is essential with acute hallux rigidus that the predisposing cause is identified and treated to prevent long-term problems with the joint function.

Chronic hallux limitus/rigidus is a slowly progressive disorder and, although it may halt at any stage, it may not become completely fixed. It may or may not be associated with pain in varying degrees. The loss or limitation of movement in the first metatarsal phalangeal joint may be associated with pain, especially after walking a distance; however, the pain may be due only to the associated lesions. The symptoms of pain will be exacerbated by wearing a higher heeled shoe. Because of

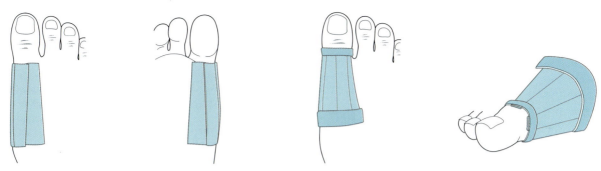

**Figure 16.23** Fan strapping for hallux limitus. May be used alone, as illustrated, or used in conjunction with a shaft pad (see Fig. 16.7).

the lack of movement at the metatarsophalangeal joint this detracts from the fulcrum action of the great toe. Pain in the first metatarsophalangeal joint may cause the patient to walk on the outer border of the foot and utilise the interphalangeal joint at the propulsive phase of gait when weight is transferred to the medial side of the foot. Secondary problems that may occur in the longer term area:

- Due to the foot functioning in a supinated position there may be the formation of corn and callus on the fifth metatarsal head.
- In a foot that adopts a less supinated position corn and callus may be evident on the second metatarsal head.
- The compensatory hyperextension that occurs at the interphalangeal joint leads to callus formation on that area.
- There may be strain of the lateral ligaments of the ankle due to the instability of the foot (supination).
- Due to dorsal lipping of the metatarsal head an adventitious bursa may develop on the dorsal aspect of the first metatarsophalangeal joint from irritation caused by footwear.

These secondary problems must be addressed with appropriate padding and footwear advice.

Pain at the first metatarsophalangeal joint that is produced on movement can be alleviated by limiting the movement at the joint. This can be achieved by means of a long shaft pad applied with rigid fan strapping. If there is insufficient room within the shoe then the fan strapping may be applied alone. This strapping utilises rigid adhesive strapping of 2.5 cm (1 inch) width (Fig. 16.23). With the first metatarsophalangeal joint held in the neutral position, the strapping is applied from a point just proximal to the interphalangeal joint of the great toe to the base of the first metatarsal. There are five pieces of strapping, which are applied in the following order: the plantar, dorsal and medial aspects of the first ray; and the final two pieces of strapping fill in the spaces between the previous three straps. This is an extremely effective method of limiting the movement in the joint. The strapping is adhered at the distal and proximal margins, as illustrated in Figure 16.22. Patients obtain great relief from padding and strapping, but at the earliest opportunity long-term orthoses should be prescribed, taking into account the biomechanical abnormality that has led to the pathological changes in the joint. When strapping is contraindicated, the joint can be immobilised by the temporary use of a leatherboard template with a shaft adhered to its undersurface made from either a thin rigid polythene material or other rigid material. The above measures will be ineffective unless advice on appropriate footwear is given and adhered to by the patient. There must be sufficient length and depth to the shoes to prevent any impaction of the proximal phalanx on the metatarsal head or pressure on an enlarged joint. The heel height should not be higher than 3 cm, and there should be a retaining medium to prevent forward movement and stubbing of the great toe. The sole should be rigid with an adequate toe spring to assist function in the propulsive phase of the gait cycle. If there is abnormal excessive pronation, the counter of the shoe

should be stiff and a patient-specific orthotic may be prescribed to prevent the pronation occurring. Adaptations to footwear, if required, consist of a rocker bar added to the outer sole of the shoe to enable the foot to 'rock' over the fixed joint. A steel stiffener may be inserted between the outer and middle sole to reduce movement and pain in a joint where complete fixation has not yet occurred. These measures can be carried out by a competent shoe repairer or cobbler. Patients who are in occupations that enable them to choose any type of footwear frequently find that clogs are extremely comfortable, and if pain is a factor it is remarkably reduced with this type of footwear. Other measures that may be adopted are stretching or balloon patching to accommodate any joint enlargement, exostosis or bursa formation (see Ch. 17).

## Plantar digital neuritis

This condition can present with or without any obvious structural abnormality and this can make the selection of padding and strapping uncertain. It should be explained to the patient that several forms of padding may alleviate the pain, and when the most appropriate padding has been determined a long-term orthotic device will be fitted. A plantar metatarsal pad with a U to the painful area is most often effective when applied with a full metatarsal strapping. Alternatively, a short-shaft pad, 2–4 plantar metatarsal pad or a metatarsal bar may be the padding of choice. All are commonly used in conjunction with digital splints to realign the toes if necessary. The patient should be reviewed after 1 week of the padding being applied in order to gauge its effectiveness.

## Plantar fasciitis

In this condition the main sites of pain are along the medial bands of the plantar fascia and, in addition, there may be localised pain over the medial tubercle of the calcaneum. Pain is felt on initial weight bearing in the morning or after a period of rest. Prolonged walking gives rise to continuous pain along the medial longitudinal arch of the foot and may be crippling. There are various causes of this condition, of which the most common biomechanical condition is excessive abnormal pronation at the subtalar joint. A change of occupation to one that involves continuous standing or unaccustomed walking may be a contributing factor, as can a sudden excessive weight gain. In addition to the use of therapeutic laser or ultrasound therapy, the application of clinical strapping followed by orthotic therapy is required. As discussed earlier in this chapter, the use of figure-of-eight strapping to invert the calcaneum, either alone or in conjunction with a tarsal platform, is helpful. When the pain is primarily along the medial longitudinal arch and there is limited sign of abnormal pronation, the use of bow strapping is effective in providing short-term relief (Fig. 16.24). This reduces the tensile stress on the fascia, and

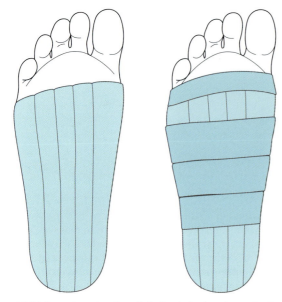

**Figure 16.24** Bow strapping for relief of pain in the plantar fascia.

therefore reduces the pain during weight bearing, and in addition takes up very little room in the shoe. Rigid strapping is used for this purpose in two widths: 2.5 cm (1 inch) for the bands running from the metatarsal head to the heel, and 3.75 cm (1½ inches) for the strapping across the plantar from the lateral to the medial sides of the foot.

## Method

- Place the foot at right angles to the leg and anchor the first non-stretch strip of 2.5 cm strapping directly over the first metatarsal head. Following the line of the metatarsal, bowstring the strapping along the medial plantar border of the foot and attach it to the medial plantar aspect of the heel and continue round the posterior aspect of the calcaneum by about 2 cm. If the foot to which the strapping is being applied is particularly broad this first strap may be 3.75 cm wide.
- This procedure is continued with a further four lengths of strapping corresponding to the second, third, fourth and fifth metatarsals. Tension must always be maintained when applying the strapping, avoiding any slackness.

- The first transverse strap is applied just proximal to the metatarsal heads, tension being applied from the lateral to the medial side of the foot. The lateral and medial margins of the strapping are attached to the dorsum of the foot over the fifth and first metatarsal shafts. The second transverse strapping is applied just distal to the medial tubercle of the calcaneum. Two further transverse strappings are required to complete the filling in process.
- The edges of the strapping are collectively adhered under an edge strapping of 2.5 cm width, which is applied in one length from the fifth metatarsal head on the dorsal aspect of the foot, along the lateral border, round the posterior of the heel, along the medial border and up to the dorsal aspect of the first metatarsal head.
- This strapping removes the tensile stress from the plantar fascia on weight bearing but, as with all adhesive strapping, its use should be limited until an orthotic device specific to the foot problem has been fitted. It is also essential with painful inflammatory conditions to consider the concurrent use of additional therapies.

## March fracture

Although this condition may require orthopaedic intervention in the form of a walking plaster, relief from pain on weight bearing can be achieved in the short term, and sometimes for the duration of the treatment, by means of a 7-mm plantar metatarsal pad with a deep U cut-out over the affected metatarsal and held in place by a strapping.

## Freiberg's infarction

Surgical intervention is rarely attempted for this condition because it requires long-term therapy consisting of removal of pressure from the affected metatarsal head for up to 2 years in order to reduce deformity to a minimum. The optimum therapy is orthotic management, which should take into account not only removal of pressure from the affected area but any biomechanical malalignments that may be present (see also Ch. 4).

In the short term the padding of choice is a plantar metatarsal pad with a U cut-out to the affected metatarsal head, combined with a metatarsal bar to remove as much pressure as possible on weight bearing. It is important that shoe length be adequate and that no back pressure from the phalanx is referred to the metatarsal head. A shoe with a low heel should be advised.

## REFERENCES

Anderson JM, Burrow JG 2001 A small scale study to determine the clinical effectiveness of electrosurgery in the treatment of chronic helomata (corns). The Foot 11(4):189–198.

Alexander NM, Nishimoto M 1981 Protein linkage, iodotyrasines in serum after tropical application of povidone-iodine (Betadine). Journal of Clinical Endocrinology and Metabolism 53:105–108.

Altman PM 1988 Australian tea tree oil. Australian Journal of Pharmacy 69:276–278.

Arca E, Tastan HB, Kurumlu Z, Gur AR 2002 An open, randomized, comparative study of oral fluconazole, itraconazole and terbinafine

therapy in onychomycosis. Journal of Dermatological Treatment 13:3–9.

Ashford R, Lagan K, Baxter D 1995 The effectiveness of combined phototherapy/low intensity laser therapy on a neuropathic foot ulcer. British journal of Therapy & Rehabilitation 2(4).

Ayme EJ, Carstensen EL 1989 Cavitation induced by asymmetric, distorted pulses of ultrasound: a biological test. Ultrasound in Medicine and Biology 15:61–66.

Baxter D 1994 Therapeutic lasers – theory and practice. Churchill Livingstone, Edinburgh.

Benett RG 1988 Fundamentals of cutaneous surgery, Mosby, St Louis, MI, pp 554, 555, 561, 570, 574, 577.

Bennett RG, Kraffert CA 1990 Bacterial transference during electrodesiccation and electrocoagulation. Archives of Dermatology 126:751–755.

Benger S, Townsend P, Ashford RL, Lambert P 2004 An in vitro study to determine the minimum inhibitory concentration of *Melaleuca alternifolia* against the dermatophyte *Trychophyton rubrum*. The Foot 14:86–91.

Benson HAE, McElnay JC 1994 Topical non-steroidal anti-inflammatory products as ultrasound couplants: their potential in phonophoresis. Physiotherapy 80(2):74–76.

Brosseau I, Welch V, Wells G 2004 Low Level Laser for Treating Osteoarthritis. Issue 3 (8) The Cochrane Library.

Broughton RS, Spencer SK 1987 Electrosurgical fundamentals. Dermatological Surgery 16(4):862–867.

Brown JS 1995 Radiosurgery: a new instrument for minor operations. The Practitioner 239:446–448.

Brown JS 2000 Minor surgery – a text and atlas, 4th edn. Chs 17 and 42. Oxford University Press, Oxford.

Broxton P, Woodcock PM, Gilbert P 1984 Interaction of some polyhexamethylene biguanides and membrane phospholipids in Escherichia coli. Journal of Applied Bacteriology 57:115–124.

Bunney MH 1982 Viral warts, their biology and treatment. Oxford University Press, Oxford.

Bunney MH, Nolan MW, Williams DA 1976 An assessment of methods of treating viral warts by comparative treatment trials based on standard design. British Journal of Dermatology 94:667–679.

Carson CF, Riley V 1993 Antimicrobial activity of the essential oil of Melaleuca alternifolia. Letters in Applied Microbiology 16:49–55.

Ceilley RI, Collinson DW 1991 Matricectomy. Journal of Dermatology Surgery and Oncology 18:728–734.

Chang F 1990 Role of human papillomaviruses. Journal of Clinical Pathology 43(4):269–276.

Charman R 1990 Bioelectricity and electrotherapy – towards a new paradigm? Part 2. Cellular reception and emission of electromagnetic signals. Physiotherapy 76(9):509–516.

Cork MJ 1997 The importance of skin barrier function. Journal of Dermatological Treatment 8:S7–S13.

Crawford JS, Lewis M 1986 Nitrous oxide in early human pregnancy. Anaesthesia 41:900–905.

Cresswell CC 1992 Introduction to electrosurgery. Journal of British Podiatric Medicine 47:11–15.

Cuiffo G 1907 Innesto positivo con filtrato di verruca volgare. Giornale Italiano delle Malattie Venere e delle Malattie della Pelle 48:12–17.

Davis GE, Francis J, Martin AR, et al 1954 1:6-Di-4´-chlorophenyldiguanidhexadine (Hibitane). Laboratory investigation of a new antibacterial agent of high potency. British Journal of Pharmacology 9:192–196.

Davis M, Marks R 1976 Studies on the effects of salicylic acid on normal skin. British Journal of Dermatology 95:187–192.

Davis MG, Vella Briffa D, Greaves MW 1979 Systemic toxicity from topically applied salicylic acid. British Medical Journal 1:661.

Dollery C (ed.) 1999 Therapeutic drugs, 2nd edn. Churchill Livingstone, Edinburgh.

Doorbar J, Campbell D, Grand RJA Gallimore PH 1986 Identification of the human papillomavirus-1a E4 gene product. EMBO Journal 5:355–362.

Donaldson D, Meecham JG 1995 The hazards of chronic exposure to nitrous oxide: an update(review). British Dental Journal 178:95–100.

Dyson M, Pond JB 1970 The effect of pulsed ultrasound on tissue regeneration. Physiotherapy 56:136–142.

Ellman International Inc. 2007 Podiatry sell sheet. Ellman International Inc., New York.

Elson JA, Paech MJ 1995 EMLA cream prior to insertion of elective epidurals. Anaesthesia and Intensive Care 23:339–341.

Emmons CW, Bunford CH, Utz JP, et al 1977 Medical mycology, 3rd edn. Lea & Febiger, Philadelphia, PA.

Farndon L, Vernon W, Potter J 2002 The professional role of the podiatrist in the new millennium: an analysis of current practice. Paper 1. British Journal of Podiatry 5(3):68–72.

Frey D, Oldfield RJ, Bridger RC 1977 A colour atlas of pathogenic fungi. Wolfe Medical, London.

Galloway DA 1989 Human papillomaviruses and carcinomas. Advances in Virus Research 37:125–171.

Gann N 1991 Ultrasound: current concepts. Electrotherapy 11(4):64–69.

Goodfield MJD, Andrew L, Evans EGV 1992 Short-term treatment of dermatophyte onychomycosis with terbinafine. British Medical Journal 304:1151–1154.

Hainer BI 1991a Fundamentals of electrosurgery. Journal of the American Board of Family Medicine 4(6):419–426.

Hainer BL 1991b Electrosurgery for cutaneous lesions. American Family Physician Nov(Suppl):81s–90s.

Hettinger D 1997 Soft tissue surgery using radiowave techniques. Journal of the American Podiatric Medical Association 87(3):131–135.

Hettinger D, Valinky MS, Nuccio G, Lim R 1991 Nail matrixectomies using radio wave technique. Journal of the American Podiatric Medical Association 81(6):317–321.

Holden C, English J, Hoare C 2002 Advised best practice for the use of emollients in eczema and other dry skin conditions. Journal of Dermatological Treatment 13:103–106.

Howley PM 1988 The human papillomaviruses: an overview. American Journal of Medicine 85:155–158.

IEC 2009 Medical electrical equipment – Part 1: General requirements for basic safety and essential performance. IEC 60601-1, Edition 3.0. International Electrotechnical Commission, Geneva.

Kitchen S 2002 Electrotherapy: evidence based practice. Churchill Livingstone, Edinburgh.

Laughlin SA, Dudley DK 1992 Electrosurgery. Clinics in Dermatology 10:283–290.

Lehmann JF, DeLateur BJ 1990 Therapeutic heat. In: Lehmann JF (ed.) Therapeutic heat and cold, 4th edn. Davis, Philadelphia, PA, pp 417–581.

Lelliott PE, Robinson C 1999 A retrospective study to evaluate verrucae regrowth following electrosurgery. British Journal of Podiatry 2(3):84–88.

Lowbury EL, Lilly HA 1973 Use of 4% chlorhexidine detergent solution (Hibiscrub) and other methods of disinfection. British Medical Journal 1:510–515.

Magnetopulse Systems Manual. Magnetopulse Systems Ltd, Northampton.

Maness WL, Roeber RF et al 1978 Histological Evaluation of Electrosurgery with Varying Frequency and Wave Form. Journal of Prosthetic Dentistry 40:304.

Martindale 1999 The Extra Pharmacopoeia, In: Parfitt K (Ed.) The Pharmaceutical Press, London.

Maxwell L 1992 Therapeutic ultrasound: its effects on the cellular and molecular mechanisms of inflammation and repair. Physiotherapy 78(6):421–426.

McHenry PM, Williams HC, Bingham EA 1995 Management of atopic eczema. Joint Workshops of the British Association of Dermatologists and the Research Unit of the Royal College of Physicians of London. British Medical Journal 310:843–847.

Niamtu J 2001 Making Waves. Plastic Surgery Products. pp 52-58.

Oakley EM 1987 Dangers and contraindications of therapeutic ultrasound. Physiotherapy 64(6):173.

Payne J 1891 On the contagious rise of common warts. British Journal of Dermatology 3:185.

Podiatry Now 1999a The aftermath of Woolf. Editorial. Podiatry Now 2(7):219.

Podiatry Now 1999b A cautionary tale. Editorial. Podiatry Now 2(8):255.

Read PJ 1978 An introduction to therapeutics for chiropodists. Actinic Press, London.

Robertson VJ, Ward AR 1996 Limited interchangeability of methods of applying 1 MHz ultrasound. Archives of Physiotherapy, Medicine and Rehabilitation 77:379–384.

Sebben JE 1988a Electrosurgery: high frequency modalities. Journal of Dermatological Surgery and Oncology 14(4):367–371.

Sebben JE 1988b Electrosurgery principles: cutting current and cutaneous surgery – Part 1. Journal of Dermatologic Surgery and Oncology 14(1):29–31.

Sebben JE 1989 Cutaneous electrosurgery. Year Book Medical Publishers, Baltimore, OH.

Shupp DY, Schroeter AL 1986 An unusual case of salicylate toxicity. Journal of the American Academy of Dermatology 15:300–301.

Spencer WG 1961 Cornelius of Celous (AD 25) De Medicina (English trans. from original

Italian), Vol. II. Heinemann, London, pp. 160–163.

Stedman's Medical Dictionary 1990 25th edn. Williams and Wilkins, Baltimore, OH, p. 498.

Strauss, MJ, Bunting MD, Melnick JL 1950 Virus like particles and inclusion bodies in skin papillomas. Journal of Investigative Dermatology 15: 433.

Tupker RA, Willis C, Berardesca E 1997 Guidelines on sodium lauryl sulphate (SLS) exposure tests. A Report from the Standardisation Group of the European Society of Contact Dermatitis. Contact Dermatitis 37:53–69.

Turner J, Hode L 2002 Laser therapy – clinical practice and scientific background. Prima Books, London.

Valinsky MS, Hettinger DF, Gennett PM 1990 Treatment of verrucae via radio wave surgery. Journal of the American Podiatric Medical Association 80,(9):482–488.

Walsh LJ, Longstaff J 1987 The antimicrobial effects of an essential oil on selected oral pathogens. Periodontology 8:11–15.

Watts WD 1968 An unoriginal treatment for plantar warts. The Chiropodist 23(12):454–455.

Whinfield A, Forster M 1998 The effect of electrodesiccation on pain intensity associated with chronic heloma durum. The Foot 7: 224–228.

Wilkinson AN, Kilmartin TEA 1998 Study into the long term effectiveness of electrosurgery for the treatment of corns. British Journal of Podiatric Medicine 1(4):138–141.

Wynne A, Whitefield M, Dixon AJ, Anderson S 2002 An effective, cosmetically acceptable, novel hydrogel emollient for the management of dry skin conditions. Journal of Dermatological Treatment 13:61–66.

Wyre HW, Stolar R 1977 Extirpation of warts by a loop electrode and cutting current. Journal of Dermatologic Surgery and Oncology 3(5):520–522.

Wyss O, Strandskov F 1945 The germicidal action of iodine. Archives of Biochemistry 6:261–267.

Young SR, Dyson M 1990 Macrophage responsiveness to therapeutic ultrasound. Ultrasound Medical Biology 16:809–816.

Zuber TJ 2002 Ingrown toenail removal. American Family Physician 65:2547–2550, 2551–2552, 2554, 2557–2558.

## FURTHER READING

Watson T 2008 Electrotherapy: evidence based practice, 12th edn. Churchill Livingstone, Elsevier

Robertson V, Ward A, Low J, Reed A 2006 Electrotherapy explained. Principles and practices, 4th edn. Butterworth Heinemann, Edinburgh.

# Chapter | 17 |

# Orthoses

*James A Black and Ian Mathieson*

**KEYWORDS**

CAD-CAM
Casted insoles
Chairside technique
Digital appliances
Functional orthoses
Heel orthoses
Hot-water plastics
Insoles
Low-temperature moulding
Non-casted insoles
Orthoses
Orthotic laboratories
Prefabricated orthoses
Proprioceptive paradigm
Prostheses
Rapid remoulding
Replaceable pads
Root paradigm
Sagittal plane paradigm
Shoe modifications
Silicones
Thermoplastics
Tissue stress paradigm

Whilst podiatrists commonly use a variety of clinical therapies, there is one particular therapeutic technique with which podiatry, and podiatrists, have become almost synonymous: orthoses. Although patients and the public probably think of some insole derivative when they hear the term 'orthosis', it actually encompasses a broader range of devices, which includes silicone orthodigita, digital covers, latex shields and replaceable pads as well as the functional devices that dominate the literature concerning orthoses. Historically, these devices were manufactured by podiatrists themselves. Modern clinicians, however, have a range of good-quality, mass-manufactured

**435**

devices at their disposal, which has reduced their reliance on their own manufacturing skills. The devices available range from silicone digital and plantar pads to prefabricated functional orthoses. The availability of such devices has perhaps led to some marginalising of skills of manufacture, for perfectly understandable reasons.

While this chapter will provide insight into some key issues surrounding functional orthoses – including emerging paradigms that influence orthosis design and the role of prefabricated devices – it is also written for those practitioners who still derive much professional satisfaction from manufacturing a range of individually designed orthotic devices that allows them to exercise close personal management of their patients' condition. This management ranges from the initial consultation to either partial or complete resolution of the condition. The inclusion of partial resolution recognises that in many cases (e.g. the chronic rheumatoid foot) resolution is not possible but restoration of some functional capacity and improvements in pain is the best that can be achieved. It is hoped that this exposure to a variety of historical techniques will inspire a new range of practitioners to become involved in manufacturing orthoses themselves, not necessarily on a permanent basis, but so as to facilitate a deeper understanding and awareness of the range of devices that a skilled clinician can use to their patients' benefit.

The use of orthoses is based on the premise that most foot problems have some mechanical factors involved in their aetiology or symptomatology. This might be some congenital variation in the structure of the foot and leg, be that bony or soft tissue, the result of a disease process such as rheumatoid arthritis, or due to neuropathy. In all cases the basic treatment philosophy remains the same: pain or pathology resulting from abnormal foot mechanics can be controlled only by mechanical means. This may be achieved by altering structure by surgical intervention to realign bones or to improve soft-tissue function, for example through gastrocnemius release to enhance ankle dorsiflexion and 'rocker' function, or through the use of an orthosis to actively optimise the biomechanical function of the foot and lower limb. There is a growing awareness that, in many situations, combined surgical and orthotic management provides the best treatment plan, and indeed podiatrists are now routinely involved in interdisciplinary musculoskeletal clinics where, for example, a surgeon may operate to create an environment where the orthosis provided by the podiatrist has a better chance of success in the long run, and where this likelihood is increased by enhancement of postoperative function through physiotherapy.

While the derivation of the word 'orthosis' seems obviously associated with the Greek 'orthos' meaning 'straight', Rose (1986) asserts that the origin of the word is actually more obscure. Accepting the term 'prosthesis' as an older word of 'respectable' Greek origin meaning 'in addition', and defining a device that is a replacement or substitute part, he suggests 'orthosis' to be a portmanteau derived from the terms 'orthopaedics' and 'prosthesis', in much the same way that 'smog' is a combination of 'smoke' and 'fog'. Whatever the origin of the term it is widely used and accepted' and it is more important that a definition be provided. The recent focus on functional orthoses may lead to the type of definition provided by Philps (1995) or Anthony (1991), but these can only be applied to functional devices, and so are too exclusive. By contrast, Rose (1986) adopted an inclusive definition, which encompasses a broader range of devices and is much more appealing:

> *A device applied direct and externally to the patient's body with the object of supporting, correcting, or compensating for an anatomical deformity or weakness, however caused. It may be applied with the additional object of assisting, allowing or restricting movement of the body.*

(Rose 1986, pp 6–7)

This definition may be applied to all forms of appliances that have a corrective function, but also to those devices that primarily accommodate and protect deformities without correcting them, for example a hallux abducto valgus shield. Although there is a temptation to divide orthoses into the categories *functional* and *palliative*, many devices combine these functions according to the nature of the pathology and the severity and duration of the mechanical abnormality, such that this division becomes somewhat arbitrary and artificial. An appliances that replaces missing parts, whether this be due to disease, trauma or surgery, is termed a *prosthesis*.

Where correction is possible, even if only partial, the corrective element should take precedence over the protective element, and this consideration determines the choice of materials. Considerable force is often required to correct even a simple deformity, such as a hammer toe, or to manage major deformation, such as abnormal pronation, from occurring under load. The more rigid the material the better its splinting properties, but the lower its tolerance to wear by the patient; it must be remembered that a 100% corrective orthosis is perhaps desirable to the practitioner, but if resigned to the back of the cupboard it will be 100% ineffective, and the practitioner must bear this in mind. It is good practice to build up the wear of an orthosis gradually, but if problems persist despite a prolonged break-in period it may have to be acknowledged that too ambitious an orthosis has been selected.

The plastics used in functional orthoses can be simply classified according to their ability to resist stress according to their thermoforming temperature. The higher the temperature at which they become malleable, the stronger they are; the lower the temperature, the more likely they are to deform under load. However, the thickness of the plastic is also of considerable importance and there is a direct association between rigidity and thickness. More recently introduced are carbon fibre composite materials that offer the practitioner a light, thin and flexible alternative. However, they are difficult to use, requiring a higher forming temperature and a shorter working time, so that the vacuum former must have a rapid action.

Orthoses need to be designed so that they are both tolerable in wear and optimally effective in their therapeutic design. Accommodative appliances, such as latex shields, are used in established deformities to protect vulnerable tissues from trauma and, to some extent, to limit painful movement. They may not correct the underlying fault, but they make it tolerable by relieving painful symptoms and controlling secondary lesions. They are more flexible than rigid, and usually can be well tolerated from the beginning. In some cases it may be useful to use an accommodative orthosis first before moving onto a more functional, corrective one.

Orthoses are worn either on the foot or within footwear and, as such, no matter how well designed and accurately prescribed, manufactured and fitted they may be, their effect is dependent on appropriate footwear. Orthoses and footwear must be considered together if the optimal outcome is to be achieved. The footwear must be of the correct size and shape, have adequate internal volume in the right places, and be correctly balanced both mediolaterally and anteroposteriorly. Modifications to footwear may be necessary to ensure these points. It is a sound principle that patients purchase their shoes after the orthosis is fitted. Heel height is of critical importance when fitting a functional orthosis. If heel height is such that the normal relationship between the forefoot and rearfoot is disturbed, then the shoe is totally unsuited for use with the orthosis. The range of stock orthopaedic shoes now available is such that an attractive shoe at a reasonable cost offers the opportunity to provide a comprehensive orthosis and shoe regimen for many pathologies and situations. Stock shoes have the added advantage that they often come with an insole system that can be removed to facilitate the fitting of prescribed orthoses. A review of footwear is provided in Chapter 18.

Orthotic technology is constantly developing as new materials and techniques are introduced and a greater understanding of foot mechanics evolves. Only a brief summary of its main aspects is possible here, and further reading is recommended to develop a comprehensive understanding of the subject.

## PRINCIPLES OF MANAGEMENT

It is essential that practitioners develop a sound working knowledge of the materials and techniques available in order to offer their patients a complete service, even if this is to be provided by an orthosis manufacturing laboratory. At the outset of treatment a management plan should be devised in consultation with the patient, and this should encompass the rationale for orthosis therapy and also the concept that other treatments are likely to be necessary, many of which require the active participation of the patient. This includes, for example, accepting advice on footwear, undertaking exercises such as stretching and strengthening, modification of activity, undergoing anti-inflammatory therapies such as ultrasound or low-power laser treatment, and losing weight, to name some. The way that all these treatments fit together must be explained in the context of the pathology that is present, and the role of the orthosis should be emphasised. In a 'prescription culture', the orthosis can take the place of the pill, and other advice ignored in the hope that all that is really required is to wear something or slip something into a shoe. Patients have a right to know what the practitioner has in mind for their treatment, and they should have a clear indication of how long this might take, the extent of improvement in the condition and, in the private sector, the costs involved. Prescribed functional orthoses can cost as much as designer spectacles and the practitioner has a duty of care to maximise the chances of success.

If this is accepted as a reasonable principle of patient management, then it is incumbent upon the practitioner to be able to offer the best possible treatment advice. If the practitioner is unable to provide this the patient should be referred to a clinician with the necessary equipment and skills. Not every patient needs an orthosis, but where this is an integral part of the treatment, patient management and patient awareness of the treatment plan and any possible sequelae must be explained. This is particularly important with regard to the emergence of new paradigms of foot function influencing orthosis design, which has resulted in variations in practice. It is more vital than ever that the management plan and its rationale are explained fully to the patient in order to maximise the chance of success and minimise the risk of dissatisfaction, which can lead to claims of medical negligence.

Before embarking on the treatment plan, certain considerations are important. The physical characteristics of the patient must be assessed, including height, weight and mobility, and also the presence of physical disability that might preclude the use of certain types of orthoses. For example, if the patient is blind he or she may find it difficult to position the orthoses or move them between shoes. In such circumstances a 'locator' might be required, to enable the patient to differentiate left from right and to position the orthosis correctly in the shoe by touch. Should the patient have any physical disability that prevents him or her from reaching the feet, orthoses that require careful positioning would also be unsuitable. In such circumstances a full-length orthosis that shares the same dimensions of the shoe insole would be easier to fit.

A summary of the points to consider when prescribing orthoses was provided by Anthony (1991), and these key questions remain relevant and should be considered every time orthotic therapy is considered:

1. Are you confident that there is a relationship between the presenting pathology and the foot function abnormality you are correcting with orthoses? If not, then how can you justify your approach?
2. Can the foot dysfunction be controlled enough to influence symptoms? Some more severe foot function abnormalities will be extremely difficult to control fully and the amount of control required to improve symptoms should be considered.
3. Will the patient's footwear accommodate the orthoses? As discussed earlier, the orthosis can be enhanced by the correct footwear and fatally compromised by the wrong footwear. Whenever the practitioner is concerned over the suitability of footwear, a more appropriate style should be recommended and the advice recorded in the notes. Failure to comply with such advice explains the failure of orthotic therapy in many cases.
4. Is the patient likely to comply with your advice – fully? Many of our patients pick and choose what advice to pay attention to and it is vital to work with patients to ensure that all recommendations are followed to ensure the optimal treatment outcome.
5. Does the patient have unrealistic expectations? If a tendon has been painful for 2 years then it is unlikely that it will be asymptomatic within 4 weeks when training for that next marathon needs to commence. Providing information on tissue turnover times can help to reinforce this concept: if the patient knows that tenocyte turnover time is more than 50 days it helps them to understand the length of rehabilitation period required.
6. Are any additional measures required? Orthoses should not be viewed as a 'silver bullet' that in isolation can manage a range of disorders. Rather, they should be seen as one of a series of treatments that in combination can help to reduce pain and symptoms and improve function.

In addition to these questions, the effect that the materials may have on the patient's foot warrants consideration, given the hostile in-shoe environment and the length of time for which shoes and orthoses will be worn. The potential for irritation and allergy, and the stability of the material in its working environment all influence material choice, as exemplified in the case of neuropathy. When all these factors have been considered, then orthotic therapy can be initiated, and this may involve a range of devices, from simple padding to full functional orthoses.

## REPLACEABLE PADS

The simplest extensions of padding and strapping to more permanent orthoses are replaceable pads. These devices take many forms and are usually held in place with elasticised bands positioned around the toes and/or foot (Figs 17.1-17.3). Before embarking on the use of a replaceable pad, the practitioner will usually try to design the clinical padding and assess its potential effectiveness. The role of clinical padding in this form is often undervalued, and substantial biomechanical control can be achieved with the skilful use of clinical padding materials either attached to the foot or positioned in the shoe. Manufacture is straightforward, and devices may be made in a variety of materials, depending on the physical properties required. A device may be required simply to replace atrophied fatty padding. Such devices are protective in nature and a material is selected on the basis of its ability to resist compression over time. Newer viscoelastic foams are much more effective in resisting compressive stress than materials derived from rubber. Table 17.1 lists some materials and

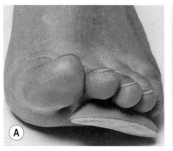 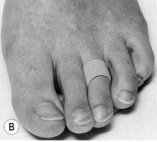

Figure 17.1 (A, B) Replaceable long prop.

**Table 17.1** Percentage strain of a variety of padding materials used in orthoses and prostheses[1]

| Sample | Load (kg) | % Strain | Load (kg) | % Strain |
| --- | --- | --- | --- | --- |
| PPT | 20 | 87.10 | 40 | 98.39 |
| Poron | 20 | 75.61 | 40 | 87.80 |
| Grey latex foam | 20 | 61.29 | 40 | 80.65 |
| NCCR | 20 | 80.39 | 40 | 98.04 |
| Clocell | 20 | 70.00 | 40 | 78.33 |

[1]All the samples were 7 mm thick and tests were carried out for 3 hours in an Instron, a device used to quantify the elasticity of materials. The percentage strain indicates the degree of deformation of the material under stress.

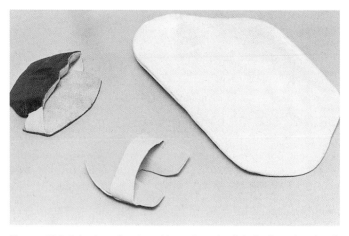

Figure 17.2 Selection of replaceable pads: orthodigital splint; dorsal pad for interphalangeal joint; Hexcelite valgus support covered in latex foam.

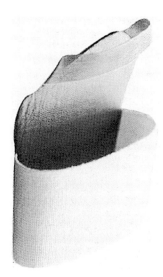

Figure 17.3 Metatarsal brace with toe-loop.

illustrates their compressibility and percentage relaxation under compressive stress.

Forces acting on the foot can be managed in one of two ways: (a) by absorbing force in such a way that the material decelerates the rate at which the forces act on the foot – this is shock absorption; (b) by increasing the surface area to which the force is applied. It must be remembered that the orthosis should be placed in such a position that during foot-flat and heel-off the maximum area is in contact with the ground.

Technological advances in materials have provided a new range of viscoelastic products that provide effective cushioning or dampen ground reaction forces. These materials, such as Sorbothane and Viscolas or silicone polymer, allow podiatrists to provide the patient with high-quality shock absorption without recourse to cutting, shaping or covering replaceable orthoses. However, such viscoelastic materials can be heavier than traditional cushioning materials, and this could be important if supplying orthoses to sports people or those with established rheumatoid foot disease. Sheets of silicone rubber are now available in varying thicknesses and have proved most effective in the treatment of plantar keratomas or lesions over pressure areas on the toes.

Replaceable digital orthoses may also be manufactured by the same process as used for plantar devices. However, practitioners may find that the effectiveness of digital orthoses is governed by their ability to remain in place, and secure anchoring is essential. Figure 17.1 illustrates a long prop; it is important that an assessment of the amount of movement in the interphalangeal and metatarsophalangeal joints is assessed before embarking on manufacture. Digital devices may conform to virtually any shape, provided the principle has been first assessed with conventional padding.

## ELASTIC ANKLETS AND BRACELETS

An elastic anklet is useful as an alternative to figure-of-eight strapping when continuing support is required for an unstable rearfoot. Commercial devices are readily available and, while quality and price vary, there are some excellent products available. They may be used with a tarsal platform or tarsal cradle fitted into the shoe or onto an insole. A buttressed heel may also be indicated for greater ankle stability.

A metatarsal brace is an elastic bandage encircling the metatarsus, and it usually includes a plantar metatarsal pad. Commercial varieties are limited by the ability of standardised dimensions to match satisfactorily the anatomy of individual patients. However, such braces can be easily manufactured using elastic webbing or elastic net. Both materials are available in various widths, and it is advantageous to be able to design both brace and padding according to individual needs. The metatarsal brace may often be combined with a toe loop or with orthodigital splints where correction and/or protection of the digits is also desired (Fig. 17.3).

There is now available a plethora of elasticised supports specifically designed for use in sport. As people become more intent on improving their fitness and using sport as a means to better health, sportswear manufacturers have met the demand by producing supports for all joints that could possibly be stressed by sporting activity. These are usually available from pharmacists or sports shops. The most popular range of supports are those manufactured from neoprene, but care is required when fitting these devices.

## INSOLES

Virtually any pathological condition affecting the plantar surface of the foot can be controlled by appropriate insoles, provided that sufficient depth is available in the footwear. It is essential that this requirement be considered whenever specially made footwear is ordered. With normal footwear, every effort must be made to save bulk by the choice of material, and by stopping the insole just behind or just in front of the metatarsal heads, depending on requirements. There are two basic types of insole:

- simple, non-casted, insoles, which essentially act as longer term padding
- contoured orthoses made to individual or averaged casts or models of the foot.

### Non-casted insoles

Non-casted insoles are manufactured in such a way that they form part of the shoe. The first prerequisite is the production of a template to the size and shape of the insole of the shoe. From this template the base material of the insole is then shaped accordingly and placed in the shoe. The anatomy to which the padding will conform must be transferred onto this base, and this can be done in various ways. Firstly, the anatomy can be palpated and coloured and the patient then allowed to walk in their shoes without socks for a few minutes so that marks are transferred to the base material. This provides a quasi-static impression, which may not be far enough forward. Therefore, if this method is used, the padding should be moved slightly further forward to allow for the greater elongation that occurs during more vigorous dynamic activities. A better technique involves taking a dynamic impression where a material such as leatherboard is used for the insole and the patient asked to walk for up to 2 weeks in them to transfer the pressure points to the insole. Whichever technique is used, template fit to the shoe is critical, because any movement will compromise the location of padding in relation to the foot and may compromise treatment success. From the wear marks provided on the template, appropriate padding can be designed that conforms exactly to the required anatomy. This is then adhered to the base, covered with a leather or synthetic covering and fitted to the shoe. Figure 17.4 shows the construction of a simple insole, without its top cover. It is also possible simply to remove the insole from the shoe, incorporate appropriate padding and replace the insole into the shoe. This technique helps ensure appropriate fit and padding placement.

### Casted insoles

Insoles made to a cast may be accommodative orthoses, which are designed to support and protect feet that have deformities that cannot be corrected, or functional orthoses, which are designed to encourage improved mechanical function of the foot and lower limb.

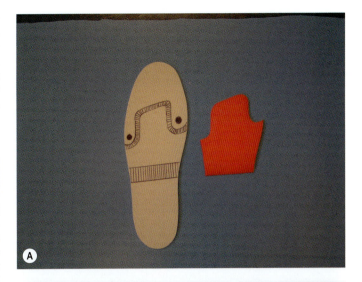

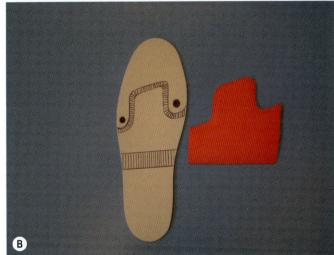

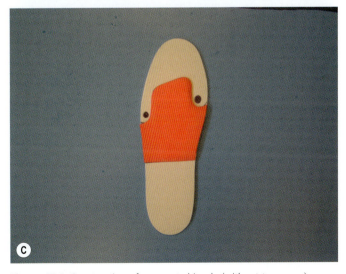

**Figure 17.4** Construction of non-casted insole (without top cover).

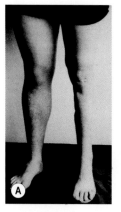
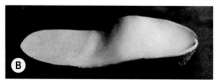
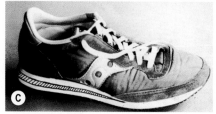

**Figure 17.5** Casted insole. (A) A 1.5-inch (3.8 cm) shortening of the left leg after an accident. (B) Orthosis in cork/latex compound gives 1-inch (2.5 cm) heel raise. (C) Orthosis is worn in running shoe fitted with additional raise to the midsole (hatched).

Accommodative orthoses are normally prescribed for conditions where joint pathology renders correction impossible. A large number of acquired and congenital deformities fall into this category. Figure 17.5 shows an accommodative insole manufactured for a patient injured in a motorcycle accident. His knee is fused and he presents with an ankle equinus and shortening of one leg by 3.8 cm (1.5 inches). The object of the insole is to load the maximum amount of foot surface contact area by filling in the exaggerated arch with a cork/latex compound. Birko cork and ethyl vinyl acetate (EVA) foams are excellent materials for this purpose. They provide a flexible support and also incorporate forefoot padding to reduce pressure under the first and fifth metatarsal heads. In the case of a cork orthosis, a mix of cork, leather dust and fine wood flour are mixed with latex to produce a porridge, which is then spread onto the cast and, after curing, is ground to the required dimensions to fit the foot and the shoe. This is an older technique, and in contemporary practice EVA would be heated to its thermoforming temperature and then vacuum formed over the cast – a much less messy technique. In the case illustrated the orthosis was fitted into a running shoe because such shoes have the features characteristic of a good shoe. The midsole has an extra piece added to it to reduce the limb-length difference further, as only small deficits can be addressed inside the shoe due to space constraints.

EVA seems to be the material of choice for most accommodative orthoses, either on its own or laminated with other materials, as it is cheap, easy to work, has a good thermoforming temperature and is available in a range of densities and thicknesses. This offers the practitioner the ability to provide light, durable, low-cost devices. Such devices are particularly useful for treating the established rheumatoid or diabetic foot, or for sporting situations where full-length devices are required, such as in skiing.

## FUNCTIONAL ORTHOSES

Functional orthoses are very popular, and are in routine use in the management of a whole host of disorders of the foot, ankle, lower limbs and even more proximally. Historically, there has been an emphasis on 'motion control', this concept originating from the perception that excessive motion, typically pronation, should be controlled aggressively to address symptoms fully. This approach has its origins in the Root model of clinical biomechanics (Root et al 1971,

1977), which promoted the control of abnormal motion as the means by which to reduce symptomatology.

The Root model has dominated clinical practice for a number of years, and has influenced research efforts that have attempted to identify the influence of orthoses on, for example, variables such as maximum calcaneal eversion and eversion velocity (Novick & Kelley 1990), and patellar glide position (Klingman et al 1997). Novick and Kelley (1990) identified significant changes in these variables, while Klingman et al (1997) found that patellar position was influenced by rearfoot posting, and this was assumed to represent the mechanism by which orthoses exerted their function. However, the importance of motion control has been challenged, and a body of research with conflicting findings has built up. For example, Zammit and Payne (2007) investigated the relationship between the degree of frontal plane rearfoot control and changes in symptoms. Despite finding a significant relationship, the actual change in the amount of motion taking place was small and suboptimal, leading to the conclusion that changes in rearfoot control are insufficient to explain the extent of symptom reduction observed. They suggested that orthoses may exert their influence via another mechanism. This conclusion is supported by other research findings. For example, Johansen et al (1994) found that an unposted orthotic shell reduced the extent of pronation by just as much as orthoses posted at rearfoot, forefoot or both. Such contradictions led Heiderscheit et al (2001) to claim that, while orthoses are an accepted and acknowledged part of the treatment of a variety of disorders, the bigger question relates to how they function.

This issue of how orthoses function was considered by Lee (2001), who discussed at length the different paradigms of foot function that currently exist. In this context a paradigm is a model, or clinical system of approach, which explains, amongst other things, mechanical foot function, how it integrates with the lower-limb kinetic chain, the origins and consequences of abnormal function, and the means by which to correct this function. Popular paradigms worthy of discussion are the Root, sagittal plane, proprioceptive (preferred motion pathway) and tissue-stress paradigms. It should be noted that, consistent with the remit of this book, what follows is merely a brief introduction to what is a complex and extensive subject, and the interested reader should gather the references cited to begin to develop a wider appreciation of the issues involved. These references provide accounts of the individual paradigms; they do not necessarily represent the first published account of the technique.

## The Root paradigm

The Root paradigm focuses on the importance of the subtalar joint functioning around the neutral subtalar joint position in promoting optimal function of the foot and lower-limb musculoskeletal chain. While acknowledging that abnormal function may arise from a variety of neuromusculoskeletal abnormalities such as motor neuropathy, gastrosoleus ankle equinus or tibia varum, the model has become closely associated with the influence of bony alignment on foot function. Frontal, transverse and sagittal plane anomalies at various segments (e.g. forefoot, rearfoot, ankle, lower leg and knee) that were thought to influence foot function were described. A biomechanical examination technique was developed to assess each segment so that abnormality could be identified and an orthosis designed, and this examination still heavily influences clinical practice. The focus of the orthoses manufactured according to this paradigm characteristically incorporates frontal plane posting to influence the rearfoot and midfoot.

Problems with the Root paradigm include the importance of neutral subtalar joint function and the validity and reliability of the measurements associated with the biomechanical assessment (Keenan 1997).

While problems associated with goniometry are associated with every discipline that utilises such techniques of clinical assessment, the value of the subtalar joint neutral position is of greater interest. The Root model asserts that in normal subjects the subtalar joint functions around the subtalar joint neutral position, but this is not supported by a series of recent research studies that tracked rearfoot motion in normal, healthy subjects (Cornwall & McPoil 1999, McPoil & Cornwall 1994, Pierrynowski & Smith 1996). These studies have repeatedly identified that normal subtalar joint motion – as represented by frontal plane calcaneal function – involves eversion from an initial inverted position, and a failure to reinvert until after heel lift. It should now be accepted that promoting a *less* pronated, as opposed to neutral, functional position should be the goal the majority of the time. A notable exception is in the case of early rheumatoid arthritis, where Woodburn et al (2002) identified that aggressive orthoses may control the development of the valgus hindfoot, which is central to the pro-found problem of foot pathology in this disease. This concept may be transferable to other destructive arthropathies and tendinopathies.

## The sagittal plane paradigm

The sagittal plane paradigm is based on rocker theory, proposed by Perry (1992), which asserts that forward progression is dependent on optimal sagittal plane function around three pivot points (rockers) in the foot (Fig. 17.6): the posterior aspect of the calcaneus, the ankle joint, and the metatarsophalangeal joints. The paradigm proposes that it is through the sagittal function about these three fulcrums that the centre of mass of the body is efficiently transported forward. Bojsen-Moller (1979) developed this model when he realised that the normal metatarsal parabola, formed because the normal second metatarsal is longer than the first, results in two forefoot axes that cannot be used simultaneously (Fig. 17.6). His experiments to determine the

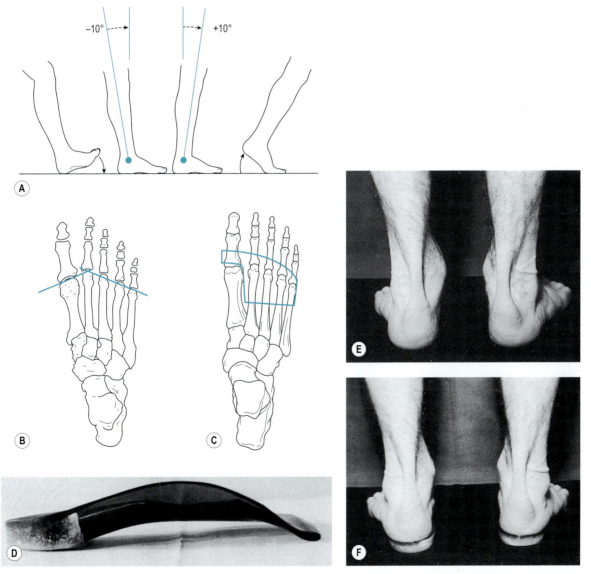

**Figure 17.6** Sagittal plane and Root paradigm orthoses. Diagram a demonstrates the three Rockers which facilitate efficient forward motion. In diagram b the two possible propulsive axes that can be used in the forefoot are shown. The transverse axis – connecting MTPJt's 1 & 2 – is associated with stable and efficient propulsion, and the blue pad outline shown in c illustrates a pad that will permit 1st ray plantarflexion, which is coupled with 1st MTPJt dorsiflexion, thereby encouraging transverse axis function. Orthoses made using the Sagittal plane paradigm are less aggressively posted that those focusing on frontal plane correction, and example of which is shown in d. The aim of such orthoses is shown in diagrams e and f, whereby the relaxed calcaneal stance position is moved towards neutral by the frontal plane posting applied.

functional differences between these two forefoot, propulsive rockers suggested that when load is transmitted medially through the first and second metatarsophalangeal joints there are a number of benefits. These include a more efficient windlass mechanism due to the larger diameter of the first metatarsal head leading to more effective resupination and stabilisation of the calcaneocuboid joint. The model was developed further by Dananberg (1993a,b), who suggested that normal first metatarsophalangeal function was vital to normal hip extension, which preserves the normal energy exchange between the upper limbs and the lower limbs that occurs through reciprocating pelvic motion. Dananberg (1995) also designed an orthosis expressly aimed at encouraging normal first metatarsophalangeal joint function, on the basis that this motion helps to restore various 'auto-support' mechanisms that are vital to optimal gait function. These orthoses are useful where a normal range of first metatarsophalangeal joint motion is present during non-weight bearing, but not used dynamically, a situation referred to as functional hallux limitus. Where there is a structural hallux limitus such orthoses are of no benefit, but rocker-bottom shoes may instead be useful. It is interesting that footwear that encourages improved sagittal plane function is now available, in the form of Masai Barefoot Technology footwear and Nike Free Trainers. This may reflect wide acceptance of this model of foot function, and certainly helps its profile.

## The proprioceptive, preferred-motion-pathway paradigm

Perhaps the most revolutionary paradigm is the proprioceptive, preferred-motion-pathway paradigm proposed by Nigg (2001). In this model, impact forces are considered as input signals that 'tune' muscles to modify their activity in the subsequent step to minimise soft-tissue vibration and reduce joint/tendon loading. This paradigm directly challenges motion-control approaches, stating that although orthoses aim to realign the skeleton they produce only small changes, and the important factor is the influence that these orthoses, or shoes, have on muscle activity in terms of their ability to reduce energy cost. This energy-cost reduction is the common characteristic of a successful orthosis. The model can be summarised as follows (adapted from Nigg (2001)):

- forces acting on the foot during stance act as input signals
- muscles respond to these signals by modifying their function in the subsequent step
- the cost function of these adaptations may increase or reduce stress on specific tissues
- for an intervention to be successful it should support the preferred-motion pathway; that is, it should reduce the energy cost and decrease the stress on tissues
- therefore, orthoses or shoes affect general muscle activity, and thus fatigue, comfort, work and performance.

This paradigm is interesting because it potentially explains the apparent success of a range of different orthoses manufactured using different materials and employing different theoretical principles. As such, it deserves further investigation.

## The tissue-stress paradigm

The tissue-stress paradigm was first proposed by McPoil and Hunt (1995) in response to deficiencies in the Root paradigm that they felt insurmountable. These deficits were described as: (a) the reliability of the measurement procedures, (b) the criteria for normal foot alignment, and (c) dynamic subtalar joint function. Taking an entirely pragmatic perspective, they suggested that the focus of treatment should not be dominated by a mechanical model, but rather should

focus on the presenting pathology, based on the assumption that excess stress was being placed on a tissue and the optimal treatment strategy involves reducing this stress by a variety of means. Although the process set out contains several steps, it can be summarised briefly as follows:

1. Identify the tissue that is painful. This is the tissue that is having excess stress applied to it.
2. If it is a mechanical-based problem, then footwear modifications and/or orthoses may be useful. However, these should not be made expressly to control motion, but rather to reduce the stresses being applied to the painful tissues. A good example is the management of medial knee osteoarthritis, where laterally posted orthoses, which may further pronate the foot, are suggested to be useful (Sasaki & Yasuda 1987).
3. In addition to orthoses, other treatments are likely to be indicated. This includes optimising muscle strength, balance and flexibility, and using physical therapies to enhance the healing process. Activity modification and a subsequent staged return to activity is also likely to be required.

The tissue-stress approach asserts that orthoses are part of a wider treatment approach, and an important point is that any orthoses used should provide only the control that is required to reduce stress on the affected tissue to a tolerable level so that healing can take place – as opposed to the pursuit of a theoretically ideal position.

While various other paradigms exist, those discussed above represent the main competing theories. Others, such as Kirby's medial subtalar axis model (Kirby 2001), may have been referred to as a paradigm but essentially represents a technique by which frontal plane subtalar joint control can be enhanced. It therefore represents a development of the Root paradigm. There is an overlap between Kirby's work and that of Close et al (1967), who presented a 'classification of the foot based on the medial deviation of the subtalar axis', which not only mirrors Kirby's thoughts but also describes the normal foot as being 'somewhat pronated', pre-empting the findings of McPoil and Cornwall (1994, 1999) and Pierrynowski and Smith (1996), and further strengthening the argument that normal subtalar joint function does not hinge on the neutral position. What goes around comes around!

## Paradigms in practice: reconciling the controversy of foot function paradigms

The existence of various paradigms fuels deep and prolonged debates amongst enthusiastic academics and clinicians, but may alienate many others. There is clearly a need to resolve these issues in a pragmatic manner that enhances clinical practice. What follows is a simple clinical guide that may help the clinician reconcile some of the issues and encourage him or her to prescribe orthoses utilising a variety of concepts.

1. The tissue-stress paradigm provides an overarching concept that should be central to practice. Focus on the presenting pathology, diagnose and understand it, and critically evaluate its association with the abnormal foot function present in the individual patient.
2. Identify the plane of origin of the abnormal foot function. This critical step is based on the premise that abnormal foot function can result from abnormalities that exist in various body planes.
3. If the primary influence on foot function is a frontal plane abnormality, for example a tibial varum, then the compensation for that deformity is abnormal pronation. The Root paradigm seems useful here. Orthoses posted in the frontal plane seem logically to be the way to control this abnormal motion.

4. If the primary influence on foot function is a sagittal plane abnormality, for example ankle equinus, then this is the factor driving abnormal foot function. Such compensations manifest in midstance, when ankle dorsiflexion is required to permit forward progression of the centre of mass. In such cases, excess pronation can be secondary to disrupted sagittal plane progression. Facilitating sagittal plane motion seems most appropriate here, and this might involve an orthosis incorporating a heel raise to enhance the ankle rocker and a first-ray cut-out or kinetic wedge (a device patented by Dananberg that is used to encourage first metatarsophalangeal joint function), as well as ankle and foot mobilisations to encourage free motion.

5. An overarching principle is that orthoses should be part of a wider treatment strategy and adjunctive therapies should be used. For example, in Achilles tendinopathy it would be negligent to fail to provide information on eccentric heel drops (Alfredson & Cook 2007).

6. The importance of achieving neutral or near-neutral subtalar joint function should be de-emphasised, given that the normal foot does not appear to function in this position (McPoil & Cornwall 1994, 1999, Pierrynowski & Smith 1996) and the mechanism of action may be different (Nigg 2001). A prominent example is the use of laterally posted orthoses in medial compartment knee osteoarthritis, which act to pronate further a foot that may already be pronated, to unload the joint (Sasaki & Yasuda 1987).

7. It is perfectly acceptable to mix paradigms: patients rarely present with isolated abnormalities in individual planes. A patient can be seen with medial tibial stress syndrome, where a tibial varum, a soleal ankle equinus and a functional hallux limitus are all present. A suitable orthosis might provide some frontal plane control but also incorporate a heel raise and first-ray cut-out or kinetic wedge to enhance sagittal plane function to holistically tackle the abnormal foot function. Stretches would also be required, and some anti-inflammatory medication or therapy and activity modification may also be useful.

The process of identifying the plane of origin of abnormal foot function may be enhanced through the use of digital video gait analysis, which also permits identification of the subphase of stance in which the abnormal foot function develops.

## Material choice and casting techniques

The manufacture of casted orthoses demands that an impression of the foot be taken from which the orthosis can be manufactured. This commonly involves heating a shell material and vacuum forming it to the cast. The choice of materials depends on various factors, including the patient's age, weight and occupation, the chronicity of the condition and the preferred style of footwear. Furthermore, in the case of the sports person, the nature of the sport must be considered. For example, it might involve running, jumping, physical contact, or sharp or sudden changes of direction. Materials range from rigid to flexible. It is important not to think of a rigid orthosis as necessarily providing a higher level of control: even if subtalar neutral function is less important it may still be desirable to use a rigid material, but with less posting, as this will deliver this reduced control over a longer period of time. Conversely, a less rigid material with higher posting might be more comfortable for and better tolerated by specific patients.

Carbon fibre composites, graphite, polypropylenes and polyethylenes make up the most popular range of materials. Hexcelite, Aquaplast and the new range of fibreglass fracture splinting materials can produce orthoses that can last for many months. It is possible to manufacture temporary orthoses in situ on the foot using these splinting materials because the skin on the sole of the foot can tolerate their thermoforming temperature. Children normally tolerate semi-rigid or flexible orthoses better than those of the rigid variety.

Custom functional orthoses are manufactured to a model of the patient's foot. The mould or cast is taken using one of a variety of techniques. The traditional technique involves lying the patient prone with their foot hanging off the end of the couch. A supine technique can also be used, but control of the foot, which is plantar flexing due to gravity, is more difficult. Plaster slabs (double thickness to increase strength) are draped over the calcaneus and extended down to the forefoot, and brought over the front of the foot and brought up and smoothed into the rearfoot splint. They are smoothed together and the foot then placed in the neutral subtalar joint position, where it is held until the plaster is dry, when it can be removed. In light of the questionable requirement for the subtalar joint to function in neutral, it may be that all that is required is a cast of the foot moderately less pronated than the functional position. An alternative technique is to use an oasis-foam impression box. The patient sits in a chair and the clinician places the foot in a neutral or less pronated position before applying controlled pressure to deform the foam so that it captures the contours of the patient's foot. Like the plaster cast in the traditional technique, the impression is then filled with plaster of Paris, which when set provides a model of the foot over which the orthosis can be formed. When plaster models are used various plaster additions are incorporated, including: a lateral expansion to permit soft-tissue spread from the non-weight-bearing casting position, to enhance fit; a forefoot platform, which provides functional correction; and a medial addition, which blends the correction platform into the device. In relation to orthosis manufacture, useful laboratory guides providing detailed information on the manufacturing process have been provided by Anthony (1991) and Philps (1995).

Children present particular difficulties when casting, and for this reason it is best to use the prone position as the child is then less likely to interfere with the process – it can be difficult to stop a child from wriggling their toes when their foot is being tickled by plaster of Paris. While casting might be required in some cases, there is a rationale for generally using prefabricated devices. In addition to a reduced cost of treating a growing foot that may require serial casted devices at considerable cost, the need for casting is removed, as is the time requirement, and all these factors may increase concordance.

Many companies now produce plastics in pre-cut template sizes ready for heating, and these eliminate the need to buy large sheets that need to be reduced to the appropriate size using a band saw. Once heated and malleable, the plastic is trimmed to its rough shape and moulded by vacuum forming until the plastic cools and conforms exactly to the shape and contours of the plantar surface of the foot. Different plastics require heating at different temperatures and for different lengths of time (Table 17.2). Prior to manufacture, it should be decided whether intrinsic or extrinsic posting is required, based on the presenting condition, range of joint movement available and the degree of correction required. Posts are best described as platforms added to the plastic shell to provide correction. An intrinsic post is one that is applied to the cast in the form of a plaster addition, so that when the shell is pressed the posting is incorporated in the shell. An extrinsic post involves the addition of material to the bottom of the shell. Irrespective of which technique is used, the principle is the same. Rigid or high-density materials, such as dental acrylic, Tensol (liquid plastic), high-density polyethylene or Birkocork, may be used for posting. These posts or wedges hold the foot in the corrected position under load, restrain it from deforming as it would otherwise do, and help restore the normal time sequence of events occurring in the foot during the gait cycle. If some accommodation is

**Table 17.2** Working temperatures and thermoforming times for plastics in common use

|  | Temperature (°C) | Time (min)[1] |
|---|---|---|
| Hexcelite | 72 | 3 |
| Aquaplast | 100 | 3 |
| Pacton | 110 | 5 |
| Evazote | 130 | 6 |
| Plastazote | 140 | 8 |
| Polythene | 140 | 10 |
| Ortholene | 165 | 14 |
| Polypropylene | 165 | 15 |
| Rohadur | 170 | 18 |
| TL61 (carbon fibre composite) | 180 | 20 |

[1]Times are based on the oven being at working temperature. All materials were 3 mm thick. Thicker materials take longer to become malleable.

required, posts will be made of a material that will 'give', such as high-density rubber.

A rearfoot post consists of a shaped wedge placed under the heel of the shell and tapered off on the lateral side to the required angle. This controls abnormal subtalar joint pronation. Forefoot posting may be either varus or valgus, as required, for either inversion or eversion control, respectively. A bar of material is placed 0.5–1 cm behind the metatarsal heads, tapering off to the medial or lateral sides to the required angle.

Rigid orthoses thus incorporate all the required correction. However, complete functional control may not always be tolerated at first, and the orthosis should be worn for short periods, increasing daily until they can be worn all day. As an alternative to rigid orthoses, semi-rigid devices can be used, and a whole range of patients may find these more tolerable.

## Custom versus prefabricated orthoses

One of the more recent introductions to the range of available functional orthoses is a rapidly growing range of prefabricated devices. These are available in a range of generic sizes that may satisfy the requirements of patients who have a relatively normal foot size with no or only minor deformity. They come with a moderate amount of intrinsic control (e.g. 4–6° of rearfoot varus posting), although most ranges have a variety of additions (e.g. rearfoot and forefoot wedges, heel raises and metatarsal domes) available that the practitioner can apply to produce an orthosis that provides a degree of customised control. Long-established prefabricated orthoses are supplied by Vasyli (previously known as AOL – Australian Orthotic Laboratory) and Formthotic. Newer ranges include those available from Talar Made, SALTS Healthcare, Algeo's First Phase Orthotics and the Salford Insole. Each manufacturer claims that their devices are superior in terms of effectiveness and cost. A majority of these devices can be heat moulded, and it is difficult to recommend one range in particular. Those interested in prefabricated orthoses should attend a podiatry conference, where they will be able to see the ranges and speak to representatives from the manufacturers. Sceptics should consider the

evidence that is emerging concerning prefabricated orthoses. For example, in a well-designed, randomised controlled trial Landorf et al (2006) found that after 1 year there was no difference in the effectiveness of prefabricated versus custom orthoses prescribed for the treatment of plantar fasciitis, and at 3 months the prefabricated devices were more effective. This was attributed to less difficulty in accustoming to the prefabricated device. In a case series, Davis et al (2008) found that there was no difference in rearfoot motion control and comfort between custom and semi-custom devices. These findings were echoed in a recent study that evaluated the influence of custom and prefabricated orthoses on plantar pressure distribution and found small, non-significant differences in only a few variables (Redmond et al 2009). Prefabricated orthoses would seem to offer potential, and certainly should not be ignored.

## CAD–CAM orthoses

The computer-aided design and manufacture (CAD-CAM) of functional orthoses is now recognised by many in the profession as the way forward, enabling practitioners to prescribe and supply their patients with devices that are produced to much finer tolerances than those produced using the traditional hand-crafted methods. The ability to accurately match the flexibility of the device to the patient's body weight, numerically apply expansions and postings, and apply a range of special accommodations has enabled practitioners to supply their patients with devices that are fit for purpose and much more easily accommodated within reasonable footwear.

The shells are produced on a computer numerically controlled (CNC) milling machine from solid blocks of polypropylene, thus avoiding any changes to the molecular structure of the material, as there is no heat moulding involved in the process. This enables the manufacturer to produce devices that do not bottom-out and carry a lifetime guarantee against breakage in normal use. Hand finishing produces devices with excellent aesthetic qualities that do not require covers unless the prescription calls for additional extensions.

The data for the design are obtained from a neutral plaster cast of the patient's foot. Good-quality casts of the type best suited to the laboratory's specification are essential, as is the quality and clarity of the prescription, to enable the manufacturer to produce the correct devices. The continual development of the software has created many more prescription options. The prescription data are retained on the laboratory's database, enabling repeat prescriptions to be produced at any time. Most laboratories are willing to provide expert help to practitioners with regard to their casting technique and prescription writing.

Practitioners who manufacture their own orthoses would find it difficult to produce a product that so closely matches the requirements of the prescription.

## Prescription writing for CAD-CAM direct-milled orthoses

The development of CAD-CAM direct-milled orthoses that have top and bottom surfaces designed independently has brought with it the opportunity to produce much more accurate and effective devices, as many of the inaccuracies inherent in the orthoses produced using traditional hand-crafted techniques are eliminated. With this comes the opportunity for innovative prescription writing. It is worth noting that there are a number of different CAD-CAM systems in operation, each with its own programme, and each offering a wide variety of types and quality of orthoses, not all of which are direct milled. The following information is representative of the technique involved. The skill and experience of the practitioner in making the prescription will have a marked bearing on the type of prescription selected.

The outcomes sought by the practitioner can be divided into three categories: high, medium and low levels of control.

- *high-level control* – for those patients who can cope with aggressive change to their foot function
- *medium-level control* – for patients with conditions that will not respond as well to aggressive change
- *low-level control* – for patients with pathologies that indicate a more accommodative type of device.

Examples of patients who will respond well to high-level control are:

- children, with hypermobile flat feet, hallux valgus, in-toeing/out-toeing gait, leg or knee pain, or other musculoskeletal problems
- healthy adults, with a wide range of pathologies; for example, plantar fasciitis, plantar heel pain, posterior tibial tendinopathy, lateral ankle instability, plantar digital neuritis, hallux valgus, metatarsalgia, nail pathologies, including involution and onychocryptosis, and musculoskeletal problems, as well as patients in the early stages of rheumatoid arthritis and diabetes.
- Active sports people, including elite athletes.

Examples of patients requiring medium-level control are:

- older patients with chronic pathologies, including posterior tibial dysfunction, peripheral neuritis or vascular disease
- many post-foot-surgery cases
- more advanced conditions of rheumatoid arthritis.

Examples of patients requiring low-level control are:

- rigid foot types
- genetic abnormalities, such as example talipes equino varus
- significant osteoarthritic changes
- very elderly patients.

Other factors that have a bearing on the chosen prescription include:

- *Footwear*. This is often a problem for female patients who require to wear dress or court shoes for social or occupational reasons. It is best dealt with by supplying a second pair of devices specially modified to suit the footwear, such as dress or Cobra orthoses. It is important to emphasise that such modifications will compromise the effectiveness of the devices. Certain types of sports footwear, such as soccer boots, ski boots and ice-skating boots, may require customised devices.
- *Occupation*. The requirement to wear safety footwear must also be considered.

## Types of orthosis

- *Standard* – normal shell incorporating all postings and accommodations
- *Dress* – extra-low-bulk device, 5% narrower than standard, more suitable for ladies' dress shoes
- *Cobra* – a significantly modified device that is more suitable for ladies' court shoes
- *gait plate* – the distal edge of the device is extended beyond the fourth and fifth metatarsal heads, to function as a counterirritant; some practitioners use these to treat gait problems.

Figure 17.7 shows various types of CAD-CAM orthoses.

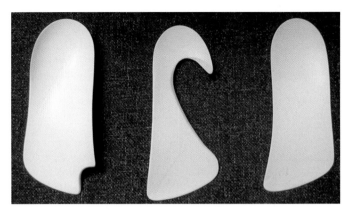

**Figure 17.7** Types of CAD-CAM orthoses: standard, Cobra and dress. In the gait plate the distal edge of the device is extended beyond the fourth and fifth metatarsal heads.

## Prescription variations

### Flexibility

The thickness of the shell determines the degree of flexibility and is calculated to produce either, rigid, semi-flexible or flexible devices, based on the patient's body weight. This produces the same degree of flexibility for each patient, irrespective of his or her weight. Occupations or sports that involve carrying or moving additional weight should be taken into account.

### Heel-cup height

This ranges from 9 mm to 25 mm and is usually determined by the style of the device and the size of the foot. Children with hypermobile feet require extra-deep heel cups to establish greater control. Heel-cup heights are:

- *low* (9 mm) – used for Cobra or dress devices
- *medium* (13 mm) – used for children and for women
- *high* (17 mm) – used for children when greater control is required and for men
- *extra high* (25 mm) – used for very large feet.

### Width

The scanning equipment reads the width of the foot accurately, and therefore only in cases of exceptionally large feet, where shoe fitting is a problem should a *narrow* device be prescribed. For sports footwear such as soccer boots, a device that is narrower in the mid-section, *narrow-mid*, can be used. It is sometimes advisable to send the patient's shoes to the laboratory to have the devices customised to fit them exactly.

## Postings

All postings are applied using numerical science, with no human intervention in the fabrication stage; they are therefore guaranteed to be correct as prescribed.

*Forefoot posting* can be applied intrinsically or extrinsically, or as a combination of both.

An *intrinsic post* allows the forefoot to come down to the ground, as in 'forefoot supinatus' conditions.

An *extrinsic post* is applied to the bottom surface at the distal edge, to bring the ground up to the foot.

The degree of posting used is dictated by the angle between the heel and the forefoot, together with the level of control being sought.

A *bar post* is added to the bottom surface of the distal edge, creating greater lateral column stability. Bar posts can range in thickness from 2 mm to 5 mm.

*Rearfoot posting* is applied extrinsically as an integral part of the shell. The degree of posting is dictated by the angle between the bisection of the calcaneum and the midline of the leg, together with the level of control being sought.

All these measurements are taken with the midtarsal area held in its most stable position, normally referred to as 'subtalar neutral'.

In *Blake-style* posting the distal edge of the forefoot is aligned parallel to the bottom surface of the rearfoot post. This produces a less forgiving device.

## Accommodations

*First metatarsal cut-out* – a section of the shell is cut away behind the head of the first metatarsal. This reduces the risk of jamming at the first metatarsophalangeal joint by providing space for the sesamoid bones, and facilitates sagittal plane motion.

*Low first* – a groove incorporated into the shell below the first metatarsal shaft, to accommodate a plantar-flexed first ray. It can range from 2 mm to 5 mm in depth.

*First-ray cut-out* – a section of the shell is cut away from below the first ray. It is used by some practitioners to facilitate greater first-ray movement. The kinetic wedge is a development of the first metatarsal/first-ray cut-out.

*Fascial groove* – a groove incorporated into the shell below the planter fascia to reduce the pressure between the foot and the shell. It is used where there is a tight band of fascia or a prominent flexor hallucis longus tendon.

*Flange out* – extends the shell on the medial side, to provide extra support for the medial longitudinal arch area. It is used in conditions such as posterior tibial dysfunction.

*Morton's extension* – the distal edge of the device is extended beyond the first metatarsophalangeal joint to limit movement of the joint and transferring motion to the interphalangeal joint.

*Lateral clip* – extends the lateral side of the heel cup distally for increased control. It may be used in conjunction with high heel cups for children when greater control is required.

*Heel skives (Kirby skive)* – the Kirby skive (Kirby 1992) is a cast modification that involves angulating the medial third of the heel cup to produce a heel cup that is inclined, to provide an effective antipronatory force. The angle and the depth of skives should be specified.

*Heel raise* – can be incorporated into the device during the milling process or added in PORON or EVA.

## Problem solving

### Devices do not fit shoes

This is usually found when patients do not wear the proper type or size of shoes. The devices are made to accurately match the size of the foot, and patients have a responsibility to ensure that their shoes accommodate the devices neatly. The importance of the shoe gripping securely in the midfoot area by means of a lace or strap must also be stressed.

### Devices cut into the lateral side of the heel

This is due to the sagittal plane blockade not being completely overcome, therefore causing the foot to torque and rub against the heel cup. The prescription may need to be revised.

### First metatarsal irritation

Orthoses can often cause irritation to the distal plantar first metatarsal. Where this occurs there can be a temptation to decrease or flatten the orthosis in this area. However, this can indicate that greater control is required, and by adding a small amount of rearfoot posting the first metatarsal declination angle can be influenced to reduce contact with the shell. Therefore, increasing, not decreasing, control is the solution.

### Devices are too tight at the heel

Soft-tissue expansions are calculated as a percentage of the size of the heel. Patients that have very large fatty heel pads may produce a greater amount of expansion and encounter this type of problem. Such cases require a wider than normal heel cup.

### Irritation in the area of the medial longitudinal arch

This is relieved by adding a fascial groove or dell to the shell.

### Insufficient control

Control can be increased via the addition of an extrinsic post, or through a posteriorly placed valgus pad applied to the dorsum of the orthosis. Alternatively, the prescription will have to be revised.

## EEC DIRECTIVE ON THE MANUFACTURE OF ORTHOSES

Directive 93/42 EEC, which came into effect on 14 June 1998, requires all manufacturers of medical devices, who place these on sale, to have registered with the competent authority (in the UK the Medical Devices Agency (MDA)).

The regulations require all such devices to display the CE mark of conformity, with the exception of custom-made devices, devices intended for clinical investigation and systems that comprise only CE-marked parts.

From a practitioner's perspective, therefore, prefabricated devices will already comply with the directive. Those practitioners who supply their own manufactured orthoses should be registered with the competent authority and their devices should carry the CE mark of conformity. The guidance issued by the Society of Chiropodists and Podiatrists (UK) on who should or should not be registered is given in Box 17.1.

This legislation is complex and those requiring further information on interpretation of the legislation in the context of particular clinical/orthotics laboratory practices should seek expert help.

## SILIPOS

This company produces a range of insoles manufactured in a cross-linked, three-dimensional polymer gel. Its structure reduces shearing stress, while the USP mineral grade oil softens and lubricates the skin. The material is also available in a range of digital pads, which protect a variety of pressure points, and in sheet form for use in the production of chairside appliances. It is important to stress that Silipos digital pads must be removed every evening and not left in position, as ulceration can occur if they are left on the foot continuously.

## HEEL ORTHOSES

There are a number of orthoses that may be made specifically for conditions affecting the heel. A heel cup may be fabricated on a cast of the heel using the plastics already described or fibreglass. Such devices are well tolerated because they take up little room and can be worn in a wide variety of shoes. Wedges or posts may be incorporated in such devices, either at the time of manufacture or at a later stage. The devices are corrective in nature. However, palliative heel orthoses may be required for lesions on the plantar aspect of the heel, such as calcaneal bursitis, and for the area around the insertion of the Achilles tendon where the bursae are often subject to irritation from footwear. Skaters are particularly vulnerable to retrocalcaneal bursitis because of the rigidity of the counter surrounding the heel of skating boots. These heel orthoses can be manufactured on casts or made directly onto the heel using silicone.

Painful intractable hyperkeratotic lesions frequently occur on the area of the heel following trauma. The formation of scar tissue in such cases leaves the practitioner no other course than to rely on palliative orthoses. Most often, these devices are best fabricated in latex for wear on the foot. However, simple heel pads can also be made to fit into the shoe and can be removed for use in other shoes as required.

## LATEX TECHNIQUE

Deformities of the toes, such as hallux abducto valgus and hammer toes, are often chronic and require protection more or less permanently. In such cases, devices made in latex are often the most effective type of orthosis. Such techniques are now rarely used, but represent a rewarding technique for the patient and podiatrist alike. Irrespective of the area involved, the principle of manufacture is the same. For the purposes of illustration, the fabrication of a hallux abducto valgus shield is described, but the technique is suitable for digital orthoses as well.

The most important feature is the accuracy of the negative cast. This may be taken in a variety of materials but the most effective are the elastic impression compounds. Dental impression materials are ideal for this purpose, and the most cost-effective of these is dental alginate.

The negative is then filled with plaster, and when this has set the alginate is stripped, bit by bit, to ensure that the positive remains intact. Any blemishes on the positive are removed with fine sandpaper, and, if necessary, porosities may be filled in with a thin mixture of plaster. The positive is then allowed to dry. Care must be taken not to overheat the cast as this might reverse the chemical process, causing the cast to become crumbly.

The positive is then dipped in latex, each layer being allowed to dry, until several layers have been built up on the cast. At this stage, the correct type of pad is applied according to the therapeutic function required. If an open-cell foam is used, the pad is first covered with adhesive. This seals the pad and prevents latex from permeating into the foam, and it also traps air within the open-cell structure, thereby improving the physical properties of the material. The cast is then dipped twice more to complete the process before being removed from the cast and trimmed. In some cases, it is preferable to cover the cast in a layer of soft leather such as chamois to provide a soft lining for the appliance. If this method is employed, the edges of the leather must be sealed and the appropriate adhesive used, otherwise degradation of the leather may result, due to interaction with the solvents used to stabilise the adhesives.

It is sometimes necessary or convenient to speed up the process for latex orthoses. This may be done either by heating the cast before dipping or by using a hot-air blower such as a hair dryer to dry each dip. In this way it is possible to manufacture a latex orthosis from start to finish in 15 minutes. A variety of latex digital shields are shown in Figure 17.8.

## DIGITAL APPLIANCES FOR THE LESSER TOES

All necessary designs of digital appliances for the lesser toes can be produced by any of the methods previously outlined for hallux abducto valgus shields. The necessity for negative and positive casting when the latex technique is used, coupled with the smaller size of digital appliances, lends great advantages to the direct moulding techniques utilising silicone rubbers or thermoplastic materials. Silicone rubbers are well proven as the most suitable materials for digital orthoses. They can also be fabricated from orthotic plastic, but it is then usually necessary to line them with softer material for good tissue tolerance. Plastics used for this purpose are designed for finger-splinting, as they are soft and malleable. This combination increases the corrective effect of an appliance while maintaining patient tolerance.

The principle of reciprocal dorsoplantar padding is the most effective basis for digital appliances, and this has been previously described.

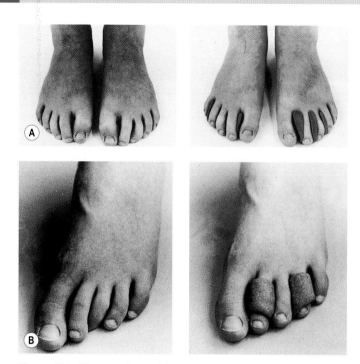
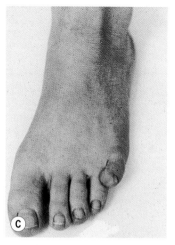
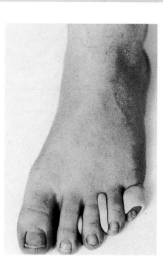

**Figure 17.8** Silicone orthoses. (A) Multiple prop for congenital curly toes. (B) Corrective sling for congenital claw toe. (C) Corrective sling for digitus quintus varus.

When moulded in silicones or thermoplastics, orthodigital splints are infinitely adjustable to individual needs. They may be either full or partial. When full, they completely cover the dorsum of the proximal phalanges and the plantar surfaces of the intermediate and distal phalanges of the middle three toes. When partial, they are reduced in size to fit one or two toes only, or to form a long prop. Maximum effect is thus obtained with minimum bulk. Deformities and lesions of the fifth toe are particularly amenable to well-designed partial splints in silicones or thermoplastics.

## SILICONES

The use of silicone elastomers in orthoses and prostheses is probably the most significant advance in this field for many years. In the short time since their introduction, rapid progress has resulted in new opportunities of treatment for digital deformity in both the old and the young. The silicones used in podiatry are derivatives of the elastomers used in dentistry, although in recent years materials designed specifically for podiatry have become available.

Silicones are generally presented as a putty to which a catalyst is added. After a period, the putty is transformed into a flexible solid. The material, while undergoing its change of state, maintains a putty-like consistency for a period of 2–8 minutes, depending on the putty/catalyst ratio and the room temperature. This space of time allows the practitioner to fabricate the device. After final setting, the material must be able to withstand repeated functional loading without dimensional change or fracture. There is a wide variety of possible formulae, but the practitioner must be aware of any alterations that he may make as they will directly affect the properties of tension and compression, and setting time, and therefore the subsequent usage of the material.

By far the most rewarding application of this material lies in the correction of congenital digital deformities in children. The same techniques may be used to correct toe deformities in older patients, if sufficient motion is present in the affected joints, and the same methods have been applied to the maintenance of correction following corrective digital surgery. Basically, the splint is fashioned around the toes and, as the silicone sets, the toes are held in their corrected position until the elastic properties of the material are strong enough to withstand the deforming forces. Figures 17.9 and 17.10 illustrate a variety of basic techniques for correcting the common congenital toe deformities, and Figure 17.11 shows silicone toe prostheses.

When using these materials in the field of postoperative maintenance, one must work closely with the surgeon who performed the operation. It is essential that the podiatrist has a good knowledge of the surgical techniques that have been employed so that any splint manufactured for the patient acts as an integral part of the patient's therapy. Figure 17.11 shows a silicone orthosis that was fitted 2 weeks after the patient had undergone a Keller's arthroplasty and capsulotomy of the second and third toes. Assessment of the inherent strength of the lesser digits is important if attempting to manufacture a splint to maintain the position of the hallux, in order to avoid moving the lesser digits laterally.

## THERMOPLASTICS

Thermoplastic materials are usually products of additional polymerisation. They will soften on heating and harden once cooled without any chemical change taking place. Polymers that are thermoplastic can be moulded to a desired shape when heat and pressure are applied. The most common thermoplastic materials used in podiatry are derivatives of polyethylene, although polypropylene materials are also used.

This range of synthetic materials has four main areas of application: (1) firm splinting, (2) impression medium, (3) moulded lining, and (4) modelling and construction.

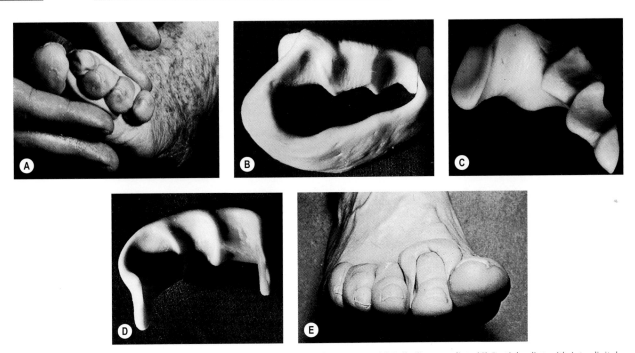

**Figure 17.9** Silicone orthodigital splints. (A) Moulding splint at first stage of correction. (B) Full silicone splint. (C) Partial splint with interdigital wedge for first cleft. (D) Silicone long prop. (E) Single dorsoplantar splint for hammer toe.

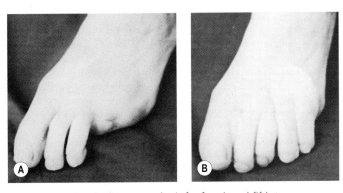

**Figure 17.10** (A, B) Silicone prosthesis for fourth and fifth toes.

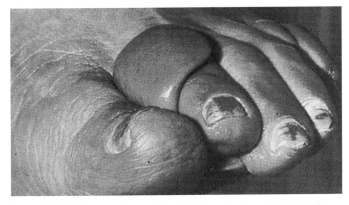

**Figure 17.11** Silicone prop and interdigital wedge to maintain position of hallux after Keller's arthroplasty.

The firm splinting material is polyethylene sheet, which is not expanded in manufacture and consequently contains no pockets of gas. It is used for direct moulding to positive casts in the production of orthotic shells.

The impression material is the expanded polyethylene which, when inserted into the shoe as a template insole, provides an accurate dynamic impression of pressure areas. The template can then be built up with appropriate padding to produce a permanent insole.

As a lining material, the thermoplastic may be expanded polyethylene or expanded vinyl acetate. After the material is heated, moulding is carried out directly on the foot and additional padding and outer layers are added in sequence. This method can be used for hallux abducto valgus shields and similar appliances (e.g. heel cups for bedridden patients to prevent bed sores).

These materials may also be used for taking negative casts. However, if they are to be used for this purpose, care has to be taken to ensure there is no deformation of the cast after removal from the foot, and it is sometimes of help to mould a rigid material around the thermoplastic to retain its shape and dimension.

The softer of the two materials is the expanded vinyl acetate (Evazote), which looks identical to expanded polyethylene (Plastozote) but feels much smoother and softer and has a lower tensile strength. Quite complex curvatures can be achieved by moulding these materials, and one of the benefits is that a seamless lining is obtained.

Footwear that conforms accurately to the shape of the foot can be simply constructed by using the various densities and thicknesses of expanded polyethylene. One style is that of the clog with an enclosed front and no heel counter. The sole block is first cut out with a leather knife or on a band saw and the foot is placed on top. The upper is then shaped and covered in an appropriate material (e.g. Yampi). It is then moulded round the foot with the foot in place on the sole block, and the upper is adhered around the edge of the base. An outer sole can then be added and trimmed. The pair of clogs may weigh no more than 200 g, an important consideration in many cases.

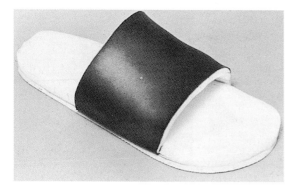

**Figure 17.12** Thermoplastic mule made directly onto the foot.

An even lighter style is that of the sandal with a block sole and two or three straps to hold it onto the foot. More complicated styles can also be produced, which, when compared with traditional surgical footwear, are extremely attractive in terms of weight, fitting, style and price.

Almost any shape can be produced by cutting, heating, moulding and buffing thermoplastic materials (Fig. 17.12). To produce a moulded article, the material is heated in an oven at about 130°C until it is soft enough to mould. It cools in a minute or two and retains its moulded shape, at which stage adhesive can be applied. In some cases, the adhesive may be applied before heating, so that the moulding and fixing is done in one stage. Synthetic contact adhesives are suitable for fixing these thermoplastics. Good surface finishing is achieved easily, particularly when this is done on a grinding machine. When heating thermoplastics, it should be remembered that they are all inflammable, giving off strong toxic fumes, if allowed to get too hot. An oven with thermostatic controls is advised and a fire extinguisher should always be at hand.

## Hot-water plastics (Polyform, Aquaplast Hexcelite, X-Lite Plus)

These orthotic splinting plastics are of particular use when an immediate appliance is required, and this technique is of great value in saving practitioner time. Its essential features are as follows: low temperature moulding; chairside technique; production time of a few minutes; rapid remoulding of part of or the whole device; no waste material, small offcuts are reusable; and readily adjustable thickness, as the material can be built up or thinned out as required.

### Low-temperature moulding

In standard thickness (3 mm) the material can be softened in boiling water (100°C) for between 1 and 3 minutes to become completely workable and thinned out to an extremely thin layer. At 65–70°C it becomes workable in about 54–60 seconds, but the moulding characteristics are not as precise as with the 100°C softening temperature. The plastic will not soften below 60°C.

The material should be dried on a towel before being moulded; it will remain workable for about 3–5 minutes. Fingers should be moistened to maintain a good 'slip' feeling on surface moulding. When moulding, any excess material can be trimmed away easily with scissors. Most patients have good tolerance to the hot material directly on the skin, but an intermediate layer of expanded thermoplastic can be included if thought advisable. Cooling can be speeded up by immersion in cold water. If the material is thinned out when moulding, and cooled in ice-water, the hardened state can be expected in about 10–15 seconds.

### Chairside technique

The whole device can be produced in as little as 2 minutes but should not normally take more than 10 minutes, allowing for modifications and adjustments.

### Rapid remoulding

The advantage of this plastic over silicone rubber is that it can always be remoulded and reshaped by heating part or all of the device. As conditions respond to the orthosis, so the device can be adjusted to correspond to such correction.

### No waste

Any small pieces can be reheated and moulded into one new piece. The new material can be flattened into a new sheet of any thickness on a smooth worktop. It will retain its cohesive properties after being heated and dried. Cold material is easily bonded to warm material by using a non-flammable Polyform adhesive. A finished device can be completely remade by placing it back into hot water. If the material has been thinned out while moulding, then in order to obtain the original or greater thickness, it will be necessary to fold over and double the material or to add other sheets.

### Complex construction

Where more complex structures are required, and trial and error may be necessary to achieve optimum results, small balls of the plastic may be added, such as under the longitudinal axis of a three-quarter length valgus insole, to gain the desired degree of spring. A valgus insole is very quickly made and can be altered at any time with ease. Heel cups are also easily made and, by careful stretching of the material, can be produced quickly and accurately. Double curvatures are not difficult to make as long as the material is well heated. Combinations of Polyform with silicone rubbers or expanded thermoplastics give good results.

Where a soft appliance lacks strength, Polyform can be added to the original device as a reinforcement or cradle. An analogy is the gumshield worn by boxers, which consists of a strong plastic shell lined with soft material that has been moulded directly to the interior of the mouth. Expanded thermoplastics can be stuck to the Polyform sheet prior to heating and moulding to give an excellent fit when finished. Individual areas of the material can be heated using a hot-air gun, and additional moulding or alterations can be performed.

### Hexcelite (X-Lite Plus)

This is a remouldable plastic impregnated over soft cotton. The material forms a mesh and, as such, combines features of excellent moulding with ventilation. It is self-bonding, light and has considerable strength. It is a relatively inexpensive material and can be heated in water at 72°C. It sets in 3 minutes and, when malleable, it will bond whether wet or dry. It has many uses and the podiatrist need only to use imagination to provide a wide array of semi-rigid orthoses. It can be used to manufacture night splints for hallux abducto valgus and it can also be used to splint lesser toes following surgery. By bonding several layers together, functional orthoses can be made in a matter of minutes. These insoles may be made directly on the patient's foot or manufactured on a cast. Posts may be added in the same material. The Hexcelite should be moulded together by rolling with a rolling pin. Any synthetic contact adhesive is suitable for use with Hexcelite.

## CONCLUSION

As can be seen from the number of techniques described, it is inappropriate to think of the term 'orthosis' as describing a narrow range of devices dominated by simple and functional insoles and silicone wedges. Podiatrists have a rich history of skilful manufacture of a range of devices and it is vital, for the management of idiosyncratic and challenging patients and rewarding practice, that practitioners embrace a range of techniques.

## REFERENCES

Alfredson H, Cook J 2007 A treatment algorithm for managing Achilles tendinopathy: new treatment options. British Journal of Sports Medicine 41:211–216.

Anthony RJ 1991 The manufacture and use of the functional foot orthosis. Karger, London.

Bojsen-Moller F 1979 Calcaneocuboid joint and stability of the longitudinal arch of the foot at high and low gear push off. Journal of Anatomy 129:165–176.

Bojsen-Moller F, Lamoreux L 1979 Significance of free-dorsiflexion of the toes in walking. Acta Orthopaedica Scandinavica 50(4):471–479.

Close, JR, Inman VT, Poor PM, et al 1967 The function of the subtalar joint. Clinical Orthopaedics and Related Research 50:159–179.

Cornwall MW, McPoil TG 1999 Three-dimensional movement of the foot during the stance phase of walking. Journal of the American Podiatric Medicine Association 89(2):56–66.

Dananberg HJ 1995 Lower extremity mechanics and their effect on lumbosacral function. Spine: State of the Art Reviews 9:389–405.

Dananberg HJ 1993a Gait style as an etiology to chronic postural pain: Part 1. Functional hallux limitus Journal of the American Podiatric Medicine Association 83:433–441.

Dananberg HJ 1993b Gait style as an etiology to chronic postural pain. Part II. Postural compensatory process. Journal of the American Podiatric Medicine Association 83:615–624.

Davis IS, Zifchock RA, DeLeo AT 2008 A comparison of rearfoot motion control and comfort between custom and semicustom foot orthotic devices. Journal of the American Podiatric Medicine Association 98(5):394–403.

Heiderscheit B, Hamill J, Tiberio D 2001 A biomechanical perspective: do foot orthoses work? British Journal of Sports Medicine 35:4–5.

Johansen MA, Donatelli R, Wooden MJ, et al 1994 Effects of three different posting methods on controlling abnormal subtalar pronation. Physical Therapy 74(2):149–161.

Keenan AM 1997 A clinician's guide to the practical implications of the recent controversy of foot function. Australasian Journal of Podiatric Medicine 31:87–93.

Kirby KA 1992 The medial heel skive technique: improving pronation control in foot orthoses. Journal of the American Podiatric Medicine Association 82:177–188.

Kirby KA 2001 Subtalar joint axis location and rotational equilibrium theory of foot function. Journal of the American Podiatric Medicine Association 91:465.

Klingman RE, Liaos SM, Hardin KM 1997 The effect of subtalar joint posting on patellar glide in subjects with excessive rearfoot pronation. Journal of Orthopaedic & Sports Physical Therapy 25(3):185–191.

Landorf KB, Keenan AM, Herbert RD 2006 Effectiveness of foot orthoses to treat plantar fasciitis. Archives of Internal Medicine 166:1305–1310.

Lee WE 2001 Podiatric biomechanics: a historical appraisal and discussion of the Root model as a clinical system of approach in the present context of theoretical uncertainty. Clinics in Podiatric Medicine and Surgery 18(4):555–684.

McPoil TG, Cornwall MW 1994 Relationship between neutral subtalar joint position and pattern of rearfoot motion during walking. Foot and Ankle International 15:141.

McPoil TG, Hunt GC 1995 An evaluation and treatment paradigm for the future. In: Hunt GC, McPoil TG (eds) Physical therapy of the foot and ankle, 2nd edn. Churchill Livingstone, Edinburgh.

Nigg BM 2001 The role of impact forces and foot pronation: a new paradigm. Clinical Journal of Sport Medicine 11:2–9.

Novick A, Kelley DL 1990 Position and movement changes of the foot with orthotic intervention during the loading response of gait. Journal of Orthopaedic & Sports Physical Therapy 11(7):301–312.

Perry J 1992 Gait analysis: normal and pathological function. Slack, Thorofare, NJ.

Philps JW 1995 The functional foot orthosis, 2nd edn. Churchill Livingstone, Edinburgh.

Pierrynowski MR, Smith SB 1996 Rear foot inversion/eversion during gait relative to the subtalar joint neutral position. Foot and Ankle International 17:406.

Redmond AC, Landorf KB, Keenan AM 2009 Contoured, prefabricated foot orthoses demonstrate comparable mechanical properties to contoured, customised foot orthoses: a plantar pressure study. Journal of Foot and Ankle Research 2:20.

Root ML, Orien WP, Weed JH, et al 1971 Biomechanical examination of the foot, Vol. 1. Clinical Biomechanics Corp, Los Angeles, CA.

Root ML, Orien WP, Weed JH 1977 Biomechanical examination of the foot, Vol. 2. Normal and abnormal function of the foot. Clinical Biomechanics Corp, Los Angeles, CA.

Rose GK 1986 Orthotics: principles and practice. Heinemann Medical, London.

Sasaki T, Yasuda K 1987 Clinical evaluation of the treatment of osteoarthritic knees using a newly designed wedge insole. Clinical Orthopaedics and Related Research 221:181–187.

Woodburn J, Helliwell PS Barker S 2002 A randomized controlled trial of foot orthoses in rheumatoid arthritis. J Rheumatol 29:1377–1383.

Zammit GV, Payne CB 2007 Relationship between positive clinical outcomes of foot orthotic treatment and changes in rearfoot kinematics. Journal of the American Podiatric Medicine Association 97(3):207–212.

# Chapter | 18 |

# Footwear

*J Douglas Forrest and Wendy Tyrrell*

## KEYWORDS

Assessing fit of footwear
Backstay
Bars
Boots
Bottom fillings
Bunion pocket
Contralateral wedges
Derby shoe
Features of a good-fitting shoe
Flared heel
Flares (floats)
Heel-to-ball fitting
Insole
Lateral sole wedges
Length
Medial sole wedges
Measurements
Moccasin
Modular footwear
Outsole
Oxford shoe
Quarters
Rocker soles
Sandals
Shank
Shoe raises
Sizing systems
Sole
Sole and heel wedges
Stock surgical footwear
Therapeutic footwear

Thomas heel
Toe box
Toe cap
Tongue
Upper
Vamp
Wear marks in diagnosis
Welt
Width

## INTRODUCTION

The examination of a patient attending for podiatry treatment cannot be considered complete until assessment has been made of the footwear. It must also be remembered that footwear worn on the day of the examination may not reflect that which is typically used by the patient, and it is therefore necessary for the podiatrist to question the patient about their footwear preferences and habits.

To establish the cause of a foot complaint a thorough case history and examination of the feet during stance, gait and non-weight bearing is required (see Ch. 1). Application of podiatric skills and knowledge, including the normal parameters of gait and the range and direction of joint motion, leads to a clinical judgement to determine the presence, or absence, of any abnormality that accounts for the patient's symptoms. The outcome of this examination process may lead the practitioner to determine that no significant abnormality is present. The conclusion may then be made that there is no intrinsic cause of the patient's symptoms, and therefore attention must be focused on what extrinsic influences are placed on the feet and consideration given to the effects of these influences on normal foot function and gait. Frequently, footwear plays a major extrinsic role in the development of, or contribution to, a patient's foot symptoms. Failure to formally appraise the footwear presented renders the practitioner incapable of fully understanding what can be a complex source of foot discomfort. Footwear appraisal also provides the ideal opportunity to discuss with the patient the relationship between the dynamic foot and footwear.

For the patient to receive maximum benefit from the consultation, and gain an understanding of how they can positively contribute to the management of their own foot condition, discussion regarding footwear must take place. This also allows the podiatrist to advise the patient regarding specific features they require in footwear to achieve maximum foot function and comfort. While this point is easily made, the issue of the provision of footwear advice can present with one of the greatest patient education and communication challenges of the podiatrist's professional life.

Examination of footwear necessitates the podiatrist to reflect on how the normal foot functions in footwear. When managing the abnormal foot the podiatrist must consider how any identified abnormality within the foot being examined may manifest itself within the footwear during stance and gait. To achieve a successful management outcome it is often necessary to address the issue of the presenting intrinsic structural pathologies with the prescription and application of functional or accommodative orthoses while also making specific recommendations about footwear.

Examination of the wear marks appearing on footwear often reveals information about the gait of the wearer. This can significantly contribute to the practitioner's understanding of the patient's symptoms. In addition, comparing the wear marks on the patient's footwear with that which is considered 'normal' can often assist in early diagnosis of conditions that previously have been asymptomatic.

## FUNCTION OF FOOTWEAR

### Primary function

The wearing of footwear by man at an early stage of civilisation is confirmed (McDowell 1989) by the discovery in Spain of paintings dated between 12,000 and 15,000 BC that depict a man wearing boots made of skin and a woman wearing boots made of fur. The existence of footwear can be traced back to the Ice Age, when basic foot coverings were made from animal skins. In the early and simple form this footwear provided protection principally to the plantar aspect of the foot. With the development of more sophisticated foot coverings the protection provided to the plantar aspect of the foot was extended to the dorsal aspect of the foot and the lower leg. This dorsal extension provided greater protection to the lower limb from extremes of weather, barbed plants and rough terrain. Today, even with the many influences on shoe design and manufacture, protection is still regarded as the primary function of footwear.

### Secondary functions

Footwear is also considered to have a number of secondary functions. Appreciation of the secondary functions of footwear enables the podiatrist to question the patient and establish to what extent these secondary functions influence footwear selection, style and wear time. The shoes worn to attend the podiatrist for consultation may not typify those worn on a day-to-day basis. It is extremely important that the podiatrist has a clear understanding of each patient's footwear preference and wear habits before consideration can be given to any influence the footwear choice may have on the patient's presenting symptoms. In addition, the full footwear history and habits can have a significant influence on the clinical examination outcome and the management plan. Failure on the part of the podiatrist to establish a clear and current footwear history may cause significant disadvantage when conducting a clinical examination, and may result in an inability to adequately manage the patient.

### Completing a fashion

There are many functions of footwear that may be considered secondary to the primary function of protection. The fashion industry plays a major role in dictating what style of footwear is in vogue. Female footwear styles are particularly influenced by the fashion industry. A cursory look into any woman's fashion magazine will confirm the close relationship between clothing style and footwear style. The frequent changes in fashion clothing trends invariably dictate a change in the height and breadth of the heel and the shape of the toe box of the shoe. Footwear therefore plays a significant role in completing a fashionable 'look'. This function of footwear is also applicable to specific occupations where the wearing of a particular style of shoe is a requirement of a company on its employees in order to comply with a particular corporate image. For example, some companies within the airline industry require both male and female employees to wear a particular style of shoe in order that corporate identity is preserved. This preservation of image is often at the expense of efficient foot function and the comfort of the employee.

## Conducting specific tasks

Specific types of footwear are worn in order that the wearer can perform particular tasks. It would be impossible for a ballet dancer to perform on stage without wearing custom-made ballet shoes that allow the dancer's foot to adopt precise positions and rapidly change direction of motion while looking graceful and elegant. Similarly, the ability of the combat soldier to march long distances would be impaired if the typical army boot were not worn. Incorporated within the construction of the army boot is a high toe spring and rigid outsole. The combination of these two features minimises foot fatigue when walking long distances and reduces the motion required at the metatarsophalangeal joints during propulsion. A further function of footwear can therefore be identified as a means of assisting the foot to perform a specific task.

## Compensating for an abnormality

Footwear may also assist the wearer to overcome a lower-limb abnormality. Significant limb-length discrepancy may be overcome through adaptation of traditional footwear with the addition of a raise to the outsole to the value of the discrepancy. For example, a limb-length discrepancy of 4 cm may be compensated for through the addition of a 4-cm raise to the outsole of the shoe. The rigidity and consequent inflexibility of the modified outsole would be offset by the incorporation of an exaggerated toe spring to facilitate a more natural and efficient toe-off during the propulsive phase of gait. Simple adaptations may be carried out by a traditional cobbler, while more sophisticated adaptations will be provided by a bespoke shoe maker.

## PARTS OF A SHOE

Shoes and footwear in general are made in a variety of styles and are manufactured using a wide selection of natural and synthetic materials. Shoe design is largely dependent on the function for which the shoe is intended. A significant influence on the design of the shoe is the targeted retail market and the anticipated price range of the shoe. Although shoes vary immensely in appearance and function all shoes have some common features which, when combined during the manufacturing process, create the completed footwear.

To gain an appreciation of the relationship of one part of the shoe upper to another, examination of the traditional Oxford shoe provides a good example (Fig. 18.1). The Oxford shoe exhibits the many individual shoe parts that are combined during the shoe manufacturing process. In its traditional format, the Oxford shoe is proven to be a robust, hardwearing and long-lasting shoe. Although not singularly reserved for males, historically the Oxford shoe was the favoured shoe worn by professional men. Today, with the influence of fashion and cheaper shoe manufacturing techniques, the Oxford shoe is no longer

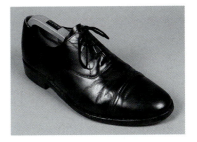

**Figure 18.1** The traditional men's Oxford Shoe.

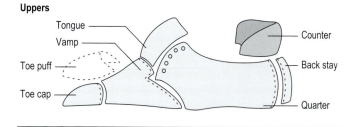

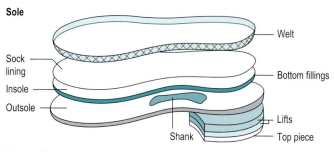

Figure 18.2 Parts of a shoe based on the traditional Oxford shoe.

reserved for businessmen and the style, or variations of it, is frequently seen in high-street shops. Variations in style, shoe manufacturing processes and the cost of footwear will undoubtedly alter the manufacturing process and ultimately the final appearance of the shoe. However, all footwear examined by the podiatrist will display some of the elements seen in the Oxford shoe.

Shoes are traditionally made on lasts that are developed by shoe designers. The last can be made of wood or plastic and is the mould on which the shoe is made. The design of lasts varies depending on the style of footwear to be manufactured. Traditionally, the various parts of the shoe used in the manufacturing process are grouped under the headings of upper, sole and subsidiary parts (Fig. 18.2).

## The upper

The upper of the shoe comprises the shoe parts brought together during the shoe manufacturing process to form that part of the shoe which embraces the dorsal aspect of the foot and the medial, lateral and posterior borders of the foot. Depending on the design of the footwear, uppers may consist only of single or multiple straps, as seen in some women's sandals. At the other extreme, where greater protection is required or as dictated by fashion, uppers may extend to the leg in the form of knee- and thigh-length boots. The typical upper of a shoe comprises all or many of the parts detailed below.

### The toe box

The toe box is the space found at the most anterior part of the shoe. This provides accommodation for the toes, and any inadequacy in the design of the last results in poor breadth or depth of the toe box, which can lead to lateral compression of the digits or compression on the nail plate. The toe box is often lined with a 'toe puff' or 'stiffener'. The object of the toe puff is to maintain the shape of the toe end of the last within the shoe following its production. This preserves the final appearance of the shoe and, with care, will maintain the anterior shape for the lifespan of the shoe. In this context, the toe puff does not offer toe protection properties; this can be achieved only by the incorporation of steel toe protectors, as seen in some industrial footwear.

### The toe cap

The toe cap is the layer of material in the upper that is applied to the toe end of the shoe. This forms the most anterior part of the upper and encloses the toes within the toe box of the shoe. In the traditional Oxford shoe, the toe cap is an additional piece of hard-wearing leather that is applied to the anterior end of the upper at the toe box and stitched posteriorly to the vamp. It is used to provide decoration and added strength and wear to the area. As with the toe puff, it should not be confused with the protective steel toe cap that is incorporated in industrial shoes to provide protection for the toes against impact. In traditional, everyday footwear the protection provided by the toe cap is negligible.

### The vamp

The term 'vamp' refers to the upper piece of material that forms the part of the shoe immediately above the metatarsophalangeal joints. In the Oxford shoe it is attached anteriorly to the toe cap and posteriorly to the medial and lateral quarters.

The metatarsophalangeal joints form the fulcrum point of the foot during propulsion; therefore, the vamp is frequently subjected to much flexion during gait – particularly during propulsion to allow the necessary dorsiflexion at these joints. The vamp is required to be made of a flexible but hard-wearing material capable of withstanding repeated stress. Good-quality flexible leather is ideal for this purpose. Cheaper shoes made from synthetic materials frequently show early signs of wear and tear at the vamp, which becomes cracked and eventually may break under the strain.

### The tongue

The tongue of a shoe, incorporated in lacing shoes, is an important part of the design. This is a shaped piece of material, usually leather. In the Oxford shoe it is attached on the inside of the shoe to the posterior surface of the vamp. In other styled, lacing shoes (e.g. the Derby shoe) the tongue is formed through a posterior extension of the vamp. In either case, the tongue is positioned in such a way that the dorsal aspect of the foot, particularly the area of the tarsometatarsal joints, is protected from the pressure of the laces and eyelets in the medial and lateral quarters of the shoe. This protection is particularly necessary when the foot is held firmly within the shoe and is efficiently tied with the laces, thereby effectively retaining the foot within the shoe. To successfully perform this protective function, the tongue of the shoe should be well positioned over the dorsal aspect of the foot. It should also be thick enough to provide the necessary absorption of pressure. Some manufacturers incorporate a robust cushioning material between the outer leather of the tongue and its inner lining. This additional piece of material maximises the protection to the dorsal aspect of the foot and encourages an effective lacing technique by the wearer. The absence of an effective tongue in lacing shoes discourages the wearer from lacing the shoes firmly on the feet – mainly because of the uncomfortable pressure of the laces and eyelets on the dorsal aspect of the feet. In response to this discomfort the wearer either discontinues wearing lacing shoes altogether or prefers to wear them loosely tied. The former option may result in the alternative style offering, at best, inadequate retention of the foot within the shoe and, at worst, a shoe that is too small. The latter option results in the creation of physical stresses within the foot as it is no longer held securely during gait and stance. Due to the poor retention, the foot is permitted to move mediolaterally and anteroposteriorly. Over a period of time this repeated motion and lack of security of the foot within the shoe can result in a plethora of foot conditions and strain on the joint ligaments and tendon insertions, giving rise to chronic foot strain and other soft-tissue pathologies.

## The quarters

The quarters form the posterior part of the shoe. The medial and lateral quarters of the shoe cradle the hindfoot and should provide a close fit of the shoe to the tarsal and metatarsal regions of the foot. The quarters are joined anteriorly with the vamp and are stitched together at the back of the shoe. To accommodate the medial longitudinal arch of the foot the medial quarters are higher than the lateral quarters. In lacing shoes, the anterior part of the quarters gives rise to the facings that accommodate the eyelets of the shoe. The material from which the quarters are made needs to be hard-wearing and must be able to endure the strain placed on it by the laces while maintaining the eyelets in their correct position. In good-quality footwear the quarters are reinforced to add strength to the area with the addition of a counter located between the quarters and its lining. The combination of close-fitting quarters, the counter and the correct use of the laces serves to hold the foot firmly within the footwear and to minimise any undesirable anteroposterior movement of the foot within the shoe during gait. Similarly, the elimination of mediolateral movement of the heel of the foot within the rear of the shoe is vital to maximise normal foot and joint function during stance and gait. Failure of any shoe to minimise these movements results in stress that can, in time, produce a variety of bone and soft-tissue pathologies within the foot.

## The sole

The composition of the sole of shoes varies greatly and is controlled by numerous factors. Sole construction is influenced by the quality and style of the footwear, the material used during manufacture, the manufacturing process and the projected cost of the footwear. Varied use of the basic sole unit components may be seen in modern footwear. Typically, the men's Oxford shoe consists of the elements detailed below.

## The insole

The insole of the shoe is the innermost part of the sole unit and is the platform upon which the foot rests. The material used in insole manufacture must be robust while providing a smooth surface. Any irregularities in the surface of the insole are potential irritants to the plantar aspect of the foot and can result in discomfort to the wearer and the formation of skin pathology. The importance of the quality and integrity of the insole is well demonstrated when considering the effects of a poor-quality, rough insole on the neuropathic foot. While the traditional material for the insole is leather, a variety of synthetic materials is also used. The insole is usually lined with a fine 'sock lining', which serves to provide extra smoothness and improve the appearance of the inner part of the shoe. The sock lining may be full length or only three-quarter length, covering the waist and heel seat of the insole. It is usual for the manufacturer to incorporate their name or logo on the sock lining.

In modern footwear, manufacturers often incorporate removable full-length insole liners, many of which are manufactured from synthetic foam materials. The removal of the manufacturer's insoles permits replacement with commercially available or bespoke insoles.

## Bottom fillings

Traditionally made Oxford shoes incorporate bottom fillings within the sole construction of the shoe. The bottom fillings are an infill material used to level out the surface of the lasted shoe once the shank is positioned between the insole and the attached outsole. The bottom fillings found in traditionally manufactured Oxford shoes are typically made from granulated cork. With wear of the shoe, the bottom fillings sustain a mild compression that permits an accommodative depression in the tread area of the insole immediately below the metatarsal heads. Many modern shoe manufacturers do not need to incorporate bottom fillings as they rely on the direct moulded method of sole construction to eliminate irregular contours on the undersurface of the lasted shoe.

## The welt

Incorporated in the outsole of the traditional Oxford shoe, and in many other more expensive shoes, the welt serves as a joining material uniting the lasted upper to the outsole. The welt is a narrow piece of leather sewn to the perimeter of the upper of the lasted shoe and projecting slightly outwards. The outsole is then attached to this projection and then attached by a further stitch around the entire surface of the welt, providing a strong attachment of the outsole to the upper of the shoe. The use of the welt in shoe sole construction provides a means of easily removing the outsole when it is worn and attaching a new one, thereby significantly increasing the lifetime of the shoe.

## The outsole

The outsole of a shoe is the section that is in direct contact with the ground. Traditionally, it is made of specially treated hard-wearing leather; current methods of sole construction utilise rubber, crepe or other synthetic hard-wearing material. The outsole is required to withstand much wear and tear, and must be tough while retaining the necessary flexibility to permit propulsion during gait.

Leather outsoles are typically found on Oxford shoes. They are hard-wearing and flexible enough to achieve efficient propulsion; they are not, however, particularly good for shock absorption. Manufacturers have commonly replaced the use of leather with hard-wearing synthetic materials that are light in weight and adequately flexible. They will provide shock absorption and protect the foot and skeletal tissues against impact and ground reaction force from hard unyielding surfaces.

Outsoles are attached to the lasted upper by a variety of methods of sole construction, the most commonly used being direct moulded, cemented and welted.

## The subsidiary parts

In addition to the main parts of the shoe that are found within the upper and the sole, the subsidiary parts may be incorporated in the manufacture to enhance shoe structure and function; they are not necessarily found in all examples of footwear.

## The heel

The heel of the Oxford shoe consists of layers of leather, termed 'lifts', attached together providing the required heel height. On the outermost part of the heel, which is in direct contact with the ground when the shoe is worn, a top piece is applied. The top piece is so named because as the lasted shoe reaches its final stage of manufacture it is presented to the shoemaker in the inverted position with the sole facing upwards. This is the final component placed on the shoe before the last is removed. This top piece is made of hardwearing leather and is easily removed when worn and can be replaced. Frequently in modern day shoe manufacture the heel unit is fully integrated with the sole unit and is a composite part of the outsole created through the direct moulding method of sole construction.

## The shank

The shank is inserted between the insole and the outsole at the waist of the shoe to form a reinforcing bridge between the heel and the forepart of the shoe. Shanks are traditionally made of a narrow strip of steel or wood and provide support to the non-weight-bearing part of the outsole of the shoe. The former is usually reserved for women's shoes and the latter for men's shoes. The shank is particularly necessary in women's shoes that incorporate a higher heel, preventing the shoe from snapping at the waist during wear.

## The counter

The heel counter is a moulded cup-shaped piece of leatherboard or thermal plastic material that may be inserted at the rear of the shoe between the medial and lateral quarter and its lining. The counter is responsible for preserving the shape of the rear medial and lateral quarters during wear and preserving a close relationship between the quarters and the rear part of the foot.

## The backstay

The backstay is a narrow strip of leather that is attached to the rear of the shoe and acts as reinforcement to the joint of the medial and lateral quarters. The backstay protects this vulnerable part when the last is removed from the completed shoe and also during wear when the foot is placed in the shoe. The backstay is recognised as an additional strip of leather attached externally at the junction of the rear quarters; alternatively, it may simply comprise a discreet overlay of the upper part of the rear lateral quarters on the medial quarters.

## FEATURES OF A GOOD-FITTING SHOE

To achieve maximum benefit from podiatric treatments, patient compliance with footwear advice and a commitment to wearing appropriate shoes on a regular basis is fundamental. It is necessary for the practitioner to be aware of footwear fashion trends, the quality and characteristics of footwear manufactured by individual companies, and local suppliers of footwear. Unfamiliarity with such information renders the podiatrist ill prepared to provide important advice to patients. This may result in a significant reduction in the benefit from both short- and long-term care received by the patient and the full treatment potential will not be realised. Achieving patient compliance with footwear advice is fraught with difficulty. Female patients may present particular resistance to the adoption of footwear advice. They often, incorrectly, anticipate that the podiatrist is recommending 'old ladies'' shoes and, as a consequence, reject the advice and quickly respond with an excuse as to why they cannot wear that type of shoe. There may be an incorrect perception of the type of shoe that the podiatrist is recommending. As a result, the patient invariably interrupts the delivery of the advice and fails to hear accurately the facts within the information given. Male patients tend to be more receptive to footwear advice. Male footwear styles are less varied and, in general, provide better accommodation for the foot and permit a more natural foot function.

The delivery of footwear advice may be more successfully achieved if it is provided through the podiatrist exploring with the patient what qualities and level of comfort they would like to achieve when purchasing footwear. Careful questioning of the patient can provide the podiatrist with information that can later be reflected back to the patient when recommending specific features about an appropriate shoe. An explanation of how specific footwear features will meet the individual patient's requirements suggests to the patient that they have remained in control of the footwear selection. The information supplied by the podiatrist regarding specific features of footwear and relating the desirable features to specific manufacturers and styles is invariably more positively received than is a more dictatorial, uncompromising approach.

Normal foot function is described (Merriman & Tollafield 1995) as being pain-free and energy-efficient. Rossi (2003) distinguished between the terms 'normal gait' and 'natural gait'. The former term may be applied to shoe-wearing societies, while the latter can be applied to barefoot societies. It is suggested that the use of the term 'normal' may be defined as the accepted standard, mean or average. In contrast, the term 'natural' is reserved for what is 'pristine, the ideal state, the ideal form and function stemming from nature itself'. The difference between the two terms is summarised by: 'The difference between normal and natural is essentially the difference between what is and what can or ought to be.' (Rossi 2003).

When this definition is applied in the context of wearing footwear, it can be considered that those who wear shoes will not have a natural gait, as is seen in those who live within shoeless societies, but they will have the potential for a normal gait, the features of which will demonstrate the accepted parameters of normal shoe-assisted gait. Ideally, therefore, any footwear worn to assist walking on hard unyielding surfaces should function in a manner that maximises the potential for more natural gait and that ensures natural foot function is subjected to the minimum of interference. It is desirable that any shoe will work in harmony with and permit the foot to function as naturally as it can.

When advising patients on footwear, attention should be drawn to the desirable features discussed below. Footwear advice must take into account the function for which the footwear is to be used. The features required in footwear to be worn for a busy working day differ from those used for less-active social occasions.

## Good retaining medium

A 'good retaining medium' refers to any device that retains the foot within the shoe and eliminates undesirable forward movement of the foot within the shoe. Lacing devices are the best means of achieving this. A minimum of three pairs of eyelets with laces is recommended. Although lacing devices are the retaining mechanism of choice, unless the shoe is laced correctly retention can be significantly compromised. The correct way of lacing a shoe is to hold the foot at approximately 45° from the floor surface with the heel of the foot firmly pressed into the rear of the shoe (Fig. 18.3). While maintaining this position the laces should be firmly adjusted from the lowest pair of eyelets to the uppermost and then tied firmly. This method mimics the position the foot adopts when it is placed on the fitting stool used by reputable shoe retailers. For patients with back pain or those who find it difficult

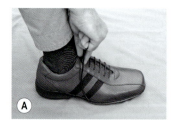
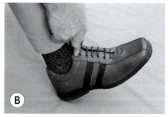

**Figure 18.3** (A) Incorrect foot position when tying shoelaces. Note the poor security of the heel at the posterior counters. (B) Correct foot position when tying shoelaces, with the heel secured.

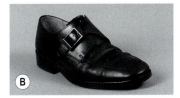

**Figure 18.4** Alternative effective retaining mechanisms. (A) T-bar shoe for women. (B) Monk-style shoe for men.

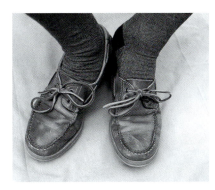

**Figure 18.5** Habitual insertion and removal of the foot from the shoe without untying laces leads to breaking down of the quarters and poor retention of the foot in the shoe, and results in chronic foot strain.

to stoop down to lace shoes in this manner, the heel of the foot may be placed on a stool or step. Any discomfort anticipated from the firmness of tied laces should be removed by ensuring that the shoe has a good pressure-absorbing tongue. Shoes that do not have this feature may be adapted through the application of a cushioning tongue pad applied to the inner surface of the shoe's existing tongue and extending to a point just anterior to the vamp.

An alternative to laces, particularly in women's shoes, may be the incorporation of a strap that is attached anteriorly at the shoe quarters crossing the forefoot from the medial to the lateral quarters. It is typically held in position using a buckle or hooks and loop attachments. To be effective in retaining the position of the foot this strap must be broad enough and must be attached when the foot is held in the same position as when lacing. In women's footwear a variation of the forefoot strap is the T-bar strap. The monk-style shoe for men, in which the shoe is retained in position by a side buckle attaching an extension of the medial quarter to the lateral quarter, may be a suitable alternative to lacing shoes (Fig. 18.4).

## Close-fitting medial and lateral quarters

A comfortable close fit of the medial and lateral quarters of the shoe will complement the retaining mechanism provided by either laces or strap. The close fit of the quarters around the tarsal region of the foot will also reduce the incidence of the heel sliding medially or laterally and creating frictional stress on the plantar and posterior aspects of the heel. The quarters, ideally reinforced with counters, are required to embrace the rear of the foot and permit normal subtalar, midtarsal and ankle joint function. When examining the weight-bearing foot, with the shoe correctly retained on the foot, the examiner should not be able to identify any gap between the medial and lateral aspects of the foot and the quarters. The medial quarters are positioned slightly higher on the foot than the lateral quarters. This reflects the higher medial longitudinal arch and ensures a good fit around the anterior tarsal and metatarsal region of the foot. They should be shaped to reflect the narrower shape of the hindfoot below the medial and lateral mallelous when compared to the relatively wider plantar aspect of the heel. On the shod foot the quarters should be shaped and positioned in order not to cause irritation to the malleoli or the Achilles tendon. In a shoe that is worn correctly there should be no mediolateral or anteroposterior drift of the foot during gait. Similarly, there should be no evidence of the rear part of the shoe slipping off the heel area of the foot.

The quarters of the shoe must be robust enough to withstand the frequent insertion and removal of the foot from the shoe. This is achieved by the selection of good-quality materials, the incorporation of an effective counter and the utilisation of a backstay. It should be noted that poor, slovenly habits used to insert or remove the foot from the shoe without undoing the retaining mechanism rapidly result in destruction of the quarters. This results in poorly fitting footwear with inadequate retention of the foot, giving rise to potential foot strain and many other pathologies (Fig. 18.5).

> ### CASE STUDY 18.1 THE IMPORTANCE OF ESTABLISHING TYPICAL EVERYDAY FOOTWEAR HABITS AND PRACTICE
>
> A retired woman aged 67 years attended the clinic complaining of a pain in both feet of at least 6 months duration. She stated that she felt less able to carry out her domestic chores and physical activities, and had become reliant on her husband to do the shopping and tend to the garden, etc. The pain was initially described as 'aching all over both feet'. On questioning, it was established that, while the pain was now present on weight bearing and at rest, at the time of onset the pain was localised to the medial aspect of the rearfoot of both feet and occurred only after weight bearing. Further questioning established that the 'general' pain was now bilaterally focused in the region of the talonavicular joint, plantar heel pad, metatarsal heads and posterior aspect of the lower leg. Rest provided mild relief, but further weight bearing increased the intensity of the pain. Using a visual analogue scale (VAS) the pain was reported to be at its best 4 and at its worst 8.
>
> The patient's general health was good; all pedal pulses were steady, strong and palpable. There were no sensory or motor deficiencies; the skin was mildly anhidrotic. Non-weight-bearing examination revealed some hypermobility of the subtalar joints. The metatarsophalangeal joint motion was unrestricted and within the normal range. Examination of the ankle joints revealed a bilateral ankle equinus, and a maximum dorsiflexion of the ankle being restricted to approximately 3° of plantar flexion. There were no other significant structural abnormalities.
>
> Weight-bearing examination revealed lowering of the medial longitudinal arch, with associated abduction of the forefoot, mild clawing of the lesser toes and prominence of the talonavicular joint. Current medication consisted of an anti-inflammatory drug that had been prescribed by the patient's family doctor when she presented with her initial symptoms. The footwear worn was lacing, with adequate heel height, shock absorption and toe-box accommodation. It was noted, however, that the shoes had been removed prior to the examination without undoing the laces.
>
> The patient reported that prior to developing the symptoms she enjoyed walking, participated in weekly swimming sessions and was a keen gardener. As a result of her foot pain she had noticed that she had increased in weight, and she blamed this on her relative inactivity. Her main activity now was housework; leisure walking was now minimal due to the pain. On asking the patient what she wore on her feet when working in the house she explained she always wore her slippers as they were 'roomy' and felt very comfortable. Frequently, to avoid having anything on her feet, she would be barefooted and conduct her household chores in this manner, as she assumed it was better to have nothing on her feet rather than be restricted in footwear.

Following the examination and history taking, a diagnosis of chronic foot strain was made. It was concluded that the presence of ankle equinus, in the absence of any other significant structural abnormality, had resulted in compensatory pronation at the subtalar joint. This rendered the feet inefficient, not only as a lever during gait but also as a mobile adaptor. Initially this resulted in a local tensile stress on the calcaneonavicular ligament. In association with the hypermobility of the subtalar joints, this resulted in poor foot posture during stance and gait, rendered the forefoot hypermobile, and gave rise to overloading of the metatarsal heads in addition to chronic ligamentous strain in the rearfoot and forefoot joints. The failure of the patient to lace correctly the shoes worn outside resulted in rearfoot instability and forefoot hypermobility, giving rise to chronic ligamentous strain. A further contributing factor was the wearing of slippers that offered no significant support to the hindfoot and offered little to compensate for the ankle equinus or permit functionally uncompromised weight bearing for the heel. This was compounded when the feet were unshod during significant weight-bearing indoor activity.

The first line of management was to explain, in lay terms, the cause of the foot strain and have the patient understand that a significant cause of her discomfort was a result of poor use of what were satisfactory outdoor shoes and the inappropriate wearing of slippers, or going barefooted, while in the house. The poor lacing practice was addressed by demonstrating the correct method of shoe lacing, with the foot on the ground in a dorsiflexed position and the heel firmly at the back of the shoe with the quarters closely fitting. The need for the foot to be supported while indoors and performing household chores and activities was emphasised. It was recommended that the patient used a pair of shoes, similar to the ones she wore to the consultation, but dedicated to wearing in the home when working and weight bearing. Reinforcing this recommendation, she was advised that slippers should be worn only when physically resting or when weight bearing for only a very short interval.

The patient was reviewed 6 weeks later and having followed the advice given stated that the pain had all but resolved (when present it was only after significant period of activity) and was scored as 1 on the VAS. She was now doing her shopping and other outdoor activities in comfort, and habitually kept shoes on while carrying out her chores indoors. She reported that she no longer went barefooted and reserved her slippers for relaxation while watching television or reading.

This case demonstrates the need to consider not only the appropriateness of the footwear presented to the podiatrist at consultation, but also to confirm that footwear is being used and retained on the foot correctly. It also demonstrates the importance of questioning the patient with regard to footwear habits while indoors, and making appropriate recommendations. Finally, the case highlights the importance of identifying and managing the source of the patient's complaint.

## Adequate width and depth in the toe box

Normal toe function during gait with efficient intrinsic and extrinsic muscle action requires unrestricted toe movement. During stance and gait the toes should not be in direct contact with the toe end of the shoe and the toe puff should not exert pressure directly onto the nail plate. Adequate toe-box width and depth is often difficult to ascertain, and in used shoes is best examined by the practitioner feeling directly into the toe box of the shoe to identify any depression or wear of the lining material within that area. If wear or tear is present this is often the result of direct and repeated impact of a toe into the toe box. When width and depth are inadequate, examination of the outer toe box also reveals a distension of the upper material as the toe presses on

the upper of the toe box. The presence of these abnormal features may confirm inadequate width and depth of the toe box, but consideration must also be given to the possibility that shoes that are too long, or poorly retained in position, may result in a forward shifting of the foot within the shoe during gait and may result in toe box impact. A similar outcome may also result from wearing shoes that are too short.

There is no standard amount by which any shoe should extend beyond the longest toe. The amount of room provided by shoe manufacturers is variable and is dependent on many factors, including the style and shape of the forepart of the shoe. It is important that the practitioner, through examination of the foot and questioning of the patient, can establish that during gait under normal walking circumstances the shoe provides the necessary accommodation to ensure that the toes are not in direct contact with the toe box.

## Correct length

Shoe designers and manufactures consider many factors that influence the length of shoes, including the style of the shoe, the toe shape and the growth allowance for children's shoes. The podiatrist is interested in the length of shoe relative to the adequacy of the accommodation it provides relative to normal foot function. The result of wearing shoes that are too short or too long is particularly seen in the digits, where impact within the toe box gives rise to toe abnormalities, hypertrophic nail pathologies, an increase in the transverse curvature of the nail plate and articular damage to the joint surfaces of the toes and metatarsophalangeal joints.

The appropriate length of a shoe is determined by the use of a shoe-fitting device (a variety of which are currently in use), the skill and knowledge of the experienced shoe fitter about the footwear, and the response of the wearer of the shoes on trial. People may have subtle differences in the length of the right and left feet, and the shoes provided should accommodate the larger foot unless significant size differences are encountered. The smaller foot may be better accommodated within the shoe through the use of a pad applied to the inner surface of the tongue. Commercially available heel grips are of limited value as they may cause a widening of the quarters, reduce the close fit at the rear foot and serve to push the foot forward into the toe box of the shoe.

The use of a measuring device is not considered by reputable shoe retailers as the definitive means of identifying the correct size of shoe required. Similarly, it is unwise to consider that if one pair of shoes of, for example, a size 7 provides a comfortable fit then all shoes sized 7 will also give a comfortable fit. Subtle differences in the shoe and last design, manufacturing process, the sizing system in use and the country of origin of the shoes may all influence the ability of the shoe to accommodate the foot adequately. It is recommended that when purchasing footwear some time should be spent on ensuring that the correct length (and breadth) is achieved and that the services and advice of a reputable shoe retailer and fitter are sought.

The podiatrist may test to confirm that the length of a shoe is satisfactory by examining the shoe on the foot of the patient. When the shoe is correctly applied and laced there should be no gaping at the medial, lateral and posterior quarters. On palpation, the position of the metatarsophalangeal joints should coincide with the broadest part of the shoe at the tread line. The toes should be able to move freely within the toe box and the hallux should be able to be extended before pressure from the inner surface is noted. The toes should not be in direct contact with the end of the shoe. Finally, gentle depression on the toe box area should reveal approximately 10–12 mm of available toe space beyond the longest toe (Fig. 18.6). To assist in determining the suitability of the length of the shoe, examination of the hosiery worn by the patient whose shoes are too short frequently reveals a hole in the area accommodating the apex of the longest toe.

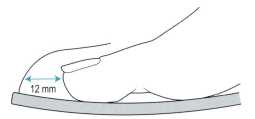

**Figure 18.6** Diagram indicating the toe clearance allowance of 12 mm beyond the longest toe.

Questioning of the patient may also reveal that the appearance of holes in hosiery occurs rapidly and repeatedly. It must be remembered that in many cases the longest toe is the second toe.

## Correct width fitting

Adequate width fitting is of equal importance to length fitting. The correct width fitting of a shoe is achieved when the foot is accommodated in such a way that the toes are straight, unrestricted and maintain the normal relationship of one to the other during gait.

Many foot-measuring devices give a fitting scale measurement based on the measurement seen between two parallel lines that represent the widest part of the foot. This measurement is usually given an identifying letter. For example D is considered to be an average width, while B is narrow and G is broad. (Between each increase in full size of shoe there is a corresponding increase of approximately 6 mm in the girth measurement of the shoe. Some manufacturers produce shoes of the same size but with a range of girth measurements or fittings that accommodate both the narrow and broad foot within one length fitting.) The widest part of the foot is normally transversely between the first metatarsophalangeal joint and the fifth metatarsophalangeal joint. This measurement, when used in association with the length measurement, suggests the most appropriate width fitting for a particular pair of feet. While this is an important measurement, attention should also be drawn to the part of the shoe distal to the metatarsophalangeal joints. If this part tapers too greatly, the first and the fifth toes, and the other lesser toes can frequently be subjected to damaging pressure.

Examination of the foot relative to the width available in the forepart of the shoe will indicate whether there is any inadequacy on the medial, lateral or both aspects of the forepart. This will dictate the shape of the forepart of the shoe best suited to the foot in question. It is often found that the recommendations made by the podiatrist regarding the shoe shape and shoe width are in stark contrast to the shape preferred by the patient.

Examination of the forepart of the shoe when on the patient's foot to establish the appropriateness of the width should not evidence medial or lateral forced stretching of the quarters and vamp over the outsole of the shoe. Similarly, neither the hallux nor the fifth toe should be seen to exert undue pressure on or distort the upper of the shoe. Tightness to the vamp is suggestive of inadequate width. Examination of the shoe internally may reveal an indentation of the upper where the compressed digit is forced to stretch the upper in an attempt to achieve better accommodation. Conversely, if the vamp area is loose, excessively creased and puckers easily when the thumb is run across the forepart of the shoe, the shoe is too wide.

## Adequate heel seat

Shoes are largely reliant on the retaining mechanism and the close fit of the quarters to ensure security on the foot. To function in harmony with the foot and eliminate undesirable movement shoes must be firmly attached around the rear of the foot and the tarsometatarsal region, and permit the toes at the metatarsophalangeal joints to function normally in an unrestricted manner.

The rear quarters must be narrow enough to hold the rear of the foot firmly. It is necessary for the designer of the last to ensure that the heel seat of the shoe is wide enough to accommodate the relatively broad heel of the foot. The relationship of the heel seat to the posterior medial and lateral quarters on cross-section forms a triangular-like shape when correctly designed. This acknowledges the narrowness of the foot below the malleoli and the breadth at the plantar surface of the heel. This shape at the rear of the shoe, which may be described as 'wedging' the rearfoot in position, contributes to the retention of the foot within the shoe.

The heel seat must accommodate the heel of the foot. If it is too wide it may allow the heel to drift during wear, making the foot insecure within the shoe. This repeated drifting of the heel may result in the formation of diffuse callus on the plantar aspect of the heel or, in severe cases, the development of plantar calcaneal bursitis. Poor retention of the hindfoot within the shoe may lead to chronic strain on the joints and ligaments of that area, and may contribute to the development of chronic foot strain. In time, secondary to the poor retention of the foot within the shoe, a variety of symptoms may be experienced in the forefoot. A heel seat that is too narrow will cause the soft tissue on the plantar aspect of the heel to be effectively wedged into the junction of the heel seat with the quarters, and may cause a ridge of tightly packed callus to form on the peripheral aspect of the heel.

Examination of the foot within the correctly applied shoe where the heel seat is too broad may reveal a gaping of the medial and lateral quarters. The examiner's finger may be able to be inserted between the rear foot and the quarters, making contact with the heel seat. Where the heel seat is too narrow, a tightness and forced stretching of the rear quarters will be noted and the patient will describe a feeling of fullness in the rear of the shoe. Dense callus may form on the peripheral borders of the heel.

## Heel height no greater than 2 inches (5 cm)

Heels are a fashion accessory to footwear, rather than contributing to 'natural gait' during wear. No other part of a shoe is subjected to such change and variety by shoe designers as the heel. Examination of footwear available from shoe retailers reveals a variety of heel heights, widths and shapes. Shoe heel height is variable. Consideration of the concept of 'natural' gait opposed to 'normal' gait leads to the realisation that the presence of a heel is not necessary for natural foot function. Any footwear worn should allow the foot to function as naturally as possible, and therefore the conclusion is that the absence of a heel from a shoe could be a distinct advantage. The inclusion of heels on footwear is well established and today they are considered to be an integral part of footwear design. Heels can contribute to an imbalance in body-weight distribution between the forefoot and the hindfoot. An increase in heel height can transfer greater body weight to the forefoot. An increase in heel height causes an increase in the angulation of the heel seat from the horizontal, which causes an increase in the thrust of the forefoot into the toe box of the shoe. The higher the heel the more anteriorly positioned is the centre of gravity of the body. As a consequence, the wearer of high-heeled shoes must extend the lumbar spine to maintain upright posture and good balance. This can result in lower back discomfort in addition to the local foot pathologies (e.g. ankle equinus) that may result from the modified, unnatural way the foot is required to function if held in this abnormal position.

To prevent significant overload of the forefoot it is recommended that the heel height should not exceed 5 cm.

## Broad heel base in contact with the ground

It is vital to consider the surface area of the heel in contact with the ground during stance and gait. Many women's shoes may have an acceptable height of heel but a narrow heel breadth offers little stability to the body due to the small area of the heel in contact with the ground at heel-strike. Some women's fashion shoes offer as little as 1 cm$^2$ of heel contact area. In such cases the outer part of the heel in contact with the ground is made of steel or other hard-wearing plastic material. During heel-strike the efficient transmission of body weight to the weight-bearing heel is significantly jeopardised due to the poor traction properties of the outer part of the heel coupled with the inadequate ground surface contact provided by the narrow heel. Frequently this type of heel results in inversion strains and can lead to fractures at the styloid process of the fifth metatarsal or to more severe ankle fractures.

Ideally, the ground contact surface of the outer part of the heel should be broad and, where possible, extend beyond the parameters of the heel seat of the shoe.

## Upper material made of leather or other natural material

The upper of any shoe is subjected to flexion and extension, particularly over the area of the vamp corresponding to the metatarsophalangeal joints. To withstand the wear at this area the material must be hard-wearing and maintain the necessary flexibility to permit the required movement. The plasticity of the material during the shoe-making process (i.e. its ability after distortion, or moulding around a shoe last, to retain the new shape produced) makes leather the most suitable material from which to manufacture the shoe upper. Leather provides the benefits of being plastic when moulded; however, when stretched over the last only a residual amount of the plasticity remains within the material. The remaining plasticity allows for minor adaptations by the material when the shoe is worn and effectively accommodates the foot allowing the shoe to 'give' or 'break-in'.

Leather also provides elastic properties during wear (i.e. the ability to completely recover shape after distortion such as stretching and compression). Bending of any material, as occurs on the vamp of the shoe, requires the stretching of the layers on the outside of the bend and the compression of the layers on the inside of the bend. Failure of the upper to provide elastic properties results in a shoe that does not provide a close fit around the foot and rapidly loses its shape and proportion.

The permeability of shoe leather is important. The ability of the upper to transmit water, air and vapour is an important quality to achieve maximum foot comfort. The perspiring foot relies on the absorption and evaporation of moisture to ensure maintenance of healthy skin. Many synthetic materials are not permeable and therefore result in the accumulation of perspiration on the foot. Prolonged use of footwear incorporating this type of material frequently leads to local hyperhidrosis and the associated skin pathologies that result from a reduction of the skin's natural resistance to tensile stress. Failure to perform rigorous foot hygiene may result in the decomposition of the sweat and sebum and give rise to bromidrosis.

## FOOTWEAR AND LAST TERMINOLOGY

When examining or recommending footwear it is necessary to consider important elements of last design and footwear construction that

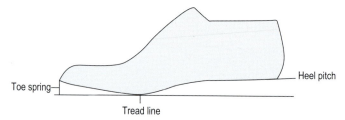

**Figure 18.7** A last standing correctly on the tread line, displaying the corresponding heel pitch and toe spring.

may influence how well or naturally the foot functions when shoes are worn.

## Tread line

The term 'tread line' refers to the part of the shoe that is in direct contact with the ground surface at the forepart of the shoe when the heel height, pitch and the toe spring are correct (Fig. 18.7). The tread line lies at an oblique angle across the forepart and runs from the first metatarsal head to the fifth metatarsal head. As the term suggests, the tread line corresponds to the widest part of the forefoot at the metatarsal heads. With normal wear, and in a well fitting shoe, it is this area of the forepart of the outsole where the greatest amount of wear occurs. It is at this point the foot bends when walking. The vamp is the part of the upper subjected to flexion and extension as the foot bends at the metatarsophalangeal joints and is located in the upper above the tread line.

It is important that, where possible, the mildly oblique angle created by the position of the first relative to the fifth metatarsophalangeal joint of the foot matches that of the tread line of the shoe. In reality this often differs slightly, which results in compression of the fifth toe by the upper of the shoe distal to the tread line. This is due to a reduction in the angle of the tread line relative to that of the metatarsophalangeal joints. The dynamic foot flexes slightly distally to the tread line, and this may contribute to compression of the lesser toes. Similarly, people with a relatively long medial longitudinal arch may find that in some shoes the tread line is positioned too far posteriorly and that, while the shoe appears to be the correct length in relation to the toes, accommodation within the shoe is poor across the metatarsophalangeal joints and as a result compression of the forefoot occurs.

## Toe spring

The toe spring of a shoe or last is defined as 'the elevation of the toe end of the last from a horizontal surface when the seat is raised to its correct height (pitch) so that the last is standing correctly on its tread line' (Ceeney 1958). The toe spring of the shoe will reflect the same elevation as that incorporated in the design of the last on which the shoe is made.

The toe spring reduces the resistance to flexion that the shoe will place on the foot when it is flexed at the metatarsophalangeal joints and while the heel is raised during the propulsive phase of gait. Effectively, the presence of the toe spring at the toe end of the shoe serves to reduce the amount of flexion required at the metatarsophalangeal joints to produce propulsion and reduces foot fatigue when walking a distance. The toe spring also helps to reduce the amount of wear and tear that occurs at the vamp.

The amount of toe spring incorporated in the design of a last (and shoe) is dependent on the level of resistance to flexion that will be encountered by the shoe when worn. A number of factors influence

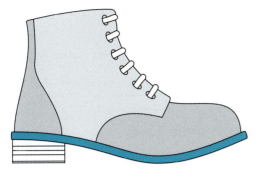

**Figure 18.8** Rigid-soled boot demonstrating a high toe spring.

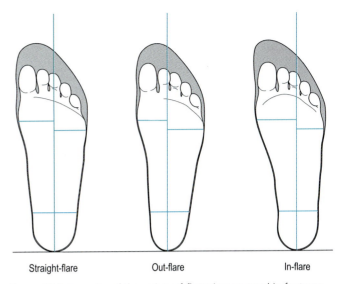

Straight-flare  Out-flare  In-flare

**Figure 18.9** Examples of the variety of flares incorporated in footwear. Note the relationship of the centred heel to the accommodation available in the forepart of the shoe relative to the forward extension of the centred heel line.

the height of the toe spring, including the rigidity of the outsole, the style of shoe, heel height and heel pitch.

## Rigidity of the outsole

The more rigid the outsole of a shoe the greater the effort required for the foot to flex the outsole to permit propulsion. Footwear incorporating rigid outsoles (e.g. the army boot) always incorporates a high toe spring to reduce the effort required by the foot to flex the outsole and to compensate for the shoe or boot's resistance to flexion (Fig. 18.8). An extreme example of a high toe spring is seen in the traditional wooden clog where no flexion is available. The incorporation of an exaggerated toe spring allows the wearer to effectively 'rock' forward on the shoe using the forward shift of the body's centre of gravity to create the rocking effect on the outsole of the clog and permit propulsion. In contrast, shoes with thin outsoles that offer little resistance to flexion have significantly less toe spring incorporated in the design of the shoe.

## Style of shoe

Court shoes and slippers usually incorporate flexible outsoles that offer little resistance to flexion. This suggests that there is no need to incorporate a toe spring in the design of the shoe. However, in the absence of any retaining mechanism in these types of shoe the manufacturer often incorporates a higher than necessary toe spring. This is done to ensure that downward pressure of the toes within the toe area of the shoe during wear will effectively reduce the toe spring and result in the quarters of the shoe being pulled against the rear foot and ankle, thereby providing a more secure fit. This tends to work best when the shoes are new.

## Heel height

The height of the heel also dictates the height of the toe spring. The foot subjected to a higher heeled shoe is automatically placed in a position where the metatarsophalangeal joints are held in a dorsiflexed, propulsive position. The lasts created to manufacture high-heeled shoes only incorporate a small elevation as a toe spring, the function of which is to prevent the toe end of the shoe scuffing against the ground during gait.

## Heel pitch

The term 'heel pitch' refers to the angle of elevation of the heel seat of the last from the horizontal surface, when the last is standing correctly on its tread line. The heel pitch is largely dependent on the heel height, and fluctuates relative to the heel height of the shoe. An over-

short heel relative to the heel pitch results in an increased toe spring, and causes the shoe to fall backwards during stance or when the shoe is standing on a horizontal surface. When the foot is placed in such a shoe the metatarsophalangeal joints flex and extend at a more posterior position relative to the tread line of the shoe. If the heel is too high, the shoe is tilted forward, with a corresponding decrease in the toe spring. When the shoe is worn, the metatarsophalangeal joints flex and extend in a more anterior position than the shoe's tread line. An incorrect relationship between the heel pitch and the heel height results in an unbalanced shoe and a reduction in comfort during wear.

During stance the centre of the body weight falls slightly anterior to the ankle joint. Any significant increase in heel pitch, and consequently the height of the heel, results in the centre of the body weight being positioned more anteriorly. To compensate for this and to maintain balance there is a need to extend the lower back. The greater the heel pitch or height, the more the ankle joint is held in plantar flexion and the subtalar joint in an inverted position during the stance phase of gait. The potential for normal foot function is compromised, and prolonged walking in this position may give rise to a variety of foot pathologies and skeletal symptoms affecting the lower back.

## Flare

The term 'flare', sometimes referred to as 'form', refers to the shape of the last or shoe relative to the position that the centre of the heel seat occupies in relation to the forepart. Examination of the relationship between the undersurface of the forepart of the shoe to the centre of the heel in a last or a shoe produced for an adult shows that there is a greater forepart tread width on the inner medial side of the shoe compared to the lateral side. A line from the centre of the heel seat projected forward to bisect the tread line in the forepart reveals the relationship between the medial and the lateral aspect of the tread (Fig. 18.9). A greater tread area on the medial border of the line indicates that a shoe is 'in-flared'. Tread width that is equal on either side is 'straight-flared', and if the lateral tread has a greater surface area the shoe is 'out-flared'.

If a similar examination is made of feet it will be noted that there can be a wide variation in the relationship of the forepart to the central heel. This variation is clearly shown when comparing a pes plano valgus with a pes cavus. The former reflects an out-flared structure, while the latter is more suggestive of a straight-flared structure. A typical healthy adult foot displays little variation on either side and is more in keeping with a straight-flare or a slight in-flare.

If a foot is subjected to a shoe that does not have a corresponding flare it is poorly accommodated and is subjected to considerable stress. If a pes plano valgus foot is subjected to an in-flared shoe, in addition to the distortion that will occur at the hind part of the shoe, the lesser toes, due to the abduction of the forefoot, will be subjected to considerable pressure from the lateral aspect of the forepart of the shoe. This abnormal pressure will be seen in the shoe by distortion of the lateral aspect of the toe box, which may overhang the outsole.

The podiatrist should always consider what extrinsic influences might affect the foot. Frequently, footwear, and in particular the flare of the shoes being worn, is unsuitable and may be directly responsible for the patient's symptoms.

## DESIRABLE FEATURES OF FOOTWEAR FOR SPECIFIC FOOT CONDITIONS

The podiatrist is required to make footwear recommendations according to the specific foot condition with which the patient presents. The standard recommendations stated above may require to be supplemented with some additional and specific features associated with the nature and severity of the patient's complaint.

It is acknowledged that the severity of some foot conditions necessitates the provision of bespoke or semi-bespoke footwear. Before the patient's condition advances to this stage it is often possible to recommend specific commercially available shoes that will offer the required level of comfort and accommodation for the foot without the expense of custom-made shoes. Below are listed a variety of foot types and the desirable features that may be incorporated within the footwear worn by the patient. The podiatrist must have good knowledge of the various suppliers of a wide range of commercially available specialist footwear and advise patients on how this may be acquired.

### Hallux abducto valgus

- Additional 'bunion pocket' to accommodate joint abnormality.
- Seam-free uppers with the absence of stitching that may irritate the prominent first and fifth metatarsophalangeal joint.
- Deep toe box to accommodate associated lesser toe abnormalities.

### Hallux limitus/rigidus

- Seam-free uppers with an absence of stitching in the forepart of the upper to eliminate the possibility of irritating the enlarged dorsal aspect of the metatarsophalangeal joint.
- Thick outsole with exaggerated toe spring to compensate for the reduced first metatarsophalangeal joint function.
- Removable manufacturer's insole to facilitate supply of bespoke insole.
- Deep toe box to accommodate enlarged first metatarsophalangeal joint.

### The short, broad foot

- Derby-style shoe with wide opening anterior quarters.
- Broad, padded tongue under eyelets.
- Thick microcellular, shock-absorbing outsole.

- Exaggerated high toe spring.
- Good heel-to-ball fitting.
- Good quarter and forepart depth to shoe.
- Well-rounded toe box that adequately accommodates digital formulae.
- Removable manufacturer's insole to facilitate supply of bespoke insole.

### The long, mobile foot

- Frequently requires a narrow fitting.
- Close-fitting rear quarters and counters.
- Robust retention mechanism.
- Good heel-to-ball fitting.

### The highly arched foot

- May require slightly higher heel than standard footwear.
- Derby-style shoe with wide opening anterior quarters.
- Fully adjustable retaining medium joining the medial and lateral quarters (e.g. adjustable tarsal strap or 'hook and loop' straps).
- Broad, padded tongue under eyelets.
- Deeper toe box that is also well rounded and adequately accommodates digital formulae.
- Thick, microcellular, shock-absorbing outsole.
- Exaggerated high toe spring.
- Good posterior and forepart depth to shoe.
- Good 'heel-to ball' fitting.
- Removable manufacturer's insole to facilitate supply of bespoke insole.

### The foot of the patient with rheumatoid arthritis

- Broad heel base with medial buttress.
- Upper and outsole of a light robust construction.
- Wedged outsole.
- Lightweight, thick, pressure-absorbing outsole.
- Often straight-flare is required (out-flare in advanced stages).
- Seamless forepart to uppers with the absence of stitching that may cause irritation.
- Self-adhering 'hook and loop' type broad retaining strap.
- Well-cushioned tongue that is an extension of a seamless vamp.
- Well-lined, close-fitting quarters with appropriate counters.
- Removable manufacturer's insole to facilitate supply of bespoke insole.
- Soft, smooth, hardwearing inner lining to uppers.

### The foot of the patient with diabetes

- Removable, thick, pressure-absorbing insoles to permit the insertion of bespoke insoles.
- Seam-free uppers with an absence of stitching.
- Removable manufacturer's insole to facilitate supply of bespoke insole.
- Upper and outsole of a light robust construction.
- Good functional retaining medium; laces, broad tarsal strap or 'hook and loop' type strap.
- Well-padded tongue that is a continuation of vamp.
- Soft, smooth, hardwearing inner lining to uppers.
- Thick, pressure-absorbing outsole.

## SIZE SYSTEMS AND SYSTEMS OF MEASUREMENT

A size system is a method of measuring the length of feet, lasts and shoes using a specific unit of measurement. When measured a descriptive size number is allocated; this is known as the 'notation'. In the UK two principal size systems are in use: the English size system and the Continental size system. Each has its own unit of increase between sizes and its own notation.

A measurement system that facilitates a regular increase in girth measurements relative to an increase in length measurements, and provides a range of girth measurements for individual sizes, is known as a 'girth measurement system'. Where shoes of one size are available in different girth measurements this is known as 'fittings'. Fittings are identified by letters; for example, A denoting a narrow fitting and E denoting a broad fitting. There are significant design, manufacture and production costs to providing shoes in different fittings, and consequently the availability is limited to some of the more established manufacturers of both children's and adults' shoes.

A 'heel-to ball' measuring system measures the distance from the posterior aspect of the heel to the first metatarsophalangeal joint in addition to the heel-to-toe measurement. The scale used in this system gives a shoe size that is considered appropriate for feet with the particular heel-to-ball measurement. This system is based on the observation that the length of the typical foot from the heel to the first metatarsophalangeal joint is seven-tenths that of the heel-to-toe length. When using this system the desirable outcome is that feet measured from heel-to-toe and heel-to-ball should arrive at the same measurement, albeit from the different scales used for each measurement. When this ideal outcome is achieved, the corresponding shoe size fitted will accommodate the widest part of the foot and will bend correctly at the tread line. Problems may arise when the heel-to-ball measurement of the foot is longer than the heel-to-toe measurement. If the heel-to-toe measurement is used to fit the shoes, the widest part of the shoe will not correspond to the widest part of the foot and this will result in pressure on the forepart of the foot beyond the metatarsal heads. In addition, the shoe is designed to bend at the tread line, which, in the case highlighted, will be positioned slightly posteriorly to the corresponding widest part of the foot. This may lead to undue pressure on the foot and give rise to discomfort.

### The English size system

This well-established size system has a unit of increase of one-third of an inch (8.5 mm) between full sizes. Therefore, within a 1-inch measurement there are three full sizes. The English size system includes half sizes, one-sixth of an inch (4.25 mm) between that of the full size. The notation that allocates a size number to the measurement made commences at size 0 (zero), which is four inches (102 mm) in length. Size 1, therefore, is four and a third inches (110 mm) in length, size 2 is four and two-third inches (118 mm) and size 3 is five inches (127 mm). The notation is continuous up to size 13, following which it is repeated from size 1, giving rise to the adult sizes. The repetition of the notation can give rise to confusion in sizes and it is usual to identify the size with the prefix 'children's' or 'adult's'.

### The Continental size system

The Continental size system is arguably the simplest system and is commonly used. The unit of increase in this system is two-thirds of a centimetre; this unit is referred to as the 'Paris point'. Within a measurement of 2 cm there are three Paris points. Due to the smallness of

**Table 18.1** Adult shoe size conversion table

| English | Continental |
|---------|-------------|
| 5 | 38 |
| 6 | 39 |
| 7 | 41 |
| 8 | 42 |
| 9 | 43 |

the unit of increase there are no half sizes in the continental size system. The notation is simple in its application, with size 1 being 1 cm in length. It is continuous, without any repetition in the adult size range (Table 18.1).

## COMMON FOOTWEAR STYLES

Examination of the stock held by any shoe retailer will confirm that the choice of shoe style is varied in the ranges for both men and women. Cost, fashion and proposed activity frequently dictate the type of footwear selected. Within each broad category of footwear are assortments of styles and designs from which a particular pair of shoes may be selected. These variations permit the manufacturer to reflect fashion trends. For example, court shoes, so popular with women, may be manufactured with high heels, low heels, backless and sling-backed.

### Tie lace

The tie-lace shoe, although worn more frequently by men for business, is also available to women. The adjustable retaining mechanism offered by the laces, when correctly used, serves to minimise undesirable drift of the foot within the shoe and makes this the preferred style of shoe recommended to patients by podiatrists.

### The Oxford shoe

The Oxford shoe is distinctive by a decorative toecap attached to the distal end of the upper over the toe box. The vamp is stitched posteriorly to the quarters. The anterior medial and lateral quarters of the shoe, when laced correctly, closely oppose each other over the dorsal tarsal area of the foot. The quarters house the eyelets through which the laces are threaded. Typically, the Oxford shoe has five pairs of eyelets. The potential for pressure on the dorsal aspect of the foot from the laced quarters is reduced by the provision of a tongue. In the Oxford shoe this is attached separately and is stitched anteriorly to the undersurface of the vamp. A more decorative variation of the Oxford shoe is seen in the brogue. The upper of this shoe is pinked and has numerous perforations. The more fashionable brogue shoe worn today is derived from the practical origins of the shoe. Originally a footwear style favoured by Irish land workers, the perforations in the upper material allowed for the evacuation of water when walking in the wet marshy ground of the Irish bog lands. The brogue shoe is very popular and is styled in versions for both men and women. The need for a close apposition over the tarsal region of the foot of the anterior end of the quarters when the shoe is laced means that the Oxford shoe may not be suitable for a foot with a high arch.

## The Derby shoe

Often referred to as a 'Gibson shoe', the Derby is a variation of the tie-lace shoe. It is simple in design, with the vamp extending under the anterior medial and lateral quarters to form the tongue of the shoe. Unlike the Oxford shoe, the anterior quarters of the Derby do not directly oppose each other when tied correctly. When untied and the quarters are loosened and pulled back there is greater accessibility for the foot to the inside of the shoe. These features are important when shoe recommendations are made for people with broad feet or highly arched feet. In contrast with the Oxford shoe, it is usual for the Derby shoe to have only three pairs of eyelets (Fig. 18.10).

## The moccasin-style shoe

This popular style of shoe is based on the traditional North American Indian footwear. Typically made of buckskin, the sole of the shoe and the medial and lateral borders are composed of one piece of material drawn from the plantar aspect of the foot over the dorsal aspect of the forefoot. An 'apron' front, which is attached by stitching, covers the toes and the dorsal aspect of the midfoot.

Modern tie-lace and slip-on shoes made in the moccasin style (e.g. loafers) are popular and tend to be worn for more casual occasions. Many people with healthy good functional feet find the shoes comfortable, as they can exhibit many of the desirable features of a good-fitting shoe. However, care should be taken when recommending this style of shoe. If worn by individuals who have prominence of joints, as in hallux abducto valgus or lesser toe abnormalities, care must be taken that the stitching of the apron front to the upper of the shoe and the resultant internal seam does not cause pressure on the skin over the prominent joints (Fig. 18.11). In quality moccasin style shoes, manufacturers frequently

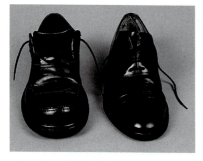

**Figure 18.10** The Derby (left) and Oxford (right) shoe. Note, compared with the Oxford, the wider parting anterior quarters in the Derby shoe permit easier access for the broad foot.

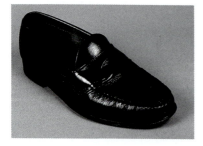

**Figure 18.11** A moccasin shoe showing the typical apron front.

incorporate linings that protect the forefoot from the seam of the apron attachment.

## The sandal

The sandal, with its simple design and openness, was the standard footwear style of warm Mediterranean countries. The basic sandal provided a simple method of protecting the sole of the foot. As the use of the sandal moved further north with the advancement of the Roman Empire, adaptations were made to provide greater protection to the foot and lower leg, and gave rise to the development of the shoe and boot. The first crafted foot covering, the simple sandal, has provided shoe designers with an opportunity to create endless variations of this basic shoe design. Sandal design can be very simple, creating a means of protecting the sole of the foot. Retention is achieved by the incorporation of various foot and ankle straps that arise from the sole. In contrast, the basic sandal design can be transformed by fashion shoe designers to an elegant foot covering worn by fashion-conscious women as an integral part of a designer outfit. While sandals vary widely in appearance they can be categorised into three distinct styles.

- Strapless sandals, a variation of which is the mule sandal, are predominately worn by women, although some men's sandals may be effectively backless. The retention of footwear on the foot relies on a strap of varying widths over the dorsal aspect of the forefoot.
- Sling-back sandals of different heel heights feature straps of various breadth that are retained around the ankle to provide, albeit limited, retention of the foot in the shoe. These straps are usually seen in addition to straps around the forefoot. Women's sandals tend to incorporate fine straps. This style of sandal is adapted for men, in which case the heel is low, the outsole is more robust than in the women's version and the retention straps are more robust and effective. These sandals frequently fail to adequately retain the foot in position and give rise to shearing stress. If worn habitually the resultant stresses applied to the foot give rise to callus formation on the plantar aspect, particularly over the heel area or around the periphery of the heel. As the callus accumulates it is frequently subjected to tensile stress and results in fissuring. The high-heeled strapless and sling-back sandals worn by women jeopardise the stability of both the ankle and subtalar joints, leaving the wearer vulnerable to inversion and eversion ankle strains.
- Enclosed sandals are worn by men and women and vary greatly in appearance. They are enclosed at the back, where a full rear quarter and frequently a counter are incorporated. There is usually an effective retention mechanism over the dorsal aspect of the forefoot. This may take the form of straps, buckles or laces. The forepart of the sandal is usually structured to permit the circulation of air around the foot, with the toes frequently exposed. This is the preferred style of sandal. When purchasing sandals, careful selection will ensure that many of the desirable features of a shoe may be incorporated.

## The court shoe

The term court shoe (referred to in North America as a 'pump') is thought to have originated in the reign of Henry VIII who had chronic gout and needed to wear footwear that readily and easily accepted a swollen and painful forefoot. Royal courtiers were commanded to wear a similar style of footwear when in the King's presence in order that attention was not drawn to the King's foot disorder. The conse-

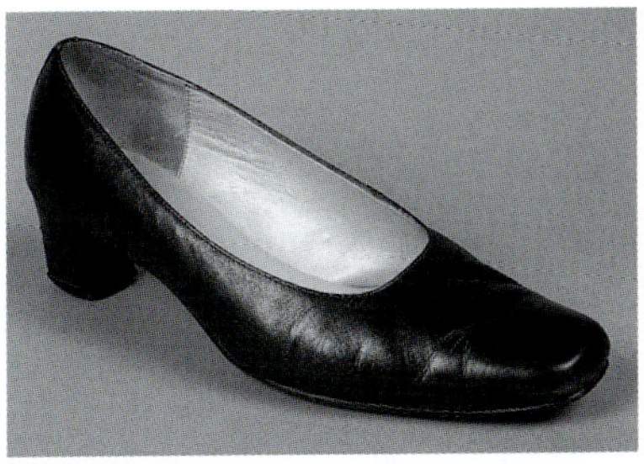

**Figure 18.12** A women's court shoe.

quence of this royal decree was shoes that slipped onto the feet with a typically squared off broad forefoot, referred to as 'court shoes', which are commonly worn today. Male versions are slip-on style shoes, while women's court shoes have various styles and appearances, ranging from simple slip-ons to more elegantly designed and expensive dress shoes.

Court shoes must rely on a close fit to the foot for retention; many have a higher than necessary toe-spring that is depressed by the pressure from the toes, resulting in a closer, although temporary, fit of the shoe around the posterior, medial and lateral borders of the heel (Fig. 18.12). Prolonged wearing of a slip-on shoe often results in poor retention of the shoe on the foot because of the tendency of the quarters to stretch and gape away from the medial and lateral borders of the foot.

## Sports shoes

Sports participants require footwear with a range of features that permit performance of activities with maximum efficiency. A wide variety of sports shoes are commercially available, each with particular features specific to the sporting activity for which they are intended. In general, sports shoes have many desirable features that the podiatrist would recommend for regular wear. It must be remembered, however, that sports shoes suit more leisurely attire. When making footwear recommendations the podiatrist should be conscious that not all patients will accept the concept of wearing trainers nor be realistically expected to wear them to business. It is necessary for the podiatrist to consider what features of the sports shoe are required for the individual patient, and be knowledgeable about current footwear styles and trends in order to direct the patient to an appropriate traditional footwear brand that also exhibits desirable features. (See the discussion of sports shoes in Ch. 13.)

## Boots

Boots were originally reserved almost exclusively for wear by men, with the exception of riding boots. Fashion boots are now popular with both sexes, but are also utilitarian and worn by the armed forces, land workers, tradesmen, and fire service and police personnel. Wellington boots are worn by many and are frequently worn by farmers or are reserved for wear in inclement weather or for walking in wet and marshy ground.

The various styles of boot, including the ankle boot and the knee-length boot, are usually retained on the foot and lower limb by a variety of mechanisms. To be retained in position fashion boots frequently rely on the proximity of the material of the upper around the foot and lower limb. Frequently in the more fashionable women's knee-length boots the inclusion of a zip, usually found on the inside of the boot, may contribute to retention of the foot and lower limb.

The more practically styled boots invariably have laces to provide firm retention of the foot.

## WEAR MARKS AS AN AID TO DIAGNOSIS

Examination of the wear marks occurring on the upper and the sole of shoes can give the podiatrist an insight to the structure and function of the foot and the features of the gait adopted by the individual. Careful examination of the shoe worn by the patient can serve to confirm a diagnosis of structural abnormalities of the foot. Often by the examination of shoe wear a diagnosis can be made of a potential abnormality before it becomes clinically apparent.

When examining the wear marks occurring on a shoe the practitioner must consider normal foot function and gait and how they influence the development of normal wear marks. This benchmark reference must then be contrasted with the wear observed on the shoes of patients with foot and gait abnormalities. Examination of the shoe should give consideration to the wear on the outsole and heel, the insole, the lining of the upper and the upper itself. No clinical examination should be considered complete until the footwear worn by the patient has been fully examined. The podiatrist must also ascertain that the footwear presented is that which is normally worn by the patient. Questioning the patient should reveal whether any other style of shoe is regularly worn. It is not unusual for patients to wear their 'best' shoes for the first visit to a podiatrist, which can be misleading when relating the footwear to the subjective symptoms. With experience and the application of anatomy and biomechanics theory the podiatrist can examine shoe wear and identify areas of abnormality and relate abnormal wear to gait alterations and presenting symptoms.

Wear marks should not be considered as standard; however, certain abnormalities and gait patterns do tend to present with typical patterns of wear. As a guide, typical wear patterns seen in the 'normal' foot and contrasted with those seen in association with common foot abnormalities are summarised below.

## Normal wear

### The outsole and heel

- Posterior/lateral heel wear.
- Heavier wear across the forepart of the sole at the tread line becoming more apparent in the area of the first and second metatarsal head.
- Heavier wear distal to the first metatarsal head corresponding to the final toe-off by the hallux.

The insole (sock lining)

- Uniform discoloration of the heel seat only slightly greater on the posterior/lateral border.
- Lateral discoloration of the waist of the insole corresponding to the soft tissue of the lateral longitudinal arch.
- Discoloration and some indentation, due to compression of bottom fillings, at the metatarsal heads. This may be slightly more evident under the central and first metatarsal heads.
- Distal discoloration corresponding to the pulps of the toes approximately 1 cm from the distal end of the shoe.

### The lining of the upper

- The lining at the posterior aspect of the quarters, corresponding to the backstay, and that of the medial and lateral quarters should be evenly discoloured. There should be no evidence of

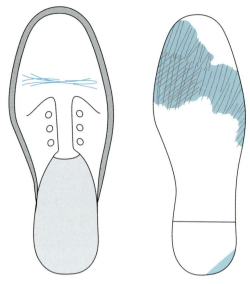

Figure 18.13 The typical 'normal' wear patterns seen in footwear.

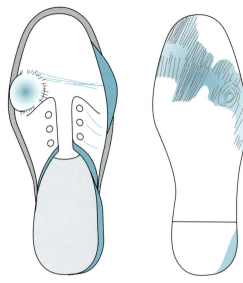

Figure 18.14 Typical shoe-wear patterns seen in cases of chronic hallux limitus.

excessive wear secondary to excessive unrestricted movement of the foot within the shoe.

- The lining of the distal end of the toe box and the toe puff should be smooth, with no evidence of indentation or undue wear.

## The upper

- In welted shoes, when viewed directly from above, no part of the upper of the forepart should obscure the welt.
- The main transverse crease across the vamp should be mildly oblique corresponding to the metatarsal formula and be consistent with the appearance of the tread line of the outsole.
- Anterior quarters should be parallel and directly oppose one another.
- Medial and lateral quarters should be symmetrical.
- The material of the upper should be essentially smooth and evenly contoured, with no obvious distortion (Fig. 18.13).

## Wear marks seen in association with common foot disorders

### Hallux limitus/rigidus

*The outsole and heel*

- Excessive posterior/lateral heel wear.
- Extreme wear under the fifth metatarsal head. This may display evidence of internal rotation of the limb through the appearance of wear marks appearing as concentric rings.
- Wear under the second metatarsal head may be exaggerated.
- Minimal wear under the first metatarsal head may be noted.
- The height of the toe spring may be reduced.
- Excessive wear may be evident on the undersurface corresponding the distal phalanx of the hallux.

*The insole (sock lining)*

- Excessive discoloration may be noted on the lateral border of the heel seat.
- Heavy discoloration and depression of bottom fillings may be present in the region of the fifth metatarsal head; may also present as excessive wear of insole material.

- Heavy discoloration and depression of bottom fillings may be apparent under the central metatarsal heads, particularly the second.
- Minimal discoloration and depression under the first metatarsal head.
- Deep depression and discoloration under the distal phalanx of the hallux; may also present as excessive wearing of insole material.
- Deep depression and discoloration of the insole from the toe pulp of the lesser toes may be evident.

*The lining of the upper*

- The lateral lining of the quarters may exhibit excessive wear.
- Excessive wear of the lateral lining of the vamp in the region of the fifth metatarsophalangeal joint may be evident.
- Excessive wear of the lining of the medial/dorsal vamp may be evident and consistent with excessive wear in the area from osteophyte formation at the first metatarsophalangeal joint.

*The upper*

- Evidence of bulging of the posterior/lateral quarters over the outsole at the heel.
- The lateral vamp may bulge over the outsole, consistent with prolonged inversion of the hindfoot and forefoot.
- Shallow dorsal creasing of the vamp is diagonal from the fifth metatarsophalangeal joint to a point just lateral to the first metatarsophalangeal joint.
- Diagonal dorsal creasing of the vamp gives way to dorsal bulging of the upper to accommodate dorsal exostosis formation at the first metatarsophalangeal joint.
- The throat of the shoe may appear to drift laterally (Fig. 18.14).

### Pes cavus

*The outsole and heel*

- Heavy transverse wear at the posterior aspect of heel.
- Heavy wear across the tread line.
- Minimal wear proximal and distal to the tread line.
- The toe spring of the shoe may be exaggerated.

### The insole (sock lining)

- Heavy discoloration and wear on the heel seat.
- Extreme discoloration, depression of bottom fillings and excessive wear across the area in contact with the metatarsal heads.
- If claw toes are present there may be a deep discoloration and depression corresponding to the toe pulps.

### The lining of the upper

- The lining of the medial, lateral and posterior quarters may show evidence of excessive wear.
- The lining of the tongue may be depressed and show evidence of excessive wear due to the prominent tarsal bones.
- The lining of the upper toe box may show excessive wear due to the pressure applied by the clawed or retracted toes and the retraction of the hallux.

### The upper

- The posterior quarters may bulge over the outsole due to the fullness of the heel.
- The anterior quarters may show evidence of stretching due to the prominence of the tarsal region; when the shoes are on the feet there may be a failure of the anterior quarters to parallel and correctly oppose one another.
- There may be a deep transverse crease across the vamp.
- Bulging of the upper anterior to the vamp may be evident, accommodating the severely clawed or retracted toes.
- The tongue may not display evidence of eyelet compression; only lace marks may be evident due to failure of anterior quarters to adequately oppose one another. Consequently, the dorsal aspect of the foot is not adequately protected from the eyelets (Fig. 18.15).

## Pes plano valgus

### The outsole and heel

- Posterior/lateral heel wear.
- Anterior/medial heel wear.

- The waist of the shoe may collapse and be in ground contact.
- The shank may break and penetrate the waist of shoe.
- Excessive wear under the second, third and fourth metatarsal heads.
- Excessive wear to the anterior/medial aspect of the forepart of the shoe.

### The insole (sock lining)

- Excessive wear of insole and sock lining under the second, third and fourth metatarsal heads.
- Wear on the insole may be more apparent on the medial aspect at the waist of the shoe compared to on the lateral aspect.
- Excessive wear may be noted at the forepart of the insole relative to the pulps of the lesser toes; in particular the third, fourth and fifth toes, as they are forced into a clawed position through impact against the toe box due to the associated abduction of the forefoot.

### The lining of the upper

- Excessive wear of the lining of the lateral toe box may be noted.
- Excessive wear of the anterior/medial aspect of the toe box lining due to impaction of the hallux.
- The posterior medial and lateral quarters may demonstrate excessive wear.

### The upper

- Medial drifting of the throat of shoe.
- The posterior and lateral quarters appear excessively wide and rounded.
- The medial quarters bulge over the outsole.
- Shallow transverse crease marks on the vamp.
- If secondary hallux abducto valgus is present, bulging of the quarters on the medial side of the vamp will be noted. Bulging of the lateral toe box is secondary to clawing of the lesser toes of the abducted forefoot (Fig. 18.16).

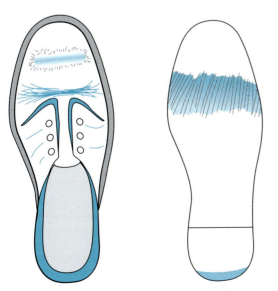

**Figure 18.15** Typical shoe-wear patterns seen in cases of pes cavus.

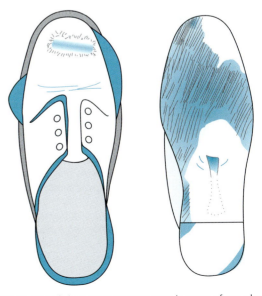

**Figure 18.16** Typical shoe-wear patterns seen in cases of pes plano valgus.

## THERAPEUTIC FOOTWEAR

### Introduction

Footwear is a valuable aid to any therapy designed to improve foot health. Footwear alone can resolve the consequences of many biomechanical anomalies, aid joint function, and reduce friction and pressure to which the foot might otherwise be subjected.

Effective footwear advice and prescription requires an understanding of the presenting foot pathologies and how footwear features are used to meet the needs of management. Assessing the foot for signs of trauma, deformity and limitation in function is part of the podiatrist's professional role, and that expertise is employed when prescribing orthoses. The same criteria should be applied to the appropriateness of footwear with consideration of the features of the individual component parts of the shoe. Practitioners automatically examine footwear for signs of abnormal wear, creasing and suitability, but must also evaluate the fit and functionality of footwear and the way in which the various elements contained within the shoe or boot may be modified to improve foot function.

### Indications for therapeutic footwear

The need for therapeutic footwear is indicated by a number of local or systemic conditions or if the feet are outside the normal size and fitting range of retail footwear. Therapeutic footwear is costly but often is the only option available or the most effective way of treating a condition (White 1994). Therapeutic footwear is indicated for a wide range of foot pathologies and many respond positively to the prescription of therapeutic/orthopaedic footwear. These vary from localised pathologies, including digital deformities, to multisystem conditions, such as diabetes mellitus. The diagnosis of pathologies does not necessarily indicate that therapeutic footwear prescription is required, rather the extent and severity of the condition is the guide for prescription.

Conditions that may benefit from therapeutic footwear prescription include:

- patients whose foot shape and function vary from the normal due to congenital abnormality, trauma or surgical intervention. Therapeutic footwear designed to fit each foot and containing features such as sole modifications can be helpful in overcoming any gait anomalies that may develop.
- patients with scarring as a result of leg ulcers, burns, tissue grafts and muscle flap repairs to debriding injuries may develop contractures and thus may have an altered gait pattern. Prescription footwear can improve gait and reduce discomfort.
- bulky dressings or the lower limb or foot oedema can lead to difficulty in finding accommodative footwear, and the additional width and depth available in therapeutic footwear may be required.
- in patients with a limb-length discrepancy a raise can be added to the shoe of the shorter limb to provide symmetry, aid gait, improve mobility and minimise the lower back pain that often results from this condition.
- peripheral vascular disease may lead to atrophy of skin and nail in the foot, and may cause severe pain. Appropriately prescribed footwear can help to insulate the foot and minimise trauma to vulnerable feet.
- in patients with diabetes when the complications of the disease have affected the feet. Footwear may be used to redistribute areas of high plantar pressure and provide a non-irritant environment for neuropathic feet.

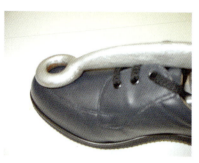

**Figure 18.17** A ball-and-ring stretcher being used to stretch the upper of a shoe to accommodate a hammer toe deformity.

- abnormal gait and impaired mobility may be helped by the prescription of therapeutic footwear. These conditions include multiple sclerosis and cerebral palsy.
- common foot pathologies such as hallux valgus, hallux rigidus, pes cavus, and triggered, hammered or severely clawed toes may be better accommodated within prescribed therapeutic footwear. The painful superficial lesions that often develop in such cases are resolved by removing the pressure caused by inadequate footwear.
- all types of connective tissue disorder, such as arthritis, from generalised osteoarthritis in small joints to rheumatoid disease, where joint function is impaired.

Prior to prescribing therapeutic (orthopaedic) footwear, foot size, foot shape and biomechanical function is assessed. Footwear purchased from a retail outlet should be considered for modification. If the footwear is of a suitable style and material, a number of adaptations can be made. For example, a ball-and-ring stretcher can be used to stretch leather uppers to accommodate problems such as toe deformities and hallux abducto valgus; tongue pads and heel grips can be included to improve fit. Despite these options, there will be a small number of patients whose foot health needs can only be accommodated in specialist footwear (Fig. 18.17).

### CASE STUDY 18.2 ROLE OF FOOTWEAR IN MANAGEMENT OF CHRONIC HALLUX LIMITUS

An otherwise healthy 52-year-old man presented complaining of pain from both first metatarsophalangeal joints. On questioning he confirmed that the joints had sustained no significant trauma and that the onset of the pain had been some considerable number of years prior to his attendance. Previously a keen walker, walking was now uncomfortable, mainly because of the pain in the affected joints. At its worst, the patient scored the level of pain as 8 on a visual analogue scale (VAS). In addition, he complained of pain from corns that had developed on the plantar aspect of both second metatarsal heads, and from callus on the plantar aspect of both fifth metatarsal heads and on the plantar surface of the interphalangeal joint of the first toes. On questioning, the patient stated that he experienced muscle pain in the posterior aspect of his lower leg, and occasionally strained the lateral border of both his ankles. These symptoms were experienced particularly when he walked a distance. A previous recommendation for orthopaedic surgery had been declined, and the patient was keen to explore what conservative methods of treatment were available.

On examination, the relaxed calcaneal stance position revealed long, narrow feet, excessive subtalar joint pronation with associated lowering of the medial longitudinal arches, abduction of the forefoot, and clawing of the lesser toes. Both first metatarsophalangeal joints

**(A)** Sole wear seen in the shoe of a patient with chronic hallux limitus.

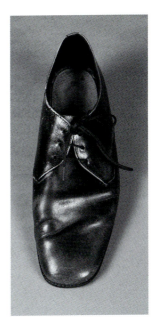

**(B)** Upper wear seen in the shoe of a patient with chronic hallux limitus.

were enlarged on the dorsal aspect. Non-weight-bearing examination of passive joint motion revealed a range of motion of 40°, with a direction of motion of only 20° dorsiflexion from the neutral position of the right first metatarsophalangeal joint. The left first metatarsophalangeal joint was similarly affected. Subtalar neutral examination revealed no significant hindfoot to forefoot structural abnormality; however, hypermobility of the joints of the rearfoot and at the lesser metatarsophalangeal joints was evident.

Examination of the patient's footwear revealed a pair of Derby, lacing shoes. It was established that when wearing lacing shoes they were never laced firmly, the patient preferring to be able to slip them on and off. The upper at the toe box was both narrow and shallow, and a bulging of the upper, coinciding with the enlarged first MTPJ, was noted (see A). The outsole was thin, well worn and showed little evidence of a viable toe spring. Excessive wear was demonstrated on the lateral aspect of the heel. Examination of the forepart of the outsole displayed heavy tread wear at the second to fifth metatarsal heads and at the interphalangeal joint area of both first toes. In contrast, reduced wear was noted under the first metatarsal head (see B). The patient stated that an alternative shoe style was a slip-on shoe that he tended to wear for leisure.

The conclusion was made that the patient suffered from chronic hallux limitus. In view of the general joint hypermobility, the excessive subtalar joint pronation and the patient's preference to wear either poorly tied or slip-on style shoes, it was considered that, combined, these elements served to cause repeated minor damage to the first metatarsophalangeal joints, which resulted in the chronic hallux limitus. The pain experienced in the posterior compartment of the leg was a result of overuse of the tibialis posterior muscle inverting the hindfoot during midstance and propulsion in order to direct load away from the painful first metatarsophalangeal joint, thereby overloading the fifth and second metatarsal heads and causing lesions. This avoidance gait and the continued use of inappropriate shoes also contributed to the lateral ankle strains. An overpull of the flexor hallucis longus provided the patient with a distal fulcrum point during the modified propulsive phase of gait, leading to a heavy callus on the plantar aspect of the interphalangeal joint of the hallux.

The inadequacy of the retaining medium on the footwear permitted the hypermobile foot to slip forward during use, resulting in repeated impact of the first metatarsophalangeal joint into the toe box of the shoe, causing osteoarthritic lipping on the dorsal aspect of

the joint. The narrow and shallow toe box served to irritate the dorsal lipping and contributed to the clawing of the lesser toes. The thin outsole failed to provide any significant protection to the plantar aspect of the metatarsal heads, while the less than effective toe spring served to exacerbate the painful first metatarsophalangeal joint symptoms. The reduction in toe spring height negated any protective function, and it may have contributed to the painful first metatarsophalangeal joint in reducing the extent of dorsiflexion necessary for normal gait.

Careful explanation was given to the patient regarding the complexity of the causes of his symptoms and lesions. Conservative care was provided, with bespoke neutral casted orthoses to manage the hypermobility and excessive subtalar joint pronation. To accommodate the joint abnormality and promote a more normal gait, plain-fronted footwear incorporating laces, a broad and deep toe box, and a firm thick outsole with a high toe spring was advocated. It was stressed that, to receive maximum benefit from the proposed orthoses and footwear, the correct method of lacing must be adopted. The advice was well received.

At review, following the purchase of appropriately styled footwear and the fitting of the orthoses, the patient reported a significant improvement in symptoms and foot comfort. Posterior compartment muscle pain had been eliminated and no further lateral ankle sprains were reported. On questioning regarding the level of pain, a score of 2 was now reported on a VAS.

## CLASSES OF THERAPEUTIC FOOTWEAR

Therapeutic footwear may be grouped into several categories:

- normal retail footwear – modified as required
- stock surgical footwear
- modular footwear
- bespoke footwear.

Stock surgical, modular and bespoke footwear is also often referred to as 'orthopaedic' footwear.

## Stock surgical footwear

Several manufacturers provide stock ranges of therapeutic footwear available for immediate delivery at a relatively low cost. Colours are basic, usually black or brown, but shoes are made in a wide range of sizes and fittings. Catalogues are provided by each manufacturer, with fitting details. The measurements given include size length, width at the metatarsophalangeal joints, girth at the metatarsophalangeal joints and instep girth. The width and girth measurements are in millimetres, and the length is given usually in the English size system. When measuring length, the gauge used must correspond to the manufacturer's length units. Measuring sticks are available as foot-length sticks or as shoe-size sticks. Shoe-size sticks should correspond to the shoe size provided by the manufacturer, although each make of stick varies slightly in the readings given. Foot size sticks require that an additional allowance (generally two sizes) is added to the reading to establish the required shoe size. The sticks should be calibrated against the manufacturer's sizing system prior to measuring.

Stock surgical footwear is available on a sale or return basis. This allows the practitioner to fit and advise without a commitment to purchase. A high percentage of patients requiring therapeutic footwear are fitted from stock. When a good-fitting shoe is identified, further pairs from the same last may be ordered in a different style and colour, but these are non-returnable and require to be paid for on ordering. Stock surgical footwear may be used when a raise is required to compensate for a limb-length discrepancy if the raise required is 1 cm or less. A higher raise requires alteration to the heel-height/toe-spring relationship on the last, and a bespoke prescription is required to meet individual requirements.

## Modular and bespoke footwear

Feet outside the dimensions of shoes available from stock ranges require prescription of modular or bespoke footwear. Complex prescription is required and precise, detailed instructions must be given to the shoe manufacturer. Modular footwear relies on the modification of a manufacturer's existing last, but modifications are limited to ensure that the existing shoe upper pattern pieces are large enough to include modifications. Additional width, girth (up to a total of 2 cm can be accommodated within existing patterns), height and length can be added to an existing last at specific points. Examples are: the inclusion of additional girth to accommodate an exostosis of the first metatarsal head, additional toe-box depth to accommodate deformed toes, the inclusion of additional depth in the tarsal region, an alteration in the height of the quarters to prevent irritation on prominent malleoli.

A range of foot deformities can be accommodated within the modular approach but, despite this facility to adapt lasts, there will be foot shapes or deformities so severe that modification to existing lasts will not suffice. Fully bespoke footwear requires a last to be made by taking plaster of Paris impressions of the feet and lower legs and charting a diagram of the foot outline, with length, width and girth measurements identified at specific points on each foot. British Standard 5943 exists for this process (British Standards Institution 1980) and the measurement system provided in the Standard must be followed for a successful outcome.

Modular and bespoke footwear is available at a fitting stage, and footwear can be fitted to the feet before the shoes are completed. At this stage, the uppers have been prepared and attached to the innersole, and excess upper material is wrapped under the innersole and is available for re-lasting and modification if required (Fig. 18.18).

Any modifications required are illustrated by marking the upper material at the exact location where modification is required using a

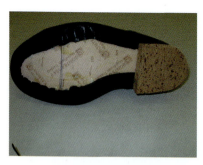

**Figure 18.18** Footwear received at the fitting stage. Note the upper material attached to the innersole and the temporary heel. The upper material can be adjusted to include any change required in the dimensions of the shoe before the outsole is attached.

special effaceable pen. If required, the footwear can be refitted once the modifications have been completed, but once the outsole has been added no further modifications can be made. It is essential to obtain an exact fitting with modifications before the outer sole is attached.

## Features of the therapeutic shoe upper

Once foot measurements have been taken and the dimensions of the 'frame' of the footwear derived, the features of the footwear components need to be considered. This is true for each of type of footwear – stock, modular or bespoke. The shoe should contain a fastening capable of holding it onto the foot, preferably laces but a Velcro fastening is acceptable when mobility is a problem.

The vamp (the front part of the upper) should be seam-free, and any pattern or decoration should be added externally as internal seams may irritate. The quarters (the back part of the upper) should be made from one piece of material with no back seam, which might irritate the retrocalcaneal area. Leather is the most popular material and the one that suits most foot pathologies, but occasionally there is a need to use an extensible material such as neoprene. Lining material may be leather, nylon, cotton, synthetic fabric or shearling (sheepskin). Selection of the lining depends on the internal climate of the footwear during wear and the external environment in which the footwear will be used. Shearling is indicated for cold climates; nylon is cheap but wears quickly; cotton or cambrelle is best for moist feet, as these materials have a wicking property; and leather is good in temperate climates but not for hot weather. Sweaty feet may cause leather linings to become hard and crack, as the foot moisture level affects the tanned leather.

Without any stiffening the shoe will collapse, crease and cause damage to the feet. Without heel counters the shoe quarters will collapse and the shoe may slip off the foot. The extent of the heel counter and the degree of support offered by it should be evaluated. Patients with ankle instability may find a boot helpful, with heel counters additionally stiffened and extended proximally through the quarter. In a midfoot deformity, particularly a valgus deformity, the quarters may be extended distally through to the waist of the shoe. This will minimise deformation of the shoe during gait and can also be used to reinforce the action of an orthotic device.

The properties required in the toe puff should be carefully considered. A toe rim that holds the shoe up over the toe area is required. This may be a standard toe puff that covers the area at the front of the vamp as far proximally as the interphalangeal joints, or a reinforced toe puff to give additional protection against trauma from external objects. In the presence of toe deformities, sensory neuropathy and the environment in which the footwear will be worn should be considered and should inform the prescription. Where there is sensory neuropathy and deformed toes, a rim toe puff is indicated. This will hold up the front of the shoe but will not extend proximally over the dorsum of the toes. In this case the stiffening of the vamp provided by the toe puff in the very front part of the shoe will stop short of the position of the toe deformities in order not to irritate them. The toes will be protected by the upper and lining material without the added hardness of toe puff material in this area. However, if a patient works in an environment where materials may possibly drop onto the feet, a full-size, reinforced toe puff will be beneficial, provided the toe box is of adequate depth to accommodate the toes.

## Features of soling in therapeutic footwear

The type of sole and heel required is also significant. Historically, outsole and heel units were made of leather. However, leather has some disadvantages: it has poor slip resistance, especially in wet conditions; it tends to have little effect in reducing the magnitude of ground reaction force against the foot (Perry 1995); and it absorbs and retains water when wet underfoot conditions are present. Advances in technology have made available a range of materials more suitable for outsole units with varying properties specifically indicated for certain types of activity. Modern sole materials include polymers, most commonly polyurethane, thermoplastic rubber and EVA. The construction of these materials makes them particularly good at shock absorption due to air flow through interconnecting air cells within the materials. These materials are viscoelastic, but the overall effectiveness in reducing plantar pressure is dependent on the thickness of the material, the durability of its elasticity and the speed of recovery of the outsole following deformation under body weight during gait (Even-Tzur et al 2006). Both viscosity and elasticity are important factors in reducing the magnitude of the ground reaction force against the foot. A highly elastic interface will return stored energy to the foot, generally resulting in an increased force between the foot and the ground, whereas a highly viscous interface will absorb most of the energy of the impact caused by the foot hitting the ground. However, if a material is too viscous and is not elastic, it will fail to recover its previous shape after impact and remain flattened, and thus be ineffective during subsequent strides. An element of elasticity is required in soling material to promote material recovery before the next step is taken (Whittle 1999).

All sole materials should keep the foot dry, tolerate a range of external temperatures, be durable and possess a coefficient of friction high enough to prevent slipping but low enough to allow movement across the ground surface without any adherence to it. This coefficient of friction of the outsole material is important. The sole material should allow the foot to move easily across the surface without slipping but also without gripping too firmly to the ground surface, when the body's momentum is likely to cause the body to continue to move forward while the feet stay still, causing a fall.

EVA is generally the preferred sole and heel material. Occasionally, polyurethane or leather topped with rubber to prevent slipping is used. The durability of EVA is determined by its shore value; with a low shore value EVA wears out very rapidly. Footwear made with extra-durable material may be requested from any manufacturer. Recent developments include the use of injection moulding and preformed sole and heel units in polyurethane and thermoplastic rubber for therapeutic footwear. However, because of the costs involved, these sole and heel units are in predetermined sizes and can be used only where the sole required is within a specified length and width range. It is generally unavailable for bespoke footwear, which may be

well outside the normal size range. When prescribing bespoke footwear, soling units may need to be cut from sheets of material and the choice is limited to certain grades and sole patterns of EVA and leather.

The sole material should be appropriate for the lifestyle and activity levels of the wearer. Footwear success is dependent on the choice of sole material and the type of environmental conditions in which it is worn. Studies on safety footwear (Rowland et al 1996) have shown that the wear characteristics of the floor–sole combination must be considered. The wearer's occupation and activities must be considered when prescribing. A rough terrain requires commando soles with additional grip. Some chemicals may damage soling materials, and advice needs to be given if the shoes may come into contact with chemical spillage on the work floor. A lightweight and smooth-surfaced outsole and heel is ideal for a lightweight person with a shuffling gait (Menz et al 2001). Heel and sole prescription is required when combating postural instability. A wide heel base provides greater stability than narrow heels, which are implicated in falls (Rubenstein et al 1988). Certain features can be added to the heel to increase stability. A leg-length discrepancy may require a raised sole on the shorter side. Rocker- or roller-bottom soles increase the rapidity of the midstance phase of the gait cycle and limit the movement at the metatarsophalangeal joints (Wu et al 2004). A rocker or roller sole is beneficial only if the sole of the shoe is inflexible.

## HEELS

### Heel height

There is a relationship between forefoot loading and heel height. The higher the heel, the greater the forefoot loading and the lighter the heel loading. This must be taken into account when considering footwear as a therapy for the treatment of foot pathologies (Broch et al 2004). Normal heel height for therapeutic footwear is 2–4 cm and averages at 2.5 cm (1 inch). Certain pathologies require the prescription of a higher than normal heel height. Consideration is given to the effect of surgical intervention on ankle mobility. Ankle joint fixation may vary from the normal 90°, and the required heel height will be determined by the angle of fixation.

## HEEL MODIFICATIONS

In the solid ankle cushion heel (SACH) the posterior portion has been replaced by a softer material (Fig. 18.19). This reduces shock at heelstrike and is used to compensate for reduced ankle joint motion. A SACH can add a cushioning effect at heel-strike if ankle joint motion is restricted (Wu et al 2004).

A lateral SACH (the lateral portion of the heel is softer) is sometimes used in cases of hyperpronation to bring the subtalar joint to the neutral position, particularly in adolescents.

### Thomas heel

The Thomas heel (Fig. 18.19) is extended anteromedially by 0.5 inch. It is designed to give additional support to the sustentaculum tali and medial longitudinal arch. A *lateral* or *reverse* Thomas heel supports the cuboid and tends to rotate the foot externally.

If additional support is needed, the heel can be wedged on either the medial or lateral side only, or across its width. The wedges stabilise

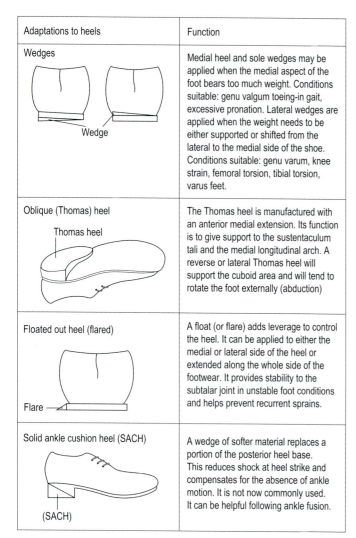

| Adaptations to heels | Function |
|---|---|
| Wedges | Medial heel and sole wedges may be applied when the medial aspect of the foot bears too much weight. Conditions suitable: genu valgum toeing-in gait, excessive pronation. Lateral wedges are applied when the weight needs to be either supported or shifted from the lateral to the medial side of the shoe. Conditions suitable: genu varum, knee strain, femoral torsion, tibial torsion, varus feet. |
| Oblique (Thomas) heel | The Thomas heel is manufactured with an anterior medial extension. Its function is to give support to the sustentaculum tali and the medial longitudinal arch. A reverse or lateral Thomas heel will support the cuboid area and will tend to rotate the foot externally (abduction) |
| Floated out heel (flared) | A float (or flare) adds leverage to control the heel. It can be applied to either the medial or lateral side of the heel or extended along the whole side of the footwear. It provides stability to the subtalar joint in unstable foot conditions and helps prevent recurrent sprains. |
| Solid ankle cushion heel (SACH) | A wedge of softer material replaces a portion of the posterior heel base. This reduces shock at heel strike and compensates for the absence of ankle motion. It is not now commonly used. It can be helpful following ankle fusion. |

Figure 18.19 Heel modifications.

the weight distribution and, when used on one side only, offer added support to a given area.

## Flared heels (floats)

A flared heel (Fig. 18.19) adds leverage to control the heel. A grossly inverted heel-strike may be helped by a lateral flare to stabilise the ankle and subtalar joint. A medial heel flare will help if the strike is too everted. A flared heel will add to that stability and can prevent excessive pronation (with a medial heel flare) or excessive supination (with a lateral heel flare).

## Combined heel and sole modifications

### Flares (floats)

Flares may be extended along the entire length of the sole and heel unit, but in order to achieve this a wedged sole and heel unit is preferred (see below). These combined sole and heel flares are useful if the foot is excessively inverting (lateral flare) or everting (medial flare). They increase the ground surface contact area and stabilise the foot.

## Wedges

Medial heel and sole wedges (Fig. 18.19) are prescribed when the medial aspect of the foot bears too much weight, and are considered in cases of hyperpronation or depression of the medial longitudinal arch.

Lateral heel wedges with anterior extensions transfer weight off the fifth metatarsal shaft. The apex of lateral heel and sole wedges should not extend beyond the fifth metatarsal head as this stiffens the shoe and causes two main problems: in time the toe will curl upwards, causing the foot to roll more to the lateral side; and the stiffness of the shoe encourages the shoe to slip off the heel during gait.

## Contralateral wedging

Contralateral wedging includes a medial heel extension or wedge (e.g. Thomas heel) and a lateral forefoot wedge. This combination was traditionally used to reduce pronation, but has become less popular as the technology underpinning orthotic therapy has advanced.

## Through-sole and heel wedging

This type of wedging gives greater stability during gait. The shoe remains flexible but the ground surface contact area is increased and the central portion of the shoe is strengthened.

## MODIFICATIONS TO THE SOLE

### Lateral sole wedges

These are used when weight needs to be transferred from the lateral to the medial side of the shoe.

### Medial toe wedges

These discourage in-toeing, but should be used with caution.

### Bars

Metatarsal bars may be added posterior to the metatarsal heads on the outer sole of shoes in a line that reflects the angle between the first and fifth metatarsal. This helps to offload pressure from the metatarsal heads and moves the tread line more proximally.

### Rocker soles

The rocker shoe is characterised by a rigid sole that restricts movement at the joints, particularly dorsiflexion of the metatarsophalangeal joints. This limitation of movement decreases plantar pressure by preventing anterior displacement of the soft-tissue cushioning of the submetatarsal head and distributes forefoot load over a larger area (van Schie et al 2000). Walking in the rigid shoe is possible because the shoe tips forward when the centre of pressure moves distal to the rocker fulcrum.

Rocker soles eliminate the propulsive phase of gait. Schaff and Cavanagh (1990) suggest that the mechanism of unloading in the rocker-soled shoe may be a combination of the following effects:

- a redistribution of the load over a larger area
- an increase in the loading time for the regions of the foot in contact with the rigid shoe

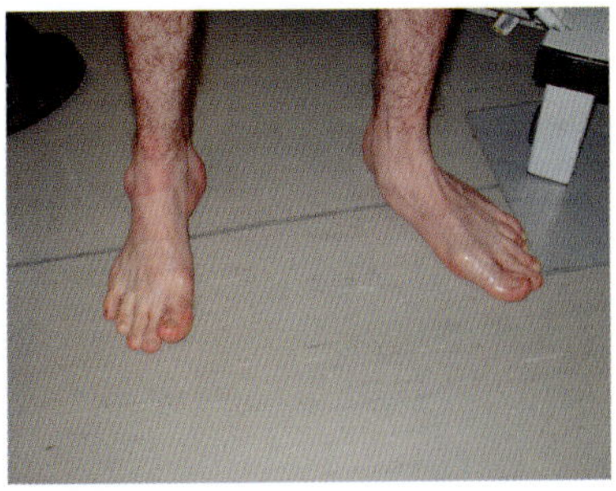

**Figure 18.20** A patient with a limb-length discrepancy. Note that the left foot (longer leg) is pronated and the knee is flexed, while the right foot (shorter leg) is supinated, with the patient failing to make heel contact.

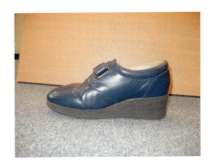

**Figure 18.21** A shoe with a through raise.

- a change in the function of the foot due to the restriction of motion, particularly at the metatarsophalangeal joints
- a change in the patterns of motion of the lower extremity due to the altered geometry and rigidity of the shoe
- a reduction in shear pressure on the plantar surface.

## Adding rockers to existing footwear

When adding a rocker sole to existing footwear the effect on the heel height of the shoe must be considered. The typical metatarsal rocker added to the tread-line area of the shoe significantly raises the height of the toe spring, which in turn distorts the balance of the shoe and reduces the relative heel height. In some cases this can lead to a negative heel, where the heel is functioning at a lower level than the tread-line foot position.

## Shoe raises

Shoe raises added to the outer sole are the most effective means of compensating for limb-length discrepancy (Alexander 2004). Length discrepancy may be caused by congenital anomalies, traumatic injuries, or nerve or muscle damage (Fig. 18.20). Measurement of the length of both limbs is essential to establish the discrepancy and to calculate the height of the raise required. Measurements are taken from the anterior superior iliac crest to the medial malleolus, with the patient supine. Additional measurements should be taken from the ziphoid process to the medial malleolus of each limb, and both these measurements are used to check the discrepancy, which should be used as the first basis for calculation of the raise required. Other factors to be taken into account are hip flexibility, knee flexion and the available range of motion at the ankle, all of which have an effect on functional limb length and must be accounted for in the final calculation of the raise height required.

Individuals with a limb-length discrepancy may use specific strategies to improve ambulation. Commonly they may:

- flex the knee of the longer limb
- rotate the pelvis to shorten the longer limb
- pronate the foot of the longer limb and supinate the foot of the shorter limb.

Once the discrepancy has been quantified, blocks of material equating in height to the estimated difference in limb length are placed under the shorter limb. A pelvic levelling tool, placed to rest on both iliac crests and containing a spirit level, is used to evaluate the symmetry between the length of the two limbs. Comfort relating to the height adjustment is confirmed, and any necessary adjustment made. Full compensation is not always acceptable or comfortable initially, and

it is better to underprescribe the raise height and evaluate again at a later prescription.

## Measuring for the raise

The height of the heel raise required should always be measured in the sagittal plane directly underneath the position of the malleoli and not at the back of the heel (Fig. 18.21). Raises over 1 cm in height should be tapered through the remainder of the sole of the footwear to prevent excessive pelvic tilt. The gradation ratio through the sole should be: heel raise = 1 unit; tread line (metatarsophalangeal joint) = 0.5 units; toes = 0.25 or 0 units.

A limb-length discrepancy of 4 cm should have a raise of 4 cm placed under the heel, and 2 cm under the metatarsophalangeal joints tapering to either 1 cm or 0 cm at the toe, depending on the length of the foot and the degree of angulation required for forward propulsion.

In cases of ankle joint fixation it is unwise to use a tapered raise and the ratio here will be: heel = 1 unit; joint = 1 unit; toes = 0.5 unit.

## Types of raise

Heel elevation contained inside footwear may be used where the elevation required is <1cm. The cosmetic effect of internal raises is preferred, as the raise is not obvious, but where retail footwear is being used there is seldom enough depth in the heel quarter of the shoe to use a raise of more than 5 mm. Raises may be made of cork, EVA of high shore value (70 shore) or of materials of similar density. Surgical footwear may be manufactured with deeper quarters to include the raise, but it is difficult to disguise the difference in elevation between the two shoes when raises of more than 1.5 cm are involved. It is possible to use an internal and external raise on the same shoe, splitting the height of the raise required between the internal and external raises.

External raises can be added to existing soles if the soling and heel material is suitable. They may be added to the outside of the existing unit, or the existing unit may be removed and the raise added between the shoe and the outsole. It is not advisable to add a heel raise only, as this will affect the heel-height/toe-spring relationship and the shoe will no longer stand correctly on its tread line. The shoe then acquires additional toe spring in wear, causing the front part of the shoe to become upturned and the vamp to become excessively creased. This creasing may irritate the dorsum of the foot, causing superficial lesions.

Where external raises are integrated as part of a surgical shoe they must be made of lightweight material to prevent the shoe becoming too heavy for the wearer. They can be covered with the same material as the upper of the shoe or be made to appear as part of the outer-sole unit. Limb-length discrepancy can have serious consequences for mobility. Accurate measurement and careful prescription of a shoe raise can restore relatively normal function and reduce trauma on the knees, hip and lower spine.

## ASSESSING THE FIT OF THERAPEUTIC FOOTWEAR

Whether fitting new therapeutic footwear or evaluating existing therapeutic footwear, the effectiveness of the fit should always be assessed.

Therapeutic footwear is normally provided with a selection of inlays that match the width and length of the shoe, and these provide a useful tool for assessing the dimensions of the shoe in comparison with the foot. Place the foot on the inlay, leaving a small area of the inlay visible behind the foot to allow for the heel curve. Check the overall length of the inlay, from the back of the heel to the longest toe. The inlay should be about 12 mm longer than the longest toe to allow for elongation on walking. Check the proportional length of the foot segments against the inlay. First, check the heel-to-ball length. Then, with the inlay remaining in position under the foot, check that the metatarsophalangeal joints are positioned at the widest part of the inlay, where the shoe is designed to flex. Check the ball-to-toe length to ensure that this is adequate.

If the above lengths are not appropriate the shoe will never fit properly (Fig 18.22). The point at which the shoe flexes (the tread line) must agree with the point at which the foot flexes. If the foot flexes too far proximally the shoe will acquire additional toe spring, the vamp will crease and the shank contained in the shoe will break through the outsole, destroying the integrity of the sole unit. The creased vamp material will cause trauma to the dorsum of the foot, possibly leading to lesion development. If the foot flexes too far distally, the toe spring will be depressed and the toes will be compressed within the shoe.

The inlay is also used to check the width of the shoe at the heel, the instep, the metatarsophalangeal joints and the toes.

The next assessment must be done with the shoe on the foot and containing any orthoses that are to be worn in it. The following should be noted:

- the way in which the foot slips into the shoe – this often indicates how well the shoe will fit, but the shoe must be fastened to evaluate fit
- examine for a good snug heel fit, because the way the foot is held back in the shoe determines the position of the foot within the shoe
- ensure the counter is not causing pressure on the malleoli or the back of the heel
- check the fastenings of the shoe and ensure that the facings are lined up correctly
- look at the instep area and ensure that the fit is neither too tight nor too loose
- evaluate the girth and depth at the metatarsophalangeal joints and over the toes
- ensure that there are no bony prominences visible or evident on palpation that could be damaged by a too-shallow vamp or toe area in the shoe
- the patient should walk in the shoe to ensure there is no heel slippage and that stability in gait is evident.

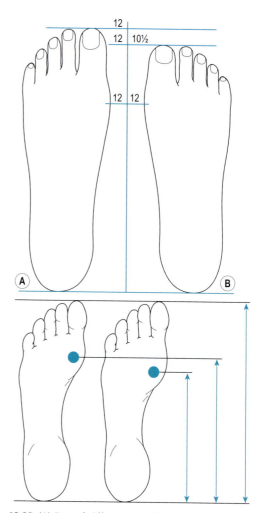

**Figure 18.22** (A) Feet of different overall length but the same heel-to-ball measurement; the right foot will be difficult to fit properly. (B) Feet of the same overall length feet but different heel-to-ball measurement; shoes will need to be of different lengths to suit the heel-to-ball lengths.

## CONCLUSION

Footwear is not only a fashion item or only a protection for the feet. In its various forms footwear can facilitate activity, improve mobility, become an effective therapy, reduce morbidity, and improve and extend quality life. To ensure that footwear is optimal, the podiatrist needs to understand how the normal foot functions when shod, how the shoe may have contributed to any pathology present and, conversely, how the various components of the shoe may be used to remedy any pathological state. Footwear should be regarded as part of both the diagnostic and the therapeutic strategy.

## REFERENCES

Alexander N, Goldberg A 2004 Gait disorders: search for multiple cause. Cleveland Clinic Journal of Medicine 72(7):586–600.

British Standards Institution 1980 BS 5943: Methods for measurement and recording for orthopaedic footwear. BSI, Milton Keynes.

Broch NL, Wyller T, Steen H 2004 Effects of heel height and shoe shape on the compressive load between foot and base. Journal of the American Podiatric Medicine Association 94(5):461–469.

Ceeney E 1958 An introduction to shoe fitting, 1st edn. Pitman, London.

Even-Tzur N, Weisz E, Hirsch-Falk Y, Gefen A 2006 Role of EVA viscoelastic properties in the protective performance of a sports shoe: computational studies. Bio-Medical

Materials and Engineering 16(5): 289–299.

McDowell C 1989 Shoes fashion and fantasy, 1st edn. Thames and Hudson, London.

Menz H, Lord SR, McIntosh AS 2001 Slip resistance of casual footwear: implications for falls in older adults, Gerontology 47:145–149.

Merriman LM, Tollafield DR (eds) 1995 Assessment of the lower limb, Ch. 8. Churchill Livingstone.

Perry JE 1995 The use of running shoes to reduce plantar pressures in patients who have diabetes. Journal of Bone and Joint Surgery 77(12):1819–1828.

Rossi WA 2003 Why shoes make 'normal' gait impossible. How flaws in footwear affect this complex human function. Available at: http://www.unshod.org/pfbc/pfrossi2.htm (September 2009).

Rowland FJ, Jones C, Manning DP 1996 Surface roughness of footwear soling materials: relevance to slip resistance. Journal of Testing and Evaluation 24(6): 368–376.

Rubenstein L, Robbins A, Schulman B, et al 1988 Falls and instability in the elderly. Journal of the American Geriatrics Society 36:266–278.

Schaff P, Cavanagh P 1990 Shoes for the insensitive foot: the effect of a 'rocker bottom' shoe modification on plantar pressure distribution. Foot & Ankle 11(3):129–140.

van Schie C, Ulbrecht JS, Becker MB, Cavanagh PR 2000 Design criteria for rigid rocker shoes. Foot and Ankle International 21(10):833–844.

White JM 1994 Custom shoe therapy. Clinics in Podiatric Medicine and Surgery 11(2):259–270.

Whittle MW 1999 Generation and attenuation of transient impulsive forces beneath the foot: a review. Gait and Posture 10: 264–275.

Wu WL, Rosenbaum D, Su FC 2004 The effects of rocker sole and SACH heel on kinematics in gait. Medical Engineering & Physics 26:639–646.

## FURTHER READING

O'Keeffe L 1996 Shoes, 1st edn. Workman, New York.

Thornton JH 1958 Textbook of footwear manufacture, 2nd edn. National Trade Press Ltd, London.

# Chapter | 19 |

# Pain control

*Michael Graham Serpell*

## KEYWORDS

Analgesics
Chronic pain
Complex regional pain syndrome
Neuropathic adjuvants
Neuropathic pain
Nociceptive pain

> 'The Lords Prayer'
> *May those that love us, love us*
> *and for those who don't love us*
> *may He turn their hearts.*
> *But if He can't turn their hearts*
> *may He turn their ankles,*
> *so we will know them by their walk.*
>
> Anon

Pain is a common cause of limp, and needs to be diagnosed and managed appropriately. Pain control is required in the acute setting, after surgery or trauma for instance. Pain is a fundamental component of the stress response to injury, and if not adequately controlled can impede the recovery process and result in complications (Table 19.1). Pain also persists in many chronic conditions that affect the foot (Box 19.1).

## DEFINITION

The International Association for the Study of Pain (IASP) defines pain as 'an unpleasant sensory and emotional experience associated with potential or actual tissue damage'. Pain is a complex interaction

**Table 19.1** Pathophysiological associations of pain

| Organ system | Potential effects |
|---|---|
| Central nervous system | Inhumane, misery, anxiety, depression, sleep disturbance |
| Cardiovascular system | ↑ Blood pressure, heart rate and vascular resistance, ↑ cardiac ischaemia |
| Respiratory system | Cough inhibition (pneumonia), hyperventilation (respiratory alkalosis) |
| Gastrointestinal system | Ileus, nausea, vomiting |
| Genitourinary system | Urinary retention, uterine inhibition |
| Muscle | Restlessness – ↑ oxygen consumption Immobility – ↑ incidence of pulmonary thromboembolism |
| Metabolic | ↑ Catabolic; cortisone, glucagon, growth hormone, catecholamines ↓ Anabolic; insulin, testosterone ↑ Plasminogen activator inhibitor (↑ blood clotting) |

of sensory, emotional and behavioural factors, and therefore its diagnosis and treatment must address all these aspects.

Pain is classified into nociceptive, neuropathic and psychogenic, all of which types can be either acute or chronic (Box 19.1). Acute somatic pain is the most common type of pain that podiatrists will deal with in clinical practice.

## ANATOMY

Pain is transmitted from the peripheral tissues to the brain cortex via three distinct levels called the primary, secondary and tertiary afferents. Peripheral pain receptors or nociceptors (Latin 'nocere' – to harm) are activated to produce an action potential (Table 19.2). This action potential then conducts along the primary afferent nerve fibres (peripheral level) to synapse with secondary afferent fibres (spinal level), which ascend up the spinal cord. The impulse then synapses to tertiary afferents within various structures in the brain (supraspinal level) (Figure 19.1). Optimal analgesia can only be obtained by utilising treatments that work via different mechanisms and pathways. This is the philosophy behind using multimodal analgesia. An example of such a regimen would be a combination of local anaesthetic infiltration into the wound and oral non-steroidal anti-inflammatory drugs (NSAIDs) (acting at the peripheral level), with oral paracetamol and opioids (acting at the supraspinal level).

## SOMATIC PAIN

*Physiological* pain, also known as first or 'fast' pain, is a protective and useful event that enables the organism to rapidly and accurately localise pain and withdraw from the stimulus in order to avoid or reduce further tissue damage. It is produced by stimulation of *high-threshold thermomechanical nociceptors* and is transmitted by fast-conducting A delta (Aδ) fibres. The Aδ primary afferent enters the dorsal horn of the spinal cord and synapses at laminae I, V and X. Conduction continues along the secondary afferent fibres via the neospinothalamic tract,

**Box 19.1 Characteristics of clinical pain**

**1. Nociceptive** (pain due to tissue damage)

|  | *Somatic* (skin, bone, muscle) (OA, RA, ulceration, infection) | *Visceral* (sympathetically innervated organs) |
|---|---|---|
| Site | – well localised, cutaneous or deep | – vague distribution |
| Radiation | – dermatomal | – diffuse, can be transferred to body surface |
| Character | – sharp, aching, throbbing, gnawing | – dull, vague (cramping, squeezing, dragging) |
| Periodicity | – often constant, also incident pain | – often periodic, building up to peaks |
| Associations | – rarely | – nausea/vomiting, sweaty – blood pressure and heart rate changes |

**2. Neuropathic** (pain due to injury of nerve fibres or tracts)

| Site of injury | Central – post-stroke central pain, phantom limb pain Mixed – plexus avulsion, post-herpetic neuralgia Peripheral – neuroma, nerve compression, neuralgias, painful diabetic polyneuropathy, complex regional pain syndrome |
|---|---|
| Character | – Burning, tingling, pricking, numb, cold, pressing, squeezing, itching – Constant and/or intermittent shooting, lancinating, electric shock |

**3. Psychogenic** Pain entirely due to psychological or psychiatric pathology is rare. One-third of medically depressed patients will have pain as one of their primary complaints but this will resolve as their depression is managed. Anxiety and depression are common sequelae of severe and chronic pain, and often contribute to the unpleasant experience of pain. They need to be managed in conjunction, as pain management will be less successful if they are not.

OA, osteoarthritis; RA, rheumatoid arthritis

**Table 19.2** Cutaneous sensory afferent receptors and fibres

| Stimulus | Nerve fibre |
|---|---|
| **Thermal** | |
| – warm, heat (noxious), sleeping (silent) | C |
| – cold | Ad |
| **Nociceptors (high threshold > 0.6 g wt)** | |
| – polymodal (mechanothermal–chemical) | C |
| – mechanical (some thermal) | Ad |
| **Mechanoreceptors (low threshold < 0.1 g wt)** | |
| – slow adapting types I, II, and C (cold) | Ab |
| – fast adapting types I and II | Ab |

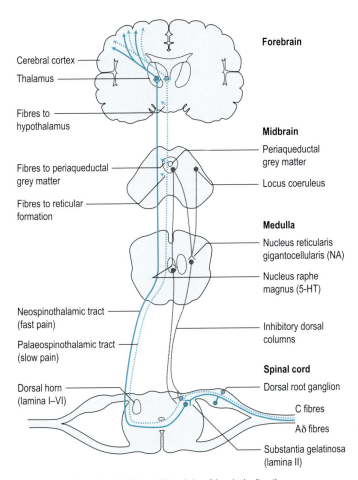

Cerebral cortex

Thalamus

Fibres to hypothalamus

Fibres to periaqueductal grey matter

Fibres to reticular formation

Neospinothalamic tract (fast pain)

Palaeospinothalamic tract (slow pain)

Dorsal horn (lamina I–VI)

**Forebrain**

**Midbrain**

Periaqueductal grey matter

Locus coeruleus

**Medulla**

Nucleus reticularis gigantocellularis (NA)

Nucleus raphe magnus (5-HT)

Inhibitory dorsal columns

**Spinal cord**

Dorsal root ganglion

C fibres

Aδ fibres

Substantia gelatinosa (lamina II)

Ascending nocireceptive fast (blue solid) and slow (blue dashed) pathways
Descending inhibitory tracts (grey)
NA, noradrenaline; 5-HT, 5 hydroxytryptamine

**Figure 19.1** Schematic diagram of the spinal and supraspinal pathways of fast and slow pain, and the dorsal inhibitory pathways that suppress pain. (From Serpell 2005.)

19.1). All are involved in producing the emotional and behavioural response to pain. They also activate the inhibitory pathway that descends the spinal cord via the dorsal columns and terminates at the dorsal horn, where the neurotransmitters noradrenaline and serotonin (5-HT) and the endogenous opioids are released to provide antinociception.

In addition to the two types of nociceptor mentioned above, there are 'silent' or 'sleeping' nociceptors (Table 19.2). These are present in the skin and visceral organs and become active under inflammatory conditions when they may respond spontaneously or become sensitised to other sensory stimuli.

## PHYSIOLOGY

### Peripheral nociceptor level

Most pain originates due to tissue damage. The release of inflammatory mediators from tissues, immune cells and sympathetic and sensory afferent nerve fibres results in an 'inflammatory soup' that bathes the nociceptors. These chemicals sensitise the high-threshold nociceptors so that they can be activated by low-intensity stimuli. When it is produced by normally non-painful stimulation, such as touch, this sensitisation to pain is called *allodynia*. It is called *hyperalgesia* when a normally mildly painful stimulus results in an exaggerated pain response. Sensitisation at the site of injury is called *primary hyperalgesia*.

Some mediators act directly on ion channels in the membrane (protons and 5-HT) but most bind to membrane receptors and act via regulatory intermediates (G proteins and second messengers) to produce changes in membrane ion channels or enzymes. These inflammatory mediators can also produce long-term sensitisation by producing genetic changes in the neuron.

### Spinal level

The dorsal horn area of the spinal cord is the site where complex interconnections occur between excitatory and inhibitory interneurons and the descending inhibitory tracts from the brain. The second-order neurons are of two types: nociceptive specific neurons located in the substantia gelatinosa, which respond selectively to high-threshold nociception; and wide dynamic range (WDR) or convergent neurons, which are located in deeper laminae (V and VI) and respond to a wide range of noxious and non-noxious input.

The gate-control theory was proposed in 1965 by Melzack and Wall in order to explain the highly variable and non-linear relationship between injury and response to pain. They proposed that primary nociceptive fibres (C and Aδ) synapse with a WDR neuron that carries the impulse onward to higher centres (Figure 19.2). This WDR neuron can also be excited by Aβ fibres (which convey non-nociceptive afferent input) under certain conditions, thus possibly explaining mechanical allodynia (a painful response to non-painful stimuli). Crucial to this theory is the presence of an inhibitory interneuron in the substantia gelatinosa, which prevents activation of the WDR neuron. This interneuron can be activated by Aβ fibre firing and inhibited by the small Aδ and C nociceptor fibres. The theory proposes that pain is 'gated-out' by stimulating the large Aβ fibres in the painful area. The mechanism by which transcutaneous electrical nerve stimulation (TENS) works for pain control is by electrical stimulation of the large Aβ fibres, which act to close the 'gate' for pain transmission (Figure 19.3).

Excitatory amino acids and neuropeptides are the neurotransmitters involved in the nociceptive transmission through the dorsal horn.

which is monosynaptic as it ascends to the *posterior thalamic nuclei* (Figure 19.1). From there it synapses with tertiary afferents to the somatosensory postcentral gyrus at the cortex. If this short duration stimulus does not result in tissue damage, the pain disappears when the stimulus stops.

*Pathophysiological* pain, sometimes called second or 'slow' pain, is responsible for the delayed pain sensation that occurs after tissue injury and encourages tissue healing by eliciting behaviour to protect the damaged area. This is the type of pain that occurs after surgery, trauma and inflammation, and is the kind that health carers strive to manage in the clinical setting. It originates from stimulation of the *high-threshold polymodal nociceptors* (free endings) present in all tissues. The nociceptors respond to mechanical, chemical and thermal stimuli that are transmitted via slow-conducting C fibres, which synapse at laminae II and III (substantia gelatinosa) of the dorsal horn. Secondary afferents ascend cranially, mainly via the paleospinothalamic tract and a polysynaptic dorsal column tract to the *medial thalamic nuclei* (Figure 19.1). The paleospinothalamic tract has collaterals that also project to the midbrain, pontine and medullary reticular formations, the periaqueductal gray (PAG), and the hypothalamus, where they synapse onto neurons that in turn project to the forebrain limbic structures. This system is primarily involved with the reflex responses concerned with respiration, circulation and endocrine function (Table

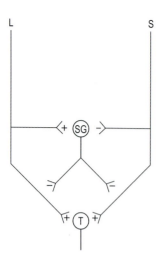

Figure 19.2 Schematic diagram of gate control theory. Both the primary nociceptive small (S) fibres (C and Aδ) and large (L) non-nociceptive Aβ fibres synapse with a wide dynamic range (T) neuron, which carries the impulse onwards. The inhibitory interneuron in the substantia gelatinosa (SG), is inhibited (–) by the S fibres, thus allowing onward pain transmission. However, it is stimulated (+) by the L fibres, which prevents activation of the wide dynamic range neuron, and so impedes pain transmission.

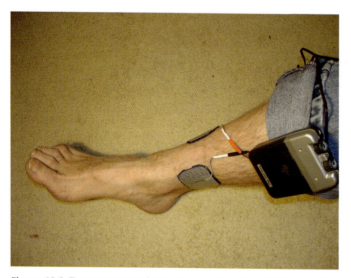

Figure 19.3 Transcutaneous electrical nerve stimulation (TENS) applied to the skin overlying the shin to provide pain relief in the foot.

They activate several receptors on the WDR neurons, but it is the NMDA (*N*-methyl-D-aspartic acid) receptor that, once activated, results in long-term sensitisation of the nociceptive pathway, resulting in *secondary hyperalgesia* (sensitisation outwith the area of tissue injury) and allodynia.

## Supraspinal level

The supraspinal organisation and function in nociception is highly complex, but it is commonly agreed that the perception of pain is associated with changes in activity of the thalamus, primary and secondary cortex, and particularly the anterior cingulate cortex. Various regions of the brain are involved in stimulating the descending inhibitory dorsal column pathway. Opioid receptors are fundamental in stimulating this pathway, predominantly via the mu (μ) and delta (δ)

**Table 19.3** Opioid receptors and their specific actions

| | OPIOID RECEPTORS | | |
| --- | --- | --- | --- |
| | **mu** | **delta** | **kappa postsynaptic only** |
| Density on spinal cord % | 70 | 24 | 6 |
| Endogenous ligand | endomorphin endorphin | enkephalin endorphin | dynorphin |
| Exogenous ligand | morphine | none | enadoline |
| Action | opens K | opens K | closes Ca |
| Analgesia | good | good | poor |
| CNS effects | Respiratory depression | Respiratory stimulation | Psycho-mimetic |
| constipation | yes | no | no |

opioid receptors (Table 19.3). Endogenous opioids such as endorphins and enkephalins are produced in this region of the brain and stimulate these receptors under normal circumstances. However, the only practical way of activating these receptors in the clinical setting is by using exogenously administered opioids such as the μ agonist morphine.

The descending inhibitory dorsal column pathways originate at the level of the cortex and thalamus, and are mediated via relay stations in the brainstem such as the PAG, nucleus raphe magnus (NRM) and locus coeruleus–subcoeruleus complex (LC/SC).

## Neuropathic pain

Neuropathic pain occurs following damage to the neural structures. Nervous system activity depends on the overall balance between the excitatory and inhibitory components. Complete transection or damage of a nerve fibre results in complete loss of sensation and motor power. When the damage is only partial, gross motor and sensory function can be preserved, and nerve activity can often be increased. This can result in subtle abnormalities such as altered temperature sensation, unusual or unpleasant feelings, or even pain. In the feet this may occur after surgery on the toes, resulting in an interdigital neuroma, or with medical conditions such as diabetes or shingles. The common treatments used for neuropathic pain work by suppressing neural hyperactivity (see later).

Patients often find neuropathic pain symptoms difficult to describe, but some of the words commonly used include burning, tingling, numb, pressing, squeezing and itching (Box 19.1). The pain can be constant or intermittent, and may be associated with electric shooting sensations. Examples of neuropathic pain affecting the lower limbs include painful diabetic neuropathy, postoperative neuromas, entrapment neuropathies, some types of complex regional pain syndrome (CRPS – see later) and spinal radiculopathies (frequently involving compression of the fifth lumbar or first sacral nerve root).

It is important to identify any treatable aetiology of pain in order to prevent progression of the underlying disease. For example, good normoglycaemic control will delay deterioration of painful diabetic neuropathy, and surgical laminectomy may correct radicular pain. However, this is not always possible, and treatment of pain should commence as soon as pain is experienced.

## PRINCIPLES OF PAIN MANAGEMENT

The general principle of pain management is based on managing the component parts of the condition, namely the nociceptive and neuropathic constituents. It would be too simplistic to regard pain as being caused by either one or other of these two mechanisms; rather it is often a combination of the two. As complete analgesia is rarely achievable in chronic pain, the primary goals are to improve pain as much as possible and, most importantly, to optimise physical function and coping with any residual pain.

Pain symptoms are managed using techniques that fall into four main groups: pharmacological, regional analgesia, physical therapy, and psychological therapies. The exact order of implementation of therapies depends on local availability, the side-effect profile of the treatment, and the preference of the patient (some patients prefer to avoid medications or injections).

This chapter deals primarily with pharmacological treatments, but the reader should be aware of the importance of the other modes of management.

## THE WORLD HEALTH ORGANIZATION (WHO) THREE-STEP ANALGESIC LADDER

The WHO analgesic ladder was developed in the early 1980s to manage cancer pain (Figure 19.4). It is successful in controlling pain in over 80% of cancer patients who suffer from pain, and has subsequently been adopted for use with all other types of pain. Pain treatment is initiated using the drugs for mild to moderate pain listed on the first step, with progression to steps 2 and 3 for severe pain (Table 19.4). The approach utilises conventional analgesic drugs and adjuvant drugs. Adjuvant drugs are predominantly targeted at neuropathic pain, and include drugs such as antidepressants, anticonvulsants and antiarrhythmics.

### Step 1

Non-opioid analgesics are derived from three types of compounds: aniline derivatives, such as paracetamol; aspirin and other acidic non-steroidal anti-inflammatory drugs (NSAIDs); and non-acidic pyrazole drugs such as phenylbutazone and dipyrone.

Paracetamol works at the supraspinal level by an as yet unknown mechanism. It is well tolerated by most patients and can be as effective as the NSAIDs in managing pain. There is little effect on the liver when taken at normal recommended doses (maximum dose 4 g/day). It is indicated for mild to moderate pain, but has been shown to reduce the requirements for more potent analgesic drugs in severe acute pain.

There are over 20 different NSAIDs. They are a heterogeneous group of drugs exhibiting many different chemical structures and biological profiles. They all inhibit the cyclo-oxygenase (COX) mediated production of prostaglandins, prostacyclins and thromboxanes (Figure 19.5). This mechanism is responsible for their analgesic effect, as prostaglandins sensitise the peripheral nociceptors. Unfortunately, the decreased production of these compounds is also responsible for their side-effects (Table 19.5). These drugs are very useful for musculoskeletal pain and incident (movement related) pain. It would be appropriate to start with the drug that has the least side-effect profile first, and then move on to other drugs. Consequently, most patients will be tried on ibuprofen first, followed by voltarol or mefenamic acid. These drugs are commonly taken by the oral route, but side-effects can be reduced if administered topically (ibuprofen) or rectally (diclofenac). Some NSAIDs (diclofenac, ketorolac) can be injected by the intramuscular or intravenous route if a rapid effect is required.

When NSAIDs are used for longer than a few weeks, the side-effect profile increases. They are responsible for 20% of hospital admissions for upper gastrointestinal perforation or haemorrhage, and 20% (2500) of these patients will die each year. This problem has led to the development of a new generation of NSAIDs, the COX 2 inhibitors, that have a reduced incidence of side-effects. COX 2 inhibitors, such as celecoxib and etorocoxib, provide analgesia by blocking the action of the COX 2 isoenzyme, which produces the prostaglandins mainly responsible for pain. They do not significantly block COX 1, which can still produce the beneficial endoperoxides, thus reducing the side-effect problems. COX 2 inhibitors have absolutely no effect on platelet function and a reduced incidence (50%) of gastrointestinal effects. However, they still have the same incidence of problems with the other side-effects, and both NSAIDs and COX 2 inhibitors seem to increase the risk of myocardial infarction and stroke.

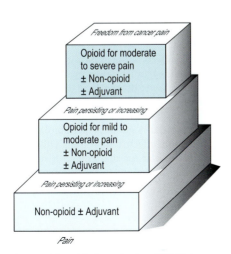

Figure 19.4 The World Health Organization (WHO) three-step analgesic ladder.

**Table 19.4** The World Health Organization (WHO) three-step analgesic ladder

| Step | Drugs |
|---|---|
| Step 1 | Paracetamol<br>NSAIDs or COX 2 inhibitors |
| Step 2 | Codeine, dihydrocodeine, often prescribed as co-analgesics<br>Co-codamol (compound of codeine 30 mg/paracetamol 500 mg) |
| Step 2 → 3 | Tramadol |
| Step 3 | Morphine, diamorphine, pethidine<br>Methadone, fentanyl<br>Oxycodone, hydromorphone |
| Adjuvants | Antidepressants – amitriptyline<br>Anticonvulsants – gabapentin, pregabalin, carbamazepine<br>Antiarrhythmics – lidocaine, mexilitine<br>Miscellaneous – ketamine (NMDA antagonist)<br>– clonidine (alpha 2 agonist)<br>– capsaicin |

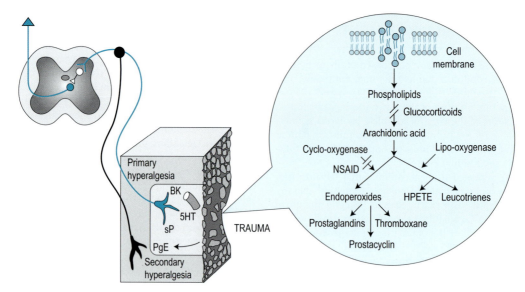

**Figure 19.5** Action of non-steroidal anti-inflammatory drugs (NSAIDs) on cyclo-oxygenase (COX). NSAIDs inhibit the production of prostaglandins, thromboxanes and prostacyclins.

**Table 19.5** Side-effects of non-steroidal anti-inflammatory drugs (NSAIDs)

| System | Side-effects |
|---|---|
| Gastrointestinal | – Nausea, dyspepsia, diarrhoea<br>– Peptic ulceration, perforation, bleeding |
| Renal | – Fluid retention, renal failure, papillary necrosis, interstitial fibrosis |
| Respiratory | – Bronchoconstriction, pulmonary eosinophilia, alveolitis |
| Coagulation | – Reduced platelet aggregation, increased bleeding time |
| Skin | – Severe allergic reactions such as Steven–Johnson syndrome, toxic epidermal necrolysis or angio-oedema |
| Visceral | – Congestive heart failure, hepatitis, pancreatitis, aseptic meningitis |

**Table 19.6** Side-effects of opioids

| System | Side-effects |
|---|---|
| Central | Depressant: analgesia, sedation, ↓ basal metabolic rate (↓ temperature), cough, respiration, vasomotor (↓ blood pressure)<br>Excitatory: euphoria, hallucinations, convulsions, miosis (small pupils), slow heart rate via stimulation of vagus nerve, nausea/vomiting via chemoreceptor trigger zone and vestibular nucleus<br>Endocrine: release of ADH resulting in water retention, inhibition of ACTH, FSH and LH – unknown long-term effects |
| Peripheral | Ileus, constipation, urinary retention<br>Histamine release, bronchospasm, erythema, flushing |

ADH, antidiuretic hormone; ACTH, adrenocorticotrophic hormone; FSH, follicle stimulating hormone; LH, luteinising hormone.

Aspirin is rarely used as an analgesic because it has a higher incidence of the side-effects common to NSAIDs (Table 19.5). It causes irreversible inhibition of COX, and so its effects do not subside with a reduction in plasma level of the drug, but have to await new production of prostenoids from new cellular production, which may take several days.

Phenylbutazone, the only pyrazole available in the UK, is restricted for use in resistant ankylosing spondylitis due to the incidence of aplastic anaemia and agranulocytosis.

The issue of adjuvant drugs was discussed previously in this chapter in the section on neuropathic pain.

## Step 2

The less potent opioids, such as codeine and dihydrocodeine, are commonly used. These drugs act at the supraspinal level and can produce the same side-effects as the more potent opioids (Table 19.6). In practice, however, they cause fewer problems because they are weaker and are used in lower doses. These drugs are usually taken in combination with paracetamol (usually 500 mg). This limits the daily dose of opioid that can be taken as the patient is restricted to eight tablets per day (maximum 4 g/day paracetamol). The use of compound analgesics is more effective than using either drug alone, and makes consumption simpler for the patient. It may, however, limit the opioid from being titrated up to the optimal dose, and is often much more expensive.

## Step 2 to 3

Tramadol is a drug that has dual mode of activity. One-third of its activity is via an opioid action, but two-thirds of its activity is due to a supraspinal effect, like with amitriptyline, which potentiates the dorsal column inhibitory pain pathway in the spinal cord. It is truly a multimodal drug, which is in keeping with the underlying principle of current pain-management strategies.

Tramadol has been proposed as a drug that bridges the gap between step 2 and step 3. It can be administered by the oral, intramuscular or intravenous routes. It is as potent as pethidine but has fewer opioid-type side-effects. However, it can cause nausea, sedation and, in excessively high doses, predisposes to convulsions.

## Step 3

Potent opioids are required for severe acute pain and cancer pain. Morphine is the standard drug, and is usually the first choice (Table 19.4). The oral route is the most common and simplest route of administration, and is recommended for stable conditions. However, for severe acute pain, where rapid onset of action of the drug is often required, it is usually given by intramuscular, or preferably, by intravenous injection.

There are several other opioid drugs now available, which can be used if morphine produces side-effects. For instance, oral oxycodone or transdermal application of fentanyl or buprenorphine patches are as effective and seem to cause less constipation and sedative side-effects. Pethidine is rarely used, as it has a short duration of action and produces toxic metabolites that can induce convulsions.

Potent opioids can be used for chronic non-cancer pain conditions, but it is best to have the patient assessed at a specialist pain clinic first. The pain clinic will try other treatments that can be used instead of or in combination with potent opioids, and they will be able to screen the patient to exclude any psychological risk factors for addiction.

## ADJUVANT ANALGESICS

Conventional analgesics used for nociceptive pain are often not effective for neuropathic pain, and so adjuvant analgesics are used (Table 19.4). The adjuvant analgesics share a common action – they are usually membrane stabilisers and they can suppress the excessive neuronal activity that results from neuropathic pain.

## ANTIDEPRESSANTS

The tricyclic antidepressants are the most effective. They work by inhibiting the reuptake of the neural transmitters noradrenaline and 5-HT, and so potentiate the dorsal inhibitory pathway that terminates in the dorsal horn of the spinal cord. The analgesic effect is separate from, and usually occurs sooner and at lower doses than, that required for depression. Not all antidepressants are effective, and it appears that the serotonin selective reuptake inhibitors (SSRIs) are not regarded as useful, and therefore are seldom used.

Amitriptyline is the gold standard antidepressant. It is started at a low dose (10 or 25 mg) at night and gradually increased up to 50–100 mg to allow the patient time to tolerate the side-effects. These may include sedation, dry mouth, constipation, urinary retention, weight gain, low blood pressure and increased heart rate. Analgesic benefit may occur after 2 weeks, but often the drug must be taken for at least 8 weeks before it can be said to have been given a fair trial. Compliance is poor because patients often experience side-effects early on without any benefit.

In addition, if the patient has not been given an adequate explanation of the rationale for prescribing an antidepressant, they may feel that their pain is not being taken as genuine and lose trust in the doctor. One in three patients will get greater than 50% pain relief with an antidepressant, which is regarded as an excellent result for a chronic pain condition.

## ANTICONVULSANTS

Anticonvulsants have been used successfully for neuropathic pain. They have many varied mechanisms of action, but all result in suppressing neural excitability. The older drugs, such as carbamazepine and phenytoin, generally produce more side-effects, such as sedation, and induce liver enzymes that can affect the metabolism of other drugs. This is particularly important if patients are taking other medications. Carbamazepine can also give rise to more severe idiosyncratic reactions such as allergy and liver and bone marrow suppression.

Gabapentin and pregabalin are modern anticonvulsants that are licensed specifically for neuropathic pain. They are often used as first-line anticonvulsant therapies because they are as effective as the others but have fewer side-effects.

## ANTIARRHYTHMICS

Lidocaine (lignocaine) and mexilitine block sodium channels and therefore can suppress excessive neuronal activity. Lidocaine can only be given intravenously, as it undergoes extensive first-pass metabolism when administered orally. Oral mexilitine is an alternative. Both drugs can slow the heart rate, and so an electrocardiogram must be taken before commencing taking these drugs to ensure there are no contraindications to their use.

## TOPICAL DRUGS

These have the advantage that they are not taken systemically and so have fewer side-effects. However, for topical drugs to be suitable, the pain symptoms need to be located predominantly in a small and accessible cutaneous area.

Capsaicin is a nerve toxin that inactivates small C pain fibres. It needs to be applied 3–4 times daily for up to 8 weeks before a decision on its effectiveness can be made. Capsaicin comes as 0.075% for neuropathic pain, and 0.025% for arthritic pain. The 0.075% strength can cause an uncomfortable burning sensation, but this often recedes after a week. This problem can be reduced by mixing the drug with lidocaine gel, glyceryl trinitrate ointment or titrating the dose up gradually from the 0.025% strength.

Lidoderm 5% patch (containing lidocaine) is applied for 12 hours/day. The systemic levels absorbed are very low, as it works via a local mechanism.

## NMDA RECEPTOR ANTAGONISTS

Ketamine can block the NMDA receptor and so reduce allodynia and hyperalgesia. It can be useful either given alone or to potentiate the effects of an opioid. It can be taken orally or as an intravenous or subcutaneous infusion. However, it produces unpleasant side-effects of hallucinations, sedation and amnesia, and therefore its clinical use is reserved for particularly problematic cases.

# REGIONAL ANALGESIA

Regional analgesia comprises the injection of a mixture of pharmacological agents into the painful tissue. The injection can be placed either around an inflamed joint or around a nerve. This has the advantage of needing only a small dose of drug, with the consequent low risk of side-effects. For inflamed tissue, the drugs often used to reduce inflammation are a mixture of local anaesthetic and steroid, such as bupivacaine 0.5% with depomedrone 40 mg. The same mixture can be used for perineural injections. However, various other alpha drugs are often used to reduce pain fibre activity, such as alpha 2 agonists (clonidine) and NMDA antagonists (ketamine). For major nerve blocks, when you want to avoid producing profound numbness and weakness, more dilute local anaesthetic solutions (bupivacaine 0.1%) can be used. This will block the pain fibres but often spare the sensory and motor fibres, resulting in an 'analgesic' versus an 'anaesthetic' block. While this is not a long-term cure, these blocks often have a beneficial response outlasting the pharmacological action of the drugs. They can provide benefit for days to weeks, and can be a useful component in conjunction with other therapies in the management of the pain.

Neurolytic blocks (using alcohol, phenol, cryotherapy or radiotherapy) destroy nerves permanently but do not have a permanent effect. The neural system usually regenerates and adapts after 3–6 months and the pain can return or even be worse, with permanent sensory and motor deficits, and deafferentation pain. These procedures are usually reserved for the terminally ill patient who will not survive long enough to experience these complications. However, there are some conditions for which this approach is more appropriate (e.g. neurolytic lumbar sympathectomy for small-vessel peripheral vascular disease). This procedure blocks the sympathetic supply to the leg and can dramatically improve peripheral circulation and ischaemic leg pain.

# PHYSICAL THERAPY

Physical therapy includes a whole array of treatments such as good foot hygiene, physiotherapy, heat, cold and ultrasound therapy, braces and splints, aromatherapy and many others. It also includes the local application of treatments such as transcutaneous electrical nerve stimulation (TENS) (Figure 19.3) and acupuncture.

Acupuncture involves the use of very small needles to stimulate certain channels or trigger points. There are various theories for its mode of action, but most evidence indicates that it results in a local tissue response and systemic release of endogenous opioids. Its effects can be antagonised by opioid antagonists. Both TENS and acupuncture have a low risk of side-effects and should be tried early if pain is persistent.

# PSYCHOLOGY

It is inappropriate to see pain as either physical or psychological, it is always both, as stated in the IASP definition. The gate control theory was hypothesised to account for some of the clinical observations made about pain. Such observations include the fact that pain sometimes occurs without apparent cause or does not occur despite obvious injury (e.g. a wounded soldier on the battlefield), or often persists after tissue healing or fails to respond to appropriate treatments. The theory proposed that there were mechanisms in the spinal cord (see above) that increase or decrease pain signals. An example of this is the placebo response, whereby a 'sham' treatment can produce good pain control. The converse of this is the nocebo response, where pain can be experimentally induced despite there being no nociceptive stimulus, only a suggestion of one.

The pain experience and amount of suffering is dependent on many psychological parameters such as anxiety, past experiences, the meaning to the patient of the pain, injury or illness, their beliefs about treatment and medications (fear of dependence, addiction, tolerance, organ damage, etc.) and self-management strategies. This applies equally to acute as it does to chronic pain and so health care providers should screen patients to address any critical psychological issues as an integral component of appropriate medical management.

One of the most commonly used techniques is cognitive–behavioural therapy. Briefly, the patient is trained to behave differently in the pain experience by a combination of preparatory information, diaphragm breathing, muscle relaxation, guided imagery and/or hypnosis which all lead to greater self control. Motivation and positive attitudes can be just as important to pain control and recovery as medical interventions.

# SPECIFIC CHRONIC PAIN CONDITIONS OF THE LOWER LIMB

## Complex regional pain syndrome

The term 'complex regional pain syndrome' (CRPS) has now replaced terms such as reflex sympathetic dystrophy and causalgia, which were used previously for this condition. CRPS predominantly affects the younger age group, presumably because the young are more prone to trauma, and there is a female/male predominance of 3 to 1. It is often a mild and transient condition that resolves spontaneously; some cases stabilise into a mild disorder, while a small subset become chronic and severely disabled.

There are two types of the syndrome:

- CRPS I – symptoms are preceded by a tissue injury. It is more common than CRPS II, the incidence being about 1–2% following a fracture of a limb, but it can occur with trivial injuries.
- CRPS II – as above but occurs after nerve injury, and the incidence is around 1–5%.

Both types can be further subdivided into sympathetically mediated pain (SMP) or sympathetically independent pain (SIP). Patients with SMP (about one-third of all cases) are diagnosed either by obtaining an analgesic effect from a sympathetic block or by increasing the pain by sympathetic stimulation (i.e. total body cooling). The proportion of SMP declines over time, which may explain why sympathetic nerve blocks are more effective in the early stages of pain.

Signs and symptoms may begin at the time of injury or may be delayed for weeks. CRPS is manifested by a collection of sensory, vasomotor, sudomotor and motor/trophic disturbances. Typically, the pain is described as constant, burning, shooting, or aching localised deep in the somatic tissues, and often increases when the limb is dependent. All patients suffer from hyperalgesia to mechanical stimuli or on joint movement. Patients can have a sensory deficit, which is often non-dermatomal and which can progress proximally. Sensory deficits of temperature and proprioception are usually the first to appear. Sensory deficits are more common in CRPS II, due to the accompanying nerve lesion.

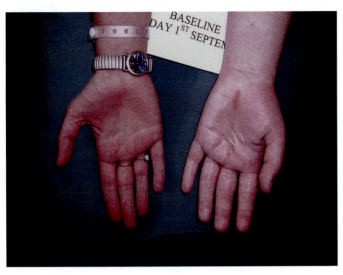

**Figure 19.6** Complex regional pain syndrome of the left hand, showing diffuse swelling, vasoconstriction and the glossy appearance of skin.

The vasomotor effects include colour (vasodilatation – red; vaso-constriction – cyanosed (blue) or white) and temperature (hot or cold). The sudomotor signs include hyperhidrosis/hypohidrosis (excess or decreased sweating) and oedema. All these changes can be spontaneous or induced by movement or other stimulation.

Trophic changes present as abnormal hair and nail growth, fibrosis, thin glossy skin and osteoporosis (Figure 19.6). If a limb is cold at the onset, the condition is associated with increased trophic disabilities, and warrants aggressive management. The motor changes can be secondary to disuse atrophy or due to trophic changes in the tendons and muscles. These result in limb weakness, restricted range of movement and impaired coordination.

Treatments include the general measures described above (the WHO ladder and adjuncts), with emphasis on multidisciplinary pain management and restoration of full function. In addition, sympathectomy blocks can be performed on the lower limb, including lumbar sympathectomy and intravenous regional sympathetic blockade (IVRA).

Finally, remember there are many reasons why a person may limp, and there are even more ways in which to treat it.

## REFERENCES

Serpell MG 2005 Physiology, pharmacology and psychology of pain. Anaesthesia and Intensive Care Medicine 6 (1):7–10.

## FURTHER READING

Netherlands Society of Rehabilitation Specialists 2006 Guidelines. Complex regional pain syndrome type 1. Available at: http://pdver. atcomputing.nl/pdf/CRPS_I_Guidelines.pdf (accessed 19 September 2009).

Moore A, Edwards J, Barden J, McQuay H 2003 Bandolier's little book of pain. Oxford University Press, Oxford.

Symposium on Mechanisms of Pain 1995 British Journal of Anaesthesia 75:1–200.

Wall PD, Melzack R (eds) 1999 Textbook of pain. Churchill-Livingston, London.

# Chapter 20

# Local anaesthesia

*Jeffrey Evans and Robert James Hardie*

## KEYWORDS

Choice of anaesthetics
Digital nerve trunk blocks
Drug interactions
Infiltration
Liver function
Safety considerations
Sepsis
Techniques of administration
Toxicity
Vasoconstrictors

## INTRODUCTION AND BACKGROUND

> Note:
> While it is appreciated that individual countries will have legislation pertaining to the access to and use of local anaesthetic agents, this text, in terms of a legal context, is directed to those who practise in the UK.

The purification and synthesis of cocaine by Niemann in 1860 led to its subsequent use by Köller for anaesthesia of the eye, and the first nerve block was carried out by Halsted in 1884. In 1904, Einhorn synthesised procaine, which was introduced to clinical practice by Braun in 1905, and the rest, as they say, is history. The following century saw the introduction of a number of new local anaesthetic agents, with the most recent being ropivacaine, which was available for clinical use from 1996 (Ruetsch et al 2001).

Access to local anaesthetic for podiatrists in the UK was first approved by the Chiropodists Board in 1972 (Dagnall 1995) to include specifically lidocaine, mepivacaine, bupivacaine and prilocaine. Subsequent amendments to the 1968 Medicines Act by Statutory Instruments has seen the addition of lidocaine and bupivacaine with 1 : 200 000 epinephrine in 1997 (Order 1830 Department of Health), and most recently the addition in 2006 of levobupivacaine and ropivacaine (Order 2807 Department of Health). Dosage calculation is incumbent on the practitioner and is variable up to the maximum safe dose (MSD). Local anaesthetics are available as amino amide and amino ester solutions, but the esters, while available for medical and dental use, are not normally accessible for podiatric use in the UK.

## BASIC CHEMISTRY AND PHARMACOLOGY

Local anaesthetics are weak bases that are insoluble in water, which are combined with a strong acid to provide a water-soluble salt. They have a lipid-soluble hydrophobic aromatic group linked by an intermediate chain (which determines the class of drug) to a charged amine lipophilic group (Fig. 20.1).

In practice, they are all supplied as hydrochloride solutions. At normal body pH of 7.4 they exist as both ionised and unionised forms. The proportions of each are dependent on the pKa (the acid dissociation constant) of the drug molecule, which is the pH at which the drug is 50% ionised. This is given by the Henderson–Hasselbach equation

$$pK_a = pH + \log_{10}([HA]/[A^-])$$

where the square brackets denote concentration. The pKa determines the onset of action. Ionisation of the drug is in reference to the fact that most drugs have a mixture of molecules, some of which are uncharged, or unionised, and some of which have a negative or positive charge (i.e. are ionised). Only the unionised form of the drug is able to penetrate the membrane barriers, but it will revert in the lower pH of the axoplasm to an ionised form (Tetztaff 2000).

Amino amides have significant advantages over the amino esters, because they are more stable than esters. Esters are more easily hydrolysed than amides, particularly if solutions are autoclaved or exposed to alkaline solutions. Consequently, they are prepared in acidic solutions and so they are more stable in an ionised soluble form; however, they do not store as well and cannot be autoclaved. The pH of esters is 2.7–5.5 and that of amides 4.1–6.5. With a higher pH there is more rapid penetration at sites of action. Esters are far more likely to cause a sensitivity, or allergic reaction, because in their metabolism they

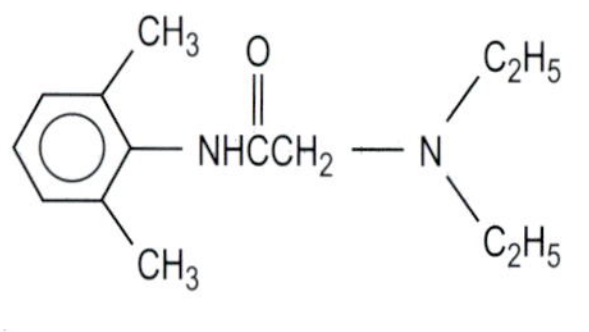

produce *para*-aminobenzoate (PABA). The onset and duration of action of amides is also superior.

The molecular weights of local anaesthetic agents vary and there is some evidence to indicate that this may affect the absorption of the drug (Wildsmith et al 1987).

Lipid solubility is the primary determinant of the potency of a local anaesthetic. Higher lipid solubility is accompanied by a greater degree of protein binding, with similar implications for potency and duration of action of the anaesthetic effect. Aqueous solubility is another important physiochemical property, and is directly related to the extent of ionisation (and therefore decreases as the pH is raised) and inversely related to its lipid solubility.

*Stereoisomerism* describes the existence of molecules that have the same structure but different spatial arrangements around an atom. This becomes relevant when one considers that bupivacaine has two stereoisomers, known as the *R* and *S* forms. Bupivacaine has been developed into a single stereoisomer, known as levobupivacaine (Calvey & Williams 2008).

## Membrane electrophysiology

Local anaesthetic solutions exert their primary pharmacological action by interfering with the excitation–conduction process of peripheral nerve fibres and endings, decreasing the rate and degree of depolarisation of the nerve membrane such that the threshold potential for transmission is not achieved and the nerve ceases to conduct (de Jong 1994). There is no effect on the resting or threshold potentials, but prolongation of the repolarisation phase and refractory period may also play a role in anaesthetic action. All excitable tissues possess special voltage-sensitive channels (Morgan & Johnson 2000).

Most of the clinically useful anaesthetic is likely to act by displacement of the calcium ions ($Ca^{2+}$) from a lipoprotein receptor site on the interior of the nerve cell membrane. This will block the sodium ion ($Na^+$) channels. Potassium ion ($K^+$) channels are also blockable, but are less sensitive than the sodium channels. However, potassium channels are important in regulating the resting potential. The voltage-sensitive channels can be open, closed or inactivated. It is also possible that the local anaesthetic binds at some receptor sites intracellularly, called G-protein receptors (Scholz 2002).

Local anaesthetics are use or state dependent; that is, the degree of block is proportional to the rate of nerve stimulation (i.e. the more rapidly firing neurons are more susceptible than the slower ones) (Wildsmith 2007). Nerve fibres may be of one type or mixed; however, it is generally the smaller C diameter fibres which are more sensitive than larger myelinated A fibres. Thus, a differential block can be achieved where the smaller pain and autonomic fibres are blocked while coarse touch and movement fibres are spared (Strichartz & Ritchie 1987).

## CHOICE OF LOCAL ANAESTHETIC AND DOSAGE

The choice of local anaesthetic is primarily determined by the practitioner's preference, experience, the characteristics of the drug (e.g. protein binding and metabolism) and the procedure to be carried out. Minor procedures, such as toenail avulsion with phenolisation, that are quickly completed and which are associated with little postoperative pain can be successfully undertaken with lidocaine. If there is a known allergy or sensitivity to a local anaesthetic, then choosing the least chemically similar local anaesthetic is the best alternative. Longer and more postoperatively painful procedures can be best dealt with

(A) Lidocaine HCl

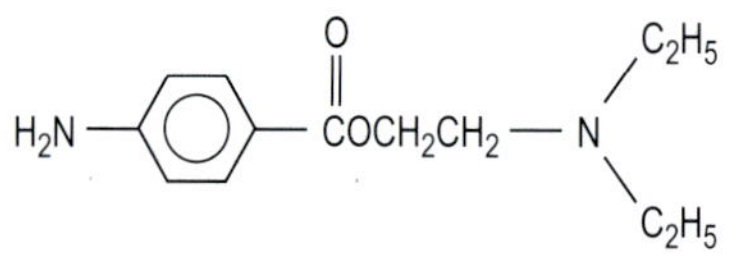

(B) Procaine HCl

**Figure 20.1** An example of (A) an amide and (B) an ester local anaesthetic.

using a longer acting anaesthetic such as bupivacaine or levobupivacaine (Thompson & Lalonde 2006). However, the availability of local anaesthetic agents may not always simply be a matter of practitioner choice, but may be influenced by the access that the individual practitioner has to these agents. For example, as previously mentioned, in the UK esters are not available to podiatrists. There may be a Health Trust protocol/policy that limits 'open' access to all the amide agents. Hospital and Trust chief pharmacists may not permit access to 4% Citanest® as this is only licensed for dental use (see below). Etidocaine hydrochloride, while available in the USA, is not currently available to UK podiatrists. Whichever agent is chosen, it should conform to what are often regarded as the ideal characteristics (Uddin & Reilly 2008) and these are summarised below:

- *Complete reversibility* (also known as *regression time*) – this may be fairly quick, as with lidocaine, or much longer, as with bupivacaine. Whichever drug is used, there needs to be a re-establishment of sensation and motor function. Nerve damage may occasionally result in a temporary or permanent numbness.
- *Rapid onset* – generally, the quicker the onset the better. However, in podiatric surgical units it may be advantageous to anaesthetise all the patients with a slower onset, longer-acting agent before the surgical list commences, ensuring they have anaesthesia by the time they enter theatre.
- *Sufficient and predictable duration* – generally in podiatry all the agents provide satisfactory duration. However, in longer surgical procedures, or where delay has occurred, the local anaesthetic may be metabolised and there may be a need for a 'top-up' injection.
- *Low tissue and systemic toxicity* – see below.
- *Distribution/action confined principally to nerve tissue* – loss of proprioception and effects on musculature will be seen with more proximal and profound blocks.

Figures for the MSD are not universally accepted, and variation occurs between countries and formularies. Indeed, the traditional methods of dose calculation are sometimes challenged:

> *In most cases there is no scientific justification for presenting exact milligram doses or mg/kg doses as maximum dose recommendations. Instead, only clinically adequate and safe doses (ranges) that are block specific are justified, taking into consideration the site of local anesthetic injection, and patient related factors such as age, organ dysfunctions, and pregnancy, which may influence the effect and pharmacokinetics of the local anesthetic.*

> (Rosenberg et al 2004)

Readers are advised to consult their home formularies (e.g. the *British National Formulary* and *Martindale's*). Whatever the suggested safe dosage, it is incumbent on the practitioner to consider factors such as the patient's general health and age, the integrity of their vasculature, the type of procedure to be undertaken and the anatomical site, as the effect of large doses is fairly meaningless unless the site of injection is considered, with the more peripheral injection sites being less of a risk than core areas such as the head and neck (Lagan & McClure 2004).

In general in the UK, the podiatrist calculates the MSD based on body weight, by multiplying the agent in milligrams (mg) by the body weight in kilograms (kg). Many drug calculations can be based on surface area, and the *British National Formulary* has an online calculator to enable this. It is deemed prudent to consider this only to a maximum body weight of 70 kg and as a '24-hour' dose (Hardie & Lorimer 2006).

A simple way to arrive at a MSD dose is as follows. First, calculate the MSDs:

MSD (mg) = weight (kg) × MSD for the local anaesthetic
For a patient weighing 65 kg and having 2% lidocaine administered this would be: 65 kg × 3 mg/kg (the MSD for lidocaine) = 195 mg.

To convert this to the volume, remember that there are 10 mg per 1% solution:

MSD (ml) = MSD (mg)/s ÷ (local anaesthetic % × 10)
Therefore, in our example of the 65-kg patient, the maximum injectable volume is 195/(2 × 10) = 9.75 ml.

It is not unusual in podiatric surgery to use more than one local anaesthetic agent, whereby a fast-acting drug such as lidocaine is followed by a longer acting agent such as bupivacaine. This will sustain the anaesthesia throughout the procedure and possibly extend postoperative pain relief. The maths is a little more involved, but not difficult. For example, if your 65-kg patient has received 5 ml of 1% lidocaine and now requires levobupivacaine 0.5% to complete the procedure:

MSD for lidocaine = 3 mg/kg = 65 × 3 mg/kg = 195 mg.
The patient has had 5 ml of the drug, therefore: 5 ml of 1% lidocaine = 5 × 10 = 50 mg.
So the remaining 'available' MSD is: 195 − 50 = 145 mg.
Now, dividing this remaining 145 mg by the 3 mg/kg figure for lidocaine gives: 145/3 = 48.3 per kg.
The MSD for levobupivacaine is 2 mg/kg, so: 48.3 × 2 mg/kg = 96.6 mg.
Converting his figure to a volume: 96.6/(0.5 × 10) = 19.3 ml.

The patient could therefore receive 19.3 ml of 0.5% levobupivacaine in addition to the 5 ml of 1% lidocaine before being considered as over the MSD. Alternative ways to calculate the MSD are available, and some podiatrists refer to a chart of MSD values (Butterworth & Dockery 1992, Hardie & Lorimer 2006, Uddin & Reilly 2008) (Table 20.1).

*Note*: in general, the MSD is increased in solutions that have vasoconstrictors added.

**Table 20.1** The maximum safe dose (MSD) of amide local anaesthetic agents

| Generic name | Common brand names: | MSD in plain solution |
|---|---|---|
| Bupivacaine hydrochloride | Marcain Sensorcaine | 150 mg (2 mg/kg) |
| Lidocaine hydrochloride | Xylocaine | 200 mg (3 mg/kg) |
| Levobupivacaine hydrochloride | Chirocaine | 150 mg (2 mg/kg) |
| Mepivacaine hydrochloride | Scandonest/Scandocaine Carbocaine | 400 mg (6 mg/kg) |
| Prilocaine hydrochloride | Citanest | 400 mg (6 mg/kg) |
| Ropivacaine hydrochloride | Naropin | 200 mg (4 mg/kg) |
| Etidocaine hydrochloride (USA) | Duranest | 300 mg (6 mg/kg) |

## Bupivacaine

Bupivacaine, a homologue of mepivacaine and ropivacaine, is a very stable hydrochloride and has been used for its long duration, which may be up to four times that of lidocaine (McClure & Rubin 2005). It is reported to be four times as potent as lidocaine and mepivacaine – a 0.5% solution is approximately equivalent to a 2% solution of lidocaine. It is available in concentrations of 0.25–0.75% and can be acquired with 1 : 200 000 adrenaline added. If the latter agent is used, it would be prudent to retain the same MSD of 150 mg (Mather et al 2005). A disadvantage of bupivacaine is that it does have a slow onset time. There is more likelihood of cardiac toxicity with this drug; for example, cardiac arrhythmias and reduced myocardial contractility, often resulting in a resistant ventricular fibrillation (Royse & Royse 2005), and patients who suffered this were difficult to resuscitate. Bupivacaine may also increase the toxicity of certain drugs that are metabolised by plasma cholinesterases. In podiatry it is more often used in the surgical field.

## Levobupivacaine

The great advantage of levobupivacaine over bupivacaine is its reduced cardiotoxicity, while it retains the desirable qualities of being long acting and virtually as potent. Levobupivacaine is the S-enantiomer of racemic bupivacaine (McLeod & Burke 2001). It is available as a 0.25%, 0.5% or 0.75% solution. It is not available in cartridges for dental syringes. The MSD is the same as for bupivacaine (i.e. 150 mg; 2 mg/kg). Levobupivacaine is contraindicated for a Bier's block in those with severe hypotension, as it has been associated with cardiac shock and serious cardiac arrhythmias. There is little research to show that it is unsafe in other situations or with certain drugs, but it is best avoided in those taking antiarrhythmic drugs such as mexiletine (Burlacu & Bugg 2008). Patients given levobupivacaine should be warned not to drive and/or operate machinery afterwards, and while no time is specified on the data sheet 12 hours seems a sensible recommendation (Foster & Markham 2000).

## Etidocaine

This agent is used predominantly in the USA, particularly by the dental profession. It is has a rapid onset and medium to long duration of action of approximately 4 hours. Generally available in concentrations of 1% and 1.5%, it is also available with 1:200 000 adrenaline added (Wynn 1995). Currently, this agent is not available to UK podiatrists, but it has been used for a long time by some American podiatrists (Caputo et al 1982).

## Lidocaine

Since its introduction to clinical practice in 1948, lidocaine has become one of the most widely used local anaesthetics (Winstanley & Walley 2002). It is a fairly fast-acting local anaesthetic, with a variable duration of action, which may be as long as 3 hours. It is usually used in plain solutions by podiatrists, but from 1998 was available with adrenaline 1:200 000 added as a vasoconstrictor to certified podiatrists in the UK. The MSD is 200 mg (3 mg/kg). In solutions with adrenaline, the MSD is increased to 7 mg/kg to a maximum of approximately 490 mg. It is available in a number of concentrations from 0.5% to 4%; however, the higher concentrations are usually for intrathecal injection, while the 1% and 2% solutions are the favoured strengths for peripheral nerve block anaesthesia. It is usually supplied in ampoules, but may sometimes be available in a cartridge format that fits into the dental syringes much favoured in podiatry.

There are other medical uses for lidocaine, such as in the management of cardiac ventricular arrhythmia, in this case marketed as Xylogard, this use being due to its marked membrane-stabilising properties. However, for this reason high doses should be avoided in patients with hypovolaemia or heart block problems (Smith, 2007). There are also some pharmacological interactions to be considered, for example: propranolol (Inderal), a beta blocker used in patients with angina, which slows hepatic clearance; cimetidine, which is widely used for peptic ulceration, also interferes with hepatic clearance; and ranitidine, also an ulcer treatment, requires the same consideration. However, these are all considered relative contraindications, and in the main will not be a problem with small dosages (www.astrazeneca.co.uk).

Lidocaine is also used in topical creams, the most relevant of which is EMLA® (eutectic mixture of lignocaine and prilocaine), a cutaneous gel applied to the skin under a dressing for up to an hour to facilitate pain-free injections. This is particularly useful with nervous children.

## Mepivacaine

Known under the brand names of Carbocaine, Scandonest and Scandicaine, mepivacaine is related to bupivacaine and ropivacaine and was introduced into clinical practice in 1957 (Ruetsch et al 2001). It is less toxic than lidocaine, particularly to neural tissues. Mepivacaine has a less pronounced vasodilator effect than lidocaine, probably because of its slower clearance. It has a longer duration and quicker onset of action than lidocaine. Because of its slower clearance its use is not advised in obstetric anaesthesia (Kuczkowski 2004). The MSD is 400 mg based on 6 mg/kg, thus enabling a larger dose to be given than with lidocaine. It is available in cartridges for use with dental or disposable syringes. It is available in concentrations of 0.5–4%. In podiatry, solutions up to 3% are used, with Scandonest 3% (plain solution) being the choice in the UK. While this drug is not licensed for the treatment of children, its use in podiatry is indemnified by the Society of Chiropodists & Podiatrists. The law allows podiatrists who hold a certificate of competence in local anaesthesia to administer the substance without any requirement that such administration must be in accordance with the terms of the licence.

*The Society would consider the administration of Scandonest, suitably dose adjusted for children, to be acceptable professional practice. This would not of course preclude any civil liability should something go wrong, but this would be the situation whatever treatment was being administered.*

(Ashcroft 2003, p. 6)

## Prilocaine

Prilocaine was introduced into clinical practice in 1960, after being synthesised by Löfgren and Tegnér in 1959 (Ruetsch et al 2001). This agent has an MSD of 400 mg, and is most commonly available in concentrations of 1–4%. It is also available with the addition of octapressin or adrenaline for use in dentistry. It is available in ampoules or in dental cartridges in the higher concentrations. While the effectiveness and duration of action are only slightly greater than those of lidocaine or mepivacaine, its safety profile is superior to both due to its rapid clearance (Arthur et al 1987). Being a toluidine derivative its metabolism will produce *ortho*-toluidine, and in large doses (usually exceeding 600 mg) it may produce methaemoglobinaemia. This is a cyanotic condition and the patient will develop a bluish hue. It occurs because there are ferric rather than ferrous ions in the haematin in the haemoglobin, so the oxygen is unable to combine with ferric ions and transport the oxygen. It is not generally considered a serious condition in otherwise healthy individuals, but some authorities recommend not using prilocaine in the early stages of pregnancy, or in cases where there is severe anaemia or circulatory impairment (Haas & Carmichael 2007).

> **Note:**
>
> Citanest 4% has been a very popular with British podiatrists for many years, but can sometimes be difficult to obtain because of its license status. The producer, Astra-Zeneca, has advised against its use at the 4% strength in digital nerve blocks. The company advise the lower concentration of 1% or 2%, as they feel the 4% strength has led to injection-site necrosis on a number of occasions (Jones, 22 December 2000, personal correspondence). They emphasise that its licence is specifically for dentistry (Spires-Lane, 11 December 2000, personal correspondence ). The fact that the drug is licensed specifically for dentistry does not make it illegal for the podiatrist to use it; however, it does mean that the practitioner is willing to take responsibility for its use off licence, and should any mishap occur they would have to defend their use of that agent (Ashcroft, 11 January 2001, personal correspondence). The final decision remains with the podiatrist.

## Ropivacaine

Although synthesised in the late 1950s by Ekenstam, Naropin was not used clinically until 1996 (Whiteside & Wildsmith 2001). It was made available to appropriately qualified UK podiatrists in November 2006 (Order 2807 Department of Health). It is produced as a single-enantiomer drug, unlike bupivacaine and mepivacaine, to which it is closely related. Bupivacaine and mepivacaine are analogues of ropivacaine. However, ropivacaine is marketed as a single stereoisomer, while bupivacaine and mepivacaine are sold as equal mixtures of the two possible stereoisomers. Ropivacaine was created for its long-term efficacy, having a duration of action about 10% less than that of bupivacaine, but with a much safer profile. It also has a more discrete separation between motor and sensory block (McClure 1996). The evidence for the side-effects of and contraindications to ropivacaine is sparse. There is no evidence for dangers in pregnancy and it is used for epidural deliveries. Its use on patients with hypotension should be avoided. There is no direct evidence to indicate that patients should not drive after receiving the drug, but good sense should prevail. Prolonged administration in patients on Faverin (a serotonin reuptake inhibitor/antidepressant) should be avoided (Hansen 2004). It is available in 10 ml polypropylene blister packs, in concentrations of 0.25%, 0.5% and 0.75%. The MSD is not clearly defined by the manufacturer, but the suggested volumes would indicate approximately 4 mg/kg with a maximum dose of 300 mg (Astra-Zeneca 2001). Unlike most other anaesthetic agents, the addition of adrenaline has little effect on the drug's onset or duration.

## LOCAL AND SYSTEMIC COMPLICATIONS AND TOXICITY

### Local effects

The following is not exhaustive list, and in most circumstances the risk should be minimised by best clinical practice and attention to detail.

- There is always the possibility of needle breakage. However, with the silicon-coated needles used in conjunction with dental cartridge systems this should be very unlikely. If using the ordinary non-dental Luer or Microlance needles, it is best practice to avoid inserting to the hub of the needle. Deliberately bending the needle prior to injecting is also to be avoided, as this may be construed as negligent, making the needle unfit for purpose.
- Intravascular injection may pose a clinical risk. If arterial puncture occurs, for example in the posterior tibial artery, the high pressure in the vessel will result in a 'blow back' of blood into the syringe, requiring withdrawal, renewal of the delivery system and repositioning for injection. Bruising may be evident as a consequence. Injection into a large vein with a bolus of 10 ml or more of local anaesthetic poses a systemic risk, as it may decrease the conductivity and contractility of the cardiac muscle, with a subsequent drop in blood pressure and possible loss of consciousness (Mulroy 2002). Intravascular injection is best avoided by aspiration, and is recommended for those injection sites where large blood vessels run in close proximity to the nerves. It is the authors' opinion that aspiration is unnecessary for superficial infiltrations and digital blocks, where a 'moving-needle' technique, the small size of the vessels and the anatomy of the area should preclude the deposition of large quantities of intravascular local anaesthetic.
- A number of other unwanted local sequelae may occur following injection, ranging from tissue trauma, bruising, damaging the skin excessively and inclusion cysts, to nerve damage (Hardie & Lorimer 2006). Infection at the injection site is also possible, but most of the above are usually the result of poor procedure and a breakdown in best clinical practice. Avoiding injecting into infected or inflamed tissue is paramount in avoiding spreading an infection, or negating the local anaesthetic's function because of the more acidic pH of these tissues.

## Systemic effects

Local anaesthetics are very safe, and in the doses used in standard podiatric practice are unlikely to cause problems. However, when larger doses are used, as in podiatric surgery, the risks increase (Maher et al 2008). Even larger volumes are used in orthopaedics and other disciplines, where patients may have a line access for continuous input of the anaesthetic (Wiegel et al 2007).

All local anaesthetics can cause systemic toxicity but, as mentioned above, some have a greater potential for specific problems (e.g. bupivacaine and cardiotoxicity). The patient's ability for hepatic metabolism and renal clearance of amide anaesthetic agents has to be considered. Those agents that have a more rapid clearance will be safer than those that have a longer half-life and slower clearance. Acute toxicity following administration of anaesthetic solution is very rare, but recent advances have seen the introduction of Intralipid as an intravenous treatment for cardiac arrest following local anaesthetic reaction (Clark 2008). This has prompted the suggestion that patients undergoing foot surgery under popliteal blocks and large volumes of local anaesthetic should have an indwelling cannula in case of emergencies arising during the procedure (Maher et al 2008).

It is incumbent on the practitioner to assess the patient's suitability for the anaesthetic and subsequent procedure (Crausman & Glod 2004). A full medical, medication and social history should be completed, and if there are doubts about the patient's suitability for local anaesthesia the best practice would be to consult the patient's medical practitioner or medical consultant.

The following areas are highlighted for particular consideration:

### Central nervous system (CNS)

Local anaesthetics have an intrinsic ability to cause irritation of the CNS as they readily cross the blood–brain barrier. They stimulate the cerebral cortex but will then depress the medulla, particularly the vasomotor and respiratory centres (Finucane 2007). It would be considered very bad practice to administer excessively high doses of local anaesthetic to a patient, but if this occurred the patient may show one or more of the following signs/symptoms: restlessness, or general irritability, dizziness/blurred vision, and possibly tinnitus and numbness in the mouth region. It is then possible that they may feel nauseous and begin trembling and twitching, and possibly convulsing. Drowsiness, leading to unconsciousness may follow and, finally, this could lead respiratory failure. This could ultimately impact on the cardiovascular system, which in turn would also collapse. Specific conditions, such as patients with epilepsy, may need special consideration, especially if they are not stabilised well by their medication. However, it is often the 'situation', rather than the local anaesthetic that heightens tension and could precipitate a convulsion.

## Cardiovascular system

Although higher doses of local anaesthetic are required to cause toxicity in the cardiovascular system than in the CNS, an initial increase in peripheral vascular resistance has been noted, probably because of the effects on vascular smooth muscle (Rang et al 2003). The main cardiovascular effects in very high doses would be depression of the myocardium, systemic hypotension due to a generalised vasodilatation and a decrease in myocardial contractibility. This would lead to a fall in cardiac output. Bradycardia and arrhythmias may then occur, ultimately leading to ventricular fibrillation and cardiac arrest. Bupivacaine has been noted for its cardiac toxicity (Casati & Putzu 2005) but the newer pure S-isomers levobupivacaine and ropivacaine have a much better safety profile with regard to cardiotoxicity.

## Allergic reaction

A patient having a known allergy or hypersensitivity to a local anaesthetic will constitute an absolute contraindication. While fatalities due to an allergic reaction (e.g. due to a full-blown anaphylactic reaction) are extremely rare, a number of non-life-threatening situations may arise. For example, there may be an urticarial reaction or difficulty in breathing due to oedema in the laryngeal pathway. The number of cases of allergy, and in particular anaphylactic shock and death, are sometimes quoted as approximately 1 in 200 000, but the reliability of these statistics may be dubious (Finucane 2003).

Systemic toxicity is far more likely to occur when the anaesthetic is injected intravenously and in large doses. Good practice reduces these chances and leaves one time to deal with the 'lesser emergencies' caused by psychogenic reactions.

## Hepatic and renal function

The metabolism, by hydroxylation and conjugation within the liver, of amide local anaesthetics relies on an adequately functioning hepatic system. In those patients suffering from any liver disorder, such as cirrhosis or hepatitis, care will be needed. A history of alcohol abuse may be an underlying factor. The clearance of the drug relies on kidney function, with up to 86% of drug being excreted via this channel (Malamed 2004).

## Pregnancy

There is a dearth of research and literature pertaining to the use of local anaesthetics in pregnancy. There also appears to be a divergence of opinion on whether these drugs are safe to use in non-obstetric surgery, although many feel that their safety is established (Kuczkowski 2004). Known adverse affects, such as fetal bradycardia, have been documented in the literature. However, the caution that applies to the use during pregnancy of mepivacaine and bupivacaine in particular refers to data collected in animal teratogenic studies (Briggs et al 1990). That said, as it is known that these agents cross the placenta it seems sensible to avoid local anaesthetics in the first trimester, and as most foot surgery is elective the procedure may be delayed until after delivery. In emergency situations this debate may not arise.

## Drug interactions

Individual interactions have been noted above under each of the local anaesthetic agents. However, it is worth emphasising that any drugs that compromise the liver's ability to carry out detoxification by inhibiting the action of the hepatic microsomes, in particular the microsomal cytochrome P450 enzymes, may present a clinical problem (Smith 2007). For this reason, drugs such as the monoamine oxidase inhibitors and the procarbazines will require noting. The action of some drugs may be affected by the systemic action of the local anaesthetic rather than by a true pharmacological interaction; for example, by slowing the patient's heart rate and with a generalised vasodilatation, patients taking diuretics and other antihypertensive agents may experience hypotension. Furthermore, one should be aware that summation interactions may occur where drugs have similar receptor sites. However, in the main, and particularly in podiatric practice, local anaesthetics have proven to be extremely safe.

# LOCAL ANAESTHETICS IN PRACTICE

Safe use of local anaesthetics and the associated equipment is paramount. Not only has the patient's health to be assessed, but also the safety of the practitioner.

Any injectable anaesthetic being used should be confirmed as the agent of choice and have its expiry date and batch number noted. These details should be entered into the patient's record and kept with the consent forms for the administration of the agent and the subsequent procedure.

From the practitioner's perspective, a needlestick injury poses the primary risk. Resheathing needles constitutes over 50% of needlestick incidents in the UK (Royal College of Nursing 2003). Other incidents occur during disposal, suturing and the procedure itself. The risk of associated blood-borne viruses is obvious (Gabriel 2009), and these injuries are preventable. A number of strategies may be employed to reduce this risk (Raghavendran et al 2006). Firstly, never resheath needles. For disposable systems, a needle guard may be used (Fig. 20.2). However, disposing of the whole system into a sharps container would be the best option. If reusable dental cartridge syringes are being used it is possible to use the Safe-Point system (Fig. 20.3), or to remove the needle using locking forceps. Several dental safety systems are available that can accept an anaesthetic cartridge and are ready fitted with a 27- or 30-gauge needle in either long or short format. On completion of the injection the needle is not disconnected, but a sliding protector sleeve is moved forward and covers the needle entirely; the whole apparatus is then disposed of.

To administer local anaesthetics successfully it is necessary to consider the anatomy of the area and the site of injection. Note any physical/anatomical barriers, such as scar tissue, skin lesions, superficial blood vessels and infected areas, that might impede the movement of the needle or cause damage to the tissues. Histologically, the myelin sheath will absorb varying amounts of the anaesthetic, and the diameter of the fibres in the area will also influence the outcome. There will often be a need to redirect the needle. Some 8–10 mm of

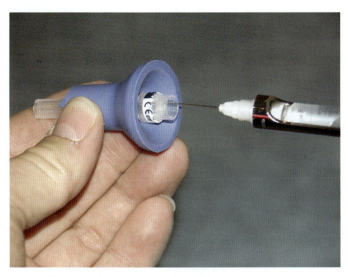

**Figure 20.2** The Safe-Point automatic needle remover.

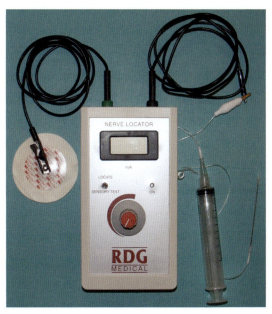

**Figure 20.4** Nerve locator apparatus.

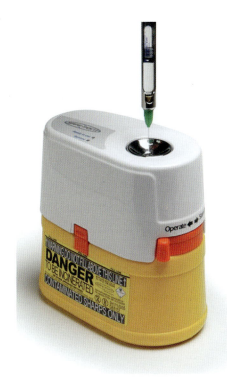

**Figure 20.3** An example of a needle guard in use.

nerve fibre will need to be affected by the local anaesthetic for anaesthesia to occur (de Jong 1994). Even with meticulous planning and procedure, anaesthetic failure can occur. This may be due in some cases to poor anatomical knowledge, anatomical variation or the patient's psychological state, and, rarely, to specific conditions such as hypermobility syndromes (Hakim 2005).

The scope of anaesthetic practice varies within podiatry. All UK podiatry students are trained in infiltration, and digital and ankle block techniques, but there is a wide variation in the actual use of these skills in practice. The technique most frequently used by UK podiatrists is the digital block, facilitating nail surgery. In the surgical field, podiatrists routinely perform ankle and popliteal blocks. With the larger and more proximal nerve blocks accurate identification of the site of the nerve may be difficult. This technique is augmented by the use of a nerve locator/stimulator (Fig. 20.4) or, increasingly, utilisation of ultrasound-guided injections. The use of the nerve stimulator requires insertion of a relatively blunt insulated needle deep into the tissues in the proximity of the nerve. The needle is supported by the use of the nerve stimulator, which emits an audible signal, allowing for adjustment of current on the stimulator. The muscle will twitch on stimulation and the current is then reduced until twitching stops. The process can be repeated until the operator is confident that the needle is in close proximity to the nerve, and the current is reduced to approximately 0.5 on the readout (Hardie & Lorimer 2006). The anaesthetic can then be introduced from the syringe via the cannula. The use of the stimulator is an efficient way of introducing relatively large amounts of anaesthetic into the popliteal fossa and, while there are some limitations to the process, the use of the nerve stimulator has been described as the gold standard for this type of anaesthesia (Jochim et al 2006). The use of the ultrasound-guided anaesthetic injection is developing and has been used in more proximal lower limb blocks (Peterson et al 2002). Furthermore, the combination of a nerve stimulator and ultrasound guidance seems to offer the least traumatic approach, and may assist in avoiding nerve damage (Moore et al 1994).

## SPECIFIC SITES

### Local infiltration

This is the simplest of the techniques and requires the deposition of the anaesthetic around and subcutaneously beneath the lesion (Fig. 20.5). It may be used for a variety of skin lesions, such as warts, basal cell carcinoma and various minor excrescences, and is ideal where electrocautery, curettage or scalpel excision is to be used (Koay & Orengo 2002).

### The digital block

Perhaps the most widely used local anaesthetic procedure in podiatry, the digital block is administered to block the hallux and any of the

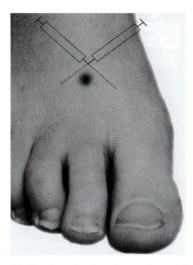

**Figure 20.5** Local infiltration, showing the needle positions around the lesion.

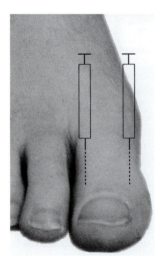

**Figure 20.6** Digital nerve block technique.

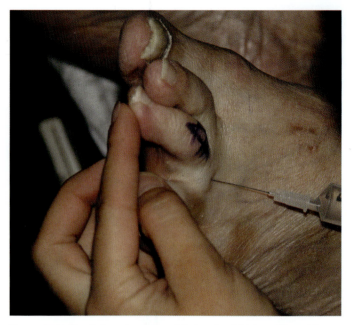

**Figure 20.7** The "triangular approach" showing initial needle position.

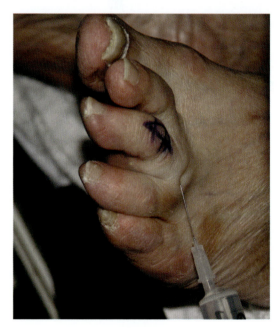

**Figure 20.8** The "triangular approach" showing secondary needle position.

lesser digits (Fig. 20.6). There are a number of variations to this technique, with each practitioner favouring their own. In its basic form the needle is directed from dorsal to plantar at an angle of 80–90° to the skin surface and slightly distal to the webbing line. The needle is advanced and local anaesthetic deposited en route and on the plantar side of the digit. The needle may be withdrawn slightly, without leaving the skin, and redirected so that the points of the needle converge towards the plantar surface, forming a 'triangular approach' (Figs 20.7 and 20.8). It is the authors' practice to keep injecting the solution as the needle advances. This technique does not require aspiration, as the needle is moving and there are no large vessels in this area; however, this remains a decision for the individual practitioner to make. Some podiatrists will also direct the needle laterally across the dorsum of the toe (Uddin & Reilly 2008). In the hallux, the four digital nerves will be anaesthetised. The plantar nerves arise from the medial plantar nerve and these traverse the apex of the toe. Dorsally, the deep peroneal (fibular) will supply the medial border of the hallux and the medial dorsal cutaneous branch of the superficial peroneal (fibular) nerve will have some input along the lateral side. Anaesthesia can normally be achieved with approximately 2–4 ml of solution; occasionally there may be a need to use rather more. Lesser toes rarely require more than 1–2 ml. The main problems with this

procedure arise if excessive amounts of solution are forced into an area where distension cannot occur (see earlier reference on personal communication). Digital blocks can be uncomfortable, especially in children or those with low pain thresholds. The use of a needleless system has been considered (Dialynas et al 2003), but has not found widespread use in podiatric practice. Furthermore, each practitioner has their own preferred delivery systems and technique, and novel methods are sometimes used as they may be less painful or use less local anaesthetic (Ouzounov 2005). The use of vasoconstrictors (e.g. adrenaline 1 : 200 000) in end organs and digits is generally advised against (Dollery 1999). However, there is little evidence to support its avoidance when using the amide anaesthetics (Wilhelmi et al 2001), and extensive literature searches have highlighted only 50 cases of digital gangrene since the turn of the last century, and none involving

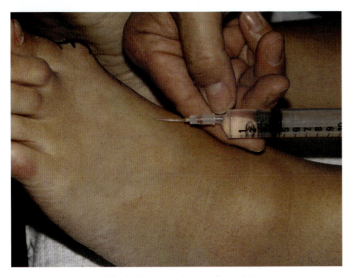

Figure 20.9 The ray block, showing the needle positions.

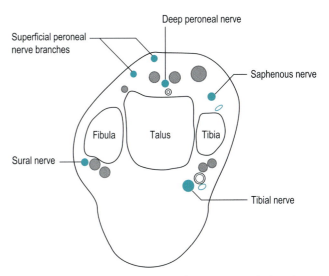

Figure 20.10 The anatomical positions of the posterior tibial, saphenous, sural, deep and superficial peroneal nerves.

lidocaine with adrenaline (Denkler 2001). It might be that other factors, such as the use of digital tourniquets or infection, heighten the risk of necrosis. It should also be noted that much of the evidence pertains to the fingers, not the toes. Vasoconstrictors may also have adverse systemic effects, such as increased heart rate, tremors and palpitations.

## The ray block

This is usually associated with the first (Mayo block) and fifth rays and is a highly effective technique for anaesthesia of the forefoot, for example for bunion, lesser ray procedures and neuroma. The needle is advanced at a proximal point in the metatarsal interspace and from a dorsal start and is then directed plantarly, where additional anaesthetic is deposited. The needle is then withdrawn and redirected medially and, if required, laterally so that there is a 'collaring' of the ray (Fig. 20.9). Anaesthesia of the other rays follows a similar pattern to the Mayo block. This can be a very effective technique, with a low failure rate of less than 1% (Worrell & Barbour 1996).

More extensive anaesthesia is achieved by blocking the nerves around the ankle. Only rarely is it necessary to block all the nerves at the same time. The nerves involved are the posterior tibial, saphenous, sural, deep and superficial peroneal (Fig. 20.10). All, with the exception of the saphenous nerve, which is a terminal branch of the femoral nerve, are branches of the sciatic nerve. The practicality of these injections is aided by having a relaxed and comfortable patient. All injections may be done with the patient supine, and rotating the leg into an accessible position. However, some practitioners would have the patient in a prone position for the posterior tibial and the sural blocks; it really depends on operator preference and to some extent the patient's comfort.

## Posterior tibial nerve

This is the larger of the two branches of the sciatic nerve (root index L4, L5 and S1, S2, S3). At the ankle it runs medially in the neurovascular bundle behind the posterior tibial artery. It passes behind the medial malleolus and flexor retinaculum, and then gives off calcaneal branches before dividing into the medial and lateral plantar nerves. As with all anatomy, there may be individual variations. This may be the reason for failure to achieve anaesthesia in some patients. The most useful indicator for finding the nerve is to palpate the posterior

tibial pulse (McGlamry et al 2001). The usual way to approach this injection is to palpate the posterior tibial artery and introduce the needle at the medial aspect of the Achilles tendon. Advance the needle in an anterior direction to the posterior surface of the tibia, and then withdraw very slightly and aspirate before injecting. Whether you choose to actively cause a paraesthesia is again a matter for debate. It is advisable to inform the patient of possible paraesthesia. You should then withdraw slightly and aspirate, and this should result in a good anaesthesia. An alternative method is to go about 4 cm above the medial malleolus, direct the needle deeply to the medial border of the Achilles tendon and then inject into the neurovascular channel. A nerve stimulator may be used to locate the nerve. Although unlikely, putting too much local anaesthetic into the bundle could cause a pressure necrosis, as the nerve lies between the tibial and flexor retinaculum. Aspiration avoids intravascular injection. Approximately 5–10 ml of anaesthetic will be required, and there may be a time lag before full anaesthesia is achieved.

## The sural nerve (root index S1/S2)

This nerve, also known as the lateral cutaneous nerve, continues down the posterior calf and runs behind the lateral malleolus with the short saphenous vein. It is a cutaneous nerve supplying the lateral aspect of the foot and the fifth toe. While not particularly difficult to anaesthetise, ultrasound guidance has been used to improve the success rate (MacFarlane & Brull 2009, Redborg 2009).

Insert the needle lateral to the Achilles tendon and at a right angle to the lateral malleolus (Fig. 20.11). Advance needle to lateral malleolus and then withdraw slightly. Aspirate and inject. It is possible to inject, with a fanning action, about 1 cm above the lateral malleolus and this tends to take out the small branches or one can raise a wheal from the Achilles tendon to the lateral malleolus.

## Saphenous nerve (root index L3/L4)

This nerve, which is the sensory terminal branch of the femoral nerve, passes down the anteromedial aspect of the leg and enters the dorsum of the foot (accompanying the long saphenous vein) about one finger's width from the medial malleolus (Fig. 20.12). Enter the needle between the tendon of the tibialis anterior and the long saphenous vein. Advance to the medial malleolus, aspirate and inject. Aspiration is essential due to the close proximity of the vein.

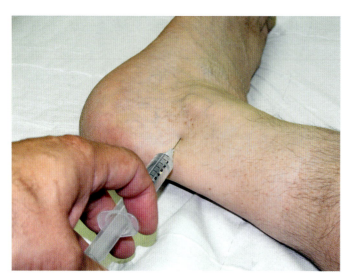

Figure 20.11 Sural nerve location and sensory distribution.

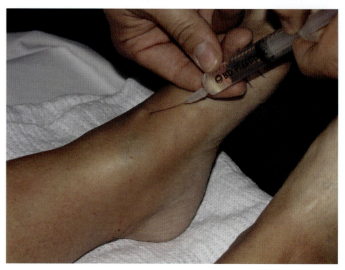

Figure 20.13 Medial branch of the superficial peroneal nerve and its distribution.

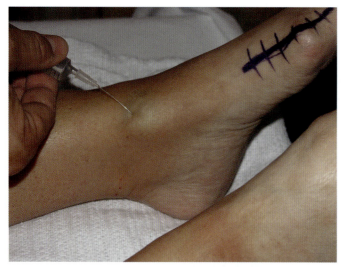

Figure 20.12 Saphenous nerve location and sensory distribution.

## The superficial peroneal (fibular) nerves (root index L4/L5, S1)

One of two terminal branches of the common peroneal (fibular) nerve. It becomes cutaneous between the middle and distal thirds of the leg and divides into two branches, medial and lateral although the point of division varies from person to person. The medial branch supplies the skin of the mediodorsal aspect of the foot, medial aspect of the hallux and adjacent sides of the second, third and fourth toes (Dhukaram & Senthil 2004). The lateral branch supplies the intermediate and lateral skin on the dorsum of the foot, the adjacent sides of the third and fourth toes and the medial aspect of the fifth toe.

The medial branch is centrally located between the malleoli as it crosses the extensor digitorum longus (EDL) tendons. If you ask the patient to dorsiflex the foot, and then palpate the EDL tendons, you should be able to roll the nerve with your index finger. Insert the needle on either side of the nerve. It is not vital to aspirate for this procedure (Fig. 20.13).

The lateral branch can be palpated lateral to the peroneus (fibularis) tertius muscle between the malleoli. Ask the patient to dorsiflex the

foot, and then palpate the peroneus tertius or lateral edge of the EDL muscles. Rolling the nerve will elicit a slight paraesthesia. Inject slowly, there is no need to aspirate. Alternatively, a wheal of anaesthetic may be deposited subcutaneously across the anterior aspect of the ankle.

## The deep peroneal (fibular) nerve (root index L4/L5, S1/S2)

This enters the dorsum of the foot between the tendons of the tibialis anterior and the extensor hallucis longus (Kopka & Serpell 2005). It is covered by the superior and inferior retinaculum and runs deep, roughly following the course of the anterior tibial artery. It supplies opposing sides of the hallux and the second toe. Insert the needle between the two tendons and advance until you make contact with the bone, aspirate and inject. Anaesthesia will be over the superolateral foot (Fig. 20.14).

## The popliteal block

The use of this block is expanding in podiatric surgery (Rees & Tagoe 2002). The technique is suitable for more extensive, long-duration forefoot and midfoot operations and for more involved rearfoot procedures where general and spinal anaesthesia is best avoided. In practical terms, both the saphenous nerve on the medial aspect of the knee and terminal portion of the sciatic nerve in the popliteal fossa will need to be blocked (Donohue et al 2004). In an anatomical sense this means that the tibial and common peroneal nerves, which share a common epineural sheath, will be anaesthetised.

This technique does mean that the patient is less mobile for some time following the procedure until motor function returns. However, this block allows a long postoperative anaesthesia, which helps with pain management and allows for a painless application of a midcalf or ankle tourniquet (Reilley et al 2002).

Because it is not possible to palpate these nerves, the use of a nerve stimulator/locator is required. In addition, a Doppler flowmeter may be used to identify the position of the popliteal artery.

Various techniques have been developed to approach the popliteal fossa. Donohue et al (2004) refer to the 'classic' approach, which is a posterior injection where the needle is introduced 1 cm lateral to a line drawn from the borders of the semimembranosus medially, the

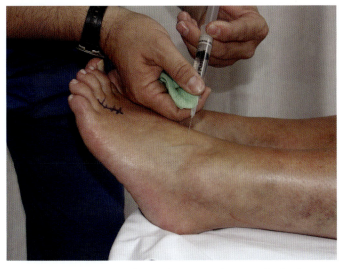

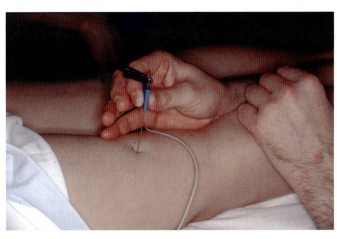

Figure 20.15 Deep popliteal nerve location and sensory distribution.

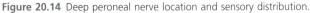

Figure 20.14 Deep peroneal nerve location and sensory distribution.

biceps femoris laterally and a line about 5 cm above the popliteal crease. However, they say that this has been superseded by an inter-tendinous approach that 'calls for needle insertion midway between the semimembranosus and biceps femoris tendons and 5 cm above the popliteal crease' (Donohue et al 2004, p. 370) (Fig. 20.15).

An alternative lateral approach may be used with the patient either sitting with the knee flexed or in a supine position. In this technique, the needle is passed from the lateral side of the thigh along the anterior border of the biceps femoris tendon, about 5 cm proximal to the popliteal crease. The saphenous nerve may also be anaesthetised by injecting along a line drawn from the tuberosity of the tibia to an intersection of the anterior and medial borders of the gastrocnemius muscle. Fairly large volumes (10–20 ml) of 0.5% lev-obupivacaine, 0.5% bupivacaine or 0.75% ropivacaine may need to be used.

The success of these procedures is likely to see their increased usage in podiatric surgery. However, while the procedure does have signifi-cant advantages in some scenarios, as highlighted above, the ankle block remains a very effective technique for most forefoot surgery (Miques et al 2005).

## REFERENCES

Arthur BR, Wildsmith JAW, Tucker GT 1987 Pharmacology of local anaesthetic drugs. In: Wildsmith JAW, Armitage EN (eds) Principles and practice of regional anaesthesia. Churchill Livingstone, London.

Ashcroft D 2003 Statement of indemnity for Mepivacaine. Podiatry Now 6.

Astra-Zeneca 2001 Naropin (ropivacaine hydrochloride). Product monograph/data sheet.

Briggs GG, Freeman RK, Yaffe SJ 1990 Drugs in pregnancy and lactation: a reference guide to fetal and neonatal risk, 3rd edn. Williams & Wilkins, Baltimore, OH.

Burlacu CL, Bugg DJ 2008 Update on local anesthetics: focus on levobupivacaine. Therapeutic Clinical Risk Management 4(2):381–392.

Butterworth RF, Dockery GL 1992 Forefoot Surgery. Mosby, St Louis, MI.

Calvey N & Williams NE 2008 Principles and practice of pharmacology for anaesthetists 5th ed. Wiley-Blackwell: London.

Caputo LJ, Hembree JL, Dobbs BM 1982 Two long acting anesthetics: etidocaine HCL, bupivacaine HCL. Journal of the American Podiatry Association 72(4):186–190.

Casati A, Putzu M 2005. Bupivacaine, levobupivacaine and ropivacaine: are they clinically different? Clinical Anaesthesiology 19(2):247–268.

Clark MK 2008 Lipid emulsion as a rescue for local anaesthetic related cardiotoxicity. Journal of Perianesthesia Nursing 23(2):111–121.

Crausman RS, Glod DJ 2004 Perioperative medical assessment of the podiatric surgical patient. Journal of the American Podiatric Medical Association 94:2:86–89.

Cavaliere RG, Pappas E 2001 Anesthesia. In: Banks AS, Downey MS, Martin DE, Miller SJ (eds) McGlamrys' Comprehensive Textbook of Foot and Ankle Surgery. 3rd ed. vol 1. Lippincott Williams and Wilkins, Philadelphia.

de Jong RH 1994 Local anesthetics. Mosby, St Louis, MI.

Dagnall C 1995 History of the Society 1945–1995. Journal of British Podiatric Medicine 50:21–27.

Denkler K 2001 A comprehensive review of epinephrine in the finger: to do or not to do? Plastic & Reconstructive Surgery 108(1):114–124.

Dhukaram V, Senthil KC 2004 Nerve blocks in foot and ankle surgery. Foot and Ankle Surgery 10(1):1–3.

Dialynas M, Hollingsworth SJ, Cooper D, Barker SGE 2003 Use of a needleless injection system for digital ring block anesthesia. Journal of the American Podiatric Medical Association 93(1):23–26.

Dollery C 1999 Therapeutic drugs, 2nd edn. Churchill Livingstone, Edinburgh.

Donohue CM, Goss LR, Metz S, et al 2004 Combined popliteal and saphenous nerve blocks at the knee. Journal of the American Podiatric Medical Association 94(4):368–374.

Finucane B 2003 Allergies to local anesthetics: the real truth. Canadian Journal of Anesthesia 5:869–874.

Finucane B 2007 Complications of regional anesthesia, 2nd edn. Springer-Verlag, Berlin.

Foster RH, Markham A 2000 Levobupivacaine: a review of its pharmacology and use as a local anaesthetic. Drugs 59(3):551–579.

Gabriel J 2009 Reducing needlestick and sharps injuries among healthcare workers. Nursing Standard 23(22):41–44.

Hakim AJ 2005 Local anaesthetic failure in joint hypermobility syndrome. Journal of the Royal Society of Medicine 98(2):84.

Hardie RJ, Lorimer DL 2006 Local anaesthesia. In: Lorimer DL, French GJ, O'Donnell M, Burrow JG, Wall B (eds) Neale's disorders of the foot, 7th edn. Churchill-Livingstone, Edinburgh.

Haas DA, Carmichael FJL 2007 Local anaesthetics. In: Kalant H, Roschalu WH (eds) Principles of medical pharmacology. Churchill Livingstone, London.

Hansen TG 2004 Ropivacaine: a pharmacologic review. Expert review. Neurotherapeutics 4(5):781–791.

Jochim D, Iohom G, Diarra DP, et al 2006 An objective assessment of nerve stimulators used for popliteal nerve blocks. Anaesthesia 61(6):557–564.

Koay J, Orengo L 2002 Application of local anaesthesia in dermatologic surgery. Dermatological Surgery 28:143.

Kopka A, Serpell MG 2005 Distal nerve blocks of the lower limb. Continuing Education in Anaesthesia, Critical Care and Pain 5(5):166–170.

Kuczkowski KM 2004 Non-obstetric surgery during pregnancy: what are the risks of anesthesia? Obstetrical & Gynecological Survey 59(1):52–56.

Lagan G, McClure HA 2004 Review of local anaesthetic agents. Current Anaesthesia & Critical Care 15:247–254.

MacFarlane A, Brull R 2009 Ultrasound guided ankle block. The Journal of the New York School of Regional Anaesthesia (NYSORA) 12:1–5.

McClure JH 1996 Ropivacaine. British Journal of Anaesthesia 76:300–307.

McClure HA, Rubin AP 2005 Review of local anaesthetic agents. Minerva Anestesiol 71:59–74.

McLeod GA, Burke D 2001 Levobupivacaine. Anaesthesia 56:331–341.

Maher AJ, Metcalfe SA, Parr S 2008 Local anaesthetic toxicity. The Foot 18(4):192–197.

Malamed SF 2004 Handbook of local anesthesia, 5th edn. Mosby Year Book, New York.

Mather E, Copeland S, Ladd L 2005 Acute toxicity of local anaesthetics: underlying pharmacokinetic and pharmacodynamic concepts. Regional Anaesthesia and Pain Medicine 30:553–566.

Miques A, Slullitel G, Vescovo A, et al 2005 Peripheral foot blockade versus popliteal fossa nerve block: a prospective randomised trial in 51 patients. Journal of Foot & Ankle Surgery 44(5):354–357.

Moore DC, Mulroy MF, Thompson GE 1994 Peripheral nerve damage and regional anaesthesia (editorial). British Journal of Anaesthesia 73:435–436.

Morgan R, Johnson M 2000 Pharmacology for podiatrists. Blackwell-Science, Oxford.

Mulroy M 2002 Systemic toxicity and cardiotoxicity from local anaesthetics: incidence and preventative measures. Regional Anesthesia & Pain Medicine 27:556–561.

Ouzounov KG 2005 New nail block technique. Journal of the American Podiatric Medicine Association 95(6):589–592.

Peterson MK, Millar FA, Sheppard DG 2002 Ultrasound guided nerve blocks (editorial). British Journal of Anaesthesia 88(5): 621–623.

Raghavendran S, Bagry HS, Leith S, Budd JM 2006 Needlestick injuries: a comparison of practice and attitudes in two UK district General Hospitals. Anaesthesia 6(9): 867–872.

Rang HP, Dale MM, Ritter JM, Moore PK 2003 Pharmacology. Churchill-Livingstone, Edinburgh.

Redborg KE, Sites BD, Chinn CD, et al 2009 Ultrasound improves the success rate of a sural nerve at the ankle. Regional Anesthesia and Pain Medicine 34(1):24–28.

Rees S, Tagoe M 2002 The efficacy and tolerance of local anaesthesia without sedation for foot surgery. The Foot 12:188–192.

Reilley TE, Gerhardt MA 2002 Anaesthesia for foot and ankle surgery. Clinics in Podiatric Medicine and Surgery 19(1):125–147.

Rosenberg P, Veering B, Urmey W 2004 Maximum recommended doses of local anesthetics: a multifactorial concept. Regional Anesthesia and Pain Medicine 29(6):564–575.

Royal College of Nursing 2003 Monitoring sharps injuries: what can the RCN EPInet surveillance study tell us? RCN, London.

Royse CT, Royse AG 2005 The myocardial and vascular effects of bupivacaine, levobupivacaine and ropivacaine using pressure volume loops. Anesthesia and Analgesia 101:679–687.

Ruetsch YA, Boni T, Borgeat A 2001 From cocaine to ropivacaine: the history of local anaesthetic drugs. Current Topics in Medicinal Chemistry 1(3):175–182.

Safe-Point Healthcare Ltd. Safe-Point – the automatic needle remover for dentists and podiatrists. Available at: http:www.safe-point.co.uk (18 September 2009).

Scholz A 2002 Mechanisms of (local) anaesthetics on voltage gated sodium and other ion channels. British Journal of Anaesthesia 89:52–61.

Smith T 2007 Systemic effects of local anaesthetics. Anaesthesia and Intensive Care Medicine 8(4):155–158.

Strichartz GR, Ritchie JM 1987 The action of local anaesthetics on ion channels of excitable tissues. In: Strichartz GR (ed.) Local anaesthetics: handbook of experimental pharmacology. Springer-Verlag, Berlin, pp 21–52.

Tetztaff J 2000 The Pharmacology of local anesthetics: Anesthesiology Clinics of North America 18(2):217–233.

Thompson CJ, Lalonde DH 2006 Randomised double blind comparison of duration of anesthesia among three commonly used agents. Plastic and Reconstructive Surgery 118(2):429–432.

Uddin A, Reilly I 2008 Ropivacaine and levobupivacaine: potential uses in podiatric medicine and surgery. Podiatry Now 11(4):22–28.

Whiteside JB, Wildsmith JAW 2001 Developments in local anaesthetic drugs. British Journal of Anaesthesia 87(1):27–35.

Wiegel M, Gottschalt U, Hennenbach R, et al 2007 Complications and adverse effects associated with continuous peripheral nerve blocks in orthopaedic patients. Anesthesia & Analgesia 104(6):1578–1582.

Wildsmith AW 2007 Local anaesthetic agents. In: Aitkenhead AR, Smith G, David J, et al (eds) Textbook of anaesthesia. Churchill Livingstone, Edinburgh.

Wildsmith JA, Gissen AJ, Takman B, et al 1987 Differential nerve blockade: esters versus amides and the influence of pKa. British Journal of Anaesthesia 59:379–384.

Wilhelmi BJ, Blackwell SJ, Miller JH, et al 2001 Do not use epinephrine in digital blocks: myth or truth? Plastic & Reconstructive Surgery 107(2):393–397.

Winstanley P, Walley T 2002 Medical pharmacology, 2nd edn. Churchill Livingstone, Edinburgh.

Worrell JB, Barbour G 1996 The Mayo block: an efficacious block for hallux and first metatarsal surgery. American Association of Nurse Anesthetics 64(2):146–152.

Wynn R L 1995 Recent research on mechanisms of local anesthetics. General Dentistry 43(4):361–368.

## FURTHER READING

British Medical Association: http://www.bma.org.uk (19 September 2009).

British National Formulary: www.bnf.org (19 September 2009).

Martindale's: The 'Virtual' Pharmacy, Pharmacology & Toxicology Center: www.martindalecenter.com (19 September 2009).

New York School of Regional Anesthesia (NYSORA): http://www.nysora.com (19 September 2009).

Ashcroft D Personal correspondence by email, 11 January 2001, SOCAP.

Jones G Personal correspondence by email, 11 December 2000, Astra-Zeneca.

Spires-Lane V Personal correspondence by email, 22 December 2000, 361–368, Astra-Zeneca.

# Chapter | 21 |

# Nail surgery

*Peter Madigan*

## KEYWORDS

Esmarch bandage

Frost's procedure

Matricectomy

Partial avulsion

Phenol

Phenolisation

Sodium hydroxide

Subungual exostosis

Terminal Syme's amputation

Total avulsion

Winograd's procedure

Zadik's procedure

The most common problems for which patients seek the assistance of a podiatrist are disorders of the toenails (Krautz 1970). The disorders that are seen most commonly include those of congenital, traumatic, infectious, inflammatory, acquired and neoplastic aetiology (Shereff 1994). However, it has long been acknowledged that the ingrown toenail (Fig. 21.1) is the most common abnormality of toenails seen in orthopaedic practice, and that ingrowing toenails are a common cause of pain, disability and absence from work (Bartlett 1937, Bose 1971, Dixon 1983, Fowler 1958, Murray 1979). Matricectomy is now the most common surgical procedure performed on the foot (Boberg et al 2002, Espensen et al 2002). For many years the most widely used operation was the wedge excision, as described by Cheyne and Burghard in 1912. However, this method of treatment gives considerable discomfort and has a high recurrence rate (Palmer & Jones 1979, Sykes 1986).

## PHENOLISATION

Removal of part or the entire toenail with phenolisation of germinal tissue has become a common procedure with high levels of patient satisfaction and very low regrowth rates, particularly when carried out by podiatrists (Bostanci et al 2001, Gabriel et al 1979, Islam et al 2005, Laxton 1995, Morkane 1984). In a comparison of matrix excision and phenolisation, Bos et al (2007) found significantly better results in the phenolisation group. As a method of treatment the phenol and alcohol matricectomy remains pre-eminent in the radical treatment of painful nail conditions.

### Phenol

Phenol ($C_6H_5OH$, carbolic acid) was originally isolated from coal tar by Friedlieb Runge in 1834. Although naturally occurring as a by-product of decomposition it is a largely man-made product synthesised for use in the manufacture of phenolic resins.

Phenol is uniquely both hydrophilic and lipophilic. It is poorly soluble in water but is highly soluble in isopropyl alcohol, glycerine, ketones and esters (Boberg et al 2002). It has a sweet and acrid odour

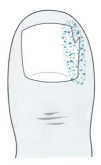

**Figure 21.1** Onychocryptosis (ingrowing toenail), showing a splinter of nail within the sulcus and overlying granulation tissue.

in its liquid form. Liquefied phenol is colourless, and is particularly stable when stored in an airtight container and protected from light. The solution becomes pink when left exposed to air and light but loses none of its potency or concentration.

Phenol has long been used as a chemical agent against bacteria and fungi and as an anaesthetic in many medicinal preparations (Espensen et al 2002). In 1865, Joseph Lister reduced the mortality rate in amputation surgery by two-thirds by disinfecting his theatre in Glasgow Royal Infirmary with an airborne spray of dilute phenol. Phenol is toxic and has the potential to cause serious local and systemic effects if absorbed or ingested. Reported effects include fluctuating body temperature, cardiac and respiratory changes, convulsions and, ultimately, death. The medical use of phenol has been shown to be very safe, and no systemic complications have been reported in relation to its use in matricectomy (Boberg et al 2002). However, the UK Health and Safety Executive issued a Hazard Alert Notice in 2000 following concerns regarding phenol. This imposed on employers a legal obligation to protect staff by using control measures to limit exposure to phenol or, preferably, to prevent exposure entirely by using a different substance or method.

In the UK, the Medicines and Healthcare products Regulatory Agency (MRHA) considers that phenol as applied to the skin is a medicinal product, and as such is classified as an unlicensed medicine. As only medical and dental practitioners are legally entitled to use an unlicensed medicine, the use of phenol by podiatrists in the UK must be considered illegal. The MRHA has, however, approved a commercial product called EZ Swabs, which is a method of containing and applying phenol, as a Class 11b Medical Device. Approving it in this way enables podiatrists to continue to use phenol within the law. Other regulations may apply in other parts of the world.

## History

The use of the procedure of phenolisation of symptomatic toenails has grown since Boll first described it in 1945. In 1962, Suppan and Ritchling combined the use of phenol with the more traditional technique of wedge resection of the nail plate, bed and matrix by suggesting that phenol should be applied for 5 minutes without pressure following the resection. Greene (1964) considered that the alcohol used to wash out the phenol delayed healing, may have increased postoperative pain and was unnecessary as it did not neutralise the action of the phenol, which was in effect self-limiting. The need to apply the phenol with pressure was stressed in 1956 by Nyman, who used alternate applications of phenol and alcohol, finishing with an alcohol-soaked dressing postoperatively. In the early 1970s Yale (1974) presented a paper at West Point Military Academy describing the results of 500 phenol and alcohol matricectomies. The study had been carried out over a 2-year period on soldiers who were able to

return to light duties on the day of surgery and full duties within a week. He stressed the need for the use of fresh phenol and strict haemostasis. The requirement for the procedure to be carried out in a bloodless field was further stressed by Dagnall in 1981. Bostanci et al (2001) reported a series of 350 phenol matricectomies with a mean follow-up of 25 months. The success rate was found to be 98.8%. Subsequent authors have reported results of varying the length of time of application of phenol and alternative dressing regimens (Dovison & Keenan 2001, Dunlop 1998, Drago et al 1983, Rinaldi et al 1982).

## THE PHENOLISATION TECHNIQUE

The phenol and alcohol technique is not an invasive procedure, and therefore does not require a full operating-theatre protocol. However, it should be carried out with a local sterile field around the foot and using sterile instruments and dressings. Following local anaesthesia, normally a digital block (see Ch. 20), and a pre-surgical scrub to the toe and forefoot, a tourniquet is applied to enable the procedure to be carried out in a bloodless field. The tourniquet should be broad and flat, such as an Esmarch bandage, to minimise damage to underlying structures. Using an elasticised bandage style of tourniquet will give good exsanguination of the toe, as it is applied from distal to proximal and allows the application of the phenol in a bloodless field. A long length of Esmarch bandage may appear unsightly when applied, and subsequently 'dangling', but it becomes virtually impossible to apply a postoperative bandage whilst leaving the tourniquet in place. This is a useful fail-safe procedure.

The Esmarch bandage is applied in the following manner. One end is doubled back for approximately 2 cm and applied to the digit distally, with the doubled end appearing as a tab. The bandage is then wound around the toe with the material stretched so that each layer overlaps and secures the preceding layer. This overlap should be used for all further layers of the bandage down to the base of the toe, ensuring that the material is stretched so that the pressure prevents the blood from entering the toe. On reaching the base of the toe the bandage and its tension is secured and maintained using forceps. Using the tab at the distal end of the toe, the bandage is loosened to uncover the nail and most of the distal phalanx. This end of the bandage is also secured. The distal end of the toe should now be completely exsanguinated. The time for which a tourniquet is in place should be kept to a minimum so that the risk of swelling after its release is minimised. Ideally, this should be less than 30 minutes.

Currently there are commercially produced devices for exsanguinating the toe and providing a tourniquet effect. One of these is Tournicot.

The time of application of the tourniquet, the time of its release and the return of the blood to the digit after the nail procedure must be noted in the patient's case record.

## Total nail avulsion

A narrow spatula or elevator is used to separate the eponychium from the nail plate. Using steady pressure an elevator is inserted below the nail plate and moved, parallel to the long axis of the toe, until there is separation of the nail plate and the nail bed and matrix (Fig. 21.2A). Under the eponychium the instrument is out of sight and the separation is felt as a sudden reduction in resistance. Care must be taken to ensure that the elevator is inserted into each proximal corner of the posterior nail fold by reinserting the instrument until the nail plate is fully separated. The nail plate is removed by locking mosquito forceps or a haemostat onto the plate half way between the sulcus and the midline of the toe, and rolling the instrument dorsally towards the midline (Fig. 21.2B). A similar procedure will release the other side of the plate and the nail can normally be lifted in one piece.

## Partial nail avulsion

A partial nail avulsion is designed to remove the involuted section of nail, which is causing painful symptoms within the sulcus. The remaining nail plate should be flat and must be sufficiently wide to give an acceptable cosmetic appearance. It is entirely possible to carry out partial nail avulsions in both sulci and leave a nail plate with good cosmesis.

The toe is prepared as for a total nail avulsion and a fine spatula inserted to free the eponychium from the nail plate. There should be as little separation as necessary to limit the tracking of the liquid phenol. A narrow elevator is inserted below the nail plate to separate it from the nail bed, as with a total avulsion, but being careful to separate only the section of nail to be avulsed (Fig. 21.3A). The section

of nail plate to be removed is split by introducing a pair of Thwaite's single-bladed nail nippers (Fig. 21.3B), a nail chisel, or a combination of both. The nippers are moved proximally to split the nail with as few cuts as possible and, preferably, if possible, only one. Alternatively, a nail chisel may be used with gentle controlled force. In either case, the most proximal part of the cut takes place below the eponychium, out of sight of the operator, and care must be taken to avoid damage to the underlying distal phalanx. A pair of mosquito or artery forceps is locked onto the full section of nail, to reduce the possibility of splintering, and rotated dorsally towards the midline of the toe (Fig. 21.3C).

The proximal edge of the nail plate must be checked to ensure that all the plate has been removed and to exclude the possibility that fragments have been left in situ. The proximal nail fold and sulci must also be checked for fragments that would interfere with the phenolisation procedure and become a focus for infection.

The destruction of the nail matrix is best achieved using liquefied phenol BP, although a number of alternatives have been used with acceptable results. There has been much debate surrounding the application of the phenol, but it is now generally acknowledged that a rigid adherence to time of contact is not sufficient. The liquefied phenol should be fresh, free from contamination and colourless, and can be used as a saturated solution of 80% BP or 89% USP. It is best to apply the phenol with a cotton wool bud lightly moistened with the liquid and discarded after each application (Fig. 21.3D). Care should be taken to limit the quantity of phenol used, as it is can be absorbed and cause tissue toxicity (Shepherdson 1977). The phenol is worked into the nail matrix, sulcus and bed with pressure. For partial nail avulsions it may be necessary to remove much of the cotton wool from the bud to facilitate its insertion below the eponychium. It is important to avoid phenol tracking onto adjacent tissue and, although with judicious use this is unlikely, the application of tincture of benzoin compound or petroleum jelly to the surrounding tissue may prevent unnecessary skin contact. As a general guide, the phenol should be applied for three separate 1-minute applications. However it is normally the case that older tissue will respond more quickly than younger, moister tissue and that chronic toenail dystrophies that exhibit increased fibrous tissue will require longer application. There is a change in the colour of the nail bed and matrix tissues from pinkish to a dirty white, and in texture from firm to softer during phenolisation, and the observation of these changes should be used as the main determinant of the total time of application. The site is flushed with alcohol, taking care to avoid contaminating the surrounding area, to wash out the phenol, although it

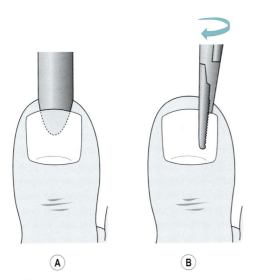

**Figure 21.2** (A) The instrument to separate the nail plate from the nail bed is inserted under the nail in a central location. The nail is completely detached from the nail bed, with the elevator moving towards the sides of the nail plate. (B) The forceps are used to grip the detached nail plate and apply a rolling motion towards the midline of the toe.

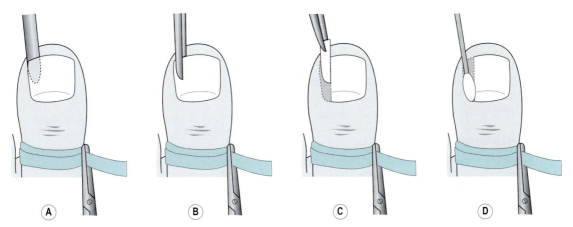

**Figure 21.3** (A) Separation of the section of nail plate to be removed using a fine elevator. (B) Cutting the section of nail using Thwaite's nippers. (C) Removal of the section of nail using fine artery forceps. (D) Application of phenol using a fine cotton wool bud.

should be noted that this does not neutralise or terminate the action of the acid. The area is dried and the tourniquet removed, with the return of arterial blood flow being noted when the colour returns to the digit.

Sodium hydroxide has been used with success for many years. The nail plate is removed in a similar manner as in the phenolisation technique, with a pellet of 10% sodium hydroxide being rubbed into the nail bed and matrix until the capillaries are seen to coagulate. Travers and Ammon (1980) observed this to take from 3 seconds to 3 minutes, depending on the patient. Kocyigit et al (2005) experimented with application times of 30, 60 and 120 seconds. Their success rates of 71%, 93% and 94%, respectively, indicate that a single application of 30 seconds is insufficient, but they noted a prolonged healing time with the 2-minute applications as a disadvantage. Those who advocate the use of sodium hydroxide report it to have a higher success rate, lower recurrence rate, less drainage and faster healing time when compared with phenolisation. However, Cumming et al (2005)compared phenol and sodium hydroxide matricectomies and found no significant differences between the groups in terms of healing time, postoperative pain, regrowth or satisfaction rates. Travers and Ammon (1980) analysed the results of 1000 sodium hydroxide procedures carried out over a 6-year period. They reported 15 (1.5%) cases of regrowth, of which 12 required revision.

Several authors (Abbott & Geho 1980, Gardner 1958, Polokoff 1935, Zuber 2002) have reported the successful use of negative galvanism, with little postoperative infection or pain. The direct current when applied to the nail bed and matrix causes sodium ions to migrate towards the negative pole and chlorine ions towards the positive pole. When the sodium ions reach the negative pole they break down to form sodium hydroxide and hydrogen gas, producing an alkali chemical burn and cauterisation of the germinal tissue. The effect at the positive pole (anode) is negated by using a flat dispersive plate with a large surface area (in excess of $150 \text{ cm}^2$). The negative pole (cathode), in contrast, concentrates its current by using an electrode of 2-5 mm. Despite its reported success, negative galvanism is not widely used as experience is required to adopt an adequate current and length of application. In addition, there is the potential electrical hazard to both the patient and the operator.

Yang and Li (2002) attempted to assess the effectiveness of a carbon dioxide laser for matricectomy. In a small-scale study of 18 partial matricectomies (14 patients) they found that use of the SharPulse $CO_2$ laser had a high cure rate, short postoperative pain duration and low risk of postoperative infection. Orenstein et al (2007) treated 40 patients and achieved 94% success when measuring the recurrence rate. Laser, however, remains an expensive option in the management of ingrown toenails.

Radiosurgery (radiowave surgery, high-frequency electrosurgery) is a relatively new modality in the surgical management of skin lesions, including ingrowing toenails. By using high-frequency radiowaves at 4 MHz, and using the tissues rather than the electrode to provide resistance, the electrode tip remains cool and causes less damage to surrounding tissues than traditional electrocautery. The resulting wound heals faster and with less postoperative pain (Sperli 1998).

## Postoperative management

It is essential that the patient is given clear verbal and written advice regarding the signs (and symptoms) of immediate postoperative problems. The written advice should contain a contact telephone number so that the patient can speak to a podiatrist in case of emergencies (see Ch. 27).

Patients must be advised to expect some postoperative bleeding, and indeed this is a good indication that the wound is freely draining.

Elevation of the limb(s) should be encouraged for the remainder of the day to minimise any bleeding and local swelling.

There is normally little postoperative pain if phenol is used because of its neurolytic action on local nerve endings, and discomfort can be controlled by the patient's preferred choice of analgesics obtained over the counter in any pharmacy.

The first redressing should be carried out at 3–5 days. Earlier redressing does not allow the wound to epithelialise and later can cause the postoperative dressing to harden and irritate the wound.

Strict antiseptic precautions, a 'no-touch' technique and sterile dressings must be employed. There should be evidence of early granulation and a serous exudate, which occurs as a result of the chemical-burn effect of the phenol. The discharge will be noted for 2–6 weeks. Nails that were locally infected before the procedure drain for a slightly longer period postoperatively. Prolonged drainage may be caused by individual hypersensitivity to phenol, the use of too much phenol, matrix or nail spicule left in situ, the formation of an epidermoid inclusion cyst or indolent infection (Yale 1987).

Opinions vary as to whether the toe should be kept dry or bathed in saline. In either case, however, ointments or pastes, which impede wound drainage, are contraindicated. Dovison and Keenan (2001) found there to be no clinical difference between dressings of povidone iodine and amorphous hydrogel in terms of rate of healing or infection. However, other complications such as hypergranulation were more likely in the amorphous hydrogel group.

Patients can be taught to redress their toe by taking time at the first redressing to explain each step of the procedure and by giving written instructions, which must include a contact telephone number for help or advice.

Redressing by the patient should be carried out every 5–7 days whenever 30 minutes of uninterrupted time is available. Using a basin, lined with a polythene bag or bin liner to reduce the chances of cross-infection, enough tepid water to cover the foot is added. A tablespoon of household salt (sodium chloride) is dissolved and the foot immersed. After 10 minutes the foot is removed and dried, but care is taken not to dry the toe, which should be left to dry in the air before covering with a clean gauze dressing using a minimal-touch technique. Redressing should continue until there is no staining on the dressing when it is removed.

In a 1998 audit of post-phenolisation wound care, Dunlop suggested that patients should be seen 1, 2 and 4 weeks postoperatively. In the study the vast majority of patients required either shorter or longer periods between their appointments, demonstrating the flexibility that is required and the individuality of patient needs.

Several studies (Felton & Weaver 1999, Giacalone 1997) have sought to add evidence to the debate surrounding the use of phenol in patients with diabetes. The theory would suggest that such patients cannot tolerate the chemical burn and would have difficulty healing, with increased infection and postoperative complications. However, no significant difference has been noted in healing time or postoperative infection rate in studies to date. Felton and Weaver (1999), however, noted a 10.3% infection rate in their diabetic group (12.2% in non-diabetic group) and the potential for serious complications must be considered in preoperative planning.

## SURGICAL PROCEDURES

Phenol and alcohol ablation of the nail matrix is noted for its considerable advantages. However, the potential for an increased rate of infection and delayed wound healing must be borne in mind. Thus,

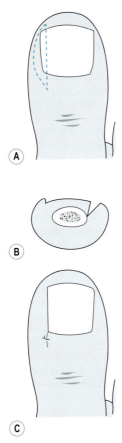

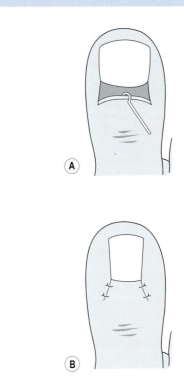

**Figure 21.5** (A, B) Stages in Zadik's total matricectomy procedure.

**Figure 21.4** (A–C) Stages in the Winograd partial matricectomy procedure.

there remains a place for incisional matricectomy in patients whose history or circumstances do not favour phenol ablation.

## Winograd procedure

The Winograd procedure, originally described in 1929, allows the excision of the medial or lateral nail sulcus with its adjacent nail plate, bed and proximal nail root matrix. A linear incision, from the free edge of the nail plate to about 5 mm beyond the eponychium, is deepened to bone (Fig. 21.4A). A narrow elevator is inserted distally to proximally to free and remove the border of the nail plate. A second elliptical incision joins either end of the first incision, creating a wedge of tissue that includes any hypertrophied soft tissue, nail bed and nail matrix (Fig. 21.4B). Following removal of the wedge, non-absorbable sutures or skin closures are used to approximate the wound edges (Fig. 21.4C).

## Zadik's procedure

In the belief that excision of the nail bed was not necessary to prevent regrowth of the nail, Zadik described a procedure in 1950, which involved excision of the nail matrix only. Using an elevator the nail plate is removed and a full-thickness flap created by extending oblique incisions from both corners of the proximal nail fold. This flap allows good access to the matrix, which is carefully excised from the bone. Regrowth of spicules of nail is a common consequence of inadequate dissection, and the periosteum should be removed to ensure complete removal of nail matrix cells. For closure, the eponychial flap is replaced and the lateral incisions sutured (Fig. 21.5).

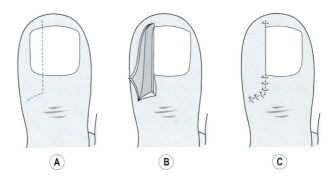

**Figure 21.6** (A–C) Stages in Frost's partial matricectomy.

## Frost procedure

In a development of Winograd's procedure, Frost (1950) used the initial incision of the original operation to which he added an incision posteriorly to give an L-shaped tissue flap for better exposure of the nail matrix (Fig. 21.6A,B). With deep dissection the nail plate, bed and matrix are excised. Sutures or skin closures may be used for closure. Tissue necrosis of the flap has proved to be the most common complication, and a number of modifications have been developed in an effort to reduce damage to the blood supply of the flap by altering the right angle of the L to give a curved or diagonal incision (Fig. 21.6C).

## Terminal Syme's amputation

In 1951 Thompson and Terwilliger described an amputation of the distal half of the distal phalanx that significantly reduced the rate of recurrence following toenail surgery. Using an elliptical incision around the entire nail plate and matrix, which is deepened to bone, the nail folds are excised. The distal phalanx is cut distal to the insertions of the long tendons and released from the soft tissue pulp of the toe in a similar fashion to that used when the calcaneum is dissected in a Syme's ankle amputation (hence the name 'terminal Syme's amputation'). The soft tissues are sutured to give good pulp cover of the remaining bone. There remains a potential for recurrence, and complications include growth of nail spicules and inclusion cysts at the suture line. Some women regard the resultant shortening of the hallux as cosmetically unsatisfactory, and women particularly should be counselled thoroughly preoperatively (Fig. 21.7).

## AVULSION USING UREA

Not all patients are suitable for surgical treatment of symptomatic nail conditions, and the use of urea has advantages, particularly in cases of uncontrolled diabetes, vascular disease or in the immunosuppressed. The urea softens the nail plate while also dissolving the bond between the nail bed and the nail plate. Its use, however, is time consuming and requires good patient compliance in the application of the urea and in maintaining a dry dressing. With the surrounding skin protected, 40% urea is applied to the nail plate and occluded with adhesive tape and/or a finger cut from a surgical glove. The patient is instructed to change the dressing and reapply the urea once or twice a week, with the necrotic nail being debrided at regular visits until symptomatic relief is obtained (Faber & Smith 1978, Port & Sanicola 1980, South & Faber 1980).

## TREATMENT OF SUBUNGUAL EXOSTOSIS

A subungual exostosis is a small outgrowth of bone under the nail plate or near its free edge. It generally occurs singly and unilaterally and will most frequently affect the hallux. While the aetiology is not fully understood, it is associated with either a single traumatic event or, more likely, multiple minor trauma. The lesion is slow growing, rarely exceeding 5 mm in diameter, and becomes progressively more painful as it increases in size. It is more commonly seen in patients aged 20–40 years, with a female/male ratio of 2:1 (Dochery 1987, Evison 1966).

In the later stages tenderness is experienced when even mild pressure is exerted over the nail plate. The epidermis covering the exostosis, which becomes stretched and thinned and takes on a bright red colour, will blanch with the application of pressure and will present a hard resistance upon palpation. These observations are useful in the differential diagnosis with subungual heloma durum and other soft-tissue lesions, including glomus tumour, pyogenic granuloma, subungual verruca and inclusion cyst. Accurate diagnosis of subungual exostosis is by means of a lateral-projection radiograph with the involved digit isolated (Fig. 21.8).

Temporary relief may be obtained with the use of protective padding or avulsion of the nail plate. More permanent relief is afforded by surgical excision, either using a minimal incision distally (fish mouth) or by an incision at the hyponychium and raising a proximally based flap. In either case, the lesion is removed and its base curetted.

In addition to regrowth of the exostosis, subsequent nail deformity must be considered as a possible postoperative complication.

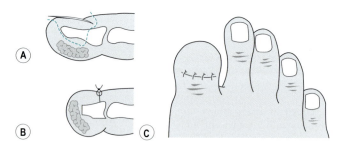

**Figure 21.7** (A) The fatty pulp of the toe is retained to cushion the stump. (B) Terminal Syme's amputation. (C) Patients should be warned about the shortening of the hallux following the procedure.

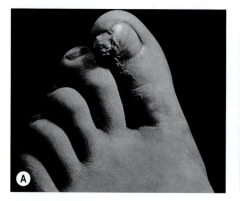 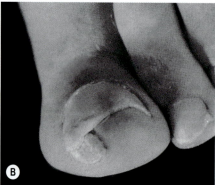 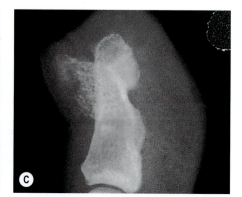

**Figure 21.8** Subungual exostosis. (A, B) Physical appearance. (C) Radiographic appearance.

## REFERENCES

Abbott WW, Geho H 1980 Partial matricectomy via negative galvanic current. Journal of the American Podiatry Association 70:239–243.

Bartlett R 1937 A conservative operation for the cure of so-called ingrown toenail. JAMA 108:1257.

Boberg JS, Frederiksen MS, Haron FM 2002 Scientific analysis of phenol nail surgery. Journal of the American Podiatric Medical Association 92:575–579.

Bos AM, van Tilburg MW, van Sorge AA, Klinkenbijl JH 2007 Randomized clinical trial of surgical technique and local antibiotics for ingrowing toenail. British Journal of Surgery 94:292–296.

Bose B 1971 A technique for excision of nail fold for ingrowing toenail. Surgery, Gynecology and Obstetrics 132:511.

Bostanci S, Ekmekci P, Gurgey E 2001 Chemical matricectomy with phenol for the treatment of ingrowing toenail: a review of the literature and follow-up of 172 treated patients. Acta Dermatologica Venereologica 81:181–183.

Cumming S, Stewart S, Harborne D, Smith J, Broom H, Abbott A, Barton A, 2005 A randomised controlled trial of phenol and sodium hydroxide in nail surgery. British Journal of Podiatry 8(4):123–127.

Dagnall JC 1981 The history, development and current status of nail matrix phenolisation. Chiropodist 36:315–324.

Dixon GL 1983 Treatment of ingrown toenail. Foot and Ankle 3:254–260.

Dochery GL 1987 Nails: fundamental conditions and procedures. In: McGlamry ED (ed.) Comprehensive textbook of foot surgery. Williams & Wilkins, Baltimore, OH, pp 5–10.

Dovison R, Keenan A 2001 Wound healing and infection in nail matrix phenolisation wounds. Journal of the American Podiatric Medical Association 91:230–233.

Drago JL, Jacobs AM, Oloff L 1983 A comparative study of postoperative care with phenol nail procedure. Journal of Foot Surgery 22:332–334.

Dunlop GM 1998 Clinical audit of a patient teaching programme in the care of wounds following toenail removal. The Foot 8:85–88.

Espensen EH, Nixon BP, Armstrong DG 2002 Chemical matricectomy for ingrown toenails. Journal of the American Podiatric Medical Association 92:287–295.

Evison G, Price CHG 1966 Subungual exostosis. British Journal of Radiology 39:451.

Faber EM, Smith DA 1978 Urea ointment in the nonsurgical avulsion of nail dystrophies. Cutis 22:689.

Felton PM, Weaver TD 1999 Phenol and alcohol chemical matricectomy in diabetic versus nondiabetic patients. Journal of the American Podiatric Medical Association 89:410–412.

Fowler AW 1958 Excision of the germinal matrix: a unified treatment for embedded toenail and onychogryphosis. British Journal of Surgery 45:382.

Frost L 1950 Root resection for incurvated nail. Journal of the National Chiropractic Association 40:19.

Gabriel SS, Dallas V, Stephenson DL 1979 The ingrowing toenail; a modified segmental matrix excision operation. British Journal of Surgery 66(4):285–286.

Gardner P 1958 Negative galvanic current in the surgical correction of onychocryptotic Nails. Journal of the American Podiatry Association 48:555–560.

Giacalone VF 1997 Phenol matricectomy in patients with diabetes. Journal of Foot and Ankle Surgery 36:264.

Greene AA 1964 A modification of the phenol–alcohol technique for toenail correction. Current Podiatry 13:20–23.

Islam S, Lin EM, Drongowski R, et al 2005 The effect of phenol on ingrown toenail excision in children. Journal of Pediatric Surgery 40:290–292.

Kocyigit P, Bostanci S, Ozdemir E, Gurgey E 2005 Sodium hydroxide matricectomy for the treatment of ingrown toenails: comparison of three different application periods. Dermatologic Surgery 31:744–747.

Krautz CE 1970 Nail survey (1942–1970). British Journal of Chiropody 35:117.

Laxton C 1995 Clinical audit of forefoot surgery performed by registered medical practitioners and podiatrists. Journal of Public Health and Medicine 17:311–317.

McGlamry ED (ed.) 1987 Comprehensive textbook of foot surgery. Williams & Wilkins, Baltimore, OH.

Morkane AJ, Robertson RW, Inglis GS 1984 Segmental phenolisation of ingrowing toenails: a randomised controlled study. British Journal of Surgery 71:526–527.

Murray WR 1979 Onychocryptosis: principles of non-operative and operative care. Clinical Orthopaedics and Related Research 142:96.

Nyman SP 1956 The phenol–alcohol technique for toenail excision. Journal of the New Jersey Chiropodists Society 5:4.

Orenstein A, Goldan O, Weissman O, et al 2007 A comparison between CO2 laser surgery with and without lateral fold vaporization for ingrowing toenails. Journal of Cosmetic Laser Therapy 9:97–100.

Palmer BV, Jones A 1979 Ingrowing toenails: the results of treatment. British Journal of Surgery 66:575–576.

Polokoff M 1935 Negative galvanic current used to destroy nail matrix. Cited in McGlamry (1987).

Port M, Sanicola KF 1980 Non surgical removal of dystrophic nails utilising urea ointment occlusion. Journal of the American Podiatry Association 70:521–523.

Rinaldi R, Sabia M, Gros J 1982 The treatment and prevention of infection in phenol–alcohol matricectomies. Journal of the American Podiatry Association 72:453.

Shepherdson A 1977 Nail matrix phenolisation, a preferred method to surgical excision. Practitioner 219:725–728.

Shereff MJ 1994 Disorders of toenails. In: Gould JS (ed.) Operative foot surgery. WB Saunders, Philadelphia, PA.

South DA, Faber EM 1980 Urea ointment in the nonsurgical avulsion of nail dystrophies. A reappraisal. Cutis 25:609–612.

Sperli AE 1998 The use of radiosurgery in plastic surgery and dermatology. Surgery Technology International 7:437–442.

Suppan RJ, Ritchlin JD 1962 A non-disabilitating surgical procedure for ingrown nail. Journal of the American Podiatry Association 52:90.

Sykes PA 1986 Ingrowing toenails: time for critical appraisal? Journal of the Royal College of Surgeons Edinburgh 31:300–304.

Thompson TC, Terwilliger C 1951 The terminal Syme's operation for ingrown toenail. Surgical Clinics of North America 31:575–584.

Travers GR, Ammon RG 1980 The sodium hydroxide chemical matricectomy procedure. Journal of the American Podiatry Association 70:476.

Winograd AM 1929 A modification in the technique of operation for ingrown toenail. JAMA 229–230.

Yang KC, Li YT 2002 Treatment of recurrent ingrown great toenail associated with granulation tissue by partial nail avulsion followed by matricectomy with SharPulse carbon dioxide laser. Dermatologic Surgery 28:419–421.

Yale JF 1974 Phenol–alcohol technique for correction of infected ingrown nail. Journal of the American Podiatry Association 64:46–53.

Yale JF 1987 Yale's podiatric medicine, 3rd edn. Williams and Wilkins, Baltimore, OH.

Zadik FR 1950 Obliteration of the nail bed of the great toe without shortening the terminal phalanx. Journal of Bone and Joint Surgery (British Edition) 32:66–67.

Zuber TJ 2002 Ingrown toenail removal. American Family Physician 65:2547–2558.

# Diagnostic imaging

*Jeffrey Evans*

## INTRODUCTION

Röntgen's (usually written as Roentgen) accidental production of x-rays in 1895 and the first ever x-ray image (radiograph) of living human tissue, his wife's hand, served to advance the course of medical investigation and diagnosis, with ensuing benefits for patients. Diagnostic imaging continues to be one of the most dynamically evolving fields of medicine (Yester & White 2006). Advances in imaging have gathered pace with, for example, the use of multiplanar image reconstruction, ever increasing resolution in tomography and the developments in fifth-generation magnetic resonance imaging (MRI) scanners.

The production of three-dimensional imaging data improves visualisation. The development of new radioisotopes may enable the visualisation of inflamed and damaged synovia (Fleming et al 2005). Advances in arthroscopic examination and surgery allow for the evaluation of conditions such as synovitis, impingements and obscure fractures (Katz & Gomoll 2007). While the traditional plain radiograph may still have precedence for most initial imaging, its production and storage is now likely to be digital rather than analogue. The latter format may be converted to a digital format using laser scanners, and then stored electronically, and sent almost anywhere in an instant using the Picture Archiving & Communication System (PACS). Thus 'teleradiology' is an increasing phenomenon (Körner et al 2007). The nature of investigation has also developed, so that there is often a physiological component to imaging as well as the usual anatomical context, and the next move will be at the molecular level.

> The first hundred years of imaging have looked at structure, while the next hundred will concentrate on function.
>
> (Cassar-Pullicino 2002:58)

Podiatrists' access to radiography and other modalities varies greatly. For some, particularly those involved in surgery, it will be routine to request, and be involved in the interpretation of, radiographs and other imaging modalities, while for others there may be little opportunity for direct contact with these specialities. However, changes in legislation in the UK have facilitated the possibility of more practitioners, including extended-scope podiatrists, referring directly to radiology departments. Even practitioners not directly involved with imaging require a basic knowledge of the key features of these modalities to enable effective understanding within their practice. To that end, the main aim of this chapter is to provide an introduction that will enable podiatry students and practitioners to appreciate each of the imaging modalities, their advantages and disadvantages, and their specific uses in the foot and ankle. More detailed information should be sought in specialist texts.

## IMAGING MODALITIES

Radiographs provide a considerable amount of information for the assessment of osseous, and in some cases, soft tissues. The plain radiograph remains the most widely used of the imaging modalities. However, other technologies are also available to aid diagnosis. These are usually 'second-line' investigations, partly because some are very expensive, and partly because they require highly specialised application and interpretation. The radiologist will choose the most appropriate modality for assessing the pathology under investigation. The patient's and the operator's safety is of paramount importance when utilising imaging modalities, which are based on ionising radiation, and there needs to be a justification for each exposure. Non-ionising imaging modalities do not constitute the same known risks. However, because no long-term damage has been noted, does not mean that it does not exist.

## MAGNETIC RESONANCE IMAGING

MRI has minimal complications or contraindications, does not rely on ionising radiation and can provide highly detailed, multiplanar images. Despite the relative expense of the equipment, there is an increasing availability of MRI scanners, including open machines, which ameliorate the 'fear factor', and those developed specifically for limb investigations. Together with reducing capital costs, there has also been a significant drop in the per capita costs to NHS Trusts, and increasing options for relatively low-cost private investigations. However, in the majority of cases MRI would be regarded as a second-line option (McGonagle et al 2002). MRI is considered a safe modality, and only a small number of patients are at risk from the powerful

magnetic force of the machine. However, considering the relative newness of this modality, long-term bioeffects and operator and patient safety cannot be completely discounted (Bassen et al 2005). It is only those patients with cardiac pacemakers, cerebral aneurysm clips, or implanted electromagnetic devices who are absolutely contraindicated. Pregnant patients, and those with prosthetic heart valves, or orthopaedic metalwork, may undergo an MRI scan if there is a defined clinical need.

When a patient, or part of a patient's anatomy, is placed in a strong magnetic field of approximately 1 tesla (T) and subjected to electromagnetic pulses, magnetic resonance images will be generated. A tesla is defined as the field intensity generating one newton of force per ampere of current per metre of conductor (Rowlett 2004). One tesla is an extremely powerful magnetic force and many times that exerted by the Earth's own magnetic flux at its surface (50 μT). The hydrogen atoms within the patient's body align themselves in the direction of the magnetic field. This is because hydrogen atoms have their own magnetic property, known as the 'nuclear magnetic moment'. Normally, protons have their own random orientation, but in a strong magnetic field they will align in parallel. In order to excite the hydrogen atoms, radiofrequency electromagnetic pulses are directed at the patient, usually at 43 megahertz (MHz). The pulses have the same frequency as the protons, enabling them to acquire energy from the pulse, and this is known as 'resonance'. The protons will alternately relax and realign, and they will emit radio waves that can be detected and, via a complex processing of signal transmission, reception and reconstruction, magnetic resonance images will be built by the computer (Yester et al 2006).

Choosing different radiofrequency pulse sequences can alter tissue contrast. The most commonly used MRI sequences are T1 weighted (T1W) and T2 weighted (T2W), and short T1 inverse recovery (STIR). The 'T' refers to a time factor where the alignment of the atoms follows a logarithmic curve, and T1 indicates the point at which 63% of the maximum possible alignment has been reached. T2 indicates the time it takes the signal to die down to 37% of its original intensity. T1-weighted images give good definition of the anatomy because fat-containing structures have a high signal, seen as white on the scan, while water-bearing tissues will appear much darker. T2-weighted images are better for showing pathologies, because of the presence of water/swelling.

The scan can be done in 3–5 mm sections, and in any plane – the thinner the section, the greater the subtle detail (Heron 1993).

The best resolution is found in the soft-tissue contrast; for example, tendons, muscles, blood vessels, and hyaline cartilage. T1-weighted images will show healthy bone marrow as white, because of its hydrogen content, but if the fat is selectively suppressed (STIR) a much darker, almost black image of the healthy marrow is formed.

In podiatry, MRI is useful for normal anatomy and for pathologies involving tendons, ligaments and infections, including osteomyelitis. It can also be used to image compartment syndromes and tumours. In addition, it has a high sensitivity and specificity for Morton's neuroma (George et al 2005). MRI is superior to computerised tomography (CT) scans and ultrasound imaging for all soft-tissue and marrow investigations, but the CT scan will be required when examining the bony cortex and for any bone erosion (Traughber 1999) (Fig 22.1). Intravenous gadolinium is used a contrast medium when a definitive diagnosis of osteomyelitis is needed.

## ULTRASOUND

Ultrasound is based on the use of inaudible high-frequency sound waves to produce images. Similar to radar, these sound waves are sent

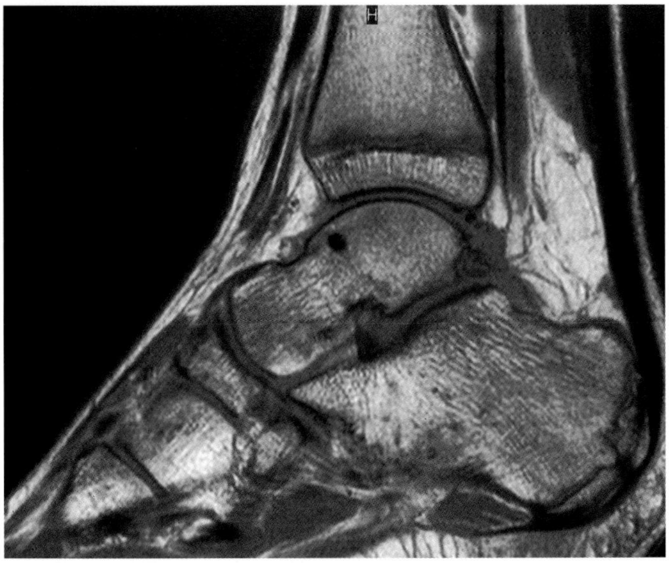

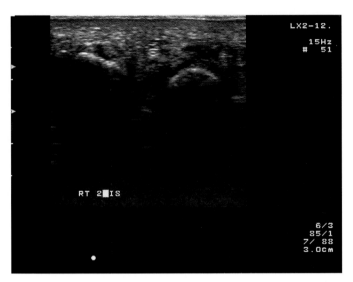

**Figure 22.1** Sagittal MRI image of the normal foot.

**Figure 22.2** Ultrasound scan of a neuroma.

as pulses. The sound waves enter the body, where some are absorbed and others are reflected back. The pulses are transmitted via a scan head, which has a number of transducers (i.e. piezoelectric crystals), which convert electrical pulses to sound waves. Typical frequencies are 3–10 MHz, but 6–10 MHz are the most often used frequencies used in pedal examinations (Mendicino & Rockett 1997). The ultrasound pulses are attenuated by tissues, and they are almost totally reflected by bone. Fluids do not reflect signals and are termed 'anechoic', but firmer tissues, for example tendon and muscles, will produce reflections and are called 'echogenic'.

Sonography may be used to image any of the soft tissues in the foot. It can be used to identify soft-tissue tumours and trauma (e.g. a torn tendon). One of its major uses for podiatrists is, for example, in identifying a Morton's neuroma (Fig. 22.2) and perhaps establishing a differential diagnosis from a bursa. However, obtaining a completely accurate diagnosis is based on the skill of the operator and adherence to a defined technique (e.g. scanning the foot both dorsally and plantarly). The actual neuroma may lie in an adjacent intermetatarsal

space to the one identified on the scan, necessitating the surgical investigation of the adjoining interspace (Betts 2003). The use of this modality in musculoskeletal investigation, by a variety of health professions, including podiatry, is likely to continue to expand as the costs become more affordable. However, it does require an extremely well-trained operator to translate the images, particularly as it is a 'real-time' modality and, although 'capturable', the images are transient. Quantitative ultrasound has been used as a diagnostic examination of the calcaneal bone for osteoporosis (Cryer et al 2007). This technology is also employed in basic and advanced Doppler examinations (Chambers 1995). To date, no known safety problems or bioeffects have been recorded, but this does not ensure that none will emerge (Hachiya 2006).

## IMAGING MODALITIES UTILISING IONISING RADIATION: SAFETY AND LEGISLATION

Everyone is exposed to background radiation to a greater or lesser extent. This may be from natural sources or man made, with the majority of the latter received from medical exposures. The use of 'high-load' (in dosage terms) procedures is increasing (Picno 2004). However, it must be appreciated that radiation does have a damaging effect on tissues, including genetic damage and the development of cancers, and therefore the uncontrolled use of ionising radiation would not be acceptable (Berrington De Gonzalez & Darby 2004). The public are protected by legislation that requires *justification* for exposure to these modalities. The ALARA principle (i.e. As Low as Reasonably Achievable) is still regarded by national and international bodies, such as the International Commission on Radiological Protection (ICRP), as the optimum approach. Specific information about dose levels and the effects on biological tissue are beyond the scope of this text; suffice it to say that all exposures will need justification that the benefits outweigh the costs (Martins 2003).

The current UK and European Union regulations, Ionising Radiation (Medical Exposure) Regulations 2000, is the statutory instrument and came into force on 13 May 2000 (Journal of the European Communities 1997). The central tenet of the new regulations is that all medical exposures are fully justified.

In practice, precise definitions are used to identify those referring, taking, or making a clinical decision on whether and what imaging is required, and that there is a net benefit to the patient. Podiatrists could be categorised in one or all of these designations, depending on their working environment. The definitions are:

- *The Operator* – that person carrying out the exposure. The operator will be responsible for all practical aspects, comply with employer's procedures and cooperate with medical specialists and other medical staff.
- *The Practitioner* – the primary responsibility of this practitioner is to justify and be clinically responsible for each medical exposure. Furthermore, they will comply with the employer's procedures and cooperate with other staff where necessary. Thus it is required that this person has full knowledge of the benefits of such an exposure. The act does acknowledge 'certain health professionals' acting as the practitioner, particularly in the case of radiographs of the extremities.
- *The Referrer* – as with practitioners, the decision as to who may act as a referrer can be taken at a local level by the employer (e.g. the NHS Trust and a consultant podiatric surgeon). However, it is stated that the referrer may be restricted; for example, a podiatrist may be able to refer for a plain radiograph

of the foot, but would be required to consult on the need for a complex CT scan. The referrer must provide sufficient clinical information to justify the exposure.

- *The Employer* – this may be an NHS Trust, a private company or, possibly, a self-employed podiatrist using his or her own radiography unit. It is a requirement that the employer ensures that all operators and practitioners have been adequately trained and that all records are kept up to date.

In practical terms, there will obviously be a great variation in the number of patients that podiatrists will refer for radiographs. The patient's general practitioner will probably remain the first referral point for most podiatrists. However, those in private practice may purchase radiographic services for their patients, and those in hospital situations may have direct access to the radiology department via local rules and protocols. There may be a small number of podiatrists who may have their own radiography unit. In this scenario, and if self-employed, they may fulfil the role of employer, practitioner, referrer and operator. The use of a radiography unit outwith a medically controlled hospital setting will necessitate the podiatrist notifying the Health & Safety Executive and establishing a link with a radiation-protection advisor, usually a physicist, who will advise on all aspects of the radiography setup.

## COMPUTERISED TOMOGRAPHY

The CT scan offers major advantages over the standard radiograph. In particular, the limiting quality of the two-dimensional radiographic image is replaced by a technique that can, ultimately, with the use of computer technology, produce three-dimensional images of body tissues through all planes. The scan may be done in a plain format or by using a contrast medium, which can be introduced into the patient's body orally or via a vein.

A CT scanner will usually consist of a gantry that holds the x-ray tube and a series of up to 1200 detectors, and this will be connected to an x-ray generator. There will be connection to a computer for the analysis of the data and production of the images. The patient will be placed in the desired position and moved slowly through the apparatus. The x-ray tube can rotate continuously around them by up to 360°, emitting a narrow beam of x-rays in a fan-shaped configuration. This beam is picked up by the detectors and fed back into the computer. As the data are acquired in a spiral manner, the term 'spiral CT' is used (Sutton 1997).

A CT scan is an individual slice or section of data ranging from 1.5 mm to 10 mm. A larger number of thin sections will produce better data for diagnosis. The 2-mm sections are probably the most useful for the foot and ankle (Oloff-Solomon & Solomon 1988). The digitised images are displayed on a monitor. Advances in software permit three-dimensional surface reconstructions.

Fundamentally, as the x-rays pass through the body tissues they are attenuated, and this enables absorption coefficient values to be calculated. These values are expressed in Hounsfield units (HU) and are normalised to water: water is scored as 0 HU, air at –1000 HU and bone at 1000 HU. Compact bone will appear white, while air will appear black on the subsequent image (Fig. 22.3). Manipulation by the operator will produce the desired image quality of the part under investigation.

The main advantages of the CT scan are its spatial precision, excellent contrast and three-dimensional image. The main disadvantages are that the patient is exposed to relatively large doses of ionising radiation and that soft-tissue differentiation is far inferior to that obtained with MRI. CT scans are particularly valuable for examining cortical bone (but not the bone matrix), periosteal reactions, calcifica-

tion of tissues, osteomyelitis (particularly valuable in the diabetic foot) and tarsal coalitions (Loredo & Metter 1997). CT scans have been described as the gold standard for cross-sectional imaging of the leg and ankle (Oloff-Solomon & Solomon 1988).

## FLUOROSCOPY

Fluoroscopy, first used in 1896, is an x-ray technique with the same safety considerations as all techniques utilising ionising radiation. In modern units the x-rays strike a fluorescent plate that is linked to a computer, which sends the data to a monitor where real-time images are displayed. In some podiatric surgery facilities a C-arm fluoroscopy unit is used to ascertain the position of pins, screws and, possibly, joint implants. The exposure rate must be kept as low as possible, and this can be achieved by means of taking time-delayed images and safe practice.

The freedom to position the fluoroscopy unit and the fact that 'real-time' images are available makes fluoroscopy a valuable, although expensive, tool. Modern machines use lower exposure than standard images using radiographic film, but the resolution of the image is inferior (Sanders et al 1993). Fluoroscopy is used in a variety of situations, including endoscopy, imaging the gastrointestinal tract and in a process called digital subtraction angiography (DSA).

Dual energy x-ray absorptiometry (DEXA) is another use of ionising radiation, where evaluation of the bone mass is usually made at the femoral neck and spine, but the whole body can be imaged. It provides a more accurate assessment of whether the bone is osteoporotic than do plain radiographs, where operator variability may compromise their validity (Walker 2008). Another technique, x-ray radiogrammetry (DXR), is also used and this may be valuable in quantifying bone loss, particularly in rheumatoid disease. The use of an ultrasound scan for an assessment of calcaneal bone has not proved to be as accurate in identifying osteoporosis (Böttcher et al 2006).

## NUCLEAR MEDICINE IMAGING

Nuclear medicine (NM) imaging is a long-established imaging modality, originating in the 1940s (Sutton 1997), that continues to evolve in sophistication with the development of new radioisotopes and increasingly powerful computers. While not a first-line modality, radioactive isotopes are used in a variety of clinical situations where plain radiographs may have failed to identify pathology. Their original use in identifying tumours, particularly metastases (Loredo & Metter 1997), has expanded and radioisotopes are now very valuable for the identification of osteomyelitis, soft-tissue infections, trauma and degenerative changes found in neuroarthropathy, particularly in the diabetic foot.

NM imaging differs from the other techniques in that it may be considered a physiological, as well as an anatomical, modality. NM techniques are much more sensitive to changes in the bone tissue; for example, osteomyelitis can be detected much earlier, at some 2–3 days, unlike the several weeks associated with a standard radiograph (Schauwecker 1992). Stress fractures can also be identified very early, within 24–48 hours, which may be critical for an elite athlete in training or competition.

The three mostly widely used and tested agents are technetium-99m ($Tc^{99m}$) phosphate, gallium-67 ($Ga^{67}$) citrate and indium-111 ($In^{111}$).

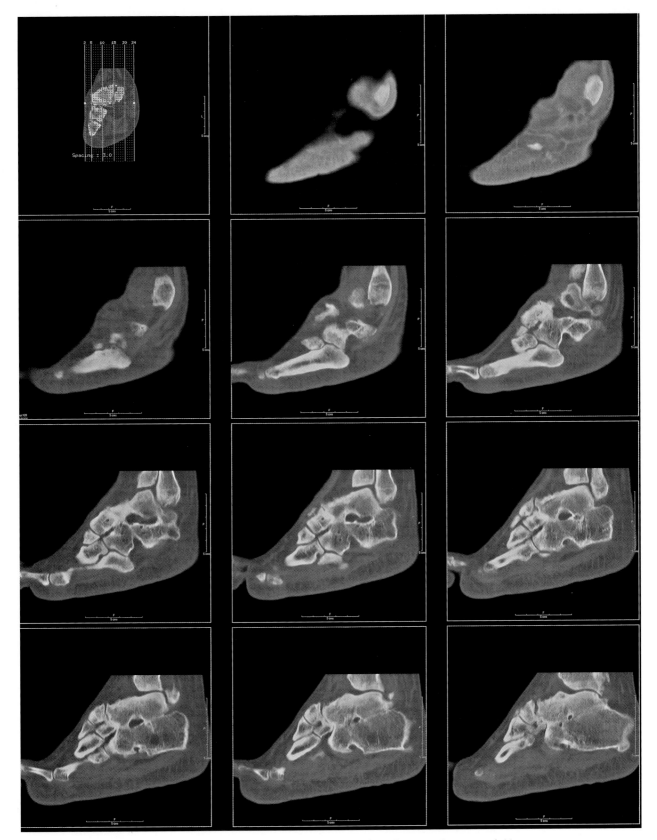

**Figure 22.3** CT scan illustrating multiple sections through the foot in the sagittal plane, demonstrating osteoarthritis.

Technetium-99m and gallium-67 are introduced via intravenous injection, while indium-111 requires a more time-consuming technique, involving extraction of blood from the patient and preparation by fractionating and labelling the leucocytes, which are then reinjected into the patient (hence the name, 'labelled leucocyte scan'). However, while this latter method has greater sensitivity and specificity, the technetiumc-99m remains the most frequently used agent (Brown & Holder 1996).

The triple-phase bone scan (TPBS) utilises radioactive technetium-99m, which following intravenous injection is first taken up by the blood (flow phase), and may be imaged serially in 60 or more sections at 1- to 10-second intervals. It is then taken up by the soft tissues (blood pool phase) and may be imaged at 3–6 minutes. Finally, it is taken up by bone, and may be scanned 4–6 hours later (delayed phase or metabolic phase). The technetium-99m has a short half-life (6 hours), and within 3 hours approximately 35% of the injected dose will have been excreted via the kidneys. Bone will take up 30–40% of the technetium-99m. It is regarded as a safe procedure for the patient in terms of exposure to radiation, comparing favourably with a standard radiographic exposure.

Imaging is undertaken using either a gamma scintillation camera or by means of a specialised CT scan. The camera uses a sodium iodide scintillation crystal that is able to detect the gamma photons given off by the radioisotope. The apparatus electronically converts the energy into a light scintillation, and ultimately an electric signal that produces the anatomical image, or scintigram. However, technetium-99m will only give off one gamma ray or photon at a time, and these can be recorded in a CT scan by a process known as 'single photon emission tomography' (SPECT). Another radionuclide is fluorine-18; this will emit positrons when in contact with electrons. The two photons produced by the positron emitters travel in opposite directions. Detectors in a ring formation are able to detect and scan the positrons. This process is known as 'positron emission tomography' (PET) (Collier et al 1996).

Gallium-67 citrate is particularly good for identifying osteomyelitis, malignant melanoma, metastases and inflammation, but it is used far less than technetium-99m. It has a half-life of 3 days and will be excreted by the kidneys initially, but then via the intestinal mucosa.

Indium-111 scans are the least used because of their higher cost, greater complexity and the fact that they may give false-positive results (Alazraki 1995). However, it is particularly sensitive for identifying acute osteomyelitis and soft-tissue infections of the foot. Scintiscans can also demonstrate a 'hot spot' in an arthritic condition (Fig. 22.4).

## PLAIN RADIOGRAPHY

*The plain radiograph is still an indispensable tool and should form the cornerstone of imaging protocols. It is quite cheap, enjoys the highest spatial resolution, and is easily reproducible.*

(Cassar-Pullicino 2002, p. 58)

Accelerating electrons across a high-voltage vacuum tube from the cathode to the anode produces x-rays, albeit that only approximately 1% of the energy will be converted to x-rays, with the remaining energy being converted to heat. These rays strike the patient, with some being absorbed and others scattered. Some rays will pass through the foot and strike a cassette, which in addition to holding the photographic film may also contain rare-earth intensifying screens, which in practice reduces the dose of x-rays required to produce an image. When developed, the film provides a negative image of the tissues (Dattner 1999). Although not as frequently used, Polaroid radiography is available. However, the image obtained with this process is reversed, with a black image against a white background (Fig. 22.5). Plain radiography is widely used in the diagnosis of a number of conditions affecting the feet. These pathologies may be of a local origin, as a result of trauma, or as a consequence of some systemic disease. Radiographs may be utilised in the pre- and postsurgical assessment of patients and for biomechanical charting. This latter use may be difficult to justify in terms of best practice, as the benefits would need to outweigh the costs of exposing individuals to ionising radiation.

## COMMON RADIOGRAPHIC PROJECTIONS

A radiographic *projection* refers to the direction in which the x-ray beam travels through the body. This term describes a positioning technique, and not the radiological image that is created. *Position* refers to that part of the body that is closest to the radiographic film. It includes such factors as whether the radiograph is taken when weight bearing or non-weight bearing, or by defining the angle (e.g. 'non-weight-bearing, lateral oblique' would serve to refine the basic anatomical position). A radiographic *view* refers to the image and is not a directional factor. There is sometimes confusion regarding these terms, with 'projection' and 'view' often interchanged when they should not be (Christman 2003).

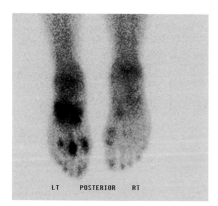

**Figure 22.4** Scintigram scan illustrating inflammatory reaction in rheumatoid arthritis.

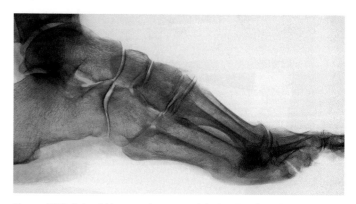

**Figure 22.5** Polaroid image of a non-weight-bearing foot, lateral projection.

**Table 22.1** Projection techniques

| Projection/technique | Weight bearing/non-weight bearing | Technique |
|---|---|---|
| Dorsoplantar projections | Weight on or off | Vertical or 15° cephalic |
| Oblique positions | Weight on | Medial<br>Lateral |
| | Weight on | Lateromedial oblique projection<br>Mediolateral oblique projection |
| Lateral positions | Weight on or off | Lateromedial projection<br>Mediolateral projection |
| Individual toe positions | Weight on or off | Lateromedial projection<br>Mediolateral projection<br>Dorsoplantar projection<br>Oblique positions |
| Sesamoid positioning techniques | Weight on or off | Posteroanterior axial projection<br>Anteroposterior axial projection<br>Lateromedial tangential projection |
| Tarsal positioning techniques | Weight off | Dorsoplantar calcaneal axial projection |
| | Weight off | Plantodorsal calcaneal axial projection |
| | Weight on | Harris–Beath (calcaneal axial view) |
| | Weight off | Broden |
| | Weight off | Isherwood |
| Ankle positioning techniques | Weight on or off | Anteroposterior projection<br>Mortise position<br>Oblique positions (internal/external)<br>Lateral positions (lateral/medial projections) |

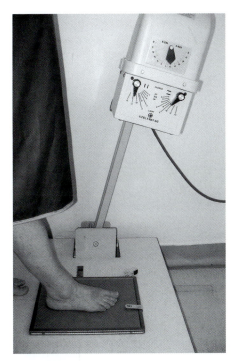

**Figure 22.6** Photograph illustrating positioning for a dorsoplantar projection.

There are over 20 possible projections of the foot and ankle (Table 22.1), but in daily practice only a small number of these projections are used. It is the individual practitioner who determines how many views are required. Some will take views of both feet, so enabling a comparison to be made. Others may choose to image just one foot. In many cases the two-dimensional image provided by the radiograph will yield inadequate information, thus necessitating two different projections to be made. For example, a fracture may not be evident on one view, but may show up on a view recorded from a different angle. When looking at the first metatarsophalangeal joint prior to surgery, a dorsoplantar and a lateral or lateral-oblique projection may be the best options.

## The dorsoplantar projection (also known as the anteroposterior view)

This is the most frequently used projection for the foot, and one that is best done on weight bearing. The beam is directed 15° cephali-cally, thus eliminating any distortion caused by the natural declination of the metatarsals. This projection is particularly valuable for demonstrating the phalanges, metatarsals and midfoot. However, the 'useful beam' may be collimated (limited) to a more particular area under investigation. This centring and collimation of the beam will highlight the area for greatest detail on the exposure (Figs. 22.6 and 22.7).

## Lateromedial oblique projection

This projection is used frequently for podiatric presurgical evaluation. If weight bearing, the tube head is angled at 45°, and if non-weight bearing the foot is angled to 45° while the tube head remains vertical. This projection gives good visualisation of the phalanges, metatarsals and sesamoids (Figs. 22.8 and 22.9).

## Mediolateral oblique projection

There is some variation of the angle, with some texts quoting 45° (Christman 2003), while others may reduce it to between 25° and 30° (Fig. 22.10). This projection is valuable for evaluating the first ray and associated structures prior to bunion surgery.

*Note*: oblique projections will give a much distorted impression of the foot, as they elongate the image, even more so if weight bearing.

## Lateral projections

These projections may be weight bearing or non-weight bearing, but in both cases the tube head is angled at 90° to the foot. This projection is valuable for showing the whole foot in profile, but some superimposition will obscure certain features, such as the midtarsal joint (Figs 22.11 and 22.12).

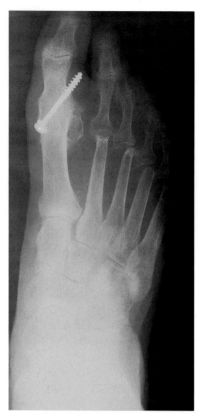

Figure 22.7 Radiograph illustrating an anteroposterior view in a patient with rheumatoid arthritis.

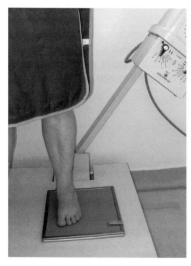

Figure 22.8 Positioning for a lateromedial oblique projection.

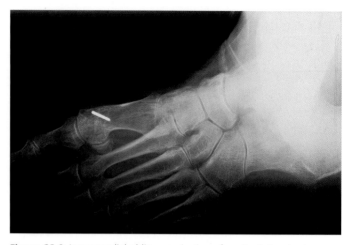

Figure 22.9 Lateromedial oblique projection of an Austin's osteotomy 1 year postoperatively.

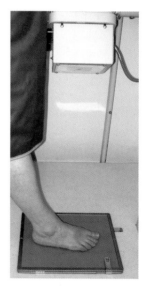

Figure 22.10 Photograph illustrating positioning for a mediolateral projection.

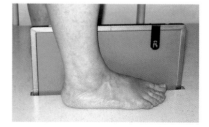

Figure 22.11 Positioning for a lateral projection.

## Digital projections

The lateromedial projection is particularly good for identifying subungual exostoses. The hallux, or any lesser toe, can be raised above its neighbours. This may be achieved either by placing a pad of material under the toe, or by placing tube gauze or bandage around the toe and then distracting it dorsally. Less often, latero-

medial and mediolateral projections may be utilised (Figs 22.13 and 22.14).

## Sesamoid positioning

The axial projection is most commonly used for isolating and defining the sesamoids. It is possible to take this view either weight bearing or

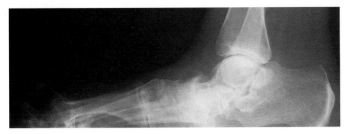

Figure 22.12 Radiograph of patient with pes planus following systemic lupus erythematosus.

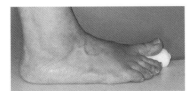

Figure 22.13 Positioning for a weight-bearing lateral digital projection.

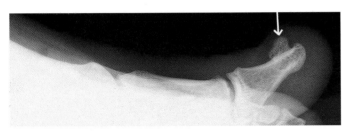

Figure 22.14 Radiograph of 15-year-old male with subungual exostosis.

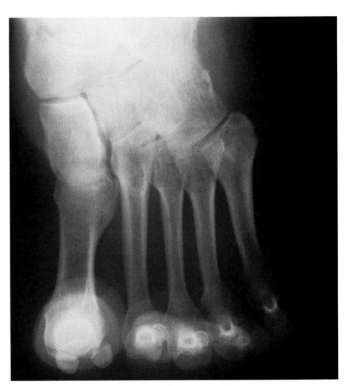

Figure 22.16 Weight-bearing axial sesamoid radiograph.

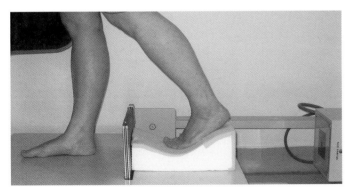

Figure 22.15 Positioning for a weight-bearing axial sesamoid projection.

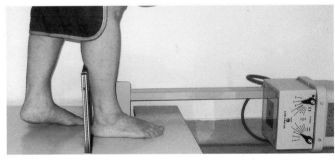

Figure 22.17 Positioning for an anteroposterior projection of the ankle.

non-weight bearing, and the foot can be positioned on a felt of foam pad to enhance the image (Figs 22.15 and 22.16).

## Tarsal and ankle projections

There are a large number of possible techniques for visualising the rearfoot and ankle. The most commonly used projections for the ankle would be the anteroposterior lateral and mortise techniques (Figs 22.17 and 22.18). The mortise technique is favoured to the straight anteroposterior projection as it allows better visualisation of the articular surfaces. The various tarsal projections can be used to highlight the relationships between the joints of the rearfoot (e.g. the talocalcaneal joint and the subtalar joint) or to view the sustentaculum tali or the calcaneus. The axial calcaneal projection involves directing the beam at the posterior aspect of the calcaneus at 45° (Figs 22.19 and 22.20). This view is primarily used for assessing the calcaneus for trauma. The Harris-Beath projection is very similar to the axial calcaneal one, but the patient is asked to bend at the knees as if preparing to jump. The central ray is aimed at the posterior of the ankle joint and the operator may make the exposure at between 35° and 45°. To a large extent, CT scanning has taken over from this technique (Weissman 1988).

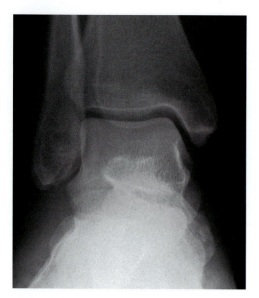

**Figure 22.18** Anteroposterior radiograph of the ankle.

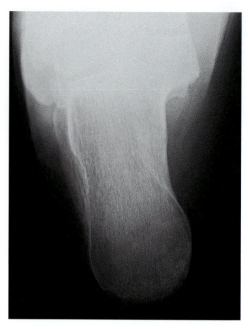

**Figure 22.20** Weight-bearing radiograph of the right heel from an axial calcaneal projection.

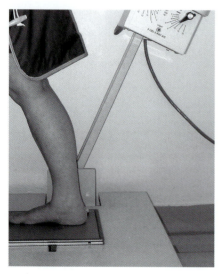

**Figure 22.19** Positioning for a weight-bearing axial calcaneal projection.

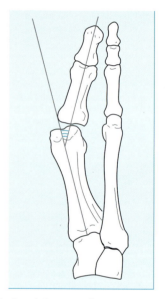

**Figure 22.21** The hallux abductus angle.

## RADIOGRAPHIC CHARTING

It is probably true to say that the majority of radiographs requested or taken by podiatrists are weight-bearing views, and usually in the angle and base of gait, as the foot is then in a functional position (Shereff et al 1990). However, if the patient is referred to a radiography department, it will usually be necessary to ask specifically for weight-bearing views.

Radiographic charting is the process of employing standardised marking and measurement techniques on the radiographic film to enable comparisons and conclusions to be drawn on a number of features. These features will involve the relationships of the osseous structures, and may be used for presurgical evaluation or for biomechanical factors, such as the classification of foot type (Street et al 1980). However, the use of charting for biomechanical examination is rather difficult to justify in most situations, as best practice would

be to not expose the patient to unnecessary amounts of ionising radiation. Whether the benefit outweighs the cost in such situations is open to debate. However, some basic measurement and charting may be used in certain areas of orthopaedics and trauma surgery. The use of presurgical radiographs allows the surgeon to assess the position of the bones and their relationship with their neighbours. It also gives an indication of the quality of the bone tissue (e.g. whether there is any localised osteopenia) and the state of the joints involved. The use of preoperative charting for hallux valgus surgery has been widely used by the podiatric fraternity, particularly in the USA (Kaschak & Laine 1988). The main reference lines and angles used are the intermetatarsal angle and the hallux valgus angle (Figs 22.21 and 22.22). Calculating the proximal and distal articular set angles assesses the

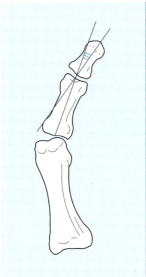

**Figure 22.22** The hallux interphalangeal angle.

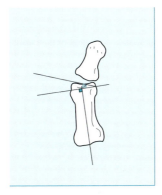

**Figure 22.23** The proximal articular set angle.

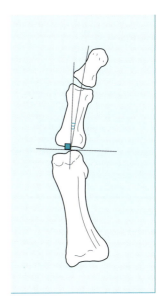

**Figure 22.24** The distal articular set angle.

congruency of the first metatarsophalangeal joint (Figs 22.23 and 22.24).

There is some debate as to the reliability of the measurements. A number of factors may operate to confound the reliability of radiographic charting. Variations in technique, error of measurement, poor landmark selection and patient movement are some of the factors that may give rise to inaccurate results. Furthermore, intra- and interobserver reliability will need to be confirmed (Astor et al 2004, Saltman et al 1994, Traughber 1999).

In terms of the biomechanical evaluation of radiographs, most charting can be done utilising dorsoplantar (Figs 22.21 to 22.28) and lateral views (Figs 22.29 to 22.31). The dorsoplantar view will provide for analysis in the transverse plain, and the lateral views will enable comparison in the sagittal plane. The angles demonstrated in the diagrams represent some, but certainly not all, of the measurable angles.

## RADIOGRAPHIC ASSESSMENT AND INTERPRETATION

Any radiograph must be read and assessed accurately. There is a logical and sequential method to this process. If the overall quality of the

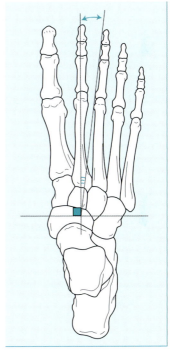

**Figure 22.25** The metatarsus adductus angle.

radiograph is poor, it may require the patient having further exposures, and this does not fit with best practice.

First the technical quality of the radiograph is assessed for *detail* (Gambol & Yale 1975). Are the structural components (i.e. the bones) clearly discernible? Is there a defined *contrast* (i.e. is there a clear profile of the part being examined)? Is there sufficient *density*, or is the radiograph clearly grey or black enough for the image to stand out? And, finally, is the film of sufficient overall *quality* and not marred by handling or processing faults?

The next stage involves the medical interpretation of the image. Christman (2003) uses the following terminology, but others have

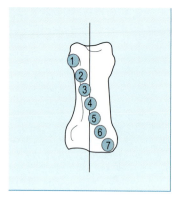

**Figure 22.26** The tibial sesamoid position.

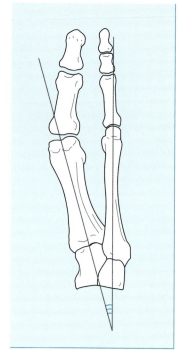

**Figure 22.27** The metatarsus adductus primus angle.

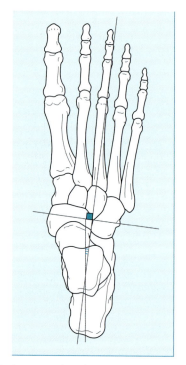

**Figure 22.28** The lesser tarsal angle.

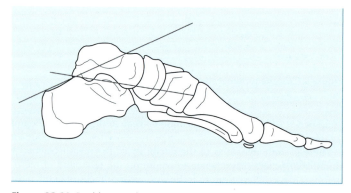

**Figure 22.29** Boehler's angle.

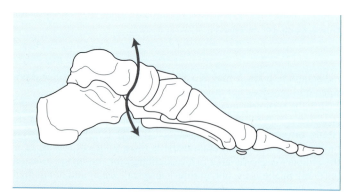

**Figure 22.30** The *CYMA* line.

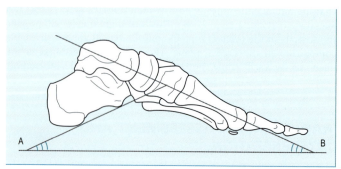

**Figure 22.31** The calcaneal inclination angle and the talar declination angle.

their own preferences. *Position* encompasses specific features (e.g. the alignment, apposition and angulation of the bone(s)); it can also refer to the joint, where there may be subluxation or dislocation. *Form* refers to the basic shape of each osseous component; it is useful for looking at the length, girth and general contour of the bone.

Whether one examines the foot from proximal to distal or from distal to proximal is not that important. What is important is that a consistent method is used for the analysis of each radiograph. Each of the major osseous components can be examined in turn, but care will be needed not to confuse normal structures. It is only through regular examination of radiographs that interpretation becomes an accurate and reliable process.

If the examination begins at the rearfoot, start by looking at the talus and calcaneus. In a dorsoplantar projection one would find the superimposition of the talus on the calcaneus. Indeed, superimposition will occlude much rearfoot detail. It is only possible to see the talus fully on a lateral view; the calcaneus may be seen in its entirety on lateral or medial oblique views. It should be noted that the relationship of the bones of the rear foot will vary depending on the foot type (i.e. whether it is pronated or supinated) and this would be most evident from a dorsoplantar projection. Lateral views give good information on joint relationships and the angulation of the components. The cuboid can be fully appreciated on a medial oblique view, while the navicular is visible on most views. Obviously, it is possible to vary the projection to enable a more 'refined' view of a particular aspect of these bones. The cuneiforms are best visualised on a dorsoplantar view, as they tend to be superimposed on other views.

Moving distally, the lesser metatarsals are best seen from a medial oblique view. This also serves to most clearly demonstrate the fifth metatarsal, which can also be seen on a dorsoplantar view. The first metatarsal is usually best seen on lateral and dorsoplantar views, but sometimes a medial oblique view is also taken (e.g. before a surgical procedure).

Dorsoplantar views are usually chosen for the phalanges and hallux, but occasionally an oblique view will be required. The sesamoids are best visualised on an axial view.

*Architecture* is described by Christman (2003) in two ways: the internal architecture, encompassing the structure of the cortices and the trabeculae; and the external architecture, which encompasses the margin of each bone, the subperiosteal surface and subchondral bone plate. Continuity of the cortex can be visualised along the shafts of the long bones, where it may be 1–2 mm thick. The cortices are far less well defined in the tarsal bones. The trabecular patterns are evident at the base and head of the long bones and are well demonstrated in the calcaneus. These trabeculae are 'stress-line indicators', and relate to the maximising of the bone's internal architecture to cope with stress and loading.

*Density*, or bony mineralisation, is a very good indicator of certain pathologies. The density relates to how black the film is and how white the bone appears (this is reversed with Polaroid radiographs). The bone may show increased or decreased density. Increased density (i.e. increased whiteness of all or part of the bone on the radiograph) may be referred to as increased radio-opacity, sclerosis or eburnation. Increased density may be associated with increased osteoblastic activity, and this is a feature of certain pathological conditions such as a fracture site or neoplastic activity. Paget's disease exhibits marked sclerosis, together with cortical thickening, osteolysis and decrystallised, coarsened trabeculae. It may also be associated with the development of a very painful osteogenic sarcoma. The rapid increase in the bone production and resorption has a disruptive effect on the normal structure of the bone, and may result in deformity and fractures. Radioisotope scans will demonstrate the extent of the disease, but plain radiographs are also very informative (Resnick 1996).

Osteopetrosis (Albers–Schönberg disease) is a rare, inherited condition wherein there is a defect in resorption of bone by the osteoclasts, and all bones show increased density. Band-like areas of denser bone appear below the epiphyseal lines and in the vertebrae. The bones are more prone to fracture. Melorheostosis is another rare dysplasia, in which small areas of the bone are affected, often following the course of the sclerotome. There is a proliferation of new bone at the cortices (Berquist 2000). Increased density may also be seen in hypoparathyroidism and a number of fairly rare pathologies; for example, osteopoikilosis, an inherited skeletal dysplasia, is characterised by many small foci of bone sclerosis, which mimic solitary bone islands. They may be found in the tarsal bones.

Decreased bone mineral density is also known as increased radiolucency, osteopenia or rarefaction. The term *osteoporosis*, once used in a general qualitative sense with regard to decreased density, is now used only as a pathologic descriptor (Raisz 2005). Decreased density may be associated with generalised or localised osteopenia. Osteoporosis is a common bone pathology characterised by a low bone mass, and in the UK it affects about 1.2 million people. Both sexes lose bone mass as they age, but this is more dramatic in women after menopause (Scottish Intercollegiate Guidelines Network 2003). Plain radiographs will not detect osteoporosis until approximately 30% of the bone mass has been lost. However, a dual energy x-ray absorptiometry (DEXA) scan provides information, usually from the hip and spine, on the bone density (Compston et al 1995). Radiographically, the appearance is characterised by thinning cortices, prominent primary trabeculae, subperiosteal bone resorption and sometimes a 'spotty' moth-eaten appearance in the cancellous bone (Fig. 22.32) (Ralston 1997). If it is in an individual bone, the osteopenia may be associated with a neoplasm or an osteomyelitis. As the disease advances, small stress fractures of the vertebrae may be visible on the radiograph.

Regional pain syndrome, often called reflex sympathetic dystrophy (RSD) or Sudek's atrophy, is also associated with loss of bone mass (Knobler 2000). This condition may arise for no apparent reason, or may be seen following a surgical procedure or trauma to the foot. The underlying pathology is not fully understood. The radiological evidence is patchy juxta-articular osteopenia giving a mottled effect, deossification in the metaphyseal ends of the toes, and subchondral deossification, eventually leading to a widespread osteoporosis. The use of advanced imaging modalities offers no great advantage over plain radiographs (Mayer & Kabbani 2003). Decreased density of bone may also be seen in deficiency disorders; for example, the lack of vitamin D in osteomalacia and rickets. In addition to the loss of bone mass, there is retardation of bone growth, causing a softening of the bones due to the inadequate mineralisation of the osteoid

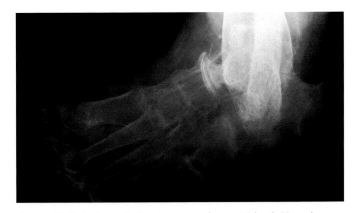

**Figure 22.32** Radiograph showing severe rheumatoid arthritis and osteoporosis.

**521**

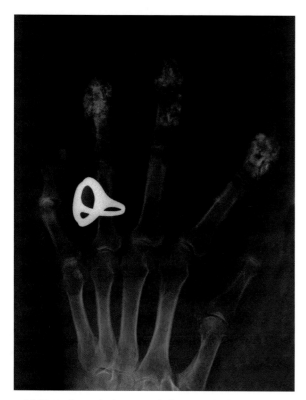

Figure 22.33 Radiograph showing calcification of soft tissues in a patient with progressive sclerosis.

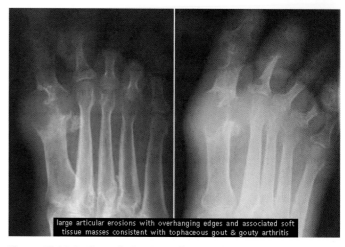

large articular erosions with overhanging edges and associated soft tissue masses consistent with tophaceous gout & gouty arthritis

Figure 22.34 Radiograph showing soft-tissue changes in gout.

framework. In children, there may be widening and cupping of the metaphyses, while in adults there is osteopenia and possibly, in later stages, pseudofractures, often called Looser's zones.

Lack of vitamin C, or scurvy, hyperthyroidism, hyperparathyroidism, thalassaemia and hypopituitarism will all demonstrate osteopenia.

The structure of the joints may also be examined, and one would seek a clear, dark, demarcation line in a healthy joint with good spacing between the opposing bones. Any closure of this space, loss of parallelism, or erosion and discontinuity of the joint surfaces or periarticular bone could indicate pathology (see the discussion of arthritides later in this chapter).

Finally, the *soft tissues* are appraised. This is not the main point of recording a radiograph, but a trained eye will often spot atypical features; for example, there may be calcification or ossification within the tissues. Calcification can occur in muscles, veins, arteries and even in bursae. For example, in long-standing diabetes there may be calcification of the smaller arteries (Loredo & Metter 1997). Calcification differs from ossification in that it has no cortex or trabeculae, and is often more irregular in outline (Fig. 22.33). Ossification is more defined with the development of trabeculae and a cortex. Ossification within the tissues may be seen following trauma, or it may be associated with neoplasia or venous insufficiency. It can often be seen associated with the Achilles tendon.

In gout, tophaceous material may show as a whitened mass around the joint margins. It is sometimes possible to see a shadow of some soft-tissue lesion or swelling, and it would be important to be able to delineate this from the surrounding normal tissue (Fig. 22.34). Oedema will also give an increased density.

*Infection* may be evident as a diffuse or localised swelling, which may also involve the production of gas within the tissues (Newman 1995). Foot infections may involve aerobic or anaerobic organisms,

which may lead to a non-suppurative type infection with local abscess formation. Unresolved infections may go on to involve bone, resulting in an osteomyelitis. Initially, this may involve just the periosteum, but later may affect the cortical and medullary bone. In children, the epiphyseal growth plate may temporarily halt the spread of the infection.

The classification of osteomyelitis may be based on the route of entry of the organism. Haematogenous infection is via blood-borne bacteria. These have a predilection for the highly vascular metaphyseal bone and are more common in children. A second course of entry could be following puncture wounds to soft tissues, or the implantation of screws, wires and plates following foot surgery. The final pathway may be from an extension of soft-tissue infection and ulceration. Once established, the infection will traverse acute, subacute and chronic phases. In the acute stages plain radiographs would be of little value, as for the first 10–14 days they would show little evidence, other than some soft-tissue swelling, blurring of the fascial planes and, possibly, a periostitis (Williams 2003). The patient would also show clinical signs such as pain, raised temperature and malaise. Later, demineralisation of the bone will occur, but this will usually need to be of the order of approximately 50% before a diagnosis can be made. In the subacute through to the chronic stage, the 'classical' signs may be evident. These would include bone lysis (destruction), with possible malformation, sclerosis, and the development of a *sequestrum* (a portion of dead and relatively sclerosed bone). An *involucrum* would also be evident. This is an envelope of new bone formation surrounding the sequestrum. A 'Brodie's abscess' may also be evident as a walled-off lytic inclusion, which resembles a bone cyst. Finally, a channel develops for the transport of pus from the site through the cortex. This is known as a *cloaca*. This should be differentiated from a sinus, which will develop within the soft tissues. Obviously, clinical examination and laboratory tests will also be necessary, and the use of other modalities, such as MRI, may be considered as part of the diagnostic process (Christman 1990). Infection is always a possibility in the compromised foot.

Patients with diabetes may develop atherosclerosis or possibly Möenckeberg's sclerosis. The former, affecting the tunica intima of the artery, is seen on radiograph as a solid column of calcification. The latter, affecting the tunica media of the artery, is seen as a less solid and often broken line of calcification. Occasionally, it is possible to see calcification of the arteries in the intermetatarsal spaces (Fig. 22.35). This may be discovered by accident when taking presurgical radiographs. These vessels rarely calcify in non-diabetic patients (Cheung et al 2002).

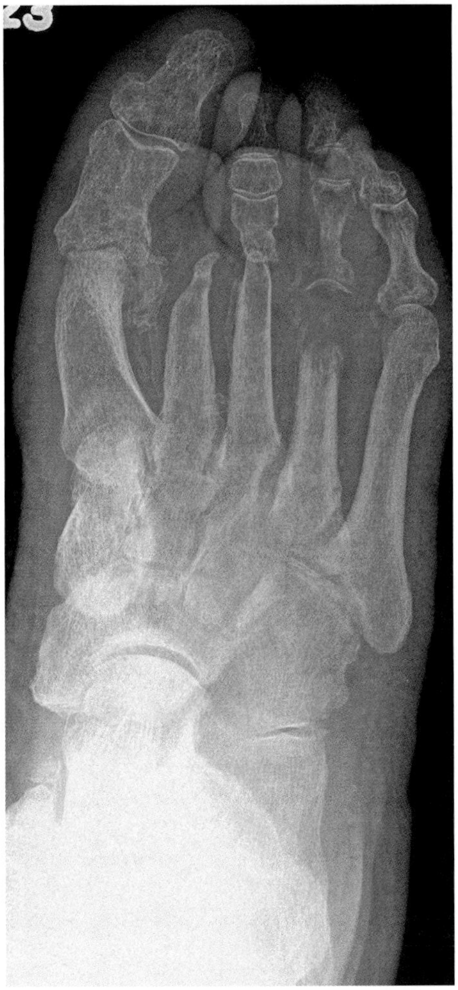

Figure 22.35 Radiograph showing osteoarthropathy.

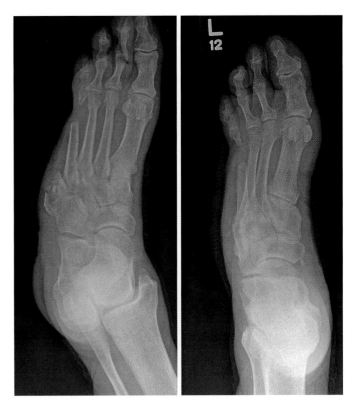

Figure 22.36 Radiograph showing salvage surgery following osteomyelitis.

## DEVELOPMENTAL VARIANTS: NORMAL AND ABNORMAL

While the adult radiograph demands specialised skills for analysis, the paediatric foot presents an even greater challenge. The clinician will require knowledge of the norms for development of the ossification centres, and the timing of their appearance and their closures. However, the appearance of the primary and secondary ossification centres varies within an accepted age range. Children rarely develop at the same pace, and bone development and maturity in girls is normally 2 years ahead of that in boys. Cartilaginous models of the tarsus are identified from approximately the seventh to ninth week of intrauterine life, and at the same time ossification is well under way in the metatarsals and phalanges. Between 24 and 28 weeks intrauterine, the tarsal bones will begin ossifying, with the talus and calcaneus being ossified at birth. By 2 years of age the lateral and medial cuneiforms are discernible, with the intermediate visible by 3 years of age, together with the navicular. The process of ossification in the foot is completed with the calcaneal apophysis and the fifth metatarsal head epiphysis; this will occur at the age of approximately 13–15 years in girls and 14–17 in boys. It is important that the developing ossification centres follow a recognised pattern in terms of their appearance, their size and shape, and their relation to their neighbouring centres (Oloff & Moore 1992). The growth plates at the epiphyses provide for increase in the length of the bone, whilst the apophyses add bulk and form to the bone. The appearance of the primary and secondary ossification centres, and the completion of ossification in the foot, is better referenced from detailed anatomical texts, for example Saraffian (1983), as there are variations of timing within the literature (Oloff 1987).

Osteomyelitis (Fig. 22.36) is sometimes confused with neuropathic osteoarthropathy (Fig. 22.35) because of the similar appearance on the radiograph. Neuropathic osteoarthropathy may be associated with a number of pathologies, such as syringomyelia, Hansen's disease, tabes dorsalis and, of course, diabetes. In diabetes it is often referred to as 'diabetic neuroarthropathy' or 'Charcot joint' (Christman 2003). The condition may affect any joint in the foot, but the general predilection is for it to manifest in the forefoot and midfoot, in particular in the metatarsophalangeal and the tarsometatarsal joints. The fundamental pathology is not fully understood, but it has been subdivided into two forms: atrophic and hypertrophic. The atrophic form is associated with loss of vascular sympathetic tone, which in turn results in a hyperaemia and an increased osteoclastic activity. This will result in a weakening of the bone by osteolysis, and possible fragmentation and fracturing. The metatarsal heads may collapse and have a 'pencilled' appearance. There may also be a periostitis. The hypertrophic form is not generally associated with loss of sympathetic innervation of the blood vessels. There is no associated hyperaemia, but there is a potential for massive bone disruption. Subluxation and dislocation may occur, as can bone fragmentation. The radiographic appearance is one of severe degenerative joint disease, with the appearance of an arthritis mutilans, similar to, but more severe than, that seen in psoriatic arthritis. A classical 'rocker-bottom' foot may be the final outcome (Loredo & Metter 1997).

Not only will the radiograph appear different from the mature foot, but also the actual method of capturing the image presents certain difficulties. For example, very young children will probably need restraining/sedating whilst the exposure is made. Finer details are obtained while non-weight bearing, and the resulting images will be of more use in cases of trauma, infections, neoplasms and bone diseases (Oestreich 1992).

*Variation* may present in a number of ways. For example, there may be variation in the size, shape or position of a bone (Fig. 22.37). There may be changes in density and architecture. There may be extra bones present. It is not unusual to find ossicles at various sites, and supernumerary sesamoids are sometimes observed under the lesser metatarsal heads. Occasionally, a part of or a whole bone may be absent. The radiologist's skill is in determining which of these features is a developmental anomaly and which is pathological (Fig. 22.38).

Bridges or *coalitions* may develop between two or more bones in the foot. These begin life as fibrous syndesmoses. They gradually become cartilaginous as synchondroses, finally becoming ossified as synostoses. They often remain undetected and symptom free until they ossify, when they become painful and restrict motion. They are usually congenital, but may arise as a result of trauma, infection, joint disease, or iatrogenically as a result of surgery. The most familiar are the tarsal coalitions, and of these the calcaneonavicular and talocalcaneal (Fig. 22.39) are the ones most frequently referred to in the literature (Blakemore et al 2000). Although rare, it is possible to see talonavicular, calcaneocuboid, cubonavicular and even multiple coalitions. Diagnosis is based on detailed radiographs employing two or more projections. However, while it may be possible to identify some bone coalitions on the radiograph, others will require MRI or a CT scan to enable complete and accurate visualisation (Keats 1988).

It is possible to identify up to 21 *accessory bones* (ossicles) within the foot (Romanowski & Barrington 1991). These are found to varying degrees, may be unilateral or bilateral, and are considered as normal variants. It is estimated that 20–30% of adults have one or more accessory bones. Generally, they appear as distinct, well-defined structures, but some (e.g. the os trigonum) may be attached to adjacent bones. They are generally asymptomatic, but occasionally they will need to be differentially diagnosed from a possible fracture.

The *os trigonum* is found at the posterior aspect of the talus and occurs in 2.5–14% of the population (Sopov et al 2000). It may be round or oval, but is most commonly triangular. Its position at the

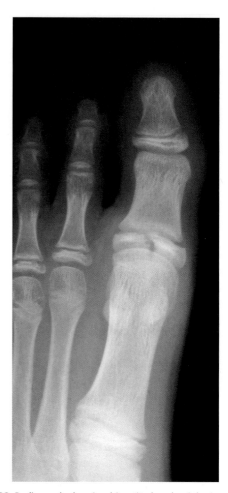

Figure 22.38 Radiograph showing bipartite basal epiphysis.

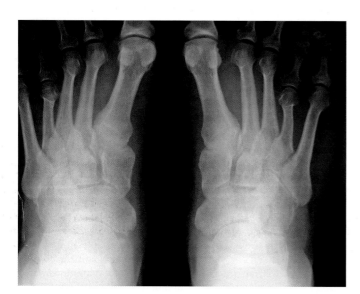

Figure 22.37 Radiograph showing congenitally short fourth metatarsals.

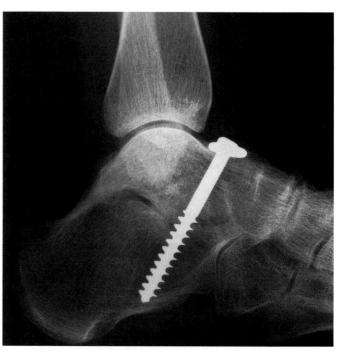

Figure 22.39 Radiograph showing fusion of the talocalcaneal joint.

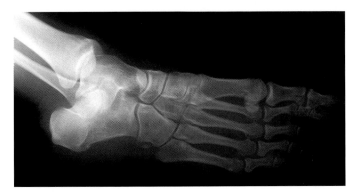

**Figure 22.40** Radiograph showing os peroneum.

posterior surface of the talus means that plantar flexion of the foot will cause it to impinge on the posterior surface of the tibia. Painful cases have been particularly associated with those sports and professions, such as football and ballet dancing, in which the feet are subjected to this extreme plantar flexion (Davies 2004).

The *os tibiale externum*, often referred to as the accessory navicular, is found adjacent to the proximal part of the tuberosity of the navicular and in association with the tendon of tibialis posterior. It is more common in women than men, and is frequently bilateral. Estimates of its incidence range from 2% to 12%. It was classically described by Lawson (1985) as having three basic forms: - accessory navicular type 1, 2 and 3. In type 1 there is a sesamoid bone in the tendon of tibialis posterior, which has no attachment to the navicular (os tibiale externum). Type 2 has an articulating accessory ossification centre with the navicular, while type 3 may be regarded as an end-stage fused accessory ossification centre. Some controversy exists as to whether types 2 and 3 need to be classified separately (Mosel et al 2004).

*Os peroneum* is another fairly common accessory bone, and it is found in the tendon of peroneus longus (Fig. 22.40). It lies adjacent to the lower border of the cuboid or calcaneocuboid joint. Its incidence is estimated at 9%. It may give rise to pain, and occasionally may be confused with a fracture (Sobel et al 1994). It is most clearly seen on a medial oblique view.

Other accessory bones are: *os vesalianum*, which is situated at the base of the fifth metatarsal and is of importance as it may be confused with an avulsion fracture of the metatarsal base; *os intermetatarseum*, which is usually found as either a separate ossicle, or a spur between the first and second metatarsals; and *os interphalangeus*, which is sometimes found lying on the inferior surface of the hallux on presurgical radiographs.

## OSTEOCHONDRITIS OR OSTEONECROSIS?

There has been a tendency to conveniently group those pathologic conditions where there is an actual osteonecrosis, and those that are merely normal variations or minor growth disturbances, under the general heading of the 'osteochondroses'. *Osteonecrosis* is bone death and is seen as part of the pathological process associated with some of the osteochondroses. However, osteonecrosis can be differentiated as an ischaemic necrosis of bone and may be associated with a variety of causes. It may be seen in gout, systemic lupus erythematosis, sickle cell disease and thalassaemias, and it may also be associated with trauma, long-term steroid therapy and alcohol abuse (Resnick 1996).

*Osteochondrosis* has been traditionally used to denote and describe those conditions that share a number of common features. They are only seen in the immature skeleton, and they may involve the epi-

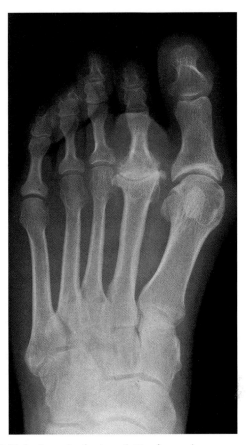

**Figure 22.41** Radiograph of osteoarthritis of second metatarsophalangeal joint following Freiberg's disease.

physes and the apophyses. Some are associated with joints, some with growth disturbance and others with trauma (Tachdjian 1990). They have a distinctive radiographic appearance characterised by a condensation of the ossification centre, increased sclerosis, fragmentation and possible collapse of that portion of bone. Generally, this is followed by 'healing' and restitution of the normal bone architecture. It is important to realise that most conditions will resolve with no residual problems (Cohen & Christman 2003). However, in some cases, for example Freiberg's disease, there may be a residual problem with the associated joint(s) (Fig. 22.41).

Table 22.2 outlines the main types and features of the osteochondroses.

## BONE TUMOURS

The following is merely offered as an overview of those neoplasms that may occasionally be found in the leg or foot and their radiographic characteristics. The incidence of neoplasia in the lower limb in general, and the foot in particular, is extremely low, with perhaps some 2–4% of all neoplasms being found in the foot (Helm & Newman 1991). Bone tumours may be benign or malignant, with the malignant varieties representing less than 1% of all tumours (Shaylor et al 2000). Some may arise directly from the bone, or from adjacent non-osseous structures. Very rarely, metastases from a primary malignancy elsewhere in the body may be discovered in the lower limb, but these are usually above knee level (Lee 2008). The authenticated

**Table 22.2** The 'osteochondroses'

| Name | Site | Pathology | Age (years) | Radiographic features |
|---|---|---|---|---|
| Sever's disease | Calcaneal apophysis | Probably a normal variation in the secondary ossification centre of the calcaneus | 10–14 | Sclerosis, fragmentation and increased density of the apophysis |
| Kohler's disease | Navicular | Extremely rare as a true osteonecrosis, rather a developmental variation | 3–7 | Sclerosis, fragmentation and bone resorption, followed by repair |
| Freiberg's disease | Usually the second, sometimes the third, metatarsal head | A true osteonecrosis, which may result in an osteoarthritic joint in the adult | 12–18 | Osteonecrosis. Flattening of metatarsal head, with subchondral bone fracture. Thickening of the cortex and neck of the metatarsal. The proximal phalanx may become moulded concavely |
| Iselin's disease | Base of the fifth metatarsal | Traction apophysitis, with no osteonecrosis | 11–15? | There may be fragmentation of the apophysis, but this is accepted as a developmental anomaly |
| Treve's disease | Affects the sesamoids | A true osteonecrosis | 15–20 | Irregular sesamoid with fragmentation and a mottled appearance |
| Buschke's disease | The cuneiforms are affected. | Not an osteonecrosis; a temporary anomaly of ossification | 11–15 | Change in the shape of the cuneiform and an increased radiodensity |
| Blount's disease | Posteromedial portion of the proximal tibial metaphysis/epiphysis | Not a true osteonecrosis. Two forms described originally: infantile and adolescent | 1–3 6–13 | Medial epiphysis is poorly developed |
| Osgood–Schlatter disease | Tibial tuberosity | Not a true osteonecrosis. May be associated with trauma, jumping and running sports. | 11–15 | Fragmentation and sclerosis of tibial tubercle |
| Sinding–Larson–Johansson disease | Patella | Not a true osteonecrosis; associated with traction/stress | 10–14 | Osseous fragmentation of the lower aspect of the patella |
| Legg–Calve–Perthe disease | Capital femoral epiphysis | A true osteonecrosis, which may predispose to osteoarthritis in the adult | 2–16 | Fragmentation and compaction of subchondral bone. Fracture of the necrotic bone. Flattening and sclerosis of the ossification nucleus. Collapse of the femoral head |
| Osteochondritis dissicans | Talar dome and lateral aspect of medial femoral condyle | Osteonecrosis | 12–18 | A defined area of subchondral bone circled by a marked radiolucent ring |

reporting of their presence in the foot barely reaches three figures (Anderson & Kakarlapudi 2000).

The identification of any neoplasm needs the expert eye of a consultant radiologist, who will usually base the diagnosis on a number of criteria. Plain radiography may not be sufficient, and other imaging modalities are likely to be employed to confirm a diagnosis. The following criteria are adapted from Shook et al (2003), and may vary slightly from practitioner to practitioner.

- Is the lesion single or multiple? Are there multiple lesions within one bone?
- What is the size of the lesion? Aggressive lesions attain a larger size more quickly then benign ones.
- What is the shape of the lesion? The cortex contains slow-growing lesions, which grow in an elongate manner along the diaphysis.

- Does the lesion have a destructive pattern or productive pattern (i.e. is it producing or destroying bone)?
- What is the degree of cortical involvement? It may appear 'moth eaten' with aggressive lesions penetrating the cortex.
- Is there a periosteal reaction, and if so to what extent? Aggressive lesions have a greater periosteal reaction.
- Anatomical site: which bone or part of the bone is involved – epiphysis, diaphysis, metaphysis, cortex, medullary or periosteal areas?
- Is there trabeculation? Not seen frequently, but may be associated with giant-cell tumours and bone cysts.
- Is there matrix production? Not seen in most tumours, but when present it may be in a solid or mineralised form.

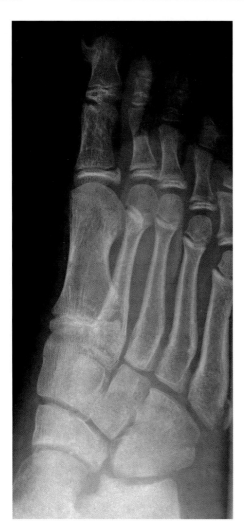

**Figure 22.42** Radiograph of a solitary osteochondroma.

The main *benign* tumours are:

- *Aneurysmal bone cyst* – mainly seen in children and young people aged 5–30 years. This is a rapidly expansile growth, often affecting the metaphyses, and is very painful. These are thought not to be neoplastic lesions, but a reactive process where blood-filled cystic cavities occur, producing a variety of possible outcomes. The lesion may: remain small; grow rapidly, destroying the cortex; expand slowly and become trabeculated; or become progressively ossified (Yeager et al 1988).
- *Solitary osteochondroma* – perhaps more familiar to podiatrists as an osteocartilaginous exostosis. These are predominantly found in the lower limb and may occur in any of the pedal bones. They are often associated with the dorsal aspect of the hallux, where they form a pedunculated shape. Surgical removal is usually necessary if they are growing aggressively and are painful (Fig. 22.42).
- *Simple (solitary) bone cysts* – these are common in children and are not thought of as neoplastic. Generally, they are not painful and are often discovered by chance. They are fluid-filled cavities lined by a thin connective tissue, or osteoid membrane, and have a sclerotic margin. They can be found in the foot, often in a metatarsal, or in the calcaneus. It is possible for them to fracture and release their serous or vascular contents. On a radiograph they appear as well-defined locular structures, which

have a sclerotic border. If there is an associated pathological fracture, it may be possible to see some periosteal reaction.

- *Osteoid osteoma* – these form approximately 11% of all benign neoplasia. They are found in long bones, but are recorded within the foot, with a predilection for the talus and calcaneus. Young people aged 5–25 years are most commonly affected (Shook et al 2003). They are osteoblastic lesions, small and circumscribed. They may be found in the cancellous, medullary or subperiosteal bone. A small, defined central area of osteoid material, classically referred to as a 'nidus', is surrounded by vascular connective tissue, and permeated with trabeculae. Non-myelinated nerves abound, and these may be associated with the severe pain that is characteristic of this lesion (Freschi & Dodson 2007). Radiographically they appear as well-defined sclerotic lesions with varying degrees of new bone formation and cortical thickening (El Rayes & El Kordy 2003). Clinically, there is pain, particularly at night, which can be relieved by the use of aspirin. Because of the risk of misdiagnosis and the fact that plain radiographs may not reveal the lesion accurately, the use of other modalities such as a CT scan is recommended (Chakrabarti et al 1995).
- *Giant cell tumour* – an uncommon tumour, particularly in the foot, which although benign may be very aggressive locally. In the leg, the distal femur and proximal tibia are the most affected, while in the foot it is the metatarsals and phalanges. Histologically, it is composed of a mixture of multinucleated giant cells together with mononuclear stromal cells (Asirvatham et al 1992). The main symptom is of a dull pain. A tender, firm swelling may be palpable. Radiological features indicate a circumscribed, radiolucent area with minimal periosteal reaction, no matrix and little cortical damage. Occasionally, these may be confused with aneurysmal bone cysts.
- *Enchondroma* – the origin of this benign lesion is cartilaginous. They are more commonly found in the phalanges of the hand, but may present in the foot and, rarely, are discovered on the axial skeleton (Shook et al 2003). They occur in the age range 10–35 years. The radiological appearance is a sharply defined, circumscribed lesion, with little cortical disruption, moderate sclerosis and an endosteal 'scalloping' of the inner cortex. Occasionally, pathological fractures may occur through the lesion.
- *Chondroblastoma* – this is an uncommon lesion comprised of immature cartilage cells. They are mainly seen in the leg around the knee, but have been reported in the foot, in particular, the talus and calcaneus (Huvos 1991). They present on the radiograph as well-defined, oval or round lesions with a border of sclerotic bone. They may be asymptomatic or present as a dull pain.

Where considered necessary, the above tumours may be removed by surgery and/or curettage.

The main *malignant* bone tumours that are found throughout the body, but are rare in the foot, are:

- *Chondrosarcoma* – like the enchondroma, these have a cartilaginous origin. They tend to affect older adults and are very rare in children. In the foot, they may be seen in any bone, but are more common in the calcaneus and talus. A dull pain and possible swelling may be the only clinical symptoms. Extremely difficult lesions to identify on radiograph, the more common indicators are: calcification of the matrix, 'scalloping' of the endosteal layer, a thinning and expansion of the overlying cortex and possible soft-tissue involvement (Bullough 1997). As it is sometimes difficult to differentiate histologically between chondrosarcoma and enchondroma, there is a need to correlate any histological findings with detailed imaging and clinical investigations (Mohammadianpanah 2004).

- *Ewing's sarcoma* – one of the most aggressive of all bone tumours, described as a non-matrix-producing, round cell tumour (Stibe & Cobb 1993). Its histological origins remain unclear. Its predilection is for the long bones of the leg, and in the foot, as with so many neoplasms, it is more common in the calcaneus. It mainly affects young people, particularly around the middle teens. There may be unremitting pain and, as the tumour enlarges, soft-tissue swelling. The radiograph shows destruction of the bone, possible periosteal reaction and, particularly in the calcaneus, there may be a rather atypical non-lytic reaction with a reactive sclerosis. The actual appearance is very similar to that of an osteomyelitis. Pathological fractures and soft-tissue involvement are also extremely likely.

- *Osteogenic sarcoma* – this highly malignant neoplasm also has a peak occurrence in younger people, within the age range 12–30 years, and it is more common in males. In the foot, it is mostly found in the calcaneus, and radiographically it presents a somewhat mixed picture. It may be lytic, densely sclerotic, or exhibit both features. There may be very distinctive periosteal reactions, often referred to as a 'sunburst' effect. There will be destruction of the internal bony architecture, giving a 'moth-eaten' appearance, destruction of the cortex, and invasion and ossification of the adjacent soft tissues (Harrelson 1991).

Because of their relative rarity, and the fact that they may be unobserved or misdiagnosed, the treatment of these highly dangerous tumours is sometimes delayed. Imaging and bone biopsies will usually confirm the diagnosis. Following this, resective surgery will be necessary to remove the primary tumour, and this may be supported by radiotherapy (Shaylor et al 2000). However, amputation of the limb may be necessary in some cases.

## BONES, JOINTS AND CONNECTIVE TISSUES

The arthritides form a complex group of joint and connective-tissue diseases, many with a predilection for the foot. In the early stages of these diseases, radiography may not be of primary importance, and clinical and laboratory investigations may be of more value. As the disease becomes more chronic, there may be an associated development of clearly defined radiological markers (Nuki et al 1999).

The disorders may be classified on the basis of the underlying pathology – whether they are inflammatory, metabolic or degenerative. Alternatively, they may be classified on the basis of specific radiographic characteristics (Christman 1991). Whatever method is used, a logical sequence of examination will be required when viewing the radiographic evidence, such as the ABCDS approach, where A refers to alignment, B to bone mineralisation, C to cartilage (joint) space, D to distal to proximal and S to soft tissue (Kaschak & Laine 1988).

The fundamental radiographic characteristics are represented by either a hypertrophic or an atrophic reaction. *Osteoarthritis* represents a hypertrophic reaction. While classically considered a degenerative disease, possibly resulting from frank trauma or mechanical overload, it is possible that there may be an underlying genetic link (Spector et al 1996). Osteoarthritis is common in the foot, particularly in the first metatarsophalangeal, the metatarsocuneiform, and the naviculocuneiform and talonavicular joints. The characteristic features associated with osteoarthritis are focal destruction of the articular cartilage and osteophytosis (i.e. the presence of osteophytes), which is particularly noticeable as 'dorsal lipping' at the first metatarsophalangeal joint (Fig. 22.43). Metatarsosesamoid involvement is also possible.

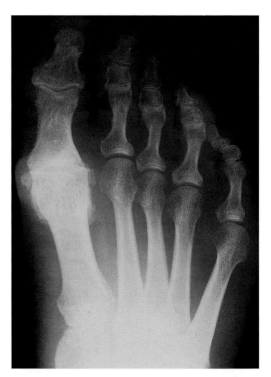

**Figure 22.43** Radiograph of severe osteoarthritis of the first metatarsophalangeal joint.

There is an uneven narrowing of the joint space, which may eventually be totally lost. Subchondral sclerosis, together with cyst formation, completes the picture in moderate to severe osteoarthritis.

*Rheumatoid arthritis* is a seropositive, inflammatory polyarthritis with various non-articular manifestations. Its course can be highly variable, as is the prognosis. However, the disease tends to follow a relapsing and remitting course in most sufferers (Walker 1996). The incidence of the disease is on the decline, but it is still the most common of the inflammatory arthritides (Helliwell et al 2007). Rheumatoid arthritis has a tendency to begin as a synovitis in the small joints of the hands and feet. The disease may attack any of the pedal joints, but it is generally associated with the metatarsophalangeal joints. Involvement of the midfoot and rearfoot joints also occurs, but whether one joint is more affected than another is uncertain (Wiener-Ogilvie 1999). Radiographs will usually provide good detail at the metatarsophalangeal joints, but imaging the rearfoot will require several views and possibly different modalities (Fig. 22.32).

The radiographic evidence will usually show early joint-space distension, which accompanies the inflammation and hypertrophy of the synovium, and is caused by effusion into the joint. Later the joint space will narrow. Periarticular osteopenia and erosion will usually follow. Eventually, there may be secondary osteoarthritic damage. There may be a much disrupted foot, with subluxations and dislocation of one or more joints. Finally, there may be ankylosis of the joint(s) (Prioli et al 1997).

*The spondyloarthropathies* are a group of seronegative arthritides that share common features:

- peripheral asymmetrical arthritis
- sacroiliitis, evident on radiograph
- seronegative for rheumatoid factor
- no nodule formation
- associated with HLA B27
- genetic transmission.

*Ankylosing spondylitis* is a chronic inflammatory disorder, mainly affecting the axial skeleton; however, involvement of the peripheral joints is not uncommon. It is most common in young males. Enthesopathy may occur at certain sites, particularly in the heel, where the inflammation affects the ligamentous attachments, eventually causing erosion of the adjacent bone (Rai & Struthers 2002). Enthesopathy also affects the spine, where healing often leaves scars and new bone formations, known as syndesmophytes, at the junction of the vertebral bodies. Diagnosis is based primarily on signs and symptoms. Recourse to laboratory tests and radiography is of little value, particularly in the early stages. As the condition progresses, changes may be discernible on radiography (e.g. marginal sclerosis at the sacroiliac joints, erosion and sclerosis of the anterior corners of the vertebrae). There may also be some osteopenia. The use of a CT scan early in the disease may reveal some evidence of osseous changes, while the use of MRI may reveal specific changes such as inflammation in the bone marrow adjacent to the joints (McGonagle et al 2002).

*Reiter's disease* is mainly seen in young males. It is normally associated with a gastrointestinal or sexually transmitted organism, and manifests as a classic syndromic triad of non-specific urethritis, reactive arthritis and conjunctivitis. Foot and lower limb involvement is high, with possible synovitis of the small foot joints, enthesopathy at the attachment of the plantar fascia and the Achilles tendon, swollen 'sausage' toes (dactylitis) and ketatoderma blennorrhagia affecting the plantar skin (Keat 1996). It would be necessary to differentially diagnose for gout, or a septic arthritis. Laboratory tests will be necessary, but imaging might only be of value in a chronic inflammatory case, where it is possible to find periarticular osteopenia, bone erosion at the calcaneus, and periostitis in the metatarsals and phalanges. There may also be a marked sacroiliitis identical to that seen in ankylosing spondylitis.

*Psoriatic arthritis* is commonly associated with psoriasis, but only approximately 6%–8% of psoriasis sufferers actually develop the arthritic condition. Five clinical patterns are observed (Nuki et al 1999):

- asymmetrical oligoarthritis (35%)
- symmetrical seronegative arthritis (30%)
- sacroiliitis/spondylitis (15%)
- distal interphalangeal joint arthritis (15%)
- arthritis mutilans (5%).

Radiological evidence consists of small-joint involvement in the hands and feet. The interphalangeal joints may exhibit marginal erosion of the bone, with adjacent areas producing a proliferation of new bone, often referred to as 'whiskering' (Wright & Helliwell 1996). Osteolysis may occur in the metatarsals and phalanges, resulting in their compaction, sometimes referred to as 'mushrooming' or 'telescoping' of the digits. In the rare, but severe, arthritis mutilans, there may be a 'pencil in cup' deformity of the metatarsal. Periostitis and erosion of the terminal phalanges is also common. As in ankylosing spondylitis and Reiter's disease, involvement of the entheses is widespread, with the calcaneus often involved. Differential diagnosis should be established between this and rheumatoid arthritis, or the spondyloarthropathies.

*Systemic lupus erythematosis* is a connective-tissue disorder with a wide range of joint and other tissue manifestations. It is an autoimmune disease and predominates in females. There will usually be a symmetrical involvement of the wrists, knees, metacarpophalangeal and metatarsophalangeal joints, and the proximal interphalangeal joints in the hand and foot. The arthritis is migratory and is not usually as destructive as rheumatoid arthritis (Fig. 22.44). In chronic cases there may be some osteopenia and erosion. Avascular necrosis of the hip or knee is a possibility.

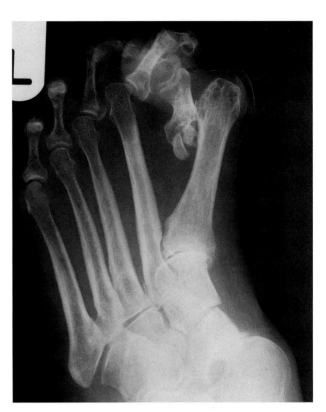

**Figure 22.44** Radiograph of aggressive systemic lupus erythematosus affecting the foot joints.

*Systemic sclerosis (scleroderma)* is a complex spectrum of disorders with wide-ranging involvement of the skin, skeleton and major organs. There may be an arthralgia, but there is little erosion in most cases. The most interesting of the radiological manifestations is subcutaneous calcification (Fig. 22.33) and possible resorption of the terminal phalangeal tufts (Black 2002).

Of the *crystal deposition* diseases, *gout* is the most frequently encountered by podiatrists. Gout actually represents a group of disorders characterised by a hyperuricaemia leading to the deposition of crystals of monosodium urate monohydrate in the tissues, which in turn leads to an inflammatory reaction. It may attack any joint, but in over 70% of cases it occurs in the first metatarsophalangeal joint. The wrist, knee, ankle and hand may also be affected. Gout is sometimes confused with the less common calcium pyrophosphate dihydrate arthropathy (pseudogout), but analysis of the synovial fluid under a polarising light microscope will allow for identification of the crystals formed in these diseases. Radiographic evaluation will not show changes in the early stages of the disease (Nuki 1998). However, if chronic and poorly managed, 'punched-out' erosions may develop at the joint margins. Some subchondral sclerosis may be evident, and secondary osteoarthritis may develop with some osteophytosis. Tophaceous deposits in the soft tissue may show on the radiograph.

## FRACTURES

The following is a general overview of the common fractures and their radiographic appearance. Further detail should be sought in a traumatology or orthopaedic text.

*A fracture is dissolution in the continuity of a bone which may be complete or incomplete.*

(Gambol & Yale 1975, p.138)

The plain radiograph will usually be excellent for the identification of most fractures, providing that one or more views are taken in different projections to confirm the diagnosis. However, it is occasionally necessary to use a different imaging modality to confirm the diagnosis where there is difficulty in identifying a suspected fracture. NM scintigrams will often show a 'hot spot' where there may be a stress fracture. CT scans can also disclose difficult-to-see fractures. Any bone in the foot is liable to fracture, and this may include an associated subluxation or dislocation of one or more associated joints (Christman 2003).

Not only are there different types of fracture, but the actual fracture line may run in a transverse, oblique or spiral manner. In a *simple* fracture there are only two segments of bone, but sometimes there will be multiple fracturing of the bone with a number of separate bone segments. This is known as a *comminuted* fracture and is sometimes seen in the calcaneus following a fall onto the heel from a height. *Impacted* fractures occur when one bone is jammed with great force against another. If the skin is penetrated and the bone exposed through the wound, the term *open* or *compound* fracture is used. If the deeper structures, together with blood vessels and nerves are involved, the fracture may be classified as *complicated*.

*Avulsion* fractures occur when there is a forceful tearing of soft-tissue structures, such as muscles, ligament, tendon, or even joint capsule, taking a portion of bone with them. These are common at the base of the fifth metatarsal (Fig. 22.45) (Ekrol & Court-Brown 2004).

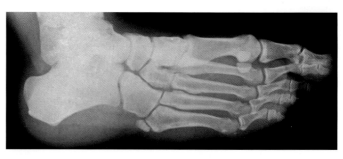

**Figure 22.45** Radiograph of an avulsion fracture of the base of the fifth metatarsal.

*Stress*, or 'overuse', fractures occur as a result of multiple or repetitive damage, as opposed to a single event. They are common in the calcaneus, metatarsals and the tibia. They are often associated with those individuals who increase the demands on their feet through unaccustomed activity levels (e.g. the march fracture associated with new recruits to the armed services).

*Pathologic* fractures occur where there is an underlying pathology (e.g. a neoplasm) or some systemic illness that has predisposed to osteoporosis.

*Greenstick* fractures are generally seen in children and are represented by an incomplete breakage through the bone. The fracture line traverses the cortex incompletely, so that the bone bends rather than snaps.

## REFERENCES

Alazraki N 1995 Radionuclide techniques. In: Resnick D (ed.) Diagnosis of bone and joint disorders. Saunders, Philadelphia, PA.

Anderson M, Kakarlapudi TK 2000 Metastatic lesion in the hallux. The Foot 10(1): 42–43.

Asirvatham R, Rooney RJ, Antonius JI 1992 Giant cell tumour of the metatarsal: a case report & review of the literature. The Foot 2(1):49–53.

Astor AS, Forster MC, Rajan RA, et al 2004 Radiographic pre-operative assessment in hallux valgus: is it reliable? The Foot 14(3):129–132.

Bassen H, Schaefer DJ, Zaremba L, et al 2005 IEEE Committee on Man & Radiation (COMAR): Technical information statement: exposure of medical personnel to electromagnetic fields from open MRI systems. Health Physics 89(6):684–689.

Berquist TH 2000 Radiology of the foot and ankle, 2nd edn. Lippincot Williams & Wilkins, Philadelphia, PA.

Berrington De Gonzalez A, Darby S 2004 The risk of cancers from diagnostic x-ray: estimates from the UK and 14 other countries. Lancet 363:345–351.

Betts RP, Bygrave CJ, Jones S, et al 2003 Ultrasonic diagnosis of Morton's neuroma: a guide to problems, pointers, pitfalls and prognosis. The Foot 13(2):92–99.

Black C 2002 Systemic sclerosis. In: Collected Reports On The Rheumatic Diseases. The Arthritis Research Campaign, Chesterfield.

Blakemore LC, Cooperman DP, Thompson GH 2000 The rigid flatfoot: tarsal coalitions. Clinics in Podiatric Medicine and Surgery 17(3):531–550.

Böttcher J, Pheil A, Mentzel HJ, et al 2006 Peripheral bone status in RA evaluated by digital XR and compared with multi-site quantitative ultrasound (QUS). Calcification Tissue International 78:25–34.

Brown M, Holder LE 1996 Miscellaneous orthopaedic applications of radionuclide bone imaging. In: Collier BD, Fogelman I, Rosenthal L (eds) Skeletal nuclear medicine. Mosby Year Book, St Louis, MI.

Bullough P 1997 Orthopaedic pathology, 2nd edn. Times Mirror International, London.

Cassar-Pullicino VN 2002 The place of imaging in rheumatological disorders. In: Collected reports on the rheumatic diseases. The Arthritis Research Campaign, Chesterfield.

Chakrabarti I, Greiss ME, Jennings P 1995 Osteoid osteoma of the os calcis: computed tomography-guided diagnosis and excision. The Foot 5(3):153–154.

Chambers J 1995 Clinical echocardiography. BMJ, London.

Cheung Y, Hochman M, Brophy DP 2002 Radiographic changes in the diabetic foot.

In: Veves A, Guirini JM, LoGerfo FW (eds) The diabetic foot: medical and surgical management. Humana Press, Totowa, NJ.

Christman RA 1990 The radiographic presentation of osteomyelitis in the foot. In: Clinics in Podiatric Medicine and Surgery 7(3):443–446.

Christman RA 1991 A systematic approach for radiographically evaluating joint disease in the foot. Journal of the American Podiatric Medical Association 81(4):174.

Christman RA (ed.) 2003 Foot & ankle radiology. Churchill Livingstone, St Louis, MI.

Cohen RE, Christman RA 2003 Osteonecrosis and osteochondritis. In: Christman RA (ed.) Foot and ankle radiology. Churchill Livingstone, St Louis, MI.

Collier BD, Fogelman I, Rosenthal L (eds) 1996 Skeletal nuclear medicine. Mosby Year Book, St Louis, MI.

Compston JE, Cooper C, Kanis JA 1995 Bone densitometry in clinical practice. BMJ 310:1510–1517.

Cryer JR, Otter SJ, Bowen CJ 2007 Use of quantitative ultrasound scans of the calcaneus to diagnose osteoporosis in patients with rheumatoid arthritis. Journal of the American Podiatric Medical Association 97(2).

Davies MB 2004 The os trigonum syndrome. The Foot 14(3):119–123.

Dattner RH 1999 Clinical radiology: the essentials, 2nd edn. Williams & Wilkins, Baltimore, OH.

Ekrol I, Court-Brown CM 2004 Fractures at the base of the 5th metatarsal. The Foot 14(2):96–98.

El Rayes MA, El Kordy S 2003 Osteoid osteoma of the talus. The Foot 13(3):166–168.

Fleming DJ, Murphy MD, McCarthy K 2005 Imaging of the foot and ankle: summary and update. Current Opinion in Orthopedics 16(2):54–59.

Freschi S, Dodson NB 2007 Osteoid osteoma: an uncommon cause of foot pain. Journal of the American Podiatric Medicine Association 97:5.

Gambol FO, Yale I 1975 Clinical foot roentgenology, 2nd edn. Krieger, New York.

George VA, Khan AM, Hutchinson HCE, Maxwell HA 2005 Morton's neuroma: the role of MR scanning in diagnostic assistance. The Foot 15:14–16.

Hachiya H 2006 The safety of ultrasonic diagnosis. The Journal of Medical Ultrasonics 33:195.

Harrelson JM 1991 Tumours of the foot. In: Jahss MH (ed.) Disorders of the foot and ankle: medical and surgical management, 2nd edn. WB Saunders, Philadelphia, PA.

Helm RH, Newman RJ 1991 Primary bone tumours of the foot: experience of the Leeds Bone Tumour Registry. The Foot 1(3):135–138.

Heron C 1993 Magnetic resonance imaging of the foot and ankle. The Foot 3:1–10.

Helliwell P, Woodburn J, Redmond A, et al 2007 The foot and ankle in rheumatoid arthritis. Churchill Livingstone, Edinburgh.

Huvos A 1991 Bone tumours: diagnosis, treatment and prognosis. WB Saunders, Philadelphia, PA.

Journal of the European Communities 1997 Directive 97/43 Euratom.

Kaschak TJ, Laine W 1988 Surgical radiology. Clinics in Podiatric Medicine and Surgery 5(4):798–804.

Katz JN, Gomoll A 2007 Advances in arthroscopic surgery: indications and outcomes. Current Opinion in Rheumatology 19(2):106–110.

Keat A 1996 Reiter's syndrome and reactive arthritis. In: Collected reports on the rheumatic diseases. Arthritis Research Campaign, Chesterfield.

Keats TE 1988 Normal roentgen variants of the foot and ankle that may stimulate disease. Clinics in Podiatric Medicine and Surgery 5(4):777–795.

Körner M, Christof H, Weber MD, et al 2007 Advances in digital radiography: physical principles & system overview. Radiographics 27:675–686.

Knobler RL 2000 Reflex sympathetic dystrophy: complex regional pain syndrome, type 1. In: Mandel S, Willis J (eds) Handbook of lower extremity neurology. Churchill Livingstone, Philadelphia, PA.

Lawson JP 1985 Symptomatic radiographic variants in extremities. Radiography 157:625–631.

Lee DK 2008 Prostate cancer metastases to the leg and foot. Journal of the American Podiatric Medicine Association 98(3):242–245.

Loredo D, Metter D 1997 Imaging the diabetic foot. Clinics in Podiatric Medicine and Surgery 14(2):235–264.

Martins B 2003 Radiation physics, biology and safety. In: Christman RA (ed.) Foot and ankle radiology. Churchill Livingstone, St Louis, MI.

Mayer DP, Kabbani YM 2003 MRI/cross sectional imaging. In: Christman RA (ed.) Foot and ankle radiology. Churchill Livingstone, St Louis, MI.

McGonagle D, Conaghan PG, Emery P 2002 Magnetic resonance imaging in rheumatology. In: Collected Reports On The Rheumatic Diseases. Arthritis Research Campaign, Chesterfield.

Mendicino SS, Rockett MS 1997 Imaging of the foot and ankle. Clinics in Podiatric Medicine and Surgery 14(2):303–311.

Mohammadian PM, Torabinezhad S, Bagheri MH, Omidvari SH, Mosalae A, Ahmadlou N 2004 Primary Sarcoma of the Foot. The Foot 14(3):159–163. Elsevier.

Mosel LD, Kat E, Voyvodic F 2004 Imaging of the symptomatic type 2 accessory navicular bone. Australian Radiology 48(2):267–271.

Newman LG 1995 Imaging techniques in the diabetic foot. Clinics in Podiatric Medicine and Surgery 12(4):75–86.

Nuki G 1998 Gout. Medicine 26:54–59.

Nuki G, Ralston SH, Luqmani R 1999 Diseases of the connective tissues, joints and bones. In: Haslett C, Chilvers ER, Hunter JAA, Boon NA (eds) Davidson's principles and practice of medicine, 18th edn. Churchill Livingstone, Edinburgh.

Oestreich AE 1992 Radiology. In: Drennan JL (ed.) The child's foot. Raven, New York.

Oloff Solomon J 1987 Computerised Radiographic Evaluation of the Pediatric Patient. In: Clinics in Podiatric Medicine and Surgery. Vol 4. Iss 1. WB Saunders, Philadelphia, pp 21–36.

Oloff-Solomon J, Solomon MA 1988 Computerised tomographic scanning of the foot and ankle. Clinics in Podiatric Medicine and Surgery 5(4):931–944.

Oloff J, Moore SG 1992 Diagnostic imaging of the paediatric patient. In: DeValentine SJ (ed.) Foot and ankle disorders in children. Churchill Livingstone, New York.

Picno E 2004 Sustainability of medical imaging. BMJ 328:578–580.

Prioli F, Bacaini L, Cammisa M 1997 Changes in the feet of patients with early rheumatoid arthritis. Journal of Rheumatology 24:2113–2118.

Rai A, Struthers GR 2002 Ankylosing spondylitis. In: Collected reports on the rheumatic diseases. Arthritis Research Campaign, Chesterfield.

Raisz LG 2005 Clinical practice screening for osteoporosis. New England Journal of Medicine 353(3):164–171.

Ralston SH 1997 Science, medicine and the future: osteoporosis. BMJ 315:469–472.

Resnick D 1996 Bone and joint imaging, 2nd edn. WB Saunders, Philadelphia, PA.

Romanowski CAJ, Barrington NA 1991 The accessory ossicles of the foot. The Foot 2:61–70.

Rowlett R 2004 How many? A dictionary of units of measurement. Available at: http://www.unc.edu/~rowlett/units/dictT.html (accessed 19 September 2009).

Sanders P, Kaval KJ, DiPasquale T, et al 1993 Exposure of the orthopaedic surgeon to radiation. Journal of Bone and Joint Surgery 75A:326–330.

Saltman CL, Braudser EA, Berbaum KS 1994 Reliability of standard foot radiographic measurements. Foot and Ankle International 15:661.

Saraffian SK 1983 Anatomy of the foot and ankle. Lippincot, Philadelphia, PA.

Schauwecker DS 1992 The scintigraphic diagnosis of osteomyelitis. American Journal of Roentgenology 158:9–18.

Shaylor PJ, Abudu A, Grimer RJ, et al 2000 Management and outcome of the surgical treatment of primary malignant tumours of the foot. The Foot 10(3):157–163.

Shereff MJ, DiGiovanni L, Beggani FJ 1990 A comparison of non-weight bearing and weight bearing radiographs of the foot. Foot and Ankle 10:306.

Shook JE, Osher LS, Christman RA 2003 Bone tumours and tumour like lesions. In: Christman RA (ed.) Foot and Ankle Radiology. Churchill Livingstone, St Louis, MI.

Scottish Intercollegiate Guidelines Network 2003 Management of osteoporosis. Report No. 71. SIGN: Edinburgh.

Sobel M, Pavlov H, Geppert MJ, et al 1994 Painful os peroneum syndrome: a spectrum of conditions responsible for lateral foot pain. Foot and Ankle 15(3):112–124.

Sopov V, Lileson A, Groshar DJ 2000 Bone scintigraphic findings of os trigonum: a prospective study of 100 soldiers on active duty. Foot and Ankle International 21(10):822–824.

Spector TD, Cicuttini F, Baker J, Loughling J, Hart D 1996 Genetic influences on osteoarthritis in women: a twin study. BMJ 312:940–943.

Stibe ECL, Cobb JP 1993 Ewing's sarcoma in the foot. The Foot 3(3):120–122.

Street MW, Johnston KA, DeWitz MA 1980 Radiographic measurements of the normal adult foot. Foot and Ankle International 15:661.

Sutton D 1997 Radiology and imaging for medical students, 7th edn. Churchill Livingstone, Edinburgh.

Tachdijian MO 1990 Tachdjian's Pediatric Orthopedics. 3rd ed. Saunders, Philadelphia.

Traughber PD 1999 Imaging of the foot and ankle. In: Coughlin MJ, Mann RA (eds) Surgery of the foot and ankle, 7th edn. Mosby, St Louis, MI.

Walker J 2008 Osteoporosis: pathogenesis, diagnosis and management. Nursing Standard 22(17):48–56.

Walker DJ 1996 Rheumatoid arthritis. In: Collected reports on the rheumatic diseases. Arthritis Research Campaign, Chesterfield.

Weissman S 1988 Standard radiographic techniques for the foot and ankle. Clinics in Podiatric Medicine and Surgery 5(4):767–775.

Wiener-Ogilvie S 1999 The foot in rheumatoid arthritis. The Foot 9:169–174.

Williams M 2003 Bone infection. In: Christman RA (ed.) Foot and ankle radiology. Churchill Livingstone, St Louis, MI.

Wright V, Helliwell PS 1996 Psoriatic arthritis. In: Collected reports on the rheumatic diseases. Arthritis Research Campaign, Chesterfield.

Yeager KK, Mitchell M, Sartoris DJ, Resnick D 1988 Diagnostic imaging of bone tumours of the foot. Clinics in Podiatric Medicine and Surgery 5(4):859–876.

Yester M, White SL 2006 Advances in medical physics. Medical Physics Publishing, Wisconsin.

# Chapter 23

# Podiatric surgery

*Robert James Hardie and Pamela M Sabine*

## KEYWORDS

Adducto varus deformity
Arthrodesis
Basal procedures
Consent
Digital amputation
Distal metaphyseal procedures
Excisional arthroplasty
Extensor substitution
Flexor stabilisation
Flexor substitution
Hallux rigidus
Hallux valgus
Lesser metatarsal osteotomies
Mallet toe
Midshaft procedures
Morton's neuroma
Patient selection for surgery
Postoperative complications
Postoperative dressings
Rearfoot surgery
Sesamoid problems
Simple bunionectomy

Skin plasties
Suture materials
Suture techniques
Tissue handling

# INTRODUCTION

This chapter presents an overview of podiatric surgery. There are many facets to the subject and the intention is to cover most of these, providing enough information to enable the practitioner to make informed decisions regarding surgery and communicate these to patients and colleagues alike. Podiatric surgery has undergone considerable development in recent years, with the recognition that podiatric surgeons are fulfilling the role of specialists within the broader field of healthcare.

With the expansion of podiatric surgery has come the increasing responsibility for the welfare of the patients being treated. This responsibility starts from the first contact with the patient and finishes at discharge at the conclusion of a treatment programme or episode. Patient management begins at the point of referral and covers many aspects, and ends at discharge. Skill is required to allow communication with all patients, ensuring that they have the required information. This will enable them to take an active role in determining their regimen of care and to give informed consent to treatment. Therefore, it is important to understand the concepts of what is required to fulfil the role and deal responsibly with each stage.

Responsibility is an issue that can weigh heavily when dealing with the patient presenting with a difficult complication after the surgery. The patient holds the surgeon responsible for the outcome and demands a solution to any complications. Careful management of the patient is required if the patient–practitioner relationship is not to break down. Poor communication and surgical result are perhaps the quickest routes to litigation.

Miller and Boegel (1992) summarise the process of surgical principles, as shown in Table 23.1. These headings indicate the stages required in undertaking surgical practice, and at all stages good communication with the patient and colleagues is a vital aspect of surgical management. Good communication is the only way of making patients understand their problems, their management and how they are involved in the decision-making process. Being responsive to the needs of the patient also means that the surgeon needs to be able to understand what they are trying to communicate, and clarity at all stages will help to avoid any misconceptions. Many patients are better informed than previously because information is now widely available and no longer the sole preserve of medical professionals. Only by adapting practices to fit around the need for good communication at all levels will the professionals be able to deliver the type of service demanded of them.

# PATIENT SELECTION FOR SURGERY

The basis of patient selection is deciding when to operate and when not by balancing risks against benefits. It is pointless undertaking complex multiple procedures on a patient who is unlikely to reap the benefits due to extreme age or infirmity or because they are wheelchair-bound. Likewise, to deprive a healthy 80-year-old a simple procedure because of age is equally wrong. It is essential to make an assessment of what the likely outcome might be and how the risks of the procedure are likely to affect the patient should they occur.

**Table 23.1** Summary of the process of surgical principles

| | |
|---|---|
| Planning | Looking at the whole patient and setting achievable goals |
| Conceptualisation | Visualisation of the foot and how the surgery will alter this |
| Antisepsis | Reducing the risks of infection with attention to preparation of the surgical site and maintaining the environment |
| Wound healing | Creating an appropriate environment for healing using an understanding of how structures heal and how the surgeon can facilitate this |
| Surgical approach | Planning the incision to allow for adequate exposure while allowing for maximal return to function postoperatively |
| Anatomical dissection | Using knowledge of the anatomy to allow for minimisation of trauma to the foot while allowing reconstruction of the anatomy with closure |
| Atraumatic technique | Gentle handling of tissues to minimise cell death |
| Haemostasis | Control of bleeding using appropriate techniques |
| Instrumentation | Using appropriate instruments in the correct manner to achieve surgical goals with the minimum of tissue trauma |
| Wound protection | Keeping cellular damage to a minimum by lavage to remove injured cells and maintain wound hydration |
| Drainage | Allowing for removal of fluids from the wound using appropriate techniques |
| Implants | Understanding the effect of implanted materials in the body and the associated risks of infection |
| Fixation | Understanding the techniques of rigid internal fixation to achieve immobilisation |
| Intraoperative analysis | Continually assessing the surgical process and making adjustments as required based on the progress of the procedure. Being aware of how the procedure is progressing in relation to the preoperative plan and how this might need to be modified in the light of what presents |
| Dressing/ bandages | Protection and immobilisation of the foot |
| Immobilisation | Allowing for protection of the foot to facilitate optimal healing |
| Postoperative management | Facilitating healing and rehabilitation |

The decision-making process is multifactorial and needs to be based on the patient's physiological, medical, psychological and podiatric status, as well as their personal circumstances.

Physiological age is an important factor in patient selection. Often a fit 70 year old may make a more suitable surgical candidate than a 50 year old with multisystem pathologies, because the 70 year old may well be physiologically 'younger' than the 50 year old. However, the notion of physiological age is a difficult one to quantify, and the surgeon needs to make an estimate.

A patient's medical status needs to be considered carefully and this becomes increasingly difficult if there are several problems. A single pathology such as diabetes is something that can be assessed and quantified as a risk. However, if that diabetic also has hypertension and a history of renal problems the risk factors begin to accumulate. Where patients have multiple pathologies affecting different body systems the risk is much more difficult to quantify. Specialist opinion should be sought to clarify the decision-making process where this is complex or if there is any uncertainty.

Psychological assessment is a difficult area, and most practitioners rely on making an assessment based on their interaction with the patient during the consultation. Patients who present with a psychological history may be open and able to discuss and rationalise it. Very young and very old patients may show more overt signs of their psychological status. However, some patients appear calm and measured at consultation but develop more overt signs of psychological abnormalities when under the stress of the surgery and during the subsequent stages in follow-up treatments. These patients pose a potential management problem and may cause problems in the follow-up clinics in that they need more time and input during recovery and rehabilitation.

Podiatric status is more straightforward. This being the practitioner's main area of expertise it should be possible to assess the risks of a particular procedure and the incidence of complications associated with it.

Personal circumstances are important. The patient's expectations as to how they will cope with the enforced rest after surgery and how quickly they will be able to return to work and other activities need to be addressed. Patients who live alone without any support from family or friends are not good candidates for day surgery. There is a strong case for these patients to be managed as inpatients or in some sort of intermediate care facility. Self-employed manual workers often pose difficulties when they are under pressure to return to work as quickly as possible. Incorporating the requirement to be off work for a certain period into the consent form is a good way to protect the practitioner against a claim for damages related to this. People's home environment, job, dependants and hobbies need to be included in assessing the patient's suitability for the proposed surgery.

All these factors must be carefully considered, and the patient informed as to the surgeon's opinion in language that they understand. With elective surgery the final decision to proceed rests with the patient. The decision not to operate lies with the surgeon.

## PATIENT CONSENT

Patient consent (see also Chs 16 and 28) is an important part of the surgical management of any patient. The need to communicate what a procedure will entail and its possible outcomes is paramount in keeping the process running smoothly without 'hidden surprises'. There is always debate as to how much a patient needs to know regarding complications, and how common a complication needs to be before it becomes mandatory for patients to know (for the purposes of informed consent) is not clear. The NHS consent forms use the phrase 'commonly occurring or serious' when referring to complications. The gravity of a particular complication is another consideration as to how important it is for a patient to be appropriately advised. A complication with only a minor risk, such as a stitch abscess, has much less impact than, for example, chronic regional pain syndrome

(CRPS), which is likely to have a much more lasting and serious impact on the patient's life.

The situation with regard to consent is not universal, and in different countries the law differs. The interpretation of 'informed consent' in the USA is quite different, and complications of a much lower risk are included in the group 'need to know' prior to surgery.

As a standard for podiatric surgery it would be best to advise patients regarding the risks of infection, swelling, thrombosis, loss of function/stiffness, recurrence of deformity (where appropriate), delayed healing, non-union and the potential to be worse off after surgery. These cover most eventualities, but risks specific to the procedure need also to be communicated to the patient. There are no set guidelines for this and the practitioner needs to judge how much to tell the patient and how far to go in advising of risks prior to surgery (Department of Health 2001).

The consent process also needs to prepare the patient for what they should expect from their surgical episode, beginning with their arrival at the hospital/surgery centre, to the theatre and home again. They need to have a good idea of what the normal postoperative course is for their procedure and how that might be modified according to their progress. If they are going to need to keep the foot non-weight bearing they need to be prepared and have crutch-walking training and practise prior to the day of surgery. If the surgical episode unfolds exactly as they were told, then they feel reassured.

Consent needs to be documented, and the final consent form signed by the surgeon and the patient. Consent should be supplemented with written information for the patient to take away so that they can read it thoroughly. The consent form should record what written information has been supplied to the patient for future reference in any dispute.

Consent by minors (patients under 16 years of age) must be made in conjunction with their parents or guardians. Minors can give consent in special circumstances (usually in emergency situations) but as podiatric surgery is elective surgery this question will not arise (see also Ch. 28). The use of written information is of considerable help in the process of gaining informed consent (see Ch. 27). It allows a patient, and their relatives, to digest information at leisure, away from the stresses of the hospital or clinic visit. Information giving detail of qualifications held, scope of practice, range of experience and status is also beneficial, plus it lets the patient know exactly who you are and your practice. It also removes the likelihood of a claim for misleading the patient if litigation should arise where the patient says that they believed you were an orthopaedic surgeon or other registered medical practitioner rather than a podiatrist.

In the UK, the Department of Health produces guides to advise practitioners with regard to consent 'best practice'. These are vital documents to help you shape your practice and can be ordered from the Department of Health or downloaded from their website.

## DIGITAL DEFORMITIES

Toe deformities may occur due to several factors. Some people are born with deformed toes, the overlapping fifth toe being one of the commoner congenital types of deformity. The majority of toe deformities are acquired and may be secondary to other forefoot problems such as hallux valgus, or secondary to injuries such as plantar plate rupture (Yao et al 1996), often leading to a hammered second toe. Generalised toe deformities, affecting all or most of the lesser toes, are more likely to be related to biomechanical dysfunction. Flexor stabilisation, flexor substitution and extensor substitution are possible causes in these instances (McGlamry 1992).

## Flexor stabilisation

Flexor stabilisation is where the flexor muscles are called in to play to attempt to stabilise an overpronated or unstable/hypermobile foot during the stance phase of gait. The phasing of the muscle contraction is extended so that the extensor digitorum longus (EDL) acts prior to the lumbricals. This results in flexion of the toes without the stabilising effect of the lumbricals at the proximal interphalangeal joint (PIP). The normal sequencing of lumbricals acting prior to the EDL is reversed. The EDL deforms the toes before the lumbricals can act, so that they become ineffective at the PIP joints.

## Flexor substitution

Flexor substitution occurs where the flexor digitorum longus is functioning to assist the plantar flexors of the foot. This occurs in the stance phase of gait at heel-lift. If the gastrocnemius–soleus group of muscles is weak and has difficulty achieving heel-lift, then the long flexors may be used to supplement this movement. However, their main function is plantar flexion of the toes and they are unable to exert their influence at the ankle until the toes are maximally plantar flexed. Any further pull can then plantar flex the foot at the ankle. Therefore, flexor substitution can be observed at heel-lift when there is clawing of the toes on heel-lift.

## Extensor substitution

Extensor substitution exhibits itself in the swing phase of gait. This occurs where the foot is struggling to dorsiflex sufficiently to clear the ground during the swing phase. The dorsiflexors are not strong enough to achieve this on their own, or the movement is anatomically blocked, and so the extensor digitorum longus is used to add power to dorsiflexion. Again, the effect around the ankle is only achievable when the toes are maximally dorsiflexed. This can be seen as excessive dorsiflexion of the toes during the swing phase of gait. This is seen in the highly arched cavoid-type foot, and is associated with a foot with an equinus or pseudoequinus deformity. The toes may deform to the degree that they may not make ground contact at all during gait (see Ch. 4).

## Adducto varus deformity

The adducto varus, or 'curly' toe, is usually seen in the fifth toe and to a lesser degree the fourth and then the third toes. The theory for this is that the pull of the flexor digitorum longus (FDL) is from the medial malleolus rather than straight in line with the toe. While the pull of the flexor accessorius (FA)/quadratus plantae (QP) is supposed to straighten the pull of the FDL, it is ineffective on occasion. This may be due to phasing, where the FDL is acting earlier and so the stabilising effect of the FA/QP is lost. In the pronated foot the effect of the FA/QP is reduced and the angle of pull of the FDL is greater as the medial malleolus is more medially displaced.

## Mallet toe

Mallet toe deformity is where the flexion deformity occurs at the distal interphalangeal joint. This occurs in a long toe or in toes where flexibility at the PIP joint is reduced, such as following PIP joint arthrodesis. The mallet toe deformity is commonly seen in the second toe secondary to hallux dysfunction. Following surgery leading to poor hallux function, such as a Keller arthroplasty or hallux amputation, the second toe is left longer and takes increased stresses.

## Surgical treatment

Surgical treatment is commonly an excisional arthroplasty or a digital arthrodesis. These are often supplemented with skin plasties and release of soft-tissue structures. A stepwise approach is advocated by McGlamry (1992) where a set sequence of release is made until the toe is in a good position.

## Excisional arthroplasty

The approach for this can be dorsal or from either side of the toe. Normally, a dorsal incision, excising out a skin lesion, gives good exposure. A longitudinal or transverse lenticular incision can be used. The removal of the excess skin helps in terms of tightening up the skin following bony resection assisting in correction of the deformity. The extensor tendon can be transected to open the joint or undermined and reflected. The head of the proximal or intermediate phalanx is then excised, depending on where the apex of the deformity is. The amount of bone removed needs to be sufficient to allow correction of the toe freely. If there is any tightness on correcting the toe position then further resection is probably required. With a more severe distal interphalangeal joint (DIP) joint deformity excision of the whole intermediate phalanx may be required to achieve sufficient correction.

Following excision of the bony fragment, the tendon may or may not need to be repaired. Contracture at the metatarsophalangeal joint (MTPJ) also needs to be assessed to determine whether any release of soft tissue is required. The Kelikian push-up test (pushing up under the metatarsal to simulate weight bearing) will allow some degree of assessment of how the toe will appear in stance. If the toe is still sitting up then the stepwise release is:

1. extensor hood resection
2. MTPJ capsulotomy
3. plantar capsular release
4. plantar skin 'clip' – skin plasty.

To enable a full release the incision may need to be extended to the MTPJ to gain sufficient exposure. Curving the incision as it crosses the MTPJ will help to reduce the risk of scar contracture redeforming the toe postoperatively.

Double arthroplasties can be performed where the deformity in the toe is affecting the DIP and PIP joint equally.

## Arthrodesis

This is usually performed at the PIP joint and not at the DIP joint. A DIP joint arthrodesis is liable to leave an unyieldingly straight toe that is likely to be a problem with closed-in-toe shoes. The approach to an arthrodesis is similar to that of the excisional arthroplasty, and a longitudinal or transverse incision can be used. The extensor tendon is transected and reflected to open the joint. The joint surfaces are resected and then can be apposed and fixated. The traditional method of fixing the arthrodesis is to drive the K-wire from the base of the intermediate phalanx out of the end of the toe, holding the DIP joint in a rectus position. The wire is then driven back across the PIP, down the proximal phalanx and into the metatarsal head. The remaining wire is cut to length and bent at the tip of the toe to prevent accidental further knocking in of the pin during the postoperative phase.

An alternative to this is the peg-in-the hole arthrodesis. A peg is fashioned from the head of the proximal phalanx and driven into a hole in the intermediate phalanx, following resection of the joint surfaces. This gives a larger surface area for bone healing and more intrinsic stability. This is usually backed up with a K-wire to increase stability. However, fracture of the peg is a common intraoperative complication. Due to the tubular nature of the phalanges the peg has to be fashioned from cortex, and so is slightly offset from the intermediate phalanx; however, the reduced risk of non-union makes this a good procedure. If the peg does fracture then the arthrodesis can still be fixed as in the traditional arthrodesis.

## Digital amputation

This is a useful procedure in the right circumstances. The crossover toe in the elderly patient with a severe but asymptomatic hallux valgus deformity is a common problem. Correction of the hallux valgus with second-toe realignment is an ideal, but is rarely justified in a patient who may take a prolonged time to recover from such a procedure. There is also difficulty in realigning a subluxed or dislocated second toe, so that corrective surgery may well be less than satisfactory. In this situation, digital amputation provides a quick and straightforward procedure with minimum recovery time. For this type of patient, wearing a shoe is usually the main reason for seeking advice when the overlapping toe protrudes and becomes painful.

The toe with chronic ulceration and associated osteomyelitis may be best amputated. A toe with a large neoplasm is also often best amputated, as skin coverage is likely to be difficult following its excision.

Caution should be exercised when considering removal of a chronically painful digit when there is little to explain the pain. Chronic regional pain syndrome may manifest in a single digit and an amputation is liable not to cure the pain but to shift it more proximally, as well as potentially exacerbating the pain.

## HALLUX VALGUS

Hallux valgus is one of the commonest problems that the podiatric surgeon meets on a regular basis. While its aetiology remains obscure, advances in surgical technique have offered patients a high level of satisfaction with surgery. However, there is still a failure rate of surgery leading to a dissatisfaction rate of about 5–10%, possibly due to the many forces operating around the first metatarsophalangeal joint. Continued research and audit will help to reduce the failure rate further.

## Procedures

### Simple bunionectomy

This is indicated where a large medial eminence is causing the patient's symptoms. It does not address the metatarsus primus varus or the position on the hallux. However, with careful patient selection it can relieve 'bump pain' without the need for osteotomies and the subsequent bone healing. There are, however, few patients where this is adequate as the sole procedure.

### Distal metaphyseal procedures

The distal metaphyseal procedures (DMOs) are perhaps the most widely used procedures for hallux valgus correction, and there are many variations (Figs 23.1 to 23.4). Straight osteotomies, such as the Wilson procedure, and angled osteotomies, such as the Austin and curved osteotomies, all have their advocates. The angled osteotomies offer more stability than the straight osteotomy. Fixation techniques also vary, and range from multiple screw fixation to K-wires. Generally, distal procedures offer a relatively rapid rate of recovery and earlier weight bearing postoperatively than do more proximal procedures, but this is also dependent on the fixation methods and postoperative

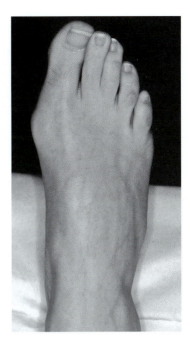

Figure 23.1 Preoperative photograph of a patient who will undergo a distal metaphyseal/Akin procedure.

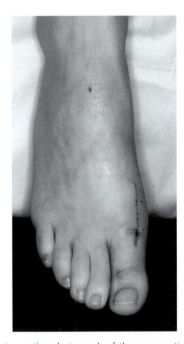

Figure 23.2 Postoperative photograph of the same patient as in Fig. 23.1.

regimen. One of the main criticisms of DMOs is the incidence of avascular necrosis. Reports vary as to its incidence, ranging from 50% to less than 1% (Wallace et al 1994, Wilkinson et al 1992). Much depends on how it is detected and, in the authors' experience, the incidence of symptomatic avascular necrosis is very low.

### Midshaft procedures

These are a good compromise between basal and distal procedures as they are capable of better degrees of correction than distal procedures

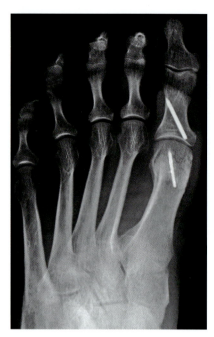

**Figure 23.3** Postoperative radiograph of a patient who has undergone a distal metaphyseal/Akin procedure.

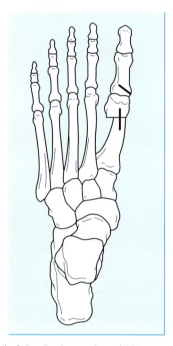

**Figure 23.4** Detail of the distal metaphyseal/Akin procedure.

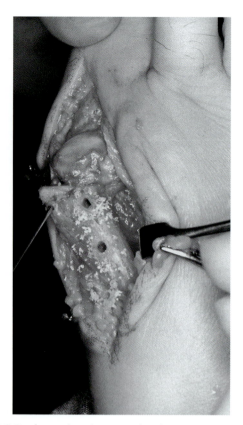

**Figure 23.5** Scarf procedure: intraoperative view.

but without the need to keep patients non-weight bearing for as long as with basal procedures. The most popular mid-shaft procedure is the Scarf osteotomy (Fig. 23.5), which gives a stable osteotomy when adequately fixed and will provide early return to weight-bearing activities, similar to the distal procedures. It is a versatile procedure that enables good control of the metatarsal head position. By judicious angulation of the cuts, the metatarsal can be lengthened or shortened, plantar flexed, dorsiflexed, as well as achieving good correction of moderate to severe intermetatarsal angles. The use of two screws giving solid fixation allows patients to begin limited weight bearing

2 weeks following surgery. The Scarf procedure (Figs 23.5 to 23.7) comprises a long Z-shaped cut (Fig. 23.6). The medial eminence is resected first by cutting the metatarsal head. Using an axis guide wire helps to decide on the degree of plantar displacement required, prior to making the bone cuts. Angling the axis guide wire towards the plantar aspect of the second metatarsal head gives a good amount of plantar displacement, with lateral rotation or transposition of the first metatarsal head. The wire should enter the metatarsal head in the dorsal half to one-third. The dorsal cut in the metatarsal head is made vertically, from the axis wire dorsally. The long cut is then made along the metatarsal. This should run from a more dorsal aspect distally to a more plantar aspect proximally, and is usually to about one-third of the metatarsal thickness from the plantar aspect. The plantar arm of the cut is then made by angling the blade forward to make an angled shelf. The direction of cut is varied depending on whether the aim is to displace the distal metatarsal or to rotate it. Transposition dictates that the distal and proximal cuts should be parallel to allow for sliding over of the metatarsal head, and for rotation angling the lateral side of the cut distally allows the metatarsal to pivot and rotate. Once positioned, the osteotomy can be fixed with two screws. The length of the osteotomy lends itself to easy placement of the screws; however, the screws need to catch the plantar shelf of bone adequately, so need to be placed where the two fragments overlap maximally. Once fixed in place, the medial side of the metatarsal can be cut to remove the overhang.

## Basal procedures

For severe hallux valgus deformity the procedure needs to be carried out more proximally along the metatarsal shaft or at the metatarso-cuneiform joint. A closing base wedge osteotomy can be used to close a severe metatarsus primus varus. This can be performed transversely

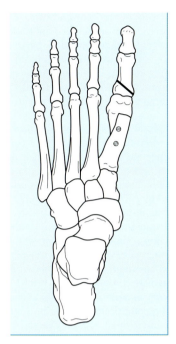

Figure 23.6 Detail of the Scarf procedure, dorsal view.

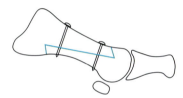

Figure 23.7 Detail of the Scarf procedure, lateral view.

or obliquely. A long oblique osteotomy borders on being a midshaft procedure. However, this is an unstable procedure and the patient needs to be maintained in a non-weight-bearing cast for 6 weeks. Weight bearing too soon on a base wedge osteotomy may lead to a potentially disastrous elevatus deformity of the first ray, which forces the first MTPJ into dorsiflexion and leads to transfer metatarsalgia. The Lapidus procedure or metatarsocuneiform joint fusion is an alternative (Fig. 23.8). This adds a degree of rearfoot stability by stiffening the medial column and thus reducing subtalar joint pronation. The Lapidus procedure (Fig. 23.8) also requires a non-weight-bearing cast for 6 weeks. There is a 10% incidence of non-union reported for the Lapidus procedure. Failure of a metatarsocuneiform fusion to unite is a difficult problem to manage. Re-fusing the joint leads to further shortening. This can be dealt with using a bone graft, but an autogenous graft is required to minimise the risk of further non-union. This means another surgical site to harvest the graft. However, it is a procedure capable of correcting the most severe degrees of hallux valgus. The level of rehabilitation following these procedures exceeds those of the more distal procedures.

## Hallux procedures

It is increasingly common for metatarsal correction to be accompanied by a closing wedge procedure on the proximal phalanx (Akin procedure) (Figs 23.1 and 23.2). The rationale is that the hallux needs to be straight, postoperatively, for the tendons to be exerting force in a straight line. Any residual deformity of the hallux will allow bow

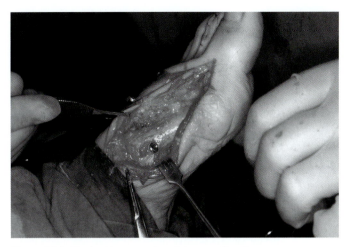

Figure 23.8 The Lapidus procedure: intraoperative view.

stringing of the extensor tendon, thus exerting a deforming force that may contribute to recurrence of the hallux valgus. The term 'cheater Akin' has been used to describe the use of the Akin procedure where there is no obvious deformity within the proximal phalanx preoperatively. However, if the hallux is not straight after the metatarsal position is corrected and the soft tissue releases are performed, then the Akin procedure is the best way to render the hallux straight. A straight toe is something that patients expect after undergoing bunion surgery and is a question commonly asked preoperatively. If a patient has residual deformity they are more likely to be unhappy with the appearance of their foot. This said, cosmesis is not the main priority in hallux valgus surgery; however, in the minds of many patients it is still very important, and if they believe it to be important then it is necessary to address this as well as relieving their pain. The Akin procedure is described in orthopaedic texts as being for the correction of hallux interphalangeus, an integral part of hallux valgus deformity and more often than not seen radiographically (Figs 23.3 and 23.4).

## Evaluation

There are many factors to take into account when selecting a procedure or technique, including: the patient's age and levels of activity; the severity of the deformity; and the degree of degenerative joint changes present, which will need radiographic assessment. The inter-metatarsal angle has been used to decide if a distal, midshaft or basal procedure is indicated. The intermetatarsal angle is perhaps of limited value in isolation as it is only one parameter. The intermetatarsal angle gives the measurement between the first and the second metatarsal angles; however, the width and length of the metatarsals is also relevant as, mathematically, the dimensional model of metatarsus primus varus is a triangle. The first and second metatarsals are two sides, and the third side is the path of displacement of the metatarsal head into a corrected position. If two sides are known and their interposing angle, then the remaining dimensions can be calculated. However, when using the intermetatarsal angle as a reference for procedure selection, there is a tendency to do so without regard to the metatarsal lengths and so the idea is fundamentally flawed.

Another method of assessing the amount of displacement necessary is to measure the width of the first metatarsal and then the amount of displacement required to move it to its corrected position. This gives a displacement ratio expressed as a percentage of the width of the metatarsal. This can then be used to assess whether a procedure is capable of offering sufficient displacement to achieve sufficient correction.

The design of an osteotomy relates to the degree of intrinsic stability. Angled bone cuts giving interlocking fragments are generally more stable than straight osteotomies. The relationship of osteotomies to the supporting surface is also relevant to their intrinsic stability. Transverse-plane-aligned osteotomies are likely to be more stable when the foot is loaded than are sagittal-plane- or frontal-plane-aligned osteotomies.

The manner in which an osteotomy is fixed is also relevant as to how stable it is: the stronger the fixation the greater displacement that can be held adequately.

The degree of intrinsic stability of an osteotomy will dictate how the patient is managed postoperatively. Unstable osteotomies usually need to be immobilised with a cast and the patient kept non-weight bearing for a period of time. Maintaining a foot non-weight bearing for a period postoperatively requires that a patient walks with crutches or uses a wheelchair. To use crutches, the patient must be fit enough and able to take the stresses on their upper limbs. This precludes many elderly patients or those with upper-limb pathologies such as arthritis. Climbing steps or stairs is also a consideration for the patient who needs to be kept non-weight bearing.

All these factors need to be assessed preoperatively; it is not simply a case of looking at the foot or the radiographs as a basis for making a decision. It may be that compromises need to be made in choosing a procedure for hallux valgus. A typical problem is the elderly patient with severe hallux valgus deformity, when a basal procedure is usually out of the question because of the need to maintain the foot non-weight bearing, and a midshaft or distal procedure may not be capable of delivering the degree of correction required. The patient's capacity to sustain bone healing must also be evaluated, along with the risk of delayed or non-union, by assessing the bone density as far as possible preoperatively.

## HALLUX VALGUS SYNDROME

Hallux valgus is described as being a disorder of the first ray, the components of the deformity being a metatarsus primus varus and hallux abductus or valgus. However, the deformity tends to be progressive and the effects of this spread to other structures, and eventually may affect the whole foot.

The association between hallux valgus and flat foot has been documented previously (Kalen & Brecher 1988). Exactly how the mechanisms join the two problems is not clear. It is possible that the hypermobility in the first ray leads to medial instability and subsequent collapse of the foot into a pronated position. Or it could be that the excessive pronation leads to first-ray dysfunction and subsequent hallux valgus. However, these two conditions often lead to a transfer of load to the second metatarsal. The foot pronates and the first ray elevates, leaving the second metatarsal to compensate with the consequent overloading of the second metatarsal head and a build up of hyperkeratosis over the area and capsulitis of the joint. The latter can progress to chronic fatigue in the capsule, leading to weakening of the capsule or plantar plate rupture. This is often a more acute condition and may in turn lead to elevation of the second toe and the formation of a hammer toe deformity. This is further progressed by the hallux moving laterally and exerting pressure against the second toe. The hammer toe adds to the problems that the patient is experiencing. Footwear is already difficult because of the hallux valgus, and now the hammered second toe is adding to the requirement for extra width and depth, which are not readily available in a normal shoe.

At this stage the patient may be walking on the lateral side of the foot to avoid the painful first and second rays. This is turn leads to pain on the lateral side of the foot and often to associated strain within the leg muscles. The midtarsus joint complex may also be starting to show early signs of degeneration due to the changes taking place in the forefoot and the overpronation in the rearfoot.

All these problems add up to a foot that is chronically painful and difficult to accommodate in a shoe. For the podiatric surgeon the question is where to start and how best to manage this type of foot.

Control of the pronation with orthoses may give some relief, although it is rare to find a patient that can accommodate orthoses in their shoes as they are already having great difficulty obtaining a shoe.

Correction of the hallux valgus surgically is often a good starting point, accompanied by correction of the hammer toe and also possibly a metatarsal osteotomy to relieve the transfer metatarsalgia.

There is also a dilemma with hallux valgus syndrome that can pose a difficult surgical choice. Should the patient, who has all the signs of but a pain-free hallux valgus/bunion, be offered the hallux valgus correction or should one simply deal with the painful areas and advise the patient that this may compromise the result? Surgery on a non-symptomatic problem may be seen as controversial, and would be harder to defend if a complication ended in litigation. However, as these problems are intertwined, a good case can be made for hallux valgus correction in conjunction with surgery to address second toe deformity and transfer metatarsalgia.

A recent unpublished departmental audit (M. Graham, 2002) indicated that the results from second-toe corrections, both arthroplasty and arthrodesis, were compromised when there was concurrent hallux valgus that was not addressed.

## CASE STUDY 23.1 REVISION SURGERY IN THE MANAGEMENT OF HALLUX VALGUS

This patient was referred for a second opinion, having previously undergone surgery for a painful bunion deformity and metatarsalgia. She had presented originally complaining of pain in the ball of her foot, at the base of the second toe. She also had a painful bunion that was severely restricting her choice of footwear and had been advised that correcting her bunion and dealing with the metatarsalgia by correcting her hammered second toe would cure the problem. Following the surgery she continued to have a painful bunion as well as the metatarsalgia.

The postoperative radiographs from the first procedure showed that she had undergone a simple bunionectomy, but the amount of bone resected from the medial aspect of the metatarsal was excessive (Fig. 1). She had also had an excisional arthroplasty to the proximal interphalangeal (PIP) joint of the second toe. This had left her with a distorted proximal phalanx and the hallux valgus deformity was still exerting a lateral deformity force onto the second toe. Her metatarsalgia was unchanged.

From the radiograph it was clear that she had significant hallux valgus deformity. She had an intermetatarsal angle of 18°, which would suggest that she might be a good candidate for a Scarf procedure. However, as she had already lost a reasonable section of her metatarsal head it was considered that this would be likely to compromise any further surgery around the metatarsal head. The patient's proximal phalanx showed angulation, with the medial side longer than the lateral side, and the second metatarsal was longer than adjacent metatarsals. However, her metatarsalgia was probably made worse as a consequence of her poor first-ray function.

The patient's second metatarsal head was tender and prominent on the plantar surface, with a degree of hyperkeratosis. Her second

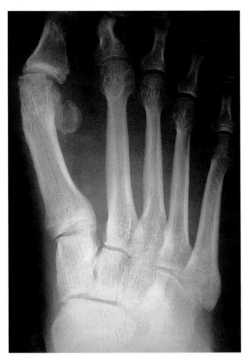

**Figure 1** Radiograph showing the Silver bunionectomy.

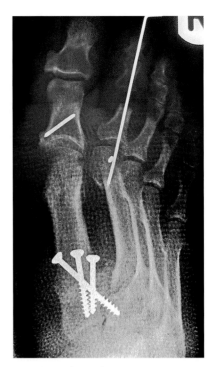

**Figure 2** Postoperative radiograph.

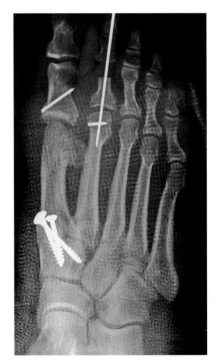

**Figure 3** Postoperative radiograph.

toe was deviated laterally at the level of the PIP joint surface and her hallux valgus was evident and the wounds had healed well. On weight-bearing examination her forefoot splayed and the foot was tending to overpronate.

Initially she was given an insole to redistribute weight to unload the second metatarsal head. An intra-articular steroid injection was also used to settle the inflammation in the second metatarsophalangeal joint. Unfortunately, neither of these actions brought much improvement and, after talking through the options with the patient, she considered that her symptoms were severe enough to go through additional surgery.

A Lapidus procedure for her hallux valgus was decided on, with an Akin procedure for the proximal phalanx. The excisional arthroplasty was re-done, to square off the end of the proximal phalanx, and a stabilising K-wire was used to hold the second toe while it was healing and to attempt to control overshortening. A Weil-type osteotomy was also carried out to address the metatarsalgia.

The surgery was carried out as a day case using a popliteal nerve block with an ankle tourniquet. The postoperative radiographs (Figs 2 and 3) showed the correction at 4 weeks, taken through a fibreglass cast. The views were not directly comparable to the initial radiographs as they were non-weight-bearing views; however, it could be seen that good correction of the hallux valgus deformity had been achieved, with the sesamoids being returned to a good anatomical position. On the postoperative views, the degree of previous resection of the medial first metatarsal is apparent, bearing in mind no further bone was removed from the metatarsal head.

The postoperative regimen was that she was kept non-weight bearing in a cast for 6 weeks. The cast was changed at her first visit at 2 weeks. At 6 weeks the cast was removed along with the percutaneous K-wire in the second toe. She was then allowed protected weight bearing in a removable Aircast boot and was encouraged to do daily range-of-motion exercises to mobilise her first metatarsophalangeal joint and to help resolve her postoperative swelling. At 3 months following surgery she had a course of low-level laser therapy to help the swelling resolve.

She did well after surgery, returning to normal footwear and activities by about 5 months, and she was discharged from the podiatric service 18 months following the surgery. However, she did return 3 years after the surgery complaining of a degree of metatarsalgia under her third metatarsal head. This has responded reasonably well to conservative treatment, and she was pleased with this result. She also had some prominence of her internal fixation, so an operation was performed to remove it.

This case history highlights the need to make a thorough assessment of the patient's complaint. The choice of surgery needs to address the symptoms as well as having to deal with the degree of deformity present. The initial choice of surgery was never going to correct the severity of the hallux valgus deformity present, and also the metatarsalgia was not managed. Had the decision been made to correct the hallux valgus with a realigning procedure, it is possible that the metatarsalgia may have resolved by placing the first metatarsal into a better functional position.

## CASE STUDY 23.2 **MANAGEMENT OF SYNDACTYLE**

A young lady presented with a congenital syndactylisation between her second and third toes. This was a problem for her psychologically rather than physically. She would never take her shoes off in public places as she found it too embarrassing. On two preoperative consultations she was advised against having surgery as there was a real potential for making the situation worse. I counselled her regarding the risks of skin-flap necrosis and failure of a skin graft to 'take'. However, she considered it would be worth the risk as the condition caused her much bother.

The desyndactylisaton procedure was carried out using a free skin graft taken from the lateral aspect of her ankle (Weinstock 1989). The incision was made around the syndactylisation to the base of the toes. From this incision, a paper template was made then opened out and the incision marked in the skin folds on the lateral side of her ankle. The midpoint of the incision was also marked to make identification easier once the graft was removed. The skin flap was then taken at full thickness. The graft was then sutured into place, using simple interrupted sutures. These were selected as they give the easiest way of adjusting the position and tension on the graft. After this was sutured, the ankle wound was closed. The toes were dressed using a saline-soaked gauze placed between the toes with a standard postoperative dressing placed over the top. Healing progressed uneventfully and the wounds settled down well. A small section of the plantar aspect healed over the skin flap. However, as this did not show too much the patient was not too concerned (Fig. 1). She was very pleased with the outcome of this and was happy to proceed with similar surgery to her other foot.

The subject of cosmetic foot surgery raises a wide range of opinions, and some surgeons will not carry out any form of cosmetic foot surgery. At what point does surgery become cosmetic? When the problem affects the patient psychologically so that it restricts their activity? If someone has a deformity that prevents them from wearing a normal shoe, but is otherwise pain free, does this offer grounds for them to undergo surgery? This is a controversial area and one where a patient's needs must be assessed on an individual basis and a suitable care programme agreed. It should be borne in mind that a patient's expectations of the outcomes of cosmetic surgery may well be higher than when the surgery is for correction of function or the relief of pain.

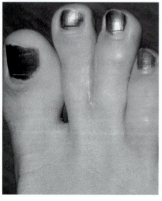

**Figure 1** Postoperative view after desyndactlylisation.

## MORTON'S NEUROMA

This is a common problem presenting with pain in the forefoot, usually described as burning and intermittent in nature (see also Ch. 4). Patients often describe the need to remove their shoe when the pain occurs. The pain often radiates into the toes, and the classic site for this is the third and fourth toes; usually, patients will have been suffering with the problem for some months before seeking advice. In most instances this is due to the fact that there is little to see and the fact that the pain is of an intermittent nature.

Treatment comprises insole therapy, steroid injections or surgical excision. The choice with regard to excision is with regard to where to place the incision. A dorsal approach avoids the problem of plantar scarring, while a plantar incision is more direct and places the incision directly over the nerve, allowing better exposure and an easier procedure. The plantar incision requires that the foot remain non-weight bearing for 3 weeks to allow healing to progress and to avoid problems with the scar. Either way the enlarged section of nerve is resected back to where it is a normal size and preferably far enough back in the foot to be off the main weight-bearing area. This helps to avoid the problem of recurrence or stump neuroma formation.

## LESSER METATARSAL OSTEOTOMIES

Lesser metatarsalgia is a problem that in many instances responds well to conservative treatment; however, when conservative treatment fails there are surgical options. A long metatarsal can be shortened or a plantar flexed, and a displaced metatarsal can be elevated. Radiographs can guide the surgeon to identify these situations; however, there are instances where the radiographs appear normal but the foot is painful and the clinical signs point to mechanical overloading. The presence of corns and callus as well as pain in the MTPJ all suggest mechanical causes. In these instances computerised pressure-measurement systems can be employed to confirm that the affected metatarsal is indeed overloaded (see Ch. 15). Other skin pathologies, such as verrucae over the metatarsal heads, can be ruled out, but this may be particularly difficult when patients have had a long history of treatment for suspected verrucae. If in doubt, a punch biopsy may be performed.

Many metatarsal osteotomies have been described over the years; however, the Weil osteotomy, and variations on this, have overcome many of the pitfalls of previous techniques, allowing for accurate control of the metatarsal position, with good internal fixation and a low incidence of non-union.

The proximal displacement osteotomy, or Weil-type osteotomy, is a valuable technique for the treatment of metatarsalgia. The metatarsal is cut just at the margin of the dorsal joint surface, with the saw as parallel to the weight-bearing surface as possible. Once the cut has been made the metatarsal head can be displaced proximally, so shortening the metatarsal. The osteotomy has a relatively large area for healing, and weight bearing tends to push the opposing bony surfaces together, allowing early weight bearing. The osteotomy can be fixed with K-wires or screws to hold it in position. One of the problems associated with the Weil-type osteotomy is a floating toe. This may occur due to scar contracture or the altered biomechanics of the joint or a combination of both. The fact that the osteotomy is never completely parallel to the weight-bearing surface means that the proximal displacement does tend to lower the metatarsal head slightly as it is displaced proximally. This has the effect of weakening the lumbrical function and so produces loss of lumbrical function on the proximal phalanx. Making a second cut into the metatarsal, to remove a thin section of the metatarsal allows the metatarsal head to elevate – countering the plantar displacement, and thus producing a good toe position and allowing it to function postoperatively.

Where a purely dorsiflexory procedure is required, in the case of a plantar-flexed metatarsal, a Schwartz osteotomy can be used. This is a dorsal, oblique closing-wedge osteotomy, leaving the plantar hinge intact. This gives a stable osteotomy with an additional point of fixation.

All metatarsal osteotomies carry the risk of either under- or overcorrection, and unfortunately there is no precise way of determining the degree of correction required preoperatively. How well the pressure is redistributed will not be known until the patient is walking again. Undercorrection may not resolve the metatarsalgia, and overcorrection will result in transferring the load to an adjacent metatarsal. Because of these factors, the patient must be advised of the risks prior to undergoing surgery.

The possibility of plantar plate rupture also needs to be taken into account. Where present, the surgeon needs to decide whether repair of this is required in isolation or in conjunction with structural realignment (Powless & Elze 2001).

## HALLUX RIGIDUS

This is a condition that ranges from the early stages of slight loss of motion at the MTPJ (hallux limitus) to a completely rigid joint. Pain is related to activity and the encroachment of footwear on the dorsal enlargement of the joint. A long metatarsal or a dorsiflexed metatarsal are thought to be aetiological factors in the development of hallux rigidus (see also Ch. 4).

Surgical treatment in the early stages is a choice between a simple cheilectomy, where the dorsal osteophytic lipping is resected, through to a metatarsal decompression osteotomy or a proximal phalangeal osteotomy. All these are carried out in conjunction with ensuring that the sesamoids are mobilised, as these will certainly contribute to loss of motion at the joint if they have become fixed to the metatarsal head. Metatarsal osteotomies have fallen from favour due to the risk of transfer metatarsalgia. Proximal phalangeal osteotomies, such as the Bonney Kessel procedure, redirect the motion at the joint into a more dorsal direction.

Once the joint range of motion has deteriorated, in conjunction with reduction of the joint space, then joint-destructive procedures are the only way to resolve the painful joint. The choices are an arthrodesis, a joint-replacement implant or a Keller procedure. The choice is determined based on the patient's age and activity levels. In a patient under the age of 60 years, a Silastic joint replacement or Keller arthroplasty are rarely advisable as primary procedures. The risks of Silastic joint failure and problems associated with a dysfunctional hallux, in the case of the Keller procedure, make them more suitable for older patients or in a salvage situation. An arthrodesis is

a tried and tested approach in patients under 60 years of age. However, the restriction this places on the wearing of heeled shoes makes this a less than ideal solution for women. Joint replacements other than Silastic joints may be an option. However, metal and ceramic joints have still to be shown to be efficacious over a long period of time.

## SESAMOID PROBLEMS

Sesamoid pathology is another cause of pain around the first MTPJ. An enlarged sesamoid may well give rise to a localised hyperkeratotic lesion. The sesamoid may be enlarged secondary to being bipartite or tripartite, or as a result of trauma or degenerative changes. The medial sesamoid is the most commonly affected.

Another factor to consider is how the sesamoid position alters with the progression of a hallux valgus deformity. As the first metatarsal moves into varus and the toe into valgus, the sesamoids move laterally in relation to the metatarsal head. The lateral sesamoid is able to move into the intermetatarsal space and move into a more dorsal position, thus becoming less weight bearing. The medial sesamoid tends to become more prominent on the plantar surface as it rides over the intersesamoidal ridge.

Evaluation of the sesamoid position can be made radiographically, from an anteroposterior view and an axial or sesamoid view. The options for surgical treatment of sesamoid problems are to remove a part, or the whole, of the sesamoid, or to reposition it into a better anatomical position. This latter option would be chosen where the sesamoid symptoms are part of a wider hallux valgus symptom complex (Fig. 23.9).

Partial removal of a sesamoid, or a sesamoid planing procedure, involves taking off approximately one-third to one-half of the sesamoid, cutting the plantar aspect off the sesamoid in a plane parallel to the weight-bearing surface. Removing too much increases the risk of the remaining bone of the sesamoid fracturing. Total sesamoidectomy is a straightforward procedure, but it is possible that removing the sesamoid may add to instability of the medial ligaments of the first MTPJ, leading to an increased risk of hallux valgus progression. Tight suturing of the capsular incision may go some way to preventing this.

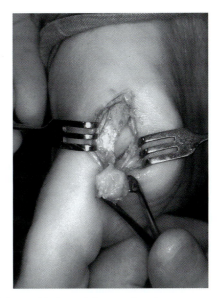

**Figure 23.9** Sesamoidectomy: intraoperative view.

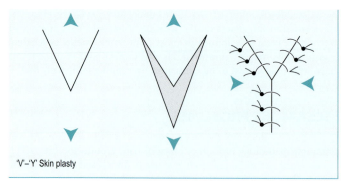

'V'–'Y' Skin plasty

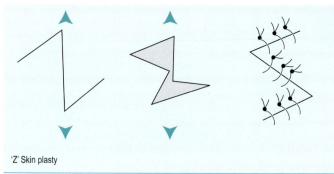

'Z' Skin plasty

**Figure 23.10** Skin plasties.

## SKIN PLASTIES

The use of skin plasties is widespread in podiatric surgery. In their simplest form, a lenticular incision over a mallet-toe correction aids in correcting the deformity by removing redundant skin. As well as removing redundant skin, the skin plasty is useful in lengthening the skin. An overlapping fifth toe is a situation where lengthening the skin aids correction of the toe position , usually in conjunction with an extensor tendon lengthening procedure. Two common techniques for this are the V-to-Y skin plasty and the Z skin plasty (Fig. 23.10). Rotational skin flaps can also be used to help close defects after skin-lesion excision. There are several variations on these approaches.

## REARFOOT SURGERY

The scope of rearfoot surgery undertaken by podiatric surgeons in the UK has increased in recent years. Rearfoot surgery is always going to be in less demand than the forefoot procedures that make up the majority of podiatric procedures. However, the realm of flat-foot reconstruction, tibialis posterior dysfunction repair and rearfoot fusions is an expanding one (McGlamry 1992).

## SUTURE MATERIALS

These can be divided into absorbable and non-absorbable, and mono-filament or braided. Monofilaments are smooth, single-stranded sutures, which slide through the tissues easily and provoke less tissue reaction. The disadvantages are that knots are less secure and they tend to be springier as the suture tends to have a degree of 'memory'. Braided sutures are woven fibres and are good for tying knots as they grip well; they are more flexible but may produce more tissue reaction.

Absorbable sutures will break down in contact with body fluids and enzymes and normally are about 30% weaker after 14 days. However, they take 90–120 days to absorb fully. A small percentage of patients will have some suture reaction, especially when absorbable sutures are used to close skin. This manifests itself as a small pustule, often with suture material expressed from it when debrided.

Non-absorbable sutures will maintain strength for much longer. However, they do need to be removed and this is often uncomfortable for the patient. Sutures are usually removed at about 10–14 days postoperatively or after 3 weeks with incisions on the plantar aspect of the foot.

Sutures come in a range of sizes and these are expressed in 0 grades. Most podiatric procedures utilise sutures in the range 2-0 (thick) to 5-0 (thin). Obviously, the thicker the suture the stronger it is. Thinner sutures produce less tissue reaction and a finer scar; however, a balance needs to be struck between the two and so a compromise is made.

The other choice to be made when selecting a suture for any given application is the needle design. The needle can be straight or curved and the point can be ground in one of several ways. Curved needles are used most commonly in foot surgery (Fig. 23.11). This is usually expressed as part of a circle, e.g. a 2/3 round needle is two-thirds of the circumference of a circle. A cutting needle is commonly used for skin suturing and in podiatric procedures. The cutting needle is ground into a triangular shape so that there are three separate sharpened edges to help the needle pass through tough tissues. The cutting needle has one of the apices of the triangular shape running around the inside circumference of the needle. This can more easily cut through the tissue and enlarge the needle hole, as the needle is pushed into the tissue. Therefore, a reverse cutting needle is to be preferred, as the apex of the triangle runs around the outside circumference and so the needle is less inclined to cut though to the edge of the wound.

The choice of sutures for different procedures is mainly dependent on preference, but within a range of possibilities. The strength of the suture combined with the type of needle needs to be matched to the purpose for which they are going to be used.

## SUTURE TECHNIQUES

Sutures are used to appose structures. How best to achieve this depends on choosing an appropriate suture material and then selecting a technique for inserting it into position (Fig. 23.11).

### Simple interrupted sutures

This is a simple loop that is tied off. Usually a row of similar sutures is used or they can be interspersed with other types of stitch, such as mattress sutures, to give additional strength to a wound. Using simple sutures allows for adjustment of tension in the suture on an individual basis. Another advantage is that if the wound starts to gape on removing some of the sutures, then some can be left in place for a longer period. Equally, if a wound is under tension, then one or two of the sutures can be removed without compromising the entire wound.

### Mattress sutures

These involve an extended loop of suture. Horizontal mattress sutures allow a wider loop and a strong everting force on the wound edges. Vertical mattress sutures also evert the wound well but allow for

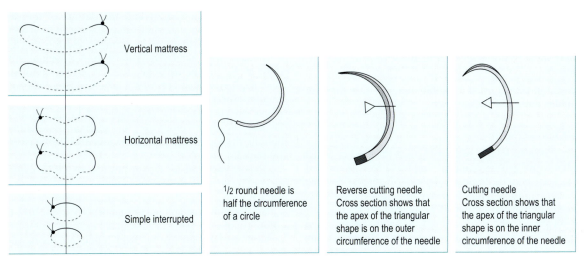

**Figure 23.11** Types of suture technique and suture needles.

stronger anchoring of the suture material, which is useful if the structures are under tension.

## Cross-over sutures

This is a double simple suture that allows for fewer individual sutures to be needed to close a wound, with the advantages of the simple suture.

## Continuous sutures

- *Running suture* – this is a continuous suture that allows for speedy closure, with knots needed at intervals or at the ends of the wound.
- *Continuous locking suture* – this is called 'blanket stitch' in embroidery terms. It is useful as it enables tension to be kept on the loops while you work along a wound.
- *Subcuticular* – this is a continuous skin closure. The suture is buried for some or all of the wound length. It can be carried out with either removable non-absorbable sutures or absorbable sutures. If non-absorbable sutures are used then periodic bridges are placed to allow easier removal of the sutures in sections. Steristrips are often used to augment a subcuticular suture to help maintain wound edges together.

There is not an 'ideal' suture technique. There is usually more than one way to repair structures or close a wound. Which technique to use will depend on preference based on experience combined with the presenting circumstances. There are few absolute rights and wrongs, but the choice of suture technique needs to be logically implemented and used in conjunction with a suitable choice of suture material.

## TISSUE HANDLING

The surgeon should always be aware of the damage that any given procedure is causing to the healthy cells within the foot. Every time an instrument grabs a piece of tissue, retracts a tendon or makes a cut, cells are being damaged. Just because this is at a cellular level and not readily visible at the time of surgery does not mean that it does not happen. The amount of swelling and inflammation postoperatively will always be greater if a procedure is carried out roughly. Thinking

physiologically, at a cellular level, will help the surgeon to visualise what is going on and appreciate how every interaction made will affect the foot. The surgeon must respect tissue and be gentle, taking care not to overstress the wound edges and the structures being retracted.

Making incisions the right size for the procedure is important – too small, and the wound needs to be stretched too much to gain access; too large, and unnecessary tissue damage occurs. Excessive undermining of the skin and dissection of the layers is likewise best avoided. The more that the inflammatory process is initiated by surgery, the more swelling will occur, placing pressure on the wound, and with it subsequent fibrosis that will bind the tissue layers together.

'Atraumatic technique' is the term used to describe careful surgical technique, and no more damage should be caused than is necessary. The concept is wide reaching in its philosophy and encompasses everything that the surgeon will do during the procedure.

Attention to positioning the foot will allow for exposure without pulling on the tissues. Incision planning is also important, and time spent accurately locating the anatomical landmarks and drawing the incision preoperatively is valuable, ensuring that the incision is located correctly. Time should be taken to do this, rather than wasting time once the clock is ticking with the tourniquet in place. A detailed knowledge of the anatomy is needed to be able to place the incision so as to locate the structures that are the focus of the procedure while avoiding structures that need to be preserved.

In summary, attention to detail and an appreciation of what is being done to the patient at a cellular level make for a better understanding of the whole process of surgery. Good tissue handling is rewarded by better outcomes from surgery and patients suffer less pain, less swelling and gain better function.

## POSTOPERATIVE DRESSINGS

The postoperative dressing (see also Ch. 10) has the following roles:

- creating an environment to encourage wound healing
- forming a barrier to prevent contamination
- maintaining antisepsis
- supporting the wound and control of swelling
- splinting the foot/toes where correction of deformity has been achieved

- ensuring absorption of blood or tissue fluid
- being small enough to allow clothes to pass over the foot and for the patient to be able to have some limited mobility
- the dressing should be non-adherent to allow for pain-free removal.

These objectives can be met using a combination of layers: the inner (contact), middle, outer and surface layers.

### The inner or contact layer

This is usually a non-stick layer such as Bactigras or Mepitel, which are sterile open-weave gauzes. Some are impregnated with an antiseptic to help keep bacteria from proliferating under the dressing. However, a balance must be struck between antisepsis and the introduction of chemicals that may inhibit cell proliferation. Clean wounds in healthy patients probably do not need antiseptic agents. These contact-layer products are usually greasy to prevent adherence to the wound.

### The middle layer

This is commonly plain gauze or a woven, woollen-type bandage such as a Velband or Softban. Several layers are used to allow the pressure applied from the outer layer to be spread evenly. This layer is also the main absorbent layer for fluids. The idea is that the dressing will rapidly soak up fluid exuded from the wound to stop it becoming macerated. Some surgeons also like to use two layers of gauze soaked in either Betadine or saline solution next to the foot. This gives a wet-to-dry type of action, and the gauze usually stiffens during the drying stage to act as a splint.

### The outer layer

This is usually an elasticated layer comprising several layers gently stretched to add an even compression over the whole surface of the dressing. Experience indicates the pressure needed. Too little pressure will lead the dressing to loosen and slip off the foot; it will also allow the foot to swell too much, which will be evident at the re-dressing appointment. If the dressing is too tight the patient will complain of excessive pain. The patient will also find any sort of ambulating considerably painful as the foot starts to swell with the foot in a dependent position.

### The surface layer

A final layer of a compressive stocking such as Tubigrip, up to just below the knee, can be used to protect the dressing as well as providing compression.

With certain procedures it is advisable to use a rigid cast to immobilise and support the foot. Casts can be either non-weight bearing or designed to allow for limited ambulating. The casts for allowing weight bearing need to be stronger to support the forces of weight bearing.

Casts are usually applied in a layered fashion. A contact layer can be either a simple stocking-type layer such as Tubigrip or a thin bandage such as Velband or Kling. Then the foot is usually protected with a soft bandage such as Velband or Softban. The thickness of this can be varied to allow for potential swelling. Extra padding around bony prominences is also useful when a weight-bearing cast is to be used.

The cast material is then applied, overlapping each turn of the material by about 50%. Too much pressure when applying the casting material will compress the padding and result in a cast that is too tight. This is usually painful and may result in vascular compromise. Massaging the material once in place usually helps to bond the layers together and smooth the outside of the cast. The foot should be positioned carefully during application of all the layers of the cast to ensure that it is comfortable and functional. A foot that is cranked from a relaxed position into a neutral ankle position (foot at 90° to the leg) once the first two layers of the cast have been applied, will end up with a large wrinkle of material across the anterior aspect of the ankle and reduced padding around the heel as this is stretched out. The end result will be an uncomfortable cast. Because of these problems, an assistant is usefully employed holding the foot in the position required while the layers of the cast are built up.

A below-knee cast for weight bearing should be reinforced with a piece of plywood or similar, and a rubber rocker applied to the plantar surface.

Patients with casts applied should be advised to check their toes for colour changes. Where a cast is applied too tightly or where the degree of swelling makes the cast too tight, it does not necessarily need to be removed totally. Removing a 2-cm strip from the anterior aspect of the cast usually releases the pressure and gives full relief without compromising the support from the cast too much.

## When to re-dress

There are a variety of opinions about how often to change a postoperative dressing. However, the work of L. Jones (unpublished) suggests a review at 12–14 days after surgery. This seems to reduce the incidence of problems, and makes the process simpler for both the patient and the practitioner. The authors has adopted this system for 5 years now and has had similar results. The patients are happier as they are more comfortable. If they have to attend for a dressing change after 5–7 days they are often still in a moderate degree of postoperative pain, which is much reduced 2 weeks after surgery. The dressing is usually easier to remove as the swelling is also often reducing. The raft of potential problems feared with re-dressing at this time point failed to materialise. Patients do need to be suitably advised regarding adverse signs to look for and be able to make contact if they have concerns.

## POSTOPERATIVE COMPLICATIONS

Complications are a fact of life; therefore, it needs to be accepted that they occur and the surgeon needs to learn how to deal with them and how to learn from them. Trying to understand complications and why they occur can help to further refine techniques to reduce their incidence to a minimum.

## Infection

This is a complication that affects any type of surgery (Figs 23.12 and 23.13). The incidence of infection in podiatric surgery is quoted at anything from 10% to less than 1%. Many factors affect infection rates, and good technique helps to reduce the risk. Good tissue handling and copious wound lavage prior to closure helps to minimise infection. The environment is also very important. Where operating theatres are used by other specialities, the rates of infection are often higher than when sole-purpose facilities are used. A high number of air changes per hour also helps to reduce the airborne transmission of bacteria to a low level. Other factors include the number of operating personnel in the theatre, as well as the length of the procedure (the longer the wound is open the greater the risk of infection).

Aspects of the patient's health may render them at a higher risk of infection. Poorly controlled diabetes, obesity, anaemia and treatment

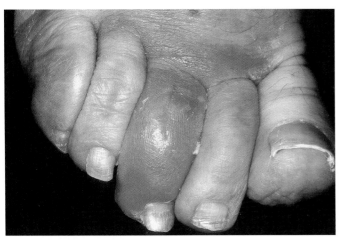

**Figure 23.12** Postoperative infections.

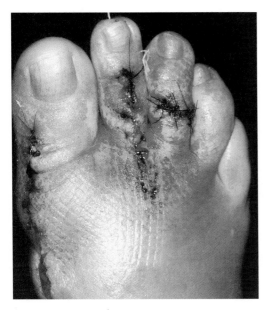

**Figure 23.13** Postoperative infections.

with immunosuppressive drugs such as steroids all need to be considered.

Infection usually becomes apparent from about 5 days postoperatively onwards, the commonest symptom of which is pain. Increased localised swelling, redness and heat are then followed by proximal spreading of the signs, with lymph-gland enlargement posterior to the knee and in the groin. Pyrexia may also develop. Discharge may be evident, striking through the dressing, and this may be malodorous.

Examination of the wound will show an acute inflammatory process, with redness and swelling beyond that which would be expected with normal wound inflammation. The wound may well be dehiscing and discharging. The discharge may be a yellow tissue fluid or pus.

Management of infection should encompass appropriate antibiosis, lavage of the wound to remove debris and pus and debridement of necrotic tissue. Frequent dressing changes are required, along with close monitoring to check for deterioration of or improvement in the infection. Microbiological analysis of a wound swab will be essential for culture of the infecting organism, with a sensitivity test to choose an appropriate antibiotic. However, immediate broad-spectrum anti-

microbial therapy should be started prior to the swab result being received, and the therapy then altered as required in the light of the results.

Localised wound infection may not need a wound swab. A 5-day course of a broad-spectrum antibiotic such as amoxicillin may be all that is required.

Blood tests to measure the white blood cell count are useful to monitor infection and aid diagnosis. The white blood cell count is raised in infection, although that is not the sole reason why it might be elevated. Blood culture can also be used to detect bacteria.

The surgeon must be alert to the possibility of infection extending to bone; some infections that may be extending to bone or are otherwise severe in nature will need urgent treatment with intravenous antibiotics.

Confirmed osteomyelitis will need treatment with appropriate antibiotics for a prolonged period. Traditionally, intravenous antibiotics have been used. However, some of the newer drugs are efficacious orally. Debridement of the infected bone is usually required. In these circumstances the debrided area may need further reconstruction in the future. This should be delayed for at least 6 months after the infection has cleared to reduce the risk of reinfection and allow optimum healing.

## Swelling

Swelling after foot surgery is to be expected, and it is perhaps the biggest problem for the podiatric surgeon. Preoperative counselling of the patient as to why swelling occurs and impressing on them the need to rest and elevate their foot is important, as is a graduated return to normal activities. Physical therapy can help to reduce swelling, but in some patients the swelling does not respond to this and it is simply a case of time to allow the swelling to resolve naturally.

Postoperative oedema is the commonest problem to be dealt with on a daily basis. The degree of swelling is not always related to the extent of surgery. Patients that are non-compliant about rest and elevation tend to develop marked swelling, and predicting how long swelling is likely to last once established is difficult. It is also true that in many cases the swelling after surgery is physiological rather than pathological. At what point it becomes a true 'complication' is a matter for debate – how long has the swelling persisted, and how much does it affect the patient? Treatment ranges from compression dressings and elevation to low level laser therapy and other physical therapies.

## Dehiscence

Dehiscence is where the wound opens postoperatively with failure of healing. This may be attributable to poor technique, with overaggressive retraction and stress on the wound margins, or infection. Low-grade infection can be difficult to differentiate from non-infective dehiscence. Dehiscence is prone to occur on areas of the wound under increased stress, such as at the main skin flexure areas. Poor compliance with inadequate resting of the foot is another cause that can usually be identified by the state of the dressing (e.g. the patient who states that they did nothing other than rest, but has a dressing that is heavily soiled from walking). In some cases it is difficult to attribute a cause. Management is cleansing and debridement of the wound and sterile dressings until healing occurs.

## Haematoma

A haematoma may form from any dead space left. If there is much potential dead space in a wound then the use of a drain will allow bleeding to exit on the surface rather than pool within the foot. Generally, good wound closure with a compressive dressing over the top will go a long way to preventing haematoma formation. If a haematoma is diagnosed soon after surgery it might be worthwhile aspirating the haematoma. If the haematoma re-forms quickly, then operating again to identify and ligate the bleeding source is indicated. However, if the haematoma is not diagnosed until some time after the procedure then the opportunity for simple aspiration will have passed. In this circumstance the choice is to wait or to reoperate to excise the haematoma. The haematoma, once formed and coagulated, is not a vascular lesion and so acts as an ideal culture medium for bacteria. Prophylactic antibiotics may help to stop the haematoma becoming infected. As the haematoma starts to resolve it might simply be a case of letting nature take its course. However, there is the potential for a haematoma to calcify, and this may lead to a degree of disability for the patient. A lot depends on the position and extent of a haematoma as to how much of a problem it proves to be.

## Joint stiffness

Any sort of joint surgery carries with it the risk of joint stiffness following the procedure. This is frustrating, especially in a patient who may have had a good range of motion preoperatively. Scarring around the joint is probably the reason for a lot of joint stiffness. Adhesion of the sesamoids in first MTPJ surgery is also a reason for limited joint range of motion after surgery. Early range-of-motion exercises and physical therapy to strengthen the muscles help to prevent this. Manipulation under anaesthesia is also an option postoperatively to try and restore a better range of motion.

## Hypertrophic scarring

Hypertrophic scarring results in raised, enlarged scars. These may be symptomatic, depending on the site. Careful history taking will go a long way to establishing whether an individual is prone to hypertrophic scars. Certainly the risk of this is low in patients who have undergone previous surgery without any problems. In known sufferers, early use of subdermal steroid injections may help to prevent the scar enlarging. Silastic gel sheeting can also help to prevent, as well as treat, hypertrophic scarring.

## Transfer metatarsalgia

Transfer metatarsalgia is a risk with any metatarsal surgery. It is generally a problem when carrying out osteotomies that will, by their very nature, bring about a certain amount of loss of bone and subsequent shortening. Compensating for shortening by using good osteotomy design and appropriate fixation will help to control the amount of shortening and allow for accurate reconstruction. The problem when assessing metatarsal position is that there is no agreed technique for preoperative evaluation. While several techniques for radiographic measurement of metatarsal length and protrusion have been described, they all have a fundamental drawback. Radiographs are only two-dimensional and so cannot show the position in three-dimensions. A short metatarsal could well be prominent on the plantar surface if it were sufficiently plantar flexed. Combining the lateral and anteroposterior radiographic views enables the assessment of the relative positions of the metatarsals in space. This technique is not readily available at present, and therefore much of the assessment is made clinically, and based on clinical experience, rather than on direct measurement. If it is difficult to assess the position preoperatively, then it is nearly impossible intra-operatively, and this is the only time when it is easy to adjust the position. Therefore, experience and good judgement are again relied upon to achieve as optimum a position as possible. It is not until the patient is sufficiently recovered from the surgery and is back to weight bearing that it can be known if the position determined at surgery is correct.

The risks of transfer metatarsalgia have to be accepted; however, warning patients preoperatively of the risks and getting them to understand the concepts helps them to accept the problem better if it should occur. Where the patient's transfer metatarsalgia occurs postoperatively, aggressive conservative treatment with weight-relieving insoles and corticosteroid injection therapy may resolve the problem without recourse to further surgery. However, it is wise to warn the patient that, if transfer metatarsalgia occurs, a further operation may be required. This will hopefully help them to accept the problem and not think of it as a failure or the result of negligent surgery.

## Avascular necrosis

Avascular necrosis is the death of bone following vascular compromise (Fig. 23.14). This is a particular problem with osteotomies. Many articles have been published on the incidence of avascular necrosis following distal metaphyseal osteotomies. The incidence seems to vary widely and much seems to depend on the sensitivity of the investigating technique. Clinically, the incidence is very low,

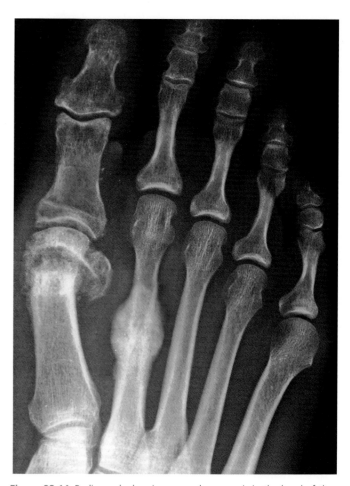

**Figure 23.14** Radiograph showing avascular necrosis in the head of the first metatarsal. There is also a stress fracture in the second metatarsal shaft.

but the use of sophisticated techniques, such as MRI, shows the incidence of avascular necrosis to be much more common. However, if the avascular necrosis is subclinical, one might question its relevance to the outcome of the procedure (Wilkinson et al 1992). Where it does occur, it can be devastating to the outcome of the procedure, with collapse of the metatarsal head. Avascular necrosis may appear several months after the procedure, and the early radiographic signs are minimal or totally absent. An increase in bone density may then occur as the bone starts to collapse inwards and distortion follows. Once detected, keeping the foot non-weight bearing will help to reduce the forces on the weakened area until such time as revascularisation occurs. Physical therapies may help to speed this along.

## Chronic regional pain syndrome

This is not a common postoperative complication but the incidence may well be higher than realised as some cases evade diagnosis. The warning features of chronic regional pain syndrome (CRPS) are pain out of all proportion to what would be expected, extending well beyond that which would be normal for the type of surgery that has been undertaken – *hyperalgesia*. Patients are generally hypersensitive and will find light touch painful – *allodynia*. Colour changes may occur, with the foot being a mottled cyanotic or erythematous colour, particularly when it is dependent. Swelling can also be present in CRPS, as can increased or decreased sweating over the affected area. Patients may also have problems moving the affected part and may develop tremors. Anxiety, depression and sleeping difficulties may also occur. Trophic problems may follow, leading to atrophy and osteoporosis. The mechanism of CRPS is not fully understood but it is considered to be of a neurological basis, and the sympathetic nerves may be responsible. These patients respond to a sympathetic nerve block. However, CRPS is best managed under the care of a pain clinic. Once a diagnosis is suspected, an urgent referral should be made to confirm the diagnosis so that treatment can be started as soon as possible.

## REFERENCES

Department of Health 2001 Good practice in consent implementation guide: consent to examination or treatment. Product code 25751.

Graham M 2002 Unpublished Departmental Audit to compare the outcomes of 2nd toe surgery, between a PIP joint arthrodesis and a PIP joint excisional arthroplasty. South-East Essex PCT.

Kalen V, Brecher A 1988 Relationship between adolescent bunions and flatfeet. Foot and Ankle 8(6):331–336.

Lehman DE 2003 Complications of hallux valgus surgery. Foot and Ankle Clinics of North America 8:15–35.

McGlamry ED 1992 Lesser ray deformities, In: McGlamry ED, Banks AS, Downey MS (eds) Comprehensive textbook of foot surgery, 2nd edn. Williams & Wilkins, Baltimore, OH, pp 321–378.

Miller S, Boegel W 1992 Perioperative considerations for foot and ankle surgery. In: McGlamry ED, Banks AS, Downey MS (eds) Comprehensive textbook of foot surgery, 2nd edn. Williams & Wilkins, Baltimore, OH, p. 181.

Powless SH, Elze ME 2001 Metatarsophalangeal joint capsule tears: an analysis by arthrography, a new classification system and surgical management. Journal of Foot and Ankle Surgery 6:374–388.

Wallace GF, Bellacosa R, Mancuso JE 1994 Avascular necrosis following distal first metatarsal osteotomies: a survey. Journal of Foot and Ankle Surgery 33(2):167–172.

Weinstock R 1989 Demonstration at cadaver workshop. Podiatry Association Annual Fellows Weekend Meeting.

Wilkinson SV, Jones RO, Sisk LE, et al 1992 Austin bunionectomy: postoperative MRI evaluation for avascular necrosis. Journal of Foot Surgery 31(5):469–477.

Yao L, Cracchiolo A, Farahani K, Seeger LL 1996 Foot and Ankle International 17:33–36.

# Chapter 24

# Principles of infection control

*Donald L Lorimer*

**KEYWORDS**

Carriers
Chief sources and reservoirs of infection
Cleaning
Colonisation
Cross-infection
Direct transmission
Disinfection
Disruption of transmission routes
Elimination of sources
Endogenous sources
Exogenous sources
HBV, HCV and HIV: implications for podiatrists
Infection
Infection control: strategies and methods
Infection control: terminology and concepts
Infective dose
Normal body microflora
Pathogens
Portals of entry
Portals of exit
Sources and vehicles of infection
Sterilisation
Transmission of infection

The prevention of all treatment-associated infection, both in patients and in staff, is an integral part of the professional responsibilities of podiatrists. An increased awareness of viral hepatitis and acquired immunodeficiency syndrome (AIDS) has heightened the concern of healthcare personnel over risks of infection. While concern over infections caused by hepatitis B and C viruses (HBV and HCV) and the human immunodeficiency virus (HIV) has focused attention on danger in clinical practice, this must be viewed in the context of infection control in general.

The basic principles and terminology of infection and its control are considered here, but because initial training, professional experience and working circumstances vary greatly, it is impossible to dictate a single infection-control regimen suitable for all practitioners.

However, equipped with a sound knowledge of the principles involved, individuals can select and implement measures most appropriate to their own practice.

## INFECTION TERMINOLOGY

The fields of infection and infection control have evolved specialised terminology but, unfortunately, there are not universally agreed definitions of all terms, and some variation in usage is demonstrated in the published literature. However, there is agreement on the essential concepts, and these are the basis of the following summary of terminology and associated information.

### Pathogen

Pathogenicity is the ability of a microorganism to invade a host and cause disease; hence, organisms that do so are termed 'pathogens'. However, it is important to realise that the original concept of there being pathogens and non-pathogens must be modified in the light of modern knowledge. While only true (virulent) pathogens may cause infection in a completely healthy host, there are many others that can cause infection if the body is weakened in some way. These opportunistic pathogens demonstrate that infection is but one outcome of a complex relationship between the body and microorganisms, infection occurring when the balance of circumstances favours a potential pathogen. Given appropriate circumstances, virtually all microorganisms are potential pathogens.

### Infection

Infection is the multiplication of microorganisms in or on body tissues, with an accompanying response by the body's immune system. Products of this immune response (e.g. antibodies against the organism) can be used to detect and diagnose infection or to monitor the progress of an infection. Note that this differs from contamination, which merely implies the presence of microorganisms, which may or may not become established.

Importantly, not all infections result in clinical infection (i.e. visible disease symptoms). Lower level infections occur in which microorganisms become established and there is an immune response but no clinical symptoms become apparent (i.e. subclinical infection is present). Even infections that eventually become overt will not show clinical symptoms in the early stages.

### Infective dose

The number of cells or particles of a microorganism that is required to establish infection is termed the infective dose. Pathogens differ in their infective dose, some requiring smaller numbers for successful invasion than others. More importantly, for any infectious agent, the greater the number contacting the body, the more probable it is that infection will become established. It follows that practical measures taken to reduce the number of microorganisms reaching the patient's tissue will reduce the likelihood of infection.

It is not possible to achieve the complete absence of microorganisms in the proximity of a patient. However, for minor non-invasive procedures, appropriate cleaning or disinfection will reduce the probability of microorganisms reaching the body in sufficient numbers to cause infection. When the body is more susceptible to invasion, such as when there has been surgery or other tissue damage, more stringent efforts must be made, by the use of sterile instruments and aseptic techniques, to minimise the numbers of microorganisms entering tissue.

### Colonisation

This differs from infection in that in colonisation an organism becomes established in or on the body but neither symptoms nor a significant immune response occur. However, colonisation may progress to infection should circumstances subsequently favour the microorganism.

### Carriers

Carriers are people who are colonised by or subclinically infected with a pathogen while showing no clear symptoms, but who are nevertheless infectious. The carrier state may be preceded by clinical infection, but not necessarily. Carrier states may be temporary or long term, even permanent. Relevant pathogens include *Staphylococcus aureus*, HBV, HCV and HIV.

### Sources of infection

A source is a site where potential pathogens can grow and multiply. A similar but more variable term is 'reservoir of infection', which has been used for sites where survival rather than growth occurs, as an alternative to the term 'source', or to describe a particular category of source. It will be used here for sites where survival or accumulation rather than growth is to be expected.

### Vehicles of infection

Many movable objects can become contaminated and transfer microorganisms to a susceptible person or body site. Some are naturally mobile because of their lightness (e.g. minute skin scales or respiratory droplets), while others are deliberately moved (e.g. instruments). Such objects are vehicles of infection that are capable of transmitting an infective dose but not usually of supporting microbial growth. Viruses, in particular, cannot multiply outside host cells, but transmission can occur via contaminated instruments (e.g. wart viruses, HBV, HCV and HIV).

The preceding points have important implications for infection control. While it is relatively straightforward to identify high-risk vehicles (e.g. instruments) and to render them safe by appropriate techniques, individual sources of infection are less easily identified. In particular, staff or patients colonised by a pathogen or in a symptomless stage of infection are sources, but they will not exhibit convenient symptoms warning of a possible infection risk. Continual awareness of the potential threat from sources, even unidentified ones, is required, and safe working practices that minimise the risk of infection from such sources must be implemented.

### Cross-infection

The term cross-infection is used in the clinical context specifically to describe the spread of infections to patients from staff or other patients. It often involves staff–patient contact or transfer of organisms via clinical equipment. Cross-infection is a significant risk to patients, and many control procedures are aimed at its prevention.

### Portals of entry

These are sites by which microorganisms gain access to the body. Most pathogens have one usual portal, although some are more versatile. Once established, organisms may remain near the entry site, causing localised infection, or spread internally to involve other areas of the body. The respiratory, gastrointestinal and genitourinary tracts are common portals of entry, but microorganisms rarely penetrate intact healthy skin.

Entry through the skin is usually via damaged areas, including minute abrasions, sites damaged by pressure, venous ulcers and areas weakened by excessive exposure to moisture. Deliberate penetration occurs in surgery, but damage may also result from other procedures such as nail reduction or treatment of keratoses and verrucae. As the skin is an important part of the body's defence, every effort should be made to avoid unnecessary damage and accidental penetration during procedures. Furthermore, any article penetrating skin or contacting damaged tissue is a potential vehicle of infection and must be free of microorganisms, which it could transport across the integument barrier.

### Portals of exit

These are sites from which pathogens exit the body and from where they are spread to other people, or other sites on the same body. Portals of entry and exit are often one and the same, for example infected wounds exuding pus, but pathogens causing systemic infections may exit from different sites. Hepatitis viruses and HIV may exit from any site where bleeding is caused by deliberate or accidental penetration of skin. Pathogens infecting superficial tissues (e.g. dermatophyte fungi, wart viruses, *Streptococcus pyogenes*) will be shed in skin particles or lesion exudates, while other pathogens whose primary target is not skin may, particularly in advanced cases, cause skin lesions containing the infectious agent (e.g. tuberculosis).

The spread of infectious material from exit sites must be minimised by, for example, the use of adequate dressings on infected lesions, safe disposal of contaminated dressings and decontamination of instruments.

### Normal flora of the body

Every human body is colonised by a large number of commensal microorganisms – the normal indigenous microflora of the body. Many species, mainly but not exclusively bacterial, occur among the flora, and different body sites support mixed populations of organisms suited to the particular conditions. The skin, mouth, upper respiratory tract and the large intestine are important sites of body flora.

The skin not only has resident flora permanently present (e.g. *Staphylococcus epidermidis*) but it is also frequently contaminated with flora from other body sites. These do not usually become established permanently on the skin but are so often present that they may be considered as transient normal flora. Above the waist, organisms from the respiratory tract often occur (e.g. *Staph. aureus*), while below the waist intestinal species may be present (e.g. *Pseudomonas* spp.). At any time additional transient contaminants acquired from the environment and other people may occur on the skin.

In health, the normal body flora is harmless or even beneficial, presenting competition to the establishment of incoming pathogens. However, it includes species that, while usually harmless in their normal sites, can be serious pathogens in wounds or damaged skin (e.g. *Staph. aureus* and *Strep. pyogenes*). In circumstances when local conditions allow excessive growth of a commensal species (e.g. erythrasma), when contamination of wounds occurs or when the body is weakened by systemic disease (e.g. venous ulcers in diabetics), many other commensal species act as opportunistic pathogens of skin tissue.

## CHIEF SOURCES AND RESERVOIRS OF INFECTION

The chief sources of infection may be categorised as:

- endogenous – sites of flora or infection in/on a person's own body
- exogenous – infected or colonised people, infected or colonised animals, environmental sources.

### Endogenous sources

Infections of wounds and damaged skin are most commonly caused by organisms from the patient's own body, which gain access to vulnerable areas on the foot. Examples include:

- *Staph. aureus* from nasal flora or, in some people, from colonised skin sites; this organism is commonly involved in external wound infections
- *Strep. pyogenes* from the throat or mouth
- *Corynebacterium minutissimum* from skin flora
- *Candida albicans*, a fungal opportunist, for example from skin or mouth
- various intestinal bacteria, including *Escherichia coli*, *Pseudomonas aeruginosa*, *Klebsiella* spp., *Proteus* spp. and *Clostridium perfringens*.

In addition to sites of body flora, any existing infected area (e.g. boils, ulcers) is a dangerous potential source from which pathogens can be transferred to damaged tissue. The importance of endogenous sources in potential wound infections means that local flora must be reduced before invasive procedures, and transmission of organisms from other body sites must be prevented.

### Exogenous sources

#### Infected or colonised people

In clinical situations, important and obvious sources of cross-infection are staff or patients with clinical infections of the skin or other accessible sites such as the respiratory tract. However, it is worth reiterating that human sources of pathogens, including *Staphylococcus aureus* bacteria, hepatitis viruses or HIV, and fungi such as *Candida albicans*, are often in symptomless states.

Commoner sources of cross-infection are sites of flora on staff or other patients which, while harmlessly colonising those people, can cause infection if transferred to vulnerable foot tissue, for example approximately 30% of patients and staff will be nasal and/or skin carriers of *Staphylococcus aureus*.

#### Infected or colonised animals

Animals can be colonised or infected by microorganisms that can cause human infections. Patients attending for treatment may have been infected from domestic animals, for example by zoophilic dermatophytes such as *Microsporum canis*. Infestation of premises by mice, cockroaches or pharaoh ants (a minute, inconspicuous species sometimes encountered in warm clinical environments) may occur. Such vermin and pests can harbour pathogens, including species acquired from clinical and human waste.

#### Environmental sources and reservoirs

Survival or growth of microorganisms outside the body is determined by their requirements and the environmental conditions. Many microorganisms associated with the human body are unlikely to grow in the environment as they have specific requirements that will be absent (e.g. complex nutrients or living host cells). All organisms need moisture for growth, and therefore even less-demanding species are prevented from multiplying by the dryness of most clinical areas. However, wet sites in clinical areas are potential sources or reservoirs, allowing the growth of some organisms and aiding the survival of others. Any body of standing water supports growth of bacteria, particularly Gram-negative bacilli which need minimal nutrients. Wet sites such as soap receptacles, leaks or spillages from pipes or equipment, and residual water in stored utensils are potential risks. Even aqueous solutions of chemicals, including disinfectants, especially if overdiluted or aged, will allow survival and even growth of microorganisms.

Dry sites are reservoirs of viable microorganisms surviving in dirt and dust. In general, Gram-negative bacteria survive poorly in dry conditions, whereas Gram-positive bacteria and fungi survive rather better. The resistance of bacterial spores to desiccation and even disinfection is well established. Protection by materials of bodily origin (e.g. dried blood, exudate and skin particles) aids survival of all types of organisms. Reduction in numbers due to cleaning procedures is counterbalanced by day-to-day contamination from staff and patients, clinical waste (e.g. skin and nail debris), and dirt or dust from clothing and footwear. Therefore, continual effort is required to restrict contamination to acceptable levels.

## TRANSMISSION OF INFECTION

For infection to occur, microorganisms from an exogenous or endogenous source must be transmitted by some means to a new host or host site. Details of transmission routes vary widely in individual instances but may be generally categorised as follows.

### Direct transmission

This involves direct physical contact with, or close proximity to, a human source or reservoir. It includes close-range transmission of pathogens in droplets or skin particles shed from the body that fall immediately onto surfaces of persons within 1–2 m (i.e. they do not become truly airborne). Those most likely to transmit exogenous infection to patients are staff who are themselves infected or colonised or whose hands and clothing have become contaminated from other patients. Staff involvement in direct-contact transmission, especially via the hands, is of major importance in clinically acquired infections.

This category can also include endogenous infection involving transmission from own-body sites, for example wound infections caused by organisms from the skin or other sites spread via the hands or clothing. Some pathogens more usually spread by direct sexual contact (e.g. hepatitis viruses and HIV) may also be transmitted by clinical contact if blood contaminates the skin or mucous membranes. Measures to prevent direct transmission in clinical situations include hand/skin cleaning and disinfection, protective clothing and 'no-touch' techniques.

### Indirect transmission routes

These usually involve intermediate vehicles of infection that transfer microorganisms from an animate (including human) or inanimate source or reservoir to a vulnerable host site. The source or reservoir is not directly involved or in close proximity, and could in fact be very distant.

### Transmission by clinical items

Any contaminated article coming into close proximity to or contact with vulnerable tissue is capable of transmitting infection. Background items, for example furniture, are relatively low risk, while articles in direct patient contact are high risk. Potential vehicles include scalpels, burrs, handpieces and other instruments, swabs, dressings and drapes, antiseptics, syringes and injected solutions. Reusable instruments and multi-use containers of pharmaceuticals are more likely to become contaminated than are single-use items. Surfaces, including trolley tops, may contaminate items placed on them. Adjustable lamps used during procedures may transfer contaminants to and from hands. Surfaces allowed direct contact with a patient's skin (e.g. foot rests if not protected by a sheet) can transfer organisms between patients.

### Airborne transmission

True airborne transmission, commonly associated with respiratory infections, should have little significance in podiatric procedures. Apart from the previously noted close-range contamination near the body, airborne contamination appears to be significant only when tissue is exposed for prolonged periods, such as during extensive surgery (Ayliffe & Lowbury 1982, Ayliffe et al 1999, Meers 1983).

However, clinic dust is a reservoir of infection and may contain remnants of skin, nail, blood, pus and lesion exudates. Various activities may render the dust airborne, and thus able to settle afterwards on exposed surfaces. Dry sweeping of skin and nail debris, vigorous movement of curtain screens, overcrowding and unnecessary human activity all increase airborne contamination. While this risk is difficult to quantify, these activities are undesirable near clinical procedures or unprotected sterile items.

### Transmission by animals

Vermin and insects may shed contaminants when feeding or defecating. They may also act simply as vehicles, transferring contamination on their body surfaces from dirty areas such as drains and disposed wastes. Either way, contamination of the clinical environment, surfaces and unprotected materials may occur.

### Faecal transmission

Faecal–oral transmission is of major importance in food and waterborne infections. While this has no direct relevance to podiatry, note that the hands and skin are often contaminated with faecal organisms, including potential wound pathogens, after toilet use, and dispersion of such contamination is more likely if diarrhoea is present.

## HEPATITIS B VIRUS (HBV), HEPATITIS C VIRUS (HCV) AND HUMAN IMMUNODEFICIENCY VIRUS (HIV) INFECTIONS

In view of current concern over these blood-borne infections, a brief overview is given below, drawing on the concepts established above. These are complex infections and only a general summary is possible here.

# Hepatitis B and hepatitis C viruses (HBV and HCV)

HBV and HCV are two important types of the several viruses that can cause hepatitis, which is characterised by inflammation and necrosis of liver tissue. Although the more recently characterised of the two, the incidence of HCV is now known to be many times that of HBV and about ten times that of HIV (Dinsdale 2004). Viral hepatitis infection may result in a range of consequences, for example:

- Subclinical infection – this is the commonest form in adults and is usually undiagnosed.
- Acute infection – after a long incubation period (1–6 months) the clinical phase usually lasts for up to a month, with mostly ill-defined symptoms (flu-like, malaise) with or without jaundice. After this, most patients with HBV recover fully – although, in rare cases, infection leads rapidly to liver failure and death. Conversely, only a minority of HCV patients recover fully after the initial illness.
- Chronic hepatitis (carrier state) – develops after initial infection in a minority of cases of HBV but in the majority of cases of HCV. Carriers may be symptomless or may undergo progressive liver damage that is eventually fatal. The carrier state may result ultimately in primary liver cancer.

As with all viruses, the components of HBV and HCV are antigenic, and these antigens together with the antibodies formed against them are used to monitor infection, to indicate the carrier state or its level of infectiousness, and to track the effectiveness of treatment. For example, the presence of the HBV surface antigen (HbsAg) indicates that the person is infected with HBV and is infectious. The antigen disappears on recovery, but its persistence longer than 6 months after infection indicates a chronic carrier state. Subsequently, the presence of HBeAg (from the HBV core) in the blood of carriers indicates that the person is highly infectious.

The latest drug therapies can reduce liver inflammation and infectiousness in HBV (in approximately 50% of cases) and are more successful in HCV, approximately 40% of cases being 'cured' as measured by virus elimination from the blood. Nevertheless, the proportion of unsuccessful treatments and the fact that many cases go untreated means that most people currently infected with HBV and HCV live with the threat of associated long-term consequences.

# HIV and AIDS

HIV (human immunodeficiency virus) causes AIDS (acquired immunodeficiency syndrome), which is the final stage of this virus's progressive attack on the human immune system. From the first described cases of AIDS in the 1980s, HIV infection has advanced to a global epidemic. There are currently tens of millions of people at various stages of HIV infection, from initial seroconversion to fully developed AIDS. Thus the likelihood of podiatrists unknowingly encountering infected people among their patients has increased greatly.

The main cellular target of HIV infection is a type of T-lymphocyte known as a CD4 (T4,-helper) cell. These cells play a vital part in controlling the body's response to infection. Any reduction in the number or function of CD4 cells leads to impaired humoral and cell-mediated immunity, with a consequent vulnerability to infection.

Initial infection by HIV causes little or no discernible illness, although the infected person is infectious. Within several weeks seroconversion (i.e. the production of anti-HIV antibodies) occurs. The person is now 'HIV-positive'. However, while these antibodies are useful in detection tests for HIV infection, within the individual they are ineffective in eradicating the virus, and the person remains permanently seropositive and infectious. The progress of the infection and the effectiveness of treatments can now be monitored by direct tests for viral load in the individual and CD4 cell counts.

Individuals who are HIV-positive present differing states of health, reflecting progressive stages (of very variable duration) of the infection:

- many remain symptomless carriers for prolonged periods (possibly several years)
- variable states of ill health short of fully expressed AIDS, which may involve persistent generalised lymphadenopathy, weight loss, diarrhoea and other symptoms, such as minor opportunistic infections (including tinea infections)
- AIDS – a drastic reduction in immune defence characterised by severe and repeated opportunistic infections (even by weak opportunists), unusual cancers and other possible developments such as wasting disease or encephalopathy (pre-senile dementia).

The exact proportion of HIV infections that results in symptoms is unknown, but from experience to date it is likely that all HIV-infected individuals develop some degree of illness eventually, up to and including AIDS. Developments in antiretroviral drug regimens have resulted in significant extension of relative well-being and life expectancy in many recipients, although these aggressive and expensive therapies are not available or appropriate for all. While an advance, these therapies are not a cure, and a vaccine remains unavailable despite extensive research.

# Implications for podiatrists

HBV, HCV and HIV are blood-borne but are also present in other body fluids, including semen and vaginal secretions – hence their association with entry of blood through mucous membranes or damaged skin, sexual transmission and mother-to-baby transfer. These infections have an increased incidence in certain high-risk-activity groups such as drug injectors sharing equipment, homosexual/bisexual men, and heterosexuals with multiple sexual partners. However, in the podiatry context it is much more relevant that these infections are *not* confined to such high-risk-activity groups and have become much more widespread in the general population. Workers in situations where blood spillage or transfer is likely (e.g. healthcare, prison personnel, police, other emergency services) are at increased risk. Patients who received blood transfusions or blood products before detection or preventive measures were available may also have become infected. Even children, seemingly unlikely risks among podiatry patients, may have been infected by maternal transmission. The crucial point is that a podiatrist will not know whether or not a patient belongs to a high-risk-activity group, and the incidence of these infections is now much more widespread among other people not in these categories.

HBV, HCV and HIV infections are all on the increase, and all have potentially serious consequences. Despite advances in treatments there are no real cures, and thus prevention of infection is the only effective strategy (Department of Health 1998).

Therefore, practitioners must treat all invasive procedures, contacts with blood/tissue fluids, and blood/tissue fluid contamination of instruments as dangerous, however unlikely it seems that the patient constitutes a risk. In effect, procedures must prevent transmission from any patient in case they are a source, while also protecting each patient from becoming a victim of clinically transmitted infection. All sharps used in procedures must be sterile, with particular care being taken with the decontamination of reusable instruments if employed. Any differences in infectiousness or hardiness between these viruses are irrelevant in most circumstances, as effective prevention must take into account the possible presence of all of them.

No vaccine is currently available against HCV or HIV infection, and although an effective HBV vaccine is now available only a minority of the general population will be protected by this in the foreseeable future. As professionals with direct patient contact, podiatrists are at risk and should seek HBV vaccination. In no way does staff vaccination reduce the necessity for other control measures, which are essential to protect patients from these and other infections.

## VARIANT CREUTZFELDT–JAKOB DISEASE

Following a large outbreak in the UK of bovine spongiform encephalopathy (BSE) in cattle, human cases of a new variant of Creutzfeldt–Jakob disease (CJD) appeared, and it is now accepted that food-borne transmission from cattle to humans occurred. The number of cases of this invariably fatal disease that will eventually develop in infected but as yet symptomless people is unknown. Although originally food-borne the danger now is that transmission via blood or tissue can occur, hence the relevance of CJD in clinical contexts. The agent is a prion protein (not a living organism as such) that is highly resistant, and it is essential that tissue traces are removed from reusable instruments by scrupulous cleaning prior to heat sterilisation to avoid its possible survival of the process. The arrival of this new threat is another reason to move towards the ideal of single-use sharps for invasive procedures wherever feasible.

## INFECTION CONTROL

The term 'infection control' reflects the realistic objective of reducing infection to the practicable minimum, rather than claiming the ideal of total prevention. Infection has always been of major concern to professionals involved in the surgery and treatment of wounds. Much is now known about prevention of infection generally and wound infections in particular. If the established principles and practices of infection control are implemented, infection following podiatric procedures should be uncommon, especially as many procedures are relatively minor in terms of tissue invasion. Infection control in clinics must encompass measures to prevent patient infections from both endogenous and exogenous sources, and also to protect staff from becoming infected by patients. As time progresses, higher standards are expected of professionals, particularly as awareness has increased of threats from blood-borne pathogens and antibiotic multiresistant bacteria such as MRSA (methicillin-resistant *Staph. aureus*).

Knowledge of infection control in clinical situations stems largely from efforts to prevent infections in hospitals, and comprehensive texts on these aspects have been produced (Ayliffe et al 1990, 1999, 2000, Bennett & Brachman 1986). In addition, the Society of Chiropodists and Podiatrists in the UK has indicated to its members recommended procedures for particular aspects of routine practice (Anon. 1987, Burrow 2004). A very important resource now available to practitioners is the information available on internet websites. Advantages of these include worldwide access, frequent updating and the availability of search facilities for the user. The following section summarises the underlying principles of infection control in the context of podiatry, and indicates how they provide a rational basis for safe procedures.

## Terminology

### Sterilisation

This is a process that renders an item free from all living microorganisms, that is it becomes sterile (British Standards Institution 1986a). There are no degrees of sterilisation; all microorganisms, including bacterial spores, must be killed or removed. Any process that does not achieve this is a disinfection and not a sterilisation process. Sterilants are chemical agents capable of sterilising, but few can achieve this in routine podiatric circumstances.

### Disinfection

Disinfection is a process by which microorganisms are reduced to a level harmless to health. In contrast to sterilisation, there are degrees of disinfection, the level of microbial reduction considered necessary being dependent on the item to be disinfected and the infection risk it presents in that situation. Bacterial spores are often little affected. Disinfection, unlike sterilisation, can be applied to living tissue, for example skin, as well as to inanimate articles.

Disinfection methods, particularly chemical disinfectants, often demonstrate a particular spectrum of antimicrobial activity, varying in effectiveness against different types of microorganisms. The terms 'bactericidal' and 'fungicidal' indicate a capability of killing bacteria and fungi, respectively. Similarly, 'sporicidal' and 'virucidal' indicate an ability to kill spores and to inactivate viruses, respectively. These properties are determined under laboratory test conditions, and such terms should not be taken to mean that disinfection so described or labelled will kill all of the specified type of microorganism under conditions of ordinary use. A term such as 'germicidal', while implying antimicrobial activity, is too vague and should not be used.

### Antisepsis

Antisepsis is the destruction or inhibition of microorganisms on living tissues, having the effect of limiting or preventing the harmful results of infection (British Standards Institution 1986a). Antiseptics are chemical agents used to achieve antisepsis; they are usually unsuitable for general use on inanimate articles, for reasons of either lower antimicrobial action or cost-effectiveness. Some antiseptics inhibit rather than kill microorganisms, this capability being described by terms such as 'bacteriostatic' or 'fungistatic'.

### Asepsis

The term 'asepsis' means an absence of contamination or, perhaps more realistically, absence of infection (sepsis) resulting from contamination. This should be the objective underlying all clinical procedures. Aseptic techniques are safe methods of working on patients by which contamination is minimised and thus infection prevented – in this context, largely by the prevention of cross-infection and the protection from contamination of damaged foot tissue. As appropriate, both sterilisation and disinfection are employed to achieve asepsis.

## STRATEGIES AND METHODS OF CONTROL

As microorganisms may be transmitted by so many routes, a similarly wide range of measures must be employed in infection control. All individual control measures stem from three basic strategies of infection control that are long-established but still relevant in the 21st century (Ayliffe et al 2000, Lowbury et al 1981):

1. elimination of sources and reservoirs of infection
2. disruption of transmission routes
3. increasing or restoring host resistance to infection.

In any particular circumstances, which will vary for individual practitioners, these strategies provide a framework for a sensible choice of suitable control measures. Strategies 1 and 2 above are especially relevant to practical podiatry and are discussed in the following sections.

## Elimination of sources and reservoirs

Important sources of infection are patients with existing clinical infections, for example septic lesions, fungal infections and verrucae. Successful treatment not only benefits that patient but also eliminates him or her as a source of cross-infection. During a course of treatment, dressings minimise the exit of pathogens from such sources. Endogenous infected sites must be covered by dressings before invasive techniques or exposing nearby tissue.

Less commonly, podiatrists providing hospital ward services may encounter source isolation. Some patients with serious infections are isolated by a variety of measures to prevent cross-infection from them to others. Essentially, both the patient and his immediate environment are considered to be contaminated, and measures are enforced to prevent transfer of pathogens from these by either personnel or equipment. Appropriate protective clothing must be donned and, after patient care, must be discarded within the isolation area. Instruments may require special arrangements for decontamination before re-use, and thorough hand cleansing after patient contact is most important. Practitioners treating such patients should familiarise themselves with, and adhere to, the isolation procedures in force at that time.

Podiatrists with clinical infections are clearly a risk to patients. Particularly relevant are infections on the hands or other exposed areas of skin, for example furuncles, infected cuts or paronychia. Covering small lesions with waterproof plasters and wearing gloves reduces the risk to patients, but such measures may not suffice to eliminate the risk, especially in procedures where glove puncture is possible. Where there is any doubt, direct contact with patients should be avoided until the infection has resolved. Infections of other parts of the body also constitute a significant risk, for example streptococcal sore throat. Skin affected by chronic skin conditions such as eczema or psoriasis may become colonised with *Staph. aureus* and lead to profuse shedding of the organism. Practitioners who become carriers of HBV, HCV or HIV are unlikely to transmit these to patients but, as personal circumstances vary greatly, practitioners should seek medical advice if in any doubt of the advisability of contact with patients, particularly with regard to invasive procedures. Other possible sources among staff include symptomless carriers of wound pathogens such as *Staph. aureus* and *Strep. pyogenes*. Routine screening of staff for such carriage is not generally justified, but it may be necessary in certain circumstances, for example to investigate an outbreak of wound infections.

Accumulations of dirt or dust anywhere in the clinical environment are reservoirs of infection and should be eliminated by cleaning, with additional disinfection if necessary. Clinical waste must not be allowed to contaminate the area and should be disposed of hygienically. Collection of patient debris at source is a sensible measure, for example by using a disposal bag underneath the foot or similar measures. Wet sites resulting from faulty equipment or plumbing can be eliminated by repair or replacement. Other wet sites need a common-sense approach to changing working procedures or choice of materials. Examples include disinfecting and drying cleaning utensils before storage, and replacing bars of soap lying in a wet dish by cleaner draining storage or, better still, by a suitable detergent/disinfectant dispenser.

Prevention of animal pest infestations is aided by maintenance of building structure (to inhibit access) and high standards of general cleanliness throughout the premises to deny them food, water and breeding sites. Should infestation occur, eradication can be difficult and professional pest-control operatives should be contacted. If the source of a patient's infection is found to be a family pet (for example *M. canis*), then successful treatment of the person may require veterinary treatment of the animal to prevent reinfection.

## Disruption of transmission routes

Essentially, this is achieved by effective decontamination of inanimate vehicles and by procedures designed to exclude contamination at the point of patient contact, the latter including hand/skin disinfection and other aspects of aseptic technique.

Decontamination of inanimate articles is based on cleaning, disinfection and sterilisation. These techniques represent increasing degrees of decontamination and are employed according to the infection hazard posed by particular articles or circumstances. As a general rule, the closer an article approaches susceptible tissue or vulnerable items such as sterile instruments, the more thorough the decontamination required. Cleaning is usually adequate for most general items, such as furniture, utensils and laundry. Disinfection is necessary when a specific infection risk is known to exist, for example articles in the vicinity of treatment procedures, blood spillages, and for articles that are unsuited to sterilisation but require more thorough decontamination than cleaning. Sterilisation is necessary for all items penetrating the body or contacting exposed tissues.

### Cleaning

The clinical environment should present a high standard of general cleanliness. Inadequately cleaned clinics will not only contain unnecessary reservoirs of microorganisms but will also reduce patients' confidence and staff morale. Cleaning should not be dismissed as a background chore that has little to do with the professional staff, but should be part of an integrated programme of clinical decontamination. In this context, it implies thorough cleaning at sufficiently frequent intervals using effective agents and appropriate, well-maintained equipment. Such cleaning is a surprisingly efficient method of decontamination and is all that is usually necessary for routine surfaces and equipment, such as floors, furniture, sinks, toilet facilities and similar items. Disinfection of these is unnecessary, firstly because such items normally present an insignificant infection risk, and secondly because recontamination is inevitable and reaches a similar equilibrium level whether or not disinfectants are used. However, disinfection is justified for such items on specific occasions of known increased risk, for example blood spillage.

In addition to preventing excessive accumulations of contaminated dirt, cleaning should not itself increase any risk of infection. Both the methods and materials employed must themselves be hygienic. There are two main dangers here: the distribution of dust-borne contamination and the growth of bacteria on wet cleaning utensils. Dry dusting or sweeping, including the sweeping up of debris after patient treatment, is not acceptable in clinical areas, and suitable vacuum cleaners (British Standards Institution 1986b) or dust-attracting mops should be used instead. Vacuum cleaners should incorporate efficient filters and/or bags, regularly checked and replaced as necessary, which retain debris and microorganisms efficiently and do not spread contamination via exhausted air. Dust-attracting mops must themselves be cleaned as soon as they are visibly dirty or at least every 1–2 days.

Wet cleaning should be done with clean water and a detergent, changed frequently to maintain effectiveness. Cloths, preferably disposable, for damp-dusting surfaces and string mops for cleaning floors are more suitable than sponge utensils, which are less easy to decontaminate after use. Utensils for wet cleaning are known to support the growth of bacteria, particularly Gram-negative organisms, if they are not effectively decontaminated after use. Ideally, items such as reusable cloths, mop heads, buckets and wet parts of cleaning machines should be cleaned after use, heat-disinfected if possible, and then stored dry. Unless their premises are serviced by a centralised hospital cleaning service, practitioners may consider this an unattainable standard, but serious efforts should be made to avoid heavy contamination of wet utensils, which in turn would contaminate the very items they are supposed to clean. Utensils should at least be cleaned in fresh hot water and detergent, and then rinsed and dried. Storage of all ancillary equipment, including cleaning materials, should, of course, be separate from the area used for patient treatment. Routine cleaning activities, even if done well, carry a risk of dust disturbance or splashing and should be completed as long as possible (ideally at least an hour) before treatment of patients, to allow airborne contamination to finish settling.

Floors, toilet facilities and furniture should be washed or damp-dusted daily, as appropriate. Sinks also require thorough cleaning daily, and additional cleaning if soiled during use, with either detergent or mild abrasive cleaning products. Sites that could harbour stagnant water, for example soap ledges, must be dried. Walls in good repair are of little significance in infection and, unless soiled, require infrequent cleaning; every few months should suffice. In contrast, adjustable lamps positioned immediately above the patient and that are handled frequently should be cleaned daily, and disinfection between patients could be recommended.

Some exceptions to daily cleaning of floors and furniture may be necessary. If there are floor areas on which patients walk barefoot there is the risk of cross-infection; careful organisation of patient movements or use of disposable coverings for floors or feet could eradicate this. As some foot conditions will render patients vulnerable to infections, while other patients may have existing infections, it is difficult to justify contact with a floor that is not at least cleaned between patients. Similarly, furniture or surfaces in the immediate vicinity of treatment procedures justify extra cleaning, and even disinfection, between patients, especially before invasive procedures.

Reusable instruments should be cleaned scrupulously after use before further decontamination and reuse. After a rinse in cold water, they may be cleaned manually using a brush and mild detergent. Rubber gloves should be worn, as thick as is consistent with dexterity, and every care taken to avoid accidental injury while cleaning, rinsing and drying sharps, because of the risk of HBV, HCV and HIV infection. Used instrument brushes should be cleaned and disinfected, preferably sterilised, and not simply left by the sink. Instruments and other utensils should not be cleaned in the same sink used for clinical handwashing, but if this is completely unavoidable the sink should be cleaned and disinfected after use for instruments. Alternatively, ultrasonic cleaning in detergent solution can be employed for instruments, in which case the manufacturer's instructions on method and suitable agents should be followed. Note that ultrasonic baths are a cleaning aid only and do not kill microorganisms – they may even disperse aerosols of microorganisms if lids are not tightly fitted. Furthermore, they should not be allowed to retain water or stagnant cleaning solution, which could support the accumulation of bacteria. For further details of cleaning methods and agents, the reader is referred to texts on clinical hygiene (Babb 1993, Maurer 1985).

## Disinfection

Many agents have been employed for disinfection in clinical situations, including steam, hot water, chemical vapours, chemical solutions and ultraviolet radiation. The agents most relevant to podiatric clinics generally are hot water and chemical disinfectants. Hot water has the advantage of being effective against all types of microorganisms except bacterial spores; it needs little expertise, leaves no residues and is inexpensive. However, it is unsuitable for very heat-labile items, cannot be used on living tissue, and is not practicable for larger items. Chemical disinfectants can be used on surfaces and furniture, and some are suitable for skin disinfection; unfortunately, as a group, they have many disadvantages – including possible toxicity, corrosiveness, variable antimicrobial effectiveness, inactivation by many materials, undesirable odours or residues, limited in-use life, and a general requirement for skilled use to be effective.

Despite the widespread use of chemical disinfectants in the past, it is now accepted that they should be used only when there is a clear need for disinfection additional to thorough cleaning, and when no practical alternative is available. If possible, hot water should be used instead, particularly as items too sensitive for heat sterilisation often withstand the lower temperatures used for disinfection.

In summary, heat disinfection is the preferred method for inanimate items of suitable size for immersion, whereas chemicals are employed for larger items and surfaces, for skin disinfection, and when heat is not practicable.

### Disinfection by hot water

Articles should be cleaned first, then fully immersed in hot water, ensuring parts are not protected by trapped air. Temperatures of at least 65°C are necessary; higher temperatures decrease the time required for effective disinfection. For routine use, the values in Table 24.1 are applicable.

Such treatments are recommended to kill vegetative bacteria on items such as heat-labile instruments (British Standards Institution 1993). Thermostatically controlled washer/disinfectors with timed cycles, and washing machines incorporating a disinfecting hot water rinse are available. Heat-resistant instruments should be immersed in boiling water for at least five minutes (Ayliffe et al 1999, British Medical Association 1989). 'Instrument boilers' need careful use as they usually lack time-controlled cycles and can also pose problems of operator safety. It must be emphasised that disinfection, even at high temperatures, is not sterilisation and it should not be used when sterility is required.

### Disinfection by chemicals

Despite their disadvantages, chemical disinfectants are required for certain tasks and are effective when used correctly. However, users should be aware of various factors that influence the efficiency of disinfectants.

The concentration of disinfectant solutions is important in determining efficiency, and the recommendations of manufacturers or

**Table 24.1** Disinfection by hot water

| Temperature (°C) | Minimum time |
| --- | --- |
| 65 | 10 minutes |
| 71 | 3 minutes |
| 80 | 1 minutes |
| 90 | 1 second |

suppliers must be followed. For this reason, in-use solutions should never be 'topped up' by the addition of more water, with or without additional disinfectant. Once prepared, in-use solutions deteriorate, resulting eventually in a lower actual concentration and thus becoming ineffective. If possible, make up fresh solutions daily; this need not be wasteful if appropriate quantities are prepared. Otherwise, it is essential to note shelf-life information and to prepare fresh solutions when required, marking the date prepared and a use-by date as appropriate. Remember that disinfectant solutions can act as sources or reservoirs of pathogens.

All disinfectants can be inactivated to some extent by various natural or synthetic materials, such as hard water, detergents, soaps, tissue or other body material, cork, cellulose (e.g. cotton wool) and plastics. This is potentially serious, as many articles used to contain or apply the disinfectants, and items for disinfection themselves, may reduce the effectiveness of the process. If required, the manufacturer's advice should be sought on these aspects.

Dirt, especially dried organic material, may inhibit disinfectants by inactivation and by presenting a physical barrier to penetration of the solution. The level of initial microbial contamination also influences the number of microorganisms surviving after a given treatment. It is important, therefore, that articles should be cleaned if possible to remove dirt and reduce contamination before disinfection.

Disinfection is not instantaneous, and adequate contact time must be allowed. This varies from seconds to prolonged soaking, depending on the agent and the item involved.

An important and very variable factor in chemical disinfection is the user, and many studies have shown that human ignorance or error is responsible for ineffective clinical disinfection. The number of different chemical agents should be kept to a minimum, and clear instructions must be available on the preparation, circumstances for use, method of use and acceptable in-use life.

## Types of chemical disinfectant

Many types of chemicals have been used in disinfection, but relatively few are suitable for clinical use. Others, while effective, have been superseded by more modern agents. The properties of the chief types in current use are summarised here.

### Phenolic compounds

These are widely effective against bacteria and fungi but have a poorer action against viruses. Organic matter has little inactivating effect, and therefore they are suitable for use in dirty conditions or on soiled items, but not when there is contamination by blood. In-use concentration is usually 1% or 2% v/v for clean or dirty conditions, respectively.

Combination with a suitable detergent (anionic or non-ionic) aids penetration of dirt, but phenolic compounds are inactivated by cationic detergents. Clear, soluble phenolics (e.g. Stericol, Clearsol and similar products) are preferred to cruder coal tar derivatives, and are used for environmental disinfection in hospitals (e.g. contaminated areas and floors, operating rooms). 'Pine'-type products, although chemically related, are often poor disinfectants and are too easily inactivated to be generally accepted for clinical use.

### Chlorine compounds

These are very effective against most microorganisms, including viruses. They are usually the agent of choice when there is risk of viral infection, including blood spillages. However, they are more easily inactivated by organic matter than are phenolic compounds, and therefore items must be cleaned first, or sufficiently high concentrations must be used to compensate for the loss. It is important to

ensure adequate activity of the in-use solution, usually expressed in terms of percentage or p.p.m. (parts per million) of available chlorine. Solutions for routine clinical use should contain 1000 p.p.m. (0.1%) and strong solutions (e.g. for blood spillage) should contain 10 000 p.p.m. (1%) available chlorine. Products may be purchased as liquid concentrates, powders or tablets, which are diluted or dissolved in water. Typical chlorine-releasing agents employed as ingredients include hypochlorites and dichloroisocyanurates (NaDCC). Product information must enable accurate calculation of the available chlorine concentration.

*Sample calculation.* Thickened liquid concentrates (e.g. Domestos) typically contain 10% (100 000 p.p.m.) available chlorine. If diluted in water, a 1% v/v solution (1 volume disinfectant to 99 volumes water) would contain 100 000/100 = 1000 p.p.m. (0.1 %) available chlorine. A cautionary note on liquid concentrates: concentration varies between brands, and degeneration can occur in storage (Coates 1988).

Dichloroisocyanurate tablets are available; these have the advantages of long storage stability and simplicity of preparing in-use dilutions of various strengths as required (Coates 1985).

### Iodine compounds

Alcoholic solutions of iodine are effective disinfectants but cause tissue irritation and staining. Improved alternatives are available. Iodophors, which are organic complexes containing iodine (e.g. povidone-iodine), are less irritant and less likely to stain. Iodophors have a wide spectrum of activity against bacteria, fungi, viruses and, unusually, bacterial spores on prolonged contact. Iodophor preparations are used for skin and hand disinfection, and wound antisepsis.

### Alcohols

Ethyl and isopropyl alcohols have a wide and rapid antibacterial action, but a poorer action against some viruses. They are most effective in aqueous solution, typical concentrations being ethanol at 70% and isopropanol at 60–70%, although higher concentrations are sometimes used. They may be used for rapid disinfection of clean skin, hands and hard surfaces, and for combination with other antimicrobial agents. Ready-to-use disposable wipes containing isopropanol are available.

### Biguanide compounds

The most widely used of these is chlorhexidine (Hibitane), which is effective against Gram-positive and Gram-negative bacteria but poorly effective against viruses. Combination with alcohol increases its effectiveness and accelerates disinfection. It is inactivated by many materials, including soaps and anionic detergents, and cannot be recommended for general environmental use. However, it is widely used for skin and hand disinfection, as it shows very little toxicity and has both immediate and residual action. It is available as both aqueous and alcoholic preparations (e.g. Hibiscrub, Hibisol).

### Triclosan (2,4,4´-trichloro-2´-hydroxydiphenylether)

This is effective against Gram-positive and Gram-negative bacteria. It has little reported toxicity, and is available as both aqueous and alcoholic preparations (e.g. Aquasept, Manusept). Several products of this type have been reported to be effective in hand disinfection, but generally chlorhexidine or povidone-iodine preparations are better.

### Quaternary ammonium compounds

These form a group of chemicals that have both surfactant and disinfectant properties, to varying degrees. Although active against Gram-positive bacteria, they are poorly effective against other microorganisms, and are too easily inactivated for clinical use. However, cetrimide is one which, in combination with chlorhexidine, provides effective wound-cleansing agents (e.g. Savlon-type products).

### Glutaraldehyde

This has been used widely for cold 'sterilisation' in podiatry, although probably only disinfection was achieved in normal practice. It is a widely effective disinfectant, with good antiviral action, and is sporicidal in certain conditions. Thorough disinfection requires 20–30 minutes of immersion (sterilisation requires 3–10 hours). As it is an irritant, disinfected items should be rinsed in sterile water. Glutaraldehyde (e.g. Cidex) still has restricted specialised use in hospitals, but its routine use in podiatry cannot be recommended (Health and Safety Executive 1998). Alternative disinfection, or sterilisation by heat, should be used for items previously treated with glutaraldehyde.

### Hexachlorophane

This once-popular compound is effective against Gram-positive bacteria but poorly effective against other microorganisms. Chlorhexidine and povidone-iodine products are more generally effective after single or repeated applications, and therefore are to be preferred.

## Disinfection of specific items

Items suitable for heat disinfection include cleaning utensils (especially if used in operating rooms or on contaminated areas), routine laundry, instrument brushes, reagent bottles before refilling, containers for antiseptics, general-purpose bowls and containers for non-sterile cotton balls, etc. Sterilisation may be preferable for some of these (e.g. instrument brushes). In the absence of sophisticated disinfection facilities, cloths and mops may be cleaned and then placed in a container to which boiling water is added, and kept immersed for at least 10 minutes before drying and storing dry. Alternatively, after cleaning they can be immersed in a 1% phenolic or chlorine-based disinfectant for 30 minutes, and then rinsed and stored dry. Note that some materials, such as plastics, may inactivate disinfectants, and that utensils should be stored dry, not in disinfectant. Clinical laundry can be cleaned in an ordinary automatic machine using a prewash followed by a wash at the highest temperature setting, unless known contamination by HBV or HCV is present.

Floors and surfaces contaminated with tissue other than blood should be cleaned and then disinfected with a 1% phenolic or 0.1% chlorine-releasing agent. Ideally, blood spillages should be disinfected before cleaning to counter any risk of hepatitis viruses and HIV; disposable gloves should be worn and the spillage covered with paper towels or other absorbent, disposable material. A chlorine-releasing agent (10 000 p.p.m. available chlorine) is then poured on and left for at least 10 minutes. The area is then cleaned, again using disposable materials. All items (gloves, towels, etc.) are then disposed of as contaminated waste. Alternatively, purpose-made packs of granular NaDCC or other antiviral agents are available for wet-spillage treatment, in which case the manufacturer's instructions should be followed. Hands should always be washed after dealing with spillages.

Small areas of clean impervious surfaces, such as trolley tops, foot rests, adjustable lamps and other hand-contact surfaces in the chair's vicinity, can be disinfected with agents that are unsuitable or uneconomic for wider environmental use. Although 1% phenolics could be used, alcohols or alcoholic chlorhexidine, as wipes or sprays, are faster acting and drying and likely to be more convenient for use between patients (e.g. Alcowipes and Azospray type products). Cartridges of local anaesthetic should be wiped with alcohol before use. Handpieces are potential vehicles of infection between patients via the operator's hands, and ideally should be sterilised. If disinfection is used, manufacturers may advise on appropriate methods; alternatively, clean thoroughly and then disinfect with alcoholic chlorhexidine.

## Skin disinfection

The hands of staff and the skin of patients both require adequate decontamination, the degree necessary being dictated by the circumstances. Whatever method is used, effectiveness depends largely on the care and thoroughness of the operator. Handwashing facilities vary, but taps operated without hand contact (e.g. foot operated) are best, and if ordinary taps are fitted they should be turned off using a paper towel.

### Hands

The main purpose of routine handwashing is to remove transients acquired from previous contacts, particularly patients. Although loosely adhering transients can be removed by washing with ordinary soaps, detergent/disinfectant preparations containing chlorhexidine, povidone-iodine or Triclosan are more effective, and on repeated use they progressively reduce the more accessible flora. Intervening washes with ordinary products eliminate this residual benefit, and, therefore, as daily case loads may include treatments that require hand disinfection, it is sensible to use disinfectant preparations for all clinic handwashing. However, choice of agent is less important than thoroughness of application (Ayliffe et al 1990, 1999). If hands are visibly clean, rapid and highly effective disinfection between patients or during procedures can be achieved with alcoholic disinfectant preparations. Handwashing with non-disinfectant products is not adequate for surgery, invasive techniques, treatment of damaged tissue or dressing changes.

Further reduction of skin contamination is required for some procedures (e.g. nail surgery). The aim is to reduce flora as much as possible on the hands and the forearms, from where organisms may also be shed. Initially, the hands and forearms are subjected to prolonged double washing with detergent/disinfectant preparations (as above), attention also being paid to cleaning the nails and nail folds. If brushing is employed to remove loose skin squames, it should be done only at the start of a clinical session. Use of an alcoholic disinfectant preparation after washing will increase the degree of this initial disinfection. For subsequent cases, these alcoholic preparations alone, well rubbed in, are very effective, although washing is necessary if hands are soiled. Note that hand disinfection is not an alternative, but an addition, to wearing gloves for aseptic procedures.

Hand cream may be employed to offset the drying effects of disinfectant products, but it should be one that is compatible, as commercial products often inhibit disinfection; pharmacists can advise on suitable products.

Recently there has been debate and discussion regarding the use of clinical dress that has sleeves reaching the wrist (Department of Health 2008). It is considered that the dress material is a possible vehicle for transporting flora. At this stage no national guidelines have been formulated, but some NHS Trusts in the UK are implementing the wearing of clinical clothing such as 'scrub suits' for all clinical procedures. This facilitates handwashing extending to the elbows.

### Patients' skin

If possible, intact skin should be cleaned before disinfection. As immediate and effective disinfection is required, alcoholic skin disinfectants are the agents of choice. Chlorhexidine is less likely to cause any reaction, although povidone-iodine has wider antimicrobial action; normally either is suitable. Friction is an important factor in skin disinfection; rubbing the site thoroughly with the agent (subject to patient comfort) is more effective than merely wiping or spraying.

Combined detergents/disinfectants (e.g. Savlon) may be used for damaged skin that requires cleaning. Injections (e.g. local anaesthetic) present little danger of infection but skin is often prepared by swabbing with alcohol.

## Sterilisation

Of the many methods of sterilisation available, only steam at increased pressure and dry heat are likely to be used directly by the podiatrist.

### Steam at increased pressure

This is generally recommended for use on clinical materials whenever possible (*British Pharmacopoeia* 1998). Steam hot enough to sterilise necessitates pressure vessels, termed 'sterilisers' or 'autoclaves'. Saturated steam sterilises the articles it contacts, the time required depending on the temperature. Minimum treatments required are:

- 15 minutes at 121°C
- 10 minutes at 126°C
- 3 minutes at 134°C.

Additional time must be allowed for heating to sterilisation temperature and for cooling after sterilisation. Saturated steam can be obtained only in the absence of air. In sophisticated equipment, air is evacuated, enabling penetration of steam even into wrapped porous materials (e.g. dressings), and evacuation after sterilisation facilitates the drying of such items. Basic units affordable by many practitioners rely on simple displacement of air by steam generated within the steriliser. Removal of air, steam penetration and subsequent drying are, therefore, not as efficient in these models. However, these small sterilisers are suitable for rapid sterilisation of instruments, either unwrapped or in steam-permeable containers. When removed, instruments must be covered immediately to prevent contamination. A sterile cloth may be used, or a lid sterilised separately in the same cycle could be clipped onto the instrument tray.

Where practicable, central sterile supplies units or similar local services should be used as a first-choice option, as these facilities should be able to guarantee sterility of products and incorporate a total quality management system. However, where such a service is not available or is not practicable, the minimum standard for clinical practice in podiatry is that instruments must be sterilised using steam pressure sterilisers. Advice on the purchase and operation of bench-top steam sterilisers is available (Medical Devices Agency 1996). In the UK, The Pressure Systems and Transportable Gas Containers Regulations 1989 set out the legal requirements for the monitoring and validation of sterilisers and must be followed. To help practitioners to comply with these regulations Health Technical Memorandum 2010 (Department of Health 1994) provides guidelines governing the maintenance, monitoring and validation of steam sterilisers. Following these guidelines will enable practitioners to demonstrate clear evidence of maintenance, monitoring and validation of their sterilisation process and procedures. The daily checks recommended by Health Technical Memorandum 2010 for sterilisers include undertaking an operational cycle at the beginning of the working day. The cycle may contain a load, provided such a load is consistently used for each daily cheek. There are also recommended weekly, quarterly and annual checks to ensure the efficacy, efficiency and maintenance of sterilisers.

To ensure the effective functioning of bench-top sterilisers there are a number of additional measures that practitioners must ensure are carried out. All instruments must be decontaminated prior to sterilisation using ultrasonic cleaning or some other suitable method. The reservoir of the steriliser must be emptied and cleaned regularly, refilling it with sterile water. The internal surfaces of the chamber of the steriliser should be cleaned using sterile water for irrigation and a lint-free cloth. The sterilising chamber should be emptied and a visual inspection of the water made to determine its colour and the presence of any debris and contaminants. Complying with these requirements will demonstrate that the instruments used have undergone a satisfactory sterilisation process. This is reinforced by the introduction of a system of audit of these processes, with documentation to show that all instruments have undergone a sterilisation cycle.

In the UK there are further legal requirements for practitioners to conform to a range of legislative requirements that come under the umbrella of the Health and Safety at Work etc. Act (1974), The Management of Health and Safety at Work Regulations (1992), The Pressure Systems and Transportable Gas Containers Regulations (1989) and The Provision and Use of Work Equipment Regulations (1992). It is a requirement of The Pressure Systems and Transportable Gas Containers Regulations (1989) that practitioners using bench-top autoclaves have third-party insurance cover and that the equipment is inspected regularly. Additional health and safety information relating to the use of bench top pressure autoclaves is given in Chapter 29.

### Dry heat

An electrical, fan-assisted, hot-air oven may be used. Microorganisms are more resistant to dry heat than to steam, and therefore higher temperatures are required for sterilisation within a practicable time (e.g. a minimum of 30 minutes at 180°C) (*British Pharmacopoeia* 1998). All items must reach sterilisation temperature before the holding time commences. As heating time varies with the load, it is often underestimated, especially for items that are wrapped or in containers; for example, individually wrapped small instruments require about 15 minutes of initial heat penetration time. Dry heat has the advantage that instruments can be packaged and it is suitable for non-stainless steel, but the longer cycle time is a disadvantage.

Sterilisers must be of a suitable design (British Medical Association 1989) and must be regularly serviced and tested. On a more frequent basis, chemical indicators that change colour when exposed to specific temperatures for sufficient time (available from medical equipment suppliers) are useful to detect failure to achieve sterilising conditions, although they are not an absolute guarantee of sterility. Such indicators are available for steam and dry heat, and their use is recommended, particularly for hot-air sterilisers, where it is very difficult to predict the time required for packaged items.

Items that should be sterilised include scalpels, files, burrs, forceps, probes, nail clippers, tissue nippers, drill handpieces (if suitable), scissors, cryosurgical probes and instrument brushes. For materials that are obtained presterilised (e.g. dressing packs) it is important to check the integrity of packaging and the sterility indicator if present, discarding any items that are suspect.

### Glass bead sterilisers

These units reach very high temperatures (235–250°C) and very short process times are suggested by manufacturers, but note that, as only part of an instrument is treated, use must be immediate and sterilising conditions cannot be checked directly. Overall, their use cannot be recommended in a modern fully effective sterilisation programme and Medical Devices Agency (1998) advises that these units cannot give the quality assurance of sterility now required for podiatric practice.

## FURTHER MICROBIOLOGICAL ASPECTS OF CLINICAL WORK

### Protective clothing

Any serious attempt at aseptic technique precludes contact of the practitioner's bare hands with damaged skin or exposed tissue (i.e.

'no-touch' techniques should be used). Routine wearing of sterile single-use gloves for such procedures should be adopted, with satisfactory tactile sensitivity achieved by the choice of an appropriate glove size and material. Apart from patient protection, there is the risk of contamination of podiatrists' skin by HBV, HCV or HIV, and gloves should always be worn, after a suitable and sufficient risk assessment, for giving injections, changing dressings, cleaning wounds and for any invasive procedure. Cuts or abrasions on the hands should be covered by waterproof plasters, even when gloves are worn. Hands require washing after gloved procedures, as not all gloves are structurally perfect.

The wearing of masks is unnecessary for minor procedures, including routine dressing changes. Situations requiring masks include nail drilling (for the podiatrist's protection) and nail surgery (where effective masks to filter/deflect organisms from the podiatrist's mouth away from the operation site are necessary). Masks must be discarded after each use and not worn around the neck to be donned at intervals. Note that drilling of mycotic nails is unwise; not all debris is removed by the drill vacuum and significant amounts escape to contaminate the clinical environment and the practitioner.

The usual clinical coat is satisfactory for many procedures but needs protection when significant debris is expected, particularly from an infected patient, to prevent cross-infection occurring via the coat. A gown, plastic apron or adequately sized impermeable paper sheet or drape would serve the purpose. Purpose-made gowns or suits of appropriate material should be used for surgical procedures, and hair should be completely covered with a surgical cap. If surgical footwear is worn, avoid contamination of previously disinfected hands.

## Aseptic technique

Initial disinfection of the patient's skin should be followed by the use of sterile instruments whenever skin is penetrated, accidental breach is likely, or previously wounded tissue is being treated. Other materials used on or near such vulnerable areas (e.g. dressings) must also be sterile. Single-use sachets of antiseptics, etc., are preferred, but if communal ones are used individual quantities should be dispensed without contaminating the remainder. For example, small quantities can be poured from bottles into sterile pots, taking care not to touch the pot with the outside of the bottle, or solutions can be transferred using bulb pipettes, which should be disposable or cleaned and disinfected before reuse.

## Sterile fields

A sterile field is an area in which contamination is kept to an absolute minimum, although it is unlikely to be fully sterile in the microbiological sense. Such a field may be established by starting with a sterile surface and thereafter taking every care to avoid contamination of that area. The surface must not be touched by bare hands, and any necessary items are transferred aseptically onto it. The initial surface may be formed by a sterile drape/towel, or the unfolded inner (sterile) wrapping of a dressing pack, placed on a disinfected trolley top. If pack wrapping is used it must be unfolded by the corners, taking care not to reach over the contents as they are uncovered because contaminants are shed from skin and clothing. Additional items may be slid gently from their sterile wrapping onto the sterile field, or transferred using sterile forceps. Outer wrappings are always contaminated and should not be opened near the sterile field.

Sterile instruments should be arranged conveniently within reach in the field. After use (i.e. when they are contaminated) they should be placed elsewhere for disposal, or on a separate secondary field (e.g. clearly to one side) for possible reuse, but not back among sterile items. (Note that reuse on a patient may be contraindicated, for example if an infected or dirty lesion is being treated an instrument used earlier may reintroduce contamination into cleaned tissue.) It may prove convenient to use a sterile, empty steriliser tray as a secondary field, which can be used later to transport used instruments. Contaminated disposable items such as swabs should be disposed of immediately and should not re-enter the sterile field. Overall, there should be a one-way movement from sterility to patient to disposal or secondary field.

## Dressing changes

Hand disinfection is necessary before commencing dressing removal, after removal of the old dressing and after completion of the treatment, and at any time during the procedure when hands become contaminated. The old dressing is removed using disposable gloves (or forceps), which are immediately carefully disposed of with the dressing. After hand disinfection, sterile gloves are worn for the remainder of the treatment.

Microbiologically clean wounds should need no further cleaning, but practice varies. Sterile saline may be used, or antiseptic preparations for contaminated areas as considered necessary. After treatment, all used and unused materials from dressing packs should be disposed of, as they are no longer sterile.

## Waste disposal

Clinical waste should be placed carefully in bags and sealed before removal to prevent contamination of the area. Bags should be colourcoded to distinguish ordinary from contaminated waste (e.g. used dressings). There is no universal code, although yellow is used in the UK to denote contaminated waste for incineration, and practitioners should check local policy. Bags should not be overfilled and must be removed from the clinical area frequently, at least daily. They should be stored safely and protected from damage, until removed by disposal personnel.

Reusable instruments should be bagged or containerised for return to a central sterile supplies unit, or cleaned before return, or cleaned and resterilised in-house, depending on individual arrangements. Disposal of sharps requires great care to protect the practitioner and others from the risk of HBV, HCV and HIV infection; they must be discarded into a rigid container meeting approved specifications such as those given in BS7320:1990 (British Standards Institution 1990), and sent for incineration.

## Operating rooms

The design of operating facilities has evolved essentially for the needs of hospital surgery. Such facilities, with positive-pressure, high-efficiency filtered ventilation systems and various ancillary support areas, may sometimes be available to hospital practitioners, and indeed access to these may be necessary for the treatment of high-risk patients. However, the infection rates associated with minor surgery and ambulatory care services are low, and such complex facilities will not always be necessary.

In general surgery, airborne contamination appears to have little responsibility for postoperative sepsis (Ayliffe & Lowbury 1982, Ayliffe et al 1999), and during minor operations of short duration true airborne contamination is unlikely. The greatest risk will be from staff and the standards of their aseptic techniques but, nevertheless, adequate ventilation is important to reduce contamination dispersed from personnel while minimising entry of airborne contamination from outside. If extraction alone is used, there is a risk that extracted air will be replaced by contaminated air from surrounding areas (i.e. an inflow of 'dirty' air to the operation area). A compromise would be extraction to the outside in combination with sufficient filtered air inlets at selected sites to replace the extracted air. Practitioners intending to expand significantly into surgery should seek expert advice on their particular facilities to ensure that adequate safe ventilation is provided.

Operating rooms should be clearly separated from the general clinic and access restricted to essential personnel. They must be large enough to allow unimpeded movement without contact contamination from other people, furniture and surfaces. Only essential equipment and surgical supplies should be stored in the room, and their use should be restricted to surgery and associated procedures, such as immediate instrument sterilisation. Initial interview and preparation of the patient should take place elsewhere, and adequate facilities for scrubbing up and dressing of surgical staff must be provided.

Thorough cleaning of general surfaces should be carried out daily and the floor cleaned after each session; routine disinfection of floors should not be necessary. Known occurrences of contamination, especially by tissue or blood, do require disinfection. Overcrowding and vigorous movements should be avoided in operating rooms, as they increase airborne contamination. Clinical waste must be removed carefully to avoid contamination of the room or associated clean facilities.

## Laboratory specimens

Podiatrists could make more use of the expertise of microbiology laboratories. Laboratory investigation of samples from skin, nails or infected wounds can confirm infection and/or identify the pathogen, thus aiding the choice of the most effective patient management. In fungal infections, where symptoms are often insufficiently specific, definitive diagnosis can only be achieved by microscopy and culture techniques.

If possible, samples should be taken before commencing antimicrobial treatment, as this may inhibit the isolation of pathogens. The receiving laboratory will advise on containers, and packaging for samples. Usually, swabs from wounds are collected into capped containers, while skin scrapings and nail clippings are collected in paper sachets that maintain dry conditions and prevent overgrowth by saprophytes. As much material as possible should be collected to increase the probability of isolating the pathogen. Specimens must be taken carefully, avoiding contamination of self, the clinical surroundings and the outside of the container. As much clinical information as possible should be provided to aid investigation.

## INFECTION-CONTROL POLICIES

Any practice, large or small, should have a written control policy. This should include instructions on the sterilisation of various items, the use and concentrations of disinfectants or antiseptics, waste disposal, the treatment of spillages, etc. For the individual practitioner this will serve as a useful aide memoire, while in larger units all staff should be able to consult it for information on agreed procedures. Health service and hospital podiatrists should ensure compliance with the local health authority or hospital policy on infection control. In units with several staff, there should be a designated person with responsibility for implementing and monitoring the control measures.

Cleaning staff must be given clear instructions on methods required and adequate facilities, and they should be given time to discharge their duties effectively.

Elaborate infection surveillance systems are not necessary, in view of the low risk associated with well-run ambulatory care facilities. However, full note should be taken of any infections that apparently result from podiatric treatment, and the overall incidence of these should be reviewed periodically. An unduly high incidence should alert staff to review control measures, and seek expert advice if necessary.

Infection-control personnel are employed by health authorities and hospitals, and these local sources are the best initial point of contact for any practitioner. Much published information is also available, including material from public health laboratories and government departments, and it is continually being augmented.

## REFERENCES

Anon. 1987 Control of cross infection. Journal of the Society of Chiropodists 42:115.

Ayliffe GAJ, Lowbury EJL 1982 Airborne infection in hospital. Journal of Hospital Infection 3:217.

Ayliffe GAJ, Collins BJ, Taylor LJ 1990 Hospital-acquired infection: principles and prevention, 2nd edn. Butterworth, Sevenoaks.

Ayliffe GAJ, Taylor LJ, Babb J 1999 Hospital-acquired infection: principles and prevention, 3rd edn. Butterworth Heinemann, Sevenoaks.

Ayliffe GAJ, Fraise AP, Geddes AM, Mitchell K (eds) 2000 Control of hospital infection – a practical handbook, 4th edn. Arnold, London.

Babb JR 1993 Methods of cleaning and disinfection. Central Service 4:227–237.

Bennett JV, Brachman PS (eds) 1986 Hospital infections, 2nd edn. Little Brown, Boston, MA.

British Medical Association 1989 A code of practice for sterilisation of instruments and control of cross infection. BMA, London.

British Pharmacopoeia 1998 HMSO, London.

British Standards Institution 1986a BS 5283: Glossary of terms relating to disinfectants. BSI, London.

British Standards Institution 1986b BS 5415-5412.2:Supplement No. 1: Safety of electrical motor-operated industrial and commercial cleaning appliances. Particular requirements. Specification for type H industrial vacuum cleaners for dusts hazardous to health. BSI, London.

British Standards Institution 1990 BS 7320 Specification for sharps containers. BSI, London.

British Standards Institution 1993 BS 2745: Washer disinfectors for medical purposes, Parts 1–3. BSI, London.

Burrow G 2004 Core update in infection control. The Society of Chiropodists and Podiatrists, London. Available at: http://www.feetforlife.org (19 September 2009).

Coates D 1985 A comparison of sodium hypochlorite and sodium dichloroisocyanurate products. Journal of Hospital Infection 6:31.

Coates D 1988 Household bleaches and HIV. Journal of Hospital Infection 11:95.

Department of Health 1994 Sterilizers. Health Technical Memorandum No. 2010. DoH, London.

Department of Health 1998 Guidance for clinical health care workers: protection against infection with blood borne viruses. HSC 1998/063. Department of Health, London.

Department of Health 2008 Clean, safe care: reducing infections and saving lives. Ref. 9278. DoH, London.

Dinsdale P 2004 Hidden threat. Public Health News 27 September.

Health and Safety Executive 1974 Health and Safety at Work etc Act 1974. HSE, London.

Health and Safety Executive 1998 Chemical hazard alert notice – glutaraldehyde. Chan. 7 (rev). HSE, London.

Lowbury EJL, Ayliffe GAJ, Geddes AM, Williams JD (eds) 1981 Control of hospital infection – a practical handbook, 2nd edn. Chapman & Hall, London.

Maurer IM 1985 Hospital hygiene, 3rd edn. Edward Arnold, London.

Medical Devices Agency 1996 The purchase, operation and maintenance of benchtop steam sterilisers. Device Bulletin 9605 (2nd reprint 1997). Medical Devices Agency, London.

Medical Devices Agency 1998 The validation and periodic testing of benchtop vacuum steam sterilisers. Device Bulletin 9804. Medical Devices Agency, London.

Meers PD 1983 Ventilation in operating rooms. British Medical Journal 286:244.

The Management of Health and Safety at Work Regulations 1992 Statutory Instrument No. 2051. HMSO, London.

The Pressure Systems and Transportable Gas Containers Regulations 1989 Statutory Instrument No. 2169. HMSO, London.

The Provision and Use of Work Equipment Regulations 1992 Statutory Instrument No. 2932. HMSO, London.

## FURTHER READING

Adler MW (ed.) 2001 ABC of AIDS, 5th edn. BMJ Books, London.

Burton GRW, Engelkirk PG 2004 Microbiology for the health sciences, 7th edn. Lippincott Williams & Wilkins, Baltimore, OH.

Fraise AP, Lambert PA, Maillard J-Y (eds) 2004 Russell, Hugo & Ayliffe's Principles and practice of disinfection, preservation and sterilisation, 4th edn. Blackwell, Oxford.

Gardner JF, Peel MM 1991 Introduction to sterilisation, disinfection and infection control, 2nd edn. Churchill Livingstone, Melbourne.

Meers P, McPherson M, Sedgwick J 1997 Infection control in healthcare, 2nd edn. Nelson Thornes, Edinburgh.

NHS Decontamination Programme: http://www.dh.gov.uk/en/Managingyourorganisation/Leadershipandmanagement/Healthcareenvironment/NHSDecontaminationProgramme/index.htm (19 September Nov 2009). Contains valuable information and links on decontamination.

Wilson J 2000 Clinical microbiology – an introduction for health care professionals. Harcourt, London.

# Chapter 25

# Medical emergencies in podiatry

*Jonathan McGhie*

## KEY WORDS

Medical assessment
Medical emergencies
Clinical monitoring resuscitation
Anaphylaxis
Local anaesthetic toxicity

Medical emergencies in the daily practice of podiatry are likely to be rare, but there are some predictable and unpredictable medical events that will occur during clinical procedures and test even the most experienced practitioner.

Predictable events are likely be those related to known comorbidities of the patient. Of these morbidities, cardiac disease and diabetic glycaemic control issues are particularly important. Unpredictable events may range from simple and recoverable situations, such as vasovagal faints, to more serious and difficult situations to manage, such as cardiac arrest and local anaesthetic toxicity. Prevention and avoidance of these events is always preferable to dealing with the consequences once they occur, and this can be achieved through careful clinical assessment to identify 'at-risk individuals. This, in conjunction with the use of good clinical monitoring, will detect untoward events earlier or avoid them entirely.

This chapter summarises both the more common and the rarer clinical situations that practitioners may face in daily practice, and highlights the red-flag signs and symptoms that should alert the podiatrist to delve further into the patient's medical and surgical history and monitor them more closely. Treatment pathways are outlined, and sources for protocols to deal with some of the more life-threatening emergencies that can occur are given.

## CLINICAL ASSESSMENT

The primary focus of the consultation by the podiatrist will relate to the podiatric complaint and the associated treatment options. However, it is important that an holistic picture of the patient's general health is gained. It is worthwhile asking a simple open-ended question such as 'Do you have any other medical problems that you get treatment for?' This can often result in a useful barrage of medical conditions and drug treatments, particularly in the elderly patient. Frequently, patients view the condition for which they have sought treatment, or are receiving treatment, in isolation, and will not freely volunteer any other disease or medical information that they view as unrelated to the consultation in hand. In this situation more direct questioning is needed, and practitioners should use their experience

**Table 25.1** Important medical conditions and symptoms to check for in the initial consultation

| System and conditions | Worrying symptoms |
|---|---|
| *Cardiovascular* | |
| Ischaemic heart disease/ myocardial infarction | Chest pain, shortness of breath on exertion |
| Hypertension | Poor control (diastolic > 95 mmHg, systolic > 160 mmHg) |
| Dysrhythmias | Slow heart rate (<60 bpm, beta blocker therapy) Faints, palpitations, shortness of breath |
| Valve surgery/cardiac stents | Check anticoagulation status |
| *Respiratory* | |
| Asthma | Shortness of breath, chest infection |
| Chronic obstructive pulmonary disease (COPD) | Current chest infection, extreme breathlessness |
| *Endocrine* | |
| Diabetes | Poor glucose control; postpone if blood glucose > 11 |
| Thyroid disease | Uncontrolled thyroid disease |
| *Hepatic/renal* | |
| Dysfunction or chronic disease | Will affect drug clearance, dosing |
| *Central nervous system* | |
| Stroke/transient ischaemic attack (TIA) | Check anticoagulant status |
| Epilepsy | Recent or uncontrolled seizures |

**Table 25.2** Baseline monitor references

| Monitor | Normal range in health |
|---|---|
| ECG | Rhythm: sinus, or sinus arrhythmia. Rate: 60–100 bpm |
| NIBP | Systolic: 80–150 mmHg Diastolic: 60–90 mmHg |
| $SpO_2$ | >95% |

## CLINICAL MONITORING

Good practice dictates that appropriate clinical monitoring should be instigated before, during and after procedural work. The duration and depth of this monitoring should be guided by local protocols and national guidelines, to which the practitioner should adhere. Deviation from these recommendations should only occur when clinical judgement and patient benefit dictate that the standard of monitoring is unnecessary. In these situations, for medicolegal reasons, the practitioner should justify and document the reasoning behind the change in practice.

If any incision or injection is required during the procedure then a baseline heart rate and blood pressure reading should be recorded before commencing treatment. In procedures where the patient remains conscious, the best monitor is always the patient themselves. The practitioner should continue verbal contact with the patient throughout the procedure, both to reassure the patient and to ensure that the intervention is being well tolerated, but also to enquire about any cardiac or respiratory phenomena that may be developing. In general, continuous echocardiography (ECG) monitoring for heart rate and rhythm, with non-invasive blood pressure (NIBP) monitoring on a 3–5 minute cycle should be used routinely during procedural work. This is especially true if there is any underlying cardiovascular disease, a history of syncope or if the patient's communication level makes clinical assessment of symptoms or signs difficult. If there is underlying respiratory disease then oxygen saturation ($SpO_2$) finger-probe monitoring should also be used. Postprocedure monitoring should measure a static blood pressure at 5–15 minute intervals until the patient is fit to leave the recovery area. ECG and $SpO_2$ monitoring can be discontinued unless symptoms suggest otherwise. Table 25.2 lists the usual accepted reference range for these monitors. Clinical values outside these ranges should stimulate further medical investigation and treatment before procedures commence.

This level of monitoring will facilitate the detection of cardiorespiratory events, including; anaphylaxis, accidental intravenous local anaesthetic injection, cardiac arrest, slow heart rate (during vasovagal syncope) and hypoxic changes. Early detection of these changes will facilitate immediate treatment to prevent spiralling deterioration of the clinical situation.

## EMERGENCY DRUGS AND EQUIPMENT

Although rare, the possibility of incidental or iatrogenic cardiac arrest exists when doing procedural work, particularly when using local anaesthetics. The ability to provide basic or advanced cardiopulmonary resuscitation (CPR) on site is needed. An emergency trolley kept in an accessible location must always be available (Fig. 25.1). It should be regularly checked and kept stocked to provide immediate

to gain information on any specific diseases of concern. As a minimum requirement, this should include questions on whether any of the following are present: heart disease, respiratory disease, metabolic complaints (of which diabetes is the most common), liver or kidney disorders and drug allergies. Table 25.1 lists some significant medical conditions and important symptoms to exclude before commencing treatment.

A list of pharmacological treatments related to these conditions should be sought and an enquiry made as to any recently commenced cardiac drugs or anticoagulation therapy. Often polypharmacy and memory impairment, due to disease, age or drug-induced side-effects, mean many patients forget their current drug treatments and doses. In this situation a prescription list, or the drugs themselves, can be most useful.

This baseline assessment of medical conditions and current therapies is so important in order to ensure the patient is optimally managed prior to commencing any treatment strategy. Poorly controlled systemic disease can result in poor wound healing, infection and bleeding problems, which may be avoidable with good holistic care. Any doubts a practitioner has about a patient's medical care or their compliance with therapy that you feel may compromise treatment options should result in a frank discussion with the patient and their primary care physician or hospital specialist, which may help to coordinate and better manage the treatment pathway.

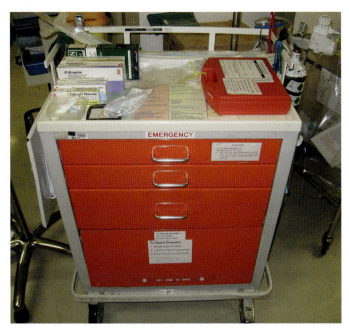

Figure 25.1 An emergency trolley.

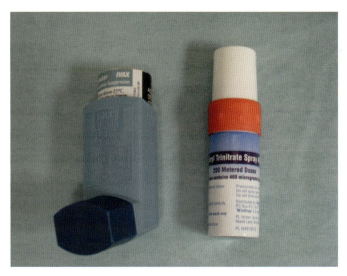

Figure 25.2 A GTN spray and sublingual tablets for angina.

airway and intravenous-access devices, as well as fluids and drugs to fulfil resuscitation protocols. Pipeline or cylinder oxygen (depending on the location of the treatment area), atropine and epinephrine (adrenaline) mini-jets and a defibrillation machine should be available. In addition, evidence for the use of Intralipid in resuscitation following local anaesthetic toxicity is increasing, and a bag of Intralipid should also be kept onsite; its use is discussed later in this chapter.

## PREDICTABLE EVENTS

### Cardiovascular: angina (ischaemic heart disease)/myocardial infarction

Coronary artery disease is the progressive occlusion of the blood supply to the heart by atheroma. This classically manifests as chest pain radiating to the left arm and jaw, with a central chest heaviness. Generally brought on by exertion, it is predictable to the patient who will generally know his or her exercise tolerance. In unstable angina the symptoms can occur spontaneously, without any provocation or warning. This occurs pathologically due to clot-type embolic phenomena. In complete occlusion of the blood vessel the heart tissue infarcts (myocardial infarct). This usually presents with a more extreme form of the angina pain, commonly with sweating and nausea, but it can occur silently without any symptoms of pain, particularly in diabetic patients. The anxiety and stress associated with a procedure or an injection can precipitate angina symptoms in some individuals.

When treating a patient with known heart disease, baseline angina symptoms and their frequency should be noted. Patients with unstable or spontaneous symptoms are at higher risk of having a heart attack and should be fully managed medically before commencing any procedures for non-life-threatening illnesses. The patient's usual medication and whether they use a GTN spray or sublingual tablet (Fig. 25.2) for their angina should be recorded.

Should an angina attack occur, all procedural work should be suspended, the patient supported to a recumbent position, and oxygen offered if breathlessness exists. Immediate use of the patient's own GTN or nitrate tablet should be offered, and this should settle symptoms within a few minutes. Repeated GTN can be used but may cause headache and hypotension (low blood pressure). If pain is unrelieved by GTN or continues beyond the patient's usual duration of symptoms the procedure should be abandoned and the patient sent to hospital immediately for medical assessment. If symptoms settle predictably it is at the discretion of the operator whether or not to proceed further. In general, it is wise to postpone therapy until the patient is more stable, so a return appointment may be the best course of action.

If a heart attack is suspected, oral crushed aspirin 300 mg should be given and an emergency ambulance called. A delay in diagnosis and treatment will worsen outcome. ECG and NIBP monitoring should be maintained until paramedics arrive. CPR may be required if cardiovascular collapse occurs.

Following a myocardial infarction a period of 6 weeks to 6 months should elapse before the patient undergoes any elective procedures, as during this time they remain at high risk of further cardiac events.

### CASE STUDY 25.1 WORSENING SYMPTOMS

A 70-year-old man with ischaemic heart disease (IHD), hypertension and diabetes attends for his initial consultation. He is flustered and sweating. He was worried about missing the appointment and is apprehensive about the treatment options. Not long into the consultation he complains of chest pain and shortness of breath. You measure his blood pressure – it is 140/90 and his heart rate is 90 bpm. He tells you his last blood glucose check an hour ago was 9. He is sweating and holding his chest.

#### QUESTIONS

1. How do you manage this?
2. What is the likely problem?
3. What do you do next?

#### ANSWERS

1. Call for help, the situation is likely to deteriorate. Assuming he remains conscious, give the patient some oxygen to breathe and sit or lie him down to rest. Continue monitoring his pulse and blood pressure. Should he lose consciousness proceed through the basic

life support (BLS) protocol. Encourage the patient to use his own GTN spray. If this does not quickly ease the symptoms, prepare to transport the patient to an acute hospital environment for monitoring and treatment.

2. The diagnosis is likely to be **angina** or **acute myocardial infarction** (MI). The latter is to be suspected if the episode is more severe and long lasting than a normal angina attack, and response to the GTN may be only temporary. If MI is suspected and time permits, give the patient some oral aspirin prior to hospital transfer.

3. Postpone the consultation and treatment until the patient has been investigated further and his cardiac therapies are better optimised.

## Hypertension

Current recommendations suggest treatment of hypertension when the blood pressure exceeds 150/90. Frequently, patients will have diet modifications or drug therapy initiated to achieve this target. Anxiety before procedures, or during the blood-pressure assessment itself, can transiently elevate blood pressure. Repeat measurements in this circumstance can satisfy the operator that it is purely an artificially elevated reading. However, if the baseline blood pressure persists above a systolic pressure of >160 mmHg or a diastolic pressure of > 95 mmHg treatment should be postponed and the patient referred to their general practitioner for further assessment and treatment. If the patient is already maximally managed then it may be acceptable to proceed, but poorly controlled blood pressure puts the patient at risk of stroke, cardiac and renal complications.

Beta blocker therapy is commonly used to treat high blood pressure. This reduces the heart rate and occasionally can result in the heart rate slowing excessively. If the baseline heart rate is below 60 bpm, postponing treatment is advised until the beta blocker therapy is adjusted.

## Dysrhythmia

Normal heart function relies on a coordinated beat of the heart chambers to optimally move blood round the body. In addition, this beating is coordinated with the breathing cycle to maximise oxygenation of the blood. When the electrical pathways are chemically or physically disrupted, abnormal heart rhythms occur. Patients may be asymptomatic or describe palpitations, faints or shortness of breath. Patients who are susceptible to abnormal heart conduction may develop an altered ECG during a procedure. Practitioners should be wary of these changes and introduce cardiovascular support as described above for symptomatic angina.

One of the commonest arrhythmias is atrial fibrillation. This, and other chronic abnormal heart rhythms, often necessitate anticoagulation to reduce the risk of stroke. Enquires should be made as to which blood-thinning drug the patient is taking, as it will increase bleeding risk during procedural work. Aspirin can usually be continued, while warfarin and clopidogrel should be temporarily ceased or changed for short-acting heparins if the patient is at high risk. Liaison with the patient's medical practitioner will be required if drug use is to be suspended around the time of the surgery, so that a balance can be found between surgical bleeding and stroke risk.

## Heart valves/stents

With improved surgical techniques and stent development, more patients with coronary artery and heart disease undergo cardiac procedures that leave non-biological tissue in the patient. These valves and stents often require permanent anticoagulation to prevent thrombosis. Should any procedures need to be done in these patients, careful assessment should be made of their anticoagulation medication and, as outlined for arrhythmia, close liaison with the patient's hospital specialist or general practitioner is essential. Anticoagulation therapy for newer drug-eluting stents must be continued for 12 months, and therefore non-essential treatments should be postponed during this period.

Antibiotic cover is also required in these patients, as the implanted stents and valves can harbour any bacteria that gain entry to the bloodstream during procedural work. The BNF (*British National Formulary*) or equivalent will give up-to-date guidance on appropriate antibiotic prophylaxis.

## Respiratory

### Asthma

This reversible disease of the airway presents with wheeze, cough and shortness of breath. It is a chronic illness, with periods of flare and control, but most patients will have an awareness of what exacerbates the condition and knowledge of how best to manage the symptoms. Conventionally this is done with inhalers that deliver a bronchodilator (salbutamol) to open up the airways (commonly known as the blue 'reliever') and a steroid that reduces inflammation (also known as the brown 'preventer') (Fig. 25.2). Occasionally, oral steroids will be needed to control symptoms. Treatment should be avoided during courses of oral steroid as these drugs reduce wound healing and can predispose to infection.

Anxiety and stress can precipitate an asthmatic attack in certain individuals. Monitoring the patient's work of breathing is the best measure of asthma severity. This is commonly done using a peak flow meter. Should difficulty arise, postponing treatment, and providing inhaled or nebulised salbutamol and oxygen by mask will usually settle symptoms. Ongoing or worsening symptoms warrant onward referral to an acute medical care centre.

### Chronic obstructive pulmonary disease

Chronic obstructive pulmonary disease (COPD) presents with similar symptoms to asthma but may not always be reversible with inhalers. In addition, some patients have productive sputum for at least 3 months of the year, and this is commonly referred to as 'chronic bronchitis'. Generally occurring in more elderly patients, secondary to cigarette or environmental toxin exposure, COPD can cause debilitating shortness of breath, and frequently necessitates antibiotic and steroid therapy. As mentioned previously, unless urgent, treatment should be avoided while steroid therapy is being used. In severe cases home oxygen is required, and in these patients a similar oxygen flow rate should be provided during treatment. If the $SpO_2$ is less than 92% on air the patient is at increased risk of developing pulmonary difficulties and should be assessed medically or undergo their treatment in a hospital environment.

## Endocrine

### Diabetes

An increasing proportion of the population is developing diabetes. Type 1 diabetes refers to endocrine pancreatic dysfunction or failure, and generally presents in childhood. It is treated by insulin supplementation. Type 2 disease is insulin resistance that develops in adulthood, and is linked to diet and obesity. It is genetically more common amongst the Asian population. This type of diabetes can initially be treated by dietary modification, but frequently requires drug therapy to boost insulin function. The increasing recognition of the importance of glucose control in preventing end-organ dysfunction means that type 2 diabetes is now frequently also managed with insulin.

Regardless of type, poor glycaemic control leads to peripheral neuropathy, skin infection, renal disease and heart disease. Very non-compliant patients can have extensive cardiac and ophthalmic complications. While the podiatrist may be primarily concerned with managing the foot disease secondary to diabetes, they should also be aware of the presentation and management of glycaemic-control problems. Most commonly in young, insulin-dependent patients this presents as hypoglycaemia. However, hyperglycaemia can occur with subtherapeutic insulin control; this is more insidious in onset and may go unnoticed initially.

### Hypoglycaemia

A drop in blood glucose to <5 mmol/l or by more than 2 mmol rapidly creates a sympathetic outflow of sweating, tachycardia and anxiety. It occurs when the amount of exogenous insulin is out of balance with food intake. If untreated it will progress to unconsciousness and coma or seizures, usually when the blood glucose is <2 mmol/l. A history of diabetes and a fluctuant or reduced Glasgow Coma Score (GCS) is cause for a blood glucose check, which can be done quickly at the bedside. If blood glucose is <5 mmol and the patient is still conscious, oral glucose should be given and regular blood glucose checks done until the patient is stable. If unconscious, intramuscular glucagon 1 mg can be given, or an intravenous glucose replacement should be administered (50-ml boluses of 10% glucose). The patient should be referred to their primary care physician for review.

### Hyperglycaemia

This is usually caused by infection or dehydration and takes a few days to a week or more to develop. Impaired intracellular transfer of glucose results in reduced energy and an osmotic build-up of glucose extracellularly. Reduced conscious level or coma, with ketotic (sweet-smelling) breath due to the metabolism of ketones can occur. Urine testing will be highly positive for sugar. It is a life-threatening condition and needs to be managed in an acute medical unit to provide glucose control and fluid and salt replacement.

## Hepatic/renal

### Renal failure

Over time renal failure causes cardiovascular changes, including hypertension. Fistulae for dialysis must be protected and, as they are usually sited in the arm, will restrict vascular access sites. Initial dosing of drugs is unchanged but repeat doses need to be given either at a lower dose or reduced frequency to prevent accumulation and toxicity. In stable disease little restriction of treatment is needed, but if there is acute or chronic deterioration of renal disease, perhaps due to infection or fluid-balance problems, non-essential treatment should be postponed.

### Hepatic disease

Autoimmune, cirrhotic or infective diseases of the liver can cause jaundice and systemic upset, and in severe cases affect blood clotting and drug metabolism. Mild liver impairment of known cause should not affect podiatry practice. As for renal diseases, new-onset or decompensated liver symptoms should be investigated and managed before treatment commences.

## Central nervous system

### Transient ischaemic attack/stroke

A patient with known cerebrovascular disease may collapse during treatment and require basic life support. In stable conditions, anticoagulation therapy may affect the treatment options, although aspirin tends to be the commonest drug used to prevent embolic events and need not be stopped. Communication and mobility issues in recovering stroke patients may pose problems during therapy and should be taken into account when planning treatments.

### Epilepsy

This is a disease characterised by minor (petit mal) or major (grand mal) seizures due to foci of neuronal excitation within the brain. In some patients symptoms can be brittle and brought on by procedural anxiety, but in most the symptoms are stable and predictable and are controlled by medication. Some patients have a warning before an attack occurs, while others are unaware until after the event.

### Minor fits

These include focal twitching of one body area, or an absence-style fit, whereby the patient stops speaking, looks vacant briefly, then returns to the conversation unaware of the event. These can occur frequently, and as long as they are no different from the patient's normal seizure events they need not affect treatment.

### Major fits

These involve a loss of consciousness, and should this type of seizure occur all procedural work must be suspended. The patient's environment should be made safe to protect them from harm. If they are on a trolley that has sidebars, these should be raised. Beds should be reduced to their lowest level in case the patient falls out. Sharp and hard objects should be removed from around the patient. Once the seizure has ended the patient should be placed in the recovery position until they regain consciousness. They may have had an episode of urinary incontinence during the seizure. Importantly, during any seizure, the patient's airway and mouth should not be instrumented in any way as this can cause injury to both them and their rescuer. During the recovery phase, routine monitoring and observation should occur until the patient is feeling better.

If the seizure lasts longer than 10 minutes an ambulance should be called, as prolonged seizure activity can have a detrimental effect on the brain.

## UNPREDICTABLE EVENTS

Although by far the commonest of these events will be vasovagal syncope, this group also includes the most life-threatening events that a practitioner may face. Cardiac arrest, anaphylaxis and local anaesthetic toxicity are the major situations that should be 'drill run' regularly, so that in the heat of the moment no time is lost trying to remember treatment algorithms.

A practitioner who has been on basic or advanced life support courses and who is up to date on current anaphylaxis and local anaesthetic toxicity treatments will best serve their patients when things go wrong, and be likely to be less stressed by the event themselves.

The designated lead for the service should ensure that all staff members are confident to deal with the following situations and should also ensure that all necessary equipment is up to date and to hand. Emergency algorithms should be clearly displayed in treatment areas and updated frequently.

## Vasovagal syncope

Dizziness and collapse can have many causes, including cardiac, neurogenic and metabolic sources, but the most common cause in an otherwise healthy individual is the simple faint or 'vasovagal' episode. This is an exaggerated reflex response to poor blood flow to the heart, which commonly occurs after prolonged standing, heat or sometimes following a large meal. Sympathetic nervous activation to stimulate the underfilled heart then triggers a parasympathetic vagal nervous reflex that slows the heart rate, resulting in faint. If monitoring is done during the event the display will show a slowing heart rate, sometimes with brief asystole (no heart beat for a few seconds), with a concomitant low blood pressure. A situational variant of this reflex occurs in some patients when they cough, micturate or are exposed to a noxious stimulus (e.g. injection or venepuncture).

In the event of a faint treatment is supportive. Lay the patient flat, or slightly head down, raising the legs to return blood flow to the heart. If the patient is sitting, get them to put their head low between their legs so that blood continues to flow to the brain; this may abolish the faint. The procedure should be postponed. When treating patients susceptible to stimuli-induced vasovagal events, the practitioner should ensure that the patient is recumbent and distracted before the noxious event to limit the severity of the faint. Patients who display postural fainting (when standing or getting up from lying) may benefit from elasticated calf stockings, and the practitioner should ensure these patients have an adequate fluid and food intake around the time of procedures.

Recurrent or unexpected fainting should be referred to the patient's general practitioner for further investigation.

---

### CASE STUDY 25.2 **SUDDEN COLLAPSE**

A 30-year-old woman, with no past medical history of note, attends for a nail bed avulsion of the second toe. The procedure is scheduled as a day-case under a local anaesthetic ring block.

Immediately after the local anaesthetic injection she loses consciousness and collapses back on the treatment bed.

#### QUESTIONS

1. What do you do?
2. What is your differential diagnosis?
3. If the patient recovers, what would you tell them?

#### ANSWERS

1. Stop the injection, if not already completed, and call for help. Lay the patient flat and assess Airway, Breathing, Circulation (ABC). If the airway is patent administer an oxygen by mask and ensure the patient is breathing adequately, if not follow the basic life support (BLS) algorithm. Check for pulse and blood pressure, if not present continue BLS until help arrives. If the patient is breathing and cardiovascularly stable, put her in the recovery position and wait for her consciousness level to improve, reassessing periodically.

2. The most likely diagnosis is **vasovagal faint**, but given the timing **anaphylaxis** to the local anaesthetic and **cardiac arrest** from inadvertent intravascular injection may have occurred. A rapid heart rate, a drop in blood pressure and feeling of 'impending

doom' may occur with the latter conditions, but a slow heart rate is more common with fainting.

3. Upon recovery, reassure the patient and postpone treatment to another time, as the autonomic system will be unstable for the next few hours. There is a risk of similar vasovagal responses at the next treatment session, so counselling and preparation to avoid this would be appropriate.

---

## Cardiac arrest

This term describes cessation of mechanical heart function and is the culmination of many catastrophic physiological events. Although usually due to an overwhelming injury to the heart itself, such as a heart attack or tamponade (fluid around the heart), it can occur due to blood clots (thromboembolism), salt imbalance (low/high potassium), shock (hypovolaemia), low temperatures (hypothermia), low oxygen (hypoxia) or collapsed lung (pneumothorax). Of these common causes practitioners are most likely come across heart attacks secondary to severe angina or local anaesthetic toxicity.

Knowledge of the likely cause of the arrest can facilitate appropriate hospital treatment to reverse the initiating pathology. However, in the interim, basic life support is needed to keep oxygenated blood going to the heart and brain. This process involves mouth-to-mouth or bag-mask-style ventilatory assists in conjunction with cardiac massage (chest compressions). The current recommendation is 30 compressions for every two breaths, but up-to-date UK resuscitation guidance for basic and advanced life support is provided by the Resuscitation Council (UK). Practitioners should familiarise themselves with local resuscitation protocols and attend simulation scenarios regularly. A nominated resuscitation officer for the service should ensure that all staff are aware of updates and undertake training.

Until definitive medical care can be given, the ongoing treatment includes 100% oxygen administration and adrenaline (epinephrine) given every 3 minutes, with treatment sustained until a spontaneous return of circulation occurs. A defibrillator (Fig. 25.3) should be attached to the patient and the ECG trace read to see if it is appropriate to administer an electrical pulse to stabilise the heart. Nowadays, automated defibrillators are more widely available and give audible instructions as well as providing cardiac rhythm interpretation. They are more user-friendly alternatives to conventional defibrillators, and

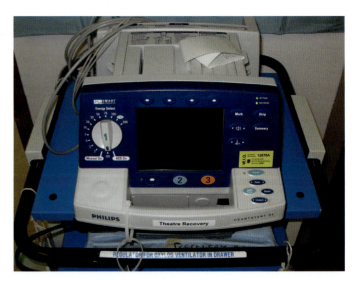

**Figure 25.3** A defibrillator.

may be useful in remote sites or where medical interpretation of ECG patterns is lacking.

## Allergy/anaphylaxis

Allergic reactions can range from innocuous itch and skin erythema due to histamine release, to antibody-mediated anaphylactic phenomena, which can lead to circulatory collapse and death if untreated.

Patients may be aware of drug and chemical allergies prior to treatment, or may only become aware of them after one or two exposures of the causal agent. Once identified, every effort should be made to avoid further precipitation of the allergic response. Local reactions are generally self-limiting and can be left to settle or be treated with oral antihistamine (e.g. chlorpheniramine). If locally severe, a topical hydrocortisone preparation can be used.

Latex allergy is an increasingly common condition noticed in medical staff and in patients exposed to multiple procedures. It is thought to be secondary to sensitisation to latex particles in disposable gloves. The use of alternative gloves and avoidance of latex plastics and rubbers in the treatment zone can limit the occurrence of this allergy in susceptible patients. Local sensitivity to adhesive in plasters can also limit the use of wound coverings in some patients.

Anaphylaxis is an antibody-mediated process whereby first exposure to the allergen causes the body to identify it as 'foreign' and create antibodies to recognise and bind it. Most frequently the reaction is associated with antibiotics, in particular penicillin. On the next exposure an immune response occurs in an attempt to exclude the allergen from the body, resulting in antibody clumping in the circulation and, ultimately, cardiovascular collapse. The newer amide-type local anaesthetics are less likely than the old ester-type local anaesthetics to provoke this response. However, allergy to the additives in the local anaesthetic ampoule can often be the precipitant. Careful questioning about previous local anaesthetic exposure may give warning of possible allergy (e.g. during dental or surgical procedures, and any unusual difficulties and drugs noted).

Clinically, anaphylaxis can present immediately with intravenous injections or be delayed by 10–30 minutes when subcutaneous infiltration is used. The patient may vocalise a feeling of 'impending doom' – a sickly dread caused by a rapid fall in blood pressure. Difficulty breathing and wheeze is common, followed by loss of consciousness and cardiac arrest. In this scenario resuscitation as per cardiac arrest protocols should be initiated, but adrenaline (epinephrine) should be given early as a 0.5–1 mg intramuscular injection (Figs 25.4 and 25.5). This can stabilise events and reverse the respiratory wheeze and hypotension. Intravenous steroids and an antihistamine should also be administered. These will assist in the recovery of the patient but take several hours to work. Airway support in the acute phase with supplemental oxygen is essential, as airway swelling and obstruction can occur from soft-tissue oedema. The patient should be transferred to a nearby hospital emergency department.

Following recovery the patient should be referred to immunology for testing to identify the true allergen before continuing with treatment. The practitioner involved in the precipitating incident should ensure that this assessment takes place and should inform the patient and their general practitioner of the result. The patient may opt to wear a 'medic-alert' bracelet to warn future clinicians, and all case-notes should be updated to reflect the patient's allergy and its severity.

## Local anaesthetic toxicity

The action of local anaesthetic agents is to reversibly block sodium ion conduction in nerve endings, thus reducing action potential trans-

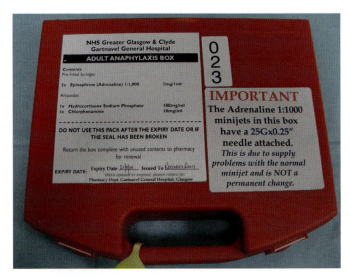

**Figure 25.4** Example of anaphylaxis kit.

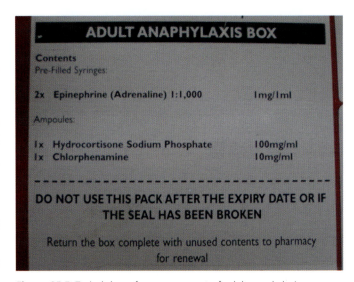

**Figure 25.5** Typical drugs for management of adult anaphylaxis.

fer through axons. While this primarily blocks pain transmission from the surgical field, should the local anaesthetic reach high concentrations in the blood stream (from inadvertent intravenous injection) the sodium channel blocking effect has deleterious effects on the central nervous and cardiovascular systems. The effect on the heart is to cause arrhythmia (heart block) by disrupting the heart's electrical conduction system. Local anaesthetics also impair sodium/calcium muscle pumping, which weakens heart contractility. In the brain the local anaesthetic block disrupts synaptic transmission and blocks higher brain functions.

Clinically, this manifests as altered heart rhythm and cardiovascular collapse followed by (or preceded by) seizures and coma. Patients may describe tinnitus (ringing in the ears), tingling or numbness around the mouth, and palpitations before the situation deteriorates.

If local anaesthetic toxicity is thought to have occurred, cease any further injection and aspirate to prevent further drug spread into the

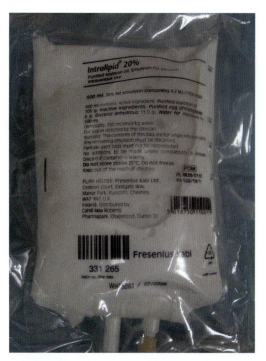

**Figure 25.6** Intralipid.

**Treatment for local anaesthetic toxicity**

- Prevent by careful injection and regular aspiration
- Limit dose of local anaesthetics to maximum dose by patient weight: lidocaine (plain) (3 mg/kg), bupivacaine (2 mg/kg), ropivacaine (3 mg/kg)
- Stop injecting and aspirate if symptoms occur
- Give 100% oxygen, establish intravenous access if not already present
- Give fluids and epinephrine in 0.1 mg intravenous boluses to support circulation
- Commence basic/advanced life support
- Administer Intralipid: 1 ml/kg up to three boluses; infuse at 0.25 mg/kg/min; maximum dose 8 ml/kg
- Prolonged resuscitation (>1 hour) may be required depending on the local anaesthetic used

Britain and Ireland (AAGBI) have also adopted Intralipid in their treatment protocol; further information can be found on their website.

## SUMMARY

Medical emergencies in podiatric practice are thankfully rare. However, both predictable and unpredictable events can occur. Through careful history taking, the identification of comorbidities and the appropriate use of clinical monitors, predictable events should be kept to a minimum or avoided entirely.

Unpredictable events will, by their very nature, catch the most experienced practitioner off guard and can be best managed by the use of practice drills and test scenarios to hone skills before the event occurs in real life. Each practitioner should ensure they are suitably up to date and familiar with algorithms for managing these emergency scenarios before treating or administering drugs to patients. With knowledge of basic and advanced life-support techniques, the appropriate use of monitoring and resuscitation equipment locally available, unexpected catastrophic events can be reversed and the patient stabilised until assistance arrives.

circulation. Continue full monitoring of the patient, ensure there is intravenous access and initiate basic life support if circulatory collapse occurs.

Lidocaine, ropivacaine and levobupivacaine are less cardiotoxic than bupivacaine but all can cause fatal reactions. Recent interest has focused on the use of Intralipid to facilitate resuscitation by sequestering the local anaesthetic in the lipid (Fig. 25.6). Case reports in humans and animal experiments suggest it is safe and effective in this regard, although there is still debate about which dose and infusion rate to use. Further information can be found online (see LipidRescue under Further Reading). Box 25.1 outlines the current treatment of local anaesthetic toxicity. The Association of Anaesthetists of Great

## FURTHER READING

Association of Anaesthetists of Great Britain and Ireland (AAGBI): http://www.aagbi.org (19 September 2009).

British National Formulary: http://www.bnf.org (19 September 2009).

LipidRescue: http://www.lipidrescue.org (19 September 2009).

Resuscitation Council (UK): http://www.resus. org.uk (19 September 2009).

# Chapter | 26 |

# Evolution and its influence on human foot function

*Donald L Lorimer*

## KEY WORDS

Adaptation
Bipedalism
Clinical disorders
Evolution
Hominin
Hominoid
Locomotion
Morphology
Ontogeny
Phylogeny
Primates

## INTRODUCTION

Among primates, humans have the unique ability of habitual bipedal posture and locomotion. However, with this activity, the human body, step by step, teeters on the edge of catastrophe (Napier 1967). This bipedal mode of walking seems potentially catastrophic because only the rhythmic forward movement of first one leg and then the other prevents the body from falling forward. Why has man developed such an apparently impractical mode of locomotion? In the past, the evolution of upright posture was viewed as a relatively easily accomplished, gradual trend, while the increase in relative brain size was considered to be all important in both its evolutionary mode and in the magnitude of its effect (Gould 1979). It is now recognised that bipedalism evolved before the relative cranial capacity of the basal hominin had developed barely beyond the range of living (extant) apes (Eccles 1989, Jablonski & Chaplin 1993, McHenry 1982). The evolution of the human foot is, therefore, a fundamental element in the adaptive transformation that produced the human lineage (Day & Napier 1964, Laitman & Jaffe 1982, Morton 1935, Olson & Seidel 1983). Erect posture and a bipedal mode of locomotion changed the lifestyle of the earliest humans and freed the upper limbs from their traditional function of supporting the body, and the structure of the human foot is fundamental to habitual bipedalism. By freeing the forelimbs from locomotion it was possible for ancestral humans to use them more extensively to interact with, manipulate and modify their environment. This may have been a significant contributing factor in the evolution of the manufacture and use of complex tools, which may have further resulted in specialisation of the neural faculties of early hominins. The utilisation of tools and the enlargement of the cerebral cortex could have also played an important role in the evolution of the human vocal tract, which allowed the evolution of more human-like language and thus improved communication between individuals (Laitman et al 1979).

Of all these evolutionary specialisations that define the human species, the foot is considered to be one of the most important, and is pivotal in allowing the evolution of the first of these changes – bipedalism (Day & Napier 1964, Jones 1944, Morton 1926, 1935, Olson & Seidel 1983). Early studies of the evolution of the human foot, such as that by Morton (1935) which is the most well-known model of human foot evolution, outlined three principal changes required to transform the hypothetical arboreal or terrestrial quadrupedal ape-like foot into the habitually terrestrial bipedal human foot. These are: (1) a transfer of locomotor function from the arms and hands to legs and feet, (2) an increase in the intrinsic base of support within the foot by a lowering of the heel to the ground, and (3) loss of grasping ability whereby the foot becomes a lever for lifting and propelling the body. Regardless of its origins, over the course of hominin development the human foot has evolved in a number of areas. These are: an elaborate plantar aponeurosis, strong plantar ligaments, longitudinal arches, enlarged musculus flexor accessorius, an adducted (non-opposable) hallux, a remodelled calcaneocuboid joint, a long tarsus, and shortened lesser toes (Susman 1983).

In reconstructing the evolutionary and adaptive transformation of the human foot in order to understand better some of the clinical disorders that affect it, there are three broad, interrelated methods of enquiry. These are the embryological, palaeontological and comparative methods. Of these, the palaeontological method usually receives the most attention as it is the only one that bases its conclusions on direct evidence of the past (Olson & Seidel 1983), typically in the form of fossils of related extinct species. The embryological and comparative methods, on the other hand, use indirect sources of data to make inferences about the history of extant forms. To place this into perspective, the fossil record of related extinct species gives us an idea of morphological and functional correlates in species that represent a transition from primitive ape to modern human. Unfortunately, due to the paucity of these specimens, particularly those of the foot, this

information, although revealing, is limited. There is, however, other evidence that might indicate modes of locomotion and locomotor diversity among early hominins. Some of the most interesting and revealing information has been gained from the interpretation of hominin body proportions in the taxa, for which there is sufficient evidence (Berger & Tobias 1996, McHenry & Berger 1998, Richmond et al 2001). The embryological methods allow us to investigate ontogenetic development which, to a large extent, reflects the transition from a primitive to a modern form. However, this is not entirely true for all parts of the body and should be considered with caution.

A comparative analysis of living forms is especially pertinent in the order of primates, which consists of primarily arboreal (tree climbing) and terrestrial animals whose evolution occurred in biodiverse tropical and subtropical forests. The basic principle in both the comparative and palaeontological methods is that phylogenetic relationships (i.e. the degree of genetic affinity) can be estimated by studying the frequency and distribution of shared anatomical specialisations in a group of organisms (Olson & Seidel 1983). If two primates – for example, a gorilla and a human – share a larger number of unique features than either does with, for example, a gibbon, then this would seem to suggest that the human and gorilla have a closer genetic relationship. This may also indicate that both the human and gorilla shared a common ancestor with each other more recently than either did with the gibbon. The pattern of morphological refinement of the feet of chimpanzees, gorillas and humans suggests a hypothetical common ancestor and a hypothetical hominin foot as postulated by Morton (1935) (Fig. 26.1). Darwin referred to this as 'propinquity of descent' (Darwin 1859). However, with the comparative method it is

**Figure 26.1** Foot skeletons from the living African apes and humans. From comparative studies a common hypothetical ancestor is presumed and it is possible to reconstruct a hypothetical 'prehuman' foot. Modified from Morton (1935).

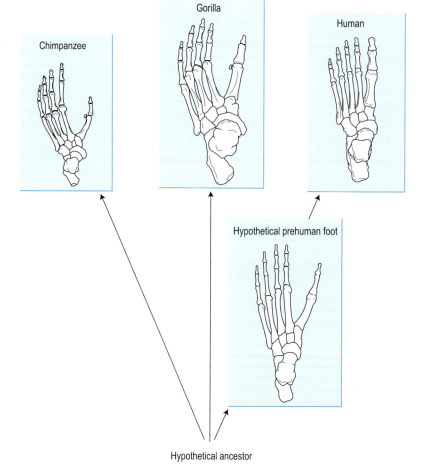

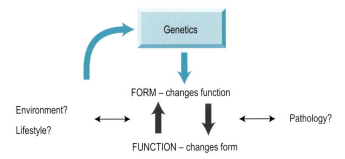

**Figure 26.2** A schematic representation of the interaction between the variables influencing morphology.

sometimes difficult to distinguish clearly between primitive features that are ancestral and specialised features that are derived. Subsequent to Morton's (1935) reconstruction of a 'hypothetical prehuman foot', a number of hominin fossils have suggested that they are very similar to this original hypothetical reconstruction. Examples of these are the reconstruction of the Stw 573 *Australopithecus africanus* (Little Foot) skeleton (Clarke & Tobias 1995) and reappraisal of the OH 8 *Homo habilis* (Olduvai Hominid) (Kidd et al 1996).

As is the case with Wolff's law of bone remodelling (Wolff 1892), the relationship between *form* and *function* is one of the most thoroughly accepted principles of biology. Thus the *form* of a biological component is closely related to its intended *function*, or functions. This also suggests that a particular function of a bone, over time, may change form (Wolff 1892). The problem in studying the exact nature of variation and differences in the form of skeletal material lies in that it may be uncertain which came first: form or function. Form, of an epigenetic nature, may result in a particular function. That function, depending on its deviation from 'normal', may in time produce modified form. Over a period of many generations, this altered form and function may in turn manifest itself as an epigenetic variant in subsequent individuals. This represents a simplified model of adaptation and transformation, which is known as evolution (Fig. 26.2).

## SOME LARGE-SCALE DIFFERENCES BETWEEN THE HOMINOIDEA

### A comparison of gait cycles

In order to test their morphologically based deductions on foot function, Elftman and Manter (1935a) and Morton (1935) in their classic work investigated the differences between human and chimpanzee walking. From these experiments they concluded that the 'immobilisation' of the transverse tarsal arch and the set of the transverse tarsal joint in a plantar-flexed position were critical factors in the evolution of the human foot. It was observed that, in their facultative bipedal walking, chimpanzees inverted the foot and placed it, heel first, immediately followed by the lateral border (Elftman & Manter 1935a). This is essentially similar to the heel contact of humans. This is where the similarity ends, and the critical functional difference lies in the way the heel lifts off the ground at the end of midstance. In humans the forefoot is much more rigid as the heel lifts off the ground and weight is transferred to the metatarsophalangeal area. Particularly noteworthy in chimpanzees is a medial shift in the centre of pressure on the foot and dorsiflexion of the midtarsal joint – known as the midtarsal break – as weight is transferred to the forefoot (Elftman & Manter 1935a).

This flexion of the midtarsal joint is immediately followed by a lateral deflection of weight over the metatarsals. At toe-off, the chimpanzee propels forward from toes 2 and 3, more lateral than humans normally do (Susman 1983). During this facultative bipedalism, there appears to be great variation in both the position and motion of the toes, often mimicking the footprint of the human pattern (Susman 1983). However, the weight distribution across the metatarsal heads is distinctive (Stern & Susman 1983). The differences in motion and morphology of the metatarsophalangeal joints are further discussed later.

## The functional adaptation of the midtarsal joint and the medial and lateral columns

The midtarsal joint has undergone intense modification during the evolution of human bipedal gait, perhaps because of its critical position at the apex of the longitudinal arch (Kidd 1993a, Kidd 1999). The shift from a mobile grasping foot (e.g. chimpanzee) to a more rigid, plantargrade lever in humans is closely reflected in a number of changes in bony morphology. During bipedal stance and locomotion, the body's centre of gravity must be concentrated within a relatively restricted base of support. In quadrupedal apes, this base is provided with an area of contact provided by the fore- and hindlimbs, but in humans this area is defined by the heel and toes. Ape feet, when engaged in bipedal stance and progression, provide a far less stable base of support than do the feet of humans (Elftman & Manter 1935a, Stern & Susman 1983). The major adaptive changes to the bony morphology of the human foot making habitual bipedalism possible include: the presence of a longitudinal arch; the shift of support from lateral to medial accompanied by pronation of the forefoot; the relative lengthening and stabilisation of the hallux; the plantar-flexed orientation of the forefoot and the stabilisation of the calcaneocuboid joint; the widening of the calcaneal tuberosity; the altered plane of the sustentaculum tali and subtalar joint; and elongation of the midfoot. The key component to these changes was the decrease in the range of motion of the midtarsal joint in bipeds compared with hominoid quadrupeds. Elftman and Manter (1935b) discuss the 'plantar-flexion set' of the talus, which lends itself to a decreased range of motion at the midtarsal joint. These modifications to the midtarsal joint are complex and beyond the scope of this chapter; apart from the reduction in range of motion, this absolute range is also dependent on the position of the subtalar joint, forming the so-called 'midtarsal restraining mechanism'. Elftman (1960) and Langdon et al (1991) stated that, when the subtalar complex is pronated, the axes of the talonavicular and calcaneocuboid joints are more or less aligned, or coincident. This means that the directions of the greatest freedom of movement of the navicular and cuboid are also aligned. By allowing the ligamentous structures to become lax during subtalar joint pronation, greater freedom of movement is gained – allowing the foot to elongate on weight bearing. This mobility affords the foot the ability to absorb shock at the initial stance phase and adapt to variable substrates.

When the subtalar complex is supinated, the talonavicular and calcaneocuboid axes are obliquely aligned. As the directions of greatest freedom of movement at the talonavicular and calcaneocuboid joints are also oblique, movement is limited (Elftman 1960). Conversely to the pronated subtalar joint, the ligamentous structures are taut and the two joints are moved one above the other in a close-packed position (Close et al 1967). This is particularly important in facilitating a rigid base necessary for propulsion at the end of the stance phase of the gait cycle. This adaptive range of motion is considered to be an essential adaptation for human bipedal gait (Inman et al 1981, Root et al 1977).

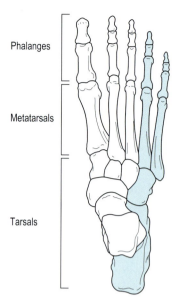

Phalanges

Metatarsals

Tarsals

**Figure 26.3** The medial and lateral columns of the foot. The shaded area represents the more stable lateral column.

In addition to the aforementioned adaptive midtarsal range of motion, another innovation of the human foot in contrast to the ape foot is that of two longitudinal segments: the medial and lateral columns (Aiello & Dean 1990). The medial column consists of the talus, navicular and medial structures distal to them. The lateral column consists of the calcaneus, cuboid and lateral structures distal to them (Fig. 26.3). As the midtarsal joint forms the apex of the arch, medially by the talonavicular joint and laterally by the calcaneocuboid joint, it does not only define the foot in terms of anterior and posterior parts, but also in terms of medial and lateral longitudinal columns. The lateral column is inherently more rigid than the medial column; the medial column is adaptive in its range of motion, allowing mobility during stance and rigidity during propulsion.

## The functional transformation of the subtalar joint

Keith (1929) and Lewis (1981) have suggested that the major differences between the human foot and the ape foot have resulted from the realignment of the human foot around the subtalar axis of the primitive prehensile primate foot. The human and ape subtalar joints appear very similar, the major differences being that the subtalar joint axis is dorsoplantarly steeper in humans than in apes. This is as a result of the disproportionately large radius of curvature of the subtalar joint surfaces in the human foot (Aiello & Dean 1990). This morphology also limits the degree of inversion and eversion in the human foot. Furthermore, the subtalar axis makes a more acute angle with the long axis of the foot in the transverse plane. It has been suggested that the adducted human great toe has been brought into line with the remaining toes as a result of the realignment of the lateral four metatarsals toward the first metatarsal and oblique subtalar axis, rather than in realignment of the first metatarsal towards the lateral four metatarsals and away from the subtalar axis (Lewis 1981). The entire foot has therefore been realigned to the subtalar axis. The angle between the talar neck and the trochlea is reduced in humans, bringing the long axis of the trochlea more in line with the subtalar axis. The angle of torsion (in the coronal plane) of the head of the talus (Lisowski 1967) or of the neck of the talus (Day & Wood 1968) is considerably smaller in the African apes than in humans. In humans

this smaller angle is partially responsible for the loss of the prehensile first ray consistent with human bipedalism (Kidd 1993a). The ontogenetic changes in talar neck angle (transverse plane) and talar head torsion (coronal plane) in both the apes and humans appear to reflect the phylogeny of talar evolution (Kidd 1993b, Lisowski 1967). This was extensively dealt with by Lisowski (1967) and Day and Wood (1968), where infant human values were similar to adult ape values and the adult human values were reduced compared to the adult ape values. This is an excellent example of *peramorphic heterochrony*. More precisely, a morphology transcends or moves beyond adult stages of its ancestors or primitive form (Shea 1983). In this sense 'ontogeny recapitulates phylogeny', meaning that embryonic development repeats the pattern of evolutionary history (Gould 1979). There is evidence for *peramorphic heterochrony* in several other areas of the foot (e.g. Lisowski 1967, Manley-Buser 1991). Curiously, this is not the case in some other parts of the body (e.g. the skull), where *paedomorphic heterochrony* has been reported. In this instance, the human foot is considered *gerontomorphic* and the human skull *neotenous* (maintaining juvenile features). This is perhaps an oversimplification of human talar ontogeny, and detailed information may be found in Scheman (1931). A number of other studies on the talus have revealed much about the evolution, function and variation of this important bone (Kidd 1995, Lisowski et al 1974, 1976).

The evolutionary morphology of the calcaneus has been studied by many authors, among whom Weidenreich (1923), Elftman and Manter (1935b) and Morton (1935) expressed the profound nature of the modifications to this bone. The human calcaneus possesses a wide, relatively long tuberosity due to its importance as a weight-bearing structure in stance and locomotion. The lateral plantar tubercle (Weidenreich 1940) and the perpendicular orientation of the sustentaculum relative to the long axis of the tuberosity (Morton 1935) are uniquely human attributes of the human calcaneus. The most profound modification is the elevation of the subtalar joint axis by elevating the anterior portion of the calcaneus, thereby forming the posterior portion of the longitudinal arch (Kidd 1999), which is represented radiographically as the calcaneal inclination angle.

## Orientation of the medial metatarsal–cuneiform joint

In humans this joint lies in a plane opposite to that characteristic in the apes. The medial edge of the human joint projects further posteriorly than does the lateral edge. The opposite condition, characteristic of the apes, accentuates the medial projection, or abduction, of the great toe in apes. The anterior articular surface of the medial cuneiform is markedly different from that of the apes with prehensile great toes (Aiello & Dean 1990). The French embryologist Leboucq, as early as 1882, had pointed out that the divergence of the first metatarsal was due to the extreme angle made by the plane of the distal articular facet of the cuneiform bone with the long axis of the foot. Leboucq (1882) studied the shape of the medial cuneiform in human embryos and found that, in 20-mm specimens, the tibial border of this bone was shorter than its fibular margin, which made its distal articular facet slope obliquely forward. This in turn induced the first metatarsal to diverge inward, away from the lesser metatarsals. As development progressed, the tibial side of the cuneiform bone grew more rapidly than the fibular border, gradually straightening the plane of the distal articular facet until, in 40-mm embryos, it assumed the position it occupied in adults. However, in contrast to contemporary literature, Leboucq made no attempt to correlate 'bunions' with the oblique setting of the medial cuneometatarsal joint. This is another example of ontogeny recapitulating phylogeny, in which the first intermetatarsal angle in the prenatal human approaches that of the adult prehensile arboreal foot of the apes.

## Relative robusticity of the metatarsals

Robusticity of the metatarsals is an expression of their absolute short-ness and relative thickness, and the dominance in relative robusticity is an important feature of bipedalism in humans. This dominance was expressed using a formula by Day and Napier (1964) in modern man as $1 > 5 > 4 > 3 > 2$, which they contrasted to the Olduvai hominid (OH8), a facultative biped from approximately 1.8 million years ago with an estimated robusticity formula of $1 > 5 > 3 > 4 > 2$. Day and Napier (1964) have suggested that this is either an individual varia-tion or represents incomplete evolution of the *Homo sapiens* pattern of metatarsal robusticity. Archibald et al (1972), in their observations of both Native American and Pongid metatarsal patterns, show the former to be the most probable interpretation. Almost half of the *H. sapiens* specimens (44%) had other than the $1 > 5 > 4 > 3 > 2$ pattern, showing eight distinct formula permutations. Five different formulae were obtained from chimpanzees (*Pan troglodytes*) and three from gorillas (*Gorilla gorilla*). The substantial variability in metatarsal robus-ticity pattern characterises both *Homo* and the apes, but in both groups a distinct gradient in relative robusticity of metatarsals 2–5 can be detected, and its direction is opposite in *Homo* and the other two genera (Archibald et al 1972). This difference is almost certainly related to different locomotor requirements. Bipedal gait delivers a substantial load on the fifth metatarsal during weight bearing and this load shifts to the first metatarsal during toe-off (Inman & Mann 1973).

## Torsion of the metatarsal shafts

In humans, the heads of the metatarsals have undergone torsion in relation to their bases to lie squarely on the ground (Fig. 26.4). In apes, the head of the first metatarsal is orientated towards the other metatarsals, with the second to fourth orientated toward the first. In humans, there is very little torsion in the first, with progressively more torsion from the second to fifth. The opposite occurs in the apes, where there is progressively less torsion from the second to fifth, allowing the forefoot to lie in an inverted position. Both the transverse and longitudinal metatarsal arch together are shaped like a half-dome with its hollow surfaces facing both downward and medially. Other primates have only the transverse arch, their feet being flat in the longitudinal direction (Aeillo & Dean 1990). Humans, by having the metatarsal torsion increase toward the lateral side of the foot, allow for the orientation of the proximal articular surfaces to be more medi-ally orientated from second to fifth metatarsal with the metatarsal heads in a plantar grade position; arches are formed in both the sagit-tal and coronal planes.

## Morphology of the metatarsal heads

In humans, the articular surfaces on the heads of the metatarsals are separated from the epicondyles by a greater distance than in apes. In animals in which the closed-packed position of the metatarso- or metacarpophylangeal joint is in *flexion*, the plantar aspect of the meta-tarsal or metacarpal head is wide (mediolateral dimension) and there is an obvious narrowing of the head near its dorsal margin. This con-figuration characterises the fingers and toes of all the apes and humans, with two notable exceptions: (1) the principal *weight-bearing* fingers of the African 'knuckle walkers', in whom the metacarpal heads are the widest on their dorsal aspect (Susman 1979); and (2) the heads of metatarsals 1–4 in humans, which are also widened dorsally (Susman et al 1984). The African apes load their fingers (principal rays 3 and 5) with the metacarpophalangeal joints in dorsiflexion; this is the closed-packed position, so that the articular surfaces are expanded mediolaterally on their dorsal aspects. Human metatarsal heads are also expanded dorsally, indicating the enhancement of dorsiflexion at toe-off and a reduced emphasis on toe flexion in human locomotion (Susman et al 1984). The significance of free dorsiflexion of the toes in human walking was established by Bojsen-Møller and Lamoreux (1979). However, in the first metatarsal head, in both humans and the apes, the superior width of the head is gener-ally narrower than the inferior width. In the apes this difference between the superior and inferior width is marked. In humans, the sides of the head are generally more 'parallel' to each other. Susman and Brain (1988), illustrate this feature by an index that compares the mediolateral diameters, superiorly and inferiorly of the first metatarsal of a Swartkrans hominin (SKX 5017) from South Africa, thought to be of *Paranthropus robustus*, to chimpanzees and humans. These two measurements in the fossil yield an index of 61.0. This value in humans is 84.8 ($n = 12$ males; SD = 3.62), in chimpanzees it is 69.0 ($n = 15$ males; SD = 7.8). Thus, while humans have a hallucal meta-tarsal that is mediolaterally broad on the dorsal (superior) surface, neither SKX 5017 nor any of the apes have a similarly broad head, indicating the uniqueness of the human metatarsal head.

Human foot-contact differs markedly from that of chimpanzees (and the other apes), which do not toe-off on the hallux (Susman 1983). Without the human toe-off mechanism, there appears to be no need for an enlarged hallucal metatarsophalangeal joint that close-packs in the dorsiflexed position (Susman et al 1984). In the chim-panzee, for example, additional dorsiflexion is achieved through a midtarsal break (Susman 1983). Another feature essential for effective dorsiflexion of the metatarsophalangeal joint is the great extent to which the articular surface continues onto the dorsum of the head. The apes in contrast, do not display a similar dorsally extended articular surface; instead, the dorsal-most portion of the metatarsal head of apes appears flat in profile (Aiello & Dean 1990, Susman & Brain 1988). Interestingly, the aforementioned hominin fossil, SKX 5017, displays a very human-like dorsally extended articular surface. This facultative bipedal hominin therefore displays functional affinities that are both ape and human. In the human lesser metatarsals there is also a result-ing sulcus, or depression, between the head and shaft (Aiello & Dean 1990). This relates to an increased potential for dorsiflexion at the metatarsophalangeal joints. This is essential to a bipedal gait, where the metatarsophalangeal joint acts as a fulcrum so that the posterior part of the foot can 'roll' over during the toe-off phase of gait.

The transverse shape of the first metatarsal head in humans is unique among the hominoids. This is evident from comparisons with the apes (Aiello & Dean 1990, Susman et al 1984) and fossil

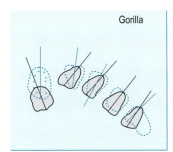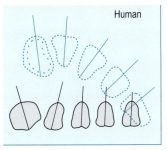

**Figure 26.4** Transverse sections through the metatarsals of a gorilla foot and a human foot. After Morton (1922). In the gorilla metatarsus, both the bases (dotted outlines) and heads (solid outlines) are elevated in line with the transverse arch of the foot. In humans the metatarsal bases are elevated but the metatarsal heads are on the ground.

hominins from, for example, Swartkrans and Hadar (Ethiopia). These apes and non-human hominins have first metatarsal heads with a highly convex surface, reflecting enhanced transverse plane mobility of the hallux suited to an arboreal or partially arboreal lifestyle (Susman & Brain 1988, Susman et al 1984).

## EVOLUTIONARY BASIS FOR SOME CLINICAL DISORDERS OF THE HUMAN FOOT

Specific clinical disorders arise from trauma, infectious disease, circulatory disturbances, developmental defects, systemic disease and biomechanical imbalances. Podiatric disorders may also be considered from the viewpoint that the human foot has evolved to its present structure and function as an adaptation to bipedal locomotion. Evolution has modified the primitive terrestrial and arboreal form into the specialised human foot that is perfectly adapted to the bipedal walking mode; this pattern has existed for almost 2 million years (Day & Napier 1964). Deviation from this adaptive pattern may result in clinical problems. Kidd (1995, 1998) has suggested that the specialist modifications pertinent to human pedal structure from that of the primitive ape-like foot took place initially in the lateral column, developing a more rigid foot specifically adapted to the stresses of walking short distances bipedally. He then went on to suggest that changes to the medial column followed later. This may well present a hypothesis as to some forefoot pathology being of ontogenetic origin. A mild delay or arrest in ontogenetic development could lead to defects on the medial side of the foot, rendering it more 'ape-like'. Such a pathological state would be characterised by the medial column possessing essentially ape-like characteristics (those of mobility), although in humans it is a function of abnormality (Kidd 1998). Typical pathologies may include bunion or hallux valgus deformity, together with a large range of motion in the talonavicular joint.

Occasionally, atavistic features occur in the first ray, and these are considered to be a variant of the normal first intermetatarsal angle (metatarsus primus varus, originally defined as metatarsus ataviticus') (Moorhead & Wobeskya 1995, Morton 1927). This feature resembles more closely that of the prehensile arboreal foot of the apes; in addition, it reflects some of the tarsometatarsal articular features of, for example, the chimpanzee, with a convex joint and extreme mediolateral orientation of the hallux (Aiello & Dean 1990, Olson & Seidel 1983, Susman 1983). They are also reminiscent of the less convex joint with a more dorsoplantar orientation of early humans and prehumans such as the Olduvai hominid (OH8) and modern Homo sapiens sapiens, as described by Susman (1983). This feature certainly makes the hypothesis suggested by Kidd (1998) seem plausible when one considers that hypermobility of the first ray appears to increase with an increase in the first intermetatarsal angle (Greenberg 1979). These features of segmental hypermobility of the medial column are also associated with increased pronation (abduction, eversion and dorsiflexion) of the foot, which, when excessive, has been assumed to

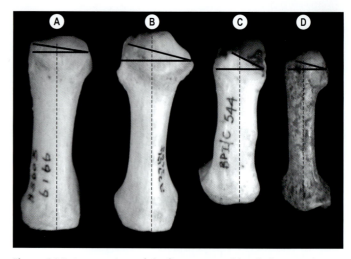

**Figure 26.5** A comparison of the first metatarsal head of a normal human (A), human with hallux valgus (B), normal gorilla (C), and normal bonobo (D). The acquired pathological human morphology is reminiscent of the normal ape morphology with an increased articular set angle.

be the underlying cause of many foot problems as expressed by, for example, Greenberg (1979) and Olson and Seidel (1983).

A laterally sloped first metatarsal head in humans has been associated with congenital hallux abducto valgus (DuVries 1973) and is also known as the 'proximal articular set angle', which, when laterally sloped, is associated with an increased hallux abductus angle (La Porta et al 1994, Landers 1992, Meyer 1979, Vittetoe et al 1994). A variation of the rounded or convex metatarsal head, often subtle, was a lateral deviation of the articular set angle. In this instance the distal articular surface lies obliquely to the lateral side, obviously indicating that the proximal phalanx will also lie laterally, in an abducted position. This morphology is reminiscent of the normal condition in the first metatarsal head of the apes. An example comparing a normal human and pathological human to a normal gorilla and bonobo is presented in Figure 26.5. This seems to suggest that when a human hallux and first metatarsal takes on a function more suited to an opposable hallux, this morphology further adapts to resemble more closely that of the ape first metatarsal head.

These are only a few examples of disorders of maladaptation. This may also happen in the form of maladaptations of arch development, first metatarsal length, metatarsophalangeal joint flexion axis and joint mobility. The structure of the human foot serves its function remarkably well. However, despite its evolutionary success, the human foot remains susceptible to clinical disorders that may be related to its development from non-human ancestors (Moorhead & Wobeskya 1995). An understanding of the evolution of the human foot can help to explain the occurrence of some foot disorders and provide a framework for understanding, explaining and planning the management of those disorders.

## REFERENCES

Aiello L, Dean C 1990 An introduction to human evolutionary anatomy. Academic Press, London.

Archibald JD, Lovejoy CO, Heiple KG 1972 Implications of relative robusticity in the Olduvai metatarsus. American Journal of Physical Anthropology 37(1): 93–96.

Berger LR, Tobias V 1996 A chimpanzee-like tibia from Sterkfontein, South Africa and its implications for the interpretation of bipedalism in Australopithecus africanus. Journal of Human Evolution 30:343–348.

Bojsen-Møller F, Lamoreux L 1979 Significance of free dorsiflexion of the toes in walking.

Acta Orthopaedica Scandinavica 50:471–479.

Clarke RJ, Tobias PV 1995 Sterkfontein member 2 foot bones of the oldest South African hominid. Science 269:521–524.

Close JR, Inman VT, Poor PM, et al 1967 The function of the subtalar joint. Clinical Orthopaedics 50:159–160.

Darwin C 1859 The origin of species. John Murray, London.

Day MH, Napier JR 1964 Hominid fossils from bed I, Olduvai Gorge, Tanganyika: Fossil foot bones. Nature 201:969–970.

Day MH, Wood JR 1968 Functional affinities of the Olduvai hominid 8 talus. Man 3:440–455.

DuVries HL 1973 Acquired nontraumatic deformities of the foot. In: Inman VT (ed.) Surgery of the foot. CV Mosby, Saint Louis, MI, pp 204–229.

Eccles JC 1989 Evolution of the brain. Routledge, London.

Elftman H 1960 The transverse joint and its control. Clinical Orthopaedics 16:41.

Elftman H, Manter J 1935a Chimpanzee and human feet in bipedal walking. American Journal of Physical Anthropology 20:69–79.

Elftman H, Manter J 1935b The evolution of the foot with special reference to the joints. Journal of Anatomy 70:56–67.

Gould SJ 1979 Our greatest evolutionary step. Natural History 88(6):40–44.

Greenberg GS 1979 Relationship of hallux abductus angle and first metatarsal angle to severity of pronation. Journal of the American Podiatry Association 69(1):29.

Inman VT, Mann R 1973 Biomechanics of the foot and ankle. In: Inman VT (ed.) DuVries' surgery of the foot, 3rd edn. CV Mosby, St Louis, MI.

Inman VT, Ralston HJ, Todd F 1981 Human walking. Williams & Wilkins, Baltimore, OH.

Jablonski NG, Chaplin G 1993 Origin of habitual terrestrial bipedalism in the ancestor of the Hominidae. Journal of Human Evolution 24:259–280.

Jones FW 1944 Structure and function as seen in the foot. Baillière, London.

Keith A 1929 The history of the human foot and its bearing on orthopedic practice. Journal of Bone and Joint Surgery 11:10–32.

Kidd R 1993a The long arch: new thoughts on the evolution of an old structure. Australian Podiatrist 27:35–43.

Kidd R 1993b Gradualistic evolution as expressed in the hominid talus. British Journal of Podiatric Medicine 48:171–174.

Kidd R 1995 An investigation into the patterns of morphological variation in the proximal tarsus of selected human groups, apes and fossils: a morphometric analysis. PhD thesis, University of Western Australia, Perth.

Kidd R 1998 The past is the key to the present: thoughts on origins of human foot structure, function and dysfunction as seen from the fossil record. The Foot 8:75–84.

Kidd R 1999 Evolution of the rearfoot: a model of adaptation with evidence from the fossil record. Journal of the American Podiatric Medical Association 89(1):2–17.

Kidd RS, O'Higgins PO, Oxnard CE 1996 The OH8 foot: a reappraisal of the hindfoot utilizing a multivariate analysis. Journal of Human Evolution 31:269–291.

Laitman JT, Jaffe WL 1982 A review of current concepts on the evolution of the human foot. Foot & Ankle 2:284–290.

Laitman JT, Heimbruch RC, Crelin ES 1979 The basicranium of fossil hominids as an indicator of their upper respiratory systems. American Journal of Physical Anthropology 51:15–34.

Landers P 1992 Introduction and evaluation of halluxabducto valgus. In: McGlamry E, Banks A, Downey M (eds) Comprehensive textbook of foot surgery, Vol. 1. Williams and Wilkins, pp 462–465.

Langdon JH, Bruckner J, Baker HH 1991 Pedal mechanics and bipedalism in early hominids. In: Origine(s) de la bipédie chez les hominidés (Cahiers de Paléoanthropologie). Editions du CNRS, Paris, pp 159–167.

La Porta DM, Mellillo TV, Hetherington VJ 1994. Preoperative assessment in hallux valgus. In: Hetherington VJ (ed.) Hallux valgus and forefoot surgery. Churchill Livingstone, New York, p. 118.

Leboucq H 1882 Le développement du premier métatarsien et de son articulation tarsienne chez l'homme. Archive Biologie 3:337–344.

Lewis OJ 1981 Functional morphology of the joints of the evolving foot. Symposia of the Zoological Society of London 46:169–188.

Lisowski FP 1967 Angular growth changes and comparisons in the primate talus. Folia Primatologica 7:81–97.

Lisowski FP, Albrecht GH, Oxnard CE 1974 The form of the talus in some higher primates: a multivariate study. American Journal of Physical Anthropology 41:191.

Lisowski FP, Albrecht GH, Oxnard CE 1976 African fossil tali: further multivariate studies. American Journal of Physical Anthropology 45:518.

McHenry H 1982 The pattern of human evolution: studies on bipedalism, mastication, and encephalization. Annual Review in Anthropology 11:151–173.

McHenry H, Berger LR 1998 Body proportions of Australopithecus aferensis and A. africanus and the origin of the genus Homo. Journal of Human Evolution 35:1–22.

Manley-Buser KA 1991 A heterochronic study of the hominoid foot. PhD thesis, University of California.

Meyer M 1979 A comparison of hallux abductovalgus in two ancient populations. Journal of the American Podiatry Association 69(1):65–68.

Moorhead J, Wobeskya L 1995 Evolutionary aspects of foot disorders. Journal of the American Podiatric Medical Association 85(4):211.

Morton DJ 1922 Evolution of the human foot. American Journal of Physical Anthropology 5:305–325.

Morton DJ 1926 Evolution of man's erect posture. Journal of Morphological Physiology 43:147–179.

Morton DJ 1927 Metatarsus ataviticus – the identification of a distinctive type of foot disorder. Journal of Bone and Joint Surgery 9:36.

Morton DJ 1935 The human foot: its evolution, physiology, and functional disorders. Columbia University Press, New York.

Napier J 1967 The antiquity of human walking. Scientific American 216(4):56–66.

Olson TR, Siedel MR 1983 The evolutionary bases for some clinical disorders of the human foot: a comparative survey of the living primates. Foot and Ankle 3(6):322–341.

Richmond BG, Begun DR, Strait DS 2001 Origin of human bipedalism: the knuckle-walking hypothesis revisited. Yearbook of Physical Anthropology 44(Suppl 33):71–105.

Root LM, Orien WP, Weed JH 1977 Normal and abnormal function of the foot, Vol. 2. Clinical Biomechanics Corporation, Los Angeles, CA.

Scheman E 1931 Die umwegige Formentwicklung des menschlichen Talus. Morphologisches Jahrbuch 67:63–105.

Shea BT 1983 Allometry and heterochrony in the African Apes. American Journal of Physical Anthropology 62:275–289.

Stern JT, Susman RL 1983 Locomotor anatomy of Australopithecus aferensis. American Journal of Physical Anthropology 60:279–317.

Susman RL 1979 Comparative and functional morphology of hominoid fingers. American Journal of Physical Anthropology 50:215–236.

Susman RL 1983 Evolution of the human foot: evidence from the Plio-Pleistocene hominids. Foot & Ankle 3(6):365–376.

Susman RL, Brain TM 1988 New first metatarsal (SKX 5017) from Swartkrans and the gait of Paranthropus Robustus. American Journal of Physical Anthropology 77:7–15.

Susman RL, Stern JT, Jungers WL 1984 Arboreality and bipedality in the Hadar hominids. Folia Primatologica 43:113–156.

Vittetoe DA, Saltzman CL, Krieg JC, Brown TD 1994 Validity and reliability of the first distal metatarsal articular angle. Foot and Ankle International 15(10):541–547.

Weidenreich F 1923 Evolution of the human foot. American Journal of Physical Anthropology 6:1.

Weidenreich F 1940 The external tubercle of the human tuber calcanei. American Journal of Physical Anthropology 23:473–487.

Wolff J 1892 Das Gesetz der Transformation der Knochen. Berlin-Verlag, Berlin (reprinted 1986: The law of bone remodelling).

# Chapter | 27 |

# Health promotion and patient education

*Anne Shirley and Jane Thomas*

## KEYWORDS

Communication

Compliance/adherence/concordance

Health promotion

Patient education

## INTRODUCTION

Health promotion developed in the 1980s and 1990s and has been described as a 'unifying concept' (Bunton & Macdonald 2002). While definitions of health promotion abound (Kickbusch 1997, Naidoo & Wills 2004, Tannahill 1985, World Health Organization 1986), it is more useful to consider the two key aspects (lifestyle and structural aspects) in relation to podiatric practice. The Department of Health (2009) has health promotion at the centre of the current 'Be active, Be healthy' strategy. This strategy focuses on England and promotes activity, critically underpinned by foot health as a key to mobility and activity. The types of activity promoted include walking and dancing and a 'can do – change for life' approach, and it sets a target of 2 million people being 'more active' by 2012. In relation to foot health, chiropody, podiatry, health promotion and patient education have value in their capacity to focus on where the difficulties lie in an enabling and empowering approach. By its very nature, in recent years the role of the podiatrist in the 'modernised' health service has evolved into a more policy-driven, collaborative and multiprofessional area of practice (Department of Health 2000a,b).

Borthwick and Nancarrow (2005) have argued for a reconfiguration of podiatric services and roles to reflect a fundamental shift in the therapeutic role to encompass health promotion. While this presents an exciting range of options for the practitioner it can change perceptions of the profession among the public and fellow professionals. Although many foot conditions and their resultant effects are amenable to health-promotion intervention, it has taken time for the health-promotion role of the podiatrist to be fully recognised. The scope to develop practice in terms of Tannahill's (1985) three domains, particularly prevention and health education, is evident, particularly through educational, behaviour-change and empowerment approaches and self-care. This is evidenced in the work by Moore et al (2003) with regard to educational programmes in self-care. The increased demand for screening and education in diabetic care (Department of Health 2000b) and the predominance of older clients in the sector exerts pressures on the service, both within the National Health Service (NHS) and in the independent sector. While empowerment approaches go some way to promoting self-care and reducing dependency, the profession is responding with tiered care provision (Moore et al 2003). Borthwick and Nancarrow (2005) assert that health promotion, facilitation and preventive care are linked closely to changing roles in podiatry and have informed the changing nature of practice.

In order to understand fully the concept of health promotion we need to understand health as a multidimensional concept. It can be regarded as a negative paradigm in terms of the absence of disease, while others see it in a positive way as a sense of well-being. The World Health Organization (WHO) (1946) in its constitution defines health as 'a state of complete physical, mental and social well-being, not merely the absence of disease or infirmity'. In later years health was redefined as a resource for everyday life not an object of living; it is a positive concept emphasising social and personal resources as well as physical capacities (World Health Organization 1984). The term 'health' is complex, imprecise and widely contested, but the various connotations must be considered and appreciated in order for health improvement to be addressed (Scriven 2005, Seedhouse 2004).

The WHO (1984) defined health promotion as 'the process of enabling people to increase control over, and to improve their health'.

In 1986, the WHO produced the Ottawa Charter, which is regarded by many as a seminal text in health promotion. The charter outlined the importance of building healthy public policies, creating supportive environments and strengthening communities. It also emphasised the need for the development of personal skills and a reorientation of health services to focus on prevention for individuals, communities and populations. Health promotion involves both environmental and political actions, and recognises the link between health and health inequalities.

# THE PODIATRIST'S ROLE AS A HEALTH PROMOTER/EDUCATOR

The importance of health promotion, health education and patient education is well documented, the emphasis being placed on educating individuals about the link between risk-taking behaviours and disease and providing the skills necessary to help them make changes (Bunton & Macdonald 2002, Naidoo & Wills 2000). Although health promotion is contemporaneous for many health professionals, it provides common ground. Key elements identified in the Ottawa Charter (World Health Organization 1986) for health promotion underpin the work of many allied health professionals. Podiatrists have the potential to enable and empower individuals to increase control over, and thereby improve, their health and well-being as recommended in the Charter (World Health Organization 1986). Podiatrists' skills in advocacy and mediation may also contribute to the creation of supportive environments conducive to health promotion. Health promotion has been included in the curriculum at schools of podiatry for many years, but some might argue it is possibly not afforded the consideration it deserves. One could argue that, as an integral part of podiatrists' work, this important topic is often overlooked. There appear to be poor levels of knowledge linking health promotion and podiatry, there being no defined syllabus or consistency of health promotion taught throughout the recognised schools of podiatry within the UK.

Feet are an overworked part of the human body, playing a major role in the everyday life of individuals. Therefore, foot afflictions have a great impact on the health and well-being of individuals so affected. Health promotion in podiatry is often regarded as addressing foot health and footwear implications (McMullan 2004), which, although relevant, comprise only a part of the holistic approach that must be embraced. For example, a large number of podiatric patients have podiatric problems associated with peripheral vascular disease, and the link between risk behaviours and disease is well documented (Hoffman 2003, Levy 1998). The role of health promotion in podiatry is essential to encourage healthful individual behaviours, especially as podiatrists have a unique opportunity of one-to-one patient contact, enhancing their ability to promote health and evaluate patient progress.

Prevention of foot and lower-limb problems, either by educational strategies or screening activities, is a key role for podiatrists, who have a pivotal role in maintaining the independence of their patients (O'Donnell 2005). This is particularly important for the elderly, where mobility is essential in everyday life (Turner & Merriman 2005). Immobility not only exacerbates pathological complications such as muscle wasting, osteoporosis and deep vein thrombosis to name but a few, but can have immense psychological implications, with loss of confidence and self-esteem, depression and isolation being attributable to a poor quality of life (Tyrrell 2006, Lorimer et al 2006). The ability of podiatrists to help keep patients ambulatory may be the dividing line between institutionalisation and remaining an active member of the community and society (Turner & Merriman 2005).

The podiatry profession, formerly known as chiropody, is depicted in the literature as a healthcare speciality devoted to the treatment and prevention of afflictions of the foot (Dagnell & Page 1992). However, while this is indeed the case, modern podiatric practice is moving away from the historical routine foot care to encompass a larger range of roles, skills and knowledge (Scriven 2005). The role of the podiatrist now includes the bigger picture, and as such health promotion and patient education are essential components of podiatric practice, particularly as the profession continues to expand its boundaries. In the current economic environment, reorganisation of health services together with associated changes in fund holding have empowered managers to explore more cost-effective treatment options. As such, podiatric surgery is now more widely recognised as being an accessible, cost-effective and efficient service (Borthwick 2000, Editorial 2002). Research also identifies the positive impact that podiatric surgery can have on patient health and well-being (Kilmartin 2000).

The ongoing development of the profession presently incorporates biomechanical expertise, foot surgery, an embryonic role in rheumatology and specialist diabetic care (Borthwick 2000, Bowen 2003, Clements 2001, Graham 2000). The podiatrist's role in childhood foot problems (podopaediatrics) is ever-increasing (Thomson & Volpe 2001). A large proportion of the podiatrist's workload is still concerned with the elderly, podiatric afflictions having many detrimental effects on the health and well-being of these individuals (Dolinis et al 1997, Menz & Lord 2001). Research shows that up to 80% of the adult population suffers some form of foot problem (Society of Chiropodists and Podiatrists 2007).

To understand why the role of the podiatrist as a health promoter/educator is so significant, the history of the emergence of the profession deserves consideration. The fundamental shift in the identity of the profession demands an increasing involvement in health-promoting strategies (Scriven 2005). Podiatry is a specialism in itself, in that the podiatrist is responsible for diagnosing and treating individuals without prior intervention by other healthcare professionals. In the 17th and 18th centuries podiatry and dentistry shared similar positions in the medical hierarchy, early chiropodists being medically qualified practitioners and regarded as foot surgeons. However, the dominance of medical interests in the 20th century limited podiatrists' scope of practice, forbidding the use of local analgesia by chiropodists/podiatrists and hence surgical interventions.

In contrast, today's podiatric practice has seen a shift back to a wide field of practice, once again encompassing not only routine foot care but also elective surgery. Legal access to local anaesthetics signalled the way forward in the development of podiatric specialisms, the use of local analgesia by podiatrists now being commonplace in everyday practice. Procedures by surgically qualified podiatrists may include forefoot surgery such as digital, metatarsal and bunion corrections, fusions and osteotomies. Digital or ray amputation, neuroma excisions, fasciotomies and rearfoot calcaneal osteotomies are also undertaken (Kilmartin 2000, Price & Tasker 2000).

These factors alone identify marked changes within the profession of podiatry. The acquisition of medical consultant posts plus associate specialist grade contracts within NHS healthcare in the UK has been the most significant achievement of the podiatry profession to date (Scriven 2005). The ever-changing role of the podiatrist encompasses a wide range of activities, and as such health promotion must complement these practices. The revision of the role of the podiatrist has also centred on patient empowerment, and the continuing benefits of this health-promotion approach are well documented (Farndon et al 2007, Laverack 2005, Moore et al 2003, Nancarrow 2003). The future of podiatry needs to remain holistic in its approach, adopting strategies identified in the Feet First report (Department of Health 1994), with expanding role boundaries, encouragement of specialisms and promotion of preventive care.

Possibly one of the most important changes in health promotion over the years has been educating people on how to manage their general health, with specific focus on key aspects. Patient empowerment as a basic right for individuals was emphasised by the WHO as an important component of health promotion (Laverack 2005). However, it can be argued that many allied health professionals may not be in a position to empower individuals, and this issue needs consideration in order to ensure that health promotion becomes an essential aspect of podiatric care, especially with podiatry entering this new specialist era.

The contribution of allied health professionals, including podiatrists, to health-promoting practice is also recognised by the UK government (Department of Health 2003). Ten key roles are identified for allied health professionals highlighting the importance of health promotion within their professional remit. The Standards of Proficiency set by the Health Professions Council (2003), with which podiatrists and other allied health professionals are registered, also reiterates the need for health promotion in professional practice. The Society of Chiropodists and Podiatrists further emphasises the importance of partnership, identifying the relevance of both clinical and educational interventions to maintain patient mobility, thereby improving health and well-being. Furthermore, podiatry education is underpinned by benchmark statements (Quality Assurance Agency for Higher Education 2001), which specifically identify the importance of health promotion within podiatry. A new White Paper 'Choosing Health: Making Healthier Choices Easier' (Department of Health 2004) encourages individuals to make choices conducive to health and encourages health workers to adopt health-promoting roles.

There is little literature relating to health promotion and podiatry, although there is a substantial evidence base relating to podiatry and diabetes (Foster 2004, Knowles 2004, O'Boyle et al 2000). The importance of the psychosocial approaches to podiatry, highlighting the need to consider the bigger picture surrounding patients' health and well-being, cannot be ignored. The literature reminds us that podiatric practice must encompass not only pathological aetiologies but also the wider determinants of health (Mandy et al 2003). Furthermore, the emergence of specialisms within podiatry requires more emphasis on the health-promoting paradigm of empowerment within podiatry.

## PATIENT EDUCATION

Podiatrists' involvement in educating their patients in preventive strategies is essential to minimise problems in the lower limb, which may be attributable to patients' lack of knowledge about their illness. This is not a new concept and it has been evidenced by many authors over the years (Bradshaw 1990, Dunlop & Baxter 2006, Valente & Nelson 1995, Wormald 1995). However, podiatrists need support to develop effective teaching techniques, conditions and communication tools (Ewles & Simnett 2003, Lockyer et al 1997). There is a range of teaching techniques, including one-to-one discussion, hard-copy information (handouts, leaflets) and DVDs, that can be used to enable practitioners to put their message across comprehensively. In addition, communication tools such as the internet and the media can assist, but these require careful management. The patient may use these routes to access information but, in the absence of practitioner input, they can create anxiety, misinformation and even undermine health. The role of the podiatrist in moderating this type of information and ensuring its appropriate use is an important aspect of patient care. While it is important to use language that is suitable to the

patient, it is also necessary to introduce the patient to relevant podiatric terminology to assist their understanding of their treatment.

Although only one aspect of podiatric care, education has important connotations in that it helps both the patient (to know about foot health and understand treatment) and the practitioner (to invest time in preventing potential complications). There are direct implications on both sides, as well as more long-term benefits to the service in terms of cost-effectiveness in an already overstretched service. Making time for patient education in a busy schedule can be difficult, as can developing the health-promotion aspects of practice. A lack of training has been recognised as one obstacle facing allied health professionals wishing to promote health as part of their professional remit (Scriven 2005). As podiatrists have a unique one-to-one access to their patients this barrier needs to be removed to encourage their role as patient educators and health promoters.

Compliance is a key issue but the term can carry negative connotations, the term 'concordance' is now used more frequently, as it is more patient-focused. Bell et al (2007) have described concordance in terms of balancing the 'power' in healthcare communication between the adviser and recipient. Phipps and Bell (2009) propose the following key points with regard to adherence to treatment:

- best practice/treatment/advice is only beneficial if recipients carry out the advice or take the treatment
- non-adherence does not lie solely with patients – poor information given by advisers, badly written information leaflets and communication breakdown may be factors
- the individual's perception of adequate information may be different from the information giver's
- working in a person-centred way, for the public health practitioner, may be the best way to support individuals in adhering to their treatment/advice regimen.

Other factors may also influence the person, such as: the level of impact of a change on their daily routine (and the cost–benefit of the change); the complexity of the change; they may not want, agree with or accept the advice/information; the timescale may be too long; and communication problems or mental health issues. Awareness of these issues is critical for the podiatric practitioner, in view of the need for concordance in all elements of podiatric intervention, as illustrated in Case Study 27.1.

---

**CASE STUDY 27.1 SELF-MONITORING BY THE PATIENT AFTER REMOVAL OF THE NAIL PLATE AND PHENOLISATION OF THE MATRIX**

Patients who have undergone nail removal and phenolisation can monitor their healing and change their dressings. Using the example of a healthy adult male patient who has had the nails of both great toes removed, let us consider his health-promotion needs. The patient would need to be advised that his participation in his care would be required in terms of changing dressings, observing the area and reporting any concerns. So, from a health-promotion and/or patient-education perspective, consider the following.

**Think about the advice you would give to the patient before nail surgery.**

On the day of your appointment for nail surgery:

- Bring a slipper or sandal to wear for the return journey home. This will allow room for the toe dressing(s), which may be bulky.
- Make transport arrangements for your return home. You will be able to walk after the operation but you should rest the foot as much as possible. You are strongly advised not to drive until the effects of the local anaesthetic have worn off. Arrange for transport home.

- If you are under 16 years old you must be accompanied by a responsible adult.
- The operation will take approximately 15 minutes, but you should expect the appointment to last for at least an hour.
- You will be required to attend the same clinic for postoperative care.

This information can be given in handout form to support verbal information.

**Now think about the advice to the patient following nail surgery:**

- Do not walk for long distances.
- Avoid driving while the toe is numb and for up to 12 hours while the systemic effects of the anaesthetic continue.
- When the anaesthetic wears off, if you are aware of any pain you should take the painkiller you would normally take.
- Try to be off your feet as much as possible for the first 24 hours after the operation. If you have to work during this time, light duties should be arranged.
- If you notice blood seeping through the dressing DO NOT remove the dressing. Apply another dressing on top and keep your foot up.
- Keep the dressing dry until your next appointment at the clinic.
- You will be seen at regular intervals until your toe has healed.
- In the unlikely event of persistent bleeding, or if you are in discomfort, contact the following number (number given).

This information should be given in written form. It is helpful to use attractive presentation, large print and clear language in patient-education materials. In this instance, the patient would be discharged with a postoperative-care sheet. The dressing would be removed at the podiatry clinic the following day, but emergency materials and phone numbers are provided in case they are needed.

*Dressing procedures*

- The dressing must be kept dry between dressing changes.
- Remove the soiled dressings and bathe your foot in warm water, adding a tablespoon of salt to a pint of water, as demonstrated. If the dressing sticks DO NOT PULL IT OFF. Soak off in the salt water.
- Keep your foot immersed in the salt solution for between 5 and 10 minutes.
- Dry the foot with a clean towel, dabbing the wound with the gauze supplied.
- Open the dressing pack and place the dressing on the toe, taking care not to touch the side of the dressing that will come into contact with the wound.
- Cover the dressing with the tubular gauze, as demonstrated, and secure with the tape provided.
- Re-dress your toe daily unless instructed otherwise.
- If you have any problems or queries do not hesitate to contact the following number (number given).

It is also important that the patient is informed of and alerted to signs of infection such as:

- pain
- swelling
- odour

The patient should be made aware of what to do and who to contact if these signs occur.

The patient should also be made aware that the toe may appear very inflamed for between 7 and 21 days and this is regarded as normal. The toe will look worse before it looks better, and may take up to 12 weeks to attain optimum improvement.

The patient would be provided with:

- the dressing procedure advice sheet (given in advance of the surgery)
- a return appointment for the following day
- a dressing pack (enough for two dressings)
- a contact number.

This mode of care will continue for a month. Not all cases will follow the plan exactly, as infection may develop or the patient may not adhere to their part in the treatment plan.

Finally, a suggestion for a multi-method approach to improving adherence (originally developed in relation to medication and older people (Bergman-Evans 2006)):

**A Assessment**: this could include assessment of the individual's capacity to understand and retain information, and of their memory function

**I Individualisation**: adherence is more likely if the treatment/advice is tailored to the individual's needs

**D Documentation**: if appropriate to the individual's needs, this helps communication between the adviser and advised, providing a focus for discussion

**E Education**: again, tailored specifically to the individual

**S Supervision**: coupled with evaluation of the regimen, so both parties can discuss what works best or is inconvenient

This model suits podiatry, with joint working between the practitioner and patient in a person-centred way.

Good communication is recognised as an essential factor in patient education, and the literature on this subject evidences a lack of these skills as being a dominant barrier. In podiatric practice the complexities of patient–podiatrist interaction, acknowledging the layout of the podiatric setting with the podiatrist based at the foot of the patient, can have a detrimental effect (Mandy et al 2003). A breakdown in patient–podiatrist communication could lead to patient non-concordance with advice, and evidence reminds us that patients respond more favourably to healthcare professionals with whom they can communicate effectively (Dunlop & Baxter 2006, Lutfey & Wishner 1999). Furthermore, some argue that the predominantly older age group of podiatric patients could limit the effectiveness of patient education (O'Boyle et al 2000). Podiatrists should therefore structure their advice to suit the target audience in terms of age and other indicators, and see this as an opportunity rather than a barrier to good communication.

It has been suggested, despite evidence to the contrary, that patient education, health education and health promotion are time-consuming activities having limited benefits (Morris 1998). Indeed, many health professionals would argue that the time allocated to an individual patient is already restricted and should be used for treatment. Research also indicates there may be scepticism amongst podiatry professionals with regard to health promotion, and such an attitude may affect the delivery of health promotion, particularly if it is felt that 'talking time' is time wasted time (Macleod Clark & Maben 1998, O'Boyle et al 2000). It could also be argued that time allocated to patient education/health promotion could have financial implications, which need to be evaluated and addressed.

However, what cannot be denied is the importance of education and prevention in healthcare, and as such these paradigms should be an integral part of podiatric practice if patient needs are to be addressed fully. Podiatrists must strive to improve concordance and adherence by using a person-centred approach, with treatment plans that are tailored around the patient's lifestyle, for maximum efficiency (Aronson 2007, Phipps and Bell 2009). Empowerment and self-care must be encouraged at all times (Farndon et al 2007, Moore et al 2003). Research identifies the impact that front-line professionals such as podiatrists can have in identifying risk factors and advising/referring accordingly, once again emphasising the need to work in partnership with the patient. An example of this would be the integration of advice to stop smoking into routine podiatry services (Gray et al 2007, Rains et al 2006).

Multidisciplinary team working and collaboration between podiatrists, health promoters and other health professionals should be encouraged to maximise health improvement. The importance of this approach is emphasised in diabetic podiatric care, where patients benefit from a range of professional expertise to address foot problems associated with the systemic disease (Gadsby & McInnes 1998, Young 2003). Podiatrists have always had a large input in diabetic care, with research identifying the importance of preventive foot-care programmes in reducing amputation rates (Robbie 2002). It has been suggested that the podiatrist's role could be enhanced further to include involvement in patient insulin dosage and patient health education regarding blood glucose monitoring (Kerr & Richardson 2000).

Collaboration is also invaluable when managing rheumatology patients, this newest specialist domain in podiatry again demanding emphasis on empowerment and self-care. The podiatrist, whether working in isolation or as part of a team, needs to work as a facilitator to ensure that patient podiatric needs are met and treated in relation to other manifestations of the disease (Woodburn & Helliwell 1997, Nancarrow 2003).

It is widely recognised that common foot problems, whether arising due to trauma, deformities or pedal complications of systemic disease, can affect the patient's lifestyle and quality of life. The role of podiatrists in public health should encompass footwear, ambulatory and activity problems, and if possible screening should be used to identify childhood foot problems as well as pedal chronic disease. However, consideration should also be given to the health determinants that affect podiatric care, in particular the relevance of income status (e.g. footwear implications), living and working conditions, social support, and genetic manifestations. The literature evidences the relationship between socio-economic status and health, arguing that a patient's needs are complex, with pathological aetiologies being only one of many factors affecting their health status (Brodie 2001, Helfand 1998, Helfand & Hausman 2001, Mandy et al 2003).

Until the last decade, the curriculum for podiatry training was based primarily on the medical model of health. While addressing podiatric complications and the restoration of physiological function is important, this model fails to consider the implications of behavioural, psychological and socio-economic influences on an individual's health or illness status. Consideration of the determinants of health, especially inequalities in health that can affect the management of the podiatric patient, is paramount (Acheson 1998, O'Donnell 2005). Some argue that health promotion in podiatry has not made much progress over the years, and suggest the development of tailor-made programmes to address this. The literature reiterates the need to provide foot and general health education to younger age groups in order to furnish individuals with the skills necessary to make informed choices (Brodie 2001).

The primary challenges for healthcare professionals are how to make change acceptable, how to tell people about it, how to make change happen and how to sustain the change. It may be helpful for podiatrists to use theoretical frameworks to enable them to address the complexities involved in behaviour change. That said, podiatrists need to recognise not only the advantages but also the disadvantages of the behaviour-change approach (Naidoo & Wills 2000). Patient vulnerability, the perceived effectiveness of any change, the opinions of significant others and the severity of underlying disease can all influence an individual's ability to change behaviour. Individuals need to have an incentive to change; they need to understand the benefits of making the changes and be empowered to confidently

make those changes. Equity and autonomy are important principles, and each patient should be encouraged to achieve their individual potential. It is crucial to avoid 'victim blaming', which can occur when dealing with patients whose behaviour may have influenced their health and/or adversely affected their care.

Mandy et al (2003) identify the need for podiatry students to develop professional skills towards autonomous practice as a basis for life-long learning, reinforcing the message that reflective practice provides the means for learning from everyday experiences (Bolton 2005). However, behaviour change cannot be guaranteed to result from the acquisition of knowledge (Davies & Macdowall 2006).

## EVIDENCE-BASED PRACTICE

The importance of evidence-based practice for healthcare professionals cannot be denied. Research identifies that podiatrists who underpin their professional practice with evidence-based knowledge can significantly contribute to the health improvement of individuals and the population as a whole (O'Donnell 2005). In the current climate of public distrust of expert knowledge podiatrists should strive not to make unvalidated or unqualified claims in health-risk advice, research identifying that it is not enough in the practice of promoting health to rely on good intentions and perceived wisdom (Dunlop & Baxter 2006, McQueen 2001, Naidoo & Wills 2005). Today's environment is such that individuals may be less inclined to readily accept advice or information given by professionals, unless supported by theory. That said, not all knowledge can be supported by evidence, but such unsupported data should nevertheless be considered (McQueen 2001).

## CONCLUSIONS

The WHO Ottawa Charter presents health promotion as a process of enabling individuals to take more control over and improve their health. The various connotations of what is meant by 'health' underpin our efforts to improve not only the physical but also the mental and social well-being of individuals (Ewles & Simnett 2003). Health can be regarded as a basic human right, an everyday resource for living, not just an objective of living, and be reiterated as a positive concept (Sidell et al 2003). As such health promotion must go beyond health-sector settings if we are to encourage healthful behaviours and lifestyles to improve well-being. The ultimate goal of health promotion is to increase not only health expectancy but to narrow the gap in health expectancy between countries and communities (Edelman & Mandle 2006). Health promotion works to reduce inequalities in health, addressing the determinants of health to achieve the greatest health gains for both individuals and the population as a whole.

Health promotion in podiatry must strive to follow the principles of the Ottawa Charter (World Health Organization 1986), and encompass a set of values that includes empowerment, equity, collaboration and participation. A bottom-up approach will encourage podiatry patients to take more control over their health. Podiatrists must avoid victim-blaming and always consider the social determinants of health underpinning patient lifestyles and behaviour. In an age where life expectancy is increasing, podiatric services are in great demand (Dunlop & Baxter 2006). In the long term, health promotion in podiatry should provide economic benefits in health services, and preventive strategies to improve long-term health gain. However, critics could argue that health promotion in podiatry may generate greater demand on an already overstretched service, and this possibility cannot be ignored.

The literature to date evidences the need for health promotion, health education and patient education in podiatry, but there is a gap in the available literature on this subject itself. The role of health promotion in podiatry should not be restricted to foot health education alone, but needs to encompass the wider variables such as behavioural and socio-economic determinants that affect the health and well-being of podiatry patients. However, although the role of health promotion and patient education is becoming more widely recognised as a requisite of podiatric care, in reality this role is still largely omitted in everyday practice. In order to address this, the podiatrists of the future need to be empowered with the necessary skills and knowledge to carry out this extended role.

Podiatrists aim to maintain patient mobility and independence, and as such patient empowerment is an essential aspect of podiatric care. The role of health promotion within podiatry is vital to ensure that podiatry patients receive the best possible care, including education in preventive strategies to help allay future health problems. The notion of making the healthy choice the easy choice is fundamental to success in health promotion, and is as relevant in podiatric care as in any aspect of lifestyle where choice applies.

In order to develop practice and improve podiatric standards, it is important to evaluate our understanding and progress. Evaluation helps us to understand the learning process more fully and can be considered in terms of process, outcome and impact. When we think about podiatric practice, the same approach can be applied to enable us to understand whether what we have done was successful in the way we did it, in the outcome it achieved and/or whether it had the intended effect. Evaluation should form an integral part of practice, encouraging reflection, which enables us to improve. With this in mind, before finishing this chapter consider evaluating your own learning:

- What have you learned from reading this chapter?
- What change might you make to your practice as a result?
- Is there anything you could pass on to colleagues?

## REFERENCES

Acheson D 1998 Independent inquiry into inequalities in health report. HMSO, London.

Aronson JK 2007 Compliance, concordance, adherence. British Journal of Clinical Pharmacology 63(4):383–384.

Bell SJ, Airaksinen MS, Lyles A, et al 2007 Concordance is not synonymous with compliance or adherence (Letter to the Editor). British Journal of Clinical Pharmacology 64(5):710–713.

Bergman-Evans B 2006 Cited in: Wilson F, Mabhala A (eds) 2009 Key concepts in public health. Sage, London, p. 231.

Bolton G 2005 Reflective Practice – Writing and Professional Development. 2nd ed. Sage Publications Ltd, London.

Borthwick AM 2000 Challenging medicine: the case of podiatric surgery. Work, Employment and Society 14(2):369–383.

Borthwick AM, Nancarrow S 2005 Promoting health: the role of the specialist podiatrist. In: Scriven A (ed.) Health promoting practice: the contribution of nurses and allied health professionals. Palgrave Macmillan, Basingstoke, pp 221–237.

Bowen C 2003 Podiatric Rheumatic Care Association conference report. Podiatry Now 6(11):32.

Bradshaw T 1990 The concept, development, anatomy and physiology of a footcare leaflet for people at risk of developing diabetic foot ulceration. Chiropodist 45(2):30–32.

Brodie BS 2001 Health determinants and podiatry. Journal of the Royal Society for the Promotion of Health 121(3):174–176.

Bunton R, Macdonald G 2002 Health promotion, disciplines, diversity and developments. Routledge, London.

Clements DJ 2001 Providing a diabetic foot care service: establishing a podiatry service. In: Boulton AJM, Conner H, Cavanagh PR (eds)

The foot in diabetes, 3rd edn. Wiley, London.

Dagnall JC, Page AL 1992 A critical history of the chiropodial profession and the Society of Chiropodists. Journal of British Podiatric Medicine 47(2):30–34.

Davies M, Macdowall W 2006 Health promotion theory. Open University Press, Maidenhead.

Department of Health 1994 Feet First: report of the joint Department of Health and NHS Chiropody Task Force. DoH, London.

Department of Health 2000a A health service of all the talents: developing the NHS Workforce. DoH, London.

Department of Health 2000b Meeting the challenge: a strategy for the allied health professions. DoH, London.

Department of Health 2003 Practitioners with special interests: bringing services closer to patients. DoH, London.

Department of Health 2004 Choosing health: making healthy choices easier. DoH, London.

Department of Health 2009 Be active, be healthy: a plan for getting the nation moving. Ref. 10818. Available at: http://www.dh.gov.uk/en/Publicationsandstatistics/Publications/PublicationsPolicyAndGuidance/DH_094358 (19 September 2009).

Dolinis J, Harrison JE, Andrews GR 1997 Factors associated with falling in older Adelaide residents. Australian and New Zealand Journal of Public Health 21(5):462–468.

Dunlop G, Baxter P 2006 In: Lorimer D, French G, O'Donnell M (eds) Neale's Disorders of the Foot, 7th edn. Churchill Livingstone, Philadelphia, PA.

Edelman CL, Mandle CL 2006 Health promotion throughout the lifespan, 2nd edn. Mosby, Philadelphia, PA.

Editorial 2002 Chiropody, podiatry and orthopaedics. Foot and Ankle Surgery 8:83.

Ewles L, Simnett I 2003 Promoting health: a practical guide, 5th edn. London: Baillière Tindall, London.

Farndon L, Vernon W, Moore M 2007 The Sheffield empowerment project: six years on. British Journal of Podiatry 10(3):104–109.

Foster A 2004 An evaluation of NICE guidelines on foot care for patients with diabetes. Nursing Times 100(22):52–53.

Gadsby R, McInnes A 1998 The at-risk foot: the role of the primary care team in achieving St. Vincent targets for reducing amputation. Diabetes Medicine. 15(Suppl 3):561–564.

Graham RB 2000 Developing the therapy professional. Presented at the Chiropody and Podiatry Conference, Royal College of Surgeons London, 10 May.

Gray J, Eden G, Williams M 2007 Developing the public health role of a front line clinical service: integrating stop smoking advice into routine podiatry services. Journal of Public Health 29(2):118–122.

Health Professions Council 2003 Standards of proficiency: chiropodists/podiatrists. Available at: http://www.hpc-uk.org/publications/standards/index.asp?id=41 (19 September 2009).

Helfand AE 1998 Podiatric medicine and public health concepts and perspectives. Special Communication 88(7):353–359.

Helfand AE, Hausman AJ 2001 A conceptual model for public health education in podiatric medicine. Journal of the American Podiatric Medical Association 91(9):488–495.

Hoffman AF 2003 Peripheral vascular considerations. Clinics in Podiatric Medicine and Surgery 20:527–545.

Kerr D, Richardson T 2000 The diabetic foot at the crossroads: vanguard or oblivion? The Diabetic Foot 3(2):70 –71.

Kickbusch I 1997 Think health: what makes the difference? Health Promotion International 12(4):265–272.

Kilmartin T 2000 Podiatric surgery in a Community Trust: a review of activity, surgical outcomes and patient satisfaction over a 27 month period. Podiatry Now 3(9):350–355.

Knowles A 2004 Diabetes care in older people. Diabetes and the feet in old age. Journal of Diabetic Nursing 8(10):382–385.

Laverack G 2005 Public health: power, empowerment and professional practice. Palgrave Macmillan, Basingstoke.

Levy A 1998 The impact of tobacco use on podiatric medicine. Journal of American Podiatric Medicine Association 88(10):517–518.

Lockyer J, Davies DM, Thivierge R 1997 Patient education materials: physicians' perceptions of their role and usefulness. Journal of Continuing Education in the Health Professionals 17:159–162.

Lorimer D, French G, O'Donnell M (eds) 2006 Neale's disorders of the foot, 6th edn. Churchill Livingstone, Edinburgh.

Lutfey KE, Wishner WJ 1999 Beyond 'compliance' is 'adherence': improving the prospects of diabetic care. Diabetes Care 22:635–639.

Macleod Clark J, Maben J 1998 Health promotion: perceptions of Project 2000 educated nurses. Health Education Research 13(2):185–196.

Mandy A, Lucas K, McInnes J 2003 Psychosocial approaches to podiatry: a companion of practice. Churchill Livingstone, Edinburgh.

McMillan C 2004 To wear or not to wear? Compliance problems with footwear advice. Southport & Ormskirk Hospital NHS Trust, England.

McQueen D 2001 Strengthening the evidence base for health promotion. Health Promotion International 16(3):261–268.

Menz H, Lord S 2001 The contribution of foot problems to mobility, impairment and falls in community dwelling older people. Journal of the American Geriatric Society 49(12):1651–1656.

Moore M, Farndon L, Macmillan S 2003 Patient empowerment: a strategy to eradicate podiatry waiting lists: the Sheffield experience. British Journal of Podiatry 6(1):17–20.

Morris DB 1998 Developing a patient education program: overcoming physicians resistance. The Diabetic Educator 24:41–47.

Naidoo J, Wills J 2000 Health promotion foundation for practice, 2nd edn. Baillière Tindall, London.

Naidoo J, Wills J 2005 Public health and health promotion developing practice, 2nd edn. Baillière Tindall, London.

Nancarrow SA 2003 Stakeholder consultation in the development of 'high risk' foot care services in the Australian Capital Territory. The Diabetic Foot 6(4):190–200.

O'Boyle PE, Hodkinson F, Fleming P 2000 Health promotion in podiatry: Podiatrists' perceptions and the implications for their professional practice. British Journal of Podiatry 3(1):21–28.

O'Donnell T 2005 In: Turner WA, Merriman LM (eds) Clinical skills in treating the foot, 2nd edn. Churchill Livingstone, Philadelphia, PA.

Phipps D, Bell S 2009 Adherence to treatment – a person-centred approach. In: Wilson F, Mabhala M (eds) Key concepts in public health. Sage, London.

Price M, Tasker J 2000 Putting the knife to the test: an audit of podiatric surgery services provided by First Community Health. Podiatry Now 3(11).

Quality Assurance Agency For Higher Education 2001 Subject benchmarks: chiropody and podiatry. Quality Assurance Agency for Higher Education, Gloucester.

Rains JC, Penzien DB, Lipchik GL 2006 Behavioural facilitation of medical treatment for headache – Part II: Implications of noncompliance and strategies for improving adherence. Headache 46(Suppl 3):S142–S143.

Robbie J 2002 Developing a diabetic foot screening service in primary care. The Diabetic Foot 5 (4):191–197.

Scriven A (ed.) 2005 Health promoting practice: the contribution of nurses and allied health professionals. Palgrave MacMillan, Basingstoke.

Seedhouse D 2004 Health Promotion: Philosophy, Prejudice and Practice. 2nd ed. Wiley, Chichester.

Sidell M, Jones L, Katz J, et al 2003 Debates and dilemmas in promoting health: a reader, 2nd edn. Palgrave MacMillan, Basingstoke.

Tannahill A 1985 What is health promotion? Health Education Journal 44:167–168.

Society of Chiropodists and Podiatrists 2007 Strategic plan 2007–2012. Podiatry Now 10(5):8–9.

Thomson P, Volpe R 2001 Introduction to podopaediatrics. Churchill Livingstone, Edinburgh.

Turner WA, Merriman LM 2005 Clinical skills in treating the foot, 2nd edn. Churchill Livingstone, London.

Valente LA, Nelson MS 1995 Patient education for diabetic patients: an integral part of quality care. Journal of the American Podiatric Medical Association 85(3):177–179.

Woodburn J, Helliwell PS 1997 Foot problems in rheumatology. British Journal of Rheumatology 36(9):932–934.

World Health Organization 1946 Constitution of the World Health Organization, 22 July 1946. WHO, Geneva.

World Health Organisation (WHO) 1984 Health Promotion: a discussion document on the concepts and principles. WHO, Copenhagen.

World Health Organization 1986. Ottawa Charter for health promotion. WHO, Copenhagen.

Wormald T 1995 Lower limb amputation in the diabetic: causation and prevention – the role of the podiatrists. Journal of British Podiatric Medicine 50(5):63–67.

Young M 2003 Generalists, specialists and super-specialists. The Diabetic Foot 6(1):6.

# Clinical governance

*Pamela M Sabine*

## KEYWORDS

Alderhey
Commission for Health Improvement
Consent
Informed consent
NICE

## INTRODUCTION

Clinical governance sits at the heart of the government's quality agenda for the National Health Service (NHS) and, indeed, the wider healthcare arena. The statutory duty now placed on everyone working in healthcare is that of overall quality improvement, year upon year, backed up by the evidence to prove it.

This is not a threat to podiatrists, any more than it is to any other healthcare professional, the majority of whom have consistently worked for the good of their patients, and in the main have provided excellent care on a very tight budget. Neither is clinical governance particularly onerous – it merely formalises that which most clinicians certainly should have been doing and usually have.

The well-publicised spate of extremely damaging and tragic cases in the late 1990s, such as Shipman, Bristol and Alderhey, brought into sharp relief the damage caused by the gross shortcomings and casual behaviour of the few, against the philosophy of the many. The government's answer to the general outcry and loss of public confidence was, in effect, clinical governance, tied in with a raft of other regulations, rules and requirements.

For the vast majority of clinicians in the healthcare arena, public or private, clinical governance actually offers a sensible way of determining priorities, developing staff and underpinning learning with experience. It offers clinicians the time to 'do things properly' in the way there has never been time before, and therefore offers an opportunity to examine activity and reflect on how that activity could be carried out differently and in a better way.

This chapter examines the evolution of clinical governance systems out of the myriad of good intentions, hard work and innovation that have always characterised the NHS. As clinical governance is now a contractual duty of all NHS employees, and its tenets underpin healthcare regulation, its presence cannot be ignored or sidestepped.

It is not just about public protection – it can be about promoting the good practice provided by clinicians throughout modern history. It places the patient at the centre of the healthcare provision and gives us the chance to prove just how we make the rhetoric live on a daily basis.

Clinical governance covers every aspect of healthcare. The quote given in Box 28.1 is taken from 'Clinical Governance in the New NHS' (Department of Health 1999) and is a full detailing of the areas affected by clinical governance requirements.

## CHRONOLOGY

In December 1997 the newly elected government published a White Paper for consultation entitled 'The New NHS – Modern and Dependable' (Secretary of State for Health 1997). In introducing the

---

**Box 28.1 Main components of clinical governance: NHS trusts (source: Department of Health 1999)**

Clear lines of responsibility and accountability for the overall quality of clinical care through:

- The NHS Trust Chief Executive carries ultimate responsibility for assuring the quality of services provided by the Trust
- A designated senior clinician responsible for ensuring that systems for clinical governance are in place and monitoring their continued effectiveness
- Formal arrangements for NHS Trust Boards to discharge their responsibilities for clinical quality, perhaps through a clinical governance committee
- Regular reports to NHS Trust Boards on the quality of clinical care given the same importance as monthly financial reports
- An annual report on clinical governance

A comprehensive programme of quality improvement activities, which includes:

- Full participation by all hospital doctors in audit programmes, including speciality and subspeciality national external audit programmes endorsed by the Commission for Health Improvement
- Full participation in the current four National Confidential Enquiries
- Evidence-based practice is supported and applied routinely in everyday practice
- Ensuring the clinical standards of National Service Frameworks and NICE recommendations are implemented
- Workforce planning and development (i.e. recruitment and retention of appropriately trained workforce) is fully integrated within the NHS Trust's service planning
- Continuing professional development: programmes aimed at meeting the development needs of individual health professionals and the service needs of the organisation are in place and supported locally

- Appropriate safeguards to govern access to and storage of confidential patient information as recommended in the Caldicott Report on the Review of Patient-Identifiable Information
- Effective monitoring of clinical care with high-quality systems for clinical record keeping and the collection of relevant information
- Processes for assuring the quality of clinical care are in place and integrated with the quality programme for the organization as a whole

Clear policies aimed at managing risks:

- Controls assurance which promote self-assessment to identify and manage risks
- Clinical risk systematically assessed with programmes in place to reduce risk

Procedures for all professional groups to identify and remedy poor performance, for example:

- Critical incident reporting ensures that adverse events are identified, openly investigated, lessons are learned and promptly applied
- Complaints procedures, accessible to patients and their families and fair to staff. Lessons are learned and recurrence of similar problems avoided
- Professional performance procedures which take effect at an early stage before patients are harmed and which help the individual to improve their performance whenever possible, are in place and understood by all staff
- Staff supported in their duty to report any concerns about colleagues' professional conduct and performance, with clear statements from the Board on what is expected of all staff. Clear procedures for reporting concerns so that early action can be taken to support the individual to remedy the situation

---

White Paper, the then Secretary of State for Health, the Right Honourable Frank Dobson, said 'This White Paper means a ten year programme of modernisation which will make the National Health Service (NHS) better every year. It will be an NHS for the next century, based on its founding principles of high quality care for all, delivered on the basis of need, and need alone.'

The Prime Minister, in his foreword to the document, was rather more explicit: 'For the first time the need to ensure that high quality care is spread throughout the service will be taken seriously. National standards of care will be guaranteed.' Chapter 3 of the document stated 'that the new NHS will have quality at its heart'.

The new measures that were proposed in order to fulfil the government's objectives were divided into three areas:

- national standards and guidelines for services and treatments
- local measures to enable the NHS staff to take responsibility for improving quality
- a new organisation to address shortcomings.

The stated aim of the White Paper was to replace the previous government's internal market with integrated care, and to reduce health inequalities. The key proposals included:

- New national standards of performance and quality measures were to be developed under the auspices of a newly established body called the National Institute for Clinical Excellence (now the National Institute for Health and Clinical Excellence, NICE). NICE was intended to give a 'strong lead on clinical and cost effectiveness'.

- National Service Frameworks (NSFs) were to be developed and introduced for particular care groups or diseases, setting out agreed standards for service delivery. The aim of these NSFs was to 'help ensure consistent access to services and quality of care right across the country'.
- The establishment of the Commission for Health Improvement (CHI) would provide support and oversee quality of clinical services at local level and 'tackle shortcomings'. The CHI was to raise standards of care by making sure that all parts of the NHS learned from and were brought up to the standards of the very best. The CHI has since become the Healthcare Commission and its role has been extended to take in standard setting for the delivery of healthcare. Wales and Scotland have established their own organisations to deal with devolved issues, and more changes are planned from 2009.
- Primary Care Groups (PCGs) were to be established, with the option of becoming Primary Care Trusts (PCTs).
- A new system of clinical governance was to be developed in NHS Trusts and primary care, to 'ensure that clinical standards are met, and that processes are in place to ensure continuous improvement'. This proposal was backed by the government's intention to give NHS organisations a new corporate statutory body for quality and clinical performance, using a system developed later under clinical governance.
- Information technology expansion was to be geared towards supporting the delivery of benefits to patients rather than towards operating the internal market.

- There was to be greater involvement of staff in service planning with greater emphasis placed on involving patients in all aspects of service delivery and ensuring that all healthcare was patient-focused.
- Strategies were to be brought forward to improve the working lives of staff and allowing ample scope for staff development.
- Health Authorities were to have an enhanced role in service planning and there were to be 'explicit quality standards in local service'.
- The establishment of NHS Direct – a 24-hour advice line manned by nurses.

The White Paper was closely followed by another White Paper entitled 'Designed to Care' in Scotland, 'Putting Patients First' in Wales and 'Fit for the Purpose' in Northern Ireland. Although there are several differences in approach between the documents, they are all heralding a period of great change in the NHS.

Thus the 'new NHS' introduced for the first time the concept of clinical governance, and advanced the notion that Trusts should be held strictly accountable for the quality of care they advanced. The objectives of health improvement and quality applied equally across the UK, and bodies such as NICE and the Healthcare Commission and others have national remits.

The standards, once set, would allow the public to judge the performance of the NHS, both nationally and locally, and all monies saved were to be redirected into front-line patient care.

In July 1998, the government took its plans one stage further with the publication of another White Paper entitled 'A First Class Service – Quality in the new NHS' (Department of Health 1998), which detailed the elements of clinical governance, bringing the concept to life, and outlining the first of several timetables for its full implementation.

The new White Paper defined clinical governance as 'a framework through which the NHS organisations are accountable for continuously updating the quality of their services and safeguarding high standards of care by creating an environment in which evidence in clinical care will flourish'. The text continues 'Clinical Governance has an important role to play in restoring public confidence in the NHS … NHS Trust Clinical Governance reports will set out progress made and demonstrate to local people that their confidence in the NHS is well placed' and then 'the requirements of Clinical Governance will be backed up by the new statutory duty for quality, which will be placed on Trusts and PCTs'.

NHS organisations now faced the enormous task of welding together systems such as clinical audit, risk management and continuous professional development (CPD) for all staff in order to produce a comprehensive measurable and implementable quality programme. The agenda was daunting, and in 1999 another White Paper 'Clinical Governance – Quality in the New NHS' moved it on again by defining the government's requirements further.

All health professionals have incessantly striven to achieve quality in their daily clinical practice, but have too often found themselves hampered by a lack of resources and time. There was, therefore, evidence of an increasing awareness of quality issues and of governance in the widest sense throughout healthcare. But for all the elements to come together, it required the impetus and imperative provided in 1997 by the government to drive clinical governance firmly into the centre of decision-making and action. In 1997, therefore, the government set out its vision for quality healthcare: 'achieving meaningful and sustainable quality improvements in the NHS requires a fundamental shift in culture, to focus effort where it is needed and to enable and empower those who work in the NHS to improve quality locally'.

Clinical governance is not in itself, wholly innovative – its components have existed for some time in most of the NHS. What is new is that the government's initiative provided the driver for the coordination of information and activity, which in turn should lead to performance improvement. Many have welcomed clinical governance as a positive and long-overdue official process. It is now a contractual requirement of all those working within the NHS, and much progress has been made towards implementation of systems to support clinical governance initiatives. However, a shortage of funding, a lack of guidance, a concern over the speed of implementation, the volume of it and the impact of mergers (of Trusts) have hampered progress. Most Trusts now have a department dedicated to coordinating clinical governance activity.

There remains a constant danger that clinical governance could be reduced to a system that looks at a series of processes and, at its best, is just a paper exercise. However, that would defeat the object of the exercise and effectively waste the opportunity we have been given to take time to stand and reflect. Clinical governance will not happen without ownership by staff – partnership between professionals and patients must develop.

The NHS comprises a multitude of highly skilled, highly motivated hard-working and creative individuals. In the past, the inevitable unpredictability that such a rich mix of talent creates sometimes encouraged organisations to design complex rules and systems, to build in check upon check – to control and command in order to safeguard. However, it is now recognised that 'the key resource for the NHS is the staff' and clinical governance offers an opportunity to bring together and value the talents and experience of those at the 'sharp end' of healthcare delivery.

It invites clinicians to ask 'Where do we want to go?' and 'How are we going to get there?' A multidisciplinary approach needs to be encouraged from the outset to ensure that every profession contributes to the implementation of clinical governance in the same way that Trust multidisciplinary teams have been established to elaborate, collate and develop initiatives. The successful implementation of clinical governance relies on team work, whether within professions, cross-boundary and/or cross-organisational.

## BACKGROUND

Quality is not a new concept. The relationship between quality improvement and organisational culture has been understood in business and industry for many years. In an organisation such as the NHS, and within the wider healthcare area, the need to 'change the way of things' was accepted long before the government's introduction of clinical governance as a named contractual requirement. But, for this to happen, time was required to think, discuss and redesign services and processes and implement the changes, then to await the effect of those changes, and in the day-to-day delivery of health and social care time is a precious commodity.

## ASPECTS

Clinical governance was founded on the NHS Act 1999 that established, among other things, a new duty of quality, a new duty of partnership and a new framework for professional recognition. The duty of quality states: 'it is the only duty of each PCT and NHS Trust to put and keep in place arrangements for the purposes of monitoring and improving the quality of healthcare which it provides to individuals'. The duty of partnership is placed on Health Authorities, Strategic Health Authorities, Primary Care Trusts and NHS Trusts to cooperate with one another as necessary for the full implementation of clinical governance.

The third strand of professional regulation is beyond the remit of this chapter, but it could be said that one of the elements of clinical governance is that clinicians employed in whatever sphere to provide health and social care must be expected to have attained a basic level of competencies in order to be able to take forward the wider issues of sound evidence-based practice.

Clinical governance comprises:

- Quality improvement processes, such as clinical audit, to be put in place and integrated with the quality programme for the organisation as a whole.
- Evidence-based practice must be in day-to-day use, with the infrastructure to support it, and guidelines and protocols should be produced.
- Leadership skills should be developed at clinical level.
- All professional development programmes must reflect the principles of clinical governance and there must be clinical education for all clinical staff.
- Problems of poor clinical performance should be recognised at an early stage and dealt with to prevent harm to patients.
- Mentoring of clinical staff must be in place to ensure that they meet professional requirements for updating or re-registration.
- Systems must be set up to ensure that lessons are learned when things go wrong – for example, via the complaints system, adverse events. Equally, all such incidents must be openly investigated and reported.
- Audit and feedback must be in place from service users and carers.
- A forum should exist for discussing all clinical practice and for agreeing/reviewing new practices. Further, that good ideas, practice and innovations, which have been evaluated, are systematically disseminated within and outside the organisation.
- Clinical risk management and redirection programmes must be put into place.
- An overall mechanism of monitoring is in place to ensure the systems are functioning well.
- Accreditation of services should be made possible.
- The quality of data collected should be good enough to allow robust evaluation of systems and services

In short, clinical governance is about making sure that all patients/clients receive high-quality healthcare. It does this by monitoring clinical quality, encouraging evidence-based practice, safeguarding high standards, encouraging clinical excellence and sharing good practice. The government's aim in 1997 and now is to tackle national differences in quality of care and help to reassure people after the adverse publicity surrounding poor clinical performance.

The elements, in short, relate to all aspects of care:

- research and development
- evidence-based practice
- continuous professional development (CPD)
- performance indicators
- patient and client improvement.

It was apparent from the inception of clinical governance as an entity that, henceforth, all health professionals were going to have to demonstrate transparently their clinical effectiveness.

Clinical governance also covers contractual arrangements made by the NHS with independent contractors, such as dental practitioners, opticians and pharmacists. In order for all parts of the NHS to act in a cohesive fashion, strategies have to be developed to link all organisational elements and establish a 'no-blame' culture that fosters ongoing learning.

## Quality planning

It is true to say that there are variations in different parts of the country as to the quality of care available. In podiatry we would go further and say that there are unacceptable variations in the availability of care across the country.

All local services plan the care they intend to provide, in liaison with the Strategic Health Authority and upwards. There are imperatives to meet, such as national targets. However, the concept of quality planning is that attention must be paid to the quality of the services at the same time as the level and type. That is, whenever it is determined during planning that a particular service will be offered, that service needs to be analysed in order to identify the deficiencies and detail the remedial action to be taken to rectify them. The skills, knowledge and experience of staff are to be used in order to assess the service's strengths and weaknesses and to plan accordingly.

Invariably, resource implications for any improvement measures must be identified, and it may not always be possible to carry out all the remedial actions in one move. The concept of looking at the planning process as a whole and as a rolling programme of improvements will allow informed and rational decisions to be made – and then publicised – about what is and what is not possible in any given time-frame.

The initial example of 'jump starting' the process of quality planning was the Health Improvement Programmes (HIMPs), which now form an integral part of each Local Delivery Plan (LDP), and these draw together all aspects of health and social care planning for the purposes of decision-making.

## Workforce planning and developing the workforce

This covers all aspects of staffing for a modern day NHS. It therefore comprises the elements shown in Table 28.1.

For some time Strategic Health Authorities devolved the responsibility for all those areas to the Workforce Development Confederations, who were set the task of drawing information together for the purposes of fulfilling the requirements of the NHS Plan. Now there are workforce leads within each Strategic Health Authority, pulling the planning of the future workforce back towards the hub of commissioning decision-making.

The theme of clinical governance, which lays great importance on the reflective practitioner, continued learning, retention of and development of skills, remains the underpinning ethos. The importance is stated again in the human resources strategy 'Working Together: Securing a Quality Workforce for the NHS' (Department of Health 1998).

However, there now also looms the stated aim of ensuring that, by 2012, the majority of the workforce is at Band 4 (the level below registration in the UK) or below, and utilising the Knowledge and Skills Framework to achieve this. There are still ongoing opportunities

| Table 28.1 | Staffing in the modern NHS |
|---|---|
| Needs analysis | Lifelong learning |
| Commissioning and funding | CPD of professional education |
| Recruitment | Skills mix |
| Retention | Extended-scope practitioners Human resources + pay + conditions |

for further training and support mechanisms to underpin these elements, such as library facilities, internet access and dedicated time for CPD, but there is also an increasing emphasis on 'step-on/step-off' mechanisms for developing lesser trained staff to undertake specified tightly defined roles.

The new professional regulatory systems also place great store by the need for clinicians to act within their assessed or learned competencies. This places the onus on each registrant to ensure that they are themselves comfortable with their ability to perform the interventions they undertake and only refer to those health professionals who are appropriately qualified. The outcome of the debates about revalidation and CPD evidencing will inform the future.

Such emphasis on continued learning and reflection is an opportunity that healthcare professionals have rarely been offered. At its best, it can mean dedicated time set aside during a working day for continued education. For private practitioners this is not necessarily as easy, but the underlying ethos of clinical governance and of regulation is quite clear. Clinicians are expected to maintain their clinical and theoretical knowledge, learn from failures, implement improvements and evaluate their interventions. However, further work is required across the country for this to become reality and to deliver the intended benefits to patients.

## Information technology

It goes without saying that any organisation requires robust, accurate and useful information to underpin its planning activity. Such information also draws comparisons to be made about the standards of services locally and nationally, and such comparisons form the basis of 'league tables'. Organisations now expect to be judged against published benchmarks, and public accountability is achieved by the publication of such information and the conclusions drawn. The results and trends can then be fed back into the planning process.

All NHS organisations are required to have in place local strategies for Information, Management and Technology, and the NHS Performance Assessment framework, with its associated set of high-level performance indicators, will be used to make comparisons within organisations. The increasing emphasis on an 'outcomes-led' commissioning strategy will be hampered by any delay in the introduction of the national IT systems.

## Research

In order for clinicians to have access to sound evidence upon which all interventions should depend, there is a need for robust, ongoing research. The government's initiatives now encourage all healthcare professionals to become actively engaged in research and audit and to develop the skills necessary for those activities. Such research is to be shared with front-line clinicians in order to support and improve high-quality clinical decision-making.

The guidelines state that: 'there needs to be a systematic approach to the collection and dissemination of evidence, within an organisation, to ensure clinicians are able to access the most up-to-date information derived from research'. To this end Trusts are encouraged to disseminate articles via bulletins and newsletters as part of their clinical governance infrastructure and to provide simple access to such national resources as the Cochrane Library, the National Research Register (which gives information about research underway in the NHS) and the NHS Centre for Review and Dissemination (CRD), which commissions and supports clinicians to undertake reviews on areas of importance to the NHS.

At the same time, of course, NICE produces and disseminates high-quality evidence-based guidance 'to support front-line staff, indicating guidelines for the management of diseases and the information on new and existing interventions'. The timescales for the production of such advice have been criticised, and NICE is now promising to reduce the time taken for decisions to be reached and disseminated.

The National Electronic Library for health has also developed swiftly in order to produce systematic reviews of primary and secondary research evidence. All NHS organisations are expected to monitor staff, usually through the appraisal system, to ensure that they are gaining access to the knowledge and evidence they need to improve the quality of their work, thus looking to an improvement in the quality of patient care. Research and audit will necessarily produce short-term restraints on already overstretched services, in pursuit of this long-term objective and the production of each new target and system reduces the time available even further.

## Poor performance

The government has acknowledged repeatedly that the percentage of poor performance in the NHS as a whole is very small. However, the adverse publicity and harm that even one isolated instance of it can cause in terms of human suffering and resources are such that specific mention is made of poor performance as an area to be monitored, reported and managed.

The systems of professional self-regulation were altered in the 1999 guidelines as 'being hitherto unsuccessful in preventing, recognising and dealing effectively with the problem of poor clinical performance'.

Reference is made to the proposed changes to be made to the regulatory systems for the professions, and nowadays it is easy to see how those now established systems dovetail with and overlap the requirements, ethos and wording of clinical governance. Of paramount importance throughout is public protection, leading to an upturn in public confidence. Regulatory processes are changing again in response to challenge about the rectitude and probity of one organisation protecting the public by carrying out the role of investigator and prosecutor of the same case, whilst also selecting, training and employing the individuals who make such decisions. An independent adjudicating body has now been established to delineate more clearly between the functions.

## Learning from experience

This is the concept of drawing together all the information pertaining to complaints, adverse incidents and service failures and examining trends, in order to identify remedial measures, thereby minimising the risk of recurrence. There is an expectation that not only will organisations learn from information about such incidents and act before similar things happen in their locality, but that they will also share good practice and adapt appropriate elements for themselves, thereby obviating the need for costly, time-consuming exercises. Out of this concept has developed the practice of peer review and validation or accreditation of whole services or parts of them, either by external agencies such as user groups or by professional bodies.

In 1999 an NHS website was set up, with a 'learning zone' to allow clinicians to share areas of good practice with others. This zone contains an NHS Trust benchmarking database to allow comparison of cost and outcomes by NHS Trusts.

Beacon services were selected, in recognition of good and innovative practice in six areas, such as waiting lists and times and services were encouraged to bid for the increased funding, offered by the Department of Health to help them disseminate their good practices to other NHS organisations.

The subsequent development of Performance Accelerator systems and Root Cause Analysis models has built on this highly important and sensitive work.

## Risk management

This is divided up into clinical and organisational. Clinical risks are defined as those risks that have a cause or effect that is primarily clinical or medical.

At the same time, controls assurance, or organisational risk management (i.e. sound financial systems and the management of non-financial and non-clinical risks) was drawn together with the clinical risk management systems to provide a cohesive approach to quality management. The division of the two is not easy because issues from either side impinge on each other.

## Consent and informed consent

Throughout the world there are many variations on the theme of consent, and the wise practitioner will seek clarification of the meaning attributed to the words in the legal framework that operates where they practise. The broad general principle that applies universally is that valid consent must be obtained before starting treatment or physical examination of a patient, based on the right of the patient to determine what happens to their own body.

Consent should be viewed as a process and not a 'once and for all' happening. It is good practice to start the process well in advance of the procedure so that there is time to respond to the patient's concerns as well as allowing the patient to give due consideration to the information about what is proposed to be done.

To give informed consent the patient must be supplied with adequate information about the nature of the procedure and the likely good and bad outcomes. So far as the latter is concerned these need to be identified clearly and the amount of risk stated unequivocally. Consent should be given freely by the patient (i.e. without any pressure to have the procedure) and on the basis of full information. The format for recording consent is also unclear, and it is generally accepted that written consent provides the best basis for the record. However, consent is only valid if the person giving the consent is in possession of all the facts and is competent to sign.

In addition, if there is to be a photographic record made of the procedure, for whatever purpose, then this must also form part of the consent process and the patient must be informed of the purpose of the photographs. This may be needed as part of a research programme and the patient should be clearly advised of the scope of the programme. These photographs should not be used for any other purpose without the express permission of the patient. The patient should also be made aware that if they refuse to be photographed this will not compromise their care.

The legal position of those aged under 18 years is complicated. The law states that those aged 16–17 years are entitled to consent to their medical treatment. This, too, should be given on the basis of full information and without pressure to accept. The major difference from adults is that a person aged 16 or 17 years who refuses to give consent could be overridden by a person with parental responsibility or by a court. The Gillick (1986) judgement made the position of children under the age of 16 years less clear, but the wise practitioner will always seek to have informed consent from the child and the parent or legal guardian before proceeding.

The law on consent is complex, and practitioners should ensure that they clearly understand the law as it applies to them. In England the Department of Health provides useful documentation.

## REFERENCES

Department of Health: www.doh.gov.uk/consent

Department of Health 1998 A first class service – quality in the new NHS. Department of Health, London.

Department of Health 1998 Guidance. Working together: securing a quality workforce for the NHS. Her Majesty's Stationary Office (HMSO), London.

Department of Health 1999 Clinical governance in the new NHS. Health Services Circular 1999/065. Available at: http://www.dh.gov.uk/en/Publicationsandstatistics/Lettersandcirculars/Healthservicecirculars/DH_4004883 (19 September 2009).

Gillick v West Norfolk and Wisbech AHA 1986 AC 112.

Secretary of State for Health 1997 The New NHS – Modern and Dependable. HMSO, London.

NHS Wales 1998 Putting patients first. Available at: http://www.wales.nhs.uk/publications/whitepaper98_e.pdf (19 September 2009).

# Chapter | 29 |

# Health and safety in podiatric practice

*Gordon Burrow*

## KEYWORDS

Control of chemicals

COSHH

Effective management

Fire safety

Legal duties

Principles of risk assessment

Risk assessment
Safe systems of work
Safety culture
Working procedures

# INTRODUCTION

Health and safety traditionally was concerned with providing technical solutions to health and safety problems, or providing items such as respiratory protective equipment to give the required protection for levels of dust exposure based on extensive dust measurements. Most accidents occur because the culture of the organisation or employees is incorrect, because production demands (increased patient numbers) create tunnel vision, or because work was 'always done that way'. In the past no one analysed the work to identify the system of work, because people were 'too busy', because insufficient attention and priority were given to health and safety, and because of the 'it won't happen to me' syndrome.

Podiatry is no exception to this traditional view of what health and safety is about. Unfortunately, health and safety is a major issue that both union members and all working people think unions should concentrate on. Within podiatry, the health, safety and welfare concerns are also high, with areas such as work-related upper-limb disorders, repetitive strain injury (RSI) and musculoskeletal problems, especially lower back and neck problems, becoming increasingly common. Stress is also an ever-increasing problem for podiatry staff. According to Williams (1999), the commonest causes of work-related stress currently are overload and bullying, and both of these are apparent in podiatry, especially in the National Health Service (NHS).

Increased patient caseloads have been imposed and met as the modern NHS strives to achieve 'target' figures with ever-decreasing resources. In podiatry, there is an increasing demand for services, alongside down-sizing in some localities and the introduction of new working practices such as decontamination of instruments. New criteria are being imposed to reduce the number of patients seeking podiatric help, and increasingly it is the high-risk patients that the NHS manages. This change brings with it increased stress and workload demands, and the requirement for higher levels of concentration and higher skills, including those of communication, manual dexterity and professionalism.

Stress should be thought of in terms of outcomes: it produces low morale and reduces productivity, and it increases both short- and long-term absenteeism as well as mistakes, which may have adverse effects on patients and potentially the podiatry service that can be delivered when litigation cases ensue. As in all areas of health and safety, the risk assessment of podiatric workplaces and practices should include stress and stress-related or stress-induced hazards and risks.

Health, safety and welfare require risk assessment, followed by management of the hazards and risks to reduce the risk factors identified to the lowest level possible. The concept of risk assessment is similar to that of clinical assessment (see Ch. 1). It is important that, in dealing with patients, practitioners consider not only the health, safety and welfare of their patients, but also their own health, safety and welfare.

Prior to the Health and Safety at Work etc. Act 1974 (HASAW Act) becoming law, health and safety legislation was retrospective – it was drafted or was enforced following accidents in an attempt to prevent recurrence. Within podiatry this has not changed, and health and safety is still seen as the poor relation, with little cognisance taken of risks and hazards (e.g. the introduction of single-use disposable instruments has been associated with an increased number of reports of RSI – something that many had suggested might happen). However, a problem identified by the National Patient Safety Agency is the low recording of accidents, incidents or near misses by all allied health professions, and an inability to distil specific podiatry information. The HASAW Act aimed to anticipate and prevent accidents before they happened, attempting to keep pace with new technology and changing working practices, assuming it was enforced. The philosophy behind the HASAW Act is self-regulation: for example, the Control of Substances Hazardous to Health Regulations 1994 (COSHH) and subsequent amendments to it; the Control of Noise at Work Regulations 2005 and the batch of six regulations that came into force at the beginning of 1993 (the 'six pack'). All these regulations are based on the premise and requirement that the employer conducts a risk assessment in each particular workplace, for each work practice, and adopts appropriate control measures necessary to deal with the hazards identified and the degree of risk assessed.

This assessment approach is philosophically different from that adopted by legislation prior to the HASAW Act. The new approach requires the employer (or private practitioner) to identify, within certain minimum legal requirements, safety standards to be achieved and control measures required. However, it is not sufficient to undertake a one-off assessment. The assessment should be set within a TQM (Total Quality Management) framework. Thus, a risk assessment is carried out, a set of aims and objectives is determined to offset the hazards and risks, and then, once that set of objectives has been achieved, the process is renewed with fresh objectives. Employers must continue attempting to reduce the level of risk to the lowest level reasonably practicable.

## CASE STUDY 29.1 RISK ASSESSMENT

| Likelihood | Severity | Risk rating | Priority |
|---|---|---|---|
| 1. Low (seldom) | 1. Slight (off work for up to 3 days) | 1 | No action |
| 2. Medium (frequently) | 2. Serious (off work for over 3 days) | 2 | Low-priority action |
| 3. High (certain or near certain) | 3. Major (death/major harm) | 3 or 4 | Medium-priority action |
| | | 6 | High-priority action |
| | | 9 | Urgent action |

| Harm | To whom | Hazard | Circumstances | Precautions | Likelihood | Severity | Risk rating | Priority | Action required |
|---|---|---|---|---|---|---|---|---|---|
| Phenol splash/ chemical burn | Podiatrist | Phenol | Phenol splashes when attempting to dry cotton bud during application to nail bed | Training in use of phenol | 1 | 2 | 2 | Low | Training and reiteration of training |
| Phenol burn | Podiatrist | Phenol spill | Phenol bottle is dropped | Limit size of phenol bottle contents – maximum size 25 ml | 2 | 3 | 6 | High | Ensure that bottles are correct size, or purchase EZswabs which are expensive but reduce risk significantly |

## EFFECTIVE MANAGEMENT

Effective management of health and safety, and thereby prevention of accidents and ill health within an organisation or practice, is important because of a whole range of factors, including:

1. Legal duties on individuals and organisations. Penalties for non-compliance can be unlimited, but for many the main deterrent is usually the adverse publicity and avoidance of a criminal record. A criminal record may exclude a practitioner from Health Professions Council (HPC) entitlement.
2. Moral responsibilities to colleagues, friends and families to ensure that they are not injured at work.
3. Good relations with employees and the public, who may be customers, patients, shareholders or influential members of the wider political community. Some businesses and practices may spend scarce resources promoting a good public image, and this would be wasted by the adverse publicity generated by a serious accident.
4. The cost of accidents and ill health. The true or total cost of an accident is generally hidden or, at best, overlooked.

Hidden costs include building and equipment damage, lost production, legal expenses, hiring replacement equipment, accident investigation time, management and administrative time, and loss of business and goodwill, etc. For example, if a bench-top autoclave were inadequately maintained and the inadequacy of maintenance resulted in an explosion, there would be considerable damage to property internally and externally.

Public disasters involving loss of life and notices in the press recalling potentially faulty consumer goods (e.g. drink bottles, food, electrical appliances) heighten public awareness that many incidents are avoidable. There is also the realisation by those injured, customers, employees, shareholders and neighbours that the key to avoidance of safety problems lies with effective management of safety. There is a growing awareness at management level of the relative costs of accidents and insurance, the requirements of legislation, and an interest in quality management systems, all considerably raising the profile of risk management with an increased need for improved health and safety practice and policies. There is also, however, an increasing risk of litigation and complaints to regulatory bodies about practitioners and their practices.

## SUCCESSFUL HEALTH AND SAFETY MANAGEMENT

The correct approach to successful health and safety management is contained in five steps. These are:

1. set your policy
2. organise your staff
3. plan and set standards
4. measure your performance
5. audit and review.

There is no specific legal requirement to adopt this system. However, it may well be that in future courts and regulatory and professional bodies will look more closely at how effectively safety was managed. Failure to provide evidence that a formal system was in operation may leave practitioners exposed to both criminal and civil law penalties if an accident occurs.

## SAFETY CULTURE

Health and safety traditionally was concerned with providing technical solutions to problems (e.g. providing guards for machinery to a specific standard). Accidents do not tend to occur because a guard was not up to standard or the dust mask was not quite technically correct. They are usually a result of there being no guard or dust mask at all. Those accidents occurred because the culture was not right, because production demands (patient numbers) created tunnel vision, because work was 'always done that way', because no one analysed work practices to identify safe systems of work, because people were too busy, and because insufficient attention and priority were given to health and safety. The problem is one of attitude. The greatest challenge to our profession is influencing and changing attitudes and behaviour. Recent research into nail dust and the hazard of dust exposure or RSI through poor equipment or poor maintenance highlights these issues for podiatrists.

## SAFE SYSTEMS OF WORK

Part of an employer's duty is to provide a safe system of work where, insofar as is reasonably practicable, the work or manner in which it is carried out is safe and without risks to health. The Health and Safety Executive (HSE) recommends five steps to a safe system of work:

- assess the task
- identify the hazards
- define safe methods or practice
- implement a system
- monitor the system.

All podiatric activities should adopt this system. Simple tasks such as nail cutting, scalpel work and routine maintenance of equipment should follow this approach, not just the more elaborate tasks such as nail surgery. This recommended analysis of work practices should ensure that guidelines or protocols are written, adopted and monitored, which may minimise risks to employees and practitioners alike.

Podiatrists need to be proactive in assessing their activities. There are problems with home visits due to poor working conditions, poor lighting, poor ventilation and poor posture. Are the problems being addressed, ensuring a rota of staff so that no single individual is solely undertaking domiciliary visits but instead spreading the risk across a number of members of staff and thus reducing the risk individually?

## LEGAL DUTIES

The most important and broad-ranging duty of care, which must be fulfilled by employers, is described by Section 2(1) of the HASAW Act:

*It shall be the duty of every employer to ensure, so far as is reasonably practicable, the health, safety and welfare at work of all his employees.*

However, this duty of care does not stop at employees – employers also have responsibility towards certain non-employees, which can include visitors, contractors and also the general public (patients and their carers). This duty of care includes their overall safety, more specific concerns, such as safe entrance and exit to the practice, as well as the provision of information (e.g. fire exits, routes or emergency procedures) and training. The employer (private practitioner) is legally obliged to undertake risk assessments. Ultimate responsibility rests with the employer, but the task of risk assessment is quite likely to be delegated; in the case of the NHS this may be to safety representatives or a health and safety manager. The general duty of care owed to employees under Section 2(1) is qualified in Section 2(2) of the HASAW Act. It includes:

**(a)** The provision and maintenance of plant (autoclaves, instruments, domiciliary cases, drills, etc.) and systems of work (lone workers policies, pregnant workers policy, young employees) that are, insofar as is reasonably practicable, safe and without risk to health.

**(b)** Arrangements for ensuring, insofar as is reasonably practicable, safety and absence of risks to health in connection with the use, handling, storage and transport of articles and substances.

**(c)** The provision of such information, instruction, training and supervision as is necessary to ensure, insofar as is reasonably practicable, the health and safety at work of employees.

**(d)** The maintenance of any place of work under the employer's control (this may include domiciliary visits or visits to residential homes, or another clinical facility) in a condition that is safe and without risks to health, and the provision and maintenance of means of access to and egress from it that are safe and without such risks, insofar as is reasonably practicable.

**(e)** The provision and maintenance of a working environment for employees that is, insofar as is reasonably practicable, safe, without risks to health, and adequate as regards facilities and arrangements for their welfare at work.

The employer has ultimate responsibility to ensure satisfactory standards of health and safety at work and their efficient management. The employer is defined as the corporate body (limited company), partnership, owner or proprietor.

The employer (private practitioner) may incur liability for health and safety in one of two ways.

1. The employer is personally liable for accidents resulting from acts or omissions of the employee.
2. The employer is vicariously liable for accidents resulting from acts or omissions of his or her employees. This liability could extend under common law to the payment of compensation to injured employees. If an employer delegates health and safety responsibility to another person, liability is not and cannot be similarly delegated.

Every employee and manager has some legal duties in this area, and these responsibilities should normally be incorporated in any job description and job title for a position within a company or practice. The delegation of responsibility should be to a competent person. Regulation 6 of the Management of Health and Safety at Work Regulations 1999 (MHSWR) defines this as 'one who has sufficient training and experience, or knowledge and other qualities, to enable him or her properly to assist in undertaking the measures needed to comply with health and safety legislation'.

Employers have a responsibility to protect the following categories of people:

1. employees
2. trainees
3. those with disabilities
4. persons susceptible to injury (e.g. female employees, pregnant workers)
5. visitors and the general public
6. contractors
7. trespassers
8. users of the company's goods or services.

To enable a practitioner to understand the practical implications of the general requirements of the HASAW Act, the practitioner will rely on regulations made under that Act and the Health and Safety Commission's Approved Codes of Practice and Guidance Notes (e.g. Essentials of Health and Safety at Work).

A large organisation such as a Trust or Board (or Local Health Care Cooperative) or Primary Care Group or Trust (PCT/PCG) may wish to appoint a member of staff as the competent person. Many employers decide to appoint an external health and safety consultant, and where such is appointed the employer (or private practitioner) will depend on the professional skill and expertise of that consultant. However, caution is needed when appointing such a person. Practitioners should ensure that the appointed consultant is competent by, for example, checking that the consultant has sufficient training, expertise, a proven track record and also adequate professional indemnity insurance.

Employers (practitioners) may legally deflect liability to an external expert should enforcement action be taken as a result of the consultant's neglect. This assumes proper documented procedures were in place to attest to the consultant's suitability as a competent person. In the event of compensation being paid to an injured employee, it may be possible for the practitioner's insurer to recover money from the consultant. Advice on the competency of consultants can be attested by contacting some of the health and safety organisations such as the Institution of Occupational Safety and Health (IOSH at http://www.iosh.co.uk; telephone 0116 257 3100).

## THE EMPLOYER'S RESPONSIBILITY TO VARIOUS PARTIES

### Employees

Section 2(1) of the HASAW Act requires the employer to ensure the health, safety and welfare of all employees, insofar as is reasonably practicable. It is necessary to consider within any risk assessment what is meant, or may be meant, by the phrase 'all employees'. The employer must consider the principle of individual assessment and incorporate individual information into the risk assessment task, as required by the MHSWR. Every employer requires, when delegating tasks to employees, to take account of each individual's capabilities with respect to health and safety and in addition provide them with the necessary information, instruction and training contained within Section 2(2)(c). The combination of these legal duties should ensure that training is provided at the following times:

- on recruitment
- when there are changes in, for example, technology, procedures, processes, systems of work, and work practices and procedures
- on a routine ongoing refresher basis (a form of continuing professional development).

Employees are also entitled to information concerning (see Case Study 29.2):

(a) the risks to health and safety
(b) the protective and preventive measures that are in force
(c) the obligations of the employee
(d) the safe systems of work that are in operation
(e) emergency procedures.

---

### CASE STUDY 29.2 AN NHS TRUST HAS BEEN FINED FOLLOWING THE EXPOSURE OF AN EMPLOYEE TO A DANGEROUS CHEMICAL, RESULTING IN OCCUPATIONAL ASTHMA

K, a healthcare worker, was employed by B Hospital NHS Trust and part of her work was decontamination of surgical instruments and medical equipment using glutaraldehyde. In the summer of 1999, K developed symptoms, including headaches, exhaustion, coughing and sneezing, a dry mouth and rashes on her arms and feet. She was diagnosed as having dermatitis and asthma as a result of working with and exposure to glutaraldehyde. K is unlikely to work ever again.

The HSE investigation concluded there were failings in the hospital's safety procedures and policy for work with the substance. Although employees had been told to use protective equipment when using the chemical, none had been given adequate training on safety procedures and/or related health risks. The hospital failed to report K's condition to the HSE until July 2000, 10 months after she became ill.

The hospital pleaded guilty and is now phasing out glutaraldehyde. Fines of £14 000 for failing to ensure the health and safety of employees were imposed, along with a £4000 fine for breach of Reporting of Injuries, Diseases and Dangerous Occurrences Regulations (RIDDOR) 1995 regulations for failing to report K's condition plus £13 000 costs.

---

### Responsibilities of employees

Employees have certain responsibilities that they are expected to fulfil under Sections 7 and 8 of the HASAW Act and the MHSWR. Employees are obliged to:

- take reasonable care for their own safety and that of others
- cooperate with the employer and competent persons
- not misuse safety devices and equipment
- use work equipment machinery, substances, personal protective equipment, etc. correctly
- report hazardous conditions and any safety shortcomings to the employer or a safety representative.

### Trainees (i.e. student podiatrists on work experience or a placement)

Employers owe a greater duty of care to trainees and inexperienced workers. Inexperienced workers may well be regarded as recent graduates who may not necessarily have the work experience of more experienced employees. Thus the risk assessment for work practices may require additional arrangements for the safety of trainees, or recent graduates (inexperienced employees) as part of looking after each employee as an individual. Non-employed trainees (e.g. students on a work placement or potential students) may require special provisions and are entitled to the degree of protection given to ordinary employees by virtue of the Health and Safety (Training for Employment) Regulations 1990.

### Health surveillance

Employers need to consider routine health surveillance, ensuring awareness of any employee disabilities. Health surveillance is a statutory requirement under the MHSWR when the following conditions are satisfied:

(a) There is an identifiable disease or adverse health condition related to the work (e.g. nail dust, or RSI from the use of nail nippers).
(b) Valid techniques are available to detect indications of the disease or condition – air monitoring, quick exposure check for risks of musculoskeletal disorders.
(c) There is a reasonable likelihood that the disease or condition may occur under the particular conditions of work (e.g. use of non-dust-extraction systems in a domiciliary setting, musculoskeletal disorders where working in residential/ nursing homes).
(d) Surveillance is likely to further the protection of the health of the employees.

Obvious examples of known disabilities may also include dermatitis, previous back or neck injury and noise-induced deafness, etc.

It may also be prudent to consider pre-employment health questionnaires; these may be used to identify existing disabilities, enabling risk assessment to be related to the individual employee.

### Visitors and the general public

Employers and practitioners have a duty to protect visitors (as non-employees) under Section 3 of the HASAW Act. The Occupiers' Liability Act 1957 suggests that the employer can be liable for compensation to visitors injured on their premises. For guidance, visitors should not be left unaccompanied and they should not, if possible, be taken into hazardous areas of the practice. (It is prudent to ask visitors to sign in on arrival and sign out on departure and, ideally, be given basic instructions on what to do in the event of an emergency such as a fire.) If visitors are accompanied at all times, then in an emergency the practitioner could lead them to safety. Constant accompaniment also enhances security and prevents unnecessary accidents – it is a form of accident prevention.

Members of the public are also owed a duty of care, ensuring that they are not put at risk by the employer's undertaking. The general duties of protection owed to visitors apply equally to the emergency services.

## Trespassers

It is generally assumed the only duty owed to trespassers is that the occupier must not intentionally cause them injury. However, under the Occupiers' Liability Act 1984, occupiers owe a duty to trespassers in respect of the state of their premises/practice and the activities undertaken if the following three conditions apply:

**(a)** the occupier knows of the risk or has reasonable grounds to believe that it exists

**(b)** the occupier knows or has reasonable grounds to believe that trespassing may occur

**(c)** the risk is one for which the occupier may reasonably be expected to offer some protection.

This does not require a practitioner to make the practice burglar-proof. However, adequate steps are required to ensure that there are no hidden, concealed or unexpected dangers on site. Warning notices or other steps to deter entry will be sufficient in most cases. Hence chemicals must be kept in a locked cupboard and clearly labelled.

## HEALTH AND SAFETY POLICY

To assist the successful management of health and safety and fulfil statutory obligations, private practitioners should consider producing a health and safety policy. Where they employ five or more persons it is a legal requirement, but it is possibly best practice to have one even where fewer employees are employed. A health and safety policy must contain the following sections.

## General statement of intent

This sets out the objectives of the health and safety at work that are applicable to and individualised to that practice. The general statement of intent may require updating on a regular basis as the objectives change. Suitable objectives will be those that include commitments to training, establishing reductions in accident rates (e.g. reducing the number of accidents with sharps; see Case Study 29.3). It may also include a standard to achieve in an externally audited system (e.g. Society of Chiropodists and Podiatrists Practice Accreditation scheme).

---

### CASE STUDY 29.3 **CHILD AT RISK FROM USED MEDICAL NEEDLES**

An NHS Trust has been fined following an accident in which a child was put at risk by a container of used needles.

A large NHS Teaching Hospital Trust failed to ensure that sharps bins containing used needles and other sharp instruments were inaccessible to members of the public at one of their hospitals. A 21-month-old girl was waiting for her father in a corridor outside the maternity ward at the hospital. She put her hand into the sharps bin that had inadvertently been left hanging from a radiator. Her father

---

then washed her hand in a sink. Hospital staff examined her and concluded that she had not suffered any puncture wounds.

The Trust failed to ensure that the sharps bin was stored in an area to which the public could not gain access. By leaving it in an unsupervised public area, the Trust had run the risk of injuring anyone who put their hand into the container. Incidents such as this could result in the contracting of diseases such as HIV or hepatitis B from used needles. The child would not have been put at risk if the sharps bin had been stored in an area away from where the general public had access.

The Trust pleaded guilty and deeply regretted the incident. Since the incident, it has commissioned independent health and safety audits to ensure that sharps bins are kept in locations where they cannot be accessed by members of the public and has produced posters to inform staff about the need to keep bins in a safe place.

The Trust was fined £3000 for a breach of Section 3(1) of the HASW for failing to ensure the health and safety of people not in employment, plus costs of £900.

---

## Health and safety at work responsibilities

A range of health and safety responsibilities needs to be allocated in the health and safety policy. In private practice it is likely that responsibilities are with the practitioner, or that some are delegated to an external competent person.

## Administration of health and safety at work

To comply with the MHSWR, a practitioner or employer must demonstrate arrangements for effective planning, organisation, control, audit and review of preventive and protective measures. The fulfilment of these items requires administration arrangements for the wide range of health and safety at work topics. These may include:

**(a)** keeping up to date with health and safety legislation (this could be achieved through the web pages of the IOSH, or through the *Health and Safety News* bulletin produced by the Society of Chiropodists and Podiatrists)

**(b)** arrangements for undertaking risk assessments

**(c)** safety training

**(d)** safety communications

**(e)** safety committee and safety representatives (where appropriate)

**(f)** disciplinary procedures – NHS rather than private

**(g)** records and registers (e.g. of all electrical equipment)

**(h)** fire safety standards – extinguisher equipment, record of maintenance

**(i)** first aid at work – first aid procedures

**(j)** accident procedures – logging of all accidents, incidents and near misses

**(k)** medical and health surveillance arrangements

**(l)** control of contractors on site

**(m)** visits by employees to other locations (e.g. home visits)

**(n)** enforcing-authority visits

**(o)** monitoring of health and safety at work.

## RISK ASSESSMENTS

Among a range of legislation, the prime example where risk assessment is required is under the MHSWR. These clearly require employers to undertake suitable and sufficient assessment of risks to health and safety arising from work activities. The range of legally required risk assessments undertaken by the practice are consolidated in the health and safety policy, or at minimum cross-referenced with the policy statement.

The exact arrangements for undertaking risk assessments are outlined in the administration of health and safety at work section, while responsibility for undertaking and recording them is contained in the responsibilities section of the health and safety policy. The actual undertaking of a risk assessment should not be seen as the end of the process – it is the beginning. It is the means of identifying steps to ensure the control of health and safety risks. Health and safety at work record-keeping requirements can arise in relation to a very wide range of issues.

## Record-keeping requirements

Practitioners need to identify the exact record-keeping requirements appropriate for their individual practice. These are just some examples and it is possible that the full list of record-keeping requirements could be greater.

1. Administration of health and safety at work
   (a) list of record keeping requirements
   (b) appointment of competent persons under the MHSWR
2. Management systems
   (a) safety committee and review meetings
   (b) health and safety monitoring and audit arrangements
3. Incidents and accidents
   (a) first aid treatments
   (b) accident and incident reports
4. Training and authorisation
   (a) machinery safety training (e.g. autoclaves, grinding or abrasive wheels for orthoses)
5. Employment records
   (a) young persons
   (b) health surveillance records
6. Monitoring procedures
   (a) occupational hygiene and COSHH surveys
   (b) noise surveys (e.g. where machinery is used)
7. Personal protective equipment (PPE)
   (a) issue and inspection of PPE (e.g. face masks, eye protection)
8. Fire and emergency
   (a) fire alarms and fire extinguishers – how often and when tested, by whom?
   (b) fire evacuation drills
9. Plant and machinery
   (a) electrical equipment
   (b) machinery guards, for example in abrasive wheels
10. Buildings and services
    (a) water treatments (e.g. for *Legionella* where appropriate)
    (b) inspection of the electrical installation.

## Safe systems of work

Related to suitable and sufficient risk assessments is the need to establish and monitor safe systems of work. The range of safety procedures and safe systems of work established may include written schemes of work for waste-disposal arrangements, sterilisation and cross-infection procedures to safeguard against hepatitis and human immunodeficiencey virus (HIV), and working alone. This may be by a poster or notice at the decontamination area stating what the procedure is in the manner of a recipe (i.e. step 1, step 2, etc.).

It is important that any working system and procedures established for employees is understood by any contractors (e.g. locums) employed for similar work in the practice. The practice manager/senior partner or practitioner should ensure that locums or students follow the practice policies and procedures when undertaking practice on their site.

## Accident procedures

The Reporting of Injuries, Diseases and Dangerous Occurrences Regulations 1995 (RIDDOR 1995) set out the legal obligations for reporting accidents and dangerous occurrences to the enforcing authority. It is each practitioner's responsibility to ensure these legal obligations are met.

The responsible practitioner should establish a clear policy in all aspects of accident and ill-health procedures, including suitable first-aid arrangements and control of health hazards such as dust. Podiatrists should ensure that musculoskeletal problems causing them to be off work for longer than 3 days are reported under RIDDOR.

## Working environment

The Workplace (Health, Safety and Welfare) Regulations 1992 are concerned with good housekeeping standards and safe storage of goods. In addition, they specify extensive standards relating to the working environment, covering such factors as ergonomic considerations and compliance with the Health and Safety (Display Screen Equipment) Regulations 1992 (as amended 2002). These regulations apply to most places of work and establish strict controls on the working environment in which display screen equipment is used.

## Control of chemicals

The Control of Substances Hazardous to Health Regulations 2002 (COSHH) require detailed risk assessment. The practitioner needs to ensure adequate attention is paid to these and, in particular, the following:

(a) hazard identification, including the establishment of an inventory of all chemicals in the practice and also those used in toilets
(b) control of chemicals and adequate storage arrangements
(c) recording of COSHH assessments, including confirmation that hazardous substances have been eliminated, insofar as is reasonably practicable. These assessments may require regular updating and satisfactory recording
(d) maintenance of control measures, including checks on extraction equipment and monitor exposure and checks that safety rules are enforced.

## Fire safety

Recent legislation (The Regulatory Reform (Fire Safety) Order 2005) altered the main approach, which is again based on risk assessment with the principle of prevention being applied. In terms of control, adequate storage of flammable and explosive materials is required. There are a number of potential substances within podiatry that fall under these headings. When fire hazards and risks are suitably controlled, then other areas, which might require attention, are:

(a) fire prevention – ensure sources of ignition are eliminated, fire doors and dampers are operational
(b) fire-fighting and fire-detection arrangements – need to be adequate and include arrangements to ensure that equipment is

provided and properly maintained by competent persons, with instructions on its use clearly displayed and known by staff

(c) means of escape and routine fire drills – these should receive attention in consultation with local fire prevention officers; the practitioner should undertake routine fire alarm checks regularly.

## Physical agents/stored energy

The main types of physical agents and stored energy of interest to the podiatrist are possibly:

(a) noise and vibration – drills, grinders
(b) electricity at work – most equipment
(c) pressure systems – autoclaves.

In all cases, there is much legislation regulating these hazards.

## Plant and equipment

There is a whole range of work equipment present in the podiatric practice, and the practice itself may require review to ensure compliance with the Workplace (Health, Safety and Welfare) Regulations 1992 and other appropriate legal standards.

The practitioner should keep a full register of work equipment with routine inspections as necessary. Arrangements for purchasing new equipment and for hiring/leasing equipment should be scrutinised, and all work equipment should be properly stored and maintained. The Provision and Use of Work Equipment Regulations 1998 (PUWER) provide a framework for the continued adequate and safe use of tools and machinery.

## Handling operations

Safe use of lifting machinery (e.g. hoists for patients), arrangements for safe manual handling (equipment and patients) and safety in storage areas are all major safety concerns. Although podiatrists do not manually handle patients in a manner such as physiotherapists do, they still need to be aware of good posture, movement, ergonomic design of workplaces, and lifting or manual handling of equipment (e.g. domiciliary cases, stools, drills).

## Risk assessment

The objective of a health and safety risk assessment is to identify or quantify the extent of risk of any activity/process/material and from that information implement measures to control or reduce the risk attached to it. An understanding of the principles and techniques of risk assessment will enable decisions to be taken about priorities in the management of risk.

Risk assessments should be 'suitable and sufficient' and must be carried out by a 'competent person'. This should allow the business to determine any measures required to allow compliance with relevant health and safety legislation. Where there are five or more employees, these risk assessments should be documented. However, it is prudent for all assessments to be documented, enabling practitioners to have proof that such an assessment was carried out.

Practitioners should regard a risk assessment as a 'reasoned judgement about the risks and extent of these risks to people's health and safety, based on the common sense application of information, which lead to decisions about how risks should be managed'. The process of risk assessment is one commonly utilised by podiatrists within normal routine practice. It is a process of reasoning skills, ending with a justifiable action plan for safety measures, which will eliminate or, at worst, minimise the risk of harm to people by the actions, operations, products or services of a podiatric practice.

## Principles of risk assessment

There is a need to define certain terms used in risk assessments. A *hazard* is defined as something with the potential to cause harm or injury. For example, a nail drill is a hazard in that it has the potential to cause harm either by the fact that electricity powers its actions, or that if it were to drop onto an unprotected toe the toe could be damaged. *Risk* is then defined as the likelihood of harm or injury resulting from the hazard. Thus, if the nail drill is checked regularly for electrical safety then the likelihood of someone coming to harm from an electrical shock is small. If the drill is not moved about unnecessarily and is on a stable base, then the likelihood of it falling and dropping onto a toe is small also. The *extent of the risk* is the number of people who might be exposed and the consequences for them. To keep the example going, the extent of the risk is that either one or two people might be affected – the operator and possibly the patient. The consequences might be severe in that in the worst case electrical shock might result in death.

Risk assessment is an extension of techniques employed by podiatrists in their daily activities. Podiatrists are used to employing clinical reasoning skills, using problem-solving and decision-making techniques to conduct examination and assessments of patients. Health and safety risk assessments employ similar techniques.

## Problem-solving and decision-making

The primary principles of risk assessment are problem-solving and decision-making and risk evaluation and control techniques. The key principles are the same as those for determining solutions to any problem, such as diagnosis of a patient's signs and symptoms:

(a) the solutions must satisfy a variety of interests – podiatrist, patient, carer, employer
(b) a united commitment to the solutions is required – patient compliance aids management planning.

Thus, the principles employ techniques similar to those used by podiatrists in practice. These are:

- involve the relevant people – communications!
- agree a definition of the problem – identify the right signs and symptoms
- solicit views and recommendations – research and continuing professional development activities, keeping up to date with techniques and practice
- agree the options for solution – outline the management of a case
- evaluate the agreed options – set out to the patient the possible management plans
- agree on a solution – the patient agrees the management plan
- agree a plan for implementing and monitoring the solution, with responsibilities and accountability clearly defined – audit and review of the case plan.

However, in terms of health and safety, the variety of interests might go further than in podiatric practice where the interests served include those of the individuals concerned:

- legal compliance – either an individual practitioner or a Trust
- the protection of people who may be at risk – high-risk patients, pregnant women
- the motivation of people who need to cooperate in such protection.
- financial management.

The problems to be addressed are the health and safety risks, with solutions being the measures designed to control or reduce the risks. The relevant people are those able to assess the risks – the practitioner or a delegated competent person; those who come into contact with the risks every day and know what can happen in practice; and those who need to invest time, money, consideration, effort or other resources to implement the measures decided upon. In all these cases the relevant person is the practitioner.

## Evaluation and expression of risk

These principles of risk assessment are found in the Health and Safety Executive (HSE) publication HS (G) 65: Successful Health and Safety Management, and in the Approved Code of Practice to the MHSWR.

The likelihood of any hazard causing harm depends on a number of factors:

1. the nature of the hazard – phenol causes burns
2. the seriousness of the harm that the uncontrolled hazard could cause – how large an area could be burned if uncontrolled spillage occurs will depend on the amount spilt
3. the events in which people could be exposed to the hazard (podiatrists – exposed through inhalation, spillage, splashing)
4. the existing controls to prevent such hazardous events (only small bottles, decant only the amount required for one procedure, air-filtration system to remove fumes)
5. the likelihood of people being exposed to the hazard (only those in nail surgery, therefore the numbers are quite controlled)
6. the number of people who would be exposed to the hazard should an event occur (how many are in nail surgery at any one time – two?)
7. the existing controls to prevent harm in cases of exposure to the hazard (see above).

## Residual risk

Once the practitioner has detailed all the relevant factors, an informed judgement is required. This leads to a decision on the likelihood of harm being caused by the hazard in particular processes, events or circumstances. The risk that results should also have taken into account existing controls – in some texts what is left is referred to as the 'residual risk'.

## Expressions to identify risk

It is difficult to give explicit information about how to undertake a risk assessment as there are no principles or standards, apart from those of language and communication, which determine how the harm, which might result, should be expressed to a third party. In cases of quantified risk assessments the principles of mathematics and statistics can apply. In some cases a numerical probability (quantitative assessment) can be designed after research, while in others a qualitative assessment is all that will transpire. Thus, in terms of a risk assessment regarding nail dust, it might be feasible to say 'it is dangerous to use a nail drill which has not been maintained' thus indicating a higher level of risk than 'it is reasonably safe to use a nail drill which has been maintained'. Similarly, 'there is a high risk of being hit by a shard of nail particle if eye protection is not worn' indicates a higher level of risk than the expression 'there is a low risk of being hit by a shard of nail if eye protection is worn'. Other means to convey the same relativity of risk include: 'Eye protection not worn – risk from dust particles in the eye = 7; risk from dust particles if eye protection worn = 3'; and, if a quantified assessment has been made: 'chance of being injured when wearing eye protection = 1 in 26 156; chance of being injured when not wearing eye protection = 1 in 10 763'. These figures are exemplars only and are not based on research, and therefore should not be used as definite figures.

The severity of the harm may be an additional factor to be taken into account when evaluating risks. Thus it is essential that a competent person use a means of expressing risk and its extent to facilitate:

(a) the making of judgements in carrying out risk assessments
(b) decisions about control using the results of the assessments.

As in podiatric practice a systematic approach to the process is useful, and provides some assurance that the decision is liable to be meaningful and consistent.

## Principles for risk control

The aim of risk assessment is to reduce or control risk. The ACOP (Approved Code of Practice) states employers should apply the following principles when deciding measures to control risks:

1. Where possible, avoid a risk completely; for example do not use a substance that is not essential and is known to be dangerous – substitute this substance for another with less risk or none at all.
2. Risks should be tackled at source. The ACOP suggests that slippery steps should be treated or replaced rather than highlighted with a warning sign.
3. Work should be adapted to the individual – not the individual to the work.
4. Technological or technical progress should be exploited – do not keep doing something if advances in technology could minimise or reduce the risk; for example there are now bagless drills on the market which do away with the need to empty the dust bags.
5. Employers should ensure risk prevention measures form part of a coherent policy and approach so that risks that cannot be prevented may be progressively reduced or avoided altogether. In RSI breaks during work reduce potential risk; therefore insist that staff take breaks.
6. Collective measures should be given priority over individual measures.
7. Employers should ensure employees understand what they need to do – need for training and education.
8. Employers should ensure and maintain an active health and safety culture encompassing the whole of the organisation.

It is good practice to reduce the risk by combating it at source if it cannot be eliminated or avoided altogether. Reliance on palliative measures (e.g. warnings, safe working procedures and personal protective equipment) is poor practice to reduce the severity of harm from the hazard or likelihood of exposure to the hazard.

## Basis for assessment

The primary basis of any technique for risk assessment is an examination of two questions:

1. What could go wrong?
   (a) What harm could result?
   (b) Whom will it harm?
   (c) What can cause it?
   (d) Under what circumstances?
   (e) What precautions have already been taken (i.e. current control measures)?
   (f) What are the chances of it happening (residual risk, this is dependent on (a)–(e))?

**603**

**2.** What measures are needed to prevent it going wrong? What additional measures are needed to prevent it going wrong?

Any technique for risk assessment needs to communicate the answers to these two questions.

## Five steps to risk assessment

### Step 1. Look for hazards

Walk around the practice identifying what reasonably could cause harm. Ignore trivial items and concentrate on significant hazards that might result in serious harm or affect several people. Ask others what they think. If you employ others, ask them and solicit views and opinions. Manufacturers' instructions and safety data sheets can help, as can the accident and illness records of any staff.

### Step 2. Decide who might be harmed, and how

Identify others who might use the premises, but may not be in contact with the hazard all the time (e.g. patients, carers, cleaners, contractors).

### Step 3. Evaluate the risks from the hazards and decide whether existing precautions are adequate or whether more is required

For the remaining hazards decide whether the risk is high, medium or low (see Figure 29.1). Ask whether you have done all that the law requires. Find out whether there are standards of clinical practice or guidelines advised by the professional body. The law requires that a practitioner must do what is reasonably practicable to keep the practice safe. The overall aim is to make all risks small by means of additional precautions. If a hazard is identified ask: Can the hazard be removed altogether? If not, how best are the risks controlled? Personal protective equipment is a last resort when there is nothing else that can reasonably be done to reduce the risk. Select hazards that can reasonably be foreseen and assess the risks arising from those hazards (see Case Study 29.4).

---

### CASE STUDY 29.4 **AN EXAMPLE OF A COSHH ASSESSMENT COMPLETED FOR DUST**

Nail dust is identified as a possible hazard that might result in occupational asthma, rhinitis or eye problems. It is a medium risk, and the following controls should be investigated:
- Do not drill any nails – is this ethical or practicable?
- Reduce exposure:
  - reduce thickened nails as much as possible with a scalpel before using a nail drill
  - use a coarse burr to reduce exposure to fine nail dust
  - take a scraping first to ensure that a fungus that should not be drilled is not present
  - drill *only* when necessary
  - ensure that the drill is well maintained
  - empty the dust bag regularly
  - fit an air-filtration system in the clinic along with dust extraction for the drill
- Safe working practices:
  - take nail scrapings and await mycology results before drilling
  - wear personal protective equipment
  - face masks to EN 149 standard
  - eye protection to EN 166

- Personal protective equipment:
  - use once and discard
  - if used more than once ensure that the internal surface does not become contaminated
  - store correctly

Date of assessment: October 2004; review: October 2005. Health surveillance required of dust monitoring samples: settle plates and air sampler, respiratory tests on staff, lung function capacity.

---

### Step 4. Record findings

Where there are five or more employees, the employer must record the assessment and the conclusions reached, as well as the plan of action to be adopted for reducing or controlling risks. The assessment required is that of suitable and sufficient, not perfect. According to the Trades Union Congress (TUC) the real points are: Are the precautions reasonable and is there something to show that a proper check was made?

### Step 5. Review assessments on a regular basis and revise when necessary

In practice, changes occur over time, and they require a corresponding change in control measures. For example, there may be a change in the design of nail nippers, which may reduce the risk of RSI. This may require a change in the risk assessment of working practice and a safe system of work for reducing toenails. Date the risk assessments, and also suggest a date for review on your records.

## Using risk factors to evaluate risk

A technique is required to evaluate the risk and quantify the risk. The HSE publication HSG65 Successful Health and Safety Management suggests that the assessment of risk involves rating two factors affecting the risk:

- the severity of the hazard
- the likelihood of an occurrence of harm from the hazard.

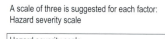

A scale of three is suggested for each factor:
Hazard severity scale

| Hazard severity scale | |
|---|---|
| Major (e.g. death/major harm) | = 3 |
| Serious (e.g. off work for over 3 days) | = 2 |
| Slight (e.g. off work for up to 3 days) | = 1 |

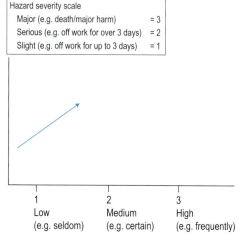

| 1 | 2 | 3 |
|---|---|---|
| Low | Medium | High |
| (e.g. seldom) | (e.g. certain) | (e.g. frequently) |

**Figure 29.1** Hazard severity rating.

**Table 29.1** The risk rating = likelihood × severity

| Likelihood of occurrence (i.e. probability) | Hazard severity (consequence) | Risk rating |
|---|---|---|
| 3 = High | 3 = Major | 1, 2, 3, 4, 6 or 9 |
| 2 = Medium | 2 = Serious | |
| 1 = Low | 1 = Slight | |

## Likelihood of occurrence rating

Risk can be calculated by multiplying the severity factor by the likelihood factor and expressing it as a number showing the significance of the risk compared with other risks. For example, the almost certain likelihood (3) of serious injuries (2) from a given hazard ($3 \times 2 = 6$) would be demonstrated by a number as a more significant risk than an unlikely (1) fatality (3) resulting from another hazard ($1 \times 3 = 3$). This value is termed the 'risk rating' (Table 29.1). It is a number (1, 2, 3, 4, 6 or 9) providing a working value of the residual risk, which helps to complete the answer to the question of what could go wrong.

## Expressing priorities for risk control

The assessment is not, however, seen as complete if it remains as only a statement of hazards and risks. It must contain conclusions about the action needed to eliminate or reduce the risk. The risk assessment therefore needs another stage beyond the evaluation of the risk. This is the step that identifies the action required (i.e. measures in addition to existing precautions, necessary to control the risk). Also, it is helpful to include a priority term, specifying the immediacy of action.

| Risk rating | Priority |
|---|---|
| 1 | no action or low priority |
| 2 | low-priority action |
| 3 or 4 | medium-priority action |
| 5 | high-priority action |
| 6 | urgent action |

A key issue in managing a risk 'insofar as is reasonably practicable' is that the employer must establish the limits of reasonable practicability.

## Limits of reasonable practicability

To establish the limits of reasonable practicability the employer (the competent person(s) appointed by the employer under MHSWR) must decide on effective control measures, having balanced the degree of risk against the cost (money, time and trouble) of eliminating or minimising risk. A risk assessment may well result in a cost–risk analysis, establishing which of various proposed control options is the most cost-effective.

## So far as is practicable

There are a few circumstances where practitioners will need to go beyond the minimum standards set by specific regulations or the limits of reasonable practicability. This is where subordinate legislation imposes a requirement qualified by the term 'so far as is practicable'. This implies that the most effective risk control that is technically feasible needs to be used, irrespective of the cost and inconvenience to the practitioner.

## Refinement of risk factors to help apply control principles

Factors affecting risk also assist in determining effective control measures. For example, when assessing the risk of podiatrists contracting HIV from a known AIDS patient the risk may be regarded as:

| Hazard | Risk |
|---|---|
| HIV | Serious |

However, the addition of the two factors 'hazard severity' and 'likelihood of occurrence' allows the judgement to be improved and to guide additional controls that might be more effective.

| Likelihood | Hazard severity | Risk |
|---|---|---|
| 2 (medium) | 3 (major) | 6 |

In this example it may not be possible to reduce the severity of the hazard, but a particular measure (good handwashing technique and disposable gloves) may reduce the likelihood of an occurrence from 2 (medium) to 1 (low), thereby reducing the overall risk.

## Checklist for risk assessments

- Date risk assessment will be carried out
- Job title
- Description of job
- Frequency of task
- Hazards – actual, potential
- Consequences of risk (low, medium, high)
- Non-routine jobs
- Other staff affected
- Workers particularly at risk (lone workers, people with disabilities)
- Other persons affected (public, contractors, carers)
- Working environment
- Legal standards that apply
- Emergency procedures
- Training
- Monitoring – control measures, health surveillance
- Recommended improvements (corrective action)
- Review date
- Signature of competent persons.

## Generic risk assessments

Generic risk assessments are termed 'model' assessments. These are designed to cover more than one work practice (e.g. a Trust may use a generic risk assessment for all podiatry clinics) in which the risks associated with particular types of workplace, work activity, plant and substance, etc. may be common.

However, caution is needed with these models. If an assessment made for one clinical facility is to be used elsewhere, whether or not the employer is in control of both sites, the employer needs to review and evaluate that assessment, making any necessary revisions to ensure that the assessment is suitable and sufficient for all the circumstances in which it is to be used. Thus the position of an employer, for example a Trust which makes model assessments for use by all its podiatry clinics, is exactly the same as that of a single-site employer who acquires copies of assessments made by a similar enterprise or recommended by a trade association or commercial publisher, etc. However, as employees differ, a generic risk assessment may have problems. For example, in the case of manual handling, generic risk assessment should be avoided as the load may be the same (i.e. domiciliary bag and content) but the individual capacity may well vary between males and females and also between individuals, which would require assessment.

Practitioners should not accept generic risk assessments without ensuring that they are suitable for the premises to which they will apply. Therefore, all generic assessments should be assessed and any necessary modifications made to adapt them to the circumstances or clinics in which they are to be used. While there are disadvantages to using generic assessments, if drawn up by competent, knowledgeable persons they may have benefits. An appropriate generic assessment can save considerable time: managers at a site can start with a generic form that includes information about hazards, risks and precautions, which they can review and make any changes needed to render it suitable and sufficient. However, an inappropriate or poorly designed generic assessment can also waste time: practitioners may waste time understanding the form and the relevance of the information in a model assessment.

## LEGAL REQUIREMENTS WHERE RISK ASSESSMENT IS SPECIFIED – SPECIFIC RISKS

### Noise at Work Regulations 2005

The level at which employers must provide hearing protection and hearing protection zones is 85 decibels (dB) (daily or weekly average exposure) and the level at which employers must assess the risk to workers' health and provide them with information and training is 80 dB. There is also an exposure limit of 87 dB, taking account of any reduction in exposure provided by hearing protection, above which workers must not be exposed.

This is potentially a problem where orthoses are manufactured, depending on the type of equipment used for grinding and buffing, as well as the size of the room and the acoustics within the room.

### Health and Safety (Display Screen Equipment) Regulations 1992 (as amended 2002)

Employers and practitioners need to assess the risks of musculoskeletal injury, visual problems and mental stress from the use of display screen equipment. This is much more likely nowadays with the use of PC-based patient record systems and computerised gait analysis systems.

### Manual Handling Operations Regulations 1992 (as amended 2002)

This area is poorly assessed within podiatry. Assessment of hazardous manual handling tasks must be undertaken, considering the interaction of the following factors: the task, the load, the working environment, the individual's capacity and any other factors. Podiatry is an occupation requiring a lot of awkward bending, rotating and lifting movements. It may not require handling of patients as is required in physiotherapy but the posture of individuals is regularly compromised by the design and set-up of the working environment.

### Personal Protective Equipment at Work Regulations 1992 (as amended 2005)

Prior to selecting personal protective equipment, employers must assess whether it is suitable, both for the nature of the hazard and for the prospective user. Facemasks have been used for a number of years when a nail drill is used. However, these are frequently inappropriate for the task, do not meet the required standard for nuisance dust and are ineffective. Similarly, eye protection is required for the aforementioned work activity and requires an individual assessment to ensure suitability of the protection for the individual practitioner due to various facial characteristics.

### Control of Substances Hazardous to Health Regulations 2002

These regulations are very important within the podiatry context. Each medicament requires an assessment of the risks to employees/practitioners through the use of and exposure to the wide range of substances or hazardous agents used or generated in the practice of podiatry. The manufacture of orthoses, the treatment regimens for verrucae and routine podiatric practice all involve the use of substances hazardous to health. The assessment must, however, relate to the system of work that the practitioner adopts.

### Management of Health and Safety at Work (Amendment) Regulations 1999

Employers are required to assess the risks to the health and safety of pregnant workers, those who have recently given birth and those who are breastfeeding, to ensure that the health and safety of these employees is not put at risk. If a risk remains, and it is not possible to remove it, employers should consider changing the employee's conditions of work or hours, or offer alternative work.

### The Regulatory Reform (Fire Safety) Order 2005

This requires an assessment of the fire risks in the premises along with appropriate emergency plans. The plans need to ensure adequate detection and warning methods in addition to suitable fire-fighting equipment. All those on the premises must be able to get out safely.

### Health and Safety (First Aid) Regulations 1981

The Approved Code of Practice (L 74) places responsibility on the employer to make an evaluation of the first aid requirements and provide necessary resources to meet the assessed need. Thus, a practitioner must assess the requirements for a first aid box and the amount of training needed, as well as decide on the number of trained first aiders required for their premises.

For the various Regulations and aspects of the HASAW and MHSAW that may apply in podiatric practice, see the Society of Chiropodists and Podiatrists website: http://www.feetforlife.org.

## REFERENCES

Williams J 1999 The evolution of stress management. Health & Safety Manager Briefing 65:2–3.

# Index

# Index

# Index

# Index